Environmental Medicine

Environmental Medicine

Jon G. Ayres BSc MBBS MD FRCP FRCPE FFOM FRCPSG
Professor of Environmental and Respiratory Medicine,
School of Health and Population Sciences,
University of Birmingham, UK

Roy M. Harrison OBE BSc PhD DSc CChem FRSC
FRMetS Hon MFPH HonFFOM
Queen Elizabeth II Birmingham Centenary Professor of
Environmental Health, Division of Environmental Health &
Risk Management, University of Birmingham, UK

Gordon L. Nichols PhD MSB CBiol FRSPH
Consultant Epidemiologist, Gastrointestinal, Emerging
and Zoonotic Infections Department, Centre for
Infections, Health Protection Agency, London, UK

Robert L. Maynard CBE FRCP FRCPath FBTS
Honorary Professor of Environmental Medicine,
University of Birmingham, UK

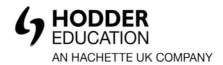

HODDER
EDUCATION
AN HACHETTE UK COMPANY

First published in Great Britain in 2010 by
Hodder Arnold, an imprint of Hodder Education,
an Hachette UK company,
338 Euston Road, London NW1 3BH

http://www.hodderarnold.com

Hachette UK's Hodder Headline's policy is to use papers that are natural,
renewable and recyclable products and made from wood grown in
sustainable forests. The logging and manufacturing processes are
expected to conform to the environmental regulations of the country of
origin.

Whilst the advice and information in this book are believed to be true
and accurate at the date of going to press, neither the author[s] nor the
publisher can accept any legal responsibility or liability for any errors or
omissions that may be made. In particular (but without limiting the
generality of the preceding disclaimer) every effort has been made to
check drug dosages; however it is still possible that errors have been
missed. Furthermore, dosage schedules are constantly being revised and
new side-effects recognized. For these reasons the reader is strongly
urged to consult the drug companies' printed instructions before
administering any of the drugs recommended in this book.

British Library Cataloguing in Publication Data
A catalogue record for this book is available from the British Library

Library of Congress Cataloging-in-Publication Data
A catalog record for this book is available from the Library of Congress

ISBN-13   978-0-340-94656-5

1 2 3 4 5 6 7 8 9 10

Commissioning Editor: Joanna Koster
Project Editor: Joanna Silman
Production Controller: Jonathan Williams
Cover Design: Lynda King
Indexer: Liz Granger

Cover images: Main and bottom right images © Science Photo Library;
bottom left © Gordon Nichols; bottom centre © Edward Arnold

Typeset in 10/12 pt Minion by MPS Limited, A Macmillan Company
Printed and bound in the UK by MPG Books, Bodmin

What do you think about this book? Or any other Hodder Arnold
title? Please visit our website: **www.hodderarnold.com**

Contents

Certain topics have been covered in shorter form, rather than as a full chapter. These are indicated in the contents list by a box symbol: ☐. These boxes occur throughout the book but are usually linked to main chapters in the same broad subject area.

Contributors

Josep M. Antó MD PhD
Director, Centre for Research in Environmental Epidemiology
(CREAL), Barcelona; Professor of Medicine, Universitat Pompeu
Fabra, Barcelona; Affiliated Researcher, Municipal Institute of
Medical Research (IMIM-Hospital del Mar), Barcelona; Director,
CIBER Epidemiología y Salud Pública (CIBERESP), Spain

Michael Aschner PhD
Department of Pediatrics, Pharmacology and the Kennedy Center
for Research on Human Development, Vanderbilt University
School of Medicine, Nashville, Tennessee, USA

Jon G. Ayres BSc MBBS MD FRCP FRCPE FFOM FRCPSG
Professor of Environmental and Respiratory Medicine, Institute of
Occupational and Environmental Medicine, School of Health and
Population Sciences, University of Birmingham, UK

Peter J. Baxter MD MSc FRCP FFOM
Consultant Physician in Occupational and Environmental
Medicine, University of Cambridge and Addenbrooke's
NHS Trust Hospital, Cambridge, UK

Paul D. Blanc MD MSPH
Professor and Chief, Division of Occupational and Environmental
Medicine, Department of Medicine and Cardiovascular Research
Institute, University of California, San Francisco, USA

Konrad E. Bloch MD
Professor, Pulmonary Division, University Hospital of Zurich,
Switzerland

Sally Bradberry BSc MD MRCP
Assistant Director, National Poisons Information Service
(Birmingham Unit) and West Midlands Poisons Unit, City
Hospital, Birmingham UK

Jon S. Brazier PhD MSc CBiol MiBiol SRCS
Consultant Clinical Scientist and Head of Anaerobe Reference
Laboratory, NPHS Microbiology Cardiff, University Hospital of
Wales, Cardiff, UK

Simon Brooker DPhil
Reader, London School of Hygiene and Tropical Medicine,
London, UK; Wellcome Trust Research Fellow, Kenya Medical
Research Institute–Wellcome Trust Research Programme,
Nairobi, Kenya

Moisés A. Calderón MD PhD
Clinical Research Fellow. National Heart and Lung Institute.
Imperial College Faculty of Medicine; and Royal Brompton
Hospital, London, UK

David Carruthers PhD
Technical Director, Cambridge Environmental Research
Consultants Ltd, Cambridge, UK

Mike Catchpole MB BS MSc FRCP FFPHM
Deputy Director, Health Protection Agency Centre for Infections,
Colindale Avenue, London, UK

John W. Cherrie BSc (Hons) PhD FFOH
Research Director, Institute of Occupational Medicine,
Edinburgh, UK; Honorary Reader, Department of Environmental
and Occupational Medicine, University of Aberdeen, UK

Robert P. Chilcott CBiol FIBiol
Professor, Principal Toxicologist and Group Leader, CBRN and
Chemical Toxicology, Centre for Emergency Preparedness and
Response, Porton Down, Salisbury, Wiltshire, UK

David Coggon OBE MA PhD DM FRCP FFOM FFPH FMedSci
Professor of Occupational and Environmental Medicine,
University of Southampton, UK

Benjamin J. Cowling PhD
Assistant Professor, Department of Community Medicine and
School of Public Health, Li Ka Shing Faculty of Medicine,
University of Hong Kong

Natasha S. Crowcroft MA MSc MD(Cantab) MRCP FFPH
Director, Surveillance and Epidemiology, Ontario Agency for
Health Protection and Promotion, Canada; Honorary Consultant,
Health Protection Agency, UK; Associate Professor, Laboratory
Medicine and Pathobiology and Dalla Lana School of Public
Health, University of Toronto, Ontario, Canada

Paul Cullinan MD FRCP FFOM
Professor in Occupational and Environmental Respiratory Disease,
Imperial College, London, UK

Sarah Damery PhD
Research Fellow, Primary Care Clinical Sciences, School of Health
and Population Sciences, University of Birmingham, UK

Finlay D. Dick MD MRCGP MFOM
Clinical Senior Lecturer in Occupational Medicine, Section of
Population Health, Division of Applied Health Sciences, School of
Medicine and Dentistry, University of Aberdeen, UK

Douglas W. Dockery ScD
Professor of Environmental Epidemiology, Chair, Department of
Environmental Health, Harvard School of Public Health, Boston,
Mass., USA

Jeroen H.J. Ensink PhD
Lecturer, London School of Hygiene and Tropical Medicine,
London, UK

Joseph O. Falkinham III PhD
Department of Biological Sciences, Virginia Polytechnic Institute
and State University, Blacksburg, Virginia, USA

John Fawell MBE
Independent consultant on drinking water

Ernest A. Gould PhD MHC
Visiting Professor, Unité des Virus Emergents, Faculté de
Médecine Timone, 13385 Marseille, France; Senior Research
Fellow, CEH Oxford, Mansfield Road, Oxford, UK

Jim Gray PhD FIBMS FRCPath
Head, Enteric Virus Unit, Virus Reference Department,
Centre for Infections, Health Protection Agency, London, UK

David R. Green
Senior Lecturer and Director of the AGT/GIS MSc Degree
Programmes, Director of the MCRM Degree Programme,
Department of Geography and Environment (Seconded to DEOM),
University of Aberdeen, UK

Brian Gulson PhD
Professor (retired), Graduate School of the Environment,
Macquarie University, North Ryde, New South Wales, Australia

David L. Hagen FFPH FRPH MD BSc
Consultant in Communicable Disease Control, Health Protection
Agency, West Sussex Office, Chichester, West Sussex, UK

John Harrison BSc PhD
Health Protection Agency, Centre for Radiation, Chemical and
Environmental Hazards, Chilton, Didcot, Oxfordshire, UK

Roy M. Harrison OBE BSc PhD DSc CChem FRSC FRMetS Hon MFPH HonFFOM
Queen Elizabeth II Birmingham Centenary Professor
of Environmental Health, Division of Environmental
Health & Risk Management, University of Birmingham,
Birmingham, UK

Mathew R. Heal MA DPhil CChem
School of Chemistry, University of Edinburgh, UK

Stephen Higgs PhD FRES
Professor of Pathology Graduate Programme, Pathology
Department, University of Texas Medical Branch, Galveston,
Texas, USA

Lisa Hill BMedSc(Hons)
College of Medical and Dental Sciences, University of
Birmingham, UK

John Hermon-Taylor MBChB MS
Division of Nutritional Sciences, School of Biomedical and
Health Sciences, Franklin-Wilkins Building, Kings College London,
Stamford Street, London, UK

Susan Hodgson BSc MSc PhD
Lecturer in Environmental Epidemiology, Institute of
Health and Society, Newcastle University, UK

Paul R. Hunter MBChB MD MBA
Professor of Health Protection, School of Medicine, Health Policy
and Practice, University of East Anglia, Norwich, UK

Fintan Hurley MA
Scientific Director, Institute of Occupational Medicine,
Edinburgh, UK

Miren Iturriza-Gómara PhD
Deputy Head, Enteric Virus Unit, Virus Reference Department,
Centre for Infections, Health Protection Agency, London, UK

Robert W. Ivens BSc (Biol)
Mole Valley District Council, Environmental Health and Housing,
Pippbrook, Dorking, Surrey, UK

Alan Johnson PhD
Clinical Scientist, Department of Healthcare-associated
Infections and Antimicrobial Resistance, HPA Centre for
Infections, London, UK

Elizabeth M. Johnson PhD
Director, HPA Mycology Reference Laboratory, The HPA Centre for
Infections, HPA South West Laboratory, Myrtle Road, Kingsdown,
Bristol, Avon, UK

Adam Kamradt-Scott BN MA PhD
Research Fellow, Centre on Global Change and Health, London
School of Hygiene and Tropical Medicine, UK

William R. Keatinge (1931–2008)
Emeritus Professor, Barts and the London. Queen Mary's School
of Medicine and Dentistry, London, UK

Frank J. Kelly BSc PhD
Professor of Environmental Health, MRC-HPA Centre for
Environment and Health, King's College London, UK

Gerald M. Kendall PhD
Honorary Senior Research Fellow, Childhood Cancer Research
Group, University of Oxford, UK

Fu-Meng Khaw MD FRCS FFPH
Director of Public Health, North Tyneside Primary Care Trust and
North Tyneside Council, North Tyneside, UK; Honorary Senior
Clinical Lecturer in Public Health, Newcastle University, UK

Leeka Kheifets PhD
Department of Epidemiology, UCLA School of Public Health,
Los Angeles, California, USA

Andrew Kibble MSc MPH
Head of Unit, Chemical Hazards and Poisons Division (Birmingham),
Health Protection Agency, Birmingham, West Midlands, UK

R. Sari Kovats BA MSc PhD
Centre on Global Change and Health, Department of Public Health
and Policy, London School of Hygiene and Tropical Medicine, UK

Om P. Kurmi BSc MSc PhD
Research Fellow, Institute of Occupational and Environmental
Medicine, University of Birmingham, UK

Ware G. Kuschner MD
Staff Physician, United States Department of Veterans Affairs
Palo Alto Health Care System, USA; Associate Professor, Division
of Pulmonary and Critical Care Medicine, Stanford University
School of Medicine, Palo Alto, California, USA

Janet A.M. Kyle BSc MSc PhD
Research Fellow, Institute of Applied Health Sciences, University
of Aberdeen, UK

John V. Lee BSc PhD FRSPH FWMSOC
Water and Environmental Microbiology Reference Unit,
Food Safety Microbiology Laboratory, HPA Centre for Infections,
London, UK

Kelley Lee BA MPA MA DPhil DLitt FHEA FFPH
Reader in Global Health, Centre on Global Change and Health,
London School of Hygiene and Tropical Medicine, UK

Giovanni Leonardi MD MSc FFPH
Consultant in Environmental Epidemiology, Centre for Radiation,
Chemicals and Environmental Hazards, Health Protection Agency.
Didcot, Oxon, UK

Gabriel M. Leung MD FFPH
Professor, Department of Community Medicine and School of
Public Health, Li Ka Shing Faculty of Medicine, University of
Hong Kong, Hong Kong

Ian Litchfield PhD
Research Fellow, Institute of Occupational and Environmental
Medicine, University of Birmingham, UK

Roger O. McClellan DVM MMS DSc IOM DABVT DABT FATS FSRA FAAAR
Advisor, Toxicology and Human Health Risk Analysis,
Albuquerque, New Mexico, USA

Francis McManus MLitt LLB (Hons) FRSPH MREHIS FHEA
Professor of Law, Edinburgh Napier University, UK

Anthony J. McMichael
Professor of Population Health, National Centre for Epidemiology
and Population Health, Australian National University, Canberra,
ACT, Australia

Geraldine McNeill MBChB MSc PhD
Senior Lecturer, Institute of Applied Health Sciences, University
of Aberdeen, UK

Robert L. Maynard CBE FRCP FRCPath FBTS
Honorary Professor of Environmental Medicine, University of
Birmingham, UK

Edwin Michael PhD
Senior Lecturer in Infectious Disease Epidemiology, Department
of Infectious Disease Epidemiology, Imperial College London, UK

Kåre Mølbak MD DMSc
Director, Department of Epidemiology, Statens Serum Institute,
Copenhagen, Denmark

Andy Moorhouse FIOA CEng
Reader in Acoustics and Director of the Acoustics Laboratories,
University of Salford, UK

Virginia Murray FFOM FRCP FRCPath FFPH
Professor and Consultant Medical Toxicologist, Centre for
Radiation, Chemical and Environmental Hazards, Chilton, Didcot,
Oxon, UK; Health Protection Agency, London, UK

Mutuku A. Mwanthi BSc MSEH PhD
Chairman, Department of Community Health, School of Medicine,
College of Health Sciences, University of Nairobi, Kenya

Isabella Myers BSc MSc
Scientific Writer, Department of Health Toxicology Unit, Imperial
College, London, UK

Gordon L. Nichols PhD MSB CBiol FRSPH
Consultant Epidemiologist, Gastrointestinal Emerging and
Zoonotic Infections Department, Centre for Infections, Health
Protection Agency, London, UK

Jonathan S. Nguyen-Van-Tam MBE BMedSci BM BS DM FFPH FRSPH
Foundation Professor of Health Protection, University of
Nottingham Medical School, UK; Honorary Consultant Regional
Epidemiologist (East Midlands), UK Health Protection Agency;
Clinical Sciences Building, City Hospital, Nottingham, UK

Yvonne Nussbaumer-Ochsner MD
Pulmonary Division, University Hospital of Zurich, Switzerland

Nara T. Orban MRCS(Eng) DLO
Clinical Research Fellow in Rhinology, ENT Specialist Registrar,
Imperial College, Royal Brompton Hospital, London, UK

Lorenzo Pezzoli DVM PhD
Fellow of the European Programme for Intervention Epidemiology
Training (EPIET), European Centre for Disease Control (ECDC),
Stockholm, Sweden; Health Protection Agency Centre for
Infections, London, UK

David H. Phillips PhD DSc FRCPath
Professor of Environmental Carcinogenesis, University of
London, UK

Roger W. Pickup BSc PhD
Bowland Professor of Biomedical and Life Sciences, Biomedical
and Life Sciences Division, School of Health and Medicine,
Lancaster University, Lancaster, UK

Geoff H. Pigott BSc PhD DipRCPath
Regulatory Affairs Manager, Nufarm Limited, Wyke,
Bradford, West Yorkshire, UK

T.L. Pitt PhD
Consultant Clinical Scientist and Deputy Director, Laboratory of
Healthcare Associated Infection, Centre for Infections, Health
Protection Agency, London, UK

Simon Pollard BSc(Hons) PhDDIC DSc FRSC CChem FCIWEM
Director, Collaborative Centre of Excellence in Understanding and
Managing Natural and Environmental Risks, Cranfield University,
Cranfield, Bedfordshire, UK

Kevin D. Privett EurIng EurGeol BSc PhD CEng FIMMM CGeol FGS CSci CEnv SiLC
Hydrock Consultants Ltd, Over Lane, Almondsbury, Bristol, UK

Sarah E. Randolph BA PhD
Professor of Parasite Ecology, Department of Zoology, University
of Oxford, UK

Glenn Rhodes BSc PhD
Centre for Ecology and Hydrology, Lake Ecosystems Group,
Lancaster Environment Centre, Bailrigg, Lancaster, Lancashire, UK

Steven Riley DPhil
Assistant Professor, Department of Community Medicine and
School of Public Health, Li Ka Shing Faculty of Medicine,
University of Hong Kong, Hong Kong

Michael O. Rivett MA(Oxon) PhD(Birm) FGS
School of Geography, Earth and Environmental Sciences,
University of Birmingham, UK

Pablo Rodriguez del Rio Mb
Allergy Department, Hospital Clinico San Carlos, Madrid, Spain

John A.S. Ross MBChB FRCA PhD HonFFOM
Senior Lecturer, Environmental and Occupational Medicine,
University of Aberdeen, UK

David Russell BSc MBBCh Dip Med Tox
Head of Unit, Chemical Hazards and Poisons Division (Cardiff),
Health Protection Agency, University of Wales Institute, Cardiff, UK

Sean Semple BSc (Hons) MSc PhD
Senior Lecturer, Department of Environmental and Occupational
Medicine, University of Aberdeen, UK

Wing Hong Seto MB BS
Head of Infection Control, Hospital Authority, Hong Kong

W. Cairns S. Smith MD PhD OBE
Professor of Public Health, University of Aberdeen, Polwarth
Buildings, Foresterhill, Aberdeen, UK

Robert M. Smith PhD
Public Health Clinical Scientist (Zoonoses), Wales, Cardiff, UK

John Swanson DPhil
National Grid, London, UK

Peter Sykes MPH
Head of the Centre for Public Protection, University of Wales
Institute Cardiff, Cardiff School of Health Sciences, UK

Allister Vale MD FRCP FRCPE FRCPG FFOM FAACT FBTS Hon FRCPSG
Director, National Poisons Information Service
(Birmingham Unit) and West Midlands Poisons Unit, City
Hospital, Birmingham, UK

Stan Venitt PhD
Emeritus Reader in Cancer Studies, University of London,
London, UK

Salim Vohra MBChB MSc PhD FRSPH
Director, Centre for Health Impact Assessment, Institute of
Occupational Medicine (London Office), Middlesex, UK

Martin Williams BSc PhD
Professor, Science Policy Unit, Environmental Research Group,
King's College, London, UK

Preface

Environment and health has increasingly become a subject of concern to the general public in recent years. With the public and governments around the world becoming increasingly environmentally aware, the need for a coherent approach to environmental issues and how they relate to health is evident. It is often difficult to establish a clear causal link between an environmental exposure and an effect upon health, and even when such a connection can be demonstrated, responsibility for addressing the problem may cut across a number of agencies. This requires a multi-disciplinary approach to situations which are often complex and sometimes of high public profile. Information is not always readily available to those who find themselves having to sort the matter, and the right mix of skills is often difficult to bring together.

The idea for this book sprang from these concerns and from the fact that there was no single volume which brought together the various threads of the subject. In the book we aim to provide a source of information that, while not necessarily covering every possible issue which could be placed under this broad title, does address methodology, key exposures and approaches to an understanding of the relationship between environment and health. As a consequence this is not a text book as such, but a resource for anyone needing to find information, who finds the area of interest or who is training in one of the many disciplines which contribute to environmental influences on health. Largely aimed at the post-graduate audience, both medical and non-medical, we believe the book will also be of help to undergraduates in the many courses which address one component or other of environmental science. In particular, we hope that departments of public health, environmental health and occupational health will find something to assist them in their work.

We are immensely grateful to all the authors who have contributed so fluently and expertly to this book and who have readily accepted our editorial suggestions and corrected us in our misconceptions. We have had to make decisions about content and approach along the way and some subjects have either not been included or are covered in less detail than some would like. This is inevitable where the breadth of subjects is so wide but we think that the resultant balance is right. All errors, whether of omission or commission, can be squarely laid at the doors of the editors and any comment on content or approach will be gratefully received.

We owe a deep debt of thanks to all staff at Hodder Arnold who have been involved in the design and production of the book over the last 5 years, but in particular Jo Koster and Jo Silman without whose advice, cajoling and encouragement, the book would not have emerged.

Jon G. Ayres
Roy M. Harison
Gordon L. Nichols
Robert L. Maynord
2010

BACKGROUND TO ENVIRONMENTAL MEDICINE

Environmental medicine in context

JON G. AYRES, ROY M. HARRISON, ROBERT L. MAYNARD,
ROGER O. McCLELLAN AND GORDON L. NICHOLS

Whoever wishes to investigate medicine properly, should proceed thus: in the first place to consider the seasons of the year, and what effects each of them produces ... the winds, the hot and the cold, especially such as are common to all countries, and then such as are peculiar to each locality.... In the same manner, when one comes into a city to which he is a stranger, he ought to consider its situation, how it lies to the winds and the rising of the sun; for its influences are not the same whether it lies to the north or the south, to the rising or to the setting sun. These things one ought to consider most attentively and concerning the waters which the inhabitants use, whether they be marshy and soft, or hard, and running from elevated and rocky situations and then if salted should be unfit for cooking; and the ground, whether it be naked and deficient in water, or wooded and well watered, and whether it lies in a hollow, confined situation or is elevated and cold....

Hippocrates

AN INTRODUCTION TO ENVIRONMENTAL MEDICINE

General context

The influence of the environment on health has been rapidly moving up the agenda in recent years, initially in relation to air quality and water quality, but latterly because of climate change. Responsibility for the management of environmental effects on health, although generally falling to public health physicians, is divided, largely because the main issue surrounding a specific situation does not fit easily into one special area of expertise. Our understanding and management of the health effects of environmental factors requires the multidisciplinary working, and consequently training and career development, that encompasses this philosophy.

Interest in and awareness of the effects of environmental pollution on health are not new. London's River Thames in

Victorian times was hugely polluted, with fish being unable to survive in its waters until high upstream in rural Berkshire. The need for a complete, integrated sewerage system for London was regarded as a health-based necessity by Bazalgette, who developed arguably one the greatest environmental health interventions of the nineteenth century. Polluted air was recognized as a source of ill-health in London from the seventeenth century onwards, the diarist John Evelyn calling for measures to reduce emissions from industrial and domestic sources alike. Interestingly, subsequent attempts in the nineteenth century to control emissions to air from specific factories usually involved in the manufacture of chemicals by legislation (the Alkali Acts) were driven by crop or vegetation loss and smell rather than by any belief that emissions were directly deleterious to health.

The turning point in air pollution control came with 'the great London smog' in December 1952, when at least 4000 (some suggest the true number was nearer to 10 000)

excess deaths occurred associated with a week-long period of pollution. This episode was remarkable not so much for the intensity of the fog (as this episode was not the most severe of of the twentieth century) but for the fact that, on this occasion, somebody decided to count the number of dead. The results were so striking that this episode led within 4 years to the passage of the first all-encompassing Clean Air Act in the world.

Environmental influences on health have thus been well recognized even where a complete causal pathway has not been identified or accepted. However, the lack of a complete chain of information along the causal pathway has often led to resistance to intervention by legislation, usually by those responsible for emissions of a specific pollutant fervently resisting the possibility that their emissions might be harmful. Such, indeed, was the case with the Alkali Acts and also, in the occupational health area, in the lead industry and in relation to asbestos production. On the other side of the coin, pressure on local or national governments by concerned groups or individuals, where an exposure is perceived to have resulted in an adverse affect on health, can influence legislation or at the very least raise media interest. The news media can play a useful role in documenting risks where reporting is done well but can sometimes, in the interests of balance, give undue prominence to minority views. This was so in the case where autism was incorrectly linked to vaccination with the measles–mumps–rubella (MMR) vaccine.

Interventions can have considerable benefits. One only has to think of the provision of clean water in response to outbreaks of infant diarrhoea in some developing countries, bridges across previously unfordable rivers to allow better access to amenities and medical care and, at a legislative level, approaches to improve air quality and water quality in order to realize that huge health benefits can occur with targeted interventions to address real health issues.

In more recent times, environment and health has occupied a much broader remit, largely due to improved methods of assessing both exposures and health impacts. Situations that previously seemed to be impossibly complex are now coming within the scope of researchers. However, it remains true that the recognition, understanding and quantification of the adverse or beneficial effects of an environmental exposure are not easy and need multidisciplinary collaboration. Epidemiologists and clinicians are required to define health outcomes (and complicating co-factors), but in order to define the relationship between specific exposures and these health end points (and subsequently to determine control interventions), expertise is needed in exposure assessment, risk assessment, risk management, disaster management, policy development and health economics, as well as in toxicology, chemistry and physiology. This is complex, and complexity is often best dealt with by developing a simple framework around which questions or strategies can be structured (Figure 1.1).

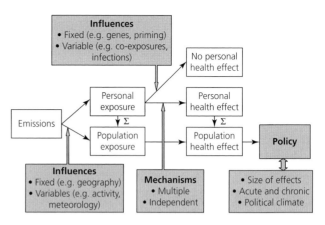

Figure 1.1   Emission, exposure, effect and control framework for the assessment of environmental exposures and their effects on health.

This simple flow diagram starts with the assumption of a potentially adverse release of an agent (e.g. a chemical) into the environment. Such an emission will result in an individual or population being exposed to that agent; those exposed may (or may not) then develop what might be perceived to be an adverse effect on health. Although understanding the mechanisms of such an effect is of both importance and interest, from a regulatory point of view the fact that it occurs at all is the important fact. Knowing that fact, quantification of the size of the effect is then needed and should take into consideration other factors that could also have contributed either directly or indirectly to the effect. Having established the burden on health, an assessment of the risk of continued exposure and finally a decision on whether an intervention is appropriate can be made.

In general, attempts at exposure or emission control can be regarded as mitigating interventions, but there are circumstances in which there may be little in terms of mitigation that can be done or in which a mitigating intervention might take a long time to have an impact. In these circumstances, adaptive interventions may need to be considered to reduce the impact of an exposure even though that exposure continues. A good example is climate change, where, whatever man might do in terms of trying to turn round the anthropogenic contributions to global warming, there is a need to find ways to adapt to the temperature rise and consequent, other, environmental changes.

The same framework can equally be used when considering a potentially beneficial effect of an environmental 'intervention'. The rationale behind an intervention usually comes from an acceptance that there is an adverse situation that needs to be changed such as the introduction of higher efficiency stoves where biomass fuels are burnt.

Finally, and having intervened, the benefit accruing from that intervention, whether by reducing emissions or reducing exposures, needs to be measured to determine whether that intervention could or should be maintained in that community, rolled out more widely or stopped.

An unsuspected adverse consequence may occasionally arise from an environmental intervention. Probably the best recognized example of this occurred in Bangladesh, where the major toll from gastroenteritis was successfully addressed by provision of clean water through standpipes. However, it became clear over subsequent years that this 'clean' water was contaminated with arsenic because the rock strata between the ground and the aquifer were naturally heavily laden with this element. As a consequence, many millions of people in Bangladesh are now suffering from chronic arsenic poisoning, and an alternative approach to providing clean water has had to be devised. Although such backfiring is not common, the potential for harm is an integral part of health impact assessment and is discussed in more detail in Chapter 63.

Interventions

Environmental legislation is becoming more ambitious. Although the various clean air acts around the world led the way in the field of environment and health, concerns about complexity, benefits and logistics as well as potential problems with the enforcement of many forms of legislation meant that only exposures associated with a clear risk became the target of Government. Sometimes the driver to control such exposures is not a human health effect. Pesticide regulation is a case in point, where the main initial driver was the effect of exposures on wildlife so graphically portrayed by Rachel Carson in her book *Silent Spring*.[1] In other situations, legislation for a totally non-health or environmental reason can have significant health implications. The Railways (Branch Line) Act of 1962 in the UK resulted in the closure of many small branch line railways on the basis that they were not economically viable. The result was the effective isolation of many small communities with reduced access to amenities and healthcare, an issue either not anticipated or ignored by the legislators.

Causation

The word 'cause' is often used when considering the health impacts of environmental exposures in an imprecise way. We will use the term to describe the initiation of a condition in an individual not previously affected, for example cigarette-smoking as a cause of lung cancer. The term also tends to be used, in our view confusingly, to describe an exacerbation of a pre-existing condition, for example air pollution 'causing' an attack of asthma. This can lead to confusion in attribution of a proportion of a health outcome in a population to a specific exposure. If

the prevalence of asthma in a population were very low, exposure to air pollution would have only a small impact as those susceptible to its effect would be few. If, however, exposure to air pollution was also associated with the *initiation* of asthma, the effect in public health terms would be much higher.

A crucial issue in environment and health research is in the determination of whether exposure A is causally related to outcome B, especially where the size of the effect may be small and other competing causal factors may be in play. Sorting out the causal pathways can at times seem impossible. This was appreciated in the 1960s by Austin Bradford Hill, a British medical statistician who produced a framework within which causation can be assessed when considering environmental influences on health.[2] This must be considered simply as a guide to tackling these issues and not, as is often incorrectly stated, as a set of criteria. The framework is remarkable in its simplicity and its proven robustness over time and, although some have reduced the component parts to a shorter list it remains an extremely useful tool. There are nine components to Bradford Hill's framework:

Strength: If there is a large effect size (a strong effect), this makes a true causal relationship more likely. There is no fundamental reason why a strong association should be more likely to be causal than a weak association. However, Bradford Hill was thinking of possible confounding factors and argued that if a strong association is *not* causal, an association with some other factor that varies closely with the factor originally suggested must exist. If the association is strong, this co-variable will be easier to recognize than if the association is weak.

Consistency: Is there evidence for the same findings from more than one study, preferably from different settings?

Specificity: Is the effect specific to the exposure? In reality this rarely occurs, and some regard this as the 'icing on the cake' when considering causal evidence. However, the specificity of a particular mechanism, if seen across a range of health end points, would meet the requirements of this component.

Temporality: This is the only absolute. Exposure must precede outcome.

Biological gradient: Is there a dose–response relationship? In addition (although not explicit in Bradford Hill's original paper), is there a threshold of exposure below which an effect is not seen?

Plausibility: Does this exposure–effect relationship make biological sense? Is there mechanistic evidence to support the likelihood that this might occur given current knowledge? Bradford Hill pointed out that this feature should not be demanded: what is implausible today may be entirely plausible tomorrow.

Coherence: Does the proposed causal association cohere with other findings? For instance, if we were concerned that a specific exposure might be related to a health effect that was based on an inflammatory response, has a similar effect been seen with other inflammatory conditions, or is an apparent effect on mortality accompanied by effects on morbidity?

Experiment: Is there evidence from experiments (involving either animals or humans, whether individually or as populations) that removal of the exposure reduces the effect?

Analogy: Are there analogous situations that would tend to support the likelihood of a causal relationship? For instance, when considering a possible teratogen, the effects of thalidomide on the developing fetus would come to mind.

This framework needs to be used intelligently rather than slavishly – it is a guide and not a checklist, but it is used at a number of places within this book. A close reading of the extended account provided by Bradford Hill in his book *Principles of Medical Statistics* is strongly recommended.

The precautionary approach

Once a possible relationship between an exposure and an effect is agreed to be likely to be causal, there is a decision to be made on whether to act to reduce exposures at an individual or a population level. There is a view that waiting for clear information on whether or not exposure A results in health effect B is unacceptable: such thinking underlies the precautionary principle. Where there is clear evidence of carcinogenicity or mutagenicity, for which thresholds of effect are regarded as unlikely to exist, the decisions are easy. The aim should be to reduce exposures as far as possible, although how that might be achieved is another issue.

The difficulty comes where the evidence is not so clear. For instance, there may be evidence of an adverse effect at high exposures (say in animal studies) that far exceed likely exposures in humans. Is that sufficient to regulate or prohibit the release of that substance into the environment? Such a hazard-based approach presents some difficulties, especially in the context of the deliberate release, for example, of pesticides. In this context, the release is associated with benefit, namely crop protection to maximize yields and thus ensure an adequate food supply to the population. So how does one balance the ecotoxicological and human toxicological effects with the health impact of reduced crop yields, possible loss of businesses and consequent unemployment in terms of population health?

Put another way, what exposures might be deemed to be 'reasonable'? Views will be expressed on both sides of the argument, views that are often based on inadequate information or understanding. One of the problems of living in the modern world, with much of the available information relatively easily accessible on the Internet, is understanding how people can live a healthy life and not be forever worrying about risks. The problem can be aggravated by scientists going to the media when, for instance, a study they have been involved in shows an apparent association between an environmental factor and a disease. There is further technical difficulty in making links between the environment and many illnesses, and in separating the effects of genetic and environmental factors. Ultimately, there may be good public health reasons for taking early action where a suspected association between a disease and a risk factor suggests that a precautionary approach is advisable in the absence of scientific certainty. The measures taken against bovine spongiform encephalopathy are a good example here.

Dealing with complexity and multiple causality

Some of the subjects covered in this book concern clear-cut exposures, some of which are in turn associated with clear-cut end points and others less so. Difficulties come from the complexity that is usually present where there are varying exposures to multiple agents without necessarily a single clear-cut effect. It is up to epidemiologists and basic scientists to try to understand and unpick key causal pathways, and only as that information becomes better understood will legislators and policy developers be able to make sensible decisions on how best to deal with environmental exposures and plan for the likely environmental impact of any development. This complexity needs to be seen within a working framework. One such is the DPSEEA (Drivers, Pressures, State, Exposure, Effect, Actions) model which has arisen largely out of a need to understand the likely impact of an environmental intervention but equally takes into consideration all the various steps in terms of emissions, exposure and the socioeconomic and other contexts in which the exposures occur (Figure 1.2).

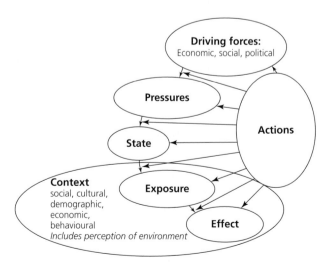

Figure 1.2   The modified DPSEEA model for assessing environmental influences on health. (Morris *et al.*, 2006.[20])

This approach allows different chains of associations to be devised. For instance, consider radon, an inert gas that decays to yield radioactive species which become attached to particles in the air. Such particles can be deposited in the lungs and cause cancer. The *state* would be radon in indoor air, the *exposure* the level inhaled by people living in that dwelling, and the potential *effect* lung cancer. *Drivers* for this would be the release of the gas from natural rocks (notably granite) and the trapping of the released gas within the building would be *a pressure. Actions* can be taken at a number of nodes, including specifying building standards to allow radon gas to escape and the provision of grants for householders affected by radon to institute radon control interventions in their home. This framework has worked well in defining such interventions in policy terms both at national level and worldwide; the World Health Organization (WHO) regularly employs this approach.

Change through international agreement

Some of the products of human activity have long-lasting effects. The general rise in atmospheric carbon dioxide levels since the start of the Industrial Revolution is rightly described as anthropogenic and is of concern in relation to its impact on climate change. The human-generated chlorofluorocarbons have had an impact on ozone depletion in the upper atmosphere that has largely been ameliorated through international agreement to restrict the use of these chemicals. Although climate change through anthropogenic 'greenhouse gas' emissions might be controlled by concerted international action, the increasing human population will make this increasingly difficult, and other anthropogenic problems from this increasing population are likely to result in the medium term, particularly if the sea level rises significantly. Measuring the impact of these changes and determining their effects on health in the future are important but not necessarily straightforward.

Radioactive strontium-90 can still be measured around the world as a marker of atmospheric nuclear tests in the 1950s, whereas the accumulation of the insecticide DDT within the natural environment has led to restrictions on its use. Although the human health impacts of these pollutants have been relatively small, they have been sufficiently important to necessitate international agreements to act.

ENVIRONMENTAL EXPOSURES

A study funded by the WHO[3] suggested the following definition of 'environment':

> The environment is all the physical, chemical and biological factors external to a person, and all the related behaviours.

The full meaning of this is not very clear, but the authors[3] note that this definition excludes behaviour not related to the environment, as well as behaviour related to the social and cultural environment, and genetics. For their study of the environmental burden of disease, the authors further restricted their definition as follows:

> The environment is all the physical, chemical and biological factors external to the human host, and all related behaviours, but excluding those natural environments that cannot reasonably be modified.

They note that this definition excludes behaviour not related to environments, as well as behaviour related to the social and cultural environment, genetics, and parts of the natural environment. This definition thus aims to cover those parts of the environment that can be modified by environmental management. Box 1.1, modified from WHO[3] gives examples of factors included or excluded from their working definition for 'environment'.

People live within both a natural and a manmade environment and are exposed, along with all other organisms, to a variety of environmental and non-environmental factors; they are also subject to the constraints of living within the social, political, religious and economic circumstances of their country. In addition to largely external constraints, most organisms have an internal environment populated by microbes, the number of bacteria living in the human gut being almost equal to the total number of cells in the human body. Microbes inhabit the oral, upper respiratory, gastrointestinal, skin and genital niches, and the microbial flora develops through our lives. We derive both nutritionally valuable organic molecules and inorganic chemicals, as well as toxic substances, through the consumption of food and water. The extent to which bodies take up and excrete these molecules affects the concentration in tissues and resulting disease. Immunity is stimulated by the presence of flora. There are a number of elements and molecules that interrupt processes essential to life, and there is a varied susceptibility to these across the plant, fungal, eubacterial and animal kingdoms.

This chapter is built on the premise that an effective and efficient control of materials found in the air we breathe, the water we drink, the food we eat and a wide array of consumer products with which we interact requires the use of appropriate procedures to identify hazardous agents, characterize the exposure, assess the risks and then manage the risks to some acceptable level.

Exposure to environmental factors

Interaction with the environment begins in early pregnancy where nutrition (e.g. vitamin B_{12}), maternal disease (e.g. diabetes), teratogenic and neurotoxic (e.g. dioxins and lead) compounds and infectious diseases (e.g. rubella,

---

BOX 1.1: Examples of factors included in, or excluded from a WHO working definition for 'environment'

Included environmental factors are the modifiable parts (or impacts) of:

- pollution of air, water, or soil with chemical or biological agents;
- UV and ionizing radiation[a];
- noise, electromagnetic fields;
- occupational risks;
- built environments, including housing, land use patterns, roads;
- agricultural methods, irrigation schemes;
- manmade climate change, ecosystem change;
- behaviour related to the availability of safe water and sanitation facilities, such as washing hands, and contaminating food with unsafe water or unclean hands.

Excluded environmental factors are:

- alcohol and tobacco consumption, drug abuse;
- diet (although it could be argued that food availability influences diet);
- the natural environments of vectors that cannot reasonably be modified (e.g. in rivers, lakes, wetlands);
- impregnated bed nets (can be considered to be non-environmental interventions);
- unemployment (provided that it is not related to environmental degradation, occupational disease, etc.);
- natural biological agents, such as pollen in the outdoor environment;
- person-to-person transmission that cannot reasonably be prevented through environmental interventions such as improving housing, introducing sanitary hygiene, or making improvements in the occupational environment.

UV, ultraviolet.

Reproduced from Pruss-Ustun and Corvalan,[2] with permission.

[a]Although natural UV radiation from space is not modifiable (or only in a limited way, such as by reducing substances that destroy the ozone layer), individual behaviour to protect oneself against UV radiation is modifiable.

Toxoplama gondii and *Listeria monocytogenes*) can influence fetal development. The fetus is to a large extent protected from the environment by the physical, immunological and chemical environment of the mother's womb. At birth, the newborn baby becomes colonized with bacteria from the mother's environment and develops a distinctive bowel flora that changes over life.

The melamine poisoning of infant formula milk in China in 2008 that resulted in 290 000 children being ill, over 12 000 hospitalized and a number of deaths highlights how exposure to the environment (in this case through food) can affect infants. The addition of melamine to milk was thought to ensure that diluted milk retained a high nitrogen content, but the result was that large numbers of children developed renal stones.

With child and juvenile development come increasing environmental exposures and insults that impact on lives. Immunity that is initially provided by maternal antibodies through breast-feeding is replaced at an early age by the immune responses to a large array of viral infections in babies and young children, many of which confer lifelong protection, such as to measles.

The main human exposure pathways are shown in Figure 1.3, which gives examples of ways in which environmental exposures to chemicals, physical factors and microbiota occur.

PROTECTING HUMAN HEALTH

The field of environmental health has developed rapidly over the past half century. It has many roots in, for example, the fields of water and food hygiene, pharmaceutical safety, occupational medicine and public health. In each of these areas, the operative adjective 'safe' was originally used, as in safe water, safe food, safe pharmaceuticals and a safe workplace. 'Safe' was typically defined as freedom from the potential for harm. It is increasingly recognized that absolute safety is seldom, if ever, possible and certainly cannot be predicted. The term 'safe' in this context might sensibly be abandoned. In some situations, 'clean' has also been used as a synonym for 'safe', i.e. clean air or a clean environment.

There is no universal agreement with regard to what encompasses the environment and the relationship of the environment to the health of individuals and populations. Consideration of Figure 1.4 provides some perspective on this matter. Some individuals may consider the five

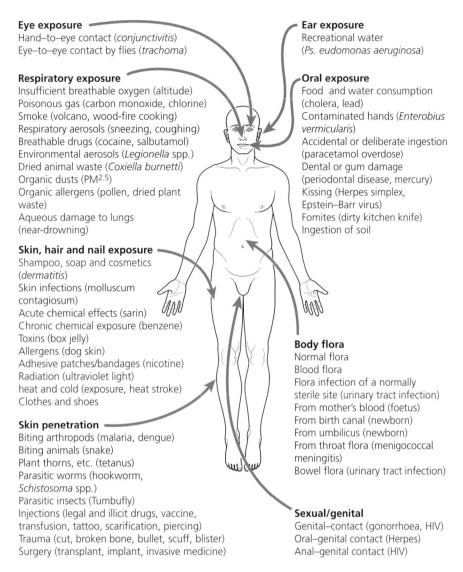

Eye exposure
Hand–to–eye contact (*conjunctivitis*)
Eye–to–eye contact by flies (*trachoma*)

Ear exposure
Recreational water
(*Ps. eudomonas aeruginosa*)

Respiratory exposure
Insufficient breathable oxygen (altitude)
Poisonous gas (carbon monoxide, chlorine)
Smoke (volcano, wood-fire cooking)
Respiratory aerosols (sneezing, coughing)
Breathable drugs (cocaine, salbutamol)
Environmental aerosols (*Legionella* spp.)
Dried animal waste (*Coxiella burnetti*)
Organic dusts (PM$^{2.5}$)
Organic allergens (pollen, dried plant
waste)
Aqueous damage to lungs
(near-drowning)

Oral exposure
Food and water consumption
(cholera, lead)
Contaminated hands (*Enterobius
vermicularis*)
Accidental or deliberate ingestion
(paracetamol overdose)
Dental or gum damage
(periodontal disease, mercury)
Kissing (Herpes simplex,
Epstein–Barr virus)
Fomites (dirty kitchen knife)
Ingestion of soil

Skin, hair and nail exposure
Shampoo, soap and cosmetics
(*dermatitis*)
Skin infections (molluscum
contagiosum)
Acute chemical effects (sarin)
Chronic chemical exposure (benzene)
Toxins (box jelly)
Allergens (dog skin)
Adhesive patches/bandages (nicotine)
Radiation (ultraviolet light)
heat and cold (exposure, heat stroke)
Clothes and shoes

Body flora
Normal flora
Blood flora
Flora infection of a normally
sterile site (urinary tract infection)
From mother's blood (foetus)
From birth canal (newborn)
From umbilicus (newborn)
From throat flora (menigococcal
meningitis)
Bowel flora (urinary tract infection)

Skin penetration
Biting arthropods (malaria, dengue)
Biting animals (snake)
Plant thorns, etc. (tetanus)
Parasitic worms (hookworm,
Schistosoma spp.)
Parasitic insects (Tumbufly)
Injections (legal and illicit drugs, vaccine,
transfusion, tattoo, scarification, piercing)
Trauma (cut, broken bone, bullet, scuff, blister)
Surgery (transplant, implant, invasive medicine)

Sexual/genital
Genital–contact (gonorrhoea, HIV)
Oral–genital contact (Herpes)
Anal–genital contact (HIV)

Figure 1.3   Routes by which chemical, radiation, radionuclides, drugs, toxins and infectious agents enter/affect the human body. HIV, human immunodeficiency virus; PM$_{2.5}$, particulate matter with a diameter of 2.5 µm or less.

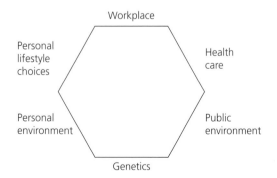

Figure 1.4   Multiple factors influencing the health status of individuals and populations.

Workplace
Personal lifestyle choices
Health care
Personal environment
Public environment
Genetics

opportunity for advancing the health of individuals and populations is when appropriate attention is given to all six components, which can, to varying degrees, be assessed and managed. Some individuals may have an exaggerated view of the role of (1) the public environment, for example air or water quality, relative to the role of (2) personal environment, for example nutrition or air quality in their home, (3) personal lifestyle choices, for example, cigarette-smoking, alcohol consumption and exercise, and (4) their workplace. In addition, in recent years the issue of access to healthcare has received increasing attention as a factor influencing the health of individuals and populations.

In this book we will focus on hazards and risks in the public environment, fully recognizing that the basic concepts are also relevant to the other factors influencing personal and public health, in particular concentrating on the usually accepted indicators of morbidity and mortality. Such an orientation focuses on disease outcomes rather

components (other than genetics) as representing the environment. Such a broad approach can mislead individuals in terms of the extent to which the various individual factors may influence their health. The best than the very broad and laudable goal articulated by the WHO[4] – 'Health is a state of complete physical, mental and social well being and not merely the absence of disease and infirmity'.

The environment in which people live and the multitude of pathways for agents that may influence their health are illustrated schematically in Figure 1.5.[5] For the majority of the world's population, a figure depicting a rural setting is not an accurate depiction of their environment. Increasingly, individuals around the world live in communities ranging in size from several hundred individuals to tens of millions of individuals.

Moreover, it is increasingly recognized that the environment depicted in Figure 1.5 is but a microcosm of the global environment in which we all live. The large-scale contamination of milk and other products adulterated with melamine in China has been demonstrated in human and animal foods in several countries, but may not have been detected in the countries lacking adequate protocols for testing imported foods. Foodstuffs grown in one hemisphere are routinely shipped to the other hemisphere, and fish harvested in one part of the world soon find their way to markets around the world. Some portion of both particulate and gaseous emissions to the ambient air in one region is circulated in the air to nearby regions and on around the globe. Water contaminated at an upstream

location may be used as drinking water in communities a few miles to a thousand miles downstream or enter the ocean and circulate long distances in ocean currents. Some emissions are primarily the result of human activity, being of so-called anthropogenic origin. Other constituents in the air and water may be of natural origin and found in raised concentrations as a result of human activity. Yet other constituents found in the environment may be of strictly natural origin without any influence from humans. Some pharmaceuticals administered to both people and animals, along with naturally occurring molecules, may be excreted in urine and be found in water downstream.

In commenting on the scope of the environment as a factor influencing health, it would be remiss not to note the increasing attention given over the last decade to the impacts of global climate change on the environment and human health.[6–8] Scientific journals are already publishing papers that project, decades into the future, changes in specific human health parameters. Many of these factors address single risk factors and specific disease outcomes. Other papers make sweeping generalizations on adverse health effects, without considering possible positive impacts.

The focus on single risk factors may do a disservice to society. The ability of society at large to make informed, science-based decisions on the impact of global climate change and alternative approaches to mitigating climate change will require that the scientific community moves beyond its current focus on individual risk factors to a more comprehensive view of risk factors influencing health in both a positive and a negative way. Kennedy[9] noted the pitfalls of focusing on individual risk factors such as those associated with a single energy source. He emphasized the need for a broad view when society is grappling with the bigger issue of global climate change that can affect health in a number of ways. Efforts to reduce the extent of climate change, for example by moving towards a wider use of nuclear power, may yield benefits for health as the use of other sources of energy decline.

We start from the premise that an effective and efficient control of materials found in the air we breathe, the water we drink, the food we eat and a wide array of consumer products requires the use of appropriate procedures to identify hazardous agents, characterize the exposure, assess the risks and then manage the risks to some acceptable level compared with the background level of risks inherent to society. These factors consequently need to be evaluated through assessing exposures and risks and managing risks to an acceptable level for agents arising from societal activities, while recognizing that the same concepts apply to both synthetic and naturally occurring substances.

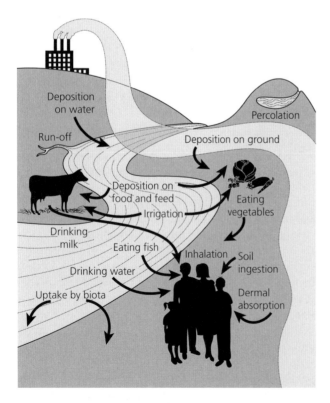

Figure 1.5 Multiple pathways for human exposure to synthetic and naturally occurring chemicals. (Adapted from Paustenbach,[4] with permission.)

Key definitions

At this point, it is appropriate to provide some definitions of terms that will be used frequently in this book.[10,11]

Hazardous, as in hazardous agent, may be defined as the potential of an agent, as a result of its intrinsic properties, to cause under some conditions of exposure an adverse effect on health. In this definition, the level or duration of exposure required to produce an adverse effect is not considered. Originally, agents were defined as hazardous based on human experience. Today, many agents may be categorized as hazardous based exclusively on data from laboratory animal studies, including studies using very high levels of exposure, indeed levels much higher than are likely to be encountered by people. In short, an agent may be classified as hazardous irrespective of whether the exposure conditions required to elicit adverse effects are relevant to human situations.

Exposure defines the extent to which a person encounters or comes into contact with a hazard. Exposure is typically characterized by both the concentration of the agent in water, food or the air and the duration of contact with the agent or intake of the agent.

Dose is the quantity of the material that actually interacts with the skin or enters the body. A robust characterization of dose will, ideally, include a description of the retention of the agent over time after intake or the retention profile of the agent and metabolites associated with repeated or prolonged intake. Dose is frequently used inappropriately as being synonymous with exposure.

Risk is defined as the probability of occurrence of adverse health effects from exposure to a hazardous agent at a specified duration and intensity of exposure. Risk may be evaluated with regard to an individual subject, i.e. the likelihood of the individual having the adverse effect, or more typically with regard to a population, i.e. the likelihood expressed as the expected outcome for a population, say of a million individuals, having the adverse health outcome, such as cancer, during the lifetime of all individuals in the population at some specified duration and intensity of exposure. When expressed on a population scale, the term 'risk' might be usefully replaced by 'impact'. The estimation of risk to an individual or population requires information on the duration and intensity of exposure *and* the potency of the agent, i.e. the agent's exposure–response relationship, for a particular adverse health outcome.

The results from epidemiological studies are frequently obtained by an analysis of data using a Cox proportional hazards model in which the risk for a specific study population exposed to any agent is evaluated relative to that observed in a reference population that is either not exposed or exposed at a lower level. The results are reported as relative risks. To derive the excess risk attributed to exposure to an agent requires knowledge of the incidence of the adverse health effect in the comparison population. In some cases, the excess risk may be related to some estimated differences in the exposure received by the two populations, for example excess risk associated with a $10\,\mu g/m^3$ increase in air concentration of an air pollutant.

Risk assessment is a process by which information is integrated to characterize the nature and magnitude of the potential adverse health effects of human exposure to hazards.

Uncertainty refers to the lack of knowledge regarding both the actual values of model input variables (parameter uncertainty) and the physical systems or relationships (model uncertainty, e.g. the shape of the concentration–response functions). In any risk assessment, uncertainty is, ideally, reduced as far as possible, but significant uncertainty often remains.

Risk management is the process by which information from risk assessments is used in concert with other kinds of information such as economics, social and political considerations to make decisions to take actions that will mitigate the risks.

Chemical and radioactive hazards and risks

The perception that certain agents are hazardous, i.e. that, at some level of intake, the agent is capable of causing adverse effects, is no doubt as old as humankind. The coal miner's use of the canary to 'test' the air provided a readily discernible link between poor air quality and acute asphyxiation. The culprit, the hazardous agent, was carbon monoxide. The food laws of ancient religions were based on an empirical and sometimes incorrect understanding that the ingestion of certain foodstuffs was bad for one's survival.

As humankind developed, it became apparent that some agents that are hazardous at some level of intake also have beneficial effects at some lower level of intake or dose. Paracelsus[12] immortalized this concept with the statement 'All substances are poisons; there is none which is not a poison. The right dose differentiates a poison from a remedy.' He advanced four fundamental concepts:

Experimentation is required for examining responses to chemicals.
A distinction should be made between the therapeutic and toxic properties of chemicals.
The therapeutic and toxic properties are sometimes closely related and distinguishable by dose.
It is possible to ascertain a degree of specificity for chemicals and their therapeutic or toxic effects.

It is apparent from the foregoing that toxicology and pharmacology are closely related fields of scientific endeavour. Pharmacology is focused on drugs, including both their effectiveness and their safety. Toxicology is concerned with all kinds of chemicals that may, at some level and duration of exposure, cause adverse health effects. Toxicological and epidemiological studies are increasingly concerned with low levels of exposure for which the effects, if any, may not be specific to the particular agent. Indeed, the observed association between exposure to the agent and the disease outcome may only be reflected in a small, statistically determined, increase in the disease or effect on health over the normal background incidence of the end point studied.

Through the first half of the twentieth century, the approaches used to minimize the risk of harm from workplace exposures to materials and the intake of pharmaceuticals or food additives made use of the concept of a *threshold* in exposure–response relationships. Adverse health effects were observed only above some threshold level of exposure observed in human or laboratory animal studies. The use of safety factors allowed the identification of some lower level of exposure that would, if achieved, ensure the safety of workers and the public. This approach is discussed in greater detail in Chapter 5.

In the mid-twentieth century, increased public concern developed over radiation and synthetic chemicals as factors influencing humankind, especially their potential for causing cancer. Concern for radiation was closely linked to the use of atomic bombs on Nagasaki and Hiroshima, and later to the atmospheric testing of nuclear weapons, Three Mile Island and Chernobyl. Opposition to the development and use of nuclear weapons soon broadened to include opposition to the development and use of nuclear power to generate electricity, with much of the concern focusing on radiation-induced cancer.

Ironically, a major research programme on the health and ecological impacts of radiation and radionuclides was a key proactive component of the Manhattan Project, the US programme initiated in World War II to develop nuclear weapons. Post-World War II, the health and ecological programme was expanded in national laboratories, universities and private institutions with increased focus on ensuring the safe use of radiation, including nuclear power. These research efforts were major contributors to a solid base of information used to develop guidance for the safe use of nuclear power. Moreover, the basic concepts developed would later support the quantitative elements of inhalation toxicology as applied to evaluating the safety of *all* kinds of airborne materials.

Many of the concepts that originated in the radiation field, such as the assumption of low dose–response linearity, have been adopted for evaluating chemical hazards and, more recently, all manner of environmental hazards. Radionuclides have played an important part in the development of molecular and cell biology, as well as in medical research. However, increased knowledge does not always equate to acceptance of technologies.

As mentioned earlier, the publication of Rachel Carson's book *Silent Spring*[1] focused public attention around the world on the impact of synthetic chemicals on human health and more broadly on impacts on the total ecosystem, of which people are just one element. Her book certainly served as a key stimulus for a wave of legislative and regulatory actions that focused broadly on the environment, with concern for clean air and water, safe food, safe pharmaceuticals, pesticides, fungicides, rodenticides and consumer products, and a safe working environment in countries around the world.

In the USA, legislative action and related administrative action in the 1970s created the US Environmental Protection Agency, the Consumer Product Safety Commission, the National Institute of Occupational Safety and Health, the National Center for Toxicological Research, the National Institute of Environmental Health Sciences and, with the National Cancer Institute, the Cancer Bioassay Programme, which evolved into the National Toxicology Programme now administered by the National Institute of Environmental Health Sciences. Similar organizations developed in many other countries around the world.

This was also a period of rapid expansion of research activities in laboratories of the pharmaceutical, food, chemical and petroleum companies. Major chemical companies working together created in 1976 the non-profit US Chemical Industry Institute of Toxicology to test commodity chemicals, investigate the mechanisms of chemical toxicity and train additional toxicologists. In the USA, the Food and Drug Administration continued its traditional dual emphasis on ensuring both the efficacy and the safety of drugs and medical devices. Government support for environmental health-related research in government and academic laboratories also increased sharply during this time period.

During this period, new international organizations emerged. The WHO Environmental Health Criteria Programme was initiated in 1973. This evolved into the International Programme on Chemical Safety, established in 1980 as a joint programme of WHO, the International Labor Organization and the United Nations Environment Program. Global concerns about cancer as a major disease, or more accurately a family of diseases, resulted in the creation of the International Agency for Research on Cancer (IARC) and the initiation in 1969 of the programme producing the IARC Monographs on the Evaluation of Carcinogenic Risks to Humans.[13]

Increasing public concern for safety and its counterpart, risk, and the resulting legislation led to the development of increasingly formalized approaches to safety and risk analyses. This included more clearly defined rules for using the results of toxicological studies, including studies with laboratory animals, to assess the safety, or conversely risk, to humans of the use of pharmaceuticals, other products in commerce and technologies. This was also an era in which more formalized approaches developed to evaluate the impacts of chemicals and other agents on the non-human aspects of ecosystems.

A number of national and international organizations have provided guidance for evaluating the risks of chemical exposure. For example, the US Environmental Protection Agency[10] has prepared a staff paper on risk assessment principles and practices. The WHO's International Programme on Chemical Safety[14] has prepared a number of Environmental Health Criteria documents that provide both general risk assessment guidance and evaluations on specific chemicals or groups of chemicals. The European Community programme REACH (the Registration

Evaluation, Authorization and Restriction of Chemicals) has begun to provide guidance documents on assessing chemical risks.[15,16] Each of these agencies has prepared documents that extend from general guidance to specific guidance for particular end points.

Physical factors affecting health

All living organisms are exposed to forms of energy that can, if encountered in sufficient quantity, cause damage to the organism. Electromagnetic energy, such as in ultraviolet radiation, and ionizing radiation provide two examples. Heat, or its relative absence, cold, is also a potent stressor, as is atmospheric pressure and, to a lesser extent, gravity. Sound waves represent a form of energy, variations in pressure of the air, that affects organisms and has effects ranging from startle responses and annoyance to physical damage to the auditory system. It is not surprising that organisms have evolved defences against these physical stressors. Such defences are sometimes regarded as adaptations: many animals avoid vigorous exercise and seek shade during the hottest times of day. In some, hibernation is a response to cold; in others fur provides protection.

The effect of these adaptations is to maintain the internal environment in what approximates to a steady state. Physiologists describe this as homeostasis and delight in quoting Claude Bernard's dictum: 'La fixité du milieu interieur est la condition de la vie libre.' This may be translated as 'The constancy of the internal environment is the (essential) condition for independent life.' The term 'independent' implies independence from environmental influences. This is seen by many as a fundamental principle of physiology, and physiological mechanisms are seen as conforming to this dictum. Sweating, seeking shade and increasing fluid intake are all physiological responses to heat. Shivering, seeking warmth and the partial shutting down of the peripheral circulation are responses to cold. The commonly perceived increase in frequency of micturition in cold weather is itself due to a movement of blood away from the periphery and to the kidneys.

Homeostatic regulation requires receptors that monitor the state of the organism, a regulator that compares the input from the receptors with a set point, and an effector system that can act in such a way as to restore normality. Such a system is described as a feedback loop. Malfunctioning of the regulator can occur: the patient with a viral infection who shivers despite a high temperature is suffering from resetting of his central thermostat and is responding, physiologically, to an error of the regulator.

Some forms of energy cannot be detected, at least not by man. Ionizing radiation provides an example. Such forms of energy thus present a greater risk than heat because they are not readily detected. This is not to say that the effects of ionizing radiation are not defended against: mutations of genetic material are repaired constantly, and cells that have acquired mutations are destroyed by the immune system. Only when these defences fail do cancer and other effects occur. Interestingly, ionizing radiation, although a stressor to the individual, may play a part in the evolutionary process: without mutations, evolution would not occur, or would at least be dependent on what we might describe as random errors in the functioning of the genes.

In lower animals, it is difficult to assess psychological disturbance in the same way as it can be assessed in man. A person can tell us that he is annoyed by noise, but for a dog we can rely only on the animal's physical response: it may move away from the source. Man is also unusual in that he exposes himself to physical stressors for pleasure. The loud music of the night-club, the intense sunlight of the Mediterranean beach and the cold water of the ocean provide examples. It is unsurprising that such exposures may cause harm; choice has overruled the capacity of evolutionary adaptation.

People vary greatly in their response to such stressors. Some are annoyed by sound levels that others would ignore or enjoy, and some put the perceived attractiveness of a tanned skin above the dangers posed by exposure to ultraviolet radiation. Illness occurs when the individual's physiological capacity to deal with stressors is exceeded. An increase in deaths from heart attacks and strokes occurs in cold weather due to changes in the viscosity and propensity of the blood to clot. In hot weather, the added stress placed on the cardiovascular system by the need to maintain a warm skin that can radiate heat can cause heart failure in those with heart disease.

The elderly are particularly at risk as their physiological reserve is reduced by ageing and their ability to cope with physical stressors is impaired. The very young are also at risk: a baby has a high surface area to body mass ratio, loses heat more quickly than an adult and is thus very sensitive to cold. Adult humans have a great advantage over non-human species in that they can understand, in a conceptual way, the effects of physical stressors and can take action to avoid them. Thus, humans have at their disposal responses beyond those provided by physiology. Rather oddly, many people fail to take sensible measures and so expose themselves to injury. Of course some humans, such as young children, those with learning difficulties and those who are physically incapacitated, may not enjoy such freedom of response.

Heat is an important physical stressor. Biological processes are exquisitely sensitive to temperature, enzyme-catalysed reactions providing an example. Heat is produced by metabolic processes, and the balance of heat production and heat loss is critical to life. This balance is described by the heat balance equation, which describes heat loss in terms of:

> Metabolic heat production
> $\pm$ Heat lost or gained by convection
> $\pm$ Heat lost or gained by radiation
> $\pm$ Stored heat
> $-$ Heat lost by evaporation

Metabolism cannot lead to anything other than production of heat, evaporation can only lead to loss of heat, but the other processes can act in either direction. People can to some extent regulate these processes. Protein stimulates metabolism and leads to heat generation to a greater extent than carbohydrate and fat (this refers to the so-called specific dynamic action of foods and not to their capacity to generate heat when being consumed during metabolic processing), and a reduction in protein intake during periods of heat stress is useful. Carbohydrate releases water during metabolic processing, and this is again useful during heat stress. Water intake can be increased voluntarily, and seeking shade is a common response to high ambient temperatures. When body temperature rises due to inadequate heat loss or excessive heat generation, physiological heat stress occurs.

Sweating is a key mechanism for losing heat. The evaporation of sweat depends on the ambient relative humidity. As long as the body surface is hotter than its surroundings, evaporation will occur even when the air is, at its own temperature, saturated with water vapour. When sweating stops, the person's temperature rises rapidly and heat stroke occurs. This is discussed in detail in Chapter 47.

Noise is another important physical stressor and has been defined as unwanted sound. Physiological defences against excessive sound energy are limited: the tiny muscles of the middle ear (stapedius and tensor tympani) contract reflexly when high pressure changes (loud noises) occur. These contractions brace the eardrum and stapes and protect the delicate mechanism of the inner ear. The reflex contraction is, however, too slow to prevent damage caused by high sound levels of short duration, so the repeated firing of a shotgun or rifle leads to damage to hearing. Such effects are described as those of impulse noise. At more ordinary noise levels, such as are encountered in the environment, physical damage to hearing is unlikely. This is not, however, the case in some occupational settings, and hearing loss due to occupational exposure to noise is an important problem.

Environmental noise causes annoyance. This is common knowledge, and complaints about aircraft noise, traffic noise, noisy dogs and neighbours are among the most common complaints received by environmental health practitioners. Sleep disturbance due to noise is also frequently complained of. This is less easy to demonstrate, and adaptation to noise is common among the majority, for example those living close to railway lines soon cease to 'hear the trains'.

In recent years, attention has been focused on the effects of environmental noise on the cardiovascular system, and there is evidence that exposure to noise leads to an increase in blood pressure and perhaps to an increased risk of heart attack. The evidence relating to effects on blood pressure is well developed in the occupational field, but the link between exposure to noise and effects on the cardiovascular system is unclear. It has been suggested that increased activity of the sympathetic nervous system (involved in 'flight and fright' responses) may play a part, and effects on plasma levels of 'stress hormones' (corticosteroids) and adrenalin have also been suggested. It is often asserted that exposure to environmental noise causes mental illness, but the evidence for this is weak. That many people dislike noise is, however, very clear.

Some attention has been paid to the effects of low-frequency noise. Care is needed here as the pressure variations of frequencies below those which stimulate the inner ear cannot be perceived as noise, even though other sensations, including the perception of tissue vibration, may occur. Wind-farms have been seen as a source of low-frequency noise, and complaints are common. There is little evidence to support the assertion that exposure to ambient levels of low-frequency sound damages health, at least not for the majority, although some individuals do seem to be unusually sensitive. The effects of noise are discussed in more detail in Chapter 57.

Biological agents affecting health

Interest in and awareness of the effects of environmental pollution on health is not new. The Greek philosopher Empedocles (490–430 BC) is credited with relieving recurring epidemics (thought to be malaria) in the Sicilian city of Selinus by joining the Selinus and Hypsos rivers and thereby draining the local marshes. Marsh draining was also used by the Roman Emperors Trajan and Hadrian, and the Roman scholar Marcus Terentius Varro suggested that tiny animals inhabiting the marshes entered the body and caused the disease. This was roughly 20 centuries before Alphonse Laveran first described the parasite (later named *Plasmodium*) in infected patients and Sir Ronald Ross demonstrated its transmission by mosquitoes. Some simple concepts of the prevention of infectious diseases through diagnosis and isolation were also understood in Biblical times.

John Snow's investigation of the Soho cholera outbreak in 1854 identified the source of the outbreak as a sewage-contaminated water source. The investigation was one of first examples of descriptive epidemiology and evidence-based public health intervention and was instrumental in undermining the prevailing 'miasma' view of disease transmission. The report was also an important demonstration of the value of mapping infectious disease data.

Since the late 1980s, there have been a number of outbreaks of cryptosporidiosis due to the contamination of mains water with *Cryptosporidium* oocysts derived from animal and human waste. The water industry has had to improve filtration at water treatment works to remove the oocysts, which are resistant to the chlorination that is usually used for disinfection. The WHO has adopted Water Safety Plans as a way of encouraging water providers to assess the risks across the whole chain of supply from catchment to tap.

Infectious diseases and their investigation differ in significant ways from chemical, radiological and physical exposures. Because pathogens grow and reproduce, there is a potential for outbreaks or epidemics and these are governed by the basic reproductive rate. The population dynamics and modelling of most microparasites such as bacteria and viruses differ fundamentally from those of macroparasites such as helminth worms, which generally grow in the host but do not reproduce. Because outbreaks occur, intervention can in theory prevent many further cases if it is directed to the right areas. This makes the timeliness of investigation of sources and transmission routes critical.

One of the most dramatic features of infectious agents is emergence. A large variety of pathogens have arisen over the last 50 years, and many of these are viruses that have moved from animal hosts to man. Human immunodeficiency virus (HIV) is a good example, in which the original source of the virus was probably African simian primates in the early 1900s. Although subsequent transmission between people has been primarily by sexual contact, the original transmission event was probably associated with the consumption of primates as 'bush meat'. Animal transmission was thought to be responsible for the outbreak of severe acute respiratory syndrome (SARS), and individual cases of human avian influenza infection and the pandemic of swine flu have been derived from bird and mammal hosts, respectively. The SARS outbreak is particularly notable in being effectively eliminated by timely international effort before it had penetrated widely in the human population.

With tuberculosis, the reduction in disease in the nineteenth and early twentieth centuries occurred before vaccination against or effective treatment for *Mycobacterium tuberculosis* had been introduced. Improvements in housing and other social changes probably contributed to this, along with a reduction in the contamination of milk with *M. bovis*. The introduction of bacille Calmette–Guérin (BCG) vaccination, mass screening and effective combined chemotherapy brought the number of cases in Western Europe down to a low level by the end of the twentieth century, but there has been a resurgence as a result of the collaspse of the Soviet Union and the HIV pandemic. This emphasizes that the social environment and national infrastructures can be important in infectious diseases.

Understanding the epidemiology of infectious diseases can be both straightforward and complicated. The ideas of contagion and hygiene are strongly developed within some cultures, but this is not universal. In getting to grips with how particular infections are transmitted, it is important to understand their sources and transmission routes. With an enteric pathogen such as *Cryptosporidium* spp., which cannot grow outside an infected animal, the sources are clearly human and animal faeces. However, the organisms can be split into species and types, and their origins from a range of domesticated animals and wild animals can be less easy to determine with confidence. The vehicle is usually water, although food and direct spread between people and from animals can occur. The transmission routes by which the infection is acquired can be diverse, such that swimming pools, farms, drinking water, nurseries, agricultural animals and pets can all contribute to infections.

Attribution is the process of estimating the relative contribution of particular sources and transmission routes of an infectious agent. Attribution can be achieved to varying degrees of accuracy using information from outbreaks, published evidence, expert elicitation, analytical studies and Monte-Carlo simulations of typing data on sources (e.g. animal contamination) and human cases. This has been particularly successful for *Salmonella* infections, where the main sources are agricultural animals and there is good typing information.

The most fundamental element in the investigation of the effects of the environment on disease is the collection of systematic data on health status, diseases and possible sources of exposure. The main historical resources in Western countries were the national registrations of deaths, with denominator data from birth and christening records, supplemented by census records. The establishment of a system that requires specified authorities to be notified of the occurrence of specified diseases (notifiable disease) provides some historical evidence for the major changes in infectious diseases that have occurred over the last century. However, because some notifications are based on clinical diagnoses rather than on the identification of infectious agents, the system is less reliable than it might be. Syndromic surveillance through primary care systems can be similarly unreliable but can give a better ascertainment of some common conditions and also information on syndromes for which laboratory diagnosis is not common. Where additional information is required, enhanced surveillance can be implemented to provide additional demographic, exposure or laboratory information.

BURDEN OF DISEASE

Worldwide, almost one in five of all deaths are of children of less than five years of age, and of every 10 deaths, 6 are due to non-communicable conditions, 3 to communicable, reproductive or nutritional conditions and 1 to injuries.[16] There are more deaths from trauma in males than females, and the leading causes of death are cardiovascular diseases, infectious and parasitic diseases and cancer.

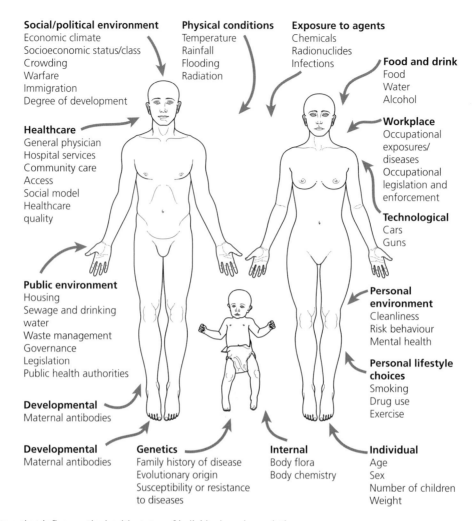

Social/political environment
Economic climate
Socioeconomic status/class
Crowding
Warfare
Immigration
Degree of development

Healthcare
General physician
Hospital services
Community care
Access
Social model
Healthcare
quality

Public environment
Housing
Sewage and drinking
water
Waste management
Governance
Legislation
Public health authorities

Developmental
Maternal antibodies

Developmental
Maternal antibodies

Genetics
Family history of disease
Evolutionary origin
Susceptibility or resistance
to diseases

Physical conditions
Temperature
Rainfall
Flooding
Radiation

Exposure to agents
Chemicals
Radionuclides
Infections

Food and drink
Food
Water
Alcohol

Workplace
Occupational
exposures/
diseases
Occupational
legislation and
enforcement

Technological
Cars
Guns

**Personal
environment**
Cleanliness
Risk behaviour
Mental health

**Personal lifestyle
choices**
Smoking
Drug use
Exercise

Internal
Body flora
Body chemistry

Individual
Age
Sex
Number of children
Weight

Figure 1.6 Factors that influence the health status of individuals and populations.

However, the disease burden differs markedly from country to country and is in part a reflection of the extent of economic development. Estimating how much of the disease burden is caused by the environment and how much is genetic or developmental in origin remains a challenge. There are many factors that influence the health status of individuals and populations, illustrated in Figure 1.6. These typically vary greatly between countries, with wealth being a major factor influencing life expectancy.

To provide an additional perspective on diseases and the role of environmental factors, it is useful to review some data from the WHO Global Burden of Disease project.[17] The causes of disease in low- and middle-income countries, high-income countries and the World are shown in Table 1.1.[17] There are stark differences associated with the income level of the countries. Communicable diseases, maternal and perinatal conditions and nutritional deficiencies dominate in low- and middle-income countries (36.4 per cent) compared with high-income countries (7 per cent). Conversely, non-communicable conditions, including heart disease and

cancer, dominate in the high-income countries (87.0 per cent) compared with the low- and middle-income ones (53.8 per cent).

A detailed tabulation of the 15 major causes of death for a high-income country, the USA, for 2005 is shown in Table 1.2.[18] The dominant role of diseases of the heart and malignant cancers, representing nearly one-half of all deaths, is apparent. Diseases of the respiratory tract, chronic lower respiratory diseases and influenza and pneumonia, account for an additional 7.9 per cent of all deaths.

An alternative analysis that tabulates deaths attributable to various risk factors (Table 1.3[17]) again emphasizes the marked differences between the role of different risk factors in low- and middle-income countries versus high-income countries. The differences in deaths due to smoking in low- and middle-income countries (6.9 per cent) versus high-income countries (18.5 per cent) is striking, especially if the latter are viewed as an indicator of what may occur in the lower-income countries as incomes rise and cigarette-smoking increases. It is noteworthy that deaths

Table 1.1   Deaths by cause – low- and middle-income countries, high-income countries and World, 2001

	Low- and middle-income deaths	High-income deaths	World deaths
All causes			
Total number (thousands)	48 351	7889	56 242
Rate per 1 000 population	9.3	8.6	9.1
Age-standardized rate per 1 000*	11.4	5.0	10.0
	Number in thousands (per cent)		
Selected cause groups			
I. COMMUNICABLE DISEASES, MATERNAL AND PERINATAL CONDITIONS AND NUTRITIONAL DEFICIENCIES	17 713 (36.4)	552 (7.0)	18 168 (32.3)
Tuberculosis	1590 (3.3)	16 (0.2)	1606 (2.9)
HIV/AIDS	2552 (5.3)	22 (0.3)	2574 (46)
Diarrhoeal diseases	1777 (3.7)	6 (<1)	1783 (3.2)
Measles	762 (1.6)	1 (<1)	763 (1.4)
Malaria	1207 (2.5)	0 (0.0)	1208 (2.1)
Lower respiratory infections	3408 (7.0)	345 (4.4)	3753 (6.7)
Perinatal conditions	2489 (5.1)	32 (0.4)	2522 (4.5)
Protein–energy malnutrition	241 (0.5)	9 (0.1)	250 (0.4)
II. NON-COMMUNICABLE CONDITIONS	26 023 (53.8)	6868 (87.0)	32 891 (52.6)
Stomach cancers	696 (1.4)	146 (1.9)	842 (1.5)
Colon and rectum cancers	357 (0.7)	257 (3.3)	614 (1.1)
Liver cancer	505 (1.0)	102 (1.3)	607 (1.1)
Trachea, bronchus and lung cancers	771 (1.6)	456 (5.8)	1227 (2.2)
Diabetes mellitus	757 (16)	202 (2.8)	960 (1.7)
Unipolar depressive disorders	10 (<1)	3 (<1)	13 (<1)
Alcohol use disorders	62 (0.1)	23 (0.3)	84 (0.2)
Hypertensive heart disease	760 (1.6)	129 (1.6)	889 (1.6)
Ischaemic heart disease	5699 (11.8)	1364 (17.3)	7063 (12.6)
Cerebrovascular disease	4608 (9.5)	781 (8.9)	5390 (9.6)
Chronic obstructive pulmonary disease	2378 (4.9)	297 (3.8)	2676 (4.8)
Cirrhosis of the liver	654 (1.4)	118 (1.5)	771 (1.4)
Nephritis and neoplasms	552 (1.1)	111 (1.4)	663 (1.2)
Osteoarthritis	2 (<1)	3 (<1)	5 (<1)
Congenital anomalies	477 (1.0)	30 (0.4)	507 (0.9)
Alzheimer's and other dementias	173 (0.4)	207 (2.6)	380 (0.7)
III. INJURIES	4715 (9.8)	471 (6.0)	5186 (9.2)
Road traffic accidents	1069 (2.2)	121 (1.5)	1189 (2.1)
Falls	316 (0.7)	71 (0.9)	387 (0.7)
Self-inflicted injuries	749 (1.5)	126 (1.6)	875 (1.6)
Violence	532 (1.1)	24 (0.3)	556 (1.0)

AIDS, acquired immune deficiency syndrome; HIV, human immunodeficiency virus.
*Age-standardized using the World Health Organization World Standard Population.
Adapted from Lopez *et al.*,[18] with permission.

attributable to environmental risk factors, including poor sanitation, represent 8.4 per cent of the deaths in low- and middle-income countries and only about 1 per cent in the high-income countries.

Estimates of the burden of disease attributable to environmental factors are very sensitive to the definition of environmental factors. It has been estimated[2] that 24 per cent of the global disease burden and 23 per cent of deaths can be attributed to environmental factors (Figure 1.7).

The discussion of the causes of deaths, and especially of deaths attributable to risk factors, is intended to provide

Table 1.2   Percentage of total deaths and death rates for the 15 leading causes of death: United States, 2005 (rates per 100 000 population)

Cause of death (based on the Tenth Revision, International Classification of Diseases, 1992)	Percentage of Total Rank*		
	Number	Deaths	Rate
United States			
... All causes	2 448 017	100.0	825.9
1 Diseases of the heart (I00–I09, I11, I13, I20–I51)	652 091	26.6	220.0
2 Malignant neoplasms (C00–C97)	559 312	22.8	188.7
3 Cerebrovascular diseases (I60–I69)	143 579	5.9	48.4
4 Chronic lower respiratory diseases (J40–J47)	130 933	5.3	44.2
5 Accidents (unintentional injuries) (V01–X59, Y85–Y86)	117 809	4.8	39.7
6 Diabetes mellitus (E10–E14)	75 119	3.1	25.3
7 Alzheimer's disease (G30)	71 599	2.9	24.2
8 Influenza and pneumonia (J10–J18)	63 001	2.6	21.3
9 Nephritis, nephritic syndrome and nephrosis (N00–N07, N17–N19, N25–N27)	43 901	1.8	14.8
10 Septicaemia (A40–A41)	34 136	1.4	11.5
11 Intentional self-harm (suicide) (†U03, X60–X84, Y87.0)	32 637	1.3	11.0
12 Chronic liver disease and cirrhosis (K70, K73–K74)	27 530	1.1	9.3
13 Essential (primary) hypertension and hypertensive renal disease (I10, I12)	24 902	1.0	8.4
14 Parkinson's disease (G20–G21)	19 544	0.8	6.6
15 Assault (homicide) (†U01–†U02, X85–Y09, Y87.1)	18 124	0.7	6.1
... All other causes	433 800	17.7	146.4

*Rank based on number of deaths.
†Indicates that they are not part of the International Classification of Diseases, Tenth Revision (ICD-10).
Adapted from Kung et al.,[19] with permission.

a context for the material covered in the remainder of this chapter and in later chapters that focuses on individual risk factors and especially the hazards and risks associated with individual chemicals. Control of the hazards and risks of individual chemicals is important. However, the most cost-effective impacts on global public health may be realized by directing attention to other risk factors such as communicable diseases, nutrition, smoking and unsafe sex.

RISK REDUCTION

Risks need to be defined before they can be reduced. Risks can be confused with hazards, and use of the two terms interchangeably can lead to confusing or misleading results. This confusion is often extended to risk and hazard reduction or removal.

Defining risk requires epidemiological rather than toxicological studies. Toxicology is very effective in identifying and quantifying a hazard in animal studies, but extrapolation from animal models to man rarely allows a confident prediction of risk. In a few areas, for example the effects of radiation, this may be possible, but a qualitative identification of hazards rather than a quantitative estimation of risks is in general more likely. Quantitative risk assessment can be undertaken with some

confidence when data from epidemiological studies are available. For example, the increase in risk of death from cardiovascular diseases associated with a long-term exposure to ambient particles is known, and from this estimates of the impact of ambient concentrations of particles on deaths from cardiovascular disease can be made. The risk is known, and the impact can be calculated.

The term 'mathematical quantitative risk assessment' tends to be used to describe the process of predicting the risks of cancer in man from data obtained in studies undertaken using laboratory animals. This process is used in a number of countries but not generally in the UK. The approach suffers from a number of uncertainties, including the impossibility of determining the accuracy of predictions at low levels of exposure. Data derived from occupational studies of the risks of cancer associated with exposure to high levels of carcinogens provide a better basis for extrapolation.

In studies of risks associated with exposure to environmental factors, such as air pollution, identification of the specific agents that are causally related to risks can be difficult. It was stated above that long-term exposure to ambient particles is associated with an increased risk of death from cardiovascular diseases, but the component or components of the ambient aerosol responsible for this effect remain unknown. Thus, although we know the increased risk associated with exposure and we can say that the ambient aerosol is a hazard, we do not know the

Table 1.3   Deaths by cause – low- and middle-income countries, high-income countries and World, 2001

	Low- and middle-income deaths	High-income deaths	World deaths
Total number (thousands)	48 351	7891	56 242
Rate per 1000 population	9.3	8.5	9.1
Age-standardized rate per 1000*	11.4	5.0	10.0
		Number in thousands (percentage)	
Risk factor			
CHILDHOOD AND MATERNAL UNDERNUTRITION			
Childhood underweight	3630 (7.5)	0 (0.0)	3630 (6.5)
Iron-deficiency anaemia	613 (1.3)	8 (0.1)	621 (1.1)
Vitamin A deficiency	800 (1.7)	0 (0.0)	800 (1.4)
Zinc deficiency	849 (1.8)	0 (0.0)	849 (1.5)
OTHER NUTRITION-RELATED RISK FACTORS AND PHYSICAL ACTIVITY			
High blood pressure	6223 (12.9)	1392 (17.6)	7615 (13.5)
High cholesterol	3038 (6.3)	842 (10.7)	3880 (6.9)
Overweight and obesity	1747 (3.6)	614 (7.8)	2361 (4.2)
Low fruit and vegetable intake	2308 (4.8)	333 (4.2)	2641 (4.7)
Physical inactivity	1559 (3.2)	376 (4.8)	1935 (3.4)
ADDICTIVE SUBSTANCES			
Smoking	3340 (6.9)	1462 (18.5)	4802 (8.5)
Alcohol use	1869 (3.9)	24 (0.3)	1893 (3.4)
Illicit drug use	189 (0.4)	37 (0.5)	226 (0.4)
SEXUAL AND REPRODUCTIVE HEALTH			
Unsafe sex	2819 (5.8)	32 (0.4)	2851 (5.1)
Non-use and use of ineffective methods of contraception	162 (0.3)	0 (0.0)	162 (0.3)
ENVIRONMENTAL RISKS			
Unsafe water, sanitation and hygiene	1563 (3.2)	4 (<0.1)	1567 (2.8)
Urban air pollution	735 (1.5)	76 (1.0)	811 (1.4)
Indoor smoke from household use of solid fuels	1791 (3.7)	0 (0.0)	1791 (3.2)
OTHER SELECTED RISKS			
Contaminated injections in healthcare setting	407 (0.8)	4 (<0.1)	412 (0.7)
Child sexual abuse	65 (0.1)	6 (<0.1)	71 (0.1)
All selected risk factors together	22 014 (45.6)	3473 (44.0)	25 488 (45.3)

*Age-standardized using the World Health Organization World Standard Population.
Adapted from Lopez et al.,[18] with permission.

specific hazards that cause the effect. Interestingly, we have identified risk before hazard. An incomplete knowledge of specific hazards leads to difficulties in the 'source-apportionment of risk', and the application of generic approaches to risk reduction is sometimes necessary. These are widely used in occupational health practice and include:

- replacement and banning (e.g. asbestos);
- reduction of exposure (e.g. air pollutants);
- protection – this is often difficult in the environmental context. For instance, the use of masks by cyclists in polluted cities, although seemingly logical, has little scientific support.

Selecting the best option can, however, sometimes lead to unexpected problems – the law of unintended consequences as touched on earlier in this chapter.

Two approaches have been developed to help in policy development. The first, cost-effectiveness analysis, is comparatively easy and leads to policies being chosen on the basis of their efficiency (cost/effect) in reducing risks. A raft of policies can be compared using this method. Effect here means reduction of hazard (and not actually risks). The second approach, cost–benefit analysis, is more difficult and involves a comparison of the costs and benefits of individual policy options. For example, retro-fitting particle traps on diesel powered vehicles is possible, but does the benefit to

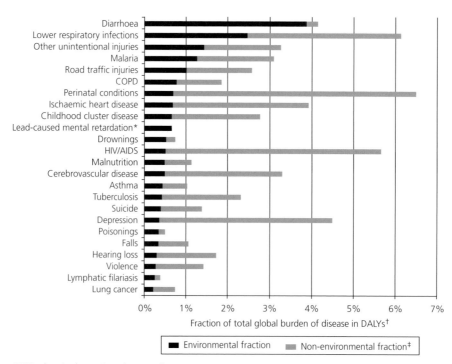

COPD, chronic obstructive pulmonary disease.
* Lead-caused mental retardation is defined in the World Health Organization list of diseases for 2002, accessed at: www.who.int/evidence.
† DALYs represent a weighted measure of death, illness and disability.
‡ For each disease, the fraction attributable to environmental risks is shown in black. Grey plus black represents the total burden of disease.

Figure 1.7   Diseases with the largest environmental contribution. AIDS, acquired immune deficiency syndrome; DALY, disability-adjusted life–year; HIV, human immunodeficiency virus. (Adapted from Pruss-Ustun and Corvalan,[2] with permission.)

health that would be produced by reducing the emission of particles justify the costs of the retro-fit exercise? How could we estimate the benefit in health terms?

Let us assume that we could (as we in fact can) calculate the reduction in the life–years lost by a population as a result of cardiovascular disease caused by exposure to particles. All we now need to do is to compare the costs with the reduction in life–years lost. But are we comparing apples with oranges and producing lemons? – we need a common metric, which could be money. That costs should be expressed in monetary terms seems self-evident, but that health benefits should be expressed in this way is less obvious and, to some, repugnant. Health economists try to value benefits in monetary terms and often use the 'willingness to pay' approach – 'how much reduction in risk are people willing to pay for?' An examination of people's behaviour with regard to avoidance of risk can also lead to useful information: the 'revealed preferences' method.

The reduction of risks to health is a laudable aspiration, but a 'risk-free society' is only an imaginary concept. Reducing risks costs money, and people vary in their attitudes to risk and thus in their views on how much should be spent to reduce risk. Some are 'risk averse' and tend to believe that society should make substantial efforts to reduce

risks, whereas others are 'risk tolerant' and would rather spend their money on other things.

This raises the difficult problem of personal compared with societal risk. A large risk for a few may, at a societal level, be regarded as substantially less important than a small risk for many. At an individual level, there remains the problem of personal choice when considering personal risk. In some instances, acceptance of risk may be voluntary, whereas in others it certainly is not. For example, a private water supply may carry an increased risk of infection or in some cases chemical contamination (e.g. pesticides), but for a rural dweller a supply of water that is cheap and tastes good is itself the most important matter in the context of health.

Finally, the ways in which the benefits from reducing risk can be expressed is a matter of some discussion. For instance, work around the many pieces of legislation worldwide aimed at reducing environmental tobacco smoke in public places has quantified benefit (e.g. respiratory symptoms in bar workers and admissions with acute coronary syndrome), but widening this to the whole community and comparing these benefits quantitatively with other public health concerns (e.g. active smoking or high blood cholesterol) carries with it a number of difficulties while appearing simple at face value.

REFERENCES

● = Key primary paper
◆ = Major review article

1. Carson R. *Silent Spring*. Boston, MA: Houghton Mifflin, 1962.
●2. Bradford Hill A. *Proc Roy Soc Med* 1965; **58**: 295–300.
◆3. Pruss-Ustun A, Corvalan C. Towards Estimation of the Environmental Burden Of Disease. Geneva: World Health Organization, 2006.
4. World Health Organization. Preamble to the Constitution of the World Health Organization as adopted by the International Health Conference, New York, 19–22 June, 1946; signed on 22 July 1946 by the representatives of 61 States (Official Records of the World Health Organization, No. 2, p 100 and entered into force on 7 April 1948).
◆5. Paustenbach DJ. The practice of exposure assessment. In Hayes AW (ed.) *Principles and Methods of Toxicology*. Philadelphia: Taylor & Francis, 2001: 387–448.
6. Parry JL, Canziani OF, Palutikoff JP, van der Linden, PJ, Hanson CE (eds); Intergovernmental Panel on Climate Change. *Impacts, Adaptation, and Vulnerability. Contribution of Working Group II to the Third Assessment Report of the Intergovernmental Panel on Climate Change*. Cambridge: Cambridge University Press, 2007.
◆7. Gamble JL, Ebi KL, Sussman FG, Wilbanks TJ (eds); Climate Change Science Program. *Analysis of the Effects of Global Change on Human Health and Welfare and Human Systems. A Report of the U.S. Climate Change Science Programme and the SubCommittee on Global Change Research*. Washington DC: US Environmental Protection Agency, 2008.
8. Environmental Protection Agency. Advance Notice of Proposed Rulemaking: Regulating Greenhouse Gas Emissions under the Clean Air Act. EPA-HQ-OAR-2008-0318, July 11, 2008.
9. Kennedy D. Risks and risks. *Science* 2005; **309**: 2137.
10. Environmental Protection Agency. *An Examination of EPA Risk Assessment Principles and Practices. Staff Paper Prepared for the U.S. Environmental Protection Agency by Members of the Risk Assessment Task Force*. EPA/100/B-04/001. Washington, DC: EPA, 2004.
◆11. McClellan RO. Human health risk assessment: A historical overview and alternative paths forward. *Inhal Toxicol* 1999; **11**: 477–518.
12. Page W. *Paracelsus: An Introduction to Philosophical Medicine in the Era of the Renaissance*. New York: Karger, 1958.
13. International Agency for Research on Cancer. *Some Inorganic Substances, Chlorinated Hydrocarbons, Aromatic Amines, N-Nitroso Compounds, and Natural Products*. Monographs on the Evaluation of Carcinogenic Risks of Chemicals to Humans, Vol. 1. Lyon: IARC, 1972.
14. International Programme on Chemical Safety. Environmental Health Criteria. Available from: http://www.who.int/ipcs/publications/ehc/en
15. Registration, Evaluation, Authorization and Restriction of Chemicals. REACH Guidance. Available from: http://ec.europa.eu/environment/chemicals/reach/research_intro.htm
●16. Williams ES, Panko J, Paustenbach DJ. The European Union's REACH Regulation: A review of its history and requirements. *Crit Rev Toxicol* 2009; **39**: 553–575.
17. World Health Organization. *Global Burden of Disease*. 2004 update. Geneva: WHO, 2008.
●18. Lopez AD, Mathers CD, Ezzati M, Jamison DT, Murray CJL. Measuring the Global Burden of Disease and Risk Factors, 1990–2001. In Lopez *et al.* (eds). *Global Burden of Disease and Risk Factors*. Oxford: Oxford University Press, 2006.
19. Kung HC, Hoyert DL, Xu J, Murphy S. Deaths: Final data for 2005. *Natl Vital Stat Report* 2008; **56**: 1–120.
20. Morris G, Beck S, Hanlan P, Robertson R. Getting strategic about environment and health. *Publ Health* 2006; **120**: 889–903.

PART 2

METHODOLOGY

2

Epidemiological methods for attributing illness

SUSAN HODGSON, FU-MENG KHAW

INTRODUCTION

Historical perspective

John Snow is widely recognized as the father of epidemiology. In his now classic text *On the Mode of Communication of Cholera*,[1] he argued a case for a 'germ theory', attributing the cause of an outbreak of cholera in 1854 to a water pump in Broad Street, London. Snow used a combination of epidemiological methods to investigate and describe the outbreak: investigation of cases and controls, exposure assessment, additional case finding, and distribution plots of cases by time and place. From his findings, he was able to make a logical link between exposure and outcome, to take immediate action to prevent further cases (removing the pump handle) and to interact with authorities to effect improvements in water supplies.

A few years previously, in May 1847, a Hungarian obstetrician, Ignaz Semmelweis, had implemented a hand-washing policy in his maternity unit. Semmelweis had observed a large difference in mortality rates from puerperal fever (bacterial infection following childbirth) between two maternity units. The only difference between the two units was the staffing arrangements: one was used for the instruction of medical students, and the other only for midwives. Semmelweis could not explain the association between medical students and puerperal fever until he attributed the cause of his friend's death from a febrile illness following an accidental injury from a medical student's scalpel during an autopsy.[2] From his observations, Semmelweis was able to explain the pathway between the source and receptor, and attribute the puerperal fever to

poor hygiene. His hand-washing policy resulted in a dramatic reduction in mortality rates.

Will Pickles, a general practitioner in the Yorkshire Dales from 1913, recognized the importance of case investigations. He meticulously recorded details of each case of infectious disease in his country practice. From these observations, and from his intimate knowledge of the lives of his patients, Pickles was able to trace the source and spread of disease in the Dale. Through careful and tactful questioning, Pickles was often able to deduce 'the short and only possible contact' between patients, allowing him to establish the incubation period and at times the period of infectiousness of each disease.[3] For example, Pickles disputed the 'wide latitude of some of the textbooks in the incubation period of measles'. Pickle's own investigations of two unconnected cases, where there was only one possible point of infection, both indicated an incubation period of 12 days.[4]

The collection of information from the observation of exposures and disease outcomes allows the development of hypotheses on aetiological factors, and is a fundamental step in attributing illness. Without such information, we cannot determine whether and how exposure to specific environmental hazards causes adverse health outcomes.

Richard Doll is arguably the father of modern epidemiology. Following a retrospective study of cases of lung cancer in London hospitals in 1950, he and his colleague Austin Bradford Hill proposed that smoking was responsible for this disease. In 1951, Doll was commissioned by the Medical Research Council to undertake a study to investigate the link between smoking and lung cancer. Doll's approach of carrying out a prospective cohort study on British doctors was ground-breaking, in terms of the scale of the project, with 40 000 participants. In 1954, the research team confirmed a dose–response relationship between smoking and lung cancer.[5]

Aims and overview

The evolution of epidemiological methodology has been stimulated by a constant quest to identify the linkage between exposure and outcome. The examples given above highlight the importance of data collection, descriptive analysis and hypothesis generation followed by analytical methods to test hypotheses.

This chapter will provide the reader with an overview of the main types of epidemiological approach for attributing illness, and will include a summary of the strengths and limitations of these epidemiological methods, a discussion of design considerations, and an approach to interpreting the findings from these methods.

EPIDEMIOLOGICAL METHODS

Categorization of studies

Our choice of epidemiological method may be based on a need to find the best available evidence. To make recommendations for evidence-based practice, it is important to consider where our approach lies in the 'hierarchy of evidence' (Figure 2.1). The strength of any recommendations for practice is based on the level of evidence.[6] As we will see, many epidemiological approaches allow us to ascertain whether there is an association between exposure and outcome, but only those approaches at the top of the hierarchy allow us to establish whether a causative link may be asserted.

Epidemiological studies may be observational or experimental (interventional) (Figure 2.2). In observational studies, the investigator measures attributes of interest (e.g. personal risk factors, exposure or health outcomes) that characterize the population of interest. Observational studies may be descriptive or analytical. Descriptive observational studies describe the occurrence of disease in a population, by characterizing the distribution according to time, person and

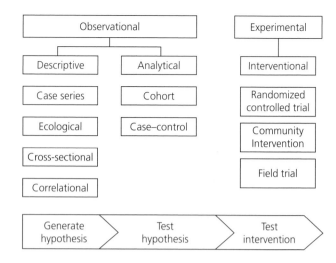

Figure 2.2 Categorization of epidemiological study designs.

place (e.g. ecological, correlation and cross-sectional studies). The findings of descriptive studies are often used to generate hypotheses. Analytical studies can test hypotheses by comparing exposures between cases that have the outcome of interest and controls that do not (e.g. case–control studies) or comparing outcomes in exposed versus non-exposed groups of individuals (e.g. cohort studies).

In experimental studies, the effect(s) of an intervention is(are) investigated by comparing an intervention group with a control (or non-intervention group) (e.g. a randomized controlled trial [RCT]).

Although there is a recognized hierarchy in epidemiological methods, our choice may be constrained for practical reasons, such as availability of study participants (cases or controls) and resources, for ethical considerations or for scientific reasons, such as bias and confounding (see the section on 'Design issues', below).

Epidemiological study design

CASE SERIES

The case series analysis is the mainstay of clinical practice, particularly during the early stages of investigating a new and emerging disease. At the outset, the investigation of cases may involve collecting exhaustive amounts of information through clinical history-taking, clinical examination and diagnostic testing. Once a set of common features has been identified among the cases, it may be possible to develop criteria for a case definition. Following this, exposure or risk factor assessment may identify the aetiology of the disease in question.

An example of the successful use of a case-series approach for attributing illness is provided by thalidomide exposure and birth defects. In 1954, the drug thalidomide was synthesized, and by 1957 it was being marketed to many countries, particularly in Europe, Asia and Australia, as a treatment for sickness during pregnancy. Although the

Systematic review/meta-analysis
Randomized controlled trial
Cohort study
Case–control study
Correlation study
Cross-sectional study
Ecological study
Case series
Expert opinion
Anecdotal evidence

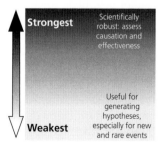

Figure 2.1 Hierarchy of evidence.

first child afflicted by thalidomide damage was born on December 25, 1956, it was not until November 1961 that an Australian gynaecologist, Dr William McBride of Sydney, reported a possible link between thalidomide and birth defects, by observing a 20 per cent incidence of congenital abnormalities among babies born to mothers who had taken thalidomide during pregnancy.[7] Meanwhile, in Germany, a paediatrician (Widukind Lenz) ascertained that 50 per cent of mothers of deformed children had taken the drug during the first trimester of pregnancy. Several years later, McBride was to discover that thalidomide affects DNA structure in fast-dividing embryonic cells, suggesting a causative link.

CROSS-SECTIONAL

A cross-sectional study assesses the exposure and outcome of interest in a 'cross-section' of the population, and usually reflects features of the population, in terms of both exposure and outcome, at a single 'snap-shot' in time.[8,9]

An example of the use of a cross-sectional approach is that adopted by the Department of Health for their Health Survey for England (HSE) studies, which commenced in 1991.[10] The HSE comprises a series of annual cross-sectional surveys that provide information on aspects of the nation's health in a representative sample drawn from those living in private households. A study by Bost et al. used HSE data from 1995 to assess blood lead and blood pressure.[11] This study found that blood lead was significantly and positively associated with diastolic blood pressure in men, but not in women, after adjustment for various confounders. Although these findings are consistent with those from other studies, they demonstrate a limitation of the cross-sectional design: where the exposure and outcome are assessed at the same point in time, the temporal sequence of the observed association cannot be established. When using a cross-sectional design, it can therefore be difficult to establish cause and effect.

Although information on exposure and outcome are gathered at the same point in time in a cross-sectional study, details of exposures occurring during an earlier, more aetiologically relevant time-point can be established using data gathered via a questionnaire. This approach can be problematic if recall of exposures differs between the members of the population with and without the disease (a phenomenon known as recall bias; see later in the text). Another approach to establishing exposure, such as that used in the example above, would be to utilize biological markers, or biomarkers, of exposure or dose (see the section on 'Exposure assessment', below), which would overcome the problem of recall bias.

The main benefit of the cross-sectional approach is that it can be carried out relatively quickly, unlike a cohort study, for which months, years or decades of follow-up may be required, and as such this approach is far less resource intensive and relatively cheap to carry out. When the prevalence, rather than the incidence, of an outcome or

exposure is of primary interest, a cross-sectional approach is ideal. However, because 'incidence' refers to the number of new cases of an outcome occurring over a specified time period, the cross-sectional approach is not suitable where incidence is the primary measure of interest.

Similarly, when investigating rare exposures or outcomes, this design may not be cost-effective as a very large sample from the population will need to be included to ensure that there is sufficient statistical power to assess any associations. For rare outcomes, a case series or case–control study may be more appropriate (see the relevant sections of the text).

ECOLOGICAL

An ecological study design uses groups of individuals as the unit of observation and analysis so assesses associations at the aggregate, or ecological, rather than individual level.[12] Because this approach assesses the relationship between exposure and outcome at the group level, caution must be applied when making inferences from ecological data about relationships at the individual level. This issue of ecological bias is often cited as a major limitation of ecological studies, and is discussed further in the section on 'Ecological bias', below.

The classic ecological approach explores differences in disease rates between population groups or geographical areas, which may be due to differences in demographic, economic or environmental factors that also vary by population group or area. For example, Armstrong and Doll's study of national cancer incidence and mortality in relation to diet found a strong correlation between fat consumption and breast cancer, suggestive of a causal role for fat in the development of this disease.[13] However, subsequent prospective cohort studies have failed to find such an association, suggesting that these early international correlations may suffer from considerable confounding by risk factors such as reproductive variables, physical activity, height and postmenopausal obesity, all of which may be associated with a country's level of affluence and development, and therefore with per capita fat consumption.[14,15]

Although ecological bias is an obvious limitation to the ecological study design, the ecological approach can be an important initial, hypothesis-generating step that can be used to help direct funds to follow-up studies using more resource-intensive, individual-level study designs.

CASE–CONTROL

The case–control study is most useful when the outcome of interest is rare (such as mesothelioma, psittacosis or new and emerging diseases), for diseases with a long latency period (many forms of cancer) and where there is a wide range of potential causative exposures (asthma and occupational exposure to inhalants). It is particularly useful during the early stages of developing an understanding of disease or outcome.

Case–control studies are almost always retrospective, in the sense that the outcome has already occurred before exposure assessment is undertaken. Hence, a major limitation to such studies is the effect of recall bias, which may contribute to the misclassification of exposure (see the section on 'Misclassification', below). The case–control study may be prospective, such as a nested case–control study, in which cases and controls are selected from an existing cohort study. The nested case–control study is of particular use where the number of cases is small and the follow-up of the larger cohort is not necessary or, indeed, cost-effective.

The selection of controls is an important consideration. A cardinal rule is that controls must be selected by virtue of absence of the outcome being assessed and independently of exposure status. The number of controls selected per case is influenced by the desired power of the study, but these details are beyond the scope of this chapter. The choice of sampling frame for controls may have an impact on findings. In a review of case–control studies of risk factors for sporadic Creutzfeldt–Jakob disease (CJD), Barash et al. found that the association observed between surgical procedure and CJD varied according to choice of control: if community controls were used, there was a significantly elevated risk of CJD for people who underwent surgery; for controls recruited from hospitals, surgery significantly reduced the risk of CJD.[16]

The choice of cases may also be subject to selection bias. In a report of intestinal infectious disease in the UK, Tam et al. suggested that cases reported to national surveillance systems were more likely to have more severe symptoms, recent foreign travel, lower educational attainment and lower socioeconomic status compared with those who did not present to their general practitioner. Where such cases are used, the recruitment of controls may have to consider educational attainment and socioeconomic status to minimize bias.[17] This may not always be possible, for example if controls are selected by a random process without access to information on education or status. An alternative is to control for these factors in the multivariate analysis.

A variant of the case–control study is the case–cohort study. Such studies are similar to nested case–control studies in which controls are sampled from an existing cohort. However, in case–cohort studies, controls are sampled from the cohort, irrespective of the outcome of interest. Hence, it is possible to calculate a direct estimate of risk. If the outcome is uncommon, the odds ratio obtained from a case–cohort study approximates the relative risk calculated from a cohort study.

COHORT

In contrast to the case–control study, the cohort study (longitudinal, follow-up or incidence study) is most useful in the following circumstances:

- where the exposure of interest is rare (such as occupational exposure);

- where the outcome under investigation is not uncommon;
- for diseases with a short latency period (as it reduces the adverse effect of loss-to-follow-up bias);
- where a wide range of outcomes may be attributed to a single exposure (air pollutants and respiratory and cardiovascular outcomes);
- where a wide range of putative risk factors may lead to a single outcome of interest (cardiovascular risk factors and coronary heart disease; such as in the 'Framingham study'[18]).

Furthermore, in a prospective cohort, where the outcomes have not occurred at the outset, a clear temporal relationship can be established between exposure and outcome. Where future outcomes are assessed in the cohort, the cohort study may also be used to estimate incidence rates, and as the population at risk is identified, the risk calculations from a cohort study (relative risk) give a direct estimate of risk.

The cohort study may be prospective, retrospective or ambidirectional. In a prospective cohort study, exposure is assessed at the start of the study and the outcome is measured at follow-up in the future, for example smoking and lung cancer in a cohort of British doctors.[5]

In a retrospective cohort study, the outcome has already occurred, and the assessment of exposure is made retrospectively. Although recall bias may affect exposure assessment, retrospective approaches are often the only option in situations where outcomes are not anticipated, such as in outbreaks of infectious disease. Friedman et al. concluded, after conducting a retrospective cohort study of guests attending 36 separate wedding functions, that a large outbreak of norovirus was associated with eating wedding cakes made by a certain bakery.[19]

In ambidirectional cohort studies, exposure assessment is made both retrospectively and prospectively. Such studies are particularly useful where short-term and long-term outcomes are expected. For example, a cohort of patients attending a sexual health clinic who are screened for Chlamydia infection may be recruited to identify the risk factors for acquiring the disease by assessing exposures retrospectively. Those who have Chlamydia infection may then be followed-up to determine the risk factors for infertility.

CASE–CROSSOVER

The case-crossover study, first proposed by Maclure, is arguably a variant of the case–control study.[20] However, in a case-crossover study, all participants have the outcome being investigated, and the controls are selected from the past experience of cases before they developed the outcome. To qualify for this approach, the following conditions must be fulfilled:

- The cases must have varying experience of the exposure over time.

- The outcome must occur soon after exposure (i.e. there is a short time lag for effect).
- The effect of the exposure must be short-lived and not have lasting cumulative effects.

There are many examples of case-crossover studies. Stafoggia *et al.* used a case-crossover design to assess the effect of high temperature on all-cause mortality in four Italian cities during 1997–2003, and reported greater mortality rates with increased temperature. They also identified that the elderly, women, widows and widowers, those with selected medical conditions, and those staying in nursing homes and healthcare facilities were more vulnerable.[21]

The case-crossover design reduces the potential for unmeasured or residual confounding, owing to the ability to assign 'internal' controls. In a study to assess the effectiveness of consistently safe condom use (i.e. without breakage or slippage) on acquisition of gonorrhoea or *Chlamydia*, Warner *et al.* compared case-crossover and cohort designs applied to the same dataset and demonstrated a statistically significant protective effect using a case-crossover approach and a non-significant protective effect using a cohort design.[22] Hence, in some circumstances, a case-crossover design may be superior to case–control studies, particularly when the case can be used as its own control.

INTERVENTION STUDIES

The RCT aims to eliminate the effects of known and unknown confounders by randomly allocating participants to receive (intervention group) or not receive (control group) an intervention. Most RCTs are clinical trials of interventions for the treatment of individuals with disease. For ethical reasons, an intervention can only be studied if there is sufficient belief that neither the control nor the intervention group is disadvantaged by either not receiving or receiving the intervention, respectively. The RCT design has a limited role in the study of aetiological factors associated with disease because it would be unethical to allocate groups to receive the exposure if it were hypothesized that the exposure causes an adverse outcome.

The preventive trial assesses whether an intervention protects against developing disease. Two variants of preventive trial exist: field trials and community intervention trials. Field trials differ from clinical trials as the study participants do not have the outcome of interest, but the preventive effect of an intervention is assessed by comparing the outcomes in two groups. The most prominent example of a field trial is the Salk vaccine trial, which assessed the efficacy of two forms of the polio vaccine.[23]

In contrast with the field trial, the community intervention trial assigns groups of individuals to receive or not receive an intervention. This approach is particularly useful to assess complex community-level interventions. In a classic example of a community trial, Dean and his colleagues assessed the effectiveness of the fluoridation of public water supplies in preventing dental caries.[24] Within a few years, they established that water fluoridation was very effective at preventing dental caries; this evidence played a pivotal role in changing dental public health policy.[25]

META-ANALYSIS

Meta-analysis is the statistical combination of results from two or more separate studies.[26] Meta-analyses are often presented as part of a systematic review, where a body of research that addresses the same research question is gathered, summarized and reviewed to provide a comprehensive and reliable overview of the results of all available relevant studies.[27] Where studies are found to be sufficiently homogeneous, a meta-analysis may be undertaken.[28,29] The meta-analytical approach employs statistical methods to combine the effect estimates from each component study, often weighted by study size and/or study quality, to provide a single, summary estimate of effect. Examples of methodologically sound systematic reviews and meta-analyses can be found in the Cochrane Library (see the end of the chapter).

The benefits of undertaking meta-analyses include increased statistical power and precision of the risk estimate, because the summary estimate of effect is based on more information than is present in any of the individual studies. In addition, by combining individual studies that have used different methodological approaches (e.g. cohort and case–control) or that involve different subsets of the population (e.g. by sex, age group or ethnicity), the consistency of the effect, as well as reasons for any differences in effect estimates, can be investigated.[26,29] For example, a meta-analysis of studies assessing the risk of breast cancer in relation to oral contraceptive use found an increased risk of breast cancer with increasing duration of oral contraceptive use.[30] However, this effect was only evident in studies looking at premenopausal women; studies that included postmenopausal women did not show this effect. Subsequent meta-analyses have confirmed a slight increase in breast cancer risk in women who have taken oral contraceptives within the previous 10 years.[31]

As can be seen from the hierarchy of evidence (see Figure 2.1, above), meta-analyses, along with systematic reviews, are considered to be among the strongest evidence available, enabling the researcher to draw conclusions about causation. Unfortunately, these approaches cannot always be adopted as they rely on a sufficient number and quality of homogeneous primary studies being available. Trying to combine primary studies that are too heterogeneous is unlikely to provide a useful summary estimate, and if sufficient consideration is not given to the study designs, within-study biases, between-study variation and missing studies (publication bias), the meta-analysis output could be very misleading. Meta-analysis can also highlight where evidence is missing in analyses of risk.

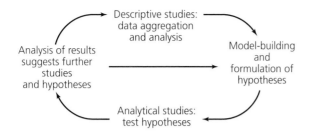

Figure 2.3 The epidemiological cycle.

Epidemiological study cycle

Attributing illness in environmental medicine often involves a multistaged, iterative approach to epidemiological investigation, involving descriptive and analytical techniques (Figure 2.3). This is especially true for new and emerging diseases, for which there may be limitations in assessing exposure or measuring outcome. In such situations, a descriptive case series can be useful to generate a hypothesis that is subsequently tested using analytical epidemiological methods. It is particularly useful to prepare an epidemic curve in outbreaks of infectious disease.

A good example of this iterative approach is the discovery of human immunodeficiency virus (HIV) infection and acquired immune deficiency disease syndrome (AIDS). In June 1981, the USA Centers for Disease Prevention and Control reported a case series of five patients with *Pneumocystis carinii* pneumonia diagnosed in Los Angeles during a period of 7 months.[32] All five cases were homosexual men aged between 29 and 36 years. Until then, *Pneumocystis* pneumonia had only been seen in severely immunocompromised patients, and its presentation in previously healthy young adult males was unusual.

Several months later, Hymes *et al.* reported a case series of eight young homosexual men with an aggressive form of Kaposi's sarcoma, a benign tumour that was known to affect older people.[33] A case-series analysis identified sexual activity between men as a risk factor and erroneously misattributed the cause of AIDS to a popular recreational drug, amyl nitrite ('poppers').[34] Subsequently, a case–control study of Kaposi's sarcoma and *Pneumocystis carinii* pneumonia in homosexual men concluded that cases had more sexual partners and were more likely to engage in anal intercourse, take illicit drugs and have a history of past sexually transmitted infections, such as syphilis. This led researchers to conclude that this was a sexually transmitted infection.[35]

By 1983, the HIV virus had been identified, and in 1985 blood tests became available to confirm the diagnosis. The ability to define a case using an objective laboratory test facilitated future epidemiological studies. It soon became clear from further case reports that this disease was not confined to homosexual men or sexual transmission; when cases among injecting drug users and haemophiliacs were identified, the role of blood-borne transmission was recognized.

Other dimensions

SPATIAL EPIDEMIOLOGY

Spatial epidemiology refers to the description and analysis of geographical variations in disease risk in relation to demographic, environmental, behavioural, socioeconomic, genetic and infectious risk factors.[36] Early spatial studies included large-scale international and regional comparisons of disease frequency, for example the International Agency for Research on Cancer's 'Cancer Incidence in Five Continents' series, established in 1966 to explore cancer frequency in different countries over time.[37]

Spatial epidemiology covers four main types of study:

Geographical correlation studies allow the exploration of disease frequency in different communities in relation to variations in environmental, demographic or lifestyle variables, at the ecological level. An example of a geographical correlation study is Armstrong and Rose's investigation of national cancer incidence in relation to dietary intake by country,[13] outlined above.

Disease-mapping, which is primarily descriptive, provides information on the spatial distribution of disease rates; one example is the *Cancer Atlas of the United Kingdom and Ireland 1991–2000*.[38]

Risk assessment studies assess disease risk in relation to putative pollution sources. These studies can help to address disease aetiology when assessing risk from a biologically plausible hazard, but can be difficult to robustly implement and interpret when the risk assessment is carried out in response to a media report or to local concerns (e.g. the reported excess of childhood leukaemia in the populations living near to the Sellafield nuclear reprocessing plant in Cumbria, UK[39]).

Cluster analyses can be carried out (with caution) to detect disease clusters – an unusual aggregation of health events grouped in time and/or space. In addition, cluster analyses can be undertaken to assess disease clustering, the tendency of cases to be distributed in a non-random spatial and/or temporal pattern relative to non-cases.[36] Such disease clustering is to be expected with infectious diseases, but has also been observed for other end points; for example, some childhood cancers have been shown to display space–time clustering.[40]

Due to issues of data availability, spatial analyses have often been undertaken at the regional, national or international level, and have proved difficult to interpret. It is often impossible to rule out ecological bias, in which factors associated with disease at the national or regional level may not necessarily be associated with disease at the individual level[41] (see Ecological bias page 35). Over the past few decades, there has been an increase in the availability of geographically linked health and population data, which has enabled the mapping and analysis of small-area variations in health risk, increasing the interpretability of these studies or allowing very local effects of point sources of pollution to be investigated.[36] Nonetheless, many spatial analyses continue to be ecological or semi-ecological in design, relying on routinely collected health data (e.g. mortality records, hospital admissions and cancer registrations) and small-area population counts (e.g. census data). Although the health outcome data may be available at the individual level, the data on potential confounders and/or exposure are often only available at the small-area level. This reliance on group-level data means that it is not possible entirely to rule out ecological bias, although by working at the small-area level, studies will be less susceptible to the component of ecological bias created by within-area heterogeneity.[36]

In studies reliant on routinely available health and population data, meaningful results will only be forthcoming if the underlying health and population data are accurate and complete. Local variations in the ascertainment of health data,[42] changes in health event recording over time,[43] intercensus population migration,[44] and inaccurate geocoding[45] may introduce spurious temporal or spatial patterns in risk. In disease-mapping studies, consideration must be given to the mapping resolution, as findings can be sensitive to changes in the scale of output (the 'modifiable area unit problem'[46]), which will influence interpretation. In a cluster analysis, care must be taken to avoid 'boundary shrinkage' or the 'Texas Sharp Shooter effect', whereby the selection of a narrowly defined underlying population at risk (in terms of study area, time frame, age and sex grouping, diagnostic categories, etc.) will give rise to a lower number of expected cases and therefore a greater estimated risk.[36]

Over the past few years, there has been considerable interest in developing 'environmental public health tracking systems' to evaluate temporal and spatial relationships between health events and environmental hazards.[47] Such networks encourage the collection and linkage of environment and health data, provide opportunity for multidisciplinary working and can be valuable in highlighting data issues and future data needs. Tools such as HealthMapper, Sistemas de Información Geográfica en Salud (SIGEpi) and the Rapid Inquiry Facility (RIF) are now available to link routinely collected health and population data to environmental exposures.[48]

GENETIC EPIDEMIOLOGY AND GENE–ENVIRONMENT INTERACTION

Most common diseases are likely to involve genetic and environmental causes as well as interactions between these risk factors.[49] Genetic epidemiology focuses on the genetic determinants of disease and the interactions between genetic and environmental factors that influence the risk of disease.[50]

Genetic variation can influence the susceptibility of an individual to a disease, and genetic markers derived from the direct analysis of DNA or from the measurement of gene products can define additional study participant characteristics for the assessment of gene and gene–environment interaction using the traditional epidemiological approaches outlined above. Other study designs have also been developed or exploited for the assessment of gene–environment interaction, including case-only and familial studies, but the description of these is beyond the scope of this chapter.

Gene–environment interactions can be assessed using case–control, cohort or cross-sectional study designs, which explore the impact of different genotypes on disease risk in environmentally exposed individuals or the impact of differential environmental exposure on individuals with a specific genotype.[51]

When attempting to attribute illness, there are several advantages to considering the gene–environment influences on disease. This approach enables the researcher to appropriately assess important genetic and environmental risk factors; in diseases where there is an influence of both, focusing only on the genetic or environmental factors would mean that important aetiological determinants would be missed.[51] In addition, these approaches can be used to identify important risk factors that confer only a small increase in risk (as is often the case with many environmental determinants) or to explore dose–response relationships at low levels of exposure by studying susceptible individuals, thus strengthening the associations observed.[49]

Other potential benefits of considering gene–environment interaction in disease include a deeper understanding of the aetiological mechanisms of disease, as well as the ability to provide individualized preventive advice or personalized treatment depending on their genetic susceptibility,[52] although this latter benefit has to date largely remained a theoretical one with respect to common, complex diseases.[53]

TIME SERIES ANALYSIS

A time series is a sequence of observations over time, such as daily air pollution levels, weekly hospital admissions, rates of infectious disease or annual healthcare expenditure.[54] Trends in health outcomes over time can be used to generate hypotheses about potential risk factors (e.g. the rise in type 1 diabetes across Europe[55]), to monitor vaccination programmes (e.g. measles, mumps and rubella vaccination uptake in the UK[56]) or to assess the consistency in health event coding over time (e.g. the impact on coding of cause of death of editions of the *International Classification of Diseases*[43]).

When trying to attribute an outcome to a specific exposure, a time series analysis can be undertaken to assess the associations between temporal trends in exposure and outcome. Because observations that are close together in time tend to be correlated, special time series methods need to be employed to take into account this correlation to produce valid inferences from the data.[54] Well-known examples of time series studies include assessing the short-term impacts of air pollution exposure on deaths and hospitalizations from respiratory and cardiac outcomes,[57,58] and the impact of heatwaves on deaths in the elderly.[59,60] Time series studies can also be used to assess the impacts of policy introductions, such as a smoking ban on coronary heart disease risk,[61] or the health effects associated with accidents, for example the risk of childhood thyroid cancer following the Chernobyl nuclear accident.[62]

Time series can be useful for modelling macroparasites, but 'SIR'-type models (compartments of susceptible, infected and recovered people) are more commonly used for modelling microparasites (most viruses, bacteria and protozoa).

DESIGN ISSUES

Availability of data and resources

Epidemiological study depends on the availability or collection of good quality and relevant outcome, exposure and confounder data. The epidemiological approach chosen will depend not only on the research question of interest, but also on the resources available to undertake the study.

Although it might be desirable to assess exposure using personal monitoring, or to utilize a sensitive biological marker of early disease development in lieu of a less sensitive measure such as mortality, these options are not always practical if a large study population is needed to provide sufficient statistical power.

Routinely collected health and exposure data may be useful for descriptive studies, such as ecological or cross-sectional studies, but bespoke data collection is usually necessary for analytical studies to allow the investigator to take into consideration the specific needs of the study, such as measurement of confounding variables.

Although prospective data collection for exposures and potential confounding variables might be considered the ideal, it might be preferable, for an outcome with a long lag period, to try in the first instance to reconstruct exposure using historical records on emissions, monitoring data, residential moves and so on, before dedicating resources to establishing a costly and time-consuming prospective cohort. For retrospective studies, a good knowledge of historical sources of information regarding exposure monitoring is important. Often, however, there are limitations in the utility of historical data as these may be subject to changes with time, such as measurement techniques and reporting protocols.

Exposure assessment

Exposure can be assessed in many different ways, with approaches often categorized as either direct or indirect. A direct approach to exposure assessment involves the measurement of each study participant's individual exposure, for instance using a personal air monitor or using biological markers of exposure. An indirect approach to exposure assessment involves assigning an exposure to each study participant based on environmental levels that may have been monitored or modelled, or ascertained from questionnaire data, for example. As with the hierarchy of evidence for epidemiological approaches, there is a hierarchy of exposure measurements (Figure 2.4), which places most weight on those direct approaches which are likely to give the best estimate of actual exposure, and least weight on indirect, proxy measures that are unlikely to describe exposure appropriately.

Although the direct approach may give the best approximation of actual exposure, it can be costly and impractical to collect personal measurements for a sizable population. In contrast, an indirect approach may lead to a degree of misclassification of exposure, but it will allow exposure to be assigned to a very large population. In many studies, there is a trade-off between ensuring that a sufficiently sizable population is included in the study such that there is sufficient power to detect an effect, and ensuring that exposure is adequately measured to allow meaningful inferences to be made from the findings. In some cases, a mixture of approaches to exposure assessment is used; for example, personal monitoring may be used to validate and inform modelled or measured environmental exposures.

As outlined above, epidemiological study designs can be categorized in different ways. One important distinction, in terms of biases inherent in the study design, is whether exposure is assessed prospectively or retrospectively relative to disease status. A classic cohort study would usually be prospective in this respect, with members of the study population being identified as exposed or unexposed at the start of the study, and disease status being followed over time. In contrast, a typical case–control study would

Types of exposure data

Quantified personal measurements

Quantified area/ambient measurements in the vicinity of the residence

Quantified surrogates of exposure

Distance from site and duration of residence

Residence in the geographical area where exposure can be assumed

Residence in the defined geographical area shared by the site

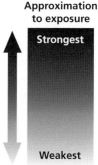

Approximation to exposure

Strongest

Weakest

Figure 2.4 Hierarchy of exposure data.

usually begin with the identification of cases and controls, and would retrospectively assess whether or not these individuals had been exposed at a time prior to disease onset. However, retrospective cohort studies are not uncommon, and nor are 'nested' case–control studies, which typically benefit from prospective exposure assessment by virtue of being embedded within a cohort study. By prospectively collecting information on exposure, a study should avoid bias caused by a incomplete or inaccurate recall of exposure. This recall or reporting bias becomes particularly important when there is a differential recall between cases and controls (see Recall bias, page 35) Although a prospective exposure assessment will avoid many of the issues associated with recall bias, this approach might require the collection of exposure data years or decades before the health events of interest are likely to be observed. In contrast, a retrospective approach can be carried out on cases that are already confirmed. Again, a trade-off between timeliness and bias needs to be made.

Guidelines on good exposure assessment practice for chemical exposures (but which apply to many types of environmental exposure) are provided by the Interdepartmental Group on Health Risks from Chemicals.[63] Discussions of issues associated with exposure assessment and recommendations for study design are provided by the World Health Organization.[64] A summary of the effect of error in exposure measurement on study efficiency is provided by Armstrong,[65] and details of advances in exposure assessment for epidemiological studies can be found in Nieuwenhuijsen et al. 2006.[66]

The investigation of cases of infectious diseases typically relies on the indirect measurement of exposure, which may include a variety of sources. The transmission of infection may be linked to contaminated food (Salmonella food poisoning from infected eggs), an infected person (sexually transmitted infections such as syphilis), a contaminated environment (norovirus on soft furnishings), an intermediate vector (e.g. mosquitoes for malaria) and contaminated objects (CJD acquired from contaminated surgical instruments). Hence, the assessment of exposure may depend on reliable information on recent food consumption, sexual activity, travel history and surgical procedures. Diseases with long incubation periods may require an exposure history that goes back several decades.

Measurement of outcome

The measurement of outcome depends on a case definition that describes the criteria that must be met before attributing the presence of an outcome. The degree of specificity of a case definition may vary according to the requirements of the epidemiological enquiry. For instance, if it does not matter whether cases have objective signs of asthma, self-reported symptoms or the receipt of a prescription for an inhaler may be sufficient. Subjective measures of outcome are frequently used for studies

involving postal questionnaires to large numbers of participants. In a comparative cross-sectional study of the prevalence of respiratory illness amongst 4860 children living near to and away from opencast coal-mining sites, Pless-Mulloli et al. used postal questionnaires to identify respiratory symptoms and the receipt of asthma medication among the participants.[67] In this study, the cost of carrying out objective tests, such as spirometry, might be prohibitive.

During outbreaks of infectious disease, the case definition may change as more information (such as symptoms and signs of the disease, positive bacterial cultures and further identification by subtyping) becomes available. Typically, as the outbreak progresses, the outcome becomes more specific or well defined.

For novel or emerging infectious diseases, initial epidemiological enquiry may depend on clinical signs and symptoms until the organism has been characterized. During the severe acute respiratory syndrome (SARS) epidemic in November 2002 to July 2003, the initial public health response was guided by clinical case definitions. On April 16th, 2003, the World Health Organization announced the identification of a previously uncharacterized coronavirus as the responsible pathogen for SARS; thereafter, a confirmed case definition could include a laboratory confirmation of infection.

Case (or outcome) definitions may change with advances in diagnostic tools and technology. Such changes may have an impact on the interpretation of epidemiological studies. For example, the diagnosis of norovirus infection has been facilitated by the introduction of more sensitive tests. Norovirus cannot be cultured and, traditionally, detection has relied on electron microscopy and serology for the presence of antibodies. However, the use of a sensitive polymerase chain reaction test can increase the detection rate of norovirus infection twofold compared with electron microscopy.[68] It is interesting that, with very sensitive polymerase chain reactions for norovirus, the detections in asymptomatic patients increase, so a more quantitative approach to detection may be appropriate. Hence, the interpretation of historical epidemiological studies also has to consider limitations in technology.

Sample size

When planning to undertake any study, it is essential that consideration is given to the sample size. Any study should have sufficient sample size to achieve its aims, i.e. to determine, with an acceptable degree of precision, the effect hypothesized to be evident.[69] This could be a difference in disease risk between exposed and non-exposed populations, or treatment effect in different legs of a clinical trial. The probability of a study correctly identifying this difference (where this exists in the populations from which the samples have been drawn) is referred to as the study power. If a study does not have sufficient power, it becomes difficult to conclude from the findings whether a lack of a significant difference between groups is due to there being no difference, or due to there being insufficient power to detect this difference. There is a clear case for avoiding undertaking an underpowered study, as well as for avoiding wasting resources on an overly large study.

To establish the appropriate study size, various factors need to be considered: the sampling variation, the effect magnitude, the significance and the power.[70,71] The variance of measurements within any sample is determined by the number of measurements made – the larger the sample, the narrower the probability distribution and the more precise the measurement. The effect size (or best estimate of the anticipated effect size) needs to be realistic and relevant; trying to assess a very small effect will require a very large study, but being too optimistic about the effect size likely to be seen may lead to an underpowered study. The significance refers to the probability of rejecting the null hypothesis incorrectly (type I error, or *P*-value) and determines how likely the observed effect is to be due to chance; by convention, this is normally set at 0.05 (or a 5 per cent probability that the effect is due to chance). The power refers to the probability of correctly identifying a difference between the two groups when such a difference exists (avoiding type II error) and is often (arbitrarily) set to at least 80 per cent. When these values have been established, tabulated values and/or formulae can be used to calculate the required sample size.[69–71] See Box 2.1 for a summary of type errors and the power of a hypothesis test.

A larger sample size is required when the variance of the measurements is large, when the significance is set to a very stringent level and when the power required is very high.[69] In addition, when the effect size is small – which is the case for many environmental risk factors – large populations are required to demonstrate a significant difference between groups.

In many epidemiological studies, several hypotheses may be tested using the same dataset. For example, in a case–control study, the association between the outcome and several putative risk factors may be explored, and/or the study population may be stratified by age, sex or other characteristics to identify high-risk groups. When such 'multiple testing' is undertaken, one may expect to see a statistically significant effect due to chance (where the significance level has been set to the conventional 5 per cent, for every 20 associations explored, one of these associations would be expected to be statistically significant simply by chance). While multiple testing can be a cost-effective means of undertaking research, careful consideration should be given a priori to the formulation of meaningful hypotheses to test.

Research governance

When undertaking epidemiological studies, the conduct of a project may be subject to research governance, and prior research ethics committee approval may be required. In the UK, there are guidelines for undertaking research that involves National Health Service patients, staff and premises.[72] Research ethics approval may be required for some epidemiological studies initiated in response to acute outbreaks of infectious disease and incidents involving biological, chemical or nuclear hazards. In the practical outbreak management of microbiological outbreaks, there is no requirement for ethical approval. Research subsequent to the outbreak that is not part of the initial investigations may require ethical approval.

In these circumstances, obtaining timely ethical approval may be a challenge if the facility for expedited ethics review is not available.

Bias

The presence of bias can be a major flaw in epidemiological studies, with significant bias leading to incorrect conclusions being drawn from the data. Measures to reduce bias need to be taken at the design stage because bias cannot be removed after data collection. There are several types of bias, some of which are associated with specific types of study.

MISCLASSIFICATION

When undertaking or interpreting the findings of a study, thought should always be given to the potential for

---

BOX 2.1: Hypothesis testing

There are four possible outcomes when testing a hypothesis, outlined in the grid below

	Null hypothesis accepted	Null hypothesis rejected
Null hypothesis true	$1-\alpha$	α Type I error
Alternative hypothesis true	β Type II error	$1-\beta$

The *significance* of the test (α) is the probability that we reject the null hypothesis when it is true, a **Type I error**, or a false positive result.

If we accept the null hypothesis when it is false (β), we make a **Type II error**, and have a false negative result.

The *power* of the test ($1-\beta$) is the probability that we correctly reject the null hypothesis.

By convention, α is usually set to 0.05 or 0.01 (meaning there is only a very small possibility of a false positive result), and β to 0.10 or 0.20 (equivalent to an 80 or 90% probability that we correctly reject the null hypothesis).

exposure measurement error (for continuous variables) or misclassification (for categorical variables). Exposure error can be non-differential or differential with respect to the case status. Non-differential misattribution of exposure will reduce study power and is likely to bias risk estimates towards the null.[65,73] Differential misattribution, where the probability of exposure error or misclassification differs between cases and controls (e.g. due to recall bias), will result in reduced study power and can lead to biased effect estimates in either direction,[65] potentially introducing an apparent effect where there is none, or falsely suggesting that there is no effect when one does exist.

Measurement error or misclassification of confounding variables can also impact on the interpretation of study findings, as any adjustment for misattributed confounders will be incomplete.[65]

RECALL BIAS

Recall bias, in which, for example, cases and controls differentially remember exposures or where exposed and non-exposed groups differentially recall symptoms, can be a significant problem where data are collected retrospectively.

The impact of prospective versus retrospective collection of exposure data on the study findings is illustrated in Bar-Oz's study of the impact of exposure to the antifungal drug itraconazole during the first trimester on congenital anomaly outcomes.[74] The rate of anomalies was assessed in two cohorts, the first consisting of 166 women retrospectively reporting itraconazole use when asked after delivery, the second consisting of 198 women prospectively reporting itraconazole use before pregnancy outcome was known. The rate of anomalies was found to be 13 per cent when exposure was assessed retrospectively, compared with 3.2 per cent (the same as in a control group) when exposure was assessed prospectively. This finding suggests that retrospective exposure assessment can introduce significant bias due to differential recall.

Blinding the study participants and researchers to the study hypothesis can help to reduce recall bias, but prospective data collection is the best way of avoiding this problem.

SELECTION BIAS

Selection bias can occur when the subjects selected for inclusion in a study fail to fully represent the underlying population from which they were drawn. There are many reasons why selection bias might be introduced, but examples include the recruitment of volunteers, non-participation and the healthy worker effect.

Self-selection bias can be introduced in a study that recruits volunteers. People who volunteer to participate in a study tend to differ from the population from which they are drawn with respect to various factors, such as health status, education, lifestyle, etc., which may also be associated with the exposures, outcomes or confounders of interest. Similarly, non-participation can also introduce selection bias if the characteristics of the non-participants differ from the characteristics of the participants with respect to their exposure distributions or other variables under study.[75]

The healthy worker effect is a form of selection bias that can be introduced into an occupational cohort study that uses a general population sample as the comparison group. Estimates of effect may be biased because the general health in an occupational group may be better than that of the wider general population, which includes those too ill to be employed.[76]

Selection bias can be introduced in any study (cohort, case–control or cross-sectional), although the case–control design is considered more susceptible to this particular bias because the underlying population at risk is not always straightforward to define.[9] To ensure that valid estimates of risk are obtained, controls must be representative of the population from which the cases were drawn. This can be achieved quite easily in a nested case–control study, where the cases and controls originate from a clearly defined study population. In contrast, in a hospital-based case–control study or other situations where there may be incomplete case ascertainment, it can be difficult to define the population group from which to draw controls.[77,78] In such a situation, the study population is often defined in terms of hospital users, with controls drawn from another patient group, but great care must be taken to ensure that the controls are not suffering from conditions that might also be associated with the exposures of interest. As highlighted above, the choice of control sample can have a significant impact on the study findings.[16]

LOSS-TO-FOLLOW-UP (ATTRITION) BIAS

Losses to follow up may occur in several ways: withdrawal of consent, death and loss of contact. In a long-term cohort study, whereby follow-up may be decades later, the number lost to follow-up may represent a significant proportion of the initial cohort. Not only will this reduce the power of the statistical analysis, but assurance will also be needed in terms of assessing whether those lost to follow-up are in any way a biased sample. Kristman *et al.* undertook a simulation study of the effect of loss to follow-up on the findings of a cohort of observations.[79] They concluded that loss-to-follow-up rates of up to 60 per cent did not significantly influence the results of the study. However, if those lost to follow-up were not missing at random (e.g. if they are significantly different from the group that were successfully followed up), it is possible that the interpretation of the findings may be flawed.

ECOLOGICAL BIAS

Ecological bias refers to making incorrect inferences about the association between an exposure and outcome at the individual level on the basis of information derived at the group level. For instance, factors associated with national or regional disease rates may not necessarily be associated with disease at the individual level.[41] Although a strong correlation was observed between fat consumption and breast cancer risk when assessed at the national level,[13] subsequent individual-level studies[14,15] failed to support this association, suggesting that the early international correlations suffered from ecological bias.

Ecological bias can be introduced into any study that uses group-level rather than individual-level data on an exposure, outcome or confounding variable. It is important to note that 'ecological' bias is not just limited to ecological (group-level) studies. In an individual-level study, the use of individual educational status as a proxy measure for dietary habits could also introduce ecological bias – although there might be a correlation between educational status and dietary habits at the group level, an individual within a specific educational group may not necessarily exhibit the dietary patterns of that group.[80]

Although ecological bias can be avoided by assessing exposures, outcomes and confounders of interest at the individual level, the ecological or contextual effect is sometimes of genuine interest. For instance, deprivation can be measured as an individual characteristic and as a community characteristic, with both potentially exerting independent effects on health.[80] In some situations, for example where the exposure of interest relates to a group property that is not an aggregate variable (e.g. social capital), an ecological study can be an appropriate way of exploring the impact of a variable not reducible to the individual level. Indeed, failure to take account of the group-level context has been suggested to lead to 'individualistic fallacy',[81] whereby major group-level determinants of health have been ignored because undue focus has been placed on individual characteristics. In such a situation, the association between the individual characteristics and health may be validly estimated, but the importance of these individual characteristics relative to the population level context cannot be assessed.[82] Just as in a population where everybody smokes one may conclude that lung cancer is an entirely genetic disease,[83] so studying homogeneous populations may wrongly lead to the conclusion that individual susceptibilities are the main or only determinants of health.

Multilevel studies are increasingly being undertaken to try to address both individual and ecological effects on health.[81,84] For example Diez-Roux explored the impact of individual and neighbourhood socioeconomic characteristics on the prevalence of coronary heart disease in a prospective cohort. After adjustment for individual-level variables, living in deprived neighbourhoods was still associated with an increased prevalence of coronary heart disease, suggesting that individual-level and neighbourhood socioeconomic characteristics are important in determining cardiovascular risk.[85]

Confounding

Confounding is an important consideration at the outset of designing an epidemiological study. If confounding variables are not measured and taken into account in the analysis, they may exert a significant influence on the interpretation of the results. Moreover, in studies where exposure assessment is made prospectively, the opportunity for reliable data collection on confounding variables is lost if such information is obtained retrospectively.

A confounding factor has the following properties:

- It must be associated with the exposure.
- It must be a causal factor for the outcome.
- It must not form part of the causal pathway between exposure and outcome.

For instance, age may be a confounding variable in the association between smoking and lung cancer if there is a dose–response relationship: age may be associated with duration of smoking, and increasing age is likely to be a risk factor for lung cancer, but smoking is not a causative factor for old age. Age, sex and socioeconomic status are common confounders.

The result of confounding is to distort the association between exposure and outcome in a positive or negative direction, by exaggerating or reducing the effect of exposure, respectively. For example, in assessing smoking as a confounding variable in the association between asbestos exposure and lung cancer, if those exposed to asbestos are more likely to be smokers, smoking will exaggerate the risk of lung cancer from asbestosis. Smoking may be a negative confounder when studying the association between smokeless tobacco and oral cancer, as individuals who use smokeless tobacco may smoke less.[86]

There are two ways to handle the problem of confounding: during either the design or the data analysis stage. The design of a case–control study may match cases and controls to 'design out' the effect of important confounding variables, age- and/or sex-matching being a commonly used technique to achieve this. In case-crossover studies, in which each case acts as their own control, many confounders are automatically designed out of the study. During data analysis, data could be stratified by the potentially confounding variable(s) to ascertain whether a similar association exists between exposure and outcome in each stratum. If this exists in each stratum, it is clear that the observed association between exposure and outcome is not influenced by the additional variable.

To enable confounders to be taken into account, all potentially confounding variables need to be measured and included as co-variates in the analysis of risk. However, confounding may be caused by unknown variables (residual confounders), particularly when there is no known evidence or hypothesis of association. To overcome the influence of this residual confounding, a randomized study design can help to ensure that such confounders are distributed randomly between the different exposure/intervention groups.

Interaction or effect modification

According to MacMahon, 'An interaction exists if the incidence rate of disease in the presence of two or more risk factors differs from the incidence rate expected to result from their individual effects.'[87] The effect may be greater than expected (synergistic) or less than expected (antagonistic). Synergistic effects may be additive or multiplicative.

The distinction between an interaction and confounding can be difficult to make. It is clear that a confounding variable has to meet the criteria described above. It is important to consider the possible effects of confounding variables as they may wholly account for the association between exposure and outcome. In an interaction, an established causative link between exposure and outcome may be modified by a third variable.

It may be invaluable to have an understanding of interaction or effect modification, as there may be implications for planning interventions. For example, the relative risk of hepatocellular carcinoma in patients with chronic hepatitis B is 7.3. For individuals exposed to aflatoxin, the relative risk of hepatocellular carcinoma is 3.4.[88] However, for those with both risk factors, the relative risk increases significantly to 59.4, suggesting a multiplicative interaction. Hence, public health measures to reduce exposure to aflatoxin might be best targeted towards communities where hepatitis B is endemic.

Relative versus absolute measures of risk

The epidemiological approaches discussed in this chapter usually result in the calculation of a measure of risk associated with the exposure of interest. Relative risk estimates are the typical measure of risk reported from a cohort study, and refer to the ratio of the incidence rates in the exposed and non-exposed groups. In case–control studies, it is not possible to calculate the incidence of disease in exposed and non-exposed groups, but it is possible to calculate the odds of exposure for the cases and controls. The odds ratio is therefore the typical measure of risk reported from a case–control study and refers to the ratio of the odds of exposure in the case and control groups. The odds ratio is an estimate of the relative risk and is generally a good estimate of this relative measure for rare diseases.

The attributable risk is an absolute measure of risk that can be calculated from epidemiological studies. The attributable risk is a measure of exposure effect that indicates how much greater the frequency of disease in the exposed group is compared with the unexposed group, assuming that the relationship between exposure and disease is causal (often a bold assumption, as detailed in the section on Causality page 38). It is the difference between the risk or rate in the exposed and non-exposed groups, and it represents the risk attributable to the exposure of interest. This measure can therefore indicate the number of cases of the disease among the exposed group that could be prevented if the exposure were reduced or eliminated.

Whereas relative risks or odds ratios (both relative measures of risk) can provide information on the strength of association between an exposure and outcome, the attributable risk can provide a measure of the impact of a risk factor in public health terms. Attributable risks are especially useful in assessing priorities for public health intervention.[89] For example, the relative risk of lung cancer associated with occupational exposure to an industrial carcinogen might be twice as great as that associated with smoking, but if more than twice as many people smoke as are exposed to the industrial carcinogen, the attributable risk from smoking will be greater, and more public health benefit might be achieved by targeting smoking rather than industrial exposure (although targeting both may be preferable!).

Attributable risks can complement relative measures of risk by providing important information about the effect of a risk factor on disease causation at the population level, but there are several limitations to consider. As alluded to above, in order to meaningfully estimate attributable risks, the relationship between the risk factor and the outcome must be established as causal. Even when causality can be assumed, the attributable risk may not represent the actual change in incidence if a risk factor were reduced or removed because risk factors are rarely independent of one another.[90] In addition, it is often difficult to generalize attributable risks to populations other than that under study because this measure is dependent on the baseline incidence of disease in the unexposed group and on the prevalence of exposure in the population.

Life–year savings

Life expectancy and mortality measures are frequently used to compare the health of different populations, regionally, nationally and internationally, but these are rather crude measures for describing the health of a population. Health-adjusted life–years allow the combined impact of mortality and morbidity to be considered simultaneously, making this a more useful measure of overall population health for comparisons of the impact of interventions or of health across a range of outcomes and populations.[91]. Several variations of health-adjusted life–year exist, for example quality-adjusted life–years, which incorporate a measure of the quantity and quality of life gained (or lost) due to an exposure or intervention, and which are primarily used for cost-effect analysis. Alternatively, disability-adjusted life–years (DALYs) measure the burden of disease in a population and provide an indication of the gap between a population's health and a hypothetical ideal. These measures of adjusted life–years are discussed in detail elsewhere.[91–93].

An example of the application of these measures is provided by the Global Burden of Disease study, which used DALYs to estimate the global burden of disorders attributable to various environmental risk factors.[94] This study found the leading causes of loss of global DALYs to be lower respiratory infections, diarrhoeal diseases and perinatal disorders, and the leading global risk factors to be malnutrition (responsible for the loss of 15.9 per cent of global DALYs), poor water supply, sanitation and personal hygiene (6.8 per cent), unsafe sex (3.5 per cent) and alcohol use (3.5 per cent).[94]

Causality

The observed relationship between exposure and outcome is assumed to be merely associative, unless certain criteria are fulfilled to demonstrate a causative link. Indeed, some associations may be spurious. For example, if the selection of cases and controls in a case–control study is based on exposure, that is if all cases were exposed and all controls were not, selection bias will have created a spurious association between exposure and outcome. An association may be an artefact of confounding, especially when the confounding variable can account wholly for the association between exposure and outcome.

In order to assess causality, the English epidemiologist and statistician Sir Austin Bradford Hill suggested nine criteria for assessment:[95]

1. the *strength* of the association, such that the risk is so large that other factors can be ruled out;
2. an association that is *consistent* in other investigations;
3. whether the exposure is associated with a *specific* disease as opposed to a wide range of diseases;
4. a *temporal* relationship between exposure and outcome, such that exposure precedes outcome;
5. a *biological gradient* whereby increasing exposure is associated with increased risk;
6. an association that is *plausible*, and the occurrence of a credible scientific mechanism to explain the association;
7. an association that is *coherent* and consistent with the natural history of the disease;
8. an outcome that may be replicated by *experimental exposure*;
9. that an *analogy* may be observed in another context.

There is an important role for epidemiological approaches to assess the strength of association and the presence of a biological gradient.

The application of these criteria to modern epidemiological approaches may require some caution. For example, the strength of association may not be compelling for attributing illness to exposure to environmental factors, or it may not be ethical to replicate the occurrence of disease following exposure to certain hazards. Notwithstanding these concerns, Hill's criteria for causation provide a useful reference point to assess whether an association is causative.

APPLICATION OF FINDINGS

Critical appraisal

Critical appraisal of epidemiological methodology is a crucial tool for assessing whether the findings of a study are sufficiently sound and robust to inform evidence-based practice. There are several critical appraisal tools available to assess the value of an epidemiological study. These tools generally take into account assessments of validity, level of bias and confounding, and generalizability to a population of concern.

Control and prevention

CONTROL OF OUTBREAKS OF COMMUNICABLE DISEASES

The investigation of outbreaks of infectious disease is important as it may be used to determine appropriate control measures for either an ongoing outbreak or future outbreaks. The identification and withdrawal of a contaminated food supply chain can have a major public health impact.

A good understanding of the epidemiology of new and emerging infectious diseases provides an important foundation on which to develop control measures and target interventions. During the early stages of the novel influenza A (H1N1, or swine flu) pandemic in 2009, early descriptive epidemiology was utilized to inform policy and public health interventions in the UK.[96]

EPISODE AND DISASTER SURVEILLANCE

Natural or deliberate disasters may have a significant adverse impact on public health. Following such events, there is an opportunity to assess the short-, medium- or long-term outcomes, with a view to identifying the health needs of affected populations. In the immediate aftermath of a disaster, the overwhelming priority response is to save lives and to provide basic life support needs. However, if this response is not informed by adequate needs assessment, it is likely that the assistance provided will be unnecessary or inappropriate. Because of the urgency of the task, an academically robust epidemiological study is unlikely to be feasible, so alternative methods need to be considered.

A rapid needs assessment may be used in circumstances where a quick, cost-effective and accurate evaluation of needs is required by emergency managers to direct and target their strategies.[97] Epidemiological methods, such as stratified cross-sectional studies and ecological studies, can inform such needs assessments.

An early example is taken from a report by Glass et al., who described how, in 1979, the rapid assessment of the health status and health protection needs of 31 000 newly arrived Cambodian refugees in Thailand, using simple epidemiological techniques, helped to influence and target healthcare delivery in the first 2 weeks after their arrival.[98] Representative cross-sectional studies were conducted at frequent intervals, and a close liaison was established with health service providers. From the community survey, it was apparent that malaria was the main cause of mortality and morbidity. Consequently, resources were directed towards the treatment and prevention of malaria, rather than vaccination for measles, cholera and typhoid, or provision of supplementary vitamins, as there was no evidence of outbreaks of these communicable diseases or of vitamin deficiency.

Remediation

Where environmental factors are found to be causally associated with health, it is good public health practice to act on these findings to minimize health risks to the population. Many examples of measures put into place to protect population health can be cited, for example the introduction of Clean Air Acts following the London fog episodes in the 1950s,[99] or the ban on the use of lead in petrol following the discovery that this was a major source of exposure for children.[100]

Although the prevention of public health problems is clearly ideal, there are some situations in which the sources of exposure remain even after good practice guidelines have been adopted or legislation has been introduced. In these situations, interventions and/or remediation may be required to prevent or minimize exposure. Using the example of environmental lead, even after legislation was introduced to minimize lead exposure (i.e. bans on the use of lead in petrol, household paint and for domestic water supplies), contamination from existing paint and water pipes in older homes persisted.[101] Household interventions have been attempted (e.g. specialized cleaning, soil abatement and repainting) to reduce exposure originating from lead paint, but none has convincingly reduced childhood exposure.[102] Where significant soil contamination is considered a potential source of exposure, remediation of the contaminated site may be required. This might take the form of dust control (e.g. by revegetation) and/or soil abatement (e.g. the addition of clean top soil and/or soil replacement).

A case study demonstrating the use of a range of legislative, intervention and remediation approaches for public health protection is provided by the Port Pirie lead smelter, South Australia. In Port Pirie, the abatement programme involved a combination of emission controls, house decontamination, soil treatment, dust control and family/community education, which led to a significant decrease in children's blood lead levels.[103] Although examples of successful remediation do exist, environmental remediation often presents a high-cost solution that can be unattractive unless the parties responsible for contamination can be identified and held to account.

Further research

Where associations are observed between an exposure and an outcome, the significance of the findings, and the potential impact of any biases and limitations, will need careful consideration. After ruling out chance, bias and confounding as possible explanations for the association, consideration can be given to the possibility of the relationship being causal. More details of the process of addressing causality are given in the relevant section above.

For many hypothesis-generating approaches, such as ecological or correlation studies, the evidence gathered from the study is usually only sufficient to highlight priority areas for further research. Such further research would usually utilize a study design higher up the hierarchy of evidence (see Figure 2.1, above) to enable the issue of causality to be addressed, and the iterative, multistaged process of hypothesis-generation and testing can be adopted (see 'Epidemiological study cycle', above). Where a convincing association is found from a strong study design (e.g. an RCT or prospective cohort study), future research could be useful to demonstrate the reproducibility of the association in other similar populations and to assess the consistency of findings across other, dissimilar populations. Ideally, evidence for a potentially important association between an exposure and outcome should be gathered using a range of epidemiological approaches and should be reproducible across different populations and over different time intervals. When such evidence has been gathered, it may be usefully summarized using systematic review and meta-analytical techniques (see above).

The investigation of fat intake as a risk factor for colon cancer provides an example of this expansion of the evidence base from an ecological, hypothesis-generating approach, through individual-level assessments using different study designs carried out over a range of populations, to the summary of these findings in a systematic review and meta-analysis. Following the finding of an association between colon cancer and per capita fat consumption from ecological comparisons,[13] there was a clear need to assess this association at the individual level, and several case–control studies were carried out. Although some of these studies supported the association, a meta-analysis of 13 case–control studies from various countries found that the relationship between fat intake and colon cancer was not generally independent of energy intake (these variables being strongly correlated).[104] Several large prospective studies have also failed to find an association between fat intake and colon cancer risk independent of energy intake.[105]

CONCLUSION

By using a variety of epidemiological methods, it is already possible to identify the causes of an increasing number of diseases, and the range of tools available to researchers in this field is growing.

Advances have been made in recent years that increase our ability to attribute disease. Improvements in computer processing power have enabled epidemiologists to manage and analyse large and complex datasets using an increasing array of statistical operations.[106] Geographic information systems,[107–109] global positioning systems,[110] remote sensing[111] and off-the-shelf packages for exposure modelling[63] have been put to use in the epidemiological setting in recent years, bringing new possibilities for exposure assessment. Biological markers of exposure, dose, effect and susceptibility are being developed and validated for a range of exposure and health outcomes,[112,113] increasing our ability to make causal inferences about exposure and effect. In addition, biobanks, such as the recently established UK Biobank,[114] will provide valuable information on baseline dose measures, as well as novel opportunities for understanding long-term determinants of health and life-course epidemiology. Such resources, along with recently developed high-throughput genotyping technologies, will provide opportunities to explore the contribution of genes, genetic susceptibility and gene–environment interactions to a wide range of important multifactorial diseases.[53]

Nonetheless, issues of data availability and limited resources will influence the approach chosen, which will in turn influence the ability to make inferences from the study. Evidence for attributing illness is often an iterative process, drawing on a range of epidemiological methods to build up a robust base of evidence of causation.

The most significant contribution that epidemiology has made to population health has been the discovery of many causes of disease, ranging from early investigations of exposures to infectious diseases to more recent enquiries on exposure to lifestyle and environmental hazards. The recent expansion in epidemiological and analytical capability has made it theoretically possible for the investigator to attribute illness for a wide range of diseases. However, the feasibility of undertaking an investigation may be influenced by constraints on resources, limitations in exposure assessment, bias and confounding, and ethical considerations. Despite advances in epidemiological methods, there remain diseases that pose significant global public health threats, such as obesity, addiction to drugs and alcohol, and chronic arthritis, for which major knowledge gaps about causation remain. There are also challenges in attributing illness associated with the wider determinants of health, such as housing conditions, crime and poverty.

REFERENCES

● = Key primary paper

◆ = Major review article

1. Snow J. *On the Mode of Communication of Cholera*. London: John Churchill, 1855.
2. Semmelweis I. *Die Aetiologie, der Begriff und die Prophylaxis des Kindbettfiebers* [*The Etiology, Concept, and Prophylaxis of Childbed Fever.*] Budapest: University of Wisconsin Press, 1983.
3. Pemberton J. *Will Pickles of Wensleydale. The Life of a Country Doctor*. London: Geoffrey Bles, 1970.
4. Pickles WN. Epidemiology in country practice. *Proc R Soc Med* 1935; **28**: 1337–42.
●5. Doll R, Hill A. The mortality of doctors in relation to their smoking habits: A preliminary report. *Br Med J* 1954; **228**: 1451–5.
6. Phillips R, Ball C, Sackett D *et al*. Oxford Centre for Evidence-based Medicine Levels of Evidence (May 2001). Available from: http://www.cebm.net/index.aspx?o=1047 (accessed January 14, 2010).
7. McBride W. Thalidomide and congenital abnormalities. *Lancet* 1962; **2**: 1358.
8. International Programme on Chemical Safety. *Guidelines on Studies in Environmental Epidemiology*. Geneva: World Health Organization, 1983.
9. Mann CJ. Observational research methods. Research design II: Cohort, cross sectional, and case-control studies. *Emerg Med J* 2003; **20**: 54–60.
10. White A. *Health Survey for England 1991*. London: HMSO, 1993.
11. Bost L, Primatesta P, Dong W, Poulter N. Blood lead and blood pressure: evidence from the Health Survey for England 1995. *J Hum Hyperten* 1999; **13**: 123–8.
12. Susser M. The logic in ecological. I: The logic of analysis. *Am J Public Health* 1994; **84**: 825–9.
●13. Armstrong B, Doll R. Environmental factors and cancer incidence and mortality in different countries, with special reference to dietary practices. *Int J Cancer* 1975; **15**: 617–31.
14. Mazhar D, Waxman J. Dietary fat and breast cancer. *QJM* 2006; **99**: 469–73.
15. Willett WC. Dietary fat intake and cancer risk: A controversial and instructive story. *Semin Cancer Biol* 1998; **8**: 245–53.
16. Barash J, Johnson B, Gregorio D. Is surgery a risk factor for Creutzfeldt–Jakob disease? Outcome variation by control choice and exposure assessments. *Infect Control Hosp Epidemiol* 2008; **29**: 212–18.
17. Tam C, Rodrigues L, O'Brien S. The study of infectious intestinal disease in England: What risk factors for presentation to general practice tell us about potential for

selection bias in case-control studies of reported cases of diarrhoea. *Int J Epidemiol* 2003; **32**: 99–105.

●18. Dawber T, Meadors GE, Moore F. Epidemiological approaches to heart disease: The Framingham study. *Am J Public Health* 1951; **41**: 279–86.

19. Friedman D, Heisey-Grove H, Argyros F *et al.* An outbreak of norovirus gastroenteritis associated with wedding cakes. *Epidemiol Infect* 2005; **133**: 1057–63.

20. Maclure M. The case crossover design: A method for studying transient effects on the risk of acute events. *Am J Epidemiol* 1991; **133**: 144–53.

21. Stafoggia M, Forastiere F, Agostini D *et al.* Vulnerability to heat-related mortality: A multicity, population-based, case-crossover analysis. *Epidemiology* 2006; **17**: 315–23.

22. Warner L, Macaluso M, Austin H *et al.* Application of the case-crossover design to reduce unmeasured confounding in studies of condom effectiveness. *Am J Epidemiol* 2005; **161**: 765–73.

23. Francis TJ. Evaluation of the 1954 poliomyelitis vaccine field trial: Further studies of results determining the effectiveness of poliomyelitis vaccine (Salk) in preventing paralytic poliomyelitis. *JAMA* 1955; **158**: 1266–70.

24. Arnold FJ, Dean H, Jay K, Knutson J. Effect of fluoridated public water supplies on dental caries prevalence. 10th year of the Grand Rapids – Muskegon study. *Public Health Report* 1956; **71**: 652–8.

25. Lennon M. One in a million: The first community trial of water fluoridation. *Bull World Health Organ* 2006; **84**: 759–60.

◆26. Higgins JPT, Green S. *Cochrane Handbook for Systematic Reviews of Interventions. Version 5.0.0 [updated February 2008]*. Oxford: Cochrane Collaboration, 2008.

27. Deeks JJ. Systematic reviews of published evidence: Miracles or minefields? *Ann Oncol* 1998; **9**: 703–9.

28. Blettner M, Sauerbrei W, Schlehofer B, Scheuchenpflug T, Friedenreich C. Traditional reviews, meta-analyses and pooled analyses in epidemiology. *Int J Epidemiol* 1999; **28**: 1–9.

29. Blair A, Burg J, Foran J *et al.* Guidelines for application of meta-analysis in environmental epidemiology. ISLI Risk Science Institute. *Regul Toxicol Pharmacol* 1995; **22**: 189–97.

30. Romieu I, Berlin JA, Colditz G. Oral contraceptives and breast cancer. Review and meta-analysis. *Cancer* 1990; **66**: 2253–63.

31. Collaborative Group on Hormonal Factors in Breast Cancer. Breast cancer and hormonal contraceptives: Collaborative reanalysis of individual data on 53 297 women with breast cancer and 100 239 women without breast cancer from 54 epidemiological studies *Lancet* 1996; **347**: 1713–27.

32. Centers for Disease Control and Prevention. Pneumocystis pneumonia – Los Angeles. *MMWR Morb Mortal Wkly Rep* 1981; **30**: 1–3.

33. Hymes K, Greene J, Marcus A *et al.* Kaposi's sarcoma in homosexual men – report of eight cases. *Lancet* 1981; **318**: 598–600.

34. Vandenbroucke J, Pardoel V. An autopsy of epidemiologic methods: The case of "poppers" in the early epidemic of the acquired immunodeficiency syndrome (AIDS). *Am J Epidemiol* 1989; **129**: 455–7.

●35. Jaffe H, Choi K, Thomas P *et al.* National case-control study of Kaposi's sarcoma and *Pneumocystis carinii* pneumonia in homosexual men. 1: Epidemiologic results. *Ann Intern Med* 1983; **99**: 145–51.

◆36. Elliott P, Wartenberg D. Spatial epidemiology: Current approaches and future challenges. *Environ Health Perspect* 2004; **112**: 998–1006.

●37. International Agency for Research on Cancer. *Cancer Incidence in Five Continents*. Vol. 1. Berlin: Springer-Verlag, 1966.

38. Office for National Statistics. *Cancer Atlas of the United Kingdom and Ireland 1991–2000*. London: ONS, 2005.

39. Gardner MJ, Winter PD. Mortality in Cumberland during 1959–78 with reference to cancer in young people around Windscale. *Lancet* 1984; **1**: 216–17.

40. McNally RJQ, Alexander FE, Bithell JF. Space-time clustering of childhood cancer in Great Britain: A national study, 1969–1993. *Int J Cancer* 2006; **118**: 2840–6.

◆41. Morgenstern H. Ecologic studies. In: Rothman KJ, Greenland S (eds) *Modern Epidemiology*, 2nd edn. Philadelphia: Lippincott Williams & Wilkins, 1998: 459–80.

42. Forand SP, Talbot TO, Druschel C, Cross PK. Data quality and the spatial analysis of disease rates: Congenital malformations in New York State. *Health Place* 2002; **8**: 191–9.

43. Anderson RN, Rosenberg HM. Disease classification: Measuring the effect of the Tenth Revision of the International Classification of Diseases on cause-of-death data in the United States. *Stat Med* 2003; **22**: 1551–70.

44. Arnold R, Elliott P, Wakefield J, Quinn M. *Population Counts in Small Areas: Implications for Studies of Environment and Health*. Report No. 62. London: Office for National Statistics, Government Statistical Service, 1997.

45. Ward MH, Nuckols JR, Giglierano J *et al.* Positional accuracy of two methods of geocoding. *Epidemiology* 2005; **16**: 542–7.

46. Openshaw S. *The Modifiable Areal Unit Problem*. Concepts and Techniques in Modern Geography No. 38. Norwich: Geo Books, 1984.

47. McGeehin MA, Qualters JR, Niskar AS. National environmental public health tracking program: Bridging the information gap. *Environ Health Perspect* 2004; **112**: 1409–13.

48. Beale L, Abellan J, Hodgson S, Jarup L. Methodological issues and approaches to spatial epidemiology. *Environ Health Perspect* 2008; **116**: 1105–10.

◆49. Hunter DJ. Gene-environment interactions in human diseases. *Nature Rev Genet* 2005; **6**: 287–98.

◆50. Burton PR, Tobin MD, Hopper JL. Key concepts in genetic epidemiology. *Lancet* 2005; **366**: 941–51.

51. Yang Q, Khoury MJ. Evolving methods in genetic epidemiology. III: Gene-environment interaction in epidemiologic research. *Epidemiol Rev* 1997; **19**: 33–43.

52. Bell J. Predicting disease using genomics. *Nature* 2004; **429**: 453–6.

53. Davey Smith G, Ebrahim S, Lewis S, Hansell AL, Palmer LJ, Burton PR. Genetic epidemiology and public health: Hope, hype, and future prospects. *Lancet* 2005; **366**: 1484–98.

54. Zeger SL, Irizarry R, Peng RD. On time series analysis of public health and biomedical data. *Annu Rev Public Health* 2006; **27**: 57–79.

55. Green A, Patterson CC. Trends in the incidence of childhood-onset diabetes in Europe 1989–1998. *Diabetologia* 2001; **44**(Suppl. 3): B3–8.

56. McIntyre P, Leask J. Improving uptake of MMR vaccine. *BMJ* 2008; **336**: 729–30.

57. Bell ML, Samet JM, Dominici F. Time-series studies of particulate matter. *Annu Rev Public Health* 2004; **25**: 247–80.

58. Schwartz J. Air pollution and daily mortality: A review and meta analysis. *Environ Res* 1994; **64**: 36–52.

59. Fouillet A, Rey G, Laurent F *et al.* Excess mortality related to the August 2003 heat wave in France. *Int Arch Occup Environ Health* 2006; **80**: 16–24.

60. Johnson H, Kovats RS, McGregor G *et al.* The impact of the 2003 heat wave on mortality and hospital admissions in England. *Health Stat Q* 2005: 6–11.

61. Khuder SA, Milz S, Jordan T, Price J, Silvestri K, Butler P. The impact of a smoking ban on hospital admissions for coronary heart disease. *Prev Med* 2007; **45**: 3–8.

62. Heidenreich WF, Bogdanova TI, Biryukov AG, Tronko ND. Time trends of thyroid cancer incidence in Ukraine after the Chernobyl accident. *J Radiol Prot* 2004; **24**: 283–93.

◆63. Interdepartmental Group on Health Risks from Chemicals. *Guidelines for Good Exposure Assessment Practice for Human Health Effects of Chemicals.* Cranfield, Beds: Institute for Environment and Health, 2004.

◆64. World Health Organization. Methodology for assessment of exposure to environmental factors in application to epidemiological studies. *Sci Total Environ* 1995; **168**: 93–100.

◆65. Armstrong BG. Effect of measurement error on epidemiological studies of environmental and occupational exposures. *Occup Environ Med* 1998; **55**: 651–6.

◆66. Nieuwenhuijsen M, Paustenbach D, Duarte-Davidson R. New developments in exposure assessment: The impact on the practice of health risk assessment and epidemiological studies. *Environ Int* 2006; **32**: 996–1009.

67. Pless-Mulloli T, Howel D, Prince H. Prevalence of asthma and other respiratory symptoms in children living near and away from opencast coal mining sites. *Int J Epidemiol* 2001; **30**: 556–63.

68. Logan C, O'Leary J, O'Sullivan N. Real-time reverse transcription PCR detection of norovirus, sapovirus and astrovirus as causative agents of acute viral gastroenteritis. *J Virol Methods* 2007; **146**(1–2): 36–44.

69. Whitley E, Ball J. Statistics review 4: Sample size calculations. *Crit Care* 2002; **6**: 335–41.

70. Florey CD. Sample size for beginners. *Br Med J* 1993; **306**: 1181–4.

71. Jones SR, Carley S, Harrison M. An introduction to power and sample size estimation. *Emerg Med J* 2003; **20**: 453–8.

72. Department of Health. *Research Governance Framework for Health and Social Care*, 2nd edn. London: Department of Health, 2005.

73. Wacholder S, Hartge P, Lubin JH, Dosemeci M. Non-differential misclassification and bias towards the null: A clarification. *Occup Environ Med.* 1995; **52**: 557–8.

74. Bar-Oz B, Moretti ME, Mareels G, Van Tittelboom T, Koren G. Reporting bias in retrospective ascertainment of drug-induced embryopathy. *Lancet* 1999; **354**: 1700–1.

75. Austin H, Hill HA, Flanders WD, Greenberg RS. Limitations in the application of case-control methodology. *Epidemiol Rev* 1994; **16**: 65–76.

76. Li CY, Sung FC. A review of the healthy worker effect in occupational epidemiology. *Occup Med* 1999; **49**: 225–9.

77. Savitz DA, Pearce N. Control selection with incomplete case ascertainment. *Am J Epidemiol* 1988; **127**: 1109–17.

78. Kopec JA, Esdaile JM. Bias in case-control studies. A review. *J Epidemiol Commun Health* 1990; **44**: 179–86.

79. Kristman V, Manno M, Côté P. Loss to follow-up in cohort studies: How much is too much? *Eur J Epidemiol* 2004; **19**: 751–60.

80. Schwartz S. The fallacy of the ecological fallacy: The potential misuse of a concept and the consequences. *Am J Public Health* 1994; **84**: 819–24.

81. Diez-Roux AV. Bringing context back into epidemiology: Variables and fallacies in multilevel analysis. *Am J Public Health* 1998; **88**: 216–22.

82. Pearce N. The ecological fallacy strikes back. *J Epidemiol Commun Health* 2000; **54**: 326–7.

●◆83. Rose G. Sick individuals and sick populations. *Int J Epidemiol* 1985; **14**: 32–8.

84. Blakely TA, Woodward AJ. Ecological effects in multi-level studies. *J Epidemiol Commun Health* 2000; **54**: 367–74.

85. Diez-Roux AV, Nieto FJ, Muntaner C *et al.* Neighborhood environments and coronary heart disease: A multilevel analysis. *Am J Epidemiol* 1997; **146**: 48–63.

86. Rodu B, Jansson C. Smokeless tobacco and oral cancer: A review of the risks and determinants. *Crit Rev Oral Biol Med* 2004; **15**: 252–63.

87. MacMahon B. Concepts of multiple factors. In: Lee DH, Kotin P (eds) *Multiple Factors in the Causation of Environmentally Induced Disease.* New York: Academic Press, 1972.

88. Qian GS, Ross RK, Yu MC. A follow-up study of urinary markers of aflatoxin exposure and liver cancer risk in Shanghai, People's Republic of China. *Cancer Epidemiol Biomarkers Prev* 1994; **3**: 3–10.

89. Walter SD. The estimation and interpretation of attributable risk in health research. *Biometrics* 1976; **32**: 829–49.

90. Anonymous. Relative or attributable risk? *Lancet* 1981; 2: 1211–12.

91. Gold MR, Stevenson D, Fryback DG. HALYS and QALYS and DALYS, Oh My: Similarities and differences in summary measures of population health. *Ann Rev Public Health* 2002; **23**: 115–34.

92. Hirskyj P. QALY: An ethical issue that dare not speak its name. *Nursing Ethics* 2007; **14**: 72–82.

93. Mullahy J. Live long, live well: Quantifying the health of heterogeneous populations. *Health Econ* 2001; **10**: 429–40.

●94. Murray CJ, Lopez AD. Global mortality, disability, and the contribution of risk factors: Global Burden of Disease Study. *Lancet* 1997; **349**: 1436–42.

●95. Hill AB. The environment and disease: association or causation? *Proc R Soc Med* 1965; **58**: 295–300.

96. Health Protection Agency, Health Protection Agency Scotland, National Public Health Service for Wales. Epidemiology of new influenza A (H1N1) virus infection, United Kingdom, April–June 2009. *Eurosurveillance* 2009; **14**(22).

97. World Health Organization. *Rapid Needs Assessment for Water, Sanitation and Hygiene.* New Delhi: WHO, 2004.

98. Glass R, Cates WJ, Nieburg P *et al.* Rapid assessment of health status and preventive-medicine needs of newly arrived Kampuchean refugees, Sa Kaeo, Thailand. *Lancet* 1980; **315**: 868–72.

99. Brimblecombe P. The Great Smog and after. In: *The Big Smoke: A History of Air Pollution in London Since Medieval Times.* London: Methuen, 1987: 161–78.

100. von Storch H, Costa-Cabral M, Hagner C *et al.* Four decades of gasoline lead emissions and control policies in Europe: A retrospective assessment. *Sci Total Env* 2003; **311**(1–3): 151–76.

101. Millstone E, Russell J. Environmental lead and children's intelligence. Britain must replace its lead pipes to meet WHO standards for drinking water. *Br Med J* 1995; **310**: 1408–9.

102. Yeoh B, Woolfenden S, Wheeler D, Alperstein G, Lanphear B. Household interventions for prevention of domestic lead exposure in children. Cochrane Database of Syst Rev 2008(2): CD006047.

103. Maynard E, Thomas R, Simon D, Phipps C, Ward C, Calder I. An evaluation of recent blood lead levels in Port Pirie, South Australia. *Sci Total Env* 2003; **303**(1–2): 25–33.

104. Howe GR, Aronson KJ, Benito E *et al.* The relationship between dietary fat intake and risk of colorectal cancer: Evidence from the combined analysis of 13 case-control studies. *Cancer Causes Control* 1997; **8**: 215–28.

105. Giovannucci E, Goldin B. The role of fat, fatty acids, and total energy intake in the etiology of human colon cancer. *Am J Clin Nutr* 1997; **66**(6 Suppl): 1564S–71S.

106. Glass RI. New prospects for epidemiologic investigations. *Science* 1986; **234**: 951–5.

107. Ward MH, Wartenberg D. Invited commentary: On the road to improved exposure assessment using geographic information systems. *Am J Epidemiol* 2006; **164**: 208–11.

108. Kistemann T, Dangendorf F, Schweikart J. New perspectives on the use of geographical information systems (GIS) in environmental health sciences. *Int J Hyg Environ Health* 2002; **205**: 169–81.

109. Nuckols JR, Ward MH, Jarup L. Using geographic information systems for exposure assessment in environmental epidemiology studies. *Environ Health Perspect* 2004; **112**: 1007–15.

110. Elgethun K, Fenske RA, Yost MG, Palcisko GJ. Time–location analysis for exposure assessment studies of children using a novel global positioning system instrument. *Environ Health Perspect* 2003; **111**: 115–22.

111. Herbreteau V, Salem G, Souris M, Hugot J-P, Gonzalez J-P. Thirty years of use and improvement of remote sensing, applied to epidemiology: From early promises to lasting frustration. *Health Place* 2007; **13**: 400–3.

112. International Programme on Chemical Safety. *Biomarkers and Risk Assessment: Concepts and Principles.* Geneva: World Health Organization, 1993.

113. International Programme on Chemical Safety. *Biomarkers in Risk Assessment: Validity and Validation.* Geneva: World Health Organization, 2001.

114. Palmer LJ. UK Biobank: Bank on it. *Lancet* 2007; **369**: 1980–2.

OTHER RESOURCES

Cochrane Library: www.cochrane.org

3

The surveillance and monitoring of diseases and agents

MIKE CATCHPOLE

PROVIDING THE EVIDENCE BASE FOR PUBLIC HEALTH ACTION

Public health surveillance has been defined as the 'ongoing systematic collection, analysis, and interpretation of outcome-specific data, closely integrated with the timely dissemination of these data to those responsible for preventing and controlling disease or injury'.[1] Surveillance outputs represent a cornerstone in the body of public health intelligence, along with research findings and information collated in a less systematic manner from other sources.

The key defining characteristics of surveillance are:

- that it is a *systematic* process of data collection, analysis and reporting;
- that its primary purpose is to prompt or inform the operation of prevention and control programmes.

The aim of surveillance is to provide information that is required to inform, and monitor the effects of, public health action. It is often part of a larger toolset used to achieve a public health outcome; surveillance outputs should be seen as an intermediate, rather than a final, deliverable in health protection. The potential roles for surveillance in informing public health actions and decisions include:[2]

- *Assessing public health status*: to inform action concerning the control and prevention of environmental hazards, exposures to potentially harmful agents and the occurrence of disease, typically through the detection of acute changes in the frequency of disease, including the detection of outbreaks, or the identification of new environmental hazards or exposures.
- *Defining public health priorities*: to inform policy and planning about the current and likely future impact of hazards, exposures and disease, typically through monitoring longer-term trends in the incidence and distribution of environmental hazards or disease and/or monitoring of outcomes.
- *Evaluating programmes*: to inform decisions regarding existing interventions, typically through monitoring longer-term trends in the incidence and distribution of disease and/or monitoring of outcomes.
- *Stimulating research*: to generate hypotheses and inform methodologies, typically through the analysis of demographic and risk factor data.

HISTORICAL PERSPECTIVE

Statistics on morbidity, and more particularly mortality, have been produced in many societies over centuries, such as the 'Bills of Mortality' produced and published in early sixteenth-century London. The information was collected by the Parish Clerk's Company of London and published weekly. Initially, these reports contained only burials, but by the 1570s baptisms were recorded, and by 1629 cause of death was given, with age distributions provided by the early eighteenth century. Although John Graunt published a statistical analysis of the Bills in 1662, their production and publication was not directly linked to public health action, and as such they are not generally cited as examples of surveillance. However, Londoners bought copies of the bills and scanned them for signs of impending disease, particularly plague, and may have made their own plans to leave the city at the first sign of rising numbers.

The first exponent of the systematic analysis of official medical statistics for disease monitoring and identifying associations between disease and demographic groups was probably William Farr, who, in the General Register Office in London, set up a system for routinely recording the causes of death in England and Wales. He collected, analysed and interpreted vital statistics, and plotted the rise and fall of epidemics of infectious disease, publishing his results in regular reports. Farr's work allowed mortality rates among different occupations to be compared for the first time. In addition, in 1864 Farr was the first to publish work containing material calculated and printed by a machine, Scheutze's Difference Engine, a forerunner of the computer.

The recognition of the microbial aetiology of infectious disease and the importance of controlling transmission led to the introduction of the notification of infectious diseases in the UK and other European countries in the late nineteenth and early twentieth century. Such notification of infectious diseases is now a global practice and the mainstay of surveillance in many countries.[3] The development of nationally organized health and microbiology services enabled further developments in surveillance during the twentieth century, with clinical reporting schemes such as that operated by the Royal College of General Practitioners in the UK[4] and laboratory reporting systems such as that established by the Public Health Laboratory Service in England.[5] More recently, advances in information technology have enabled new surveillance systems to be developed, including syndromic reporting based on calls to telephone health advice lines[6] and scanning of international media reports on the Internet.[7]

In 1965, the Director General of the World Health Organization (WHO) established the epidemiological surveillance unit in the WHO's Division of Communicable Diseases. In 1968, the 21st World Health Assembly affirmed the three main features of surveillance as the systematic collection of pertinent data, the orderly consolidation and evaluation of these data, and the prompt dissemination of results to those who need to know – particularly those in a position to take action.[8] In addition, 'epidemiologic surveillance' implied 'the responsibility of following up to see that effective action has been taken', emphasizing the cyclical nature of the surveillance process (Figure 3.1).

Surveillance is now recognized as a central component of public health systems[9] requiring the development and

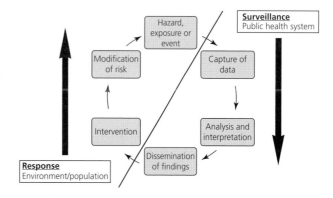

Figure 3.1 The cycle of surveillance and response.

maintenance of core public health capacities for surveillance and response.

THE SURVEILLANCE PROCESS

Data sources, operating procedures and outputs of surveillance systems need to be appropriate to meet the primary purpose of the system. The classical model of surveillance includes three major processes:

- the capture and collation of data;
- the analysis and interpretation of data (to generate information);
- the dissemination of information.

This is often shown as a cyclical process, with a fourth process of public health response (intervention), which may result in changes that will then be evaluated by the collection, analysis and interpretation of data (Figure 3.1).

Surveillance systems vary considerably in the way each of these processes is undertaken, as the scope and the design of surveillance systems are inevitably shaped by the nature of the questions that they are to address, the type of public health issue being monitored and the nature of the source (providers) of the data to be used. Surveillance system design and operation will also be affected by resource availability and the political or administrative level at which the outputs are to be used.

SCOPE

The operational scope of a surveillance system is defined by the subject under surveillance, the data sources/providers used, the level of ascertainment (either feasible or desired) and the nature of the system outputs and their intended audience. The operational characteristics of a surveillance system are defined by the nature of the core processes of data capture, data analysis and results reporting.

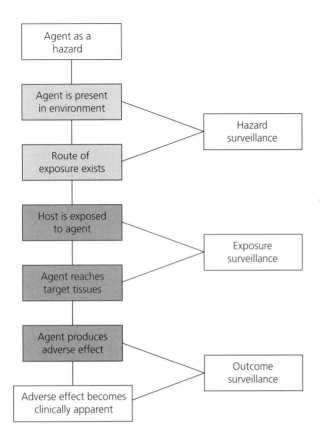

Figure 3.2 Surveillance and environmental issues. (Adapted from Thacker *et al.*,[10] with permission.)

SUBJECTS FOR SURVEILLANCE

Early surveillance approaches focused on the monitoring of explicit health events, such as the onset of disease or the occurrence and cause of death. However, such events represent the end points of a causal pathway that includes hazards (sources), exposures and host–agent interactions, each of which may represent an opportunity for control or prevention activities (Figure 3.2). The surveillance of hazards and exposures offers not only the potential for an earlier recognition of a problem requiring acute intervention, but also the potential to provide important intelligence for the design and monitoring of prevention programmes.

Surveillance activity can be regarded under three broad categories:

- *Hazard surveillance*: an assessment of the occurrence, distribution and trends over time of the levels of agents in the environment. Such agents can be physical (e.g. radon), chemical (e.g. air pollutants) or biological (e.g. *Legionella*). This category also includes microbial epidemiology, including investigation of the type, distribution and trends of organisms in the human and animal environment (e.g. the carriage rates of hepatitis B in the population) (see Chapter 5).

- *Exposure surveillance*: the monitoring of population members for the presence of an agent or its clinically inapparent effects, for example blood lead levels in children. It also includes the measurement of susceptibility in the population (e.g. immunity to a vaccine-preventable infection) and of the prevalence of risk behaviour (e.g. injecting drug use).

- *Outcome surveillance*: measuring the population effect of an agent in terms of disease morbidity and mortality, for example tuberculosis cases or cancer registration.

DATA SOURCES/PROVIDERS

The sources of data used for surveillance are many, reflecting not only the wide range of public health actions and decisions that surveillance supports, but also the variation in the organization of health services and other potential providers of data in different geographical and administrative settings. The advent of hazard and exposure surveillance, and the drive to achieve 'real-time' surveillance better to detect and respond to deliberate release incidents and emerging infectious disease, has resulted in an expansion of the sources of usable data. Advances in information technology have allowed the exploitation of new data sources, such as the Internet, for surveillance purposes, enabling the integration of data from multiple sources, thus adding value in informing decisions and actions.

The major sources of surveillance data may be broadly categorized according to the public or commercial sector in which the data providers work (Table 3.1).

Health services and vital registration authorities

The most common sources of data for the surveillance of human infection, disease and death are in the health services or in authorities responsible for the official registration of specific conditions or of deaths. The advantage of such sources is their provision of relatively rich data on the condition (aetiology, severity, etc.), its treatment and its outcome, although this is dependent upon the time and resources available. Reporting requirements may be universal or selective (sentinel surveillance) and may be mandatory, as for notifiable infectious diseases, or voluntary.

The advent of electronic patient record systems and telephone advice services has stimulated the development of syndromic surveillance, in which the reporting and analysis of data is based on reported symptoms (and sometimes clinical signs) rather than defined clinical or laboratory confirmed diagnoses. Although less specific, this can provide earlier warnings than reporting that depends on the receipt of investigations. Surveillance may also focus on interventions, such as drug prescribing or vaccination, either as an indicator of disease in the

Table 3.1   Sources of surveillance data

Source	Data examples
Mortality registration authorities	Deaths (number, cause, demographics)
Hospital admission data	Disease-specific hospital admission data
Disease registers	Cancers Congenital malformations
Clinicians Primary care Hospital/specialist	Diagnosis Syndrome Risk factors Treatment Outcome
Laboratories	Aetiological agent (infection) Antimicrobial resistance Biological markers of immunity or exposure
Pharmacies	Prescriptions
Immunization programme managers/coordinators	Vaccination uptake/coverage
The public	Knowledge, attitude and behavioural data Post-discharge surveillance of surgical site infection
Health advice telephone or Internet services	Syndrome reports
International organizations e.g. World Health Organization, European Centre for Disease Prevention and Control	Incident/outbreak reports International surveillance data
Internet press/media reports	Event reports
Animal health agencies	Veterinary data (zoonoses, antimicrobial resistance)
Animal host and vector surveys	Trapping and testing vertebrate hosts for zoonoses Trapping and testing mosquitoes for zoonotic agents Monitoring die-off of wild or domestic birds
Environmental agencies	Hazard reports
Emergency services	Incident and hazard reports
Health and safety agencies	Incident (accident) reports Occupational health data
Retail companies	Sales of medicines, groceries, etc.
Environmental samples	Radioactivity levels in airborne dust and cows' milk
Remote sensors	Land use Climate Air quality Radiation levels

population or as an indicator of susceptibility or prevention programme performance. Monitoring of vaccine uptake, particularly if combined with the serological surveillance of immunity levels in the population, can provide an early warning of the potential for epidemics as a result of falling uptake,[11] such as occurred with the measles, mumps and rubella vaccination scare in the UK.

Death registrations can be used to assess the full burden of disease, as was the case in the early days of human immunodeficiency virus (HIV) infection, when diagnoses may have been missed or may not have been reported because of concerns about stigmatization.[12] Death registrations can also provide an early warning of influenza epidemics.[13]

Emergency services and regulatory bodies

Emergency services (i.e. fire and ambulance) can provide data for surveillance of environmental contamination incidents and accidents, as can regulatory bodies responsible for environmental protection, providing data on environmental hazards and exposures.

Animal health bodies

Animals are not only a significant source of many infections, but also recently the most common source of emerging infectious diseases. The surveillance of animal disease is an important component of public health monitoring, but it is not without its difficulties. Many zoonotic diseases may not give rise to illness in animals, so will not be detected other than as an incidental finding, and not all zoonotic diseases are the subject of mandatory reporting in animals.

Collaboration between animal and human health organizations has been strengthened in recent years by a recognition of the importance of zoonoses as emerging infections, and through the development of preparedness for threats posed by bioterrorism and pandemic influenza. The surveillance of zoonotic diseases in animals may use data from veterinary surveillance, from alerts of incidents (such as the sudden die-off of poultry flocks as a potential indicator of avian influenza), from field surveys or from laboratories that may serve animal or animal and human health services.

International, commercial and media organizations

The globalization of trade and travel, and the threat of bioterrorism have driven the development of an international sharing of epidemic intelligence and real-time, or early, warning systems for the detection of new environmental hazards or disease events. The WHO has adopted an all-hazards approach to monitoring for public health events of international concern through the implementation of the 2005 International Health Regulations processes and procedures.[14] Within Europe, the creation of a European Centre for Disease Prevention and Control has provided a focus for international surveillance within the European Union and beyond. Real-time surveillance initiatives have been developed around retail sales of 'over-the-counter' medicines[15] and of media/press reports published on the Internet.[7,16]

Population and environmental surveys

Intermittent or continuous surveys of the population and environment can provide immediate surveillance data or contextual information for other surveillance systems. A number of national surveys of sexual attitudes and lifestyles have provided information on risk behaviours, test-seeking behaviours and the prevalence of disease.[17] Environmental

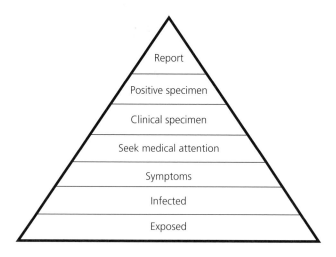

Figure 3.3   The pyramid of laboratory reporting.

surveys are increasingly being used to monitor animal hosts and vectors for zoonotic diseases.[18,19] For example, environmental sampling of the soil on Vancouver Island and adjacent areas of British Columbia, Canada, was used to monitor the distribution of the fungal pathogen *Cryptococcus gattii*.[20]

Environmental surveys are also an essential component of surveillance for certain chemical and radiological hazards. In the UK, the Health Protection Agency undertakes the sampling of airborne dust for gamma ray emitters and cows' milk for caesium-137 and strontium-90 as part of its radiological protection monitoring programme.[21] Remote sensing, using satellite imagery, is now being used for public health monitoring, for instance in the study of the distribution of schistosomiasis in Egypt.[22]

LEVEL OF ASCERTAINMENT: 'ACTIVE' AND 'PASSIVE' SURVEILLANCE

Many surveillance systems based on the universal reporting of cases (e.g. national notification systems or national laboratory reporting schemes) are subject to significant ascertainment bias, with an underrepresentation of asymptomatic and less severe cases, and a relative overrepresentation of cases in particular demographic or socioeconomic groups. Signal can be lost at various points along the pathway from the occurrence of an exposure or disease event in the population under surveillance (Figure 3.3) and needs to be minimized at each step in the pathway. In addition, operators must assess how the loss of signal might introduce bias into the data.

The completeness and consistency of reporting to surveillance systems can be affected by a range of system design and operational factors. Statutory or mandatory reporting has been used as a mechanism for achieving high reporting rates, although there is evidence to suggest that this does not guarantee complete, or even high levels of, reporting. Surveys in the UK have demonstrated very low levels of reporting of some statutorily notifiable infections,[23] with little evidence that this can be improved by increasing the payment made for reporting cases.[24] Concerns have also been raised that making some diseases notifiable may result in patients being reluctant to seek medical attention for fear of being notified, a significant factor in the decision not to make HIV or acquired immune deficiency syndrome notifiable in the UK.

Another strategy that may achieve high reporting rates is to adopt a sample-based or sentinel approach so that resources can be invested in achieving such an improvement from a smaller number of reporters, for example by providing training and support (e.g. specific software reporting). This approach is often used when it is important to include data on investigations that are not routinely ordered by clinicians or that need to be undertaken to a specified standard. Examples include surveillance for seasonal influenza virus strains in the UK[25] and the surveillance of antimicrobial resistance among gonocoocal isolates.[26,27] For rare diseases, active reporting, in which reporters are actively prompted or reminded to report cases on a regular basis, can be effective, as in the British Paediatric Surveillance Unit reporting scheme, covering a list of 10–12 conditions that are the subject of active surveillance.[28]

Surveillance systems must be capable of capturing data in a consistent and sustainable way, since fluctuations in reporting may mask or mimic genuine changes in the incidence of the disease, exposure or hazard under surveillance. Although the attainment of a measure of true disease occurrence within a population through surveillance is probably unrealistic for most situations, achievement and maintenance of high levels of ascertainment is still desirable for the early detection of outbreaks and the surveillance of uncommon diseases of public health importance and/or diseases that are the subject of elimination programmes. It also provides a level of reassurance that the surveillance system is providing a relatively representative picture of the distribution of disease within the target population. Assessment of the completeness of case ascertainment achieved by surveillance systems has been undertaken using capture–recapture methods,[29] an approach used in the UK to estimate the completeness of tuberculosis surveillance and notification levels.[30,31]

SURVEILLANCE OUTPUTS

Surveillance information is typically in the form of descriptive statistics on the frequency and distribution of cases, and temporal trends. The information on the distribution of cases may include categorization by geography, demographic characteristics, occupational and other risk factors. More sophisticated outputs may include the modelling of surveillance data or spatial analysis through geographical information systems.

In order to inform action that will result in improved control or prevention, surveillance must provide information that is both timely and accurate, and is interpreted and presented in a format and through channels that are appropriate to those who have responsibility for taking action. The range of target audiences is large but can be broadly categorized as follows:

- the public;
- clinicians, microbiologists and control of infection staff;
- public health professionals;
- environmental health professionals;
- health service managers;
- health educators and teachers;
- the government and politicians.

Of these groups, the public are often overlooked as a potential target audience for surveillance outputs, yet many public health actions that have the greatest potential for improved control and prevention, such as improved food hygiene, safer sexual practice and the uptake of vaccinations, require significant public action.

OPERATIONAL ISSUES

Operating procedures

The surveillance systems used to capture, analyse and disseminate information should be operated to agreed standards. The development and adoption of standard operating protocols and case definitions ensures that surveillance systems operate in a consistent and explicit manner over time and place. Their scope is summarized in Table 3.2. Publication of these protocols helps to make the purpose and governance arrangements for surveillance systems explicit to data providers, data subjects and the recipients of surveillance outputs.

Data capture

Surveillance system design is often based on achieving a pragmatic balance between what is desirable and what is achievable. The 'achievability' factor is particularly important in the design of surveillance systems for environmental hazards and infectious diseases, as systems need to be able to collect, analyse and report in a continuous and as near to real-time basis as possible. The sustainability and quality of data available for surveillance are likely to be higher if the data are derived from information collected for operational purposes (rather than specifically for surveillance purposes). As a general rule, surveillance systems based on the capture of data from health services are most likely to be sustainable and achieve acceptable levels of coverage of the target population where the design of the system is coherent with the infrastructure of the healthcare systems within which patients are seen. For

Table 3.2 Operating protocols: main requirements

Methodology	Reporting
Statement of purpose	Frequency of reporting
Case definitions or definitions of hazards and exposures	How reporting occurs
Laboratory investigation protocols (where appropriate)	Form and structure of electronic reporting systems
Sources of data (e.g. the type of clinical service from which the data are to be captured)	
The 'sampling' approach – universal, random or convenience sample, sentinel	
Data items to be collected (including level of person identifier required)	
Outputs	
Roles and responsibilities of those involved in the surveillance process	
Identity of the custodian or owner of the system	

Table 3.3 Dimensions of quality of surveillance systems

Dimension	Type of measure	Quality target
Completeness	Quantitative	Information should be sufficiently complete to be fit for purpose
Timeliness	Quantitative	Information should be available when it is needed
Accuracy	Quantitative	Information should be sufficiently free from error to be fit for purpose
Relevance	Qualitative	Information should be contextually appropriate
Reliability	Qualitative	Provenance, objectivity and believability
Delivery	Qualitative	Information should be formatted to satisfy users' needs

example, where specialist clinics provide the majority of care for a particular disease or group of diseases, such as is the case with sexually transmitted infections in the UK, surveillance based on data reporting from those clinics can often achieve higher quality (with regards to diagnostic validity of reports and compliance with reporting) information for a given cost than would be possible through systems based on universal reporting.

The advent of the Internet and associated new technologies presents significant opportunities for new approaches to data capture for surveillance. Browser-based forms can now be used to allow data to be recorded in a standardized way by anyone who has access to the Internet (or can be used for capturing data on hand-held devices, which can be downloaded later). This can reduce the costs and technical difficulties previously associated with deploying bespoke applications in each reporting site, often allows for a more rapid redesign of forms in response to changing data needs and can reduce training requirements. The development of software languages such as XML (extensible mark-up language) that facilitate the sharing of structured data across the Internet, particularly when used in conjunction with common coding systems (such as SNOMED), provides the opportunity to capture and combine structured data from diverse sources.

The Internet also provides unprecedented levels of access to unstructured information, including reports from national and international organizations and news items from press agencies and other sources. Scanning

these information resources and the use of analytical systems for identifying potential events has become a recognized component of surveillance and horizon scanning for emerging threats in recent years. Examples include the Global Public Health Intelligence Network system[7] and HealthMap.[16]

The quality and completeness of reporting to surveillance systems is also likely to be better where reporting makes use of data collected for operational purposes. The development of electronic patient information systems is likely to make this easier. Other opportunities for capturing data without requiring additional effort by clinical staff include making use of laboratory requesting or result-reporting data, health insurance claim forms and pharmacy records (e.g. for dispensing vaccines or disease-specific medications).

Data quality

The concept of setting quality standards for data, and measuring data against those standards, is well established for readily measurable aspects of data quality, particularly the validity, timeliness and completeness of data items. Simple quality standards in specific domains can be set (Table 3.3) and used as targets, such as maximum acceptable levels of missing items in particular data fields and the mean, median or maximum acceptable time between event detection and report to the surveillance system.

Case definitions

Harder to measure, but perhaps more important, aspects in the context of overall information quality, such as accuracy and relevance, have sometimes been neglected in the setting of standards. Relevance and reliability can be improved through the use of case definitions for reporting. These are particularly important when data are captured from diverse sources, such as when taking data from different types of healthcare setting or from more than one country, where different levels of clinical expertise or diagnostic support may exist.

Case definitions will often include different levels of likelihood (such as 'possible', 'probable' and 'confirmed'), allowing cases to be classified according to the level of diagnostic information available. For infectious diseases, the gold standard for case confirmation is usually a laboratory finding. This may require a harmonization of laboratory techniques, such as was implemented for the European surveillance networks for *Legionella* and *Salmonella* infections.[32,33] Case definitions for infectious disease surveillance in the European Union[34] and in the USA[35] have been published. The development and adoption of case definitions can have significant resource implications, particularly for training and the provision of supporting diagnostic investigations.

Case definitions used for surveillance need to be specified to achieve the desired level of sensitivity and specificity. They will often need to be more sensitive (and less specific) than those used in analytical epidemiological studies, since the purpose of surveillance is frequently to provide an early warning of the possible emergence of disease outbreaks or rising trends. Even when case definitions do exist, guidance may be required on whether cases should be reported only when they meet certain criteria (e.g. those for a confirmed case), when all exposure and risk factor data are available, or whether preliminary reporting should be made on the basis of suspected case identification and/or when only partial exposure or risk factor data are available (in which case clear mechanisms need to be defined for how more detailed information should be reported at a later date).

Data governance

The data collected should be relevant and sufficient to meeting surveillance objectives, and be restricted to items that are required to meet the objectives of surveillance. Additional, non-essential data items, which are often collected on a 'nice-to-know' basis rather than because they are justified in terms of meeting explicit objectives, place additional burdens on data providers and on the supporting information systems and, if the dataset being reported is person-identifying, may breach data protection restrictions.

Anonymized data should be used where the identification of individuals is not needed without a requirement for record linkage between different datasets. In the case of infectious disease surveillance, it is often necessary to collect person-identifying information to contact cases rapidly to undertake follow-up and contact tracing and/or outbreak investigations. When person-identifying data are used, they should be kept secure and disclosed only on a strict 'need-to-know' basis, and in accordance with data protection laws.

ANALYSIS OF SURVEILLANCE DATA

The analysis of surveillance data can range from producing simple tabulations of descriptive statistics by time, place and person, to sophisticated time-trend analyses, including their use in complex mathematical modelling, and analyses within geographical information systems (see Box 6b).

Although many significant outbreaks are first detected and reported by clinical staff or members of the public before they are identifiable through surveillance systems (largely because of the delays inherent in surveillance systems), surveillance remains an important mechanism for detecting outbreaks, particularly of uncommon infections, and diffuse outbreaks (i.e. outbreaks occurring over wide geographical areas, with relatively small numbers in any one locality). The need to be able to detect emerging epidemics or outbreaks at an early stage in their evolution is an important element of communicable disease control. A number of analytical techniques have been developed that can be applied to surveillance data to detect possible outbreaks or to assess the statistical significance of an apparent increase in reports.

Simple graphs can be used to show trends over time and to compare those trends between different geographical, demographic or exposure groups. The calculation of rates, based on appropriate denominators, and the graphing of these can similarly show changes in risks over time and between different groups. A range of statistical techniques has been applied to surveillance data, to identify outbreaks or assess the significance of observed changes in frequency, including the CUSUM technique,[36] particularly for rare events, the scan statistic[37] and more complex modelling approaches.[38]

However, surveillance systems, particularly those based on the collection of data from a single type of source, rarely achieve complete ascertainment of the hazard, exposure or event that is being monitored. Sophisticated statistical and modelling techniques have then been used to create a more complete picture of the epidemiology of a disease, such as Bayesian multiparameter evidence synthesis in the analysis of syndromic surveillance data in the USA[39] and in the UK to estimate national hepatitis C prevalence.[40] Such approaches have been used to assess determinants of incidence and the distribution of susceptibility in the population, including a Bayesian approach to investigate the contribution of unsafe injections to HIV transmission[41] and a mixture model analysis of seroepidemiological survey data on measles, mumps and rubella.[42] Methods have also been developed and applied to estimate vaccine effectiveness using routinely available data, while clinical trial and serosurvey data have been used to validate correlates of protection. This helped to identify the need for booster doses of meningococcal C and *Haemophilus influenzae* type b vaccines in the UK.[43]

The development of typing schemes, such as serotyping, phage-typing and newer molecular techniques, provides new opportunities for surveillance to detect subtype-specific outbreaks that might not be detected through clinician reporting. A good example is that of *Salmonella* surveillance, where the ability to undertake surveillance of many different serotypes and phage types of *Salmonella* has identified outbreaks that might otherwise not have been detected until considerably later, if at all. Serotyping is also an essential tool in the surveillance of vaccine-preventable diseases such as meningococcal and pneumococcal infection, for which data on the distribution and trends in serotypes have been central to the development and evaluation of vaccination policy.[44]

The exploitation of serotyping and phage-typing techniques to improve outbreak detection and inform public health policy is not the only area in which collaboration between microbiologists and epidemiologists has resulted in important advances in the field of surveillance. Monitoring of the incidence of new HIV infections, and more recently hepatitis C infections, rather than just the prevalence of diagnosed infections, was an elusive surveillance goal for many years but has now been realized through applying the serological testing algorithm of recent HIV seroconversion (STARHS) assay.[45]

Interpretation of surveillance data

As with any epidemiological dataset, interpretation must take into account issues of underascertainment and the biases that that can be introduced (see above). Although this may result in the underestimation of a true effect size, surveillance data can still, where the level of underascertainment remains consistent over time in terms of the proportion and mix of cases, provide a valid indicator of trends over time, and as such provide triggers for action and measures of the impact of interventions

The interpretation of such analyses needs to take into account issues such as the seasonality and periodicity, which may stretch over several years, shown by several diseases. Discontinuities in long-term time trends may be the result of interventions, such as the introduction of a new vaccine, but may also arise as the result of changes in factors unrelated to the true incidence of disease, such as the introduction of new diagnostic tests, changes in clinical practice that result in increased case ascertainment (e.g. the introduction of a new screening programme) or changes in coding systems (e.g. changes to the International Classification of Diseases system have resulted in significant

discontinuities in trends in deaths attributed to some causes[46]). Reporting delay can be an important factor, resulting in significant delays between the onset or detection of disease and the date of reporting to the surveillance system. This can be adjusted for if the delay varies little over time, but the data user must be aware of such delays or incorrect interpretation could result.

Appropriate presentation of data is essential when interpreting surveillance outputs. The emergence of healthcare-associated infection as a public health priority has required the development of innovative approaches to the analysis and presentation of surveillance data, to inform policy and monitor outcomes and performance, such as funnel plots to identify hospitals with outlying rates of surgical site infection allowing for a variation in sample size.[47]

A common problem in the geographical analysis of surveillance data is missing information on the geographical location of cases and the geocoding of data to the source of the report rather than the likely source of acquisition of infection. For example, an analysis of data from an outbreak of *Salmonella* infection in England and Wales in 2000 shows a considerable difference in the geographical distribution of cases and of the laboratories that submitted reports on their *Salmonella* infections (Figure 3.4).

Dissemination

Surveillance can only achieve its purpose of providing information for action if the information reaches those who have the responsibility for taking action, but the process of dissemination of the information is often given less attention.

The production of regular and timely surveillance outputs, and their dissemination in an appropriate format with relevant interpretation, requires significant investment. The development of outputs should be undertaken through close consultation with the target audience for the output, to ensure that they are fit for purpose. Some users of surveillance outputs will only require high-level summaries that focus on key messages about overall changes in the frequency of distribution, while others may require detailed line listings of cases in order to inform their own operational activities. Some users may wish to be able to manipulate surveillance data in their own systems (e.g. in their local geographical information systems), where they can undertake linkage or ecological analyses against other data that they hold. It is only through regular consultation with the relevant stakeholders that surveillance system managers can ensure that their outputs continue to meet with recipients' requirements. Such consultation should be part of the regular audit of surveillance systems against their objectives and user requirements.

Advances in information technology, particularly browser-based web technologies, provides the opportunity

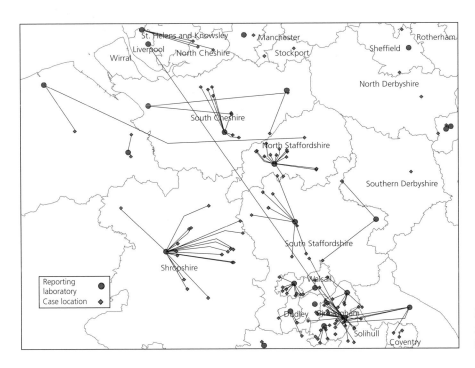

Figure 3.4 Geospatial analysis: *Salmonella* Typhimurium DT104 outbreak, England and Wales, August 2000.

of making surveillance outputs available, or even pushing them through email or technologies such as RSS, to a large audience as soon as the outputs are ready. This is clearly of benefit in terms of speed and cost of delivery, but such benefits will only be realized if the outputs are relevant and easily understood by the intended audience – if not, they are likely to be overlooked in the face of increasing information overload.

REFERENCES

● = Key primary paper

◆ = Major review article

●1. Thacker SB, Berkelman RL. Public health surveillance in the United States. *Epidemiol Rev* 1988; **10**: 164–90.

2. Teutsch SM, Churchill RE. *Principles and Practice of Public Health Surveillance*. 2nd edn. Oxford: Oxford University Press, 2000.

3. McCormick A. The notification of infectious diseases in England and Wales. *Commun Dis Rep CDR Rev* 1993; **3**: R19–25.

4. Fleming DM. Weekly Returns Service of the Royal College of General Practitioners. *Commun Dis Public Health* 1999; **2**: 96–100.

●5. Galbraith NS, Young EJ. Communicable disease control: The development of a laboratory associated national epidemiological service in England and Wales. *Community Med* 1980; **2**: 135–43.

6. Cooper DL, Smith G, Baker M *et al.* National symptom surveillance using calls to a telephone health advice service – United Kingdom, December 2001–February 2003. *Morb Mortal Wkly Rep* 2004; **53**(Suppl.): 179–83.

7. Mykhalovskiy E, Weir L. The Global Public Health Intelligence Network and early warning outbreak detection: A Canadian contribution to global public health. *Can J Public Health* 2006; **97**: 42–4.

8. *National and Global Surveillance of Communicable Disease. Report of the technical discussion at the Twenty-First World Health Assembly. A21/Technical Discussions/5*. Geneva: World Health Organization, 1968.

9. World Health Assembly. Revision of the International Health Regulations, WHA58.3.May 23, 2005. Available from: http://www.who.int/csr/ihr/IHRWHA58_3-en.pdf (accessed July 16, 2009).

◆10. Thacker SB, Stroup DF, Parrish RG, Anderson HA. Surveillance in environmental public health: Issues, systems, and sources. *Am J Public Health* 1996; **86**: 633–8.

11. Gay NJ, Hesketh LM, Morgan-Capner P, Miller E. Interpretation of serological surveillance data for measles using mathematical models: Implications for vaccine strategy. *Epidemiol Infect* 1995; **115**: 139–56.

12. Bailey NT. An improved hybrid HIV/AIDS model geared to specific public health data and decision making. *Math Biosci* 1993; **117**: 221–37.

13. Reichert TA, Simonsen L, Sharma A, Pardo SA, Fedson DS, Miller MA. Influenza and the winter increase in mortality in the United States, 1959–1999. *Am J Epidemiol* 2004; **160**: 492–502.

14. World Health Organization. *International Health Regulations*, 2nd edn. Geneva: WHO, 2008.

15. Das D, Metzger K, Heffernan R, Balter S, Weiss D, Mostashari F. New York City Department of Health and

Mental Hygiene. Monitoring over-the-counter medication sales for early detection of disease outbreaks – New York City. *Morb Mortal Wkly Rep* 2005; **54**(Suppl.): 41–6.

16. Brownstein JS, Freifeld CC, Reis BY, Mandl KD. Surveillance Sans Frontières: Internet-Based Emerging Infectious Disease Intelligence and the HealthMap Project. *PLoS Med* 2008; **5**: e151.

17. Johnson AM, Mercer CH, Erens B *et al*. Sexual behaviour in Britain: Partnerships, practices, and HIV risk behaviours. *Lancet* 2001; **358**: 1835–42.

18. Stafford KC 3rd, Cartter ML, Magnarelli LA, Ertel S, Mshar PA. Temporal correlations between tick abundance and prevalence of ticks infected with *Borrelia burgdorferi* and increasing incidence of Lyme disease. *J Clin Microbiol* 1998; **36**: 1240–4.

19. Bernard KA, Maffei JG, Jones SA *et al*. West Nile virus infection in birds and mosquitos, New York State, 2000. *Emerg Inf Dis* 2001; **7**: 679–85.

20. MacDougall L, Fyfe M. Emergence of *Cryptococcus gattii* in a novel environment provides clues to its incubation period. *J Clin Microbiol* 2006; **44**: 1851–2.

21. Widling D. *Environmental Radioactivity Surveillance Programme: Results for 2006*. HPA-RPD-039. Chilton, Oxfordshire: Health Protection Agency, 2008.

22. Malone JB, Huh OK, Fehler DP *et al*. Temperature data from satellite imagery and the distribution of schistosomiasis in Egypt. *Am J Trop Med Hyg* 1994; **50**: 714–22.

23. Cartwright KA. Meningococcal meningitis. *Br J Hosp Med* 1987; **38**: 516, 521–4.

24. McCormick A. Notification of infectious diseases: The effect of increasing the fee paid. *Health Trends* 1987; **19**: 7–8.

25. Boon AC, French AM, Fleming DM, Zambon MC. Detection of influenza a subtypes in community-based surveillance. *J Med Virol* 2001; **65**: 163–70.

26. Paine TC, Fenton KA, Herring A *et al*. GRASP: A new national sentinel surveillance initiative for monitoring gonococcal antimicrobial resistance in England and Wales. *Sex Transm Infect* 2001; **77**: 398–401.

27. Centers for Disease Control and Prevention. *Sexually Transmitted Disease Surveillance 2006 Supplement, Gonococcal Isolate Surveillance Project (GISP) Annual Report 2006*. Atlanta, GA: US Department of Health and Human Services, Centers for Disease Control and Prevention, 2008. Available from: http://www.cdc.gov/std/gisp2006/GISPSurvSupp2006Short.pdf (accessed July 17, 2009).

28. British Paediatric Surveillance Unit. *19th Annual Report 2004–2005*. London: Royal College of Paediatrics and Child Health, 2005. Available from: http://www.bpsu.inopsu.com/publications/annual_reports/annual-report_2005.pdf (Accessed July 17, 2009).

●29. Van Hest NA, Grant AD, Smit F, Story A, Richardus JH. Estimating infectious diseases incidence: validity of capture-recapture analysis and truncated models for incomplete count data. *Epidemiol Infect* 2008; **136**: 14–22.

30. Crofts JP, Pebody R, Grant A, Watson JM, Abubakar I. Estimating tuberculosis case mortality in England and Wales, 2001–2002. *Internat J Tuberc Lung Dis* 2008; **12**: 308–13.

31. Ahmed AB, Abubakar I, Delpech V *et al*. The growing impact of HIV infection on the epidemiology of tuberculosis in England and Wales: 1999–2003. *Thorax* 2007; **62**: 672–6.

32. Fry NK, Bangsborg JM, Bergmans A *et al*. Designation of the European Working Group on Legionella Infection (EWGLI) amplified fragment length polymorphism types of *Legionella pneumophila* serogroup 1 and results of intercentre proficiency testing using a standard protocol. *Eur J Clin Microbiol Infect Dis* 2002; **21**: 722–8.

33. Fisher IS, Threlfall EJ. The Enter-net and Salm-gene databases of foodborne bacterial pathogens that cause human infections in Europe and beyond: An international collaboration in surveillance and the development of intervention strategies. *Epidemiol Infect* 2005; **33**: 1–7.

34. Commission Decision of 28 April 2008 (2008/426/EC) amending Decision 2002/253/EC laying down case definitions for reporting communicable diseases to the Community network under Decision No 2119/98/EC of the European Parliament and of the Council. *OJE* 2008; **L159**: 46–90.

●35. Centers for Disease Control and Prevention. Case definitions for infectious diseases under public health surveillance. *MMWR Recomm Rep* 1977; **46**(RR-10): 1–55.

36. O'Brien SJ, Christie P. Do CuSums have a role in routine communicable disease surveillance? *Public Health* 1997; **111**: 255–8.

37. Wallenstein S. A test for detection of clustering over time. *Am J Epidem* 1980; **3**: 367–72.

●38. Farrington CP, Beale AD, Andrews NJ, Catchpole MA. A statistical algorithm for the early detection of outbreaks of infectious disease. *J R Statist Soc* 1996; **159**: 547–63.

39. Wong WK, Cooper G, Dash D, Levander J, Dowling J, Hogan W, Wagner M. Use of multiple data streams to conduct Bayesian biologic surveillance. *Morb Mortal Wkly Rep* 2005; **54**(Suppl.): 63–9.

40. Sweeting MJ, De Angelis D, Hickman M, Ades AE. Estimating hepatitis C prevalence in England and Wales by synthesizing evidence from multiple data sources. Assessing data conflict and model fit. *Biostatistics* 2008; **9**: 715–34.

41. White RG, Ben SC, Kedhar A *et al*. Quantifying HIV-1 transmission due to contaminated injections. *Proc Natl Acad Sci USA* 2007; **104**: 9794–9.

42. Vyse AJ, Gay NJ, Hesketh LM, Pebody R, Morgan-Capner P, Miller E. Interpreting serological surveys using mixture models: The seroepidemiology of measles, mumps and rubella in England and Wales at the beginning of the 21st century. *Epidemiol Infect* 2006; **134**: 1303–12.

43. Trotter CL, Ramsay ME, Slack MP. Rising incidence of *Haemophilus influenzae* type b disease in England and Wales indicates a need for a second catch-up vaccination campaign. *Commun Dis Public Health* 2003; **6**: 55–8.

44. Andrews N, Borrow R, Miller E. Validation of serological correlate of protection for meningococcal C conjugate vaccine by using efficacy estimates from post-licensure surveillance in England. *Clin Diag Lab Immunol* 2003; **10**: 780–6.

45. Murphy G, Charlett A, Osner N, Gill ON, Parry JV. Reconciling HIV incidence results from two assays employed in the serological testing algorithm for recent HIV seroconversion (STARHS). *J Virol Methods* 2003; **113**: 79–86.

46. Brock A, Griffiths C, Rooney C. The impact of introducing ICD-10 on analysis of respiratory mortality trends in England and Wales. *Health Stat Q* 2006; (29): 9–17.

47. Wilson J, Charlett A, Leong G, McDougall C, Duckworth G. Rates of surgical site infection after hip replacement as a hospital performance indicator: Analysis of data from the English mandatory surveillance system. *Infect Control Hosp Epidemiol* 2008; **29**: 219–26.

Hazard and risk: assessment and management

ROGER O. McCLELLAN

Those unfamiliar with this topic should first read Chapter 1, which provides a general introduction and definitions of key terms and concepts.

SOURCES OF INFORMATION FOR CHARACTERIZING HAZARDS AND RISKS

There are multiple sources of information, as shown schematically in Figure 4.1, for characterizing hazards and exposure–response relationships. Starting with the view

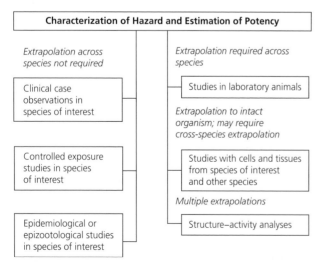

Figure 4.1 Sources of information used in characterizing hazards and estimating the potency of chemical agents.

that our primary interest is human health, it is apparent the most relevant information for evaluating hazards and risks to humans is that acquired from the study of people. If epidemiological data are available, they will be used. Unfortunately, positive epidemiological findings stand as a testimonial to the past failure of society to control human exposures to the agent(s) in question, as might have occurred in the workplace or environment, from the use of a particular technology or a specific product. Obviously, a goal is to avoid such occurrences in the future.

A major difficulty in interpreting most epidemiological data, even with regard to identifying hazards, lies in the crude indices used to describe exposure (i.e. years in a given job, a few industrial hygiene measurements in a plant, ambient measurements at a few locations, etc.). In rare studies, some more appropriate measure of dose, such as the blood levels of an agent or metabolite, may be available.

The challenges in characterizing health outcomes are equally daunting. Traditional measures of morbidity and mortality are typically used, and, increasingly, clinical parameters that are markers of disease have been used. The interpretation of many of these markers is challenging because of our incomplete understanding of disease processes. A major problem is that environmental agents typically do not have agent-specific disease outcomes that can be readily identified as distinct from diseases caused by or influenced in outcome by myriad other factors. The exceptions are rare, such as the development of mesothelioma following exposure to certain types of asbestos. However, even in the case of mesotheliomas, it has not been established that these cases are exclusively related to exposure to asbestos. Lung cancers, which are acknowledged to develop primarily in cigarette smokers, are also observed, albeit much less frequently, in non-smokers.

The statistical challenge of detecting an increase in adverse effects, such as cancer, can be appreciated by considering Figure 4.2. In this hypothetical situation, an incidence of 1 per cent for the end point of interest is assumed for the control population. It is common to conduct lifespan toxicity studies that utilize 50 animals of each gender at each exposure level. The statistical bluntness of studies of this size is apparent when it is recognized that with 50 animals, the study can only detect a 20 per cent excess incidence of the disease of interest relative to the control incidence of 1 per cent. Combining the males and females to give a group size of 100 still falls short of detecting a 10 per cent excess. To provide perspective, the relative risk of a moderately heavy smoker developing lung cancer over their lifetime is of the order of 10. In other words, if a laboratory animal species were a perfect surrogate for humans, a study of cigarette-smoking in the laboratory animal species might not detect a carcinogenic effect. The message is that caution should be exercised in interpreting a negative outcome for test substances observed in the typical experimental study.

To detect with 95 per cent statistical confidence an excess of 5 per cent compared with a background incidence of 1.0 per cent, 400 individuals must be studied in the control and test population. The detection of relative risks of the order of a few percentage points requires the study of huge populations. As the number of individuals studied in epidemiological investigations is increased, the potential for the two populations, for example smokers and non-smokers, to have differences other than the variable of interest also increases.

For some agents, it may be feasible to conduct studies with human subjects exposed under controlled conditions to the agent of interest. A key consideration is whether it is ethically appropriate to conduct the study in humans

and, indeed, use the data to evaluate human risk. This is a topic of continuing debate. Suffice it to say that, in the past, two considerations served to guide decisions on the conduct of human studies. First, is there a high degree of confidence that any effects resulting from the exposures will be reversible? Second, are humans already exposed to the agents, and if so, are the exposure levels proposed for the experimental study similar to those of individuals who may have been exposed to in the environment or workplace?

One aspect of the current debate focuses on whether human subjects should be used to test new agents, such as pesticides, proposed for introduction in the marketplace. Human studies to help ensure that appropriate exposure limits are set for the new products can be justified if assurance can be given that any anticipated effects in the volunteers will be reversible based on the results of previous studies in laboratory animals.

If the data from epidemiological studies or controlled exposure studies in humans are not adequate for assessing human hazards and risks, it is then necessary to conduct studies with intact laboratory animals, mammalian cells or tissues, cellular preparations or non-mammalian cells and to extrapolate to the human situation. It is obvious that, for new materials, human data will not be available. In such situations, the traditional approach has been to conduct studies with laboratory animals to evaluate the hazardous properties of the agent as a basis for safety/risk characterization. Both national and international agencies have provided guidance for conducting these in vivo studies.

A major issue in planning and designing toxicity studies using laboratory animals is the selection of the species to be used. Fortunately, humans and mammalian laboratory animal species share many similarities that provide a sound scientific basis for using these laboratory animal species as surrogates for humans in investigations to develop toxicity information that is applicable to humans. It is, however, important to recognize the obvious – there is no laboratory animal species that is identical to humans in all respects. Moreover, the common laboratory animal species also differ from humans in various ways that must be considered when extrapolating the findings from laboratory animal species to humans.

In recent years, there has been increased enthusiasm for using in vitro methods to replace in vivo methods. The motivation for this shift has been twofold. First, an increasing concern for animal welfare has led to encouragement to reduce the number of animals used in toxicological testing and to replace their use, as far as possible, with other methods. Second, there has been a desire to take advantage of the substantial advances made in recent years in understanding both the basic biology and pathobiology of mammals, especially at the cellular and molecular levels. Two recent reports from the US National Research Council (NRC) have reviewed advances in basic biology and how these advances can be used in toxicity testing and risk assessment.[1,2]

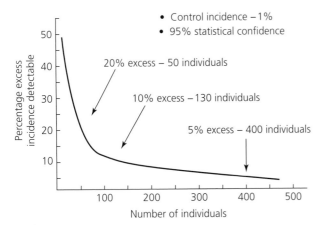

Figure 4.2 Number of subjects (humans or laboratory animals) required for detecting an increased incidence of tumours.

All toxicologists should support such activities, especially the validation of new in vitro methods using known human toxicants. It could, however, be argued that many past validation activities have been flawed because attention has focused on whether the new in vitro method is predictive of the results of in vivo laboratory animal studies. This approach fails to recognize that our primary interest is whether the in vitro methods are predictive of *human* toxicity, not that observed in rats.

Many of those experienced in respiratory toxicology are cautious in predicting near-term success in replacing many in vivo approaches with in vitro tests. The entry of material via the respiratory system poses special challenges in selecting particular cell types for use in in vitro studies and in selecting exposure (dose) levels. The respiratory tract contains over 40 different types of cell that have the potential to receive a dose of an inhaled agent. The cells lining the airways may be most directly exposed, and some cells may be exposed only to the metabolites of the inhaled agent produced in other cells. The interpretation of in vitro studies in which cells from the respiratory tract have been bathed with the test agent, typically at high concentrations, poses a special challenge. The target cells may be appropriate, but how does the dose concentration–time profile used with the cells compare with that seen by the cells from a relevant level of human exposure?

Because of these challenges, the results of in vitro studies have generally served as only a crude index of the potential inhalational toxicity of materials. It follows that the results of in vitro studies have only been moderately useful in setting exposure levels for in vivo inhalation studies and, most importantly, not particularly useful in setting exposure limits for airborne materials. The greatest value of in vitro studies relates to their use in interpreting the metabolic patterns (toxicokinetics) or biological responses (toxicodynamics) observed in intact mammals exposed by inhalation, and only then when the doses studied include exposure (dose) levels likely to result from exposures potentially encountered by people. In short, our goal is to better understand and interpret the results observed in the intact mammal, and especially humans, exposed by the relevant routes of exposure.

In summary, the design, conduct and interpretation of epidemiology and toxicity studies and the implication of the findings for human hazard and risk inevitably involve the careful consideration of a number of extrapolation issues: (1) from a specific population, such as workers who are subjects in an epidemiological investigation, to the general population; (2) from a population of healthy humans studied in the laboratory under controlled conditions to populations of individuals who are susceptible as a result of genetic differences, pre-existing disease or the influence of age; (3) from laboratory animal species to humans; (4) from high levels of exposure (dose) to the lower levels likely to be encountered by people; (e) from less than lifetime exposure to human exposures; and (5) from cellular or tissue studies to the intact human.

EMERGENCE OF A FORMAL RISK PARADIGM

The plethora of new legislation that emerged in the 1970s required the development of new standards for the workplace and the environment. For some agents and situations, it appeared that the old threshold exposure (dose)–response approach would be appropriate. However, it was apparent that cancer, as a health end point of major public concern, could not be readily dealt with using a threshold exposure (dose)–response model. This dilemma stimulated a review of the entire approach to setting standards.

> ## BOX 4.1: Common default options used by the US Environmental Protection Agency18–20
>
> 1. Laboratory animals are surrogates for humans in assessing cancer risks; positive cancer bioassay results in laboratory animals are taken as evidence of a chemical's cancer-causing potential in humans
> 2. Humans are as sensitive as the most sensitive animal species, strain or sex evaluated in a bioassay
> 3. Agents that are positive in long-term animal experiments and also show evidence of promoting or co-carcinogenic activity should be viewed as complete carcinogens
> 4. Benign tumours are surrogates for malignant tumours, so benign and malignant tumours are added in evaluating whether a chemical is carcinogenic and in assessing its potency
> 5. Chemicals act like radiation at low exposures (doses) in inducing cancer; i.e. the intake of even one molecule of a chemical has an associated probability for cancer induction that can be calculated, so the appropriate model for relating exposure–response relationships is the linearized multistage model
> 6. Important biological parameters, including the rate of metabolism of chemicals, in humans and laboratory animals are related to body surface area. When extrapolating metabolic data from laboratory animals to humans, one may use the relationship of surface area in the test species to that in humans in modifying the laboratory animal data
> 7. A given unit of intake of a chemical has the same effect, regardless of the time of its intake; chemical intake is integrated over time, irrespective of intake ratio and duration
> 8. Individual chemicals act independently of other chemicals in inducing cancer when multiple chemicals are taken into the body; when assessing the risks associated with a mixture of chemicals, one treats the risk additively.

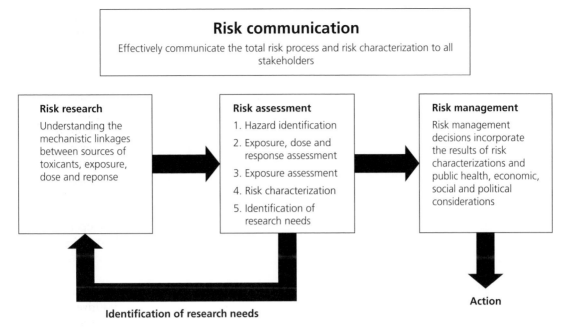

Figure 4.3   The risk paradigm that is widely used around the world.

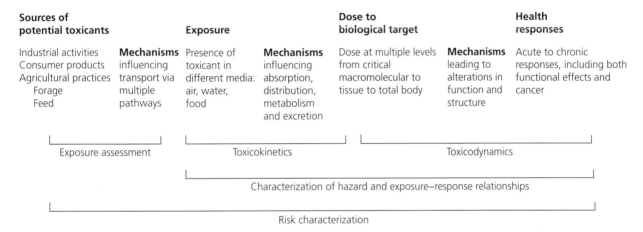

Figure 4.4   An expanded risk characterization paradigm.

The basic risk assessment paradigm that emerged, as was initially formalized in the USA, is shown in Figure 4.3.[3,4] The original paradigm, developed by an NRC Committee,[4] emphasized the four elements of risk assessment: (1) hazard identification; (2) exposure (dose)–response assessment; (3) exposure assessment; and (4) risk characterization. It also called attention to the distinction between risk assessment and risk management. Although emphasis was placed on the scientific basis of risk assessment, it was also recognized that the conduct of risk assessments inherently required that certain science policy judgements (sometimes referred to as default options) had to be made in the absence of specific scientific knowledge (Box 4.1).[4–6]

An expanded view of the risk characterization process is shown in Figure 4.4. This figure emphasizes the importance of understanding the multiple linkages that exist between a particular source of potential toxicants and, ultimately,

concern for health responses that might potentially be associated with the toxicants. Each of the mechanistic steps highlighted in Figure 4.4 can be viewed in the context of the research needs link shown in Figure 4.3.

A later NRC Committee,[6] mandated by the 1990 amendments to the Clean Air Act, directed attention to the use of both science and judgement in assessing risks. The Committee did not reach agreement on the specific criteria to be used in selecting default options and replacing them with the results of specific scientific studies (specific science). As a member of the Committee, the current author argued that specific science should be used in favour of defaults.[7] Other Committee members argued for using specific science only if the resulting assessment was more health protective, i.e. the resulting guidance values were lower. The Committee[6] also advocated a greater use of iterative risk assessments in which the identified uncertainties in a risk assessment could be used to inform

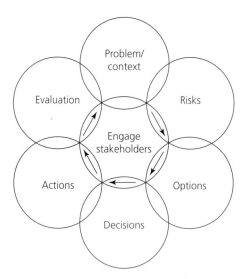

Figure 4.5   A framework for managing risks. (Adapted from Presidential/Congressional Commission on Risk Assessment and Risk Management,[8] with permission.)

the conduct of research that should, when the results were used in future assessments, serve to reduce uncertainties.

During the 1980s and 90s, it became apparent that increased attention needed to be directed to risk communication, effectively communicating the total risk analysis process and risk characterization with its uncertainties to all stakeholders. A Presidential/ Congressional Commission on Risk Assessment and Risk Management,[8] mandated by the 1990 Amendments to the Clean Air Act, conducted its work in parallel with the NRC Committee.[6] The reports of this Commission emphasized the role of the various stakeholders in the risk assessment and risk management process (Figure 4.5).[8]

The approach to risk assessment shown schematically in Figures 4.3 and 4.4 is now in general use around the world. For example, the new Registration, Evaluation, Authorisation and Restriction of Chemical Substances (REACH) law enacted by the European Community[9–12] uses quite similar risk assessment procedures. It is noteworthy that, in the REACH programme, the word 'safety', as in Chemical Safety Assessment, has been given appropriate emphasis and is used rather than 'risk'.

HAZARD IDENTIFICATION

The risk paradigm (Figure 4.3), has as an initial step of identifying the potential hazardous properties of the agent. It is important to understand that the identification of an agent as having hazardous properties does not necessarily equate to the identification of human risk. It is obvious that if the hazardous properties of the agent have been identified from human experience, the findings are directly relevant to people and the agent *is* hazardous. The situation is not as clear, however, when the categorization of the agent as hazardous is based on findings in laboratory animal studies or, indeed, from studies using tissues, cells

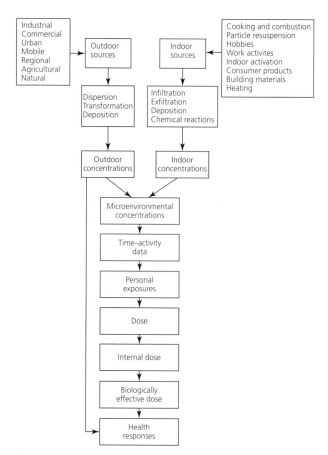

Figure 4.6   Schematic rendering of the relationship between outdoor and indoor sources, personal exposure, biologically effective dose and health responses. (Adapted from Özkaynak,[13] with permission.)

or structure–activity relationships. In such cases, the relationship between the exposures (doses) used in the laboratory studies to the exposure (dose) levels likely to be experienced by people becomes of critical importance.

It is important to recognize that the hazard identification step is essentially a qualitative characterization of any quantitative characterization of the potency of the agent, i.e. the exposure (dose)–response relationship. The various schemes used to classify agents in terms of their carcinogenic hazard potential, for example that used by the International Agency for Research on Cancer (IARC), focus on the sources of information in classifying the agents and do not address the potency of the agent for causing cancer.

EXPOSURE CHARACTERIZATION

A detailed consideration of exposure assessment is beyond the scope of this chapter. It is, however, desirable to consider some of the basic concepts involved in exposure assessment since, as already noted, the estimation of risk requires a knowledge of both exposure and the potency of the agent (Figures 4.3 and 4.4). Table 4.1 lists some of the approaches used to assess exposure.

Table 4.1 Methods of assessing exposure

Type of study	Source of information	Type of information
Epidemiological	Atmospheric models	Spatiotemporal concentration distributions from modelling emission rates, meteorology, air chemistry and geography
	Ambient (outdoor) monitoring	Ambient concentration for defined periods of time
	Indoor monitoring	Indoor monitoring for defined periods of time
	Market basket samples	Estimation of dietary intake
	Questionnaires and interviews	Occupation, personal habits, residence, diet, health status, etc.
	Personal monitoring	Personal monitoring for defined periods of time, usually in conjunction with time–activity logs
	Biological samples	Concentrations of biomarkers of exposure in human fluids, tissues and hair
Toxicological (controlled human or laboratory animal exposures)	Air or food	Measured exposure concentrations in air or food
	Biological samples	Measured or modelled concentrations in fluids or tissues

In epidemiological studies, the measures of exposure are usually quite indirect. In a study of an occupational cohort, the best indices of exposure may be the individual's job history complemented by perhaps only a few measurements of the concentration of one or a few agents in several workplace locations. Only very rarely, and then for quite small populations, are personal exposure data likely to be available. For many studies, the only estimates of exposure for populations as large as a million persons or more will be from one or a few ambient monitoring locations in a metropolitan area, frequently locations selected primarily to monitor for regulatory compliance and, only secondarily, to estimate the exposure of a particular population. This situation is illustrated schematically in Figure 4.6.[13] The solid line between outdoor concentrations and human responses indicates the relationship most typically evaluated in epidemiological studies of ambient air quality.

In controlled exposure studies with human volunteers and laboratory animals, the exposure environment can be monitored continuously to provide an accurate measure of the exposure of the subjects. In addition, measurements can be made of biomarkers of exposure, the agent and its metabolites in body fluids and tissues. In the case of studies in laboratory animals, it may be feasible to make sufficient measurements on animals killed at various times after exposure to develop very detailed models of the kinetics of the agent and metabolites, with special attention directed to concentration profiles in the target tissues. Unfortunately, very few chemicals have been studied

sufficiently to link, in a rigorous fashion, toxicokinetic parameters with the toxicodynamic parameters shown schematically in Figure 4.4.

CHARACTERIZING EXPOSURE (DOSE)– RESPONSE RELATIONSHIPS

The identification of an agent as having hazardous properties may be useful background information for taking actions that will minimize the exposure of individuals and populations, and thus minimize risk. In many situations, however, it is necessary to have information on the exposure (dose)–response relationship for the agent. Alternative exposure–response relationships, described as models, for various toxicants are shown schematically in Figure 4.7. Note that both scales in the figure are logarithmic. The horizontal scale is exposure, expressed as parts per million (ppm), ranging from very low detectable levels for some compounds to quite high concentrations. The vertical scale expresses excess risk.

It is important to recognize that for many diseases, such as cancer, the background incidence, in the absence of any chemical exposure, may be substantially greater than the added or excess risk imposed by chemical exposure. For example, in the USA as well as most developed countries of the world, about one in three individuals will be diagnosed with cancer during their lifetime, and one in four will die with cancer: these facts should be considered in relation to the data presented in Table 1.2 (see page 18).

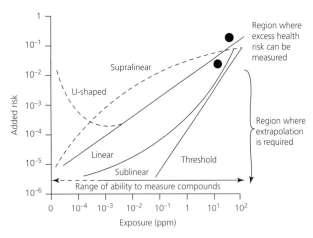

Figure 4.7 Multiple exposure–response relationships may exist for different chemical-induced end points. ppm, parts per million.

As will be discussed later, the earliest approaches to developing guidance for controlling exposure to chemicals assumed a threshold exposure–response relationship. This approach is based on a recognition that below some threshold exposure level, no added or excess adverse effects were observed. At exposures above the threshold level, the incidence of excess effect increased as exposure increased, and typically the severity of the effects also increased. The threshold exposure–response relationship has been widely accepted as applying to all kinds of non-cancer end points. However, as will be discussed, the use of a threshold model for some non-cancer end points is being increasingly challenged.

It has been recognized for some time that, for some end points, a non-threshold exposure–response model may be appropriate. The development of non-threshold models for exposure–response relationships was stimulated by findings with radiation-induced cancer. This experience with radiation-induced cancer, in turn, had a strong influence on the approach to characterization of exposure–response relationships for chemical-induced cancers, especially for chemicals that reacted directly with DNA or that had DNA-reactive metabolites.

During the last decade, there has been increased understanding of the concept of hormesis: at low levels of exposure, positive, or beneficial, effects are observed, whereas negative, or harmful, effects are observed at higher levels of exposure.[14,15] The concept of hormesis is well recognized for certain agents such as vitamins and minerals, which are essential at low concentrations for life and produce toxicity only with excess intake. Although the effects of some agents, at least on some end points, are well explained by the phenomenon of hormesis and well accepted, the value of the concept in developing approaches to the regulation of chemical exposures is less well established.

As an aside, there has been ongoing debate for decades as to whether linear exposure–response relationships, especially for cancer, are realistic, i.e. whether an added level of exposure, regardless of how small it is, results in a calculable

monotonic increase in cancer. Opponents of this view argue it is unrealistic to assume that each molecule of a chemical could have a calculable effect; certainly, normal homeostatic mechanisms must, or at least should, be operative with very low levels of exposure. Proponents of the view argue that a linear exposure–response model, especially for regulatory purposes for assessing cancer risk, is appropriate because every molecule of a new agent produces damage that is added to a background of genetic damage in somatic cells arising from multiple agents and endogenous factors.

EVALUATING THRESHOLD EXPOSURE–RESPONSE RELATIONSHIPS

The earliest approaches to developing guidance for acceptable levels of exposure to chemicals used the threshold exposure–response model from among the several models shown in Figure 4.7. An excellent example is the approach used, since 1938, by the American Conference of Governmental Industrial Hygienists (ACGIH) for limiting exposure to industrial chemicals.[16] A cornerstone of the ACGIH approach has been that, for adverse effects, a threshold is assumed to exist for exposure–response relationships such that a level of exposure could be defined below which no effect would be observed (Figure 4.8). Hence, the term 'threshold limit value' (TLV) is used, which is usually expressed as a time-weighted average for a normal 8 hour working day and a 40 hour work week. The introduction to the ACGIH TLV document[16] defines TLVs as:

> airborne concentrations of substances [that] represent conditions under which it is believed that nearly all workers may be repeatedly exposed day after day without adverse health effects. Because of wide variation in individual susceptibility, however, a small percentage of workers may experience discomfort from some substances at concentrations at or below the threshold limit; a smaller percentage may be affected more seriously by aggravation of a pre-existing condition or by development of an occupational illness. Smoking of tobacco is harmful not only because of the cancer and cardiorespiratory diseases it causes, but for several additional reasons. Smoking may act to alter the biological effects of chemicals encountered in the workplace and may reduce the body's defense mechanisms against other substances. Individuals may also be hyper-susceptible or otherwise unusually responsive to some industrial chemicals because of genetic factors, age, personal habits (e.g., smoking, alcohol, or other drugs), medication, or previous exposures.

The TLVs are based on information from industrial experiences, from experimental human and animal studies and, when possible, from a combination of these three

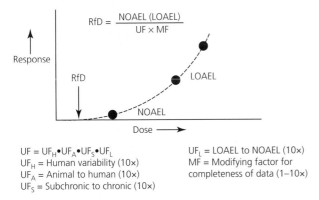

$$RfD = \frac{NOAEL\ (LOAEL)}{UF \times MF}$$

UF = UF$_H$•UF$_A$•UF$_S$•UF$_L$
UF$_H$ = Human variability (10×)
UF$_A$ = Animal to human (10×)
UF$_S$ = Subchronic to chronic (10×)

UF$_L$ = LOAEL to NOAEL (10×)
MF = Modifying factor for
completeness of data (1–10×)

Figure 4.8 Threshold exposure–response relationship traditionally used in evaluating non-cancer end points and developing guidance for controlling exposure and limiting risks. LOAEL, lowest observed adverse effect level; NOAEL, no observed adverse effect level; RfD, reference dose; UF, uncertainty factor.

sources of information (see Figure 4.1, above). The basis on which the values are established may differ from substance to substance: protection against impairment of health may be a guiding factor for some, whereas reasonable freedom from irritation, narcosis, nuisance or other forms of stress may form the basis for others. Health impairments considered include those that shorten life expectancy, compromise physiological function, impair the capability for resisting other toxic substances or disease processes, or adversely affect reproductive function or developmental processes.

The ACGIH emphasizes that the TLVs are intended for use in the practice of industrial hygiene as guidelines in the control of workplace health hazards and are not intended for other use. Despite this admonishment, many organizations and individuals have routinely made use of TLVs in developing guidance for the general population, not just workers. The ACGIH documents appropriately emphasize that the limits are not fine lines between safe and dangerous concentrations, nor are they relative indices of toxicity.

If human data of sufficient quality are available for a particular chemical, they are used to set the TLV. In many cases, however, human data are not available. This may be the result of adequate control measures such that adverse effects have not been observed in workers despite the chemical having been in commerce for many years. By definition, a newly synthesized material has not been available, so human exposure could not have occurred. In these cases, data from laboratory animals are essential for establishing a TLV for humans.

The key determinations from either the human or laboratory animal data are the establishment of a no observed adverse effect level (NOAEL) or, in the absence of such a determination, a lowest observed adverse effect level (LOAEL) (Figure 4.8). The selection of exposure levels for study dictates the specific NOAEL and LOAEL values that can be observed. To state the obvious, observations can be made

only at the exposure levels studied, and the selection of these levels can have a dramatic impact on the calculated TLV.

Extrapolations from the NOAEL or LOAEL to the TLV have traditionally been made for occupational exposures using uncertainty or safety factors. As a default assumption, laboratory animal species and humans are assumed to have similar exposure–response relationships. Thus, the addition of uncertainty or safety factors in extrapolating from laboratory animals to humans is viewed as increasing the likelihood of human safety. The US Food and Drug Administration[17] originally identified the factors as safety factors. Later, the US Environmental Protection Agency (EPA) adopted the same factors but identified them as uncertainty factors (UFs) for developing environmental exposure limits (Figure 4.8). The EPA's use of the term 'uncertainty factors' places emphasis on the uncertainty of the extrapolation, an approach that was originally intended to avoid debate over what was viewed as a more ambiguous term, 'safety'. As will be noted later, the assessment factors used in the evolving REACH programme appear to be similar.

As noted previously, the TLVs are intended to provide guidance for occupational exposure and are not intended for use in establishing exposure limits for the general population. To provide guidance applicable to the general population for evaluating the non-cancer health effects of inhaled materials, the EPA has developed a reference dose (RfD) methodology[18,19] for ingested materials and an inhalation reference concentration (RfC) methodology for inhaled materials.[18,20–23] The EPA defines an RfD as 'an estimate (with uncertainty spanning perhaps an order of magnitude) of a daily oral exposure to the human population (including sensitive subgroups) that is likely to be without appreciable risk of deleterious non-cancer health effects during a lifetime.'[23] The RfC definition is similar except that reference is made to continuous inhalational exposure.

The RfC methodology focuses on the establishment of either a LOAEL or a NOAEL as the starting point for deriving exposure limits (Figure 4.8). One criticism of the

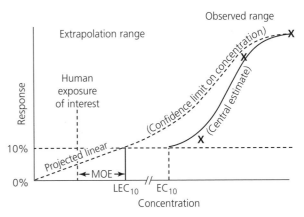

Figure 4.9 Exposure–response relationship and key metrics advanced by the US Environmental Protection Agency for evaluating both cancer and non-cancer end points. EC$_{10}$, effective concentration, 10% response; LEC$_{10}$, lowest effective concentration, 10% response; MOE, margin of exposure.

approach is that it does not make use of all the available data on a chemical. An alternative approach is to derive from the existing data an effective dose associated with a given level of response, that is, a benchmark dose (BMD) or benchmark concentration (BMC) (Figure 4.9). The BMC approach fits a dose–response curve to the data in the observed range. A lower bound on the dose causing some specified level of risk above background is calculated. In one of the early papers on this approach, Crump[24] proposed using the lower 95 per cent confidence limit on dose at a given level of response to establish the BMD. The BMC is then used as a point of departure for the application of UFs in place of the LOAEL or NOAEL. Setzer and Kimmel[25] have recently reviewed the BMD approach.

The BMD or BMC approach allows for use of a standardized measure of the dose level near the point at which responses would no longer be expected to be observed using standard experimental designs. Thus, the BMC does not depend on a single data point such as the LOAEL or NOAEL but uses the entire dataset and also accounts for sample size. By using all the data in calculating a BMC, account can be taken of the steepness of the dose–response relationship. The steepness of the dose–response curve in the dose region from which extrapolations are made can markedly influence the calculated RfC.

The EPA RfC methodology[20,21] has provision for using dosimetry data to make extrapolations. Recognizing the extent to which there are marked species differences in exposure–dose response relationships, the dosimetry adjustment provision in the RfC methodology is a significant advance over other approaches that do not have a provision for such adjustments. A wide range of dosimetric adjustments are accommodated within the RfC methodology to take into account differences in exposure–dose relationships between species. Regional differences (extrathoracic, tracheobronchial and pulmonary) are taken into account, as are adjustments for particles versus gases, and adjustments within gases for three categories based on degree of reactivity (including both dissociation and local metabolism) and degree of water solubility. Provision is also made for using more detailed, experimentally derived models if they are available. Thus, the normalization procedures are used to adjust less-than-continuous exposure data to 24 hours per day for a lifetime of 70 years.

The RfC methodology is intended to provide guidance for non-cancer toxicity, i.e. for adverse health effects or toxic end points such as changes in the structure or function of various organ systems. This includes effects observed in the respiratory tract as well as extrarespiratory effects related to the respiratory tract as a portal of entry.

CHARACTERIZATION OF HAZARDS FROM CARCINOGENS

The earliest risk assessments for cancer focused on whether a compound or occupation posed a carcinogenic hazard based on epidemiological data. Later, the carcinogen assessment process was broadened to include the consideration of data from laboratory animal studies, including inhalation studies. This gave rise to formalized criteria for evaluating the carcinogenic risks to humans such as that pioneered by the IARC, starting in 1969.[26] By the end of 2008, IARC had evaluated over 1000 agents or exposure situations.[27,28]

The IARC approach is described in the preamble to each of a long series of monographs, with individual monographs typically covering several chemicals, biological agents or occupations. The monographs, and the carcinogen categorization results, are developed by international working groups of experts. These working groups carry out five tasks: (1) ascertain that all appropriate references have been collected; (2) select the data relevant for the evaluation on the basis of scientific merit; (3) prepare accurate summaries of the data to enable the reader to follow the reasoning of the working group; (4) evaluate the results of experimental and epidemiological studies; and (5) make an overall evaluation of the carcinogenicity of the agent to humans.

In the monographs the term 'carcinogen' is used to denote an agent that is capable of increasing the incidence of malignant neoplasms. Traditionally, IARC has evaluated the evidence for carcinogenicity without regard to the specific underlying mechanisms involved. In 1991, IARC convened a group of experts to consider how mechanistic data could be used in the classification process. This group suggested a greater use of mechanistic data, including information relevant to extrapolation between laboratory animals and humans.[29,30] The use of mechanistic data can be used to either 'downgrade' or 'elevate' the carcinogenic classification of a chemical. However, a review of a summary of the classifications will find many examples of chemicals upgraded from category 2a (probable human carcinogens) to 1 (human carcinogens), and from category 2b (possible human carcinogens) to 2a (probable human carcinogens); there are very few examples of chemicals that have been downgraded based on mechanistic considerations.

The IARC evaluation process considers three types of data: (a) human carcinogenicity data; (b) experimental carcinogenicity data; and (c) supporting evidence of carcinogenicity. Definitive evidence of human carcinogenicity can only be obtained from epidemiological studies. The epidemiological evidence is classified into four categories:

- 'Sufficient evidence of carcinogenicity' is used if a causal relationship has been established between exposure to the agent and human cancer.
- 'Limited evidence of carcinogenicity' is used if a positive association between exposure to an agent and human cancer is considered to be credible, but chance, bias or confounding cannot be ruled out with reasonable confidence.
- 'Inadequate evidence of carcinogenicity' is used if the available studies are of insufficient quality, consistency

or statistical power to permit a conclusion regarding the presence or absence of a causal association.

- 'Evidence suggesting lack of carcinogenicity' is used if there are several adequate studies covering the full range of doses to which human beings are known to be exposed, which are mutually consistent in not showing a positive association between exposure and any studied cancer at any observed level of exposure.

The IARC evaluation process gives substantial weight to carcinogenicity data from laboratory animals. The IARC has concluded that 'in the absence of adequate data in humans, it is biologically plausible and prudent to regard agents for which there is sufficient evidence of carcinogenicity in experimental animals as if they presented a carcinogenic risk to humans.'[28] The IARC classifies the strength of the evidence of carcinogenicity in experimental animals in a fashion analogous to that used for the human data. The evidence of carcinogenicity from laboratory animals is classified into four categories:

- 'Sufficient evidence of carcinogenicity' is used if a working group considers that a causal relationship has been established between the agent and an increased incidence of malignant neoplasms or an appropriate combination of benign and malignant neoplasms in (a) two or more species of animals, or (b) two or more independent studies in one species carried out at different times, in different laboratories or under different protocols. A single study in one species might

be considered in exceptional circumstances to provide sufficient evidence when malignant neoplasms occur to an unusual degree with regard to incidence, site, type of tumour or age of onset.
- 'Limited evidence of carcinogenicity' is used if the data suggest a carcinogenic effect but are limited for making a definitive evaluation.
- 'Inadequate evidence of carcinogenicity' is used if studies cannot be interpreted as showing either the presence of the absence of a carcinogenic effect because of major qualitative or quantitative limitations.
- 'Evidence suggesting lack of carcinogenicity' is used if adequate studies involving at least two species are available that show that, within the limits of the tests used, the agent is not carcinogenic. Such a conclusion is inevitably limited to the species, tumours and doses of exposure studied.

Supporting evidence includes a range of information such as structure–activity correlations, toxicological information and data on kinetics, metabolism and genotoxicity. This includes data from laboratory animals, humans and lower levels of biological organization such as tissues and cells. In short, any information that may provide a clue to the potential for an agent causing cancer in humans is reviewed and presented.

Finally, all of the relevant data are integrated, and the agent is categorized on the basis of the strength of the evidence derived from studies in humans and experimental animals and from other studies as shown in Table 4.2.[28] As

Table 4.2 International Agency for Research on Cancer classification scheme for human carcinogens

Category	Human evidence	Experimental evidence
Group 1 The agent (mixture) is carcinogenic to humans. The exposure circumstance entails exposures that are carcinogenic to humans	(a) Sufficient (b) Less than sufficient	(a) No animal evidence required (b) Sufficient evidence and strong evidence in exposed humans that the agent (mixture) acts through a relevant mechanism of carcinogenicity
Group 2A The agent (mixture) is probably carcinogenic to humans. The exposure circumstance entails exposures that are probably carcinogenic to humans	(a) Limited (b) Limited (c) Inadequate	(a) None (b) Sufficient (c) Sufficient and strong evidence that the carcinogenesis is mediated by a mechanism that also operates in humans
Group 2B The agent (mixture) is possibly carcinogenic to humans. The exposure circumstance entails exposures that are possibly carcinogenic to humans	(a) Limited (b) Inadequate (c) Inadequate	(a) Less than sufficient (b) Sufficient (c) Limited, together with supporting evidence from other relevant data
Group 3 The agent (mixture or exposure circumstance) is not classifiable as to its carcinogenicity	(a) Inadequate (b) Inadequate	(a) Inadequate (b) Limited
Group 4 The agent (mixture) is probably not carcinogenic to humans	(a) Lack of carcinogenicity (b) Inadequate	(a) Lack of carcinogenicity (b) Lack of carcinogenicity consistently and strongly supported by a broad range of other relevant data

Abstracted from the Preamble of IARC Monographs, Vol. 84 (IARC, 2004).

noted, the IARC categorization scheme does not address the potency of carcinogens. A number of chemicals classified as 'carcinogenic to humans,' 'probably carcinogenic to humans' or 'possibly carcinogenic to humans' have been evaluated in terms of their carcinogenic potency with the EPA Integrated Risk Information System (IRIS) database.[31] Within each category or group, the chemicals listed vary greatly in their carcinogenic potency. This poses serious constraints on the utility of the IARC carcinogen classifications beyond hazard identification. In short, a carcinogen is a carcinogen irrespective of potency. This 'lumping' of carcinogens irrespective of potency can be misleading to non-specialists, including the lay public. The IARC is not a regulatory agency; hence its cancer classification findings are strictly advisory to other governmental organizations. However, the IARC classifications are used around the world by many national, state and local agencies.

The EPA guidelines for carcinogen risk assessment originally issued in 1986 have been updated.[32] A key feature of the most recent guidelines is to provide options for evaluating non-DNA reactive, sometimes called non-genotoxic, carcinogens versus DNA reactive, sometimes called genotoxic, carcinogens. The guidelines also include provision for evaluating the carcinogenic risk of exposures during childhood.

CUMULATIVE RISK

There is frequently a need to evaluate cumulative risk, the combined risks from aggregate exposures to multiple agents, for a particular source or receptor location. Cumulative risk assessment has been defined as an analysis, characterization and possible quantification of the combined risks to human health or the environment from multiple agents in stressors.[33]

One approach to developing cumulative risk assessments is to treat the cancer and non-cancer end points separately. The approach for carcinogenic agents is relatively straightforward if, for each agent, an estimate of exposure and an estimate of the cancer-causing potency is available. Key to this approach is the assumption that any level of exposure, irrespective of how low, is capable of causing an

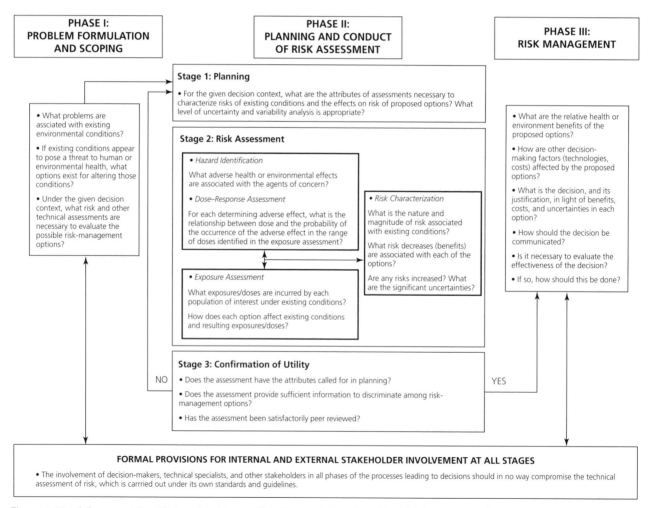

Figure 4.10 A framework for risk-based decision-making that maximizes the utility of risk assessment. (Reproduced from National Research Council,[34] with permission.)

increased risk of cancer, and that there is a linear relationship between exposure and excess cancer with the cancer potency expressed as the slope of the exposure–response curve. With this approach, the aggregate cancer risk is simply a summing of the estimates of the cancer risks of the individual agents.

The situation is more complex for agents with non-cancer end points. As discussed earlier, one approach to evaluating non-cancer end points uses a threshold exposure–response model with the identification of a LOAEL, NOAEL or BMD and their extrapolation to a lower RfD for oral exposure or RfC using uncertainty or safety factors. One approach to characterizing the risks of exposure to multiple agents causing non-cancer effects is to create for each compound an estimate of the ratio of the measured or estimated ambient exposure concentration to the RfD or RfC, and then to sum these ratio values to provide an aggregate hazard index. If the summed value is less than 1.0, it is assumed that the exposure situation does not pose an added level of risk. If the hazard index is greater than 1, it is necessary to conduct a more detailed evaluation. It is important to recall that the RfD or RfC values are levels of exposure likely to be without an appreciable risk of deleterious effects.[23]

Even as higher levels of exposure are encountered and the calculated hazard index rises above 1.0, there may be no added level of actual risk over background risk – recall the use of the uncertainty or safety factors. In conducting a more detailed analysis, it is important to examine the available exposure–response data for each specific agent to determine whether the levels of exposure are sufficiently high to have an associated risk. Obviously, if human data are available, these should be given preference over the use of laboratory animal data from which the exposure–response relationships must be extrapolated to humans.

A recent report from the NRC[34] offered suggestions for evaluating cancer end points. The Committee report expressed the view that non-cancer effects do not necessarily have either a threshold or low dose non-linearity. The current author does not agree with this view and thinks that it is likely to be challenged. The Committee, starting with this conclusion, proceeded to recommend an approach that redefined RfD and RfCs as risk-specific doses with associated information on the percentage of the population that could be expected to be above or below a defined acceptable risk with a specific degree of confidence. It will be of interest to see whether this approach proves to be helpful when an attempt is made to apply the approach to real-world situations.

The NRC Report[34] also proposes to expand the framework for risk-based decision-making, as illustrated in Figure 4.10.[34] As may be noted, the traditional risk assessment lies at the core of the proposed paradigm. The proposed approach is intended to provide for greater involvement of stakeholders. The proposed approach has many attractive features, but the key to its utility will be the extent to which it can be used effectively in a broad range of circumstances that vary widely with regard to potential or real harm. As more and more sophisticated risk analysis approaches are developed, it will be important to recognize that risk analysis is a tool, not an end in itself, and that complex analytical approaches and decision structures should not be substituted for the use of common sense in analysis and decision-making.

EXAMPLES OF HAZARD AND RISK CHARACTERIZATION

In this section, some specific examples of hazard and risk characterization taken from the EPA's IRIS system[31] are provided. The IRIS database was created by the EPA in 1995, and the IRIS staff are charged with developing new assessments and revising existing assessments. In addition, they may elect to include within the publicly available online system assessments developed by other components of the EPA when those assessments have been developed in conformance with the standards used by the IRIS staff. Individuals interested in using the assessments summarized below are encouraged to review the complete document available on the IRIS website and related electronic linkages. The following assessments have been selected to illustrate a range of hazard and risk characterization approaches. Their inclusion in this chapter does not mean that the author necessarily endorses the methodology or conclusions; they are provided only as example of work that has been done.

Vinyl chloride

Extensive documentation for vinyl chloride is reviewed in the EPA IRIS.[31] Vinyl chloride is a widely used commodity chemical whose toxicity has been intensively studied. Creech and Johnson[35] reported for the first time an association between exposure to vinyl chloride monomer and liver angiosarcoma in men employed in a plant producing polyvinyl chloride. These initial observations have been confirmed in a number of additional studies of occupationally exposed populations. Multiple studies conducted with vinyl chloride monomer administered by both the inhalational and oral routes to rats and mice show a tumour incidence response, including hepatic angiosarcomas, that is related to exposure concentration. There is sufficient evidence for the carcinogenicity of vinyl chloride in laboratory animals, and there is substantial evidence that the metabolites of vinyl chloride are genotoxic, interacting directly with DNA. The EPA has classified vinyl chloride as a human carcinogen, and the IARC has placed vinyl chloride in group 1, thus characterizing it as a known human carcinogen.[36,37]

The EPA has developed oral exposure slope factors, drinking water unit risk factors and inhalation unit risk values for vinyl chloride (Table 4.3). The oral slope factor and drinking water unit risk values were developed using

Table 4.3   Quantitative estimates of carcinogenic risk from exposure to vinyl chloride[42]

Oral risk slope factor	LMS method (per mg/kg per day)	LED$_{10}$ linear method (per mg/kg per day)
Continuous lifetime exposure during adulthood	7.2 E-1	7.5 E-1
Continuous lifetime exposure from birth	1.4	1.5

Drinking water unit risk	LMS method (per mg/L)	LED$_{10}$ linear method (per mg/L)
Continuous lifetime exposure during adulthood	2.1 E-5	2.1 E-5
Continuous lifetime exposure from birth	4.2 E-5	4.2 E-5

Risk level	Concentration (μg/L)	
	Adult exposure	Exposure from birth
E-4 (1 in 10 000)	4.8	2.4
E-5 (1 in 100 000)	4.8 E-1	2.4 E-1
E-6 (1 in 1 000 000)	4.8 E-2	2.4 E-2

Inhalation unit risk	LMS method (risk/μg per m^3)	LED$_{10}$ linear method (risk/μg per m^3)
Continuous exposure during adulthood	4.4 E-6	4.4 E-6
Continuous lifetime exposure from birth	8.8 E-6	8.8 E-6

Risk level	Concentration
E-4 (1 in 10 000)	23 μg/m^3
E-5 (1 in 100 000)	2.3 μg/m^3
E-6 (1 in 1 000 000)	2.3 E-1 m^3

LED, linear effect dose; LMS, linearized multistage model.

the tumour incidence data from a chronic oral diet intake study conducted in the Wistar rat by Feron *et al.*[38] The slope factor using the linearized multistage model is the 95 per cent upper confidence limit on tumour risk for female Wistar rats. This was applied in accordance with the EPA's 1986 Cancer Risk Assessment Guidelines – 'in the absence of adequate evidence to the contrary, a linearized multistage procedure will be employed.'[5] The updated guidelines first proposed in 1996 recommend the use of the lowest effective dose (LED) at a 10 per cent response as the point of departure and drawing a straight line from the point of departure (LED$_{10}$) to zero. The LED$_{10}$ is the lower 95 per cent limit on a dose estimated to cause a 10 per cent response. As may be noted from Table 4.3, the slopes derived using the linearized multistage and LED$_{10}$ methods are almost identical.

Human equivalent doses (HEDs) were calculated using the physiologically based pharmacokinetic (PBPK) model of Clewell *et al.*,[39,40] based on a dose metric of the daily metabolite generated divided by the volume of tissue in which the metabolite is produced, that is, milligrams of metabolite per litre of liver.[41]

In this model, the initial vinyl chloride metabolism was hypothesized to occur via two saturable pathways, one representing low-capacity, high-affinity oxidation by cytochrome P450IIE1, and the other representing higher capacity, lower affinity oxidation by other isozymes of P450. The PBPK analysis showed that when metabolites were generated with the pathway operation at low concentrations (low capacity and high affinity), the dose metric was linear with concentration. At the high concentrations used in the rodent bioassays, the second

Table 4.4   Risk guidance for non-cancer endpoints for vinyl chloride

Oral reference dose for vinyl chloride				
Critical effect	**Experimental doses**	**UF**	**MF**	**Rf D**
Liver cell polymorphism in rat chronic feeding study	NOAEL: 0.13 mg/kg per day NOAEL (HED): 0.09 mg/kg per day LOAEL: 1.3 mg/kg per day LOAEL (HED): 0.9 mg/kg per day	30	1 mg/kg per day	3E-3
Reference concentration for chronic inhalation exposure				
Liver cell polymorphism in rat chronic feeding study converted to inhalation dose	NOAEL (HEC): 2.5 mg/m^3 LOAEL (HEC): 25.3 mg/m^3	30	1	1E-1

HEC, human equivalent concentration; HED, human equivalent dose; LOAEL, lowest observed adverse effect level; MF, modification factor; NOAEL, no observed adverse effect level; Rfd, reference dose; UF, uncertainty factor.

pathway became more involved, causing the metric–concentration relationship to become non-linear. The assumption that the human response was equivalent to the rat response in the most sensitive gender (i.e. the females) and that a linear relationship between dose and response existed was grounded in the EPA's default assumption discussed earlier.[5]

Note that, based on the assumption of greater sensitivity of the young to the carcinogenic effects of vinyl chloride, the slope factors and drinking water unit risk estimates were increased by a factor of two for continuous exposure from birth relative to continuous lifetime exposure during adulthood.

The inhalation unit risk values were developed using HEDs calculated with Clewell et al.'s model[39,40] and then converted to human equivalent concentrations (HECs) using a PBPK model. The relationship between the HED and HEC was found to be linear up to nearly 100 mg/m^3.

It is of interest to note that unit risk estimates based on epidemiological observations are available.[34,39,40,42–45,46] The unit risk estimates from these studies vary by about an order of magnitude, with the upper end of the risk estimates (1.6 E-7 to 1.5 E-6) being lower than the unit risk estimates (4.4 E-6 to 8.8 E-6) developed from the animal data. A risk of 1 E-6 would represent a risk of 1 in 1 million. It is surprising that the EPA gave greater weight to the risk estimates developed by extrapolation from the rat data than to the risk estimates developed from direct human observations. It is noteworthy that the estimates based on rat and human data are within a factor of 3 to 6 of each other.

The EPA cautions that unit risk guidance for water should not be used if the water concentration of vinyl chloride exceeds 10^5 µg/L or the air concentration of vinyl chloride exceeds 10^4 µg/m^3 because the slope factors used may not be applicable at higher concentrations.

The EPA has also developed guidance values for non-cancer effects (Table 4.4). These were developed using data

from a lifespan oral intake study conducted with Wistar rats.[47,48] The PBPK model of Clewell et al.[39,40] was used to convert the administered animal dose to the HED. At the HED, the time-integrated concentration of reactive metabolites calculated by the model was predicted to be equal to or less than was achieved for the rat NOAEL or LOAEL. In developing the RfC, the NOAEL (HEC) and LOAEL (HEC) were calculated for a gas:extra-respiratory effect based on the PBPK model.

Hydrogen sulphide

Hydrogen sulphide, with a rich dataset in the EPA IRIS,[31] serves as an excellent example of use of the EPA's RfC methodology. The RfC was last revised July 28th, 2003 using the results of a subchronic inhalational study by Brenneman et al.[49] Brenneman et al. exposed Sprague–Dawley rats to 0, 10, 30 or 80 ppm of hydrogen sulphide for 6 hours a day, 7 days a week for 10 weeks. The 'critical effect' determined for this study was 'nasal lesions of the olfactory mucosa', with a NOAEL of 10 ppm. The following steps were taken by the EPA, emphasizing the results of Brenneman et al.'s study to calculate RfC for hydrogen sulphide:

- Calculation of NOAEL, conversion from ppm to mg/m^3; conversion factors and assumptions – molecular weight = 34.08, assuming 25 °C and 760 mmHg: NOAEL (mg/m^3) = 10 ppm × (34.08/24.45) = 13.9 mg/^{3}.
- Conversion of NOAEL to NOAEL (adjusted), to normalize exposures to 24 hours a day, 7 days a week: 13.9 mg/m^3 × (6 hours/24 hours) × (7 days/7 days) = 3.48 mg/m^3.
- Calculation of the NOAEL (HEC) was for the gas, hydrogen sulphide, causing a respiratory effect in the thoracic region. A regional gas deposition for the extrathoracic region (RGDR$_{ET}$) was calculated taking into account the differences in minute volumes (V) and

surface area (SA) for humans and rats to calculate the HEC for NOAEL (ADJ); $V_{E(rat)} = 0.19$ L per minute, $V_{E(human)} = 13.8$ L per minute; $SA_{rat} = 15$ cm^2, $SA_{human} = 200$ cm^2:

$$RGDR_{ET} = (V_E/SA_{ET})_{rat} / (V_E/SA_{ET})_{human} = (0.19/15) / (13.8/200) = 0.184$$

$$NOAEL (HEC) = NOAEL (ADJ) \times RGDR_{ET} = 3.48 \text{ mg/m}^3 \times 0.184 = 0.64 \text{ mg/m}^3.$$

- A UF of 300 and a modifying factor of 1 were applied to the NOAEL (HEC) to determine the RfC. The UF of 300 consisted of 10 for sensitive populations, 10 for subchronic exposure and 3 ($10^{0.5}$) for interspecies extrapolation rather than 10 because of the dosimetric adjustment already made for changing rats to humans: $(0.64 \text{ mg/m}^3) / (300 \times 1) = 0.002 \text{ mg/m}^3$.

The RfC value of 0.002 mg/m^3 represents the EPA's 'estimate (with uncertainty spanning perhaps an order of magnitude) of a daily inhalation exposure of the human population (including sensitive subgroups) [to hydrogen sulphide] that is likely to be without an appreciable risk of deleterious effects during a lifetime exposure.'[23]

Zinc

Zinc is an essential element required as part of a healthy diet. However, there is information that zinc is toxic at higher levels, as reviewed within the EPA's IRIS.[31] It has been estimated that the zinc content of a typical diet of North American adults is approximately 10–15 mg/day.[50] The recommended dietary allowances for zinc are 11 mg/day for adult males and 8 mg/day for adult women who are not pregnant or lactating.[50] Zinc can be encountered as a contaminant in the environment, and thus levels of excess intake may be of concern. The EPA has developed an RfD for chronic oral exposure to zinc.

The EPA viewed the critical effects as decreases in erythrocyte copper/zinc-superoxide mutase activity in healthy adult male and female volunteers.[51–54] The calculated average LOAEL was 0.91 mg/kg per day. An interspecies UF was not necessary for extrapolation from an animal study to humans because the observations used were from human volunteers. A UF for extrapolation from subchronic to chronic exposure was not used since it is recognized that a chronic intake of zinc is required. The database UF was not required because the database was considered to be robust. An intraspecies UF of 3 was used to account for variability in the susceptibility in human populations. This was clearly a judgement call that was recognized with the statement – 'the use of a greater UF would place some sensitive humans in the possible position of either exceeding the RfD or not obtaining sufficient zinc.'

With the use of a UF of 3, the RfD is calculated to be 0.3 mg/kg per day. Assuming that a typical adult male weighs 70 kg and an adult female weighs 50 kg, the calculated total zinc intake for individuals consuming the RfD concentration would be 21 mg/day for males and 15 mg/day for females. It is noteworthy that these values are only about twice the recommended dietary allowance of 11 mg/day and 8 mg/day for males and females, respectively.

The following comments on this recommendation are offered for consideration by the reader:

- It is encouraging that the role of zinc as an essential element has been considered.
- The end point used in setting the RfC may, however, be questioned: does the effect represent an adverse effect?

The issue of what kind of change and what level of change should be considered as adverse for regulatory purposes is deserving of critical review. This is especially the case as modern biology and medicine characterize the complexity of mammalian systems at the biochemical and molecular levels. A view held by some that any change should be characterized as adverse is, in this author's view, not tenable.

Methylmercury

An extensive review of information on the toxicity of methylmercury is contained in the EPA IRIS[31] and a report of the NRC.[55] The toxic effects of high-level exposures to mercury have been recognized for centuries. What is uncertain, however, are the effects of low-level intakes of mercury, especially methylmercury.[55]

Substantial human data are available on the disposition and effects of methylmercury. Key data are available on neuropsychological impairment related to the ingestion of organic mercury in populations ingesting fish. One large study conducted in the Seychelles Islands on mother–infant pairs yielded scant evidence of an effect of neuropsychological impairment related to in utero methylmercury exposure.[56–59] A longitudinal study[60,61] of about 900 mother–infant pairs in the Faroe Islands found methylmercury-related developmental neurotoxicity. A smaller study[62,63] conducted in New Zealand supported the conclusions drawn from the Faroe Island study.

In evaluating the Faroe Island data for setting an RfD, the EPA used a BMD approach and selected a benchmark reference level of 0.05, which would result in a doubling of the number of children with a response at the 5th percentile of the population. This is based on the recognition that a bell-shaped or normal distribution can be used to describe most human characteristics, including children's neurodevelopmental abilities. The 0.05 level was selected recognizing that children who function at or below approximately the 5th percentile are considered to be significantly compromised for specific abilities such as language, attention or memory. The BMD lower limit

(BMDL$_{05}$), the lower 95 per cent confidence limit of the BMD$_{05}$ range of 46–79 ppb in maternal blood, for different neuropsychological effects in the offspring at 7 years of age corresponds to a range of maternal daily intake of 0.857–1.472 µg/kg per day.

In calculating the RfD, the EPA elected to use a UF of 10. A UF of 3 was applied to account for pharmacokinetic variability and uncertainty in estimating an ingested mercury dose from cord-blood mercury concentration. A second UF of 3 was applied for pharmacodynamic variability and uncertainty. A UF of 10 applied to 1 µg/kg per day (range 0.857–1.472 µg/kg per day) yields an, RfD of 1 E-4 mg/kg per day. Ironically, this RfD is the same as the RfD developed earlier based on the developmental neurotoxicity observed following the ingestion of methylmercury-treated grains,[64] methylmercury having been used for many years to treat seed grain.

Before leaving the methylmercury case, it is important to note the ongoing debate over the hazards versus the benefits of ingesting seafood that may contain trace levels of methylmercury. In the discussion above, attention has focused on the hazards of ingesting methylmercury and the derivation of guidance that may serve to deter the eating of seafood. However, it is noteworthy that the ingestion of seafood also has significant benefits. Thus, there are clear trade-offs between the avoidance of a health hazard and the health benefits gained by eating seafood.

Criteria air pollutants: particulate matter and ozone

In concluding this section on evaluating non-cancer risks, it is appropriate to briefly describe the approach used in the USA in setting National Ambient Air Quality Standards (NAAQS) for criteria pollutants.[65] The case studies discussed above involve the use of rigid decision rules and are quantitatively rigorous. In contrast, the setting of NAAQS for criteria pollutants clearly involves the exercise of judgement. The criteria pollutants[65] (Table 4.5) are air pollutants that arise from multiple sources and are widely distributed, hence the need for national standards. The Clean Air Act also has provision for regulating hazardous air pollutants that may be of local concern.

For criteria pollutants, the primary standards, which are intended to protect against health effects, 'shall be ambient air quality standards, the attainment and maintenance of which in the judgement of the Administrator, based on such criteria and allowing an adequate margin of safety, are required to protect the public health.'[66,67] The primary standards are intended to protect against 'adverse effects' and not necessarily against all identifiable changes produced by a pollutant. The issue of what constitutes an 'adverse effect' has been a matter of debate. Although the Clean Air Act did not specifically characterize an 'adverse effect', it provided some general guidance. It noted concern for effects ranging from cancer, metabolic and respiratory diseases, and the impairment of mental abilities, to headaches, dizziness and nausea. To date, the NAAQS have all been set based on the intent to limit non-cancer risks.

In developing the Clean Air Act, Congress also noted concern for sensitive populations in setting the NAAQS. Specifically, it was noted that the standard should protect 'particularly sensitive citizens as bronchial asthmatics and emphysematics who, in the normal course of daily activity, are exposed to the ambient environment'. This has been interpreted to exclude individuals who are not performing normal activities, such as hospitalized individuals. Congressional guidance was given noting that the standard is statutorially sufficient whenever there is 'an absence of adverse effect on the health of a statistically-related sample of persons in sensitive groups from exposure to ambient air'. A statistically related sample has been interpreted as 'the number of persons necessary to test in order to detect a deviation in the health of any persons within such sensitive groups which is attributable to the condition of the ambient air'.

In setting the NAAQS, the EPA, while recognizing the need to consider sensitive or susceptible groups or subpopulations, has also recognized that it is impractical to set NAAQS at a level to protect the most sensitive individual. In setting the NAAQS, the Administrator must also incorporate an 'adequate margin of safety'. The margin of safety is intended to protect against effects that have not yet been uncovered by research, and effects whose medical significance is a matter of disagreement. In setting the health-based standards, the Administrator cannot consider the cost of achieving the standards. However, costs can be considered in planning for when the NAAQS must be achieved.

The Clean Air Act, in addition to requiring primary or health-based standards, demands the promulgation of secondary or welfare-based NAAQS. The welfare standards are intended to protect against effects such as damage to crops and ecosystems, soiling of buildings and impairment of visibility.

The process by which the NAAQS are developed involves the EPA's Office of Research and Development, the EPA's Office of Air Quality Planning and Standards and the EPA Administrator, who must ultimately exercise judgement in the setting of the NAAQS. Each NAAQS consists of four elements: (1) the indicator; (2) the averaging time over which ambient measurements must be made, e.g. 8 hours, 24 hours or annually; (3) the numerical level, in parts per million or mass per metre cubed; and (4) the statistical form, e.g. a 98th percentile. The indicators for the criteria pollutants identified as specific chemicals are the chemical themselves (sulphur dioxide, carbon monoxide, nitrogen dioxide, ozone, lead, etc.). For particulate matter, it is the mass by size fraction, such as particulate matter

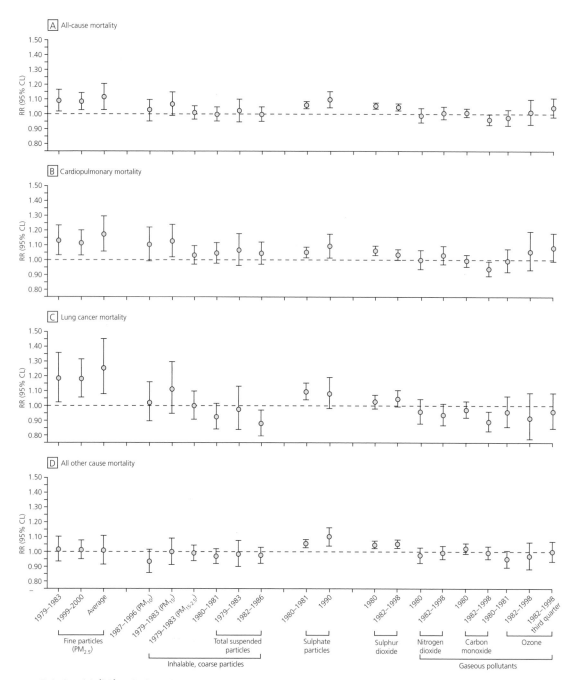

Figure 4.11 Relative risk (RR) ratio for adjusted mortality evaluated at subject-weighted mean concentrations. CI, confidence interval; PM$_{2.5}$, particles measuring less than 2.5 μm in diameter; PM$_{10}$, particles measuring less than 10 μm in diameter; PM$_{15}$, particles measuring less than 15 μm in diameter; PM$_{2.5-15}$, particles measuring between 2.5 and 15 μm in diameter. (Adapted from Pope *et al.*,[75] with permission.)

with a mean diameter of 2.5 μm or less (PM$_{2.5}$, not specified in terms of chemical composition). It is important to recognize that the level and form of the standard are linked. For example, a PM$_{2.5}$ standard set at 35 μg/m^3 never to be exceeded would be much more stringent than a standard for which attainment was based on the 98th percentile.

Extensive scientific databases, including substantial data from epidemiological, and controlled human exposure studies, and animal studies exist for all the criteria air pollutants. Readers interested in learning more about the

individual criteria air pollutants are encouraged to review the latest documentation on EPA's website.[65]

PARTICULATE MATTER

The NAAQS for PM was initially set in 1971 using total suspended PM (TSP) as an indicator.[65,68] Later, the standard was revised with the TSP indicator replaced by PM$_{10}$. PM$_{10}$ is defined as the particle size fraction collected using a device that includes 50 per cent of the particles with an aerodynamic diameter of 10 μm. A progressively smaller

Table 4.5   Summary information on criteria air pollutants as regulated by the US Environmental Protection Agency[65]

Pollutant	Sources	Key effects of concern	Subpopulations of concern	NAAQS*
Ozone	Photochemical oxidation of nitrogen oxides (primarily from combustion) and volatile organic compounds (from stationary and mobile sources)	Decreased pulmonary function, lung inflammation, increased respiratory hospital admissions	Children, people with pre-existing lung disease, outdoor-exercising healthy people	1 hour average 0.12 ppm 8 hour average 0.075 ppm
Nitrogen dioxide	Photochemical oxidation of nitric oxide (primarily from the combustion of fossil fuels) and direct emissions (primarily from the combustion of natural gas)	Respiratory illness, decreased pulmonary function	Children, people with pre-existing lung disease	Annual arithmetic mean 0.053 ppm
Sulphur dioxide	Primarily combustion of sulphur-containing fossil fuels; also smelters, refineries and others	Respiratory injury or death, decreased pulmonary function	Children, people with pre-existing lung disease (especially asthma)	Annual arithmetic mean 0.03 ppm 24 hour average 0.14 ppm
Particulate matter	Direct emission of particles during combustion, industrial processes, gas reactions and condensation and coagulation, and natural sources	Injury and death	People with pre-existing heart and lung disease, children	PM_{10}, annual arithmetic mean 50 $\mu g/m^3$, 24 hour average 150 $\mu g/m^3$ $PM_{2.5}$, annual arithmetic mean 15 $\mu g/m^3$, 24 hour average 35 $\mu g/m^3$
Carbon monoxide	Combustion of fuels, especially by mobile sources	Shortening of time to onset of angina and other heart effects	People with coronary artery disease	8 hour average 9 ppm 1 hour average 35 ppm
Lead	Leaded petrol (prior to phase-out in petrol); point sources such as lead mines, smelters and recycling operations	Developmental neurotoxicity	Children	Quarterly average 1.5 $\mu g/m^3$ Rolling 3 month average 0.15 $\mu g/m^3$

$PM_{2.5}$, PM_{10}, particulate matter with a diameter less than 2.5 and 10 μm, respectively; ppm, parts per million.
*National Ambient Air Quality Standards (NAAQS) are specified by indicator concentration, averaging time and statistical form. The latter is used to determine compliance and is too complex for coverage here. However, suffice it to note that both the specific numerical level *and* the statistical form determine the stringency of the standard.

fraction of PM mass is collected as the particle size increases above 10 μm, and a progressively larger fraction of PM mass is sampled as particle size decreases below 10 μm.

Subsequently, the standard was again changed, with $PM_{2.5}$ introduced as an indicator to complement the PM_{10} indicator. $PM_{2.5}$, the fine particle fraction, is defined as for PM_{10} with a 50 per cent cut-off point at 2.5 μm aerodynamic diameter. To state the obvious, the $PM_{2.5}$ sample is contained within the PM_{10} sample, which is contained within the TSP sample. In recent years, increased attention has been focused on the number of ultrafine particles contained within the $PM_{2.5}$ size range. There has also been interest in characterizing the health effects of the $PM_{10-2.5}$

fraction, i.e. coarse particles, and regulating this fraction with a separate NAAQS.

A detailed review of the evidence for health effects of PM is beyond the scope of this chapter. Suffice it to say that abundant data are available on the health effects of PM, characterized using different PM indicators, from epidemiological and laboratory animal studies using a range of indicators of morbidity and mortality.[68,69] In setting the PM standards, the greatest weight, appropriately, has been given to the epidemiological evidence, specifically to those studies which can provide quantitative exposure–response information.

Two large studies have yielded especially valuable information that has played a key role in the setting of the

PM NAAQS using the PM_{10} and $PM_{2.5}$ indicators. The first of these is the Harvard Six Cities study designed by Ferris and colleagues to specifically evaluate the health effects of criteria air pollutants.[70] In the current author's opinion, this is one of the best studies ever conducted of the influence of air quality on health. It involves a 14–16 year follow-up of 8000 subjects living in six communities in the USA selected to provide a gradient in several indices of air quality.[70–73] Extensive efforts were made to characterize air quality. A second air quality study made opportunistic use of data from a population of 500 000 individuals who self-enrolled in 1982–89 in an American Cancer Society (ACS) Study.[72,74] A subgroup of 240 000 of these individuals lived in 50 metropolitan areas in which $PM_{2.5}$ measurements had been made.

A review of the vast amount of information available from the Six Cities and ACS studies is beyond the scope of this chapter. However, selected data will be presented here to illustrate some of other key results that have influenced the setting of the PM NAAQS. Figure 4.11 summarizes an impressive array of information from the ACS study on all-cause mortality, cardiopulmonary mortality, lung cancer mortality and all other cause mortality.[75]

With controlling for smoking, education and national status, the controlled forward stepwise inclusion of additional co-variants had little influence on the estimated associations between fine particulate ($PM_{2.5}$ indicator) air pollution and cardiopulmonary and lung cancer mortality. As may be noted, the inclusion of cigarette-smoking attenuated the estimated relative risk of $PM_{2.5}$, which is not surprising. The relative risks for an average current smoker (men and women combined, 22 cigarettes per day for 33.5 years with smoking initiated before age 18 years) were equal to 2.58, 2.89 and 14.80 for all-cause, cardiopulmonary

and lung cancer mortality, respectively. The magnitude of these relative risks is substantially greater than that of $PM_{2.5}$ and emphasizes the critical importance of considering cigarette-smoking in any study of air pollution. The importance of including Socioeconomic Status (SES) in analysis of the relative risk of air pollution is emphasized by the findings of Steenland *et al.* They reported that for all-cause mortality, rate ratios from lowest to highest SES for men and women were 2.02, 1.69, 1.25 and 1.00 and 1.29, 1.01, 1.07 and 1.00, respectively.[76]

Moreover, it is important that investigators follow the lead of the ACS investigators and report the results of the analyses carried out for cigarette-smoking at the same time as they report relative risks for various air pollutants. These results on cigarette-smoking provide a valuable perspective for considering the results of analyses for the various air pollution indicators. A comparison of the relative risk estimates they obtain for smokers against those of other investigators serve as a 'reality check' on their analyses. Indeed, it would be useful if investigators routinely reported the relative risk for all co-variates included in the analysis. Such information would be especially useful to policy makers who must make policy judgements on acceptable risk in setting regulatory standards or guidance for air pollutants.

The results from the Six Cities study have been generally similar to those reported for the ACS study. Summary information from the two studies is given in Table 4.6,[72] with a comparison made of the risk ratios for the most polluted versus least polluted cities. For comparison, results are also shown for typical smokers. Note that, in this case, the typical smoker has been defined as about a 25 pack–year smoker, about two-thirds the value of the

Table 4.6   Comparison of mortality risk ratios (and 95% confidence intervals) for smoking and air pollution from the Six Cities and American Cancer Society (ACS) prospective cohort studies

Cause of death	Current smoker*		Particulate air pollution (Most versus least polluted city)		
	Six Cities	ACS	Six Cities (PM 2.5)	ACS (PM 2.5)	ACS (504)
All	2.00 (1.51–2.65)	2.07 (1.75–2.43)	1.26 (1.08–1.47)	1.17 (1.09–1.26)	1.15 (1.09–1.22)
Cardiopulmonary	2.30 (1.56–3.41)	2.28 (1.79–2.91)	1.37 (1.11–1.68)	1.31 (1.17–1.46)	1.26 (1.16–1.37)
Lung cancer	8.00 (2.97–21.6)	9.73 (5.96–15.9)	1.37 (0.81–2.31)	1.03 (0.80–1.33)	1.36 (1.11–1.66)
All others	1.46 (0.89–2.39)	1.54 (1.19–1.99)	1.01 (0.79–1.30)	1.07 (0.92–1.24)	1.01 (0.92–1.11)

*Risk ratios for current cigarette smokers with approximately 25 pack–years (about average at enrollment for both studies) compared with never-smokers.
Adapted from Pope and Dockery,[72] with permission.

current smoker discussed earlier for the ACS study. Interestingly, the relative risk, for example, for lung cancer mortality is about two-thirds of the value cited earlier: 9.73 versus 14.80. The range of the confidence intervals for the association between $PM_{2.5}$ and cardiopulmonary mortality, even for these studies with thousands of subjects, emphasizes the challenges faced in teasing out small effects of air pollution in developed countries.

Laden *et al.*[73] extended the observations for the Six Cities study cohort by including deaths for 1990–98 and compared those observations with the earlier time period (1974–84) and the entire period. The estimated city-specific average $PM_{2.5}$ levels were lower in the extended follow-up period in the 1990s than in 1974–89, and the mortality risk ratios were lower.

A critical issue in interpreting the data shown in Figure 4.11 is the nature of the exposure–response relationship. Pope *et al.*,[75] using the ACS cohort data, evaluated the non-parametric smoothed exposure–response relationships between cause specific and average $PM_{2.5}$ (Figure 4.12).[75] They observed that the log relative risk for all-cause, cardiopulmonary and lung cancer mortality increased across the gradient of $PM_{2.5}$ concentrations. Goodness-of-fit tests indicated that the associations were not significantly different from linear associations. The mean concentration of $PM_{2.5}$ across the ACS cohort was $14\,\mu g/m^3$.

Enstrom[77] evaluated the relationship between fine particulate air pollution and total mortality among nearly 50 000 elderly Californians for 1973–2002. He concluded that the results did not support a current relationship between fine particulate pollution and total mortality, although he could not rule out a small effect, particularly before 1983. The 2006 EPA analysis[78] used to revise the PM

NAAQS interpreted the available epidemiological data as not clearly supporting or refuting the existence of a threshold. The EPA analysis did, however, calculate added risks down to an assumed threshold of $7.5\,\mu g/m^3$, about the level of the $PM_{2.5}$ found in many US cities.

Although the estimated or excess risk for the various PM indicators is quite small, it is apparent that, when used in company with standard baseline data for specific cities with populations measured in the millions, the calculated number of excess deaths is large. The EPA Administrator can consider such quantitative risk assessment results when making a 'judgement call' in setting the standards.[94] However, the Administrator is explicitly prohibited from considering cost when setting the standard. In separate exercises, the risk assessment results are monetized in economic analyses used to estimate the benefits associated with achieving a revised standard compared with maintaining an existing standard.

Substantial controversy developed in the final stages of revision of the $PM_{2.5}$ standard announced in 2006. A majority of the EPA's Clean Air Scientific Advisory Committee's (CASAC) PM Panel recommended that the EPA Administrator reduce the $PM_{2.5}$ 24 hour averaging time standard from the previous level of $65\,\mu g/m^3$ to a level in the range of 25–$35\,\mu g/m^3$, and for the $PM_{2.5}$ annual averaging time standard reduce the standard from the previous level of $15\,\mu g/m^3$ to a level in the range of 12–$14\,\mu g/m^3$. The current author was in the minority and argued that identifying a 'specific bright line', upper bound such as $14\,\mu g/m^3$ was an issue that went beyond scientific interpretation of data to offering a judgement on acceptable risk. The Administrator ultimately revised the $PM_{2.5}$ NAAQS, 24 hour averaging time standard to $35\,\mu g/m^3$ and retained the annual standard at $15\,\mu g/m^3$.[78,79] The majority

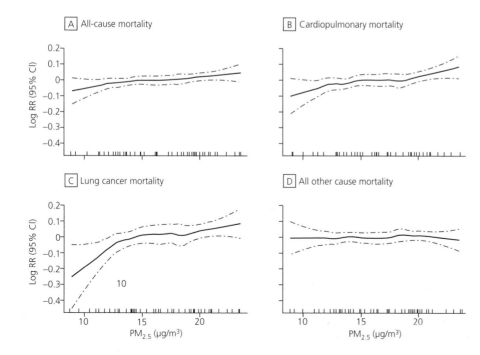

Figure 4.12 Non-parametric smoothed exposure–response relationship. Vertical lines along the x-axes indicate a rug or frequency plot of mean fine particulate pollution. CI, confidence interval; $PM_{2.5}$, fine particles measuring less than $2.5\,\mu m$ in diameter; RR, relative risk. (Adapted from Pope *et al.*,[75] with permission.)

of the CASAC committee was not happy with the Administrator's judgement call.

The 2006 revision of $PM_{2.5}$ NAAQS very quickly became a subject of several law suits. In general, environmental interest groups argued the new standards were not sufficiently stringent and industrial groups argued the new standards were overly stringent. In 2009, the District of Columbia Court of Appeals remanded the NAAQS to the EPA for reconsideration. The court ruling was complicated. A key element of the ruling was that EPA had not provided sufficient rationale for why it did not reduce the annual standard when it reduced the 24 hour averaging time standard. The EPA indicated that it was already well along in its next scheduled review of the $PM_{2.5}$ NAAQS and will address these issues in that review which is to be concluded in 2012.

OZONE

Ozone is an interesting air pollutant because it is not directly emitted from industrial sources except in rare circumstances. The majority of ozone found in the ambient environment at ground level is formed from the reactions of volatile organic compounds and nitrogen oxides in the presence of sunlight. The volatile organic compounds originate both from natural and industrial sources, and the nitrogen oxides derive largely from the combustion of hydrocarbon fuels. Ozone typically has distinct diurnal cycles because of the manner in which it is formed, with sunlight having a prominent role; the highest levels are observed at midday and the lowest concentrations at night in the summer, with lower concentrations both during the day and at night in the winter. The concern for excess levels of ozone in ambient air is a separate issue from depletion of protective ozone in the stratosphere which is considered to be protective of health since it reduces ultraviolet radiation reaching the earth.

The initial ozone NAAQS in the USA was set in 1971 using photochemical oxidants as an indicator and with a 1 hour averaging time.[80,81] The standard was later revised with ozone as the indicator. Subsequently, the averaging time was changed from a 1 hour maximum during a 24 hour period to an 8 hour rolling average maximum.

There is an abundant database on the health effects of ozone from epidemiological investigations and toxicity studies conducted in laboratory animals.[80,81] In addition, there is a substantial amount of data acquired from studies conducted with human volunteers exposed to controlled levels of ozone for short periods of time. In the setting of the ozone NAAQS, quantitative exposure–response data from human studies have been given the greatest weight. This is especially appropriate since there are well-established quantitative differences between laboratory animal species and humans in the disposition of inhaled ozone that minimize the utility of the data from laboratory animals for quantitatively estimating the human risk of ozone exposure.

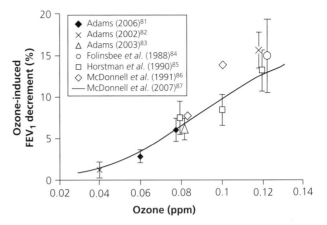

Figure 4.13 Changes in the lung function of young healthy adults following a 6.6 hour exposure to ozone. FEV_1, forced expiratory volume in 1 second; ppm, parts per million. (Adapted from Brown et al.,[89] with permission.)

The effects of ozone on the respiratory tract are well known, so it is not surprising that a consideration of these effects has had a primary influence on the setting of the ozone NAAQS. In the review, culminating with a revised standard in March 2008, the information from pulmonary function evaluations conducted on young adult volunteers undergoing moderate exercise while exposed to various concentrations of ozone for 4.6 hours played a prominent role. The key parameter evaluated, changes in the forced expiratory volume in 1 second (FEV_1), is shown in Figure 4.13.[82–89]

Data from individuals exposed to 0.08 ppm ozone and higher were considered in the previous review of the ozone standard. In the most recent review, new data were available from the studies of Adams et al.,[82] with 0.06 and 0.04 ppm exposures conducted to complement earlier studies conducted using 0.08 ppm and 0.012 ppm.[83,84,90] Adams et al.[82] interpreted the studies as showing a statistically significant effect at 0.08 ppm, effectively reproducing the effects seen in earlier studies. However, they interpreted the studies at 0.06 and 0.04 ppm as not showing statistically significant changes compared with exposure to clean air. The EPA[89] reanalysed Adams et al.'s data[82] using different statistical procedures; this EPA re-analysis was included in the final compilation of information provided to the EPA Administrator to render a judgement on the revision of the ozone NAAQS.

The EPA's CASAC recommended to the Administrator that he revise the ozone NAAQS with an 8 hour averaging time from 0.08 ppm to a level within the range 0.06–0.07 ppm. Ultimately, the Administrator exercised his judgement in revising the standard to 0.075 ppm.[91,92] The CASAC Ozone Panel expressed its displeasure at the Administrator's setting the NAAQS at a level higher than they had recommended. After the revised standard was promulgated, the EPA's statistical re-analysis[89] was published with a conclusion that Adams et al.'s data[82] had demonstrated a statistically significant, but small, biological effect at 0.060 ppm. These published findings, as well as any new data that may become available from studies conducted with human volunteers exposed to ozone at concentrations of less than 0.080 ppm, will certainly be considered in the next review and potential revision of the ozone NAAQS.

The 2008 revision[92] of the ozone NAAQS was immediately the subject of litigation. Some parties argued it was overly stringent and others argued it was not sufficiently stringent. Soon after a new Administration took office in 2009, the EPA indicated to the District of Columbia Court of Appeals that it was not interested in arguing in support of the 2008 revision and the Agency would prefer to accept a voluntary remand of the 2008 rule. The Court agreed and requested that the Agency indicate its plans for further action. The EPA in early 2010 indicated that it will reconsider the same scientific data used to set the 2008 standard and proposed a revised 8 hour standard in the range of 60 to 70 ppb later in 2010. The author remains of the opinion that the specific level and form of the standard are policy judgements, informed by science, and that only the Administrator has the exclusive authority to make these policy judgements.

The setting of both the PM and ozone NAAQS serves to illustrate the complex interplay between science and judgement in the setting of standards. In the current author's opinion, the selection of any specific numerical standard for exposure to a chemical involves both science and a policy judgement as to an acceptable level of risk associated with a specific level and form. The scientific information can identify, for a particular level of exposure, an associated level of risk and the associated uncertainty in the estimate. However, the selection of a specific level and statistical form for the standard goes beyond the science and represents a decision on an acceptable level of risk. The issue of the role of science and judgement in standard-setting is drawn to the forefront not only by the PM and ozone standards, but by chemicals that do not have clear thresholds in their exposure–response relationships. In these cases, some level of excess risk may be calculated for exposures that extend down to the ambient levels routinely observed in developed countries. In the case of Whitman vs American Trucking Association, Supreme Court Justice Breyer noted that we live in a world of risks and provided some common sense advice for setting standards, emphasizing the importance of a comparative health risk approach.[119,120]

The situation for identified thresholds is somewhat different, with the emphasis shifting to the degree of scientific confidence in the identified threshold level. The use of safety factors, UFs or assessment factors to arrive at some lower level of acceptable exposure is in fact a judgement call reflecting an added margin of safety for acceptable risk. In using the time-honoured safety, uncertainty or assessment factors, scientists should take care not to suggest or imply that these factors have a strong scientific basis.

THRESHOLD OF TOXICOLOGICAL CONCERN

Over the last half-century, remarkable advances have taken place in analytical chemistry. The capability now exists for the identification and quantification of many elements and specific molecules in air, water and various biological media at vanishingly low levels. In some cases, the chemicals being measured have been well characterized in terms of their hazardous properties, albeit typically at much higher exposure levels than are observed in the environment. In these situations, questions arise with regard to the relevance of the high exposure-level observations to estimating the risks at the lower exposure levels. Much of this chapter deals with those situations. Two approaches have been used: one when the chemical is assumed to have a threshold, and the other when a threshold in the exposure–response relationship is lacking. For the latter circumstances, an exposure level is identified that has an associated negligible risk. This is sometimes called a virtually safe level or dose.

In some situations, there is limited, or no, information available on the potential hazard of the chemical measured as a trace constituent of a drug, in food, in water or air or, indeed, found in human tissues. The question then arises of whether one should be concerned about the very low levels of exposure and associated tissue burdens revealed by ultrasensitive analytical measurements. In the absence of specific human evidence on the hazard of the chemical, it may be argued that it is necessary to acquire the necessary toxicological information. Using traditional methods, this may entail substantial costs and the use of large numbers of laboratory animals. An alternative approach using the threshold of toxicological concern (TTC) concept has been advanced. The paper by Kroes et al.[93] provides a useful review on this topic.

The TTC is a concept referring to establishment of a level of exposure for all chemicals, whether or not there are chemical specific toxicity data, below which there would be no appreciable risk to human health. The TTC concept was the scientific basis of the US Food and Drug Administration Threshold of Regulation for indirect food additives.[94] The TTC concept evolved from Munro's review of the Threshold of Regulation as applied by the Food and Drug Administration in evaluating food contact chemicals.[95] The Munro review in turn built on the classic paper by Cramer et al.[96] that proposed a decision tree approach to evaluating the hazards of chemicals, with three structural classes identified with varying hazard. Munro et al.[97,98] analysed the available chronic toxicity data for substances divided into the three structural classes advanced by Cramer et al.[96] The TTC concept was adopted by the Joint Food and Agriculture Organization/World Health Organization Expert Committee on Food Additives (JECFA) to evaluate flavouring substances,[98,99] and the approach has now been used to evaluate over 1200 flavouring substances.[100]

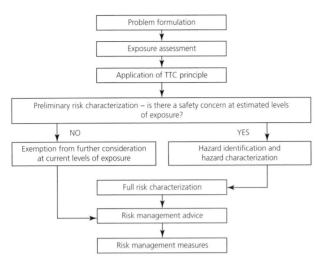

Figure 4.14 Schematic rendering of the concept of threshold of toxicological concern (TTC). (Adapted from Kroes *et al.*,[93] with permission.)

The approach used by JECFA has been extended to cover certain structural alerts for possible activity as genotoxic carcinogens.[101] The TTC concept has also been endorsed by the World Health Organization International Programme on Chemical Safety for assessing the risks of chemicals, and the European Union Scientific Committee on Toxicology, Ecotoxicology and the Environment.[102] The TTC approach has been used by the European Medicines Agency to assess genotoxic impurities in pharmaceutical preparations.[103] The European Medicines Agency, which operated from 1995 to 2004 as the European Agency for the Evaluation of Medicinal Products, has an important role in coordinating in Europe the evaluation of the safety of medicinal products. A schematic rendering of the use of the TTC concept is shown in Figure 4.14, taken from Kroes *et al.*[93]

The TTC concept is also being extended to evaluating extractable and leachable chemicals in orally inhaled and nasal drug products.[104] Extractables are compounds that can be extracted from elastomeric components, plastic components or coatings of the container and closure system when in the presence of an appropriate solvent. Leachables are compounds that leach from the elastomeric or plastic compounds on coatings of the container and closure system as a result of direct content with the drug product formulation. The approach taken has been to develop safety concern thresholds and a quantitation threshold for leachables. Below the safety concern thresholds, the identification of leachable compounds would not be necessary. Below the quantitation threshold, leachables without structural alert for carcinogenicity or irritation would not be necessary.

In summary, the TTC approach implemented in a tiered manner (see Figure 4.14)[93–104] is proving to be an efficient and effective way to minimize potential human health risks for chemicals found at very low levels in an array of products. In a broad sense, it provides a way to determine whether a chemical poses a negligible risk for risk management purposes and, if so, move forward without expending additional scarce resources to characterize the extent to which the risk is negligible. In turn, scarce resources can be applied to chemicals for which the hazards and risks are more uncertain and which will thus benefit from a more detailed toxicological evaluation, hazard identification and risk characterization.

THE REGISTRATION, EVALUATION, AUTHORIZATION AND RESTRICTION OF CHEMICAL SUBSTANCES REGULATION

On June 1st, 2007, the European Community put into force a new regulation, REACH, that will have far-reaching consequences not only in Europe, but also around the world.[9,10–12,105] Registration is required for all chemicals manufactured or imported in the European Union unless they are specifically exempted. The registration process will involve collaboration between companies. They are required to generate a dossier that includes data on the physiocochemical, toxicological and ecotoxicological properties of each chemical. If the existing data are not adequate, additional toxicological and ecotoxicological testing will be required. It will be necessary to create a Chemical Safety Report for all chemicals with a tonnage use in excess of 10 tons per year to evaluate the hazards and risks of specific chemicals.

Using the information contained in the dossier and Chemical Safety Report, the European Chemicals Agency (ECA), the European Union Member States and the European Commission will identify chemicals that may pose unacceptable hazards to human health and/or the environment, and curtail or restrict their usage. The ECA has a central role in implementing REACH. The ECA website provides access to guidance to assist industry in conducting safety assessments and preparing safety reports.[106]

The REACH regulations fully embrace the precautionary principle adopted in 1992 in Rio de Janeiro:

> in order to protect the environment, the precautionary approach shall be widely applied by States according to their capability. When there are threats of serious or irreversible damage, lack of full scientific uncertainty shall not be used as a reason for postponing cost-effective measures to prevent environmental degradation.[107,108]

By embracing the precautionary principle, the European Union regulatory structure[108] requires that information must be compiled on the potential hazards of a substance before it is allowed to be sold. This shifts the burden of compliance from regulators to industry, and industry must comply through the registration process of REACH.

Inherent within REACH is the requirement for the communication of information on hazards and risks to all stakeholders, including the public. The comprehensive nature of REACH results in its covering all aspects of the risk paradigm illustrated in Figure 4.4, above.

The data requirements of REACH continue to evolve and are linked to the marketed tonnage of the particular chemical. Studies used to fulfil the information requirements of REACH should be conducted in accordance with Organization for Economic Co-operation and Development guidelines and test method regulation guidance.[109] The REACH regulations embrace the need to minimize the use of vertebrate animals by endorsing the use of in vitro tests that have been validated by the European Centre for the Validation of Alternative Methods and in silico approaches such as quantitative structure–activity relationships.

The chemical safety assessments developed to comply with REACH registration requirements include up to six elements: (1) human health hazard assessment; (2) human health hazard assessment for physicochemical properties; (3) environmental hazard assessment; (4) persistent, bioaccumulation and toxic assessement, or very persistent, very bioaccumulative assessment; (5) exposure assessment; and (6) risk characterization. The latter two elements will only be required if a chemical is classified as dangerous under the Dangerous Substances Directive (67/548/EEC).

The goal of the human health hazard assessment is to develop a series of toxicity criteria values known as 'derived no-effect level' (DNEL) values. The DNELs are to be developed for each route of exposure (inhalational, oral and dermal) and available end points. Each DNEL is based on data (human and non-human, in vivo and in vitro) contained in the technical dossier for each chemical and focuses on key studies. A key study is described as a study that gives rise to the highest observed degree of concern, i.e. the most precautionary value.[106]

The DNELs are developed stepwise from the available data using traditional descriptors such as NOAEL, LOAEL, BMD, lethal dose for 50 per cent of the population, etc. with appropriate modification to identify a level of exposure that is thought not to represent a risk to human health. Corrected dose descriptors are developed to account for the route of exposure, differences in absorption and distribution, etc. The corrected dose descriptors may be further adjusted using assessment factors, which appear to be analogous to the safety or uncertainty factors used in the past as defaults to take into account intraspecies and interspecies differences, exposure duration, uncertainty in exposure (dose)–response relationships and the quality of the databases.

The environmental hazard assessments are developed with a goal of determining the level of each substance in the environment thought to have minimal or no impact. This level is called the predicted no-effect concentration. Predicted no-effect concentrations must be established for marine and freshwater environments, including sediments.

The ECA[106] guidance requires a separate evaluation of the persistence and bioaccumulative properties of each chemical.

The last two steps of the assessment process – exposure assessment and risk characterization – are performed only if a substance can be deemed hazardous under the Dangerous Substances Directive (67/548/EEC). The desired outcome of these steps is to establish exposure scenarios for workers, consumers and the environment such that risk management measures can be taken to control risks to human health and the environment. To demonstrate control of the potential risks, a comparison is made between the exposure concentrations modelled in the various exposure scenarios and the established DNELs and predicted no-effect concentrations to yield a risk characterization ratio. If the risk characterization ratio is less than or equal to 1, the risks are considered to be adequately controlled.

The REACH regulations call for the development of extended safety data sheets that will summarize many of the conclusions in the chemical safety assessments.

As with any new particular methodologies for evaluating hazard and risks, it is expected that the methods will evolve through practice and application. At present, the process outlined with the REACH guidance appears daunting. It is easy to envision tens of thousands of person–years of effort to integrate and summarize the existing data. Moreover, it is easy to envision similar levels of effort to develop new data that will be required to keep existing chemicals on the market or bring new chemicals to the marketplace. The experience gained over the next few years will give valuable insights into whether the new scheme is effective and efficient in regulating chemicals and protecting public health. The extent to which the new regulations actually impact on public health will probably never be known based on attributable risks from morbidity and mortality statistics; at best, positive public health impacts will have to be estimated.

Recognizing the global nature of the production, marketing and use of chemicals, it is conceivable that the REACH programme adopted by the European Community will serve as a basis for regulations in the USA and other developed countries. Even in the absence of regulatory changes in other countries, the REACH programme will have far-ranging impact on the approaches and methods used to acquire toxicological and ecotoxicological data and the practice of hazard characterization, exposure assessment, risk assessment/characterization and risk management.

RISK MANAGEMENT

Many options are available for managing risks to minimize potential harm to the environment and to people; these build on the results of the hazard and risk characterization activities discussed in earlier sections of this chapter. In some cases, there may be regulatory requirements for certain risk management activities dependent upon the hazard and risk characterization results. In other situations, individual companies may take risk management actions either to meet regulatory requirements or on a voluntary basis to conform with corporate policy. Finally, individuals may take personal action in response to public risk communication. A coverage of this range of options is beyond the scope of this chapter, but instead, a few examples will be given to illustrate risk management options.

As discussed earlier, substantial attention has been given to characterizing individual chemicals in terms of their carcinogenic potential. In many situations, the classification of a chemical as a 'human carcinogen' places severe limitations on the use of the chemical; at a minimum, it will result in the adoption of workplace strategies to minimize occupational exposure and the release of the chemical into the environment. Classification of the chemical as a 'probable human carcinogen' or 'possible human carcinogen' may also place constraints on the use of the chemical and result in actions to limit human exposures. It is apparent that the classification of a chemical with any one of the human carcinogen labels also prompts some members of the general public to take actions to limit their personal exposure to these chemicals.

In recent decades, there has been a move to classify chemicals with regard to their causing health outcomes other than cancer. Thus, one routinely sees reference in the public media, and also to some extent in scientific publications, to certain chemicals as being neurotoxicants, reproductive toxicants, developmental toxicants, respiratory toxicants, etc. In some cases, the classifications are much broader, as illustrated by the term 'endocrine-disrupting chemicals'. For example, at the time of publication there is substantial debate over the chemical bisphenol A over whether its use should be banned in certain products, such as plastic baby bottles. Such classifications and usages certainly alarm the general public and, very frequently, stimulate debate in the scientific community. Although the use of these labels may be well intentioned, a major problem with their use is that they do not take into account the level of exposure required to produce the adverse outcome. Some commentators invoke the 'precautionary principle' as supporting the use of the hazard labels; others call attention to the natural occurrence in the body of some of the chemicals being considered.

In recent years, a US government agency, the Centers for Disease Control,[110] has expanded its ongoing National Health and Nutrition Examination Survey (NHANES) to include the measurement of chemicals in the blood of a statistically representative sample of the US population.[110] The samples are analysed for a wide range of chemicals, many of which can be quantified at exceedingly low concentrations. Examples are given in the results reported by Calafat et al.[111] for bisphenol A and 4-tertiary-octylphenol.

The results of NHANES serve to document trends in the levels of the individual chemicals over time. It is important to recognize that the manner in which the NHANES survey is conducted does not allow the potential linking of these biomarkers of exposure with the health status of the individuals sampled. The NHANES data do, however, provide a valuable reference when it is necessary to interpret the significance of measurements made on an individual patient when concerns may exist over the role of a particular chemical influencing the individual's health.

As discussed earlier, use of the TTC concept[93] allows for hazard/risk characterization information based on the analysis and interpretation of a broad database on chemical toxicity, as well as chemical specific toxicity data, to make decisions that a chemical is not of concern at some estimated level of concern. This allows risk management decisions to be made in the absence of detailed hazard characterization.

In many cases, the results of detailed hazard/risk characterization activities yield quantitative estimates of risk at a particular exposure level that may be linked to a judgement on acceptable risk, such as one added cancer case per million persons over a lifetime of exposure, resulting in a limit for concentrations of the chemical in air, water or food. In short, scientific analysis can provide an estimate of the risk associated with a specific level and duration of exposure. Judgement, not science, is required to determine acceptability of the risk. A similar approach is taken for chemicals thought to result in adverse health outcomes via an exposure–response relationship with an observed threshold. In these cases, it is important to recognize that the NAAQS, RfC, RfD or ADI (acceptable daily intake) contains some non-quantified margin of safety. Having identified some acceptable concentration for air, water or food, various risk management decisions can be taken to attempt to achieve compliance with the regulatory limits on guidance values.

In considering regulatory limits or guidance values developed in different countries or by different agencies, it is important to examine critically the context of the particular value, even in situations in which the values may appear to be identical. In some situations, the value may represent a legally enforceable limit on ambient concentration. In short, this is the standard, and it shall be met or legal action will occur. In other situations, the value may be intended as guidance and be aspirational in nature. An understanding of these differences is crucial to having meaningful discussions on the differences in limits or guidance values used in different political settings.

The results of hazard/risk characterization activities have an important role in the development of new or modified commercial products. The development of new pharmaceuticals always involves concern for both the efficacy and the safety of the product. At an early stage of development, decisions must be made that the product has a high likelihood of being safe, or alternative candidates will be considered for development. The same situation is encountered with the consideration of replacement chemicals for a manufacturing process. In such cases, concern may focus on any changes required to ensure that the manufacturing process has exposure control matched to the potential hazard of the chemical.

The results of hazard/risk characterization can serve to drive the development of new products. Two excellent examples are the development of safe synthetic insulating glass fibres[112,113] and new diesel engine power trains.[113] In the 1980s, the increasing evidence that certain types of asbestos caused mesothelioma, lung cancer and other respiratory diseases cast a dark shadow of suspicion over all fibre products. In short, did synthetic fibres widely used for insulating purposes produce effects like those of asbestos? Limited animal toxicity data resulted in the decision by some manufacturers of these products to label their products as having the potential to cause cancer in humans. At the same time, a major research programme was carried out in the USA and Europe to identify the characteristics of synthetic fibres that contributed to their potential hazard. A large body of data indicated that durability and persistence in the lungs were key to producing pathological changes. Within a short period of time, methods were developed for evaluating biopersistence, and new products were developed that were not persistent when deposited in the lung.[112,113]

The decision by the IARC[115] to evaluate different kinds of fibre separately and the classification of glass wool fibres in group 3 – not classifiable in terms of human carcinogenicity – had a positive impact on the development and marketing of the new synthetic glass fibres. Most of the synthetic glass fibre insulating material sold today in Europe and the USA is of this new, non-persistent type. This is an excellent success story for toxicology and stands in contrast to many examples where the impact of toxicology stalls at the 'sky is falling' stage when adverse effects for a chemical are frequently reported without any context in terms of potential exposure.

A second example relates to concern over the exhaust emissions from diesel engines.[114] In the 1970s, attention focused on the potential for an increased use of diesel engines based on their acknowledged fuel efficiency. This, in turn, stimulated research on the health effects of diesel exhaust. The pace of this research accelerated when it was discovered that organic solvent extracts of diesel soot particles were mutagenic in the recently developed Ames assay. Lifespan studies with rodents exposed to various dilutions of diesel exhaust were conducted in laboratories in the USA, Europe and Japan. The highest exposure levels produced an increase in lung tumours in rats, but not in mice or Syrian hamsters. Later, similar high-level exposures of rats to carbon black (without any associated polycyclic organic compounds) and other poorly soluble particles also caused lung cancer in rats.[114]

Extensive research provided insight into the mechanisms involved, leading many scientists to interpret the findings of a positive cancer effect to be a high exposure, species-specific effect not likely to be relevant to humans. Other scientists took the view that, at a minimum, the findings in rats served as a warning of possible effects in highly exposed humans, but extensive epidemiological studies have not yielded convincing evidence of an excess of lung cancer in highly exposed populations.

In the face of continued debate, the EPA issued lower emission standards for both particulate matter and nitrous oxides. The lower standards, with a reduction in particulate emissions by roughly 100-fold, are being met with a multifaceted approach: (1) improved engine technology, and (2) the use of ultra-low-sulphur fuels, which in turn enable the use of (3) catalytic exhaust after-treatment devices, and (4) improved computer control of the integrated power system. Debate still continues on the human relevance of the findings concerning emissions from the traditional engines. Nonetheless, evidence is mounting that the low emissions of the new-technology diesel systems are both qualitatively and quantitatively different from the emissions from traditional diesel engines.

The success stories of both the synthetic glass insulating fibre and the new diesel technology are grounded in a close linkage being established between toxicologists and risk assessors working with technologists. Perhaps these positive examples can serve as templates for future joint activities. This will be especially important in the future as increased attention is given to developing 'safer' products and 'green technology.' In these activities, attention will need to shift from a focus on the risks of the old product or technology to whether the replacement product or technology is truly safer than the product or technology being replaced.

SUMMARY

This chapter has provided an overview of the multiple elements of risk assessment. From this overview, it should be apparent that risk assessment serves as an interface between the toxicological and epidemiological sciences and environmental health. Those sciences seek to identify and characterize the role of chemicals and other agents in causing disease or altering the incidence of disease arising from multiple factors. The scientific results from those fields that are of the greatest utility are those published in the peer-reviewed literature. Each individual paper may contain some important finding, but the information in each paper has enhanced value when it is joined with other information. Risk assessment provides a science-based process for integrating and interpreting this large body of information so that it can be used in the field of environmental health.

Although risk assessment is science-based, it is apparent that, in the absence of specific scientific information, it is necessary to make assumptions which form policy judgements. It is important that, to the maximum extent possible, these judgements must be identified and documented in terms of their influence on hazard and risk decisions. Likewise, it is important to recognize that decisions on acceptable levels of risk inherently require that judgement be exercised, with that judgement being informed by the underlying science.

REFERENCES

● = Key primary paper

●1. National Research Council. *Application of Toxicogenomic Technologies to Predictive Toxicology and Risk Assessment.* Washington DC: National Academy Press, 2007.

●2. National Research Council. *Toxicity Testing in the 21st Century: A Vision and a Strategy.* Washington DC: National Academy Press, 2007.

●3. McClellan RO. Human health risk assessment: A historical overview and alternative paths forward. *Inhal Tox* 1999; 11: 477–518.

●4. National Research Council. *Risk Assessment in the Federal Government: Managing the Process.* Washington DC: National Academy Press, 1983.

5. US Environmental Protection Agency. Guidelines for carcinogen risk assessment. *Federal Register* 1986; 51: 33992–4003.

6. National Research Council; Committee on Risk Assessment of Hazardous Air Pollutants, Board on Environmental Studies and Toxicology, Commission on Life Sciences. *Science and Judgment in Risk Assessment.* Washington DC: National Academy Press, 1994.

●7. McClellan RO. A commentary on the NRC report Science and Judgment in Risk Assessment. *Regul Toxicol Pharmacol* 1994; 20: S142–168.

8. Presidential/Congressional Commission on Risk Assessment and Risk Management. Framework for Environmental Health Risk Management. Final Report. Available at: http://www.riskworld.com/Nreports/nr7me001.htm (accessed January 21, 2010).

9. Registration, Evaluation, Authorisation and Restriction of Chemical Substances. REACH Guidance. Available at http://guidance.echa.europa.eu/guidance_en.htm

10. European Commission. Regulation (EC) No. 1907/2006 of the European Parliament and of the Council of 18 December 2006 concerning the Registration, Evaluation, Authorisation, and Restriction of Chemical Substances (REACH), establishing a European Chemicals Agency, amending Directive 1999/45/EC and repealing Council Regulation (EEC) No 793/93 and Commission Regulation (EC) No. 1488/94 as well as Council Directive 76/769/EEC and Commission

Directives 91/155/EC, 93/67/EEC, 93/105/EC and 20o01/21/EC. E.P. a.t.E. Commission. *Official J Eur Union* 30.12.2006.

11. deAvila C, Sandberg EC. REACH: Better knowledge and better use of chemicals in the European Union. *Chimia* 2006; 60: 645–50.

12. Warhurst AM. Assessing and managing the hazards and risks of chemicals in the real world – the role of the EU's REACH proposal in future regulation of chemicals. *Environ Int* 2006; 32: 1033–42.

13. Özkaynak H. Exposure assessment. In: Halgate ST, Samet JM, Koren HS, Maynard RL (eds) *Air Pollution and Health.* London: Academic Press, 1999: 149–62.

●14. Calabrese EJ, Baldwin LA. The hormesis model is more frequent than the threshold model in toxicology. *Toxicol Sci* 2003; 61: 246–50.

15. Calabrese EJ, Blain R. The occurrence of hormetic dose responses in the toxicological literature, the hormesis database: An overview. *Toxicol Appl Pharmacol* 2005; 202: 289–301.

16. American Conference of Governmental Industrial Hygienists. *Threshold Limit Values and Biological Exposure Indices for Chemical Substances and Physical Agents.* Cincinnati: ACGIH, 2008.

17. Lehman AJ, Fitzhugh OG. 100-Fold margin of safety. *Q Bull Assoc Food Drug Officials* 1954; XVIII: 33–5.

18. US Environmental Protection Agency. *An Examination of EPA Risk Assessment Principles and Practices.* Staff Paper prepared for the US Environmental Protection Agency by members of the Risk Assessment Task Force. EPA/100/B-04/001. Washington DC: EPA, 2004.

19. Barnes DG, Dourson M. Reference dose (RfD: Description and use in health risk assessments. *Regul Toxicol Pharmacol* 1988; 8: 471–86.

20. Jarabek AM, Menache MG, Overton JH Jr, Dourson ML, Miller FJ. The U.S. Environmental Protection Agency's inhalation RFD methodology: Risk assessment for air toxics. *Toxicol Ind Health* 1990; 6: 279–301.

21. Jarabek AM. Inhalation RfC methodology: Dosimetry adjustments and dose-response estimation of noncancer toxicity in the upper respiratory tract. In: Miller F (ed.) *Nasal Toxicity and Dosimetry of Inhaled Xenobiotics: Implications for Human Health.* Washington DC: Taylor & Francis, 1995: 301–25.

22. US Environmental Protection Agency. *Methods for Derivation of Inhalation Reference Concentrations and Application of Inhalation Dosimetry.* Washington DC: EPA, 1994.

23. US Environmental Protection Agency, Risk Assessment Forum. *A Review of the Reference Dose and Reference Concentration Processes.* EPA/530/P-02/002F. Washington DC: EPA, 2002.

24. Crump KS. An improved procedure for low-dose carcinogenic risk assessment from animal data. *J Environ Pathol Toxicol* 1984; 5: 339–48.

25. Setzer RW Jr, Kimmel CA. Use of NOAEL, benchmark dose, and other models for human risk assessment of hormonally active substances. *Pure Appl Chem* 2003; 75(11–12): 2151–8.

26. International Agency for Research on Cancer. *IARC Monographs on the Evaluation of Carcinogenic Risks of Chemicals to Man*, Vol. 1. Lyon: IARC, 1972.

27. Cogliano V, Baan R, Straif K *et al.* Transparency in IARC Monographs. *Lancet Oncol* 2005; **6**: 747.

28. International Agency for Research on Cancer. *IARC Monographs on the Evaluation of Carcinogenic Risks to Humans*. Available from: http://monographs.iarc.fr (accessed January 21, 2010).

29. International Agency for Research on Cancer. *A Consensus Report of an IARC Monographs Working Group on the Use of Mechanisms of Carcinogenesis in Risk Identification*. IARC International Technical Report No. 91/002. Lyon: IARC, 1991.

●30. Vainio H, Heseltine E, McGregor D, Tomatis L, Wilbourn J. Working group on mechanisms of carcinogenesis and evaluation of carcinogenic risks. *Cancer Res* 1992; **52**: 2357–61.

31. US Environmental Protection Agency. Integrated Risk Information System (IRIS). Available from: http://cfpub.epa.gov/ncea/iris (accessed January 21, 2010).

32. US Environmental Protection Agency. *Guidelines for Carcinogen Risk Assessment*. EPA/630/P-03/001F. Washington DC: EPA, 2005.

33. US Environmental Protection Agency. *Framework for Cumulative Risk Assessment*. Washington DC: EPA, 2003.

●34. National Research Council. *Science and Decisions: Advancing Risk Assessment. Committee on Improving Risk Analysis Approaches Used by the U.S. Environmental Protection Agency*. Washington DC: National Academy Press, 2009.

35. Creech JL, Johnson MN. Angiosarcomas of the liver in the manufacture of polyvinyl chloride. *J Occup Med* 1974; **16**: 150–1.

36. International Agency for Research on Cancer. *1,3-Butadiene, Ethylene Oxide, and Vinyl Halides (Vinyl Fluoride, Vinyl Chloride and Vinyl Bromide)*. IARC Monographs on the Evaluation of Carcinogenic Risks to Humans, Vol. 97. Lyon: IARC,, 2008: http://monographs.iarc.fr/

37. Grosse Y, Baan R, Straif *et al.*, on behalf of the WHO International Agency for Research on Cancer Monograph Working Group. Carcinogenicity of 1,3-butadiene, ethylene oxide, vinyl chloride, vinyl fluoride, and vinyl bromide. *Lancet Oncol* 2007; **8**: 679–80.

38. Feron V, Hendrikson CFM, Spleek AJ *et al.* Lifespan oral toxicity study of vinyl chloride in rats. *Food Cosmet Toxicol* 1981; **19**: 317–33.

39. Clewell HJ, Gentry PR, Gearhart JM *et al. The Development and Validation of a Physiologically Based Pharmacokinetic Model for Vinyl Chloride and its Application in a Carcinogenic Risk Assessment for Vinyl Chloride*. ICF Kaiser Report prepared for EPA/OHEA and OSH/DHSP. 1995. 1994. EPA/635R-090/004, Toxicological Review of Vinyl Chloride (CAS No. 75–01/04), Appendix A, U.S. Environmental Protection Agency, Washington, DC, May 2000. http://www.epa.gov/ncea/iris/toxreviews/1001tr.pdf.

40. Clewell HJ, Covington TR, Crump KS *et al. The Application of a Physiologically Based Pharmacokinetic Model for Vinyl Chloride in a Noncancer Risk Assessment*. JCF/Clement report prepared for EPA/NCEA under contract number 68-D2-0129. 1995. EPA/635R-090/004, Toxicologic Review of Vinyl Chloride (CAS No. 75–01/04), Appendix B, U.S. Environmental Protection Agency, Washington, DC, May 2000: http://www.epa.gov/ncea/iris/toxreview/1001tr.pdf.

41. Andersen M, Clewell H, Gargas M *et al.* Physiologically based pharmacokinetics and the risk assessment process for methylene chloride. *Toxicol. Appl Pharmacol* 1987; **87**: 185–205.

42. Fox AJ, Collier PF. Mortality experience of workers exposed to vinyl chloride monomer in the manufacture of polyvinyl chloride in Great Britain. *Br J Ind Med* 1977; **34**: 1–10.

43. Jones RW, Smith DM, Thomas PG. A mortality study of vinyl chloride monomer workers employed in the United Kingdom in 1940–1974. *Scand J Work Environ Health* 1988; **14**: 153–60.

44. Simonato L, L'Abbe KA, Andersen A *et al.* A collaborative study of cancer incidence and mortality among vinyl chloride workers. *Scand J Work Environ Health* 1991; **17**: 159–69.

45. Wong O, Whorton MD, Follart DE *et al.* An industry-wide epidemiologic study of vinyl chloride workers, 1942–1982. *Am J Ind Med* 1991; **20**: 317–34.

46. Chen CW, Blancato JN. Incorporation of biological information in cancer risk assessment: example-vinyl chloride. *Cell Biol Toxicol* 1989; **5**: 417–44.

47. Til HP, Immel HR, Feron VJ. *Lifespan Oral Carcinogenicity Study of Vinyl Chloride in Rats. Final Report*. TNO Report No. V83.285/291099, TSCATS Document FYI-AX-0184-0353, Fiche No. 0353. Zeist, The Netherlands: TNO–Civo Institute, 1983.

48. Til HP, Feron VJ, Immel HR. Lifetime (149-week) oral carcinogenicity study of vinyl chloride in rats. *Food Chem Toxicol* 1991; **29**: 713–18.

49. Brenneman KA, James RA, Gross EA, Dourman DC. Olfactory loss in adult CD rats following inhalation exposure to hydrogen sulfide. *Toxicol Pathol* 2000; **28**: 326–33.

50. Institute of Medicine. *Dietary Reference Intakes for Vitamin A, Vitamin K, Arsenic, Boron, Chromium, Copper, Iodine, Iron, Manganese, Molybdenum, Nickel, Silicon, Vanadium and Zinc*. Washington DC: National Academy Press, 2001.

51. Davis CD, Milne DB, Nielsen FH. Changes in dietary zinc and copper affect zinc-status indicators of post menopausal women, notably extracellular superoxide dismutase and amyloid precursor proteins. *Am J Clin Nutr* 2000; **71**: 771–88.

52. Fischer PW, Giroux A, LiAbbe MR. Effects of zinc supplementation on copper status in adult man. *Am J Clin Nutr* 1984; **40**: 743–6.

53. Milne DB, Davis CD, Nielsen FH. Low dietary zinc alters indices of copper function and status in postmenopausal women. *Nutrition* 2001; **17**: 701–8.

54. Yodrick MK, Kenney MA, Winterfoldt EA. Iron, copper and zinc status: Response to supplementation with zinc or zinc and iron in adult females. *Am J Clin Nutr* 1989; **49**: 145–50.

55. National Research Council. *Toxicological Effects of Methyl Mercury.* Washington, DC: National Academy Press, 2000.

56. Myers GJ, Marsh DO, Cox C *et al.* A pilot neurodevelopmental study of Seychellois children following in utero exposure to methylmercury from a maternal fish diet. *Neurotoxicology* 1995; **16**: 629–38.

57. Myers GJ, Davidson PW, Cox C *et al.* Neurodevelopment outcomes of Seychellois children sixty-six months after in utero exposure to methylmercury from a maternal fish diet: Pilot study. *Neurotoxicology* 1995; **16**: 639–52.

58. Myers GJ, Marsh DC, Davidson PW. Main neurodevelopmental study of Seychellois children following in utero exposure to methylmercury from a maternal fish diet: Outcome at six months. *Neurotoxicology* 1995; **16**: 653–64.

59. Myers GJ, Davidson PW, Sharmlaye, CF *et al.* Effects of prenatal methylmercury exposure from a high fish diet on developmental milestones in the Seychelles child development study. *Neurotoxicology* 1997; **18**: 819–30.

60. Grandjean P, Weihe P, White R *et al.* Cognitive deficit in 7-year old children with prenatal exposure to methylmercury. *Neurotoxicol Teratol* 1997; **20**: 1–12.

61. Budtz-Jorgensen E, Grandjean P, Keiding N *et al.* Benchmark dose calculations of methylmercury-associated neurobehavioral deficits. *Toxicol* Letts 2000; **112–113**: 193–99.

62. Kjellstrom T, Kennedy P, Wallis S *et al. Physical and Mental Development of Children with Prenatal Exposure to Mercury from Fish. Stage 1: Preliminary Test at Age 4.* Report No. 3080. Solna, Sweden: National Swedish Environmental Protection Board, 1986.

63. Kjellstrom T, Kennedy P, Wallis S *et al. Physical and Mental Development of Children with Prenatal Exposure to Mercury from Fish. Stage 1: Interviews and Psychological Tests at Age 6.* Report No. 364Z. Solna, Sweden: National Swedish Environmental Protection Board, 1989.

64. Marsh DO, Clarkson TW, Cox C *et al.* Fetal methylmercury poison in relationship between concentration in single strain of maternal hair and child effects. *Arch Neurol* 1987; **44**: 1017–22.

65. US Environmental Protection Agency. National Ambient Air Quality Standards (NAAQS). Available from: http://epa.gov/air/criteria.html (accessed January 21, 2010).

66. Clean Air Act, Public Law No. 91–604; 84 STAT. 1676, 1970.

67. Clean Air Act, Public Law No. 101–549; 104 STAT. 2399, 1990.

68. US Environmental Protection Agency. *Air Quality for Particulate Matter (October 2004).* 600/P-99/002aF-bF. Washington DC: EPA, 2004.

69. US Environmental Protection Agency. *Review of the National Ambient Air Quality Standards for Particulate Matter: Policy Assessment of Scientific and Technical Information (December 2005).* EPA-452/R-05-005a. Washington DC: EPA, 2005.

70. Ferris BG Jr, Speizer FE, Spengler JD *et al.* Effects of sulfur oxides and respirable particles on human health: Methodology and demography of populations in study. *Am Res Respir Dis* 1979; **120**: 767–79.

71. Dockery DW, Pope CA 3rd, Xu X *et al.* An association between air pollution and mortality in six U.S. cities. *N Engl J Med* 1993; **329**: 1753–9.

●72. Pope CA III, Dockery DW. Epidemiology of particle effects. In: Holgate ST, Samet JM, Loren HS, Maynard RL (eds) *Air Pollution and Health.* London: Academic Press, 1999: 673–705.

73. Laden F, Schwartz J, Speizer FE, Dockery DW. Reduction in fine particulate air pollution and mortality: Extended followup of the Harvard Six Cities Study. *Am J Resp Crit Care Med* 2006; **173**: 667–72.

74. Pope CA III, Thunm MHJ, Namboodiri MM *et al.* Particulate air pollution as a predictor of mortality in a prospective study of U.S. adults. *Am J Resp Crit Care Med* 1995; **151**: 669–74.

75. Pope CA III, Burnett RJ, Thun MJ *et al.* Lung cancer, cardiopulmonary mortality, and long-term exposure to fine particulate air pollution. *J Am Med Assoc* 2002; **287**: 1132–41.

76. Steenland K, Hu S, Walker J. All-cause and case-specific mortality by socioeconomic status among employed persons in 27 US states, 1984-1997. *Am J of Public Health* 2004; **94**: 1037-1042.

77. Enstrom JE. Fine particulate pollution and total mortality among elderly Californians, 1973–2002. *Inhal Toxicol* 2005; **17**: 803–16.

78. US Environmental Protection Agency. National Ambient Air Quality Standards for Particulate Matter: Proposed Rule. *Fed Regist* 2006; **71**: 2620–708.

79. US Environmental Protection Agency. National Ambient Air Quality Standards for Particulate Matter. *Fed Regist* 2006; **71**: 61144–233.

80. US Environmental Protection Agency. *Air Quality Criteria for Ozone and Related Photochemical Oxidant.* EPA 600/R-05/004aF. Washington DC: EPA, 2006.

81. US Environmental Protection Agency. *Review of the National Ambient Air Quality Standards for Ozone: Policy Assessment of Scientific and Technical Information.* EPA-452/R-07–007. Washington DC: EPA, 2007.

82. Adams WC. Comparison of chamber 6.6 h exposures to 0.04–0.08 ppm ozone via square-wave and triangular profiles on pulmonary responses. *Inhal Toxicol* 2006; **18**: 127–36.

83. Adams WC. Comparison of chamber and face-mask 6.6-hr exposure to ozone on pulmonary function and symptoms responses. *Inhal Toxicol* 2002; **14**: 745–64.

84. Adams WC. Comparison of chamber and face mask 6.6-hr exposure to 0.08 ppm ozone via square-wave and triangular profiles on pulmonary responses. *Inhal Toxicol* 2003; **15**: 265–81.

85. Follinsbee LJ, McDonnell WF, Horstman DH. Pulmonary function and symptom responses after 6.6-hr exposure to 0.12 ppm ozone with moderate exercise. *JAPCA* 1988; **38**: 28–35.

86. Horstman DH, Folinsbee LJ, Ives PJ, Abdul-Salaam S, McDonnell WF. Ozone concentration and pulmonary response relationships for 6.6-hr exposures with five hrs of moderate exercise to 0.08, 0.10, and 0.12 ppm. *Am Rev Respir Dis* 1990; **142**: 1158–63.

87. McDonnell WF, Kehri HR, Abdul-Salaam S *et al.* Respiratory response of humans exposed to low levels of ozone for 6.6 hours. *Arch Environ Health* 1991; **46**: 145–50.

88. McDonnell WF, Stewart PW, Smith MV. The temporal dynamics of ozone-induced FEV1, changes in humans: an exposure–response model. *Inhal Toxicol* 2007; **19**: 483–94.

89. Brown JS, Bateson TF, McDonnell WF. Effects of exposure to 0.06 ppm ozone in FEV$_1$ in humans: A secondary analysis of existing data. *Environ Health Perspect* 2008; **116**: 1023–6.

90. Adams WC. Relation of pulmonary responses induced by 6.6 h exposures to 0.08 ppm ozone and 2-h exposures to 0.30 ppm via chamber and face-mask inhalation. *Inhal Toxicol* 2003; **15**: 745–59.

91. US Environmental Protection Agency. National Ambient Air Quality Standards for Ozone: Proposed Rule. *Fed Regist* 2007; **72**: 37818–919.

92. US Environmental Protection Agency. National Ambient Air Quality Standards for Ozone: Final Rule. *Fed Regist* **73**: 16436–514.

●93. Kroes R, Kleiner J, Renwick A. The threshold of toxicological concern concept in risk assessment. *Toxicol Sci* 2005; **86**: 226–30.

94. US Food and Drug Administration. Food additives: Threshold of regulation for substances used in food-contact articles. *Fed Regist* 1993; **58**: 52719–27.

95. Munro IC. Safety assessment procedures for indirect food additives: An overview. Report of a workshop. *Regul Toxicol Pharmacol* 1990; **12**: 2–12.

96. Cramer GM, Ford RA, Hall RL. Estimation of toxic hazards – a decision tree approach. *Food Cosmet Toxicol* 1978; **16**: 255–76.

97. Munro IC, Ford RA, Kennepohl B, Sprenger, JG. Correlation of structural class with no-observed effect levels. A proposal for establishing a threshold of concern. *Food Chem Toxicol* 1996; **34**: 829–67.

98. Munro, IC, Kennepohl E, Kroes R. A procedure for the safety evaluation of flavouring substances. *Food Chem Toxicol* 1999; **37**: 207–32.

99. JECFA. *Evaluation of Certain Food Additives and Contaminants. Safety Evaluation of Flavouring Agents. Forty-first Report of the Joint FAO/WHO Expert Committee on Food Additives.* WHO Technical Report Series No. 837. Geneva: World Health Organization, 1993.

100. Renwick AG. Toxicology databases and the concept of thresholds of toxicological concern as used by the JECFA for the safety evaluation of flavouring agents. *Toxicol Lett* 2004; **149**: 223–34.

101. Kroes R, Renwick AG, Cheeseman M *et al.* Structure-based thresholds of toxicological concern (TTC): Guidance for application to substances present at low levels in the diet. *Food Chem Toxicol* 2004; **42**: 65–83.

102. Bridges J. Strategy for a future chemicals policy. The View of the Scientific Committee on Toxicology, Ecotoxicology and the Environment (CSTEE). Professor Jim Bridges, University of Surrey, UK. Available from: http://www.eutop.de/chp/Download/BridgesRe.doc . (Accessed Jan 2010)

103. EMA. European Medicines Agency, Committee for Medicinal Products for Human Use. Guideline on the Limits of Genotoxic Impurities. CPMP/SWP/5199/02, 2006. Available from: http://www.ema.europa.eu/pdfs/human/swp/519902en.pdf. (Accessed Jan 2010)

104. Ball D, Blanchard J, Jacobson-Kram D *et al.* Development of safety qualification thresholds and their use in orally inhaled and nasal drug product evaluation. *Toxicol Sci* 2007; **97**: 226–36.

105. Williams ES, Panko J, Paustenbach DJ. The European Union's REACH regulation: a review of its history and requirements. *Crit Rev Toxicol* 2009; **39**(7): 553–575.

106. European Chemicals Agency. Guidance Fact Sheets. Available from: http://echa.europa.eu/reach/fact_sheet.en.asp. (Accessed Jan 2010)

107. United Nations General Assembly. *Report of the United Nations Conference on Environment and Development. Rio de Janeiro, Brazil.* New York: United Nations, 1992.

●108. European Commission. *Communication for the Commission on the Precautionary Principle.* Brussels: EC, 2002.

109. Organization for Economic Cooperation and Development. Environmental Directorate. Series on Testing and Assessment. Adopted Guidance and Review Documents. Available from: http://www.oecd.org/document (accessed January 2010).

110. Centers for Disease Control and Prevention. *Third National Report on Human Exposure to Environmental Chemicals.* Atlanta, GA: CDC, 2005.

111. Calafat AM, Ye X, Wong LY, Reidy JA, Needham LL. Exposure of the U.S. population to bisphenol A and 4-tertiary-octylphenol: 2003–2004. *Environ Health Perspect* 2008; **116**: 39–44.

●112. Hesterberg TW, Hart GA. Synthetic vitreous fibers: A review of toxicology research and its impact on hazard classification. *Crit Rev Toxicol* 2001; **31**: 1–53.

113. Bernstein DM. Synthetic vitreous fibers: A review of toxicology, epidemiology and regulations. *Crit Rev Toxicol* 2007; **37**: 839–66.

●114. Hesterberg TW, Bunn WB, McClellan RO, Hart GA, Lapin CA. Carcinogenicity studies of diesel engine exhausts in laboratory animals: A review of past studies and a discussion of future research needs. *Crit Rev Toxicol* 2005; **35**: 379–411.

115. International Agency for Research on Cancer. *Man-made Vitreous Fibers.* IARC Monographs on the Evaluation of Carcinogenic Risks to Humans No. 81. Lyons: IARC Press, 2002.

116. International Agency for Research on Cancer. IARC Monographs on the Evaluation of Carcinogenic Risks to Humans. From http://monographs.iarc.fr. (Accessed Jan 2010).

Chemical exposure assessment

SEAN SEMPLE, JOHN W. CHERRIE

In this chapter, we aim to present an overview of the assessment of human chemical exposure in the wide range of indoor and outdoor environments we live in, and of how we can evaluate the main routes through which chemical or biological agents can enter the body. It is important for those involved in environmental medicine to have an understanding of the potential effects of chemicals on human health and have the tools to be able to investigate new or emerging associations between exposure and reduced health outcomes. We have included three case studies to illustrate the possible approaches to assessing environmental chemical exposure.

WHAT IS EXPOSURE?

Exposure is defined as contact between an individual and an agent. It is important to understand that it is the interaction between the person and the chemical rather than the presence of a contaminant in environmental media that is associated with any risk.

Exposure can occur via one of four main routes:

- inhalation;
- dermal contact;
- ingestion;
- injection.

The inhalational route is generally easy to envisage as it encompasses what we breathe, and it can be measured by attaching monitoring instruments that sample from the vicinity of the individual's nose or mouth as he or she moves around indoor and outdoor environments. The dermal route concerns contamination of the skin and then the uptake of chemicals via permeation through the skin and into the systemic circulation. Ingestion of hazardous chemicals takes account of contamination in food and water that is consumed and inadvertent ingestion via hand-to-mouth and object-to-mouth transfer. Injection is a rare exposure route that may arise from sharp tools accidentally piercing the skin or needlestick injuries.

Most investigations focus on a single route and fail to consider the interlinked nature of exposure between the environmental air, soil and water compartments. For example, it is not difficult to imagine how high levels of contamination of the air by a fine lead metal aerosol can also lead to deposition on the skin of an individual within that environment and hence inadvertent ingestion from mouthing behaviour. We can conceptualize the exposure process as shown in Figure 5.1, with various interactions and transfer processes between different human environment compartments resulting in exposure by one of the four exposure routes listed above. Figure 5.1 illustrates one example for inhalational exposure.

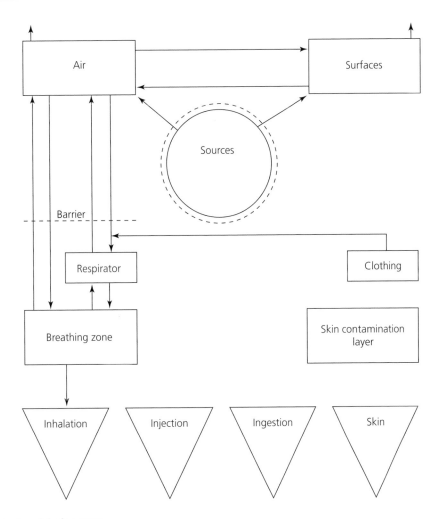

Figure 5.1 Conceptual model of exposure.

In Figure 5.1, the dotted lines are intended to represent some form of barrier; for example, around the source they may represent localized control measures such as a partial container. Contaminant passes out from the source to one or more compartments, for example the indoor air or the walls, benches, floors or tools used by the person, which are all grouped in the surfaces compartment. The triangular boxes represent the uptake of chemical contaminant into the body.

Conceptual models of this type can provide an excellent way of understanding the important determinants of exposure. For example, in the case of inhalation exposure, it is clear that both indoor and outdoor sources may be important in contributing to the inhalation of contaminant, along with deposits on surfaces that may be resuspended into the indoor air compartment. In the case of ingestion, contaminants may be deposited on surfaces and clothing before being transferred by touching to the skin-contaminant layer and then on to ingestion uptake via hand-to-mouth and object-to-mouth contacts.

Exposure is often expressed as units of concentration in the compartment being measured (air, soil or water), but more correctly it should incorporate a measure of the duration of contact between the person and the chemical in question. So, for example, where we are dealing with inhalation exposure, we often see levels quoted as mass per volume of air (e.g. μg/m^3), but exposure should really be expressed as a concentration multiplied by time equivalent (e.g. μg/m^3 per hour). It is likely that exposure will vary over time, so we often integrate the exposure over a defined averaging period to give the time-weighted average.

A simple example is provided for a person who undertakes a journey across several urban, suburban and rural areas by a variety of transport methods over the course of a day. The first exposure scenario may involve travelling by car through a busy congested urban environment for approximately 1 hour heading to a city-centre train station. During this period, the exposure to the fine particulate matter is high, with an average concentration of 65 μg/m^3. The second period involves travelling by train for a further 2 hours, when the average exposure is 25 μg/m^3, before arriving in a rural setting and cycling for 1 hour and being exposed to an average particulate concentration of 5 μg/m^3.

We can calculate the time-weighted average exposure of the traveller by multiplying the concentration by the duration of each period, summing these together and then dividing the value by the total duration of the journey event. So in this case, we have the following equation:

$$\text{Time-weighted average} = [(1 \text{ hour} \times 65\,\mu g/m^3) \\ + (2 \text{ hours} \times 25\,\mu g/m^3) + (1 \text{ hour} \times 5\,\mu g/m^3)] \\ / 4 \text{ hours} = 30\,\mu g/m^3$$

The commuter's time-weighted average exposure over the total journey is therefore $30\,\mu g/m^3$, averaged over the 4 hour period.

If the person remained in the rural setting for the remainder of the day and was exposed there to average concentrations of $2\,\mu g/m^3$ for 20 hours, the 24 hour average exposure would be $[(4 \times 30) + (20 \times 2)] / 24 = 6.7\,\mu g/m^3$.

For dermal exposure, the contact is often expressed as the mass per area of skin, primarily because this skin loading is what is simplest to measure. In reality, dermal uptake and the resulting health effects will be driven by the concentration of the chemical contaminant on the skin or dissolved in the sweat and sebum layer of the skin. The area of exposure is also key to understanding percutaneous uptake or the transfer of chemicals through the epidermis to the systemic circulation.

For ingestion, the exposure is usually easy to quantify when considering food or contaminated water, with the mass of chemical per millilitre or gram being a good surrogate for the exposure or intake. For inadvertent ingestion in which the chemical ingestion arises from hand-to-mouth or object-to-perioral contact, the methods for quantifying exposure are less clear cut. Data on transfer efficiencies and the area of the fingers or hands that are placed in the mouth, combined with skin loading and frequency of mouthing behaviour, are essential in being able to quantify ingestion exposure.

Injection exposure is, by its very nature, accidental and sporadic, so it is very difficult to gather information on exposure quantities by this route; however, the mass of chemical that enters the body by injection tends to be very small. Unless the injected material is radioactive or particularly toxic, the puncture injury itself, rather than the intake of the chemical, is more likely to be of importance.

WHAT IS ENVIRONMENTAL EXPOSURE?

For most of us, the term 'environment' brings to mind images of the outdoors, greenery, wide-open spaces, rural living or the seas and oceans. In our increasingly urban existence, however, the environment that we inhabit tends to be primarily indoors and involves the majority of our time in a mixture of home, work and vehicles, where we will come in to contact with the chemical or agent of interest via the air we breathe, the food and drink we consume and the surfaces we touch. Very little of our

environmental exposure arises while we are outdoors, although it should be recognized that outdoor air pollutants may migrate indoors. Only a small proportion of exposure to chemicals occurs in rural settings for most of the world's population.

Until recently, environmental medicine considered the effects of air, water and soil pollution on the population without also taking into account exposure to the same or similar chemicals in the workplace or through consumer exposure to products. There is a real need for science to begin to integrate the methods used in occupational, consumer and environmental exposure assessment in order to provide a more complete understanding of the effects of chemicals on human health.

The ability to subdivide exposure down to microenvironments or human exposure scenarios is essential to the exposure assessment process. 'Microenvironments' is a term used to describe the different space volumes or places where humans traditionally spend time. These may be the home, the inside of the bus or car in which they travel to work, the leisure centre or shopping complex or some other well-defined compartment. The key is that the exposure within that environment can be characterized and that the time spent within that space is easy to identify and quantify.

Similarly, human exposure scenarios are tasks or events that individuals are likely to engage in that can be clearly described and have well-understood exposure determinants. Exposure scenarios may take place in different microenvironments so, for example, the scenario of being exposed to second-hand tobacco smoke in a shopping mall will give rise to a different personal exposure than will occur with the same scenario experienced within the confined volume of a car or bus. Spraying insecticide on outdoor garden plants is likely to produce lower personal exposures than performing the same task on indoor houseplants.

CASE STUDY 1: INHALATION EXPOSURE – PERSONAL EXPOSURE TO FINE PARTICULATE AIR POLLUTION IN KUALA LUMPUR, MALAYSIA

Increases in the concentration of fine airborne particulate matter have been linked to raised respiratory and cardiovascular mortality and morbidity levels. Recent work has suggested that, at a population level in the USA, reductions in 24 hour average outdoor airborne concentrations of particulate matter less than $2.5\,\mu m$ in diameter ($PM_{2.5}$) of $10\,\mu g$ per cubic metre of air results in average increases in life expectancy of 0.61 ± 0.20 year.[1] Most of the epidemiological work that has been carried out to investigate the exposure–response relationship has used time series data from fixed-site outdoor air pollution monitoring stations and linked the data to deaths or hospital admissions.

Although the PM$_{2.5}$ concentration at fixed roadside and city-centre locations is useful in understanding emissions from sources and changes that occur as a result of meteorological conditions, it is probably of limited value in understanding the personal exposure of most individuals to fine particulate air pollutants.

Returning to the concept of microenvironments and exposure scenarios described earlier we can consider how individuals may be exposed to PM$_{2.5}$ over the course of a typical day as they move from home to work and then to the shops, a restaurant and then home again. Possible examples of high exposure are provided in Table 5.1.

As can be seen from Table 5.1, information on outdoor PM$_{2.5}$ concentrations measured at a fixed site in the centre of the city where this person lives will tell us very little about their personal exposure or how much PM$_{2.5}$ they inhale over the day in question. For our example of an individual moving from home to work, shops and a restaurant and then home again, a single city-centre located measuring device will clearly grossly under- and overestimate the exposure at various points in the day.

Improvements in technology now mean that devices that will continuously measure personal exposure to PM$_{2.5}$ are available. Instruments are now small enough to wear for extended time periods, producing a real-time record of particulate matter concentrations. Understanding how the measured concentrations relate in time and space is also important, and this can be achieved by asking the individual wearing the equipment to record their movements and activities in a time–activity diary.

Another alternative is to use satellite-tracking or global positioning systems (GPSs) or mobile-phone tracking technology to link the exposure changes to different locations and, at some level, different activities. Small, finger-sized GPS logging devices can provide highly accurate data on the wearer's movements and can be linked to software to provide time–location–exposure information. GPS technology requires line-of-sight to attain a signal from a number of satellites in order to provide an accurate fix on the user's location so tends to be limited to outdoor uses, but mobile-phone technology provides positioning even within indoor environments.

Figure 5.2 shows GPS information detailing the movements of an individual travelling around the suburbs of Kuala Lumpur between 10.20 am and 2.15 pm. Details of the speed of movement can be extracted from the GPS software to enable judgements to be made about the mode of transport or to cross-check with time–activity diaries.

Instruments capable of logging temperature and relative humidity can also be particularly instructive in deciphering movements between indoor and outdoor environments in order to enable a complete characterization of exposures to be made. It is easy to visualize methods of overlaying exposure information on to the geographical image with perhaps different colours or differently sized dots to reflect instanteous personal exposures measured along this daily journey.

The real-time PM$_{2.5}$ exposure data from much of our subject's journey, together with extracts from the time–activity diary, are presented in Figure 5.3. This output clearly shows the personal exposure of the individual varying from levels of about 20–50 μg/m^3 to

Table 5.1 Range of typical levels of particulate matter less than 2.5 μm in diameter (PM$_{2.5}$) for a selection of microenvironments

Microenvironment	Average PM$_{2.5}$ levels (μg/m^3)
Travelling in car in congested driving conditions	25–100
Eating dinner in a restaurant where smoking is permitted	100–400
At home with a smoker in the same room	300–3000
Walking in the city centre	5–40
Cooking fried food at home	500–2000
Working in a quarry	1000–20 000

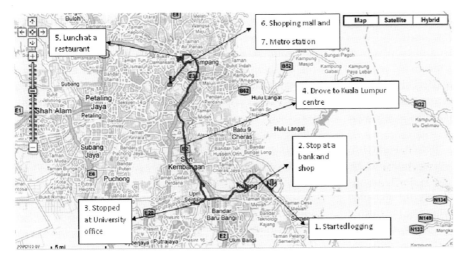

Figure 5.2 Global positioning system map of an individual's movements around Kuala Lumpur, Malaysia.

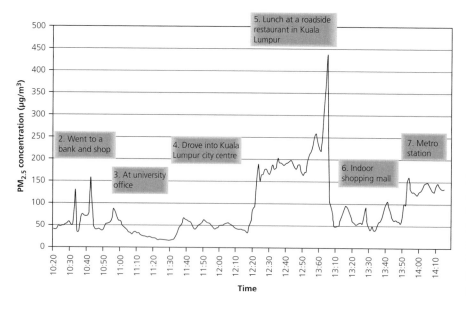

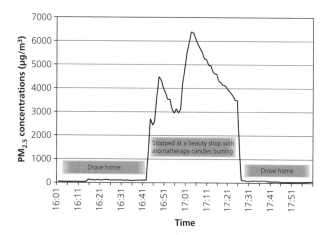

Figure 5.3   Plot of real-time concentrations of particulate matter with a diameter of less than 2.5 μm (PM$_{2.5}$) measured using a personal exposure device during a day in Kuala Lumpur, Malaysia. The graph is annotated with time–activity information that links to Figure 5.2.

Figure 5.4   Plot of real-time concentrations of particulate matter with a diameter of less than 2.5 μm (PM$_{2.5}$) measured using a personal exposure device during a visit to an aromatherapy shop in Kuala Lumpur, Malaysia. The graph is annotated with time–activity information.

peaks some 20 times this value during lunchtime. Data from the late afternoon period shown in Figure 5.4 indicate even higher exposures during time spent in a small aromatherapy shop where incense and candles were burning. Note the differences in the scale of the concentration axis on these two graphs. The exposure levels are about 10 times higher in the aromatherapy shop compared with the peaks seen at lunch in the previous chart.

Monitoring devices for measuring other air pollutants such as carbon monoxide, ozone and nitrogen dioxide are also available, and improving technology is making these devices smaller, lighter and more suitable for personal monitoring. Some devices use active sampling in which a small pump sucks air into the device to measure the chemical concentration by light-scattering, infrared

absorption or chemical reactivity with another reagent. There are often noise and battery life issues with such devices. Other instruments use passive or diffusion technology to measure concentrations via natural air movement as the wearer moves around the environment being measured.

MATCHING THE EXPOSURE METRIC TO THE HEALTH EFFECT

The variability in exposure levels seen over the course of the measurement period in Figures 5.3 and 5.4 raises another important point about environmental exposure assessment: what metric do we use to quantify exposure?

As described earlier, we generally conclude that exposure is the product of intensity and duration, and many occupational exposures are quoted as time-weighted averages over particular sampling periods such as 15 minutes or 8 hours. Shorter time periods are used for chemicals that have acute effects, whereas work-shift or 8 hour averages are employed for materials with chronic health effects. For environmental exposures 24 hour or even annual averages are often quoted. The US Environmental Protection Agency Air Quality Standards for outdoor pollutants such as PM$_{2.5}$ is set at 35 μg/m^3 averaged over a 24 hour period, but at 15 μg/m^3 when averaged over a whole year. Such a system clearly allows for some days to exceed the 15 μg/m^3 level while the area air quality remains within the annual standard, and similarly, in a given 24 hour period there may be times of the day when concentrations exceed 35 μg/m^3, but the average concentration will be below this.

Understanding the relationship between exposure and health clearly involves a knowledge of toxicity on the target organ, and pharmacokinetics and metabolism in terms of clearance of the chemical or particle from the body. For some materials, this relationship is well characterized and understood; for example, inorganic arsenic compounds are known human carcinogens affecting multiple organ sites with clear epidemiological evidence for a risk from contaminated drinking water and occupational inhalational exposure. However, the toxicological and/or epidemiological evidence is less clear cut for other environmental pollutants.

In the case of air pollution, it is difficult to determine what aspect of fine particulate pollution produces the association between exposure and increased respiratory and cardiovascular illness. Is it the inhalation of an increased mass of $PM_{2.5}$? Is it the average exposure? Is it the duration of time an individual spends in an environment where concentrations are above a particular threshold? Is it the peak exposures that people are exposed to over their day? Is it the rate of change that is harmful, with steady-state high pollution levels perhaps being handled better by the body's defences? The answer is far from clear, and we make broad assumptions that very general markers of exposure such as the time-weighted average exposure to relatively easy to measure pollutants such as $PM_{2.5}$ are appropriate to investigate exposure–health relationships and to allow us to target sources, controls and interventions.

As with most things, it comes back to what is practical and cost-effective to measure. There is little point having a comprehensive exposure assessment system if it is so costly and bulky that it allows only a small number of measurements to be made at fixed sites, while the same effort and expenditure on more simplistic methods would provide thousands of personal exposure data gathered across a wide range of microenvironments.

MEASURING EXPOSURES

Environmental concentrations are, in most cases, much lower than those experienced in occupational environments. So while there is significant overlap in the methodology used, the technology, lower limits of detection and increased sensitivity generally make environmental exposures much more difficult (because of generally more bulky equipment) and more expensive to measure.

Gravimetric analysis, in which a mass of material is collected on a pre-weighed filter paper, is the standard method of assessing occupational inhalation exposures to dusts. In environmental settings, the concentrations are several orders of magnitude lower, so direct-reading instruments are more likely to be used to quantify airborne concentrations, although the gravimetric assessment of filter samples may still be used. A direct assessment of the concentration of outdoor particulate air pollution may be made with instruments such as the tapered element oscillating microbalance used to measure PM_{10} or $PM_{2.5}$ – i.e. particulate matter with a diameter of less than 10 or 2.5 μm, respectively.

For dermal exposure, the techniques are more uniform, with methods having being developed for occupational exposure to pesticides that are equally applicable to consumers, domestic situations or the exposures experienced by people who live or happen to be within the vicinity of pesticide spraying, often termed 'by-standers'.

Dermal exposure assessment can be carried out by one of three classes of technique: interception methods, removal methods and visualization. Interception or surrogate skin methods use patches or whole-body suits to collect chemicals that would be deposited on the skin. Patch methods require extrapolation to the whole-body area and are thus susceptible to over- or underestimation depending on the pattern of exposure. Whole-body suits avoid this problem but can have issues with extraction and limits of detection due to the volume of solvent required to remove the contaminant from the suit. Removal methods use wipes, washing or tape-stripping to measure contamination on the surface or outer layers of the skin but will fail to measure material that has already been absorbed through the skin and into the systemic circulation. Visualization systems use the addition of a fluorescent tracer material to the contaminant under study. When this binds to the skin, it can then be seen under ultraviolet lighting, and image capture protocols can be used to quantify the area and mass of contamination.

All dermal exposure assessment methods also have to consider uptake, and this is related to the concentration (not the mass) of the chemical deposited on the skin, the area of skin contaminated, the chemical properties of the contaminant and other issues such as skin type, temperature, humidity and vehicle effects from chemical mixtures.

Characterizing ingestion exposure via food and water is a relatively simple process in that contaminant concentrations (mass per mass of food or mass per volume of fluid) can be multiplied by the mass or volume of food or drink digested. For inadvertent exposures, there is a need to quantify the mass of contaminant being deposited around the perioral area or transferred directly to the mouth via fingers or objects being mouthed. Methods for carrying out this quantification may include wipe-sampling of the perioral areas or direct sampling of saliva concentrations from the oral cavity to determine ingestion contamination.

BIOMONITORING

Biomonitoring is the measurement of a chemical or a metabolite within the saliva, blood, breath, sweat or urine. It offers an alternative to measuring exposure in that it allows us to measure the quantity of a material or a known metabolite that has already entered the body. Biomonitoring of blood lead levels provides a way of determining when a worker's exposure to lead is not being controlled sufficiently well. When the concentration of lead in blood exceeds certain limits, workers have to be removed from the task or job that involves lead contact until their levels reduce. Biomonitoring for arsenic in people exposed to contaminated water and soil provides a way of integrating the dermal, inhalational and ingestional exposure routes. As with all biomonitoring, there is a need to understand how exposure takes place and to position the results in the context of the task, the different exposure routes likely and the possibility of exposure and intake from sources beyond the target scenario, with a particular emphasis on dietary intake.

Biomonitoring is increasingly being used to assess the exposure of people in the general population. For example, the National Center for Environmental Health of the US Centers for Disease Control undertakes periodic national surveys for a wide range of environmental pollutants; the third report was published in 2005.[2] This report showed that there was a significant decline in exposure to second-hand cigarette smoke and continued decreases in children's blood lead levels. However, the report also showed that about 5 per cent of the US population aged 20 years and older had urinary cadmium levels close to 1 μg/g creatinine, a level that may be associated with kidney damage. Cigarette-smoking is the likely source for these higher cadmium levels.

There are potential problems in interpreting the results from biomonitoring programmes when there is an irregular episodic exposure pattern and a relatively short biological half-life for the compound in the body. In these cases, it is impossible to interpret the measurement properly unless we know something about when the person was exposed in relation to the sample collection.

Another problem with biomonitoring is that it does not provide information on the route of exposure, and is therefore less powerful in being able to target control or policy interventions to reduce uptake. We can take the example of salivary cotinine, a metabolite of nicotine and hence a well-accepted surrogate for exposure to environmental tobacco smoke (ETS) in adults, and consider measurements made in infants who have parents who smoke. An elevated result does not tell us where the exposure took place – it may have been in the child's home or at another site such as the home of relatives, or in some other public space where smoking is permitted.

The salivary cotinine level also does not tell us about the route of exposure. Nicotine-laden dust is likely to be present on the floor in the child's home and on the clothing of the smoking parents. Close contact with surfaces during crawling and mouthing behaviour will lead to ingestion of this nicotine dust; therefore, even in a home that has recently introduced a no-smoking policy indoors, the child may acquire considerable nicotine uptake via non-inhalatory mechanisms. The risk to health from ingesting ETS-generated dust is not well understood, but it is unlikely to be associated with asthma and respiratory diseases in the way that the inhalation of ETS has been clearly demonstrated to be.

EXPOSURE MODELLING

Modelling of exposure is increasingly being seen as an acceptable way of estimating exposure for regulatory purposes, for epidemiological studies and for risk assessments. The starting point for a model is often the conceptualization of the exposure process in much the same way as we have discussed at the beginning of this chapter.

Models that depend upon measured data are described as analogous models; models that seek to synthesize a precise output from a known set of variables are deterministic models. If the model provides an output that is in the form of either a probability distribution or summary statistics from a probability distribution, it is known as a probabilistic model. Probabilistic models are often built upon a deterministic or analogous model.

Exposure models can be very general in their application, seeking to provide estimates of exposure for a wide range of scenarios, or they can focus on more specific circumstances such as a specific activity or type of substance. For example, a model that is intended to estimate occupational inhalation exposure in connection with the European REACH (Registration, Evaluation, Authorisation and Restriction of Chemical substances) regulations[3] needs to be applicable to all of the situations that are covered by the legislation. A model that is intended to provide estimates for situations where paints or other surface coatings are applied can, however, be more specific in its applicability. All of these types of model have their uses, but general purpose models are most widely applicable for regulatory exposure assessment.

It is important to remember that all models are based upon assumptions and that their outputs are at best approximate and may be wrong in particular circumstances. The same can of course be said of environmental exposure measurements obtained from a small number of children on a few days at one time of year. Limited sets of exposure data provide only an indication of the true exposure. In fact, it is most appropriate to look at how models can enhance the value of measurements and vice versa.

The basic approach to most exposure modelling is to subdivide the time into a number of discrete activities or scenarios – the 'microenvironments' we discussed earlier in this chapter. The exposure level can then be estimated from existing data or from a mechanistic model, and these data can then be combined using the time-weighted averaging approach as illustrated earlier.

In this section, we describe two different modelling approaches. The first uses an extensive measurement dataset to calculate microenvironmental concentrations that are combined to estimate overall personal exposure. The second model is a general purpose model, known as ConsExpo,[4] that has been designed to estimate exposure for people using a wide variety of consumer products containing chemicals.

Delgado Saborit *et al.* measured personal exposure and microenvironmental concentrations of volatile organic compounds (VOCs – in this case 15 different compounds, including benzene, toluene, xylene and styrene) for 100 subjects on several occasions over 2 years.[5] The subjects were recruited in three areas of Great Britain. Some of the personal and microenvironmental data (75 per cent) were then used to develop the models using seven different strategies, with the remainder of the data (25 per cent) being used to validate the finally developed model.

These researchers found that when the microenvironmental data from the subject were used to develop the model for VOC exposure, the model produced reliable predictions, i.e. its estimates generally explained between 65 and 95 per cent of the variability in the measured exposures, and the bias was generally less than ± 20 per cent. The concentration in the home of each person was seen to be the dominant microenvironment, so if this approach were being used in a epidemiological study, it might be sufficient to measure the concentration in the home of each subject and to use these data as a surrogate for their personal exposure to VOCs. However, when the overall data from the microenvironments were used to estimate exposure for each person, the model explained less than about 10 per cent of the variation in the measured personal exposures, and the bias was typically between zero and -100 per cent. This approach is therefore not easily generalizable to other situations.

The consumer exposure model (ConsExpo) was developed by the Dutch National Institute for Public Health and the Environment and allows users to estimate exposure to the chemicals contained in consumer products. It has been designed to assess exposure to non-professional indoor uses of chemicals by inhalation, dermal routes and ingestion. The total exposure is determined by combining the contact, exposure and update scenarios for each route of exposure. The ConsExpo model and the associated guidance can be downloaded from the Internet.[4]

Inhalational exposure is modelled in one of two types of scenario in which:

- a compound evaporates from a surface into the room air, for example from a painted wall or a can of product;
- the compound is sprayed into the air, for example from an aerosol can.

In both situations the assessor needs to have information about the room where the exposures occur and details of the product and the way in which the product is used.

For dermal exposure, there are five different scenarios that the user can choose from:

- instant application of the product to the skin;
- a constant rate of application to the skin;
- transfer from surfaces by rubbing off;
- migration from a surface in contact with the skin;
- diffusion from a surface in contact with the skin.

In addition, dermal exposure may also occur concurrently with inhalational exposure, so selecting inhalational exposure or a scenario involving inhalation and dermal exposure automatically results in assessment of dermal exposure being selected.

For dermal uptake, there are two possible approaches to select from: either one can assume that a fixed fraction of the mass loading is absorbed, or more complex quantitative structure–activity relationship models can be used to estimate uptake. Inhalational uptake is calculated from data about the deposition of the substance in the lungs and the breathing rate of the individual.

ConsExpo has the possibility of including distributions for the model input parameters rather than point values, and it is then able to calculate the likely exposure and uptake distributions using Monte Carlo probability simulations.

There are considerable supporting data linked to the model and many default parameters that make the modelling easier for the novice user. In particular, there are several factsheets for a wide range of consumer exposure scenarios such as children's toys, cleaning products, cosmetics and DIY products.

CASE STUDY 2: ESTIMATING EXPOSURES FROM A POINT SOURCE

The following example provides an appreciation of the problems that can be encountered when estimating the non-occupational exposures resulting from a chemical release from a process plant. In this case, there is a vent pipe in a petroleum refinery that releases sulphur dioxide effluent once or twice annually for 10–20 minutes. The vent pipe is 30 m high and the estimated emission rate of sulphur dioxide is 8 g/s. The wind around this plant typically blows the emissions over a village about 500 m from the vent. There are no other residential areas within 10 km of the plant.

It should be realized that, as the pollutant disperses from the vent, it will mix with the surrounding air and dilute. This process is dependent on several factors: the wind speed, the lapse rate (the gradient of air temperature with height), the type of terrain, the temperature of the emitted gas stream, the height of the emissions and the distance from the source to the point where people may be exposed, among others. This process can be idealized as illustrated in Figure 5.5.

The rate of dispersion can be described mathematically using a Gaussian dispersion model to allow the concentration to be estimated in any circumstance. If we plot the estimated ground level concentration against the distance from the source, we get the pattern shown in Figure 5.6. The concentration between 0.1 and 1 km is less than $10\,\mu g/m^3$. Thereafter, there is a rapid increase in concentration to the maximum predicted value of $170\,\mu g/m^3$. After 10 km, the predicted concentration is

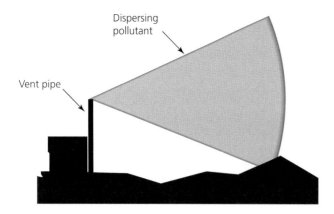

Figure 5.5   Idealized dispersion of pollutant from a stack.

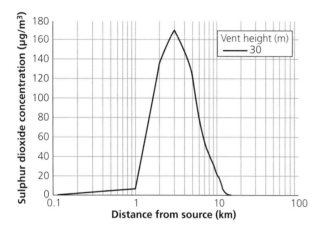

Figure 5.6   Estimated concentration with distance. Note that the horizontal scale is logarithmic.

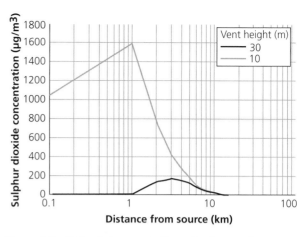

Figure 5.7   Estimated concentration with distance for two discharge heights. Note that the vertical scale is different from that of Figure 5.6, and that the horizontal scale is logarithmic.

again very low. The first section of the graph corresponds to the region where the contaminated plume is not in contact with the ground. From 10 km onwards, the pollution has dispersed to the point where it is unimportant.

Using the dispersion model, the importance of the height of the pollutant discharge above the site can be demonstrated. Figure 5.7 shows the predicted concentration profile with increasing distance from the source for the original vent height scenario (i.e. 30 m above ground) and for a much lower vent height discharging at 10 m. With the lower discharge, the plume quickly comes into contact with the ground, and the maximum concentrations are much higher than found with the other case. A more extensive discussion of air pollution and dispersion modelling can be found on the Danish National Environmental Research Institute website.[6]

The acceptable level of exposure to sulphur dioxide in workplaces is about 5000 μg/m^3, which is set on the basis of protecting workers from the possibility of chronic lung damage and from the irritant properties of sulphur dioxide. People who already suffer from asthma may be more easily irritated, and the impact of sulphur dioxide exposure may be greater for them. In addition, exercise increases the

severity of the irritant effect in the lung because of the greater volume of air inhaled and the reduced residence time of the gas in the nose, where the sulphur dioxide would normally dissolve in the mucus. Experimental studies of exercising asthma patients exposed to sulphur dioxide have demonstrated that they are generally more sensitive than healthy people. The threshold for measurable narrowing of the airways in normal healthy volunteers is about 12 000 μg/m^3. The corresponding value for asthmatics is between 700 μg/m^3 and 1500 μg/m^3, with a few individuals affected at as low a level as 275 μg/m^3.

The Department for Environment, Food and Rural Affairs (Defra), which is responsible for government policy in this area, has set up an independent medical and scientific panel to advise on such issues. This Expert Panel on Air Quality Standards contributed to the publication of the first Air Quality Strategy in 2000. On the basis of the available information for sulphur dioxide, the Air Quality Strategy decided that the UK air quality standard should be set at 266 μg/m^3, averaged over 15 minutes. This was thought to be sufficiently protective to prevent adverse health effects in most susceptible individuals.

Let us return, then, to our case study of the petroleum refinery. With the 30 m high discharge pipe, the estimated concentration of sulphur dioxide in the village would be less than 10 μg/m^3, and there should therefore be no problems. However, if the plant had been constructed with the lower pipe, the concentration in the village would probably have exceeded 1500 μg/m^3. There would then have been a strong possibility that individuals with asthma would have experienced some exacerbation of their symptoms on the days when there were sulphur dioxide emissions. In addition, if the plant had been located a little further from the village, say about 3 km away, the concentration of sulphur dioxide would have been around 170 μg/m^3 for the emission quantities described, although there could possibly still have been some health problems with slightly higher emissions.

CASE STUDY 3: ESTIMATION OF EXPOSURE TO PESTICIDES RESIDUES FROM FOOD

We have considered inhalation exposure to environmental fine particulate matter and to emissions from a point source, but it is important to remember that other routes of exposure can contribute to the total intake of a chemical. Ingestion of chemicals from food is one area that has been subject to both measurement and modelling to examine possible health effects from environmental exposure (see also Chapter 22).

Plant protection products, chemicals from within the group commonly known as pesticides, are widely used in agriculture to control pests. For example, in 2006 there were over 4.3 million hectares of arable crops in Britain; herbicides were applied to more than half, and fungicides were applied to approximately 82 per cent of the total area of crops.[7] Insecticides and nematicides (pesticides specifically for roundworms) were intensively applied to peas, with approximately 84 per cent of the area treated on average twice per year. About 85 per cent of oilseed rape and 68 per cent of beans were treated with an average of two insecticide sprays, while about three-quarters of wheat, winter barley and potatoes crops were treated with at least one insecticide.

Over 60 different pesticide compounds were used on arable crops in Great Britain, with annual usage in 2006 of 2000 tonnes of the growth regulator chlormequat, 1500 tonnes of the herbicide compound glyphosate, and 1100 tonnes of the fungicide chlorothalonil. In total, 4000 tonnes of fungicides, 8000 tonnes of herbicides and 650 tonnes of insecticides were applied to arable crops.

Despite the high usage of pesticides, the residues left on the crops when they enter the marketplace tend to be low. In the European Union in 2002, more than 46 000 samples of food were analysed for 170 different pesticides. About 92 per cent of the samples analysed were fresh or frozen fruit, vegetables and cereals, with the remainder being processed products. A total of 58 per cent of the analyses were recorded as being below the reporting limit, and a further 37 per cent had detectable residues that were less than the allowable maximum residue level, i.e. the maximum allowable concentration of pesticide in food. About 5 per cent of samples tested exceeded the maximum residue level for a given pesticide.

We eat a varied diet, so we will almost certainly consume a mixture of different pesticides from different foods. There has been some concern about exposure to mixtures of pesticides because many compounds have a similar chemistry and toxicology, so the combined effect of being exposed to several compounds may be greater than for individual compounds.[8] For example, organophosphate and carbamate pesticides all interfere with cholinesterase, an enzyme that catalyses the hydrolysis of the neurotransmitter acetylcholine, a reaction necessary to allow cholinergic neurones to return to their resting state after activation.

Exposure to mixtures is often discussed in terms of aggregate and cumulative exposure, where aggregate exposure arises from multiple sources of one active pesticide compound, for example from occupational and consumer exposure, and cumulative exposure refers to exposure to multiple pesticide compounds from multiple sources. The regulatory systems for the approval of pesticides only consider single products and not mixtures. As biological monitoring methods have limited sensitivity and because of the difficulty of obtaining a representative sample, the only practicable way to estimate the cumulative (or aggregate) exposure of the population to pesticides is through some form of modelling study.

A study performed by the Institute of Occupational Medicine in Edinburgh estimated cumulative exposure and internal dose for 16 of the most commonly used anticholinesterase pesticides in the UK.[9] Data on pesticide residues in food were obtained from the UK surveillance scheme. As we have seen, many of these data were below the laboratory detection limit, so it is possible that there was some very low level of residue present in these samples. To take account of this, a simple algorithm was developed to estimate the possible residue where it was possible that the crop had been treated with pesticide.

Where food is processed, either by a food manufacturer or by peeling or cooking at home, the residue levels may be modified. Little is know about these changes, but it is likely that it reduces the residue by some variable amount. The model accounts for this by including a random processing factor. Data on food recipes to identify food ingredients were also obtained.

Data from the National Diet and Nutrition Survey were used as the basis for linking residues with individuals in the population. These data include detailed information on the individuals taking part in the survey (a national sample of adults aged 19–64 years), which includes domicile region within the UK, social class, nutritional status, dietary preferences, obesity, blood pressure and physical activity.

The model was used to repeatedly simulate the dietary intake of an individual for each day during a year, and then repeated the process for thousands of other subjects until a stable estimate of the population exposure had been obtained. The internal dose of each pesticide compound was then estimated using a single-compartment pharmacokinetic model. As a measure of the total pesticide mixture, the total internal dose of pesticide was calculated. This measure is the sum of all the pesticides in the body for each day exposed divided by the acceptable daily intake (ADI):

$$IDX = \sum_{k=1}^{N} C_k/ADI_k$$

where IDX is a dimensionless number that provides a representation of the aggregate exposure by normalizing each internal dose estimate by the corresponding ADI,

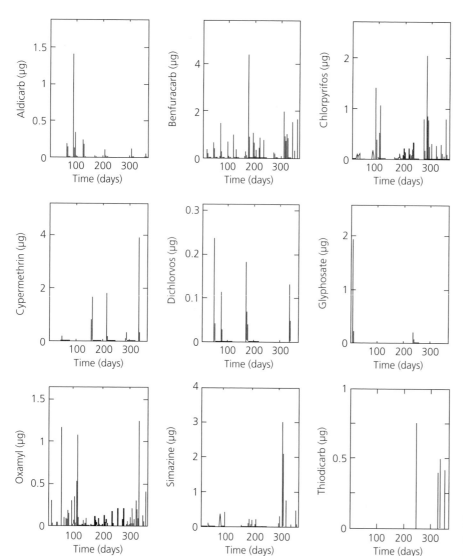

Figure 5.8 Pesticide internal dose estimates throughout the year for a single adult.

ADI_k is the acceptable daily intake for pesticide k and C_k is the internal dose estimate for the same pesticide compound.

Figure 5.8 shows the predicted daily internal dose of various pesticides associated with the fresh and fresh-processed fruits and vegetables consumed by a single adult over a year (horizontal axes) – only nine pesticide compounds are shown in this example because only these pesticides were consumed by this individual. Note that the pattern of exposure is erratic throughout the year. The results for each of the anticholinesterase compounds with positive residues are shown in Table 5.2. Note that the ADI has been adjusted to make it comparable to the internal dose estimates.

In Table 5.2, data are shown for the median daily dose for an individual over the year (i.e. 50th percentile, average dose) and for the 90th percentile of average doses for the individuals in the population. The final two columns in the table show the median and 90th percentile of the maximum daily dose during the year, i.e. the highest daily dose for any

'individual' in the simulation. From these results, it is apparent that the 90th percentile of the maximum dose for each of the individual pesticide compounds is much less than the ADI for all pesticides. The closest value is for oxamyl, but even here the difference between the ADI and the 90th percentile of the maximum dose is still over 100-fold.

Figure 5.9 shows the cumulative pesticide doses for all of the anticholinesterase pesticides combined, i.e. the cumulative exposure estimates, for adults using a log-scale, showing both the daily median and 90th percentile. On this scale -1 corresponds to a tenth of the combined ADI.

These data are reassuring in that they predict cumulative dietary exposures that are much less than any level that might be considered to be harmful and show that exposure modelling can be used to make judgements about environmental exposures. It is, however, worth reminding ourselves that the data presented here are only for dietary uptake and do not take account of the potential

Table 5.2 Summary statistics for the internal dose of pesticides for adult food consumption (mg/kg)

	Adjusted ADI dose	Average dose		Maximum dose	
		50th percentile	90th percentile	50th percentile	90th percentile
Aldicarb	10.4	0.00001	0.00004	0.0051	0.0193
Benfuracarb	20.1	0.00024	0.00040	0.0449	0.0821
Beta-cyfluthrin	3.3	0.00002	0.00003	0.0048	0.0073
Chlorpyrifos	20.4	0.00008	0.00016	0.0133	0.0258
Cypermethrin	64.8	0.00003	0.00014	0.0082	0.0374
Dichlorvos	5.1	0.00002	0.00005	0.0032	0.0069
Glyphosate	585.0	0.00008	0.00032	0.0267	0.1163
Malathion	745.0	0.00001	0.00001	0.0036	0.0080
Methiocarb	15.2	0.00001	0.00002	0.0028	0.0040
Oxamyl	2.6	0.00008	0.00014	0.0130	0.0248
Pirimicarb	57.0	0.00001	0.00012	0.0022	0.0497
Simazine	7.8	0.00008	0.00025	0.0104	0.0674
Thiodicarb	164.0	0.00001	0.00002	0.0144	0.0345

ADI, acceptable daily intake.

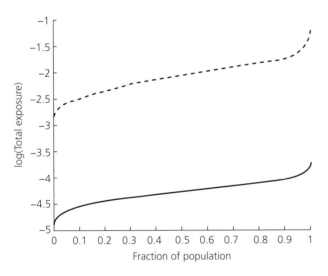

Figure 5.9 Total pesticide doses for anticholinesterase pesticides for adult non-vegetarians, distribution of daily median values and 90th percentile of the daily dose estimates. The solid line represents the median daily dose for an individual over the year, and the dotted line the maximum daily dose during the year, i.e. the highest daily dose for any 'individual' in the simulation.

human environmental exposures that may arise from occupational or hobby-related contact with pesticides.

CONCLUSION

In this chapter, we have seen how exposure to chemicals takes place through four main routes or interactions with the human body: via the lungs (inhalation), the skin (dermal and injection) and the gut (ingestion). We have identified the need to consider contributions from all of these routes when we are evaluating environmental exposures. Our perception of what constitutes the human environment needs to be broad in scope and has to bring together occupational, home-life, commuting, leisure and many other types of activity to allow an integrated conceptualization of how humans come into contact with chemicals that may have an effect on their health.

Methods of measuring exposures have developed greatly in recent years, with considerable overlap between the direct-reading instruments used for the assessment of occupational and environmental exposure. Many of these now provide real-time capability that allows a much more detailed understanding of how certain tasks or activities can influence concentrations of pollutants within the immediate vicinity of the person; they are therefore likely to help in future epidemiological studies to clarify exposure–response relationships. Tracking technology is now emerging and, coupled with small personal real-time exposure-monitoring devices, will in the coming decade transform the amount and quality of environmental exposure data that can be collected. There will be many challenges and opportunities in making best use of these data.

Not every type of environmental exposure can be measured. In some cases, the instruments are too large or bulky or the chemical analysis is prohibitively expensive. In these instances, exposure modelling can play an important role. Models are, however, only as good as the input or parameter data with which they are provided, so the conceptual stage of model development is particularly important. Going back to basics and identifying the steps involved in how exposure takes place is key to the development of any effective modelling system. A range of exposure models for a wide spectrum of occupational, consumer and environmental scenarios are now available, and most can provide exposure estimates using simple information relating to the context of the microenvironment and the activity taking place.

Bringing together exposure information across different human environments, integrating dietary, work and non-work chemical uptake and being able to consider the effect of chemical mixtures across the life-course are some of the key areas that environmental medicine has to consider in the twenty-first century.

REFERENCES

1. Pope CA, Ezzati M, Dockery DW. Fine-particulate air pollution and life expectancy in the United States. *N Engl J Med* 2009; **360**: 376–86.
2. Centers for Disease Control National Center for Environmental Health. *Third National Report on Human Exposure to Environmental Chemicals*. NCEH Publication No. 05-0570. Atlanta: NCEH, 2005.
3. European Union. What is Reach? Available from: http://ec.europa.eu/environment/chemicals/reach/reach_intro.htm (accessed January 20, 2010).
4. National Institute for Public Health and the Environment. Product Safety. Available from: http://www.rivm.nl/en/healthanddisease/productsafety/ConsExpo.jsp (accessed January 20, 2010).
5. Delgado Saborit JM, Aquilina NJ, Meddings C, Baker S, Harrison RM. Model development and validation of personal exposure to volatile organic compound concentrations. *Environ Health Perspect* 2009; **117**: 1571–9.
6. National Environmental Research Institute. Air Pollution Models. Available from: www.dmu.dk/International/Air/Models (accessed January 20, 2010).
7. Garthwaite DG, Thomas MR, Heywood E, Battersby A, for the Department for Environment, Food & Rural Affairs & Scottish Executive Environment & Rural Affairs Department. Arable Crops in Great Britain 2006 (Including Aerial Applications 2003-2006). Pesticide Usage Survey Report No. 213. Available from: http://www.fera.defra.gov.uk/plants/pesticideUsage/arable2006.pdf (accessed January 20, 2010).
8. Committee on Toxicity of Chemicals in Food, Consumer Products and the Environment. *Risk Assessment of Mixtures of Pesticides and Similar Substances*. London: Food Standards Agency, 2002.
9. Tran L, Glass R, Ritchie, P, Sleeuwenhoek A, MacCalman L, Cherrie JW. *Estimation of Human Intake of Pesticides from All Potential Pathways*. IOM Report TM/08/01. Edinburgh: Institute of Occupational Medicine, 2008.

RECOMMENDED READING

Bongers S, Janssen NA, Reiss B, Grievink L, Lebret E, Kromhout H. Challenges of exposure assessment for health studies in the aftermath of chemical incidents and disasters. *J Expo Sci Environ Epidemiol* 2008; **18**: 341–59.

Brunekreef B. Health effects of air pollution observed in cohort studies in Europe. *J Expo Sci Environ Epidemiol* 2007; **17**(Suppl. 2): S61–5.

Dahmann D, Taeger D, Kappler M *et al.* Assessment of exposure in epidemiological studies: The example of silica dust. *J Expo Sci Environ Epidemiol* 2008; **18**: 452–61.

Hellweg S, Demou E, Bruzzi R *et al.* Integrating human indoor air pollutant exposure within life cycle impact assessment. *Environ Sci Technol* 2009; **43**: 1670–9.

Jayjock MA, Chaisson CF, Arnold S, Dederick EJ. Modeling framework for human exposure assessment. *J Expo Sci Environ Epidemiol* 2007; **17**(Suppl. 1): S81–9.

Jerrett M, Arain A, Kanaroglou P *et al.* A review and evaluation of intraurban air pollution exposure models. *J Expo Anal Environ Epidemiol* 2005; **15**: 185–204.

Jurewicz J, Hanke W. Exposure to pesticides and childhood cancer risk: Has there been any progress in epidemiological studies? *Int J Occup Med Environ Health* 2006; **19**: 152–69.

Lioy PJ, Freeman NC, Millette JR. Dust: A metric for use in residential and building exposure assessment and source characterization. *Environ Health Perspect* 2002; **110**: 969–83.

Nieuwenhuijsen M. *Exposure Assessment in Occupational and Environmental Epidemiology*. Oxford: Oxford University Press, 2003.

Nieuwenhuijsen M, Paustenbach D, Duarte-Davidson R. New developments in exposure assessment: The impact on the practice of health risk assessment and epidemiological studies. *Environ Int* 2006; **32**: 996–1009.

Ramachandran G. Toward better exposure assessment strategies – the new NIOSH initiative. *Ann Occup Hyg* 2008; **52**: 297–301.

Rice PJ, Rice PJ, Arthur EL, Barefoot AC. Advances in pesticide environmental fate and exposure assessments. *J Agric Food Chem* 2007; **55**: 5367–76.

Wild CP. Environmental exposure measurement in cancer epidemiology. *Mutagenesis* 2009; **24**: 117–25.

Yantasee W, Lin Y, Hongsirikarn K, Fryxell GE, Addleman R, Timchalk C. Electrochemical sensors for the detection of lead and other toxic heavy metals: The next generation of personal exposure biomonitors. *Environ Health Perspect* 2007; **115**: 1683–90.

Zou B, Wilson JG, Zhan FB, Zeng Y. Air pollution exposure assessment methods utilized in epidemiological studies. *J Environ Monit* 2009; **11**: 475–90.

SHORT-RANGE PERSON-TO-PERSON MODELLING

DAVID CARRUTHERS

Modelling, or making quantitative predictions of concentrations of polluting material released into the atmosphere, has many applications. For regulated releases, these include calculating concentrations corresponding to air quality limits and odour thresholds. This requires consideration of a wide range of averaging times and for different emission situations – current or projected from possible future scenarios. For both regulated and accidental releases, predictions and forecasts are needed in real time to estimate over what area and for what period there may be adverse effects for people, animals or crops. In some cases, when the source location and/or source strength are not known, back calculations are also needed to estimate concentrations using, for example, meteorological and medical data as they are gathered. Where there is a potential adverse release scenario, modelling is also required so that risks and eventualities can be assessed in advance to determine whether that scenario (for instance, a development) is acceptable or to plan for emergencies.

Although many of the same basic physical and chemical processes determine the transport and diffusion of different releases, the best modelling approaches can be quite different for different situations depending on the size and complexity of the release, the scale over which the release has an impact, the nature of the underlying topography, the accuracy required, the type of scenario being considered and the time available for the calculations. Releases can be considered over short scales (see below), over large spatial scales and in urban areas (see boxes below) along with the complicating impacts of complex surface features on dispersion.

FACTORS AFFECTING SHORT-SCALE RELEASES

At the short-range or local scale (distances typically less than about 10 km downstream from the source) the key determining factors are the location, buoyancy and momentum of the source itself, the strength and direction of the mean wind and the characteristics of the turbulence between the 'source' and the 'receptor'. The momentum and the buoyancy are important in determining the initial motions of the release and its height, but mixing with ambient air generally proceeds rapidly so that material soon follows the motions of the ambient airflow. Typically, a dispersion model at short range needs to include each of these factors as illustrated in Figure 5.19, p. 100

TYPES OF MODEL

The most widely used modelling approach is the Gaussian plume model, which calculates the mean concentration assuming that the mean flow and turbulence are constant in time. The features of such a model generally include Gaussian or modified Gaussian profiles of concentration normal to the direction of the plume axis, which lies in the direction of the flow. In the simplest models of this type, the spread of the plume is related broadly to weather type or stability class, whereas more advanced approaches relate the plume spread more directly to the characteristics of the ambient turbulence by estimating its structure from parameters such as the boundary layer height and surface friction velocity. These can be estimated from standard meteorological data and surface properties including surface roughness. These simplified models can represent the considerable complexity of the processes and even estimate peak concentrations or concentration fluctuations over small time scales.

When the flow is unsteady, models require more extensive computation than the plume modelling approach and are based on methodologies similar to those used for meso-scale modelling (see boxes below). Common approaches include Lagrangian particle and Lagrangian puff modelling.

LONG-RANGE MODELLING

DAVID CARRUTHERS

Key factors determining the dispersion of toxic material close to the location of the release were discussed above. Sometimes a release is sufficiently large or toxic that it is important to model its development over larger scales (tens of kilometres or greater), and in these cases many different physical and chemical processes come into play. Examples are the release of radioactive material from the Chernobyl nuclear power station in 1985 and the fire at the Buncefield oil storage depot in the UK in 2005.

FACTORS AFFECTING LONG-RANGE RELEASES

Over these scales, it is no longer sufficient to assume that the material will be transported in the direction of the mean wind at the source and be dispersed by local turbulence. Both spatial and temporal changes in meteorology are important. Changes in the speed and direction of the wind in the vertical direction (vertical shear) can result in the dispersing cloud spreading out in different directions at different heights, as occurred at Buncefield. Horizontal spatial variations arise due to synoptic scale and smaller-scale meteorological effects and topographical influences such as hills or mountains or coastlines. The synoptic scale meteorological fields also change with time, which leads to changing patterns of dispersion.

Other processes that affect the nature of the plume over the regional scale include chemical or radioactive transformation (e.g. radioactive transformation of the Chernobyl plume) and dry and wet deposition processes. These both deplete the cloud within the atmosphere and cause accumulations of the toxic material at the earth's surface. Dry deposition results from turbulent diffusion of the material to the surface (particles and gases) and from gravitational settling (particles only). Wet deposition arises through washout of the material by rain. In addition, cloud material may be absorbed into cloud droplets, and these can deposit to the surface in the case of fog or hill cloud. Wet deposition was the principle reason why the Chernobyl accident had such an impact very far distant from the source, with the hills of north-west England and Wales receiving significant levels of radioactive material as a consequence of wet deposition from deep convective clouds. The different processes are illustrated in Figure 5.11.

MODELS USED

Modelling of the larger-scale releases uses a range of different methodologies. Most use as their starting point a numerical meteorological model (essentially a weather forecasting model) that predicts the spatially and temporally varying fields of parameters required for modelling dispersion, including mean wind, turbulence and temperature. These models provide input to the transport and diffusion models, which are generally of two types. In Eulerian models, the cloud advects and spreads through the model grid cells, the assumption being that the concentration is uniform in each cell so that gradients at higher spatial resolution are ignored. As well as dynamic effects, the concentration in each cell is subject to other physical and chemical effects such as wet deposition and radioactive decay. A Lagrangian model calculates the motions and physical and chemical changes in puffs or particles as they are advected along by the wind.

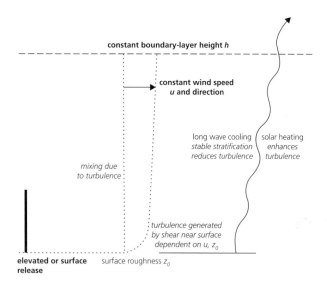

Figure 5.10 The materials emitted into the atmosphere–*the release*–may be buoyant or dense and may have initial momentum. The dispersing plume is typically within the atmospheric boundary layer.

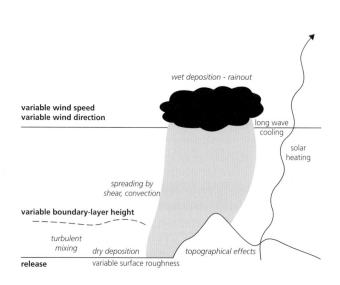

Figure 5.11 Plume often spreads to free troposphere. Meteorological variables are function of space and time.

DISPERSION IN CITIES

DAVID CARRUTHERS

In urban areas, buildings typically lie alongside open spaces, including streets and parks. There are considerable variations in the types, sizes and layouts of the buildings and streets from city to city and within individual cities. Over larger urban areas, there are usually also variations in the natural topography.

Modelling dispersion over such complex topography poses many problems, but progress can be made as urban-scale features (and hence local airflow and turbulence) typically have general characteristics on different scales. This allows different modelling approaches to be used at different scales and avoids the need for a 'one size fits all model', which may be operationally too complex and is too demanding for the available computer resources. The three scales are the building or street scale, the neighbourhood scale and the meso-scale (i.e. regional scale). As well as spatial scale, the methodologies also depend significantly on requirements for accuracy and speed of computation.

STREET SCALE

At the street scale, models need to resolve details of flow around individual buildings, including street canyons. The most accurate computational fluid dynamics models for calculating flow typically require a grid spacing of 1 m or less and a computational domain of greater than the building length scale (e.g. greater than 100 m). These models can use either Lagrangian or Eulerian dispersion models to resolve the detailed shape of the dispersing plume.

Very close to the source and before the plume has been advected or spread sufficiently for there to be interaction of the plume with the local buildings, the initial dispersion is similar to that for short-range modelling (see above) but, in this case, takes place in the higher levels of turbulence prevailing in urban areas. As the plume travels downstream, it is affected by the complex flows around the building structures, and the

details of flow around the buildings need to be well represented in the models.

Despite the large computer resources required, these most accurate models may still be overly sensitive to boundary conditions and parameterizations of turbulence at scales below the grid size. An alternative approach is to use faster approximate models where, for instance, flows around buildings are represented by 'typical' flows or where flows in street canyons are based on a semi-empirical formula.

NEIGHBOURHOOD SCALE

The neighbourhood scale represents scales up to about 5 km diameter, typical of the city centre of a large city. For these scales, numerical models use approximate representations of the buildings and open spaces, for example representing them by a porous medium or approximate shapes; they also use approximate turbulence models and input from larger-scale models for the boundary conditions. Typically, horizontal resolution is greater than the spacing between the buildings. Simpler, faster models may make use of perturbation models to calculate the change in flow from the background or upwind flow by representing buildings, open spaces, etc. with their average properties.

MESO-SCALE

At the largest urban scales, meso-scale meteorology models are used as inputs to dispersion models. These are similar to the models used for large-scale dispersion (see above) but typically use a higher resolution with grid cells of around 1–3 km over a domain of 30–100 km. Boundary conditions for these models comprise synoptic meteorological models and grids of averaged surface conditions, including surface roughness, to represent the surface features.

Mapping out the causes of infectious diseases: a case study on the multiple factors involved in *Salmonella* Enteritidis infections

GORDON L. NICHOLS

Infectious diseases can be transmitted by various transmission routes, including via food, water or air, through zoonotic contact, by direct contact with other infected people via skin, direct mucosal contact, respiratory secretions or sexual contact, from the environment within buildings including hospitals, as well as from the natural environment. Direct injection of pathogens into the body can occur from trauma, injection by syringe, biting insects or body piercing. Providing epidemiological evidence that a particular pathogen can infect people through a particular transmission route is obtained through case evidence, outbreaks and analytical studies (see Chapter 2) or through using animal models of transmission. This section examines the multiple factors that can contribute to an outbreak, using a *Salmonella* infection as an example.

Salmonella enterica serovar Enteritidis phage type 4 (SE4) has been present in the UK since the nineteenth century, and an understanding of the contamination of hens' eggs is not new.[1] The number of cases in England and Wales increased in the mid 1980s when it came to prominence as a zoonotic infection in chickens and as a cause of widespread disease in man (Figure 6a.1). As with other salmonellae, there is a regular seasonal pattern with more cases in the summer, thought to be related to warmer summer temperatures[2,3] and presumably reflecting a greater ability of the organism to grow in foods. The reason for its persistence within chicken populations is well described, as is the reason for the contamination of eggs.[4,5]

Its growth within eggs has been modelled,[6] and genes involved in the synthesis of fimbriae and flagella are important.[7,8] The structural and functional integrity of the cell wall, as well as the metabolism of nucleic acids and amino acids, appears to be important in allowing SE4 to persist in egg albumen.[9,10] A persistent problem in investigating the epidemiology of SE4 has been the clonal nature of the infections, with most isolates being identical for practical purposes.

Since the vaccination of first breeder and then layer flocks in the early 2000s, together with measures to improve on-farm biosecurity, the contamination of UK-produced chickens and eggs with SE4[11] and disease in humans[12] have both declined.

THE OUTBREAKS

In 2001, there was an increase in strains of *S.* Enteritidis phage types other than type 4 (SEN) that occurred in defined outbreaks. SEN isolates within individual outbreaks were often of a single phage type, but on microbiological sampling of the implicated eggs, several phage types were identified. The implicated eggs were imported from Spain, and the egg sampling suggested that the chicken flocks from which the eggs derived were infected with multiple types of *S.* Enteritidis. Because different locations were experiencing SEN outbreaks involving different phage types, there was a hypothesis that the outbreaks were due

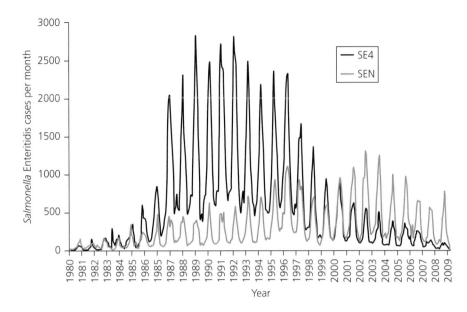

Figure 6a.1. *Salmonella* Enteritidis cases per month reported to national surveillance in England and Wales 1981–2009.*
* Cases are isolates reported to CDSC by specimen date. Cases for 2009 are provisional data that may increase with late reporting. The cases reported are those caused by *S.* Enteritidis PT4 (SE4) and those caused by all other *S.* Enteritidis (non-PT4) cases (SEN).

to a single cause and that this was eggs from Spain contaminated with a range of SEN phage types.

In developing a response to the series of outbreaks associated with SEN, there were a number of practical problems. The isolation of different SEN types from patients and eggs made the compiling of a sound evidence base difficult, as did inconsistencies in the local investigation of different outbreaks. A Public Health Investigation of eggs associated with these outbreaks was established, and eggs were sampled using a standard protocol. Specific details on the origin of the catering eggs were available for only some of the outbreaks, and this hampered the investigation. However, where information was available, it was clear that imported Spanish eggs were significantly more contaminated than UK-produced eggs from vaccinated flocks tested in previous surveys. The study also provided information on the range of SEN phage types that were found in Spanish eggs, indicating the types that might be expected to be affecting people.

IDENTIFICATION OF CONTRIBUTORY FACTORS

Investigation of the SEN problem identified that a number of possible contributory factors were playing a role in these outbreaks. These included the assumption that there was a contamination of Spanish flocks with many SEN types because these had been isolated from Spanish eggs. The reasons for this were assumed to be due to lack of vaccination of chicken flocks, and possibly poor standards of biosecurity on farms as well.[13] It was possible that there was poor temperature control of the eggs during transport that might have contributed to allowing SEN to grow within eggs, both as a result of reducing the resistance of the egg to SEN growth and through providing a suitable growth temperature for SEN. There were differences between catering and retail eggs in the rates of *Salmonella*

contamination, which could largely be attributed to the vaccination and biosecurity measures associated with the Lion Brand used on a high percentage of retail eggs in the UK. Within the catering eggs, there were large changes in the percentage of eggs imported from abroad and in the countries from where eggs were imported. Price differences were thought to be responsible for these changes.

In eggs used for catering, there was a higher than average rate of outbreaks linked to Chinese restaurants. The catering practices that may have contributed to outbreaks included:

- an incorrect storage temperature of whole eggs that allowed a breakdown of the vitelline membrane and the growth of SEN within them;[14,15]
- poor inventory control that allowed eggs to be stored for longer periods than is safe;
- the pooling of eggs so that one egg containing SEN could contaminate a large volume of raw egg;[16]
- an incorrect storage temperature of pooled egg, permitting the growth of SEN within the mixture;
- contamination of the kitchen environment with egg containing SEN;
- warmer temperatures in the summer;
- inadequate or flash cooking that did not completely kill SEN in the contaminated egg mix;
- incompletely reheating egg fried rice and storing it at room temperature, allowing SEN to regrow within the cooked egg fried rice.

Although definitive evidence of some of these factors is lacking, it is reasonable to imagine that the cause of an outbreak is not just the contamination of Spanish eggs but a variety of other less tangible contributing factors with comparatively little supporting evidence for these. Throughout the outbreak, it remained unclear whether the contamination rate of Spanish eggs sampled during outbreak investigations represented a small subset of all Spanish eggs or was common for all such eggs, with the other contributing factors causing an amplification of SEN numbers in the eggs associated with outbreaks.

ESTABLISHMENT OF AN OUTBREAK TEAM

The single most important event within the SEN outbreak was the establishment of a National Outbreak Control Team (NOCT) with a chair who was an epidemiologist from a non-gastrointestinal background and who could provide an independent evaluation of the problem. The NOCT involved people from the Food Standards Agency, the Department for Environment, Food and Rural Affairs, people involved in the individual outbreaks, staff from the Communicable Disease Surveillance Centre and the Specialist and Reference Laboratory Division, public health physicians and food-testing experts from Local and Regional Services, and experts from Scotland, Wales, Northern Ireland and the Netherlands. Information from Enternet was used to assess the impact of SEN across Europe. The NOCT provided a forum for tabling data, airing ideas and focusing on possible interventions. It also allowed evidence from the Netherlands, where an outbreak of avian flu in poultry had resulted in a large chicken cull and a need to import eggs. This was accompanied by a rise in SEN.

CONTROL MEASURES

During the course of the outbreak, a number of initiatives were undertaken to control the outbreak. Although the egg-labelling regulations were not a specific initiative of the NOCT, their implementation in 2005 led to an improvement in information about the source of eggs associated with outbreaks. The apparent absence of an SEN problem associated with eggs bought at retail (predominantly Lion Brand) meant that there was not a significant loss of confidence on the part of consumers in eggs bought at retail. However, SE4 cases and outbreaks associated with UK-produced eggs that are from non-vaccinated flocks have continued to occur. Discussions with egg importers led to action by them in temporarily sourcing eggs from other countries, with an associated reduction in SEN. There was also an initiative to inform Chinese restaurant owners of the problems associated with eggs. A dossier of evidence was submitted to the Health Protection Agency Board, Food Standards Agency and Spanish and European Authorities, and there was also an official meeting with Spanish colleagues to discuss the details of the Health Protection Agency evidence.

One concern associated with the restriction of imports of Spanish eggs was not to breach free trade rules. Another was that restricting import into the UK might result in the problem being transferred to other European countries.

There were questions about how much supporting evidence was required before communicating the risks to Spanish authorities. Because most European Union countries do not phage-type human isolates of S. Enteritidis, it is less easy to determine the rise in SEN strains. The dramatic reduction in SE4 in England and Wales has continued, and the burden of illness associated with S. Enteritidis-contaminated eggs has been recognized and acted on at a European level.

One pressure to intervene comes from the Zoonosis Directive (2003/99/EC), which requires that countries monitor zoonoses and zoonotic agents in feeding-stuffs, animals and foodstuffs along the food chain, and evidence of antibiotic resistance. They must report this to the Commission annually, along with information on food-borne outbreaks. Through the Zoonosis Directive, there is a European initiative to reduce the contamination of chicken flocks with Salmonella through regular litter sampling for Salmonella and restricting the sale of unpasteurized eggs from Salmonella-positive flocks.

There appear to be substantial differences in the risks to travellers that are thought to reflect the disease burden across Europe.[17] In trying to reduce S. Enteritidis within Europe, there need to be consistent approaches to the vaccination of breeder and layer flocks, improved subtyping and European surveillance of Salmonella isolates, and advice to the catering industry in all countries about the good and bad practices that contribute to human infection. Although it is still not practical to consider eggs as a ready-to-eat food because of the relatively high rate of contamination of some imported eggs, it is still relatively common for eggs to be used within commercial kitchens as ingredients requiring little or no additional cooking. This needs to be improved either through education or by ensuring that eggs do not contain S. Enteritidis, or both. In addition, there is strong experimental evidence that the temperature and duration of storage of eggs have a strong impact on the number of organisms that can be recovered from eggs. This suggests that temperature control throughout production, wholesale, retail and use is important, although not necessarily easy or cheap, as an intervention.

The example provided by S. Enteritidis infection highlights the potentially complex causes of infections that can result from a mixture of microbiological and host factors, agricultural, food chain, wholesale and retail practices, kitchen practices and hygiene, as well as national and international controls. Where there is an infection problem, be it an outbreak or sporadic disease, that will not respond to normal infection control measures, there is a need to get political engagement with the problem so that actions to reduce disease are possible. The political engagement can be through various government departments but can also be triggered by a particularly prominent outbreak that grabs the public attention. What is important for this is mapping out the problem using good quality information on what is causing the outbreak and what interventions are possible and likely to be effective.

In this example, the phage-typing results, together with the examination of egg contamination, and good epidemiological investigation played an important role in sorting out many of the causes. Many other European Union countries do not use phage-typing and are therefore less easily able to address the problem. The longer term control measures with the monitoring of chicken flocks across Europe and increased vaccination and improved biosecurity are likely to take some years to bear fruit. There needs to be both candor and care in how the problem is addressed politically. The resignation of Edwina Curry in December 1988 after she had caused a slump in egg sales through saying that 'most of the egg production in this country, sadly, is now affected with Salmonella' emphasizes that the public communication of scientific health messages needs to be handled carefully. The intervention to control SE4 took 10 years to implement in an effective way. In the interval between identifying the problem and effective intervention, it is possible that over half a million people in England and Wales may have been infected. The time period for SEN reduction could take a similar time.

REFERENCES

◆ = Major review article

1. Haines RB, Moran T. Porosity of and invasion through the shell of the hen's egg. *J Hyg (Camb)* 1940; **40**: 453.
2. Lake IR, Gillespie IA, Bentham G *et al.* A re-evaluation of the impact of temperature and climate change on foodborne illness. *Epidemiol Infect* 2009; **137**: 1538–47.
3. Kovats RS, Edwards SJ, Hajat S, Armstrong BG, Ebi KL, Menne B. The effect of temperature on food poisoning: A time-series analysis of salmonellosis in ten European countries. *Epidemiol Infect* 2004; **132**: 443–53.
4. Mizumoto N, Sasai K, Tani H, Baba E. Specific adhesion and invasion of *Salmonella* Enteritidis in the vagina of laying hens. *Vet Microbiol* 2005; **111**(1–2): 99–105.
5. De Buck J, Van Immerseel F, Haesebrouck F, Ducatelle R. Colonization of the chicken reproductive tract and egg contamination by *Salmonella. J Appl Microbiol* 2004; **97**: 233–45.
6. Grijspeerdt K, Kreft JU, Messens W. Individual-based modelling of growth and migration of *Salmonella*

enteritidis in hens' eggs. *Int J Food Microbiol* 2005; **100**(1–3): 323–33.
7. De Buck J, Van Immerseel F, Haesebrouck F, Ducatelle R. Effect of type 1 fimbriae of *Salmonella enterica* serotype Enteritidis on bacteraemia and reproductive tract infection in laying hens. *Avian Pathol* 2004; **33**: 314–20.
8. Cogan TA, Jorgensen F, Lappin-Scott HM, Benson CE, Woodward MJ, Humphrey TJ. Flagella and curli fimbriae are important for the growth of *Salmonella enterica* serovars in hen eggs. *Microbiology* 2004; **150**(Pt 4): 1063–71.
9. Clavijo RI, Loui C, Andersen GL, Riley LW, Lu S. Identification of genes associated with survival of *Salmonella enterica* serovar Enteritidis in chicken egg albumen. *Appl Environ Microbiol* 2006; **72**: 1055–64.
10. Lu S, Killoran PB, Riley LW. Association of *Salmonella enterica* serovar enteritidis yafD with resistance to chicken egg albumen. *Infect Immun* 2003; **71**: 6734–41.
11. Elson R, Little CL, Mitchell RT. Salmonella and raw shell eggs: Results of a cross-sectional study of contamination rates and egg safety practices in the United Kingdom catering sector in 2003. *J Food Prot* 2005; **68**: 256–64.
◆12. Cogan TA, Humphrey TJ. The rise and fall of *Salmonella* Enteritidis in the UK. *J Appl Microbiol* 2003; **94**(Suppl.): 114S–19S.
13. Liebana E, Garcia-Migura L, Clouting C, Clifton-Hadley FA, Breslin M, Davies RH. Molecular fingerprinting evidence of the contribution of wildlife vectors in the maintenance of *Salmonella* Enteritidis infection in layer farms. *J Appl Microbiol* 2003; **94**: 1024–9.
14. Chen J, Shallo TH, Kerr WL. Outgrowth of salmonellae and the physical property of albumen and vitelline membrane as influenced by egg storage conditions. *J Food Prot* 2005; **68**: 2553–8.
15. Fleischman GJ, Napier CL, Stewart D, Palumbo SA. Effect of temperature on the growth response of *Salmonella* enteritidis inoculated onto the vitelline membranes of fresh eggs. *J Food Prot* 2003; **66**: 1368–73.
16. Little CL, Suman-Lee S, Greenwood M *et al.* Public health investigations of *Salmonella* Enteritidis in catering raw shell eggs, 2002–2004. *Lett Appl Microbiol* 2007; **44**(6): 595–601.
17. de Jong B, Ekdahl K. The comparative burden of salmonellosis in the European Union member states, associated and candidate countries. *BMC Public Health* 2006; **6**: 4.

6b

Mapping the causes and transmission routes of chemicals

MATHEW R. HEAL

For people to be adversely affected by a chemical pollutant, it needs to be present in some part of the environment to which people are exposed, at a concentration sufficient to cause harm. In the most straightforward case, the pollutant is released directly into a relevant exposure environment; for example the emission of radon gas into indoor air from the underlying bedrock.

In general, however, the transmission routes between sources of pollutant and exposure of a human 'receptor' are more complex and influenced by many factors, such as transport of the pollutant away from the source, transfer of the pollutant between different compartments, or phases, of the environment (e.g. between land, water, air and biological material) and chemical transformations. These processes are controlled by physicochemical properties of the pollutant such as volatility, aqueous solubility, lipophilicity (the solubility in organic/biological material) and reactivity. If the lifetime of the pollutant is long compared with time scales for its dispersion, its distribution in the environment is determined by its partitioning between different environmental compartments (as, for example, for chemicals within the class of compounds known as persistent organic pollutants, or POPs). If the lifetime of the pollutant is short, its distribution in the environment reflects that of its sources and the local dispersion processes.

Insight into the causes and transmission routes of a given pollutant usually requires both measurements and modelling. The most basic models construct empirical relationships between source and receptor observations and assume that these relationships hold for different times and places. Process-based models seek to describe mathematically all relevant processes influencing pollutant transmission and transformation. Spatial mapping techniques may form part of the modelling process or simply facilitate spatial interpolation between point measurements or model output.

MEASUREMENT OF CHEMICAL TRANSMISSION ROUTES

Many environmental media (e.g. the atmosphere, surface and ground waters, soil and food) are subject to routine monitoring for hazardous components. The monitoring approaches involved for specific media are described in other chapters but may typically comprise fixed monitoring networks and schedules for continuous or periodic measurements at designated locations and times. The impetus for much of the measurement is often the need to check for compliance of concentrations against specified standards, but well-designed sampling regimes will provide insight into pollutant sources and transmission routes. Geostatistical techniques such as Kriging may be applied to interpolate between point measurements and produce spatially contiguous pollutant concentration maps (see the box on the application of geospatial technologies to medical studies, p. 109).[1]

Some measurement techniques provide data over a large area or volume simultaneously. For example, some portable spectroscopy systems can provide concentrations of airborne pollutants (e.g. nitrogen dioxide, sulphur dioxide or benzene) over distances of several hundred metres.[2] By scanning the angle of the receiving spectrometer above the horizontal, or using multi-axis telescopes simultaneously, it is possible to extract both vertically and horizontally resolved pollutant concentration profiles.[3] Remote sensing platforms can provide direct or indirect maps of pollutant concentrations over large areas, up to global coverage. For example, airborne gamma-ray spectrometry provides maps of surface radioactivity arising from known or accidental discharges, such as deposition of caesium-137 from the Chernobyl nuclear accident.[4] Instruments on orbiting or geostationary satellites provide an enormous variety of spatial data to map sources and movement of pollutants, including, for example, concentrations of atmospheric pollutants such as nitrogen dioxide[5] or the identification of freshwater or coastal algal blooms indicative of potential toxin exposure.[6]

Environmental biomonitors provide an indirect method of mapping hazardous pollutant burden, for example the assessment of sexual maturation in fish and other aquatic organisms as an indicator of exposure to oestrogen-like chemicals in surface waters,[7] or the health status of designated plants as a measure of exposure to air pollution.[8] Direct evidence of an individual's exposure to particular chemicals may be derived from an analysis of human biological samples; for example lead in blood, arsenic in urine or POPs in blood or breast milk.

MODELLING OF CHEMICAL TRANSMISSION ROUTES

Empirical models for associating receptor concentrations with particular pollution sources rely on deriving statistical relationships between the two. The underlying principle is conservation of chemical species. If the emission profile of all sources is known, full-source apportionment is, in principle, achievable through chemical mass balance. This 'end member' approach is widely used to determine the hydrological pathways of pollutant contamination in rivers, lakes and sediments.[9] Often, however, information on some or all of the contributing sources is lacking. In this case, modelling may use 'exploratory' multivariate statistical techniques such as principal component and factor analysis to extract correlations between species concentrations at the receptor, which may in turn reflect the commonality of contributing sources. No knowledge of the source profiles is required, although an emphasis on particular species, or 'tracers', in each factor aids interpretation of the likely physical sources. These methods have been particularly developed for source apportionment of air pollution.[10]

In a variant of the empirical approach, land-use regression modelling, a multiple regression relationship is developed between a dataset of pollutant observations and putative surrogate predictor variables for sources of that pollutant. Variables that often turn out to be significant predictors of high concentrations of air pollution, for example, include distance from the nearest major road, density of surrounding housing and altitude (the latter in an inverse sense since higher altitude usually leads on average to greater wind dilution).[11]

In process-based modelling, the transport and transformation of the pollutant through the environment are explicitly described as far as possible. The most widely deployed models of this kind are dispersion models, which are used to model the dispersal of a pollutant from discrete sources such as chimneys and roads, or effluent discharge into rivers (see the boxes following Chapter 5, p. 99). The alternative process-based approach is the grid model, in which the volume to be modelled is divided into discrete cells, each of which is subject to mass balance at each time step according to the emission, loss and chemical transformations within the cell and the transport of material across the boundaries with neighbouring cells.

These models are conventionally run forwards in time to map the transmission of pollutants through the environment from known sources. However, it is in certain circumstances possible, given observations at receptor locations, to run them backwards to derive information about the sources of pollution, a procedure known as inverse modelling. For example, the UK Met Office 'NAME' Lagrangian dispersion model has been inverted to derive annual-average source emission maps of greenhouse and ozone-depleting gases over Europe.[12] The method is best suited to locating sources of species whose lifetime is long compared with the time scale of dispersion.

A powerful approach to mapping the transmission and distribution of long-lived chemical contaminants, particularly semi-volatile organic pollutants, is 'fugacity' modelling.[13] At its simplest, fugacity modelling is an equilibrium mass-balance calculation of the propensity of a pollutant to apportion between different environmental compartments (air, water, soil, lipid material in biota, etc.), as determined by properties of the pollutant such as volatility and aqueous solubility. The volumes and physical properties of each environmental compartment in the model are set up to emulate their real-world counterparts. Increasing sophistications of fugacity modelling allow for a continuous or intermittent input of the pollutant into different compartments, the kinetics of the transport between compartments, and rates of degradation.[14] The model effectively accounts for the bioconcentration (Box 6b.1) of many pollutants (e.g. POPs) in animals, including humans, compared with the concentrations in the surrounding media of water, air or plants. The approach also explains the migration of POPs into polar regions remote from their sources.[15]

BOX 6b.1: Bioconcentration, bioaccumulation and biomagnification

Bioconcentration occurs within a food-chain level and is the increase in concentration of a chemical in an individual organism's tissues due to a greater affinity of the chemical for the tissue compared with the surrounding environment or food of the individual. Examples of chemicals that bioconcentrate included persistent organic pollutants, methylmercury, tetraethyl lead and algal toxins.

Bioaccumulation is a term often used interchangeably with bioconcentration, although it is sometimes used in respect of a kinetic explanation for the increasing concentration of a chemical in an organism due to the rate of intake exceeding the rate of excretion.

Biomagnification is the increase in concentration of a chemical in organisms higher up the food chain as a consequence of feeding on contaminated organisms lower down.

REFERENCES

● = Key primary paper
◆ = Major review article

1. Lindley SJ, Walsh T. Inter-comparison of interpolated background nitrogen dioxide concentrations across Greater Manchester, UK. *Atmos Environ* 2005; 39: 2709–24.
2. Chiu KH, Sree U, Tseng SH *et al.* Differential optical absorption spectrometer measurement of NO_2, SO_2, O_3, HCHO and aromatic volatile organics in ambient air of Kaohsiung Petroleum Refinery in Taiwan. *Atmos Environ* 2005; 39: 941–55.
3. Leigh RJ, Corlett GK, Friess U *et al.* Spatially resolved measurements of nitrogen dioxide in an urban environment using concurrent multi-axis differential optical absorption spectroscopy. *Atmos Chem Phys* 2007; 7: 4751–62.
4. Sanderson DCW, Cresswell AJ, White DC. The effect of flight line spacing on radioactivity inventory and spatial feature characteristics of airborne gamma-ray spectrometry data. *Int J Remote Sens* 2008; 29: 31–46.
●5. Toenges-Schuller N, Stein O, Rohrer F *et al.* Global distribution pattern of anthropogenic nitrogen oxide emissions: correlation analysis of satellite measurements and model calculations. *J Geophys Res* 2006; 111: D05312, doi:10.1029/2005JD006068.
6. Tomlinson MC, Stumpf RP, Ransibrahmanakul V *et al.* Evaluation of the use of SeaWiFS imagery for detecting *Karenia brevis* harmful algal blooms in the eastern Gulf of Mexico. *Remote Sens Environ* 2004; 91: 293–303.
7. Liney KE, Hagger JA, Tyler CR *et al.* Health effects in fish of long-term exposure to effluents from wastewater treatment works. *Environ Health Perspect* 2006; 114: 81–9.
8. Smith G, Coulston J, Jepsen E *et al.* A national ozone biomonitoring program – Results from field surveys of ozone sensitive plants in northeastern forests (1994–2000). *Environ Monit Assess* 2003; 87: 271–91.
9. Hyer KE, Hornberger GM, Herman JS. Processes controlling the episodic streamwater transport of atrazine and other agrichemicals in an agricultural watershed. *J Hydrol* 2001; 254: 47–66.
◆10. Viana M, Kuhlbusch TAJ, Querol X *et al.* Source apportionment of particulate matter in Europe: a review of methods and results. *J Aerosol Sci* 2008; 39: 827–49.
◆11. Hoek G, Beelen R, de Hoogh K *et al.* A review of land-use regression models to assess spatial variation of outdoor air pollution. *Atmos Environ* 2008; 42: 7561–78.
●12. Manning AJ, Ryall DB, Derwent RG *et al.* Estimating European emissions of ozone-depleting and greenhouse gases using observations and a modeling back-attribution technique. *J Geophys Res* 2003; 108: 4405.
◆13. Mackay D. *Multimedia Environmental Models: The Fugacity Approach*, 2nd ed. Boca Raton, FL: Lewis, 2001.
◆14. Wania F, Mackay D. The evolution of mass balance models of persistent organic pollutant fate in the environment. *Environ Pollut* 1999; 100: 223–40.
15. Wania F. Assessing the potential of persistent organic chemicals for long-range transport and accumulation in polar regions. *Environ Sci Technol* 2003; 37: 1344–51.

THE APPLICATION OF GEOSPATIAL TECHNOLOGIES TO MEDICAL STUDIES

DAVID R. GREEN

One way to explore spatial data and present the results of spatial analyses utilizes geographical information systems (GIS). Two-dimensional choropleth or symbol maps are the usual form of output. Increasingly, GIS functionality provides more than just a digital mapping toolbox, including the capability for spatial and network analyses, three-dimensional visualization and environmental modelling. GIS can also handle data from many disparate data sources, including remote sensing (satellite imagery and aerial photographs) and global positioning systems (GPS). The latter provide for the high-accuracy capture of spatial locations and an array of attributes including ground-based photographic records, text descriptions and environmental sensor data. Recent developments in this technology have also led to decision support systems,[1] online Internet mapping capability, mashups and real-time environmental monitoring, providing powerful and flexible ways to manage resources, access information and engage with the public.

Many GIS-based medical and health applications have been reported in the literature,[2,3] including:

mapping applications;[4] exploratory data analysis;[5] studies analysing the distribution and spread of disease;[6] proximity studies;[7,8] the study of exposure to pollution sources, for example factories, roads and airports (Figure 6B.1); cluster analysis;[9–11] identification of the significance and sources of disease outbreaks and the links between health and pollution;[12] and the use of spatial techniques such as Kriging analysis to generate surfaces.[13]

In addition, remotely sensed data have been used as a source of environmental information to correlate with health data.[14] Terrain data provide the means to consider the influence of both natural and manmade surface topography on local climate (temperature, wind direction and speed) and on observed air and noise pollution patterns. Spatial data can also be used in GIS-based pollution models.[15] Personal and environmental data can now be gathered using small GPS-based sensors to track individuals and their conditions over space and time.[16] This information can subsequently be integrated into a GIS with other spatial data that may have an explanatory role. Spatiotemporal relationships can also be studied[17,18]

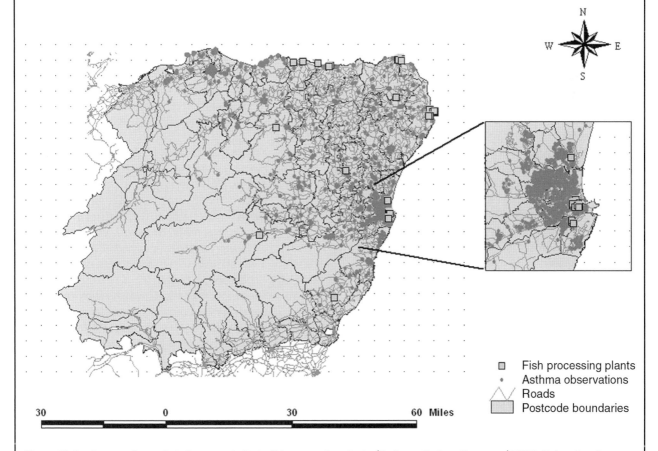

Fish processing plants
Asthma observations
Roads
Postcode boundaries

Figure 6b.1   Acute asthma admissions: proximity to fish-processing plants. (Professor Graham Devereux (DEOM, University of Abedeen) provided the fish processing plant data and asthma data used in the GIS map.)

using visualization tools[19-21] for data exploration and the generation of map animations that alert the viewer visually to any hotspots of change over time.

Although the mapping and visualization of datasets remains the most common and obvious visual (both hard- and soft-copy) output from a GIS and the related geospatial technologies, the real power of GIS lies in its potential to generate new datasets, explore datasets, utilize tools and techniques for spatial analysis, and interface with modelling and simulation tools. This is already being significantly enhanced by the addition of further utilities, specialized functionality, spatial statistics and process-based modelling tools.

References

1. Scotcha M, Parmantoa B. Development of SOVAT: a numerical–spatial decision support system for community health assessment research. *Int J Med Inform* 2006; **75**: 771–84.
2. Kamel Boulos, MN, Roudsari, AV, Carson, ER. Health geomatics: an enabling suite of technologies in health and healthcare. *J Biomed Inform* 2001; **34**: 195–219.
3. Foody GM GIS: health applications. *Prog Phys Geogr* 2006; **30**: 691–5.
4. Bautista CT, Sateren WB, Sanchez JL, Singer JE, Scott P. Geographic mapping of HIV infection among civilian applicants for United States military service. *Health Place* 2008; **14**: 608–15.
5. Bhowmick T, Griffin AL, MacEachren AM, Kluhsman BC, Lengerich EJ. Informing geospatial toolset design: understanding the process of cancer data exploration and analysis. *Health Place* 2008; **14**: 576–607.
6. Rogers DJ, Randolph SE. Studying the global distribution of infectious diseases using GIS and RS. *Nat Rev Microbiol* 2003; **1**: 231–7.
7. Royster MO, Hilborn ED, Barr D, Carty CC, Rhoneya S, Walsh D. A pilot study of global positioning system/geographical information system measurement of residential proximity to agricultural fields and urinary organophosphate metabolite concentrations in toddlers. *J Expo Anal Environ Epidemiol* 2002; **12**: 433–40.
8. Green RS, Smorodinsky S, Kim JJ, McLaughlin R, Ostro B. Proximity of California public schools to busy roads. *Environ Health Perspect* 2004; **112**: 61–6.
9. Lai PC, Wong CM, Hedley AJ *et al.* Understanding the spatial clustering of severe acute respiratory syndrome (SARS) in Hong Kong. *Environ Health Perspect* 2004; **112**: 1550–6.
10. Trooskin SB, Hadler J, St Louis T, Navarro VJ. Geospatial analysis of hepatitis C in Connecticut: a novel application of a public health tool. *Public Health* 2005; **119**: 1042–7.
11. Wen T-H, Lin N-H, Lin C-H, King C-C, Su M-D. Spatial mapping of temporal risk characteristics to improve environmental health risk identification: a case study of a dengue epidemic in Taiwan. *Sci Total Environ* 2006; **367**: 630–40.
12. Gram F, Nafsted P, Haheim LL. Estimating residential air pollution exposure among citizens in Oslo 1974–1998 using a geographical information system. *J Environ Monit* 2003; **5**: 541–6.
13. Guo D, Guo R, Thiart C. Predicting air pollution using fuzzy membership grade kriging. *Comput Environ Urban Syst* 2007; **31**: 33–51.
14. Herbreteaua V, Salema G, Souris M, Hugot J-P, Gonzalez J-P. Thirty years of use and improvement of remote sensing, applied to epidemiology: from early promises to lasting frustration. *Health Place* 2007; **13**: 400–3.
15. Cyrys J, Hochadel M, Gehring U *et al.* GIS-based estimation of exposure to particulate matter and NO_2 in an urban area: stochastic versus dispersion modeling. *Environ Health Perspect* 2005; **113**: 987–92.
16. Elgethun K, Fenske RA, Yost MG, Palcisko GJ. Time-location analysis for exposure assessment studies of children using a novel global positioning system instrument. *Environ Health Perspect* 2003; **111**: 115–22.
17. Gulliver J, Briggs DJ. Time-space modelling of journey-time exposure to traffic-related air pollution using GIS. *Environ Res* 2005; **97**: 10–25.
18. Yanosky JD, Paciorek CP, Schwartza J, Ladena F, Puetta R, Suha HH. Spatio-temporal modeling of chronic PM10 exposure for the nurses' health study. *Atmos Environ* 2008; **42**: 4047–62.
19. AvRuskin GA, Jacquez GM, Meliker JR, Slotnick MJ, Kaufmann AM, Nriagu JO. Visualization and exploratory analysis of epidemiologic data using a novel space time information system. *Int J Health Geogr* 2004; **3**: 26.
20. Koua EL, Kraak M-J. Geovisualization to support the exploration of large health and demographic survey data. *Int J Health Geogr* 2004; **3**: 12
21. Meliker JR, Slotnick MJ, AvRuskin GA, Kaufmann A, Jacquez GM, Nriagu JO. Improving exposure assessment in environmental epidemiology: application of spatio-temporal visualization tools. *J Geogr Syst* 2005; **7**: 49–66.

7

Measuring the atmosphere

MATHEW R. HEAL

As well as the familiar constituents of nitrogen, oxygen, carbon dioxide and water vapour, the atmosphere contains hundreds of other gaseous constituents that are present in very low concentrations (typically parts per billion, ppb, or less; Box 7.1) but which nevertheless have an impact on the environment and human health.[1,2] In addition, airborne particulate matter (PM) constitutes an important non-gaseous component of the atmosphere. This encompasses any solid, liquid or mixed solid–liquid material capable of remaining suspended in the atmosphere for at least a few hours (but often for days or weeks).

Some of these trace constituents may be present in the atmosphere as a result of direct emissions from natural or manmade sources ('primary' components), but the majority are 'secondary' components formed within the atmosphere by the chemical reactions of primary precursors. The lifetimes of different components in the atmosphere range from less than a few minutes to more than a century. Dispersion and transport processes within the atmosphere also contribute to determining the widely varying spatial and temporal patterns in atmospheric concentrations of different components.

A number of the trace species present in the atmosphere are identified as having the potential to cause harm to human health via exposure by inhalation.[3,4] Policy is therefore established in many countries around the world to understand and mitigate such exposure. Measurement of the atmosphere is consequently undertaken for a number of purposes:

- to understand processes affecting atmospheric composition, including provision of data for the testing and validation of models;
- to help identify and quantify human exposure to, and any adverse effects from, particular atmospheric components;
- to monitor effectiveness of air quality management policies;
- to inform the public;
- to comply with legislation.

Measurements may be undertaken through fixed networks of permanent monitors or through intensive campaigns of temporary monitoring. The ad hoc deployment of monitors may also be required in the event of accidental or intentional (e.g. sabotage or terrorism) release of hazardous components into the atmosphere.

BOX 7.1: Quantifying atmospheric abundances

Atmospheric abundances are often expressed as the volumetric mixing ratio (ppm, ppb, etc.), which is simply the fraction of molecules of the species under consideration relative to the total number of all gas molecules present. The advantages of using mixing ratio over a mass per volume expression of concentration (e.g. $\mu g/m^3$) are that it is invariant to changes in the pressure or temperature of the air, and that it is independent of the identity (i.e. molecular mass) of the species and therefore enables a direct comparison of the relative amounts of different species present at a given location. For legislation purposes, however, atmospheric trace species concentrations usually need to be quantified in mass per volume units at a specified temperature and pressure.

HAZARDOUS AIR POLLUTANTS AND AIR QUALITY STANDARDS

Evidence for an airborne hazard often derives in the first instance from experience in an occupational setting where exposures are usually higher and cohorts of individual subjects are available for detailed study. This can be particularly useful for quantifying ill-health arising from chronic exposures, for example from the inhalation of carcinogens such as benzene, 1,3-butadiene or chromium. Supplementary evidence may be derived from controlled exposure studies on animal models or human volunteers, particularly for air pollutants with acute effects such as ozone (O_3), nitrogen dioxide (NO_2) or sulphur dioxide (SO_2). Hazards may also be identified by a prior knowledge of harmful effects through other exposure routes, for example the effects on health of lead, arsenic and mercury from the ingestion of contaminated water and food.

In the ambient air pollution setting, the main approach for quantifying acute and chronic dose responses at the population scale is through time series and cohort epidemiological studies, respectively. Various expert groups worldwide, for example through the World Health Organization, have identified air pollutants whose concentrations in ambient air may cause an unacceptable morbidity and/or mortality burden, and make recommendations on ambient atmospheric concentrations to reduce or eliminate this burden.[3,4] Achievement of the latter depends on whether a threshold exposure below which there is no discernible adverse health effect exists and is practically attainable.

Recommendations may subsequently become incorporated into legislation as air quality standards (AQSs). For example, Tables 7.1 and 7.2 list ambient air pollutants specified in current European Union Directives, while Table 7.3 lists the 'criteria' air pollutants subject to US legislation. The US air quality process also includes a consideration of standards for protection of the wider environment as well as human health. The resulting legislation usually also embodies a responsibility on national and local governments to assess the quality of the air within their jurisdiction and to declare air quality management plans where the need for remedial action is identified.

Air pollutants may have more than one AQS, as with NO_2, because of evidence for an effect on health from both short-term peaks in concentration and long-term cumulative exposure. For some pollutants, a number of breaches of the headline AQS are allowed. These permitted excess values recognize the practical difficulty in sustaining 100 per cent compliance with the specified concentration, for example due to the long-range transport of a pollutant or sustained adverse meteorology, or the desire to allow occasional distinct activities to continue that might otherwise need to be banned (e.g. celebrations with fireworks). The current emphasis in air quality management on fixed-concentration AQS necessarily targets resources

Table 7.1 Limit values and target values for outdoor air pollutants as specified in European Union (EU) Directive 2008/50/EC

Pollutant[1]	Measured as	EU limit value[†]
Sulphur dioxide	1 h mean	350 μg/m^3 not to be exceeded more than 24 times a year
	24 h mean	125 μg/m^3 not to be exceeded more than 3 times a year
Nitrogen dioxide	1 h mean	200 μg/m^3 not to be exceeded more than 18 times a year
	Annual mean	40 μg/m^3
Benzene	Annual mean	5 μg/m^3
Carbon monoxide	Maximum daily running 8 h mean	10 mg/m^3
Lead	Annual mean	0.5 μg/m^3
PM$_{10}$	24 h mean	50 μg/m^3 not to be exceeded more than 35 times a year
	Annual mean	40 μg/m^3
PM$_{2.5}$	Annual mean	25 μg/m^3 (by 1st January 2015) 20 μg/m^3 (by 1st January 2020)

Pollutant	Measured as	EU target value[‡]
PM$_{2.5}$	Annual mean	20% population-weighted reduction in concentrations at urban background
Ozone	Maximum daily running 8 h mean	120 μg/m^3 not to be exceeded on more than 25 days per year averaged over 3 years

PM$_{10}$, PM$_{2.5}$, all particles in the air with a diameter of less than 10 μm and less than 2.5 μm, respectively.
[†] Legally binding parameters.
[‡] To be attained where possible by taking all necessary measures not entailing disproportionate costs, but not legally binding.
[1] The UK also has in force an objective for 1,3-butadiene of 2.25 μg/m^3 as a running annual mean.

on those 'hotspots' where AQSs are breached (see also 'Monitoring networks', below).

In addition to the 'standard' suite of ambient air pollutants listed in Tables 7.1–7.3, many other trace species may constitute a health hazard by inhalation, in particular radon, formaldehyde (HCHO), and many semi-volatile members of the generic categorization of persistent organic pollutants (POPs) such as certain polychlorinated biphenyls (PCBs), polybrominated diphenyl ethers

(PBDEs) or hexabromocyclododecanes (HBCDs). Outside occupational settings, however, the dominant atmospheric exposure to these chemicals for affected individuals is likely to be through the inhalation of indoor air where a lack of ventilation leads to accumulation.

The control of potential localized human exposure to many other airborne toxins, for example hydrogen chloride gas or other chlorinated solvents, is undertaken through the regulation and control of emissions from their limited point sources rather than through the ambient AQS/air quality management process.

AIRBORNE PARTICULATE MATTER

In contrast to the discrete nature of an individual gas pollutant, the designation of airborne PM encompasses an extremely diverse collection of condensed-phase material.[5] First, the size of suspended PM spans several orders of magnitude, from a few nanometres (nm) to several microns (μm). Second, the shape of PM is highly variable and includes spheres, crystalline fragments, needles and fluffy or agglomerated entities. Third, the chemical composition of PM varies widely depending on the contributing sources, and may include elemental carbon, hydrocarbon compounds, sodium chloride, ammonium sulphate, ammonium nitrate, bound water, metals, mineral dust and biological components such as pollen and bacteria. Some individual particles may have uniform chemical composition throughout, whereas others comprise a mixture of components.

As a consequence of this heterogeneity in characteristics, atmospheric PM can be quantified by any of several metrics: number and size distribution of individual particles, total mass concentration of particles in a given size range, or individual chemical component concentration.[6–8] An important observation for typical

Table 7.2 Target values for outdoor air pollutants as specified in European Union (EU) Directive 2004/107/EC

Pollutant	Measured as	EU target value
Benzo(a)pyrene[1] (in PM_{10} fraction)	Annual mean	1 ng/m³
As (in PM_{10} fraction)	Annual mean	6 ng/m³
Cd (in PM_{10} fraction)	Annual mean	5 ng/m³
Ni (in PM_{10} fraction)	Annual mean	20 ng/m³
Hg (total)	Annual mean	No target value specified, but 50 ng/m³ is a guideline

As, arsenic; Cd, cadmium; Hg, mercury; Ni, nickel.
PM_{10}, $PM_{2.5}$, all particles in the air with a diameter of less than 10 μm and less than 2.5 μm, respectively.
[1] As a measure of total polycyclic aromatic hydrocarbons.

Table 7.3 US National Ambient Air Quality Standards for 'criteria' outdoor air pollutants

Pollutant	Primary standards[†]		Secondary standards[‡]	
	Level	Measured as	Level	Measured as
Carbon monoxide	9 ppm (10 mg/m³)	8 h mean, not to be exceeded more than once per year	None	
	35 ppm (40 mg/m³)	1 h mean, not to be exceeded more than once per year		
Lead	0.15 μg/m³	Rolling 3 month average	Same as primary	
	1.5 μg/m³	Quarterly average	Same as primary	
Nitrogen dioxide	53 ppb (100 μg/m³)	Annual mean	Same as primary	
PM_{10}	150 μg/m³	24 h mean, not to be exceeded more than once per year averaged over 3 years	Same as primary	
$PM_{2.5}$	15 μg/m³	Annual mean	Same as primary	
	35 μg/m³	24 h mean, as 98th percentile averaged over 3 years	Same as primary	
Ozone	75 ppb (150 μg/m³)	Maximum daily running 8 h mean, not to be exceeded more than three times per year averaged over 3 years	Same as primary	
Sulphur dioxide	0.03 ppm (79 μg/m³)	Annual mean	0.5 ppm (1300 μg/m³)	3 h mean, not to be exceeded more than once per year
	0.14 ppm (370 μg/m³)	24 h mean, not to be exceeded more than once per year		

PM_{10}, $PM_{2.5}$, all particles in the air with a diameter of less than 10 μm and less than 2.5 μm, respectively.
[†] Limits to protect public health, including the health of 'sensitive' populations such as asthmatics, children and the elderly.
[‡] Limits to protect public welfare, including protection against decreased visibility and damage to animals, crops, vegetation and buildings.

outdoor PM is that, because of the cubic relationship between particle diameter and particle mass, only particles with a diameter greater than about $0.2\,\mu m$ are important in determining total particle mass concentration, whereas particles of diameter less than approximately $0.2\,\mu m$ dominate the total particle number concentration.[5]

The PM_{10} and the $PM_{2.5}$ metrics used to quantify airborne PM in AQS are mass-based concentrations ($\mu g/m^3$) nominally corresponding to all particles in the air with a diameter of less than $10\,\mu m$ and less than $2.5\,\mu m$, respectively. In practice, a sharp cut-off in particle separation is not achievable so the PM_{10} and $PM_{2.5}$ fractions are defined according to specific curves of particle sampling efficiency as a function of particle size. The PM_{10} and $PM_{2.5}$ sampling conventions are similar, but not identical, to the International Organization for Standardization sampling conventions designated as 'thoracic' and 'high-risk respirable' particles, respectively.[8]

MONITORING SITES

Exactly where to monitor depends on the component in question and on the purpose of the monitoring. The spectrum of possible monitoring locations includes sites remote from population influence, through rural, suburban and central urban sites, to sites adjacent to specific sources such as roads, airports, ports or major industrial complexes. Measurement at a range of site types provides comparative data on the concentrations and trends in background air and the perturbations to these at regional, urban and sub-urban scales.

The extent of spatial and temporal homogeneity in the concentrations of atmospheric trace species varies widely, driven principally by their lifetimes with respect to removal by chemical reactions and deposition to the surface. This in turn impacts on the spatial density and time resolution of monitoring required. If the atmospheric lifetime is short compared with dispersion, the atmospheric concentration pattern will tend to reflect the spatial and temporal patterns of the major sources. For example, nitric oxide (NO) reacts on a time scale of a few minutes so its spatial and temporal concentration patterns closely mirror those of its major sources – vehicle exhaust emissions and static combustion plants. Fast-response NO analysers at many locations are required to capture this dynamic. Benzene and carbon monoxide (CO) have atmospheric lifetimes of a few weeks so are more homogeneously distributed according to averaged atmospheric dispersion from their sources. An atmospheric pollutant with a lifetime of years or decades, such as a chlorofluorocarbon (which has an indirect impact on human health via destruction of the stratospheric ozone layer), is effectively homogeneously mixed throughout the lower atmosphere so its concentration can essentially be gauged by measurement at a single monitoring location.

The same principles apply to measurement of secondary pollutants such as O_3, which is formed within the atmosphere by photochemical reactions involving methane, other volatile organic compounds, and NO_x (the collective term for NO and NO_2). The sources and sinks of O_3 are varied and complex, and consequently its atmospheric distribution is influenced by processes operating from global scale to street scales. These include the presence of a global background due to the downward transport of O_3 from the stratosphere and its production on the time scale of months to years from the oxidation of CO and methane, superimposed upon which are summertime regional O_3 'episodes' caused by enhanced photochemical production from precursor emissions over polluted land masses (often exacerbated by stagnant high-pressure weather systems) and a localized short-term depletion of O_3 by reaction with very high NO emissions in urban areas.[9] Ozone measurements across a range of types of location are required to characterize these influences.

MONITORING NETWORKS

Many countries have centrally managed networks for the coordinated measurement of particular atmospheric components nationwide. Different networks target different aspects of air pollution, for example rural networks of monitors to quantify the deposition of acidifying and eutrophifying components to ecosystems, networks to monitor air pollutants subject to legally binding AQSs and networks that measure the individual constituents of airborne PM.

Where monitors operate continuously and unattended, automated telemetry can provide near real-time data to a single, publicly accessible web resource. This can be automated further to generate air quality status reports and targeted air pollution alerts. Data from non-automated networks must be uploaded manually in arrears. Regional or local authorities may operate their own air pollution monitors, which may or may not be affiliated to national networks, usually dependent principally on issues of data quality assurance and continuity.

Monitoring the air pollutants whose concentrations are subject to legally binding AQSs requires measurements that best emulate 'relevant' human exposure. This means siting monitors where members of the general public may be exposed to the given pollutant for a substantial portion of the duration of the relevant averaging times(s) for that pollutant (as specified in Tables 7.1–7.3). In practice, this means that the majority of monitors for AQS pollutants have inlets approximately 2 m above the ground and are located at urban centre or urban background sites distanced from primary sources such as roads, so as to be broadly representative of general urban exposure.

The current focus of air quality legislation on fixed concentration standards leads to policy action that emphasizes the identification and mitigation of pollution 'hotspots' without regard to the extent of the population affected by these hotspots. However, for pollutants for which no threshold concentration for health effect has been identified, a greater gain in population health overall may be achieved by focusing on policy that leads to reductions in pollutant concentrations across the widest areas of population, irrespective of the absolute concentrations relative to some arbitrary value. This concept of population-weighted exposure reduction is now embedded in the new European Union AQS for the PM metric of $PM_{2.5}$ (see Table 7.1). The $PM_{2.5}$ AQS has two components: a fixed maximum concentration value to ensure that extreme hotspot exposures are not ignored, and a target to deliver a defined reduction in population-weighted exposure in each member state. The Directive specifies the spatial density and location characteristics of $PM_{2.5}$ monitors required to calculate a member state's total population-weighted exposure to $PM_{2.5}$.

Temperature, relative humidity, windspeed and pressure are important physical properties of the atmosphere with direct and/or modifying and/or confounding effects on human health. Data on these parameters are collected routinely as part of meteorological networks.

MEASUREMENT OF INDIVIDUAL ATMOSPHERIC COMPONENTS

Automated analysis of standard gas pollutants

CARBON MONOXIDE

CO is measured in real time using non-dispersive broad-band infrared absorption.[10] The technique requires calibration using gas flows of known CO concentration. The typical limit of detection is less than 40 ppb (46 µg/m³) for a 60 second averaging time.

NITROGEN OXIDES (NITRIC OXIDE AND NITROGEN DIOXIDE)

Quantification of NO_x components utilizes the chemiluminescent reaction between NO and O_3.[11,12] The sample air flow is mixed with a second flow of air containing excess O_3, which is generated in situ from the oxygen in the second air stream using an electric discharge or ultraviolet (UV) lamp. The NO in the sample flow reacts rapidly with the O_3 to yield excited NO_2, which loses energy again by the emission of radiation. The intensity of this (chemi)luminescence is proportional to the NO present. Every few minutes, the incoming sample air is diverted through a heated molybdenum tube, or sometimes a photolysis lamp, to convert NO_2 to NO. The chemiluminescence recorded during this phase gives total NO_x from which the NO_2 concentration is derived by difference. The method is extremely sensitive, with limits of detection less than 0.5 ppb (1 µg/m³) for a 60 second averaging time.

OZONE

Ozone is quantified by its absorption of UV light at 253.7 nm from a mercury lamp.[12,13] The background transmitted UV intensity in the absence of O_3 is obtained by switching the incoming air flow every few minutes through an O_3 scrubber. The typical limit of detection is around 0.5 ppb (1 µg/m³) for a 60 second averaging time.

SULPHUR DIOXIDE

Sulphur dioxide is quantified in real time by directing pulses of UV radiation from a xenon lamp (in the wavelength range 195–230 nm) through the sample air flow to excite SO_2 molecules to a higher electronic state; these then emit radiation in the range 340–410 nm.[14,15] The intensity of this fluorescence radiation is proportional to the amount of SO_2 in the incoming air flow. The typical detection limit is around 1 ppb (2.6 µg/m³) for a 60 second averaging time.

BENZENE, 1,3-BUTADIENE AND OTHER VOLATILE ORGANIC COMPOUNDS

A range of hydrocarbons can be measured online by drawing air through an adsorbent medium such as activated carbon for a pre-set time, typically 30–60 minutes.[16,17] The adsorbent is then heated rapidly to transfer the trapped hydrocarbons into a gas chromatograph for separation and quantification with a flame ionization detector or mass spectrometer. The next sample is collected while the current one is being analysed. Detection limits of less than 0.5 µg/m³ for individual hydrocarbons are readily attainable.

Non-automated gas analysis by diffusive sampling

Many atmospheric gas species can be measured by passive diffusion samplers.[18] Since these require no power, they are cheap and simple to deploy, and can be exposed simultaneously at many locations or worn for personal exposure assessment. Their disadvantages include the long averaging times, sometimes of several weeks, and the generally greater imprecision compared with active monitors. The geometries of passive samplers vary widely,[19,20] but all utilize the same principle of establishing a molecular diffusion gradient between the ambient air and an adsorbent that captures the analyte for post-exposure quantification. Many different samplers, adsorbents and analyte quantification methods have been developed for a wide range of gaseous pollutants, including CO, O_3, NO_2, SO_2, HCHO, volatile organic compounds and POPs.[18]

Analysis of airborne particulate matter

The fractionation of airborne PM into broad size ranges, for example for the PM_{10} and $PM_{2.5}$ metrics, is usually accomplished by drawing the air through an impactor or cyclone in which particles smaller (and therefore lighter) than the design transmission of the inlet pass through with the air stream, while larger particles cannot follow the air flow and impact onto a surface.[7,8]

PARTICLE MASS CONCENTRATION: PM$_{10}$ AND PM$_{2.5}$

The mass of particles passing through the PM$_{10}$ or PM$_{2.5}$ size-selective inlet is determined by drawing the air through a preweighed filter for a fixed time period, typically 24 hours, and subsequent reweighing of the filter. The advantages of this approach are that it is a direct measurement of mass and provides a sample of PM that can be subjected to chemical analysis. However, it is labour intensive and provides only a time-averaged concentration, often some considerable time after the sampling. The method is also susceptible to unintended changes in mass before reweighing.

The automated quantification of PM mass is accomplished using the Tapered Element Oscillating Microbalance (Thermo Scientific, Waltham, MA, USA), in which particles in the air stream, having first passed through a size-selective inlet, are collected on a small filter attached to the end of a tapered glass tube that is free to oscillate. The decrease in resonant frequency of the element as it accumulates particle mass is converted to PM concentration in the air flow.[21]

PARTICLE NUMBER AND SIZE DISTRIBUTION

Individual particles can be counted directly from the pulses of scattered light as they pass through a laser beam focused into the air flow.[22] The intensity of scattered light as a function of scattering angle also enables the extraction of information on particle size,[23] using assumptions about particle shape and optical properties. A more direct measure of individual particle size is obtained from the particle's transit time between two closely separated laser beams.[24] A number of manufacturers supply hand-held and semi-portable devices operating on these principles, although it should be noted that optical scattering is only sensitive to particles larger than approximately 0.3 μm.

Smaller particles are enumerated using condensation particle counters in which the air is drawn through a chamber supersaturated in butanol or water.[25,26] Vapour condenses onto the particles, causing them to grow sufficiently large to be detected by a downstream optical counter. The combination of a scanning mobility analyser with a particle counter enables the determination of particle number as a function of particle size.[22] In the mobility analyser, particles in the incoming air stream are charged by an electron source and then subjected to deflection by an electric field. Scanning the electric field strength permits only particles of a certain mass at a time (taken as a proxy of particle size) to exit the electric field region into the particle counter.[27]

BLACK SMOKE AND BLACK CARBON

Black smoke was widely used as a measure of airborne PM, particularly in Europe, for many decades and consequently has been the exposure metric in many epidemiological studies of air pollution. A white-light source and photodiode are placed over a collected filter sample, and the percentage of light reflected (i.e. the inverse of optical 'darkness') is converted to a nominal black smoke concentration using a standard calibration equation.[28] Although black smoke is quoted in conventional concentration units of μg/m^3, the numerical value no longer equates to an absolute concentration, although it still indicates relative trends in the amount of black or elemental carbon present. Characterizing this remains of interest as a marker for the combustion-derived component of airborne particles.[29] A modern aethalometer instrument provides a real-time measurement of PM blackness from the optical transmission of 880 nm radiation through a slowly advancing thin quartz fibre tape onto which the PM is collected. This is converted to a black carbon concentration using a calibration mass extinction coefficient.[30]

PM CHEMICAL COMPOSITION

Samples of PM collected on filters can be subjected to a whole range of chemical characterization methods. Techniques that can be applied to particles while still retained on the filter include scanning electron microscopy,[31] X-ray fluorescence,[32] X-ray photoelectron spectroscopy[33] and proton-induced X-ray emission.[34] Although these methods provide elemental and mineralogical data, absolute quantification can be difficult to achieve.[35]

Alternatively, chemical components within the particles can be extracted into different solvents depending on the analyte(s) of interest. Extraction into water is used to prepare samples for ion chromatographic determination of cations (e.g. Na$^+$, Mg$^+$ and NH$_4^+$) and anions (e.g. Cl$^-$, NO$_3^-$, SO$_4^{2-}$ and PO$_4^{3-}$).[36] Extraction into water or different combinations of acid are used for elemental determination by conventional solution-phase methods such as atomic absorption spectroscopy or inductively coupled plasma optical emission spectroscopy[37] or inductively coupled plasma mass spectrometry.[38] Extraction into organic solvents such as acetone or dichloromethane is used when the target analytes are organic compounds such as individual polycyclic aromatic hydrocarbons[39] or particular compounds within the various categories of POP, for example PCBs, PBDEs or HBCDs.[40,41] The analytical method in these cases is either gas or liquid chromatography for analyte separation and mass spectrometry for identification and quantification.

Atmospheric radioactivity

Natural atmospheric radioactivity is dominated by radon. In continuous radon monitoring devices, air is pumped into an ionization chamber, or a scintillation cell with a photomultiplier detector.[42] The Lucas cell has internal walls coated with silver-activated zinc sulphide, which scintillates when struck by alpha particles from radon and its decay products.[43] Passive radon samplers typically consist of a vial containing activated charcoal that is left open for days or weeks. The adsorbed radon is quantified by flushing the charcoal with a scintillation fluid and counting scintillations. Alternatively, the passive sampler contains a small piece of special plastic film left exposed for several months. Damage tracks on the film caused by alpha particles are subsequently counted using a microscope or optical reader.[42]

The most versatile portable instrument for detecting radiation is the Geiger counter, which consists of a tube filled with an inert gas and a halogen that transiently becomes conducting when struck by ionizing radiation. The counter is most sensitive to alpha and beta radiation, but only detects the total intensity of radiation and not its energy. To identity the radioactive source, it is necessary to use energy-proportional alpha or gamma radiation detectors, which identify radiation energies characteristic of particular source isotopes.[44]

Bioaerosol

Viable and non-viable biological material in the atmosphere includes pollen, spores, bacteria, viruses, endotoxins and other mechanically generated fragments of biological material. Bulk samples are collected using instrumentation similar to that described above for non-biological particles,[45,46] for example: filter capture followed by optical microscopy (for pollen) or by extraction and biochemical analysis (for protein, endotoxin or biomarkers);[47,48] impaction sampling onto growth media such as agar plates;[49] or aspiration into solutions that retain viability for post-sampling assay.[50] The latter may include whole-organism culturing, biochemical assay, immunoassay or polymerase chain reaction analysis.

CONCLUSION

Air pollution science has a long history and is a mature field of research. Significant strides have been made in the developed world to identify causal links between ambient air pollutants and adverse health, and to effect measures to reduce population exposures to these pollutants. This progress has been substantially facilitated by the development of a suite of reliable measurement techniques for characterizing atmospheric composition, together with their coordinated deployment. Globally, however, a substantial ill-health burden from exposure to hazardous air pollutants remains, and future attention should also focus on indoor as well as outdoor air.

REFERENCES

● = Key primary paper

◆ = Major review article

◆1. Finlayson-Pitts BJ, Pitts JN. *Chemistry of the Upper and Lower Atmosphere: Theory, Experiments and Applications.* San Diego: Academic Press, 2000.

◆2. Hewitt CN, Jackson AV. *Handbook of Atmospheric Science: Principles and Applications.* Malden, MA: Wiley Blackwell, 2003.

◆3. World Health Organization. *Air Quality Guidelines for Europe.* WHO Regional Publications, European Series, No 91. Copenhagen: WHO Regional Office for Europe, 2000.

◆4. World Health Organization. *Air Quality Guidelines: Global Update 2005.* Copenhagen: WHO Regional Office for Europe, 2006.

◆5. Air Quality Expert Group. *Particulate Matter in the United Kingdom. Second Report of the Air Quality Expert Group.* PB10580. London: UK Department for Environment, Food and Rural Affairs, 2005.

◆6. Harrison RM, Van Grieken R. *Atmospheric Particles.* Vol. 5, IUPAC series on Analytical and Physical Chemistry of Environmental Systems. Chichester: Wiley Blackwell, 1998.

◆7. Baron PA, Willeke K. *Aerosol Measurement: Principles, Techniques, and Applications,* 2nd edn. New York: Wiley, 2005.

◆8. Vincent JH. *Aerosol Sampling: Science, Standards, Instrumentation and Applications.* Chichester: Wiley Blackwell, 2007.

9. Air Quality Expert Group. *Ozone in the United Kingdom. Fifth Report of the Air Quality Expert Group.* PB13216. London: UK Department for Environment, Food and Rural Affairs, 2009.

10. Parrish DD, Holloway JS, Fehsenfeld FC. Routine, continuous measurement of carbon-monoxide with parts-per-billion precision. *Environ Sci Technol* 1994; **28**: 1615–18.

11. Navas MJ, Jimenez AM, Galan G. Air analysis: determination of nitrogen compounds by chemiluminescence. *Atmos Environ* 1997; **31**: 3603–8.

◆12. Heard DE. *Analytical Techniques for Atmospheric Measurement.* Oxford: Blackwell, 2006.

13. Parrish DD, Fehsenfeld FC. Methods for gas-phase measurements of ozone, ozone precursors and aerosol precursors. *Atmos Environ* 2000; **34**: 1921–57.

◆14. Harrison RM, Perry R. *Handbook of Air Pollution Analysis,* 2nd edn. London: Chapman & Hall, 1986.

15. Luke WT. Evaluation of a commercial pulsed fluorescence detector for the measurement of low-level SO_2 concentrations during the gas-phase sulfur intercomparison experiment. *J Geophys Res* 1997; **102**: 16255–65.

16. Helmig D, Greenberg JP. Automated in-situ gas-chromatographic mass-spectrometric analysis of ppt level volatile organic trace gases using multistage solid-adsorbent trapping. *J Chromatogr A* 1994; **677**: 123–32.

17. Dollard GJ, Dumitrean P, Telling S *et al*. Observed trends in ambient concentrations of C-2-C-8 hydrocarbons in the United Kingdom over the period from 1993 to 2004. *Atmos Environ* 2007; **41**: 2559–69.

◆18. Brown RH. Monitoring the ambient environment with diffusive samplers: theory and practical considerations. *J Environ Monit* 2000; **2**: 1–9.

19. Tang YS, Cape JN, Sutton MA. Development and types of passive samplers for monitoring atmospheric NO_2 and NH_3 concentrations. *Scientific World J* 2001; **1**: 513–29.

20. Gerboles M, Buzica D, Amantini L *et al*. Laboratory and field comparison of measurements obtained using the available diffusive samplers for ozone and nitrogen dioxide in ambient air. *J Environ Monitor* 2006; **8**: 112–19.

●21. Patashnick H, Rupprecht EG. Continuous PM_{10} measurements using the Tapered Element Oscillating Microbalance. *Air Waste* 1991; **41**: 1079–83.

◆22. McMurry PH. A review of atmospheric aerosol measurements. *Atmos Environ* 2000; **34**: 1959–99.

23. Peters TM, Ott D, O'Shaughnessy PT. Comparison of the Grimm 1.108 and 1.109 portable aerosol spectrometer to the TSI 3321 aerodynamic particle sizer for dry particles. *Ann Occup Hyg* 2006; **50**: 843–50.

24. Volckens J, Peters TM. Counting and particle transmission efficiency of the aerodynamic particle sizer. *J Aerosol Sci* 2005; **36**: 1400–8.

●25. Stolzenburg MR, McMurry PH. An ultrafine aerosol condensation nucleus counter. *Aerosol Sci Technol* 1991; **14**: 48–65.

26. Biswas S, Fine PM, Geller MD *et al*. Performance evaluation of a recently developed water-based condensation particle counter. *Aerosol Sci Technol* 2005; **39**: 419–27.

27. Winklmayr W, Reischl GP, Lindner AO *et al*. A new electromobility spectrometer for the measurement of aerosol size distributions in the size range from 1 to 1000 nm. *J Aerosol Sci* 1991; **22**: 289–96.

●28. British Standards Institution. *Methods for the Measurement of Air Pollution. Part 2: Determination of concentration of suspended matter*. British Standard 1747, Part 2. London: BSI, 1969.

● 29. Hoek G, Brunekreef B, Goldbohm S *et al*. Association between mortality and indicators of traffic-related air pollution in the Netherlands: a cohort study. *Lancet* 2002; **360**: 1203–9.

30. Quincey P. A relationship between Black Smoke Index and black carbon concentration. *Atmos Environ* 2007; **41**: 7964–8.

31. Jones TP, Williamson BJ, BeruBe KA *et al*. Microscopy and chemistry of particles collected on TEOM filters: Swansea, South Wales, 1998–1999. *Atmos Environ* 2001; **35**: 3573–83.

32. Szilagyi V, Hartyani Z. Development of an X-ray fluorescence spectrometric method for the analysis of atmospheric aerosol samples. *Microcheml J* 2005; **79**: 37–41.

33. Qi JH, Feng LJ, Li XG *et al*. An X-ray photoelectron spectroscopy study of elements on the surface of aerosol particles. *J Aerosol Sci* 2006; **37**: 218–27.

34. da Cunha KD, Leite CVB. Metal trace analysis by PIXE and PDMS techniques. *Nucl Instrum Methods Phys Res B* 2002; **187**: 401–7.

35. Freitas MC, Almeida SM, Reis MA *et al*. Monitoring trace elements by nuclear techniques in PM10 and PM2.5. *Nucl Instrum Methods Phys Res A* 2003; **505**: 430–4.

36. Yin J, Allen AG, Harrison RM *et al*. Major component composition of urban PM10 and PM2.5 in Ireland. *Atmos Res* 2005; **78**: 149–65.

37. Robache A, Mathe F, Galloo JC *et al*. Multi-element analysis by inductively coupled plasma optical emission spectrometry of airborne particulate matter collected with a low-pressure cascade impactor. *Analyst* 2000; **125**: 1855–9.

38. Allen AG, Nemitz E, Shi JP *et al*. Size distributions of trace metals in atmospheric aerosols in the United Kingdom. *Atmos Environ* 2001; **35**: 4581–91.

39. Harrad S, Laurie L. Concentrations, sources and temporal trends in atmospheric polycyclic aromatic hydrocarbons in a major conurbation. *J Environ Monit* 2005; **7**: 722–7.

40. Harrad S, Hazrati S, Ibarra C. Concentrations of polychlorinated biphenyls in indoor air and polybrominated diphenyl ethers in indoor air and dust in Birmingham, United Kingdom: implications for human exposure. *Environ Sci Technol* 2006; **40**: 4633–8.

41. Abdallah MAE, Harrad S, Ibarra C *et al*. Hexabromocyclododecanes in indoor dust from Canada, the United Kingdom, and the United States. *Environ Sci Technol* 2008; **42**: 459–64.

42. US Environmental Protection Agency. *Indoor Radon and Radon Decay Product Measurement Device Protocols*. EPA report no. 402-R-92-004. Washington, DC: USEPA, 1992.

43. Abbady A, Abbady AGE, Michel R. Indoor radon measurement with the Lucas cell technique. *Appl Radiat Isot* 2004; **61**: 1469–75.

44. Choppin G, Rydberg J, Liljenzin JO. *Radiochemistry and Nuclear Chemistry*. Oxford: Butterworth-Heinemann, 1995.

◆45. Levetin E. Methods for aeroallergen sampling. *Curr Allergy Asthma Rep* 2004; **4**: 376–83.

◆46. Martinez KF, Rao CY, Burton NC. Exposure assessment and analysis for biological agents. *Grana* 2004; **43**: 193–208.

◆47. Menetrez MY, Foarde KK, Esch RK *et al*. The measurement of ambient bioaerosol exposure. *Aerosol Sci Technol* 2007; **41**: 884–93.

48. Lee AKY, Lau APS, Cheng JYW *et al*. Source identification analysis for the airborne bacteria and fungi using a biomarker approach. *Atmos Environ* 2007; **41**: 2831–43.

49. Lee KS, Bartlett KH, Brauer M *et al*. A field comparison of four samplers for enumerating fungal aerosols. I: Sampling characteristics. *Indoor Air* 2004; **14**: 360–6.

50. Lin XJ, Reponen TA, Willeke K *et al*. Long-term sampling of airborne bacteria and fungi into a non-evaporating liquid. *Atmos Environ* 1999; **33**: 4291–8.

8

Measuring the water and soil environments

MICHAEL O. RIVETT, KEVIN D. PRIVETT, ROBERT W. IVENS

The reliable measurement of contamination in water and soil and the quantification of risks posed to human health are critical to the safeguarding of water and food supplies and the reuse of 'brownfield' contaminated land. A lack of measurement may have dire consequences. Poorly protected water supplies may be at risk of receiving faecal waste containing microbial pathogens that may result in acute illness or death.[1] A lack of recognition of potential risks and relevant monitoring has led to many high-profile incidents. Groundwater examples include the deadly 1854 cholera epidemic in London and the pioneering work of Dr John Snow in his tracing of an outbreak to a contaminated well;[2] the widespread arsenic contamination of wells in Bangladesh;[3] the late 1970s 'Love Canal' incident in which the US government relocated 800 households amid significant health effects arising from the township being built over a former chemical dump;[4] and, in 2000, the contamination of a supply well in Walkerton, Canada by *Escherichia coli* from farm run-off that led to seven deaths and 2500 residents becoming ill.[5]

This chapter provides a summary account of contamination measurement in water and soil environments. This is an immense subject area, and the reader is referred to other texts for specific detail on water pollution,[6,7] environmental sampling and analysis,[8–10] contaminated site (subsurface) characterization,[11,12] specialist subtopics, for example sampling radiological environments,[13] and compendiums of documents, for example the US Environmental Protection Agency's (EPA's) 'SW-846 On-line', which contains over 200 sampling and analysis documents and is regularly updated.[10]

The detailed practice of soil/water measurement is not presented per se, but rather the essence of measurement approaches are incorporated within a discussion of measurement frameworks and objectives, an overview of key aspects that require consideration in measurement practice, noting in particular the challenges of uncertainty, and a summary of future research challenges. The account presented is largely within the context of contaminated land due to its all-encompassing nature and its provision of state-of-the-art soil/water measurement practice and science.[11,12] The majority of soil/water measurement programmes are associated with either the investigation, monitoring and remediation of contaminated land sites and the associated quantification of risks to human health, the water and built environments and sensitive ecological habitats, or the surveillance monitoring of key soil and water resources, for example aquifers, rivers, reservoirs and associated abstraction points for water supply, particularly of drinking water or water for other sensitive uses.

CONTAMINATION OF WATER AND SOIL ENVIRONMENTS

The conceptualization of contaminant transport and measurement in water and soil environments is illustrated in Figure 8.1. Conceptual models provide the essential 'source–pathway–receptor' framework for the effective design of measurement, risk assessment and remediation strategies. The fate of a contaminant in the environment

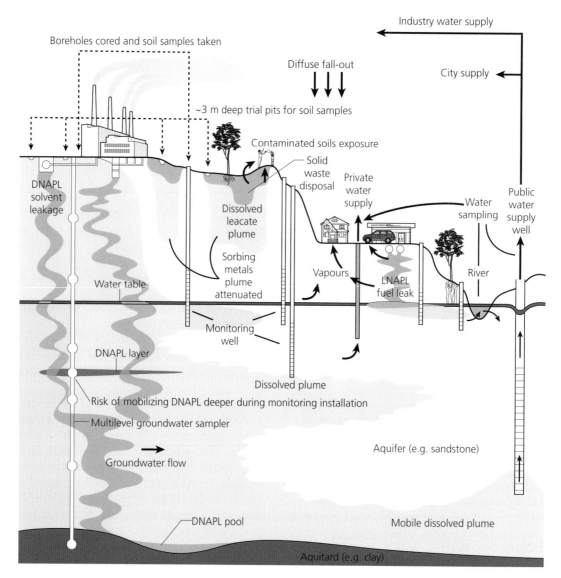

Figure 8.1 Conceptualization of the transport and monitoring of contamination in water and soil environments. DNAPL, dense non-aqueous-phase liquid; LNAPL, light non-aqueous-phase liquid.

depends on a great number of factors including its interaction with soils and water, transport mechanisms, degradation/diffusion/attenuation, etc. and uptake by potential receptors. For example, precipitation contaminated by urban emissions may infiltrate through contaminated land, picking up further industrial soil contamination, and eventually reach the underlying water table to then move laterally in the aquifer and enter a supply well, or alternatively discharge through river bed sediments to mix with surface water. People may drink the water, eat fish caught in it, eat crops grown on the land, inhale dust and vapours or simply come into direct dermal contact with contaminated media.

A vast range of chemical, radiological and pathogenic contaminants of anthropogenic or natural origin exist. The re-engineering of manufacturing processes, to cut costs and improve quality, has historically required

innumerable organic chemicals to be developed. Chemical release to the environment has occurred where handling and disposal practices have been poor or contamination risks have simply not been recognized. The physicochemical nature of these contaminants fundamentally affects their fate and transport in the environment and in turn the appropriate methods of measurement. This is exemplified in Table 8.1 for some chemical contaminants of concern in soil/water environments. The ease of measurement of the various chemical types may also vary significantly. Dense non-aqueous-phase liquid (DNAPL) chemicals, for example trichloroethene in Table 8.1, may penetrate below the water table deep into the subsurface by virtue of their immiscible and denser-than-water nature. The distribution of DNAPL in the subsurface is notoriously difficult to ascertain, even when vast sums of money, even millions of dollars, are spent on investigation.

Table 8.1 Chemical characteristics controlling the fate and measurement of some chemicals of concern in soil and water environments

Chemical	Analytical grouping	Use	Chemical characteristics controlling fate/measurement
Methyl tertiary butyl ether	Volatile organic compounds	Petroleum fuel additive (oxygenate) at 1–15% of fuel	Very water soluble with limited sorption and degradation. Extensive dissolved plumes form in groundwater from fuel spills of light non-aqueous-phase liquid (LNAPL) that accumulate on the groundwater table
Trichloroethene	Volatile organic compounds	Degreaser, dry cleaning, chemical solvent or intermediate	Dense non-aqueous phase liquid that penetrates deep into aquifers, forming large groundwater plumes subject to limited sorption and degradation. Is volatile and hence partitions from soils and surface waters to air and presents vapour plume risks.
Benzo(a)pyrene	Polynuclear aromatic hydrocarbons	Coal tar creosote component, product of incomplete combustion	Very hydrophobic, low volatility hydrocarbon of negligible biodegradability that strongly sorbs to soils. Limited transport in water, unless sorbed to mobile sediments. High concentrations occur near non-aqueous phase liquid sources of tars or sorbed within soils
Chromium (Cr)	Metals	Metal plating, steel-making, leather-tanning, naturally occurring in minerals	Relative Cr(III) and Cr(VI) occurrence depends on geochemical conditions. Toxic Cr(VI), e.g. chromate, is mobile in water but is reduced to low-solubility Cr(III) precipitates that are readily sorbed to soils and largely immobile and of low toxicity

HISTORICAL PERSPECTIVE

It is rare that the contamination of water/soils at low health-relevant concentrations can be recognized through the human senses. Many chemicals were used by industry for decades prior to their chronic toxicities being recognized, and their impacts may have gone unnoticed for decades simply because measurement techniques were unavailable. Although the acute toxicity of chemicals may have been recognized through worker exposure studies, the science and recognition of chronic toxicity affects from repeated low-level exposure were much less developed. Prior to publication of *Silent Spring* by Rachel Carson in 1962 concerning the environmental affects of the pesticide DDT, there was little appreciation of the environmental presence and significance of anthropogenic chemicals. Although knowledge of water/soil contamination was existent prior to the 1970s,[14,15] it is clear that problem recognition was largely controlled by the development and availability of chemical analysis technologies.[16] However, the ability of commercial laboratories to routinely separate and measure complex environmental chemical mixtures to low concentrations, although significantly advanced during the 1970s, was in itself insufficient to implement significant change without the appropriate national and international (regulatory) frameworks being put in place.

As the development of toxicity assessment relied upon similar analytical methods, its development inevitably paralleled that of water/soil quality standards and protocols throughout the 1970–80s and beyond. Indeed, toxicological data relating to human health remain very limited and continue to be a major limitation in assessing risks because of the large degree of uncertainty (see below). Likewise, a conceptual model understanding of transport was concurrently emerging. The DNAPL conceptualization (Figure 8.1) represented a significant paradigm shift in the late 1980s, whereupon the serious implications of DNAPL spillages and the previous inappropriate application of pump-and-treat remediation schemes became recognized.[17] Significantly too, the development of legislation was often incident, rather than problem-prediction, driven. The Love Canal incident, along with the Times Beach, Missouri case (dioxins in soils), partly led to the 1980 Comprehensive Environmental Response Compensation and Liability Act in the USA, commonly referred to as CERCLA or 'Superfund', which holds polluters accountable for their damages.

RISK ASSESSMENT FRAMEWORK

Significant legislation now exists in many countries controlling the measurement and management of contamination in soil and water environments.[18] Measurements are usually undertaken within risk-based management frameworks involving the quantification of risks for a specific source–pathway–receptor 'linkage'. For contaminated land, this typically involves assessing risks posed to (1) human health via exposure routes including ingestion, inhalation and dermal contact[18] and (2) the water environment and its associated receptors (wells etc.) via the leaching of contaminants.[19] Assessment involves a combination of desk-based data collection, on-site investigation and monitoring, and interpretation of quantitative data via contaminant transport and exposure risk assessment models. The latter quantify the risks posed and determine the contaminant thresholds considered indicative of an 'acceptable' risk to receptors.

However, the science does not exist to enable definitive clean-up levels for soils and water to be determined because of data uncertainties, and there is a balance between risk and uncertainty that involves political and socioeconomic judgement as well as scientific principles. Because toxicological data generally reflect the 'no observable adverse effect level' condition, assessments based on these data are very conservative, and it is not possible to determine with any degree of certainty the concentrations that would result in actual harm.

Risk assessment models are generally based upon analytical solutions to simplified transport and uptake models and are 'tiered' to apply increasing degrees of sophistication, which provides less uncertainty (and hence less conservatism) with increasingly higher-quality data. Although some models are deterministic, others are populated with probability distribution functions. Probabilistic modelling is generally incorporated in the risk assessment software to calculate the probabilities of exceeding standards at compliance points. Risk-based assessment criteria for contaminants are hence determined and compared with the measured site concentration data. National policy and legislation usually dictates how lower tiers of assessment, with more conservative assumptions, are used for the initial screening of a site, moving to higher tiers of more detailed assessment as the site conditions and data require.[18,19]

Although there are similarities in general approach internationally to the measurement and interpretation of soil/water data, specific differences remain, for example a variation in the approach to determining soil critical concentration. The failure to develop specific soil/water standards in some jurisdictions has led to some ad hoc international 'borrowing' of standards.[20] Specific protocols/ guidelines for the assessment of soil/water vary in terms of detail, but the sharing of international experience has led to some general consensus, albeit it with notable national differences (such as the use of slope factors for extrapolating the low-dose effects of non-threshold substances,

supported in the USA but not in the UK). Practice in less economically developed countries (LEDCs) lags behind that of developed nations. Priority attention is rightly given to the measurement of the pathogenic acute risk to water supplies,[21] and there may be limited resources to measure chemical contamination. Less strict environmental controls may, however, mean that LEDCs still contain contamination posing a significant, but unknown, risk.

INVESTIGATION AND MONITORING OBJECTIVES

The objectives of investigation and monitoring need to be carefully defined to collect cost-effective fit-for-purpose soil/water data. Inherent in this process is the initial (policy) decision on whether a site should be 'screened in' to prove it is 'clean' (as in the USA), or 'screened out' to prove it is dirty (as in the UK) – a decision influenced by risk uncertainties and the available resources. As the installation and sampling/analysis of monitoring wells and trial pits/cores are expensive and restricted by site constraints and budgets, site investigation and monitoring programmes require carefully designed clear objectives. At a practical measurement level, objectives may include the delineation of solid/liquid sources, the delineation of dissolved- or vapour-phase plumes, the establishment of on- or off-site migration, and the progression of a site's remediation. Measurement strategies need to be designed that meet the selected objectives. The sampling strategies used and the statistical manipulation of data are critical in understanding the distribution of contaminants and in creating the conceptual site model as a basis for risk assessment. A staged approach is used to essentially identify the problem and narrow it down.

The US EPA, for example, sets out an integrated 'triad approach' of systematic planning, dynamic work plans and real-time measurement technologies to plan and implement data collection and technical decision-making at hazardous waste sites.[22] A focus on overall decision quality is achieved via a data quality objectives-based approach that recognizes and manages uncertainty (a critical issue for all sites – see further below) within a tiered risk assessment approach. The method requires practitioners to synthesize and revise their conceptual model and develop a bespoke strategy of inspection, analytical testing and statistical assessment for each round of investigation. Fundamental to this approach is the development of robust decision rules for each stage.

MEASUREMENT METHODS AND PROTOCOLS

Obtaining water (millilitre-to-litre volume) or soil (gram-to-kilogram mass) samples may seem trivial to a non-specialist, but this is far from the truth. Critical decisions may be based on samples that could undergo intensive scrutiny in legal proceedings, etc. Significant efforts are hence made to ensure that quality assurance/quality control remains high.

Many sampling and analysis protocols for various sample matrices and contaminant types have been developed to ensure reliable sample acquisition, transport, preservation, non-bias, chain of custody, analysis and reporting.[23,24] A vast array of analytical determinand suites have been developed by commercial laboratories that need to be selectively used by investigators.[10,25] For example, suites for organic contaminants, which typically cover tens of individual compounds each, may include volatile organic compounds, semi-volatile organic compounds, polynuclear aromatic hydrocarbons, polychlorinated biphenyls, phenols, petroleum hydrocarbons (which may be 'total' or banded across various volatility ranges), pesticides that are typically subdivided due to their diversity to various subgroupings, for example organochlorines, organophosphates, etc., as well as newer or 'exotic' suites such as endocrine-disrupting chemicals that likewise contain subgroups that each require specialized chemical analysis methods. Crucial to the decision of what to analyse for is an understanding of the site history, as part of the conceptual site model, which can inform on the substances likely to be present.

Deciding what actually constitutes a representative sample is a much debated point. Groundwater sampling issues include: what length of monitoring well screen is appropriate; how long the stagnant well water should be purged for; what the effects of well casing or sampling device – sorption, leaching and volatilization – are; whether low-flow or passive methods can be used; whether a multilevel sampler should be used; or whether new protocol times can yield comparable samples. Much literature has been written on such nuances.[11,12] It is not just sample concentration that matters, but how the sample has been obtained. At the scale of the individual soil sample, the investigator has to decide whether to analyse, say, the clay matrix, the large lumps of rock/concrete, etc. or the whole mixture to obtain a contaminant concentration. Likewise in surveillance programmes of large aquifer resource units, should the responsible body undertake monitoring on short-screen monitoring wells or multilevel samplers that sample small, discrete packages of water, or alternatively monitor major public water supply boreholes that are extracting water at several thousand cubic metres per day yielding an integrated bulk sample? In reality, all approaches are required to give an informed, multiscaled assessment of the aquifer contamination present (see Figure 8.1, p. 120).

UNCERTAINTY

Measurement of contamination at sites is frequently associated with uncertainties that need to be recognized and managed to allow effective decision-making. The challenges of uncertainty that commonly plague site investigations and monitoring programmes are outlined below.

Site condition uncertainties

All contaminated sites are unique and contain significant uncertainties even after substantial investigation. Both contaminant distributions and geological conditions are very heterogeneous, especially where anthropogenic deposits (made ground) are present, typical of former industrial sites. Initial contaminant release conditions are typically unknown, with uncertainty of the release volumes, timing, chemical nature and polluters responsible. Based on analytical technology and environmental awareness, few contaminant-based site investigation data will exist prior to the mid-1970s and often much later (see above). Spatial densities of sampling points and temporal monitoring frequencies are still comparatively sparse, even at well-funded sites, when sample-tested volumes are compared with the overall site volume. 'Environmental forensic'-based techniques[26] are hence increasingly being used to constrain site uncertainties, and statistical techniques are used to increase confidence in sampling network design, interpolation of the site data/parameters, estimation of subsurface contaminant distributions and decision-making on soil/water volumes in need of remediation.

Contaminant uncertainties

Several sources of uncertainty may relate to the contaminants themselves. Cost and other constraints control the selection of monitoring frequencies and determinand suites.[25] There is a potential for contaminants to be missed through poor suite selection, contaminant omission from routine suites, poor sampling protocols or the non-development of analytical methods. An understanding of land use or industrial process history is vital in determining contaminant suites. There are problems with mixtures, such as petroleum hydrocarbons, which may be composed of thousands of individual compounds, very few of which have any published toxicological or physicochemical data available for risk assessment modelling. In this respect, the concept of priority pollutants or indicator chemicals is often used as a screening device for potential contamination; for example, the US EPA has identified 16 priority polynuclear aromatic hydrocarbons out of over 100 that may be present. Critical contaminant transport parameters such as degradation rates are difficult to measure and may require estimation based on the literature. Calculations of contaminant partitioning between media (e.g. the attribution of soil concentrations to aqueous, air and solid phases,[27] or uptake by vegetable crops) and risk assessment models both rely upon equilibrium constants that may be uncertain, or may be inappropriate if kinetic effects or co-contaminants modify behaviour.

Toxicological uncertainties

Returning to the framework of assessment, toxicological uncertainties, noted earlier, continue to cause concern in the assessment of risks posed by measured contaminant concentrations. In particular, uncertainties or gaps in the data, factoring to apply animal experiments to humans, factoring to interpret lowest observable to no observable effects and factoring to allow for the most critical receptors in a group all result in very low (conservative) assessment criteria (or critical concentrations) that may be less than the laboratory limit of detection or less than general background values. Problems with mixtures and the 'additivity' of effects also conspire to reduce assessment criteria. The 'clean-up value' often perceived to represent acceptable risk may be very low, and balances are required between uncertainty and pragmatism, and cost and benefit.

Innovation uncertainties

A vast armoury of site investigation and monitoring tools is now available. Advanced techniques, for example, include vertical or three-dimensional subsurface contaminant detection via multilevel sampling devices or push probes,[28] real-time four-dimensional geophysical monitoring,[29] isotope-based techniques,[30] gene-based methods,[31] direct toxicity measurements,[32] NAPL detection methods[33] and the use of field analytical methods.[34] Their routine adoption is, however, hindered by non-rigorous validation procedures and controlled field testing, method reliability, cost, acceptance by regulators and a reluctance to abandon standard methods. In short, the uncertainty surrounding innovatory measurement techniques is a barrier to their widespread use. This problem has long been recognized, by the US EPA, for example, whose 'SW-846'[10] compendium of analytical and test methods approved by their Office of Solid Waste incorporates specific 'Guidance for methods development and method validation' that facilitates the approval of innovative methods.

CONCLUSION AND FUTURE CHALLENGES

Capabilities for measuring contamination in water/soil environments have developed significantly since the 1970s. A reasonably confident assessment of contaminated sites and their associated risks can now be made given sufficient funding, a sensible application of the available monitoring tools and a consideration of the uncertainties present. Nevertheless, significant challenges remain that are the

subject of ongoing research. Examples are briefly itemized below:

- There is a perpetual need for rapid, cost-effective, high-frequency, more automated measurement techniques to generate high-resolution contamination data. Improved field-screening methods are likewise required.
- The monitoring of pathogenic viruses, bacteria and protozoa tends to be inaccurate and time-consuming, and hence indicator bacteria are commonly used to determine the relative risk of faecal contamination and pathogen presence. More rapid and specific methods are required to assess acute risks via molecular[35] or other (e.g. filtration) methods.
- There is a need for the increased availability and affordability of analytical and monitoring technology in LEDCs to avoid soil/water pollution remaining undiagnosed.
- Concentration flux measurement is often desirable over contaminant concentrations due to the interest in flux emission and receipt. Various methods are under development, for example diffusion-based and passive sorbent–tracer release methods.[36] However, most regulation is still based on concentrations rather than fluxes.
- Some regulation is based on the degree of hazard (e.g. the presence of substances in water), whereas other regulation is based on risk (e.g. the concentrations of substances in soil that equate to an acceptable dose under some exposure models resulting from a standard land use such as residential use with gardens where food may be grown). A move to risk-based regulation is taking place, for example the current two-tiered approach in the UK[37] in which the planning process is expected to prove that suspected contamination is below the threshold value yet the regulator can use a balance of probabilities, i.e. operate in the lower tail of the distribution. Dutch ground contamination law was originally based on cleaning a site for any future use, but this was abandoned and now focuses on the risks associated with a specific land use.
- More direct toxicity methods[32] need to be developed to allow confident use with or without routine concentration data.
- 'New contaminants', recent examples being endocrine-disrupting chemicals[38] and pharmaceutically active compounds, will continue to emerge. The unfortunate potential remains for analytical methods, field discovery, toxicity data and regulatory standards and management to be developed in parallel.
- There is a need for toxicological data relevant to human health that allow judgements to be made of 'safe' concentrations (indicative of a 'clean' site) and 'harmful' concentrations (indicative of a 'contaminated' site). A consequence of the uncertainty in toxicological data is that conservatism results in the derivation of assessment criteria that can be lower than the current laboratory

limit of detection. For analysis to be fit for purpose, laboratories are being driven to producing new methods with lower detection limits, with inevitable problems for quality assurance/quality control and costs.

- Physicochemical and fate-transport data are needed to support increasingly sophisticated risk assessment methods. The reliable determination of field-scale (bio) degradation rates that critically control the migration of plumes and risk-based clean-up criteria is a significant challenge.

- A greater understanding of representative sampling, statistical methods of assessment and how to estimate 'average' site conditions versus some legal assessment criterion is to be desired.

REFERENCES

1. Ferguson C, De Roda Husman AM, Altavilla N *et al.* Fate and transport of surface water pathogens in watersheds. *Crit Rev Environ Sci Technol* 2003; **33**: 299–361.

2. Price M. Dr John Snow and an early investigation of groundwater contamination. *Geol Soc Lond Special Publications* 2004; **225**: 31–49.

3. Nickson R, McArthur J, Burgess W *et al.* Arsenic poisoning of Bangladesh groundwater. *Nature* 1998; **395**: 338–8.

4. Deegan Jr J. Looking back at Love Canal. *Environ Sci Technol* 1987; **21**: 421–6.

5. Holme R. Drinking water contamination in Walkerton, Ontario: positive resolutions from a tragic event. *Water Sci Technol* 2003; **47**: 1–6.

6. Liu DHF, Lipták BG. (ed.) *Groundwater and Surface Water Pollution.* Boca Raton, Florida: CRC Press, 1999.

7. Rivett MO, Drewes J, Barrett M *et al.* Chemicals: health relevance, transport and attenuation. In: Schmoll O, Howard G, Chilton J, Chorus I. (eds) *Protecting Groundwater For Health: Managing the Quality of Drinking-water Sources.* World Health Organization Drinking-water Quality Series. Geneva: WHO, 2006: 81–137.

8. Popek EP. *Sampling and Analysis of Environmental Chemical Pollutants: A Complete Guide.* Boston: Academic Press, 2003.

9. Keith LH, *Compilation of EPA's Sampling and Analysis Methods.* Chelsea, Michigan: Lewis, 1991.

10. US Environmental Protection Agency. *SW-846: Test Methods for Evaluating Solid Waste, Physical/Chemical Methods* (SW-846 On-line). Available from: http://www.epa.gov/sw-846/main.htm (accessed July 18, 2009). Washington DC: US EPA Office of Solid Waste, 2008.

11. Boulding JR, Ginn JS. *Practical Handbook of Soil, Vadose Zone, and Ground-water Contamination: Assessment, Prevention, and Remediation.* Boca Raton, Florida: CRC Press, 2003.

12. Nielsen DM. *Practical Handbook of Environmental Site Characterization and Ground-water Monitoring,* 2nd edn. New York: CRC Press/Taylor & Francis, 2005.

13. Byrnes ME, King DA. *Sampling and Surveying Radiological Environments.* Boca Raton, Florida: CRC Press, 2000.

14. Stanley WE, Eliassen R. *Status of Knowledge of Ground Water Contaminants.* Technical Studies Program report of the US Federal Housing Administration. Washington DC: Federal Housing Administration, 1961.

15. Rivett MO, Feenstra S, Clark L. Lyne and McLachlan (1949): influence of the first publication on groundwater contamination by trichloroethene. *Environ Forensics* 2006; **7**: 313–23.

16. Travis AS. Instrumentation in environmental analysis, 1935–1975. In: Morris PJT (ed.) *From Classical to Modern Chemistry.* London: Royal Society of Chemistry, 2002: 285–308.

17. Mackay DM, Cherry JA. Groundwater contamination: limits of pump-and-treat remediation. *Environ Sci Technol* 1989; **23**: 630–6.

18. DEFRA & Environment Agency. *Model Procedures for the Management of Land Contamination.* EA R & D publication CLR 11. Bristol: Environment Agency, 2004.

19. Smith JWN. Assessing risks to groundwater from contaminated soils. *Soil Use Manage* 2006; **21**: 518–26.

20. Rivett MO, Petts J, Butler B, Martin I. Remediation of contaminated land and groundwater: experience in England and Wales. *J Environ Manage* 2002; **65**: 251–68.

21. Cronin AA, Rueedi J, Joyce E, Pedley S. Monitoring and managing the extent of microbiological pollution in urban groundwater systems in developed and developing countries. In: Tellam JH, Rivett MO, Israfilov RG (eds) *Urban Groundwater Management and Sustainability.* NATO Science Series IV: Earth and Environmental Sciences 2006; **74**: 299–314.

22. US EPA. *Using the Triad Approach to Streamline Brownfields Site Assessment and Cleanup.* Brownfields Technology Primer Series. Washington DC: US EPA Office of Solid Waste and Emergency Response, 2003.

23. British Standards Institution. *Water Quality.* Part 6: *Sampling.* Section 6.18: *Water Quality – Guidance on Sampling of Groundwater at Contaminated Sites.* British Standard BS 6068 Section 6.18: 2001 and ISO 5667–18: London: British Standards Institution, 2001.

24. American Society for Testing and Materials. *Standard Guide for the Selection of Purging and Sampling Devices for Ground-Water Monitoring Wells.* ASTM D6634–01. Philadelphia, Pennsylvania: ASTM, 2006.

25. Environment Agency. *Development of Methodology for Selection of Determinand Suites and Sampling Frequency for Groundwater Quality Monitoring.* EA Project Report NC/00/35. Bristol: Environment Agency, 2003.

26. Feenstra S, Rivett MO. Groundwater pollution: the emerging role of environmental forensics. In: Hester RE, Harrison RM (eds) *Environmental Forensics.* Issues in Environmental Science and Technology. London: Royal Society of Chemistry, 2008; **26**: 153–72.

27. Feenstra S, MacKay DM, Cherry JA. A method for assessing residual NAPL based on organic chemical concentrations in soil samples. *Ground Water Monit Rev* 1991; **11**: 128–36.

28. Environment Agency. *Guidance on Monitoring of Landfill Leachate, Groundwater and Surface Water*. EA Landfill Directive Technical Guidance LFTGN02. Bristol: Environment Agency, 2003.

29. Johnson RH, Poeter EP. Insights into the use of time-lapse GPR data as observations for inverse multiphase flow simulations of DNAPL migration. *J Contam Hydrol* 2007; **89**(1–2): 136–55.

30. Sherwood Lollar B, Slater GF, Sleep B *et al.* Stable carbon isotope evidence for intrinsic bioremediation of tetrachloroethene and trichloroethene at Area 6, Dover Air Force Base. *Environ Sci Technol* 2001; **35**: 261–9.

31. Stapleton RD, Sayler GS, Boggs JM *et al.* Changes in subsurface catabolic gene frequencies during attenuation of petroleum hydrocarbons. *Environ Sci Technol* 2000; **43**: 1991–9.

32. Sheehan P, Dewhurst RE, James S *et al.* Is there a relationship between soil and groundwater toxicity? *Environ Geochem Health* 2003; **25**: 9–16.

33. Brooks MC, Annable MD, Rao PSC *et al.* Controlled release, blind tests of DNAPL characterization using partitioning tracers. *J Contam Hydrol* 2002; **59**: 187–210.

34. US EPA. *Road Map to Understanding Innovate Technology Options for Brownfields Investigation and* Cleanup, 4th edn. EPA-542-B-05-001. Washington DC: US EPA Office of Solid Waste and Emergency Response Office of Superfund Remediation and Technology Innovation, 2005.

35. Toze S. PCR and the detection of microbial pathogens in water and wastewater. *Water Res* 1999; **33**: 3545–56.

36. Campbell TJ, Hatfield K, Klammler H *et al.* Magnitude and directional measures of water and Cr(VI) fluxes by passive flux meter. *Environ Sci Technol* 2006; **40**: 6392–7.

37. Chartered Institute of Environmental Health and Contaminated Land: Applications in Real Environments. *Guidance on Comparing Soil Contamination Data with a Critical Concentration*. London: CIEH/CL:AIRE, 2008.

38. Sarmah AK, Northcott GL, Leusch FDL, Tremblay LA. A survey of endocrine disrupting chemicals (EDCs) in municipal sewage and animal waste effluents in the Waikato region of New Zealand. *Sci Total Environ* 2006: **355**(1–3): 135–44.

SECTION **A**

Diseases from respiratory exposure to non-infectious agents

9

Deposition, absorption and mechanisms of action of gases and particles in the lung

JOHN A.S. ROSS, FRANK J. KELLY

Inhaled substances impact at all levels of the respiratory tract, the pattern of deposition affecting the probable response at a cellular level. This chapter covers how gases and particles deposit in the lung and how this relates this to mechanisms of effects.

The main function of the lungs is to provide oxygen to the body and to remove excess carbon dioxide. In order to do this, ambient air is drawn into the lung as inspiratory muscular effort is developed, and gas exchange occurs over the alveolar–capillary membrane as oxygen and carbon dioxide move down their respective partial pressure gradients. Blood and alveolar levels equilibrate, and then the gas in the lung is exhaled by recoil of the chest wall and pulmonary elasticity, with muscular effort used as breathing volume or expiratory resistance increases.

ANATOMY

The respiratory tract extends from the mouth and nose to the alveoli, and can be thought of as three functionally distinct regions:

1. The *upper airway* consists of the nose, mouth and pharynx, where air flow is generally turbulent. This region serves to warm and humidify inhaled air and to remove airborne particles. The nasal cavity has a high surface area and a relatively high resistance to air flow. During exercise (and in the presence of nasal disease such as hay fever), it is bypassed by mouth breathing. Infants, however, are obligate nose-breathers for as long as 6 months after birth.
2. Air passes turbulently between the vocal cords in the larynx and into the *tracheo-bronchial tree*, the trachea bifurcating into the two main bronchi and a further 15 generations of conducting airways, generations 11–15 being termed bronchioles. Generation 16 airways are terminal bronchioles.
3. The third functional region is that where *respiratory gas exchange* takes place. Generation 17–19 bronchioles allow gas exchange and are termed respiratory bronchioles; these further subdivide into alveolar ducts (generations 20–22) leading to numerous blind pouches (generation 23), the alveoli, where most of the pulmonary gas exchange occurs. The alveolar surface area is about 70 times the body surface area, at $70–120\,m^2$.

Gas flow in the large airways is tidal and tends to be turbulent at bifurcations. At each subdivision, gas flow and airway diameter are reduced, and gas flow becomes completely laminar as it drops below its critical velocity. By generation 17, tidal gas flow does not occur and gas movement is by diffusion only.

The walls of the conducting airway from the larynx down are supported by cartilage, which dwindles with progressive generations of bronchi and is lost completely by generation 11. From this point on, the airway is termed a bronchiole, and airway patency is maintained by the traction of pulmonary connective tissue. The conducting airway walls also contain smooth muscle down to the level of the alveolar ducts.

CELLULAR STRUCTURE

The upper airways (with the exception of the oropharynx) are lined with ciliated pseudostratified columnar epithelium, which is made up of different cell types adherent to a basal membrane. Goblet cells secrete mucus onto the luminal surface. Mucus is composed of two layers of fluid: a low viscosity (sol) phase in contact with the epithelial surface and in which the cilia beat, and an overlying gel-like layer of higher viscosity. Mucus is propelled by ciliary action towards the larynx. In adult humans, the terminal bronchioles possess non-ciliated basal or Clara cells, which have secretory and xenobiotic properties[1,2] and are the progenitor cells in small airways.[3]

The respiratory bronchioles, alveolar ducts and alveoli are lined with sheets of flat epithelial cells mounted on a basement membrane. The junctions between alveolar epithelial cells are very narrow and generally prevent the passage of fluid and large molecules such as albumin, but allow the migration of macrophages and granulocytes. The alveolar epithelial surface is covered with a predominantly phospholipid layer of low surface tension – surfactant – which serves to prevent alveolar collapse in exhalation and which is also seen in the conducting airways.[4]

Alveoli are separated by a wall consisting of two layers of epithelium, each with its own basement membrane, which enclose the interstitial space in which lie pulmonary capillaries, connective tissue, nerve endings and migrant cells. One side of the pulmonary capillary is closely applied to the epithelium, with a distance of gas to blood of less than $0.4\,\mu m$. The other side of the capillary is considerably thicker, at 1–$2\,\mu m$, with abundant collagen and elastin fibres providing a supporting structure for the lung. The junction between the endothelial cells, about $5\,nm$, is controlled to adjust for the permeability requirements of the tissue,[5] and widens in response to hypoxia and inflammation.[6,7] Fluid accumulating in the interalveolar septae drains into lymphatics between the alveolar and extra-alveolar spaces, airways and blood vessels, and is carried up to the lung hilum through several groups of lymph nodes before entering the systemic venous system.

CIRCULATION OF BLOOD THROUGH THE LUNG

The lung has two blood circulations. The pulmonary circulation, running from the right ventricle through the pulmonary capillary bed to the left atrium, is responsible for gas exchange. The bronchial circulation supplies arterial blood to the tracheobronchial tree through the bronchial arteries, which arise from the systemic circulation. Only about a third of the bronchial venous drainage returns to the right atrium for return to the pulmonary circulation for arterialization. The remaining two-thirds drains to the pulmonary veins, and this deoxygenated blood, together with some venous drainage from the coronary circulation, reduces the partial pressure of oxygen in the blood returning to the left heart, forming a shunt, blood having bypassed the pulmonary circulation.

INNERVATION OF THE LUNG

The innervation of the lung comes from the parasympathetic and sympathetic nervous systems.[8] The nerve trunks enter the lung at the hilum and are arranged throughout the lung structure in peribronchial and periarterial plexuses. Sympathetic efferents arise from the upper six thoracic segments of the spinal cord and synapse in the sympathetic ganglia. Post-ganglionic fibres innervate bronchial blood vessels and submucosal glands, but there is little noradrenergic innervation of human bronchial smooth muscle. Parasympathetic efferents run in the vagus nerve. Cholinergic parasympathetic efferents exert most of the motor control of the airways via ganglia within the airway wall, stimulation causing bronchoconstriction, mucus secretion and vasodilatation. Inhibitory non-adrenergic, non-cholinergic nerves provide a neurally mediated bronchodilator pathway. Sensory neurones may also have an efferent function since the stimulation of chemosensitive C-fibre endings can result in a local axon reflex releasing neuropeptides, among which are potent inducers of bronchial smooth muscle contraction, vasodilatation and mucus hypersecretion. The precise roles of these latter two pathways in health or disease remain unclear.[9]

There are three categories of afferent sensory pathway:[9]

1. *Slowly adapting stretch receptors* respond to changes in lung volume and pressure, and are mainly involved in the reflex control of breathing patterns.
2. *Rapidly adapting stretch receptors* are highly sensitive to mechanical stimulation and some chemical stimuli, and are important in defensive reflexes, including cough.
3. *Unmyelinated C-fibre endings* in the lung parenchyma (pulmonary) and airway mucosa (bronchial) are highly chemosensitive, particularly to capsaicin. Pulmonary C-fibres are sensitive to increases in lung volume, while bronchial C-fibres are less sensitive and unpredictable in their response. The stimulation of pulmonary C-fibres causes bradycardia, hypotension and apnoea followed by rapid shallow breathing. Stimulation of the bronchial C-fibres produces bronchoconstriction, mucus hypersecretion, extravasation of plasma and cough.

UPTAKE OF GASES AND PARTICLES BY THE RESPIRATORY TRACT

This complex subject is not easily studied, so modelled approximations are used to inform the concepts underlying environmental safety and the inhalation of therapeutic agents as aerosols. The most generally accepted model is that of the International Commission on Radiological Protection (ICRP),[10] currently under revision.[11] The more important concepts incorporated by the model are described here.

Gases

Inhaled gases distribute across the entire airway and alveolar surface. They may have local actions in the lung, in both the conducting airways and alveoli. Interactions with the conducting airways depend on the water solubility of the gas. The absorption of gases into the bloodstream is determined by the alveolar pressure of the specific gas.

Gases with low water solubility

The systemic effects of inhaled gases depend upon the potency of the agents and their arterial partial pressures (which approximate to alveolar partial pressures). Inhaled gas is rapidly humidified, so the partial pressure of an inhaled gas must be corrected for the saturated vapour pressure of water at body temperature. At alveolar level, further correction is needed for the difference between the volumes of oxygen taken up and carbon dioxide excreted. Finally, alveolar partial pressure must be corrected for the rate of uptake (or excretion) of the gas across the alveolar membrane and alveolar ventilation. Alveolar partial pressure increases with higher levels of alveolar ventilation. Uptake across the alveolar capillary increases as cardiac output and blood gas solubility rise. Alveolar partial pressure, therefore, is lower with gases of high blood gas solubility and with a high cardiac output. Accordingly, gaseous anaesthetic agents have a more rapid effect when they are relatively insoluble (e.g. nitrous oxide and desflurane) and administered with the patient at rest.

The mass of gas absorbed by the body may be more important than the immediate systemic effect for gases inhaled at a low concentration and for gases that generate their toxic effect by accumulation in the target tissues (e.g. carbon monoxide and benzene). Again, uptake is increased by raised alveolar ventilation, and the mass of gas absorbed by the body increases with cardiac output and blood gas solubility. The solubility of the gas in body tissues is also important since highly soluble agents are removed from the arterial blood, keeping the venous partial pressure low and maximizing the alveolar–capillary partial pressure gradient.

Gases with high water solubility

Water-soluble gases and fumes dissolve in the lining fluid covering the luminal surface of the respiratory tract, penetrate down to the cellular lining, subjecting the epithelium and supporting pulmonary tissues to chemical attack, and, at high concentrations, cause cellular death. Although at high concentration any corrosive gas or fume can attack the entire respiratory tract, highly soluble agents such as ammonia and hydrochloric acid mostly affect the upper airway. Less soluble agents, such as ozone and chlorine, penetrate deeply into the lungs and have the potential to cause alveolar damage. Gases with intermediate water solubility, such as sulphur dioxide, preferentially attack the bronchiolar airways. Sulphur dioxide also hydrolyses to form bisulphite, sulphite and hydrogen ions, with bisulphite being the likely intermediary for the chemical effects of sulphur dioxide in the airways. Agents with a relatively low water solubility, but which react chemically with water, behave in a similar manner. Nitrogen dioxide, for example, rapidly hydrolyses to form nitric acid.

Gases that dissolve in the airway luminal lining fluid can interact with the airway epithelium and affect the pulmonary interstitium, highly reactive gases potentially causing tissue destruction, inflammation and fibrosis. Less corrosive agents, or the same agents at a lower concentration, can interact with pulmonary nerves. Sulphur dioxide, for example, stimulates unmyelinated C-fibre nerve endings to cause bronchoconstriction.[12]

PARTICLES

Particle and fibre exposure occurs in a range of non-occupational settings. Airborne particles can be of any shape, with geometric diameters that are difficult to measure. Accordingly, particle diameter is generally expressed as the aerodynamic diameter, an expression of particle behaviour in air flow as if it were a perfect sphere with a density of $1\,g/mL$ with the same gravitational settling velocity as the original particle. It is described by the expression:

$$dpa = dps \times \sqrt{\text{particle specific gravity}}$$

where dpa is aerodynamic diameter and dps is the Stoke's diameter. Particles can be classified in terms of diameter as coarse ($2.5–100\,\mu m$), fine ($0.1–2.5\,\mu m$) and ultrafine or nanoparticles ($<0.1\,\mu m$).

The effects of particles in the lung depend upon the amount retained on the luminal surface of the airways and alveoli, or that moves into the interstitium. Particle deposition in the lung is determined by physical influences, airway gas velocity and the size of the particle.

The physical principles involved in particle deposition are inertial impaction, gravitational sedimentation,

Table 9.1 Approximate percentage of inhaled particles deposited in different areas of the lung according to particle diameter (after the model of the International Commission on Radiological Protection[10]

Particle aerodynamic diameter (μm)	Total deposition (nasal breathing)	Extrathoracic deposition (nasal breathing)	Alveolar deposition (nasal breathing)	Tracheobronchial deposition (nasal breathing)	Tracheobronchial deposition (mouth breathing)
0.001	98%	80%	0%	18%	29%
0.003	95%	40%	11%	34%	42%
0.005	90%	30%	30%	30%	37%
0.020	80%	15%	50%	15%	15%
0.2	16%	2%	14%	3%	8%
0.300	15%	3%	10%	2%	15%
5.000	97%	86%	3%	4%	22%
10	85%	85%	0%	0%	13%
20	60%	60%	0%	0%	1%
100	50%	50%	0%	0%	0%

Brownian displacement or diffusion, electrostatic precipitation and interception. High air flow velocity and turbulent air flow in the upper airway combined with obstacles to linear flow (e.g. the nasal conchae and the larynx) lead to particles inertially impacting on the airway wall by centrifugal force. This is greatest for larger particles (5–30 μm in diameter), most of which are deposited in the nasopharynx. Although individual airway diameter reduces with depth within the lung, total airway diameter increases, air flow falling rapidly so that inertial impaction decreases. As air flow velocity reduces, gravitational sedimentation becomes more important, particularly for particles over 0.5 μm.

Beyond the terminal bronchioles, air flow velocity is very low and particle movement is governed by diffusion, which is especially important for particles smaller than 0.5 μm, the effect becoming greater as particle diameter reduces below this. Residence time for small particles at this level is long, and the distance to an airway surface is short, favouring deposition by Brownian motion and diffusion. Electrostatic deposition plays a minor role since most ambient particles lose any charge naturally once inhaled. Interception happens when a particle becomes close enough to the airway surface to allow edge contact. This process requires that the particle size forms a significant fraction of the diameter of the airway and is generally only important in the deposition of fibres.

Fibres are particles with an elongated shape. The chance of a fibre being deposited in the respiratory tract depends upon its aerodynamic diameter, which is approximately three times the cross-sectional diameter for a fibre. So if a fibre has a diameter of about 3.3 μm, it will behave aerodynamically in the same manner as a particle of 10 μm diameter. Particles of diameter 10 μm are considered by international standards to be at the upper end of the range for pulmonary deposition, so fibres of a diameter of more than about 3 μm are widely considered

to be non-respirable. Long fibres with a diameter of less than 3 μm are considered highly respirable.[13]

Particles are deposited in different areas of the airway by size (Table 9.1). Deposition by particle size is biphasic, broadly following the following patterns:

- 3–4 nm and 3–6 μm in the alveoli;
- 10–20 nm and 1–4 μm in the tracheobronchial area;
- 1 nm and 2–11 μm in the extra-thoracic areas.

Deposition is influenced by whether air is inhaled through the mouth or nose. This is most important for deposition in the tracheobronchial area, which is significantly greater for both deposition peaks. In particular, a significant proportion of particles of diameter 10–20 μm become respirable if a person breathes through the mouth, as is the case during exercise and with nasal congestion due to allergy or infection. A similar consideration is required for fibres of diameter 2–7 μm, which have an aerodynamic diameter of 9–21 μm.

CLEARANCE OF GASES AND PARTICLES FROM THE AIRWAYS

Gases that are taken up into the bloodstream in the alveoli are cleared from the lung by this method, as well as by exhalation and pulmonary ventilation. Water-soluble gases and particles dissolve in the airway luminal lining fluid and are primarily taken up into the bronchial and pulmonary circulation. There is also some mucociliary clearance. Insoluble particles behave differently.

Mucociliary clearance

Inhaled particles depositing on proximal airway walls are cleared mainly by mucociliary transport, with a clearance half-life in the order of 2–4 hours for particles of a geometric diameter greater than 6.5 μm. Smaller particles and particles inhaled at low flow penetrate more deeply into the lung. Only 50 per cent of particles of a geometric diameter of 3.0 μm, for example, deposited in the proximal airway are cleared rapidly, with the rest being cleared with half-times of between 5 and 30 days.

Two mechanisms have been suggested for this effect. Particles may deposit on areas of airway surface with an incomplete layer of mucus, and particles might penetrate the surface layer of mucus onto the epithelial surface and become unaffected by mucociliary transport. Recent work in cell culture, however, suggests that transport in both layers of mucus is the same.[14,15] Phagocytosis by airway macrophages may be an important clearance mechanism in both cases. The control of mucociliary clearance has recently been reviewed.[16]

Clearance in the peripheral airway and alveoli

Although small amounts of particles deposited on respiratory epithelium may be transported to the mucociliary escalator, in man most are taken up by phagocytosis into alveolar macrophages. These migrate through the alveolar epithelium into the pulmonary interstitium, with the potential for transport to tracheobronchial lymph nodes and other interstitial sites over clearance times measured in hundreds of days.[17]

Particles that are insoluble in lung lining fluid may be dissolved within the macrophage. Particles that are not cleared from the respiratory epithelial surface may be taken up into epithelial cells or neurological tissue,[18] potentially causing cytotoxicity and genotoxicity, of relevance when considering the lung toxicity of minerals and radioactive particles. Particles taken up into the epithelium can translocate through the cells to the pulmonary interstitium, where they are phagocytosed by macrophages with the release of inflammatory and fibrogenic mediators, and potentially interstitial fibrosis.[19]

The ICRP model predicts that significant fractions of nanoparticles (100 nm or less in diameter) are retained in the alveoli and tracheobronchial tree (Table 9.1), confirmed by work in humans. The airway retention of 100 nm particles is biphasic, with mucociliary clearance removing particles within the first 24 hours, clearance from the lung periphery being much slower, most particles being retained at 48 hours. There is no evidence for translocation of particles into the bloodstream or for accumulation in the liver.[20]

Particle deposition is important not only for the intrinsic toxic properties of the particle material, but also for substances adsorbed onto the particles' surface or held within their matrix. Oil fly ash, for example, consists of particles of various sizes and shape made up of a predominantly sulphate matrix. Its pulmonary toxicity, however, is mainly related to its high content of transition metals.[21] Similarly, the toxicity of cotton dust relates to its

endotoxin content.[22] The smaller the particle, the higher its surface area and potential for the transmission of toxic materials into surrounding cellular material.[23]

DEFENSIVE MECHANISMS IN THE LUNG AND PATHWAYS OF LUNG INJURY

It is thus clear that the lung, owing to its function and large surface area, is regularly exposed to a range of substances, many of which involve direct or indirect oxidant challenge. Consequently, it is not surprising that it has developed robust antioxidant defence systems to protect the pulmonary epithelial cells from injury. Damage to the blood–gas barrier can markedly affect the gaseous exchange processes, both acutely and in chronic lung diseases.

Lung lining fluid

When a gas or particle enters the lung, the first interface it encounters is the lung lining fluid. Human lung lining fluid is a complex and regionally heterogeneous compartment ranging in depth from between 1–10 μm in the proximal airways to 0.2–0.5 μm in the distal airways and alveoli.[24] Lung lining fluid consists of secretions from underlying lung and resident immune cells, as well as plasma-derived exudates. As described earlier, it exists in the nasal and proximal airways as a two-phase structure consisting of gel and sol phases, the former consisting of thiol-rich mucopolypeptide glycoprotein or mucins. This contrasts with the distal airway and alveolar lining fluids, which are devoid of mucins but contain surfactant lipids and proteins. In addition to the mucin and surfactant components, lung lining fluid also contains a broad spectrum of low molecular weight antioxidants, as well as small concentrations of antioxidant enzymes.[25]

The low molecular weight antioxidants are present in similar concentrations to those found in blood plasma, including reduced glutathione (GSH), ascorbic acid (vitamin C), uric acid and alpha-tocopherol (vitamin E). Lung lining fluid obtained from the lower respiratory tract contains abundant amounts of GSH and ascorbate but low concentrations of uric acid and alpha-tocopherol (Table 9.2).[26]

In contrast, lung lining fluid from the nasal cavity contains uric acid in large quantities, with much smaller amounts of GSH and vitamin C. Lung lining fluid also contains antioxidant enzymes such as superoxide dismutase and catalase, as well as the metal-binding proteins caeruloplasmin and transferrin.

Oxidant challenge to the lung

Ambient air contains a range of oxidant gases and particulates, the exact combination of which varies from

Table 9.2 Lung lining fluid antioxidant defences

Type	Name
Low molecular weight	Glutathione
	Ascorbic acid
	Uric acid
	Vitamin E (alpha-tocopherol)
Enzymatic	Glutathione peroxidase
	Superoxide dismutase
	Catalase
Metal-binding	Caeruloplasmin
	Transferrin

one microenvironment to the next. Many of the individual oxidants that make up this ambient mix are free radicals, for example nitrogen dioxide, or have the ability to drive free radical reactions, such as ozone and particulates. Consequently, the exposure to a wide range of ambient air constituents causes oxidative stress within the lung, and this appears to initiate responses that are potentially dangerous to susceptible individuals.

One of these responses is the influx of inflammatory cells to the lung. This highly orchestrated series of events can lead to a second wave of oxidative stress, since activated inflammatory cells also generate and release large quantities of free radicals. In the absence of any invading organisms to kill, these free radicals attack local tissue components and cause cell injury.

Oxidant gases of particular concern

OZONE

Ozone is a highly reactive gas, and breathing concentrations of 60–120 parts per billion can result in a range of respiratory symptoms in a small proportion (10–20 per cent) of the healthy population (see Chapter 10).[27] Symptoms include decreased lung function, increased airway hyperreactivity and pulmonary inflammation. Those individuals with pre-existing conditions such as asthma and chronic obstructive pulmonary disease may experience an exacerbation of their symptoms.

As a relatively insoluble but very reactive gas, ozone uptake is directly related to reactions with substrates present in the lung lining fluid, referred to as 'reactive absorption'.[28] The uptake of ozone is thus related not only to its concentration, but also to the availability of substrates within the lung lining fluid compartment. Following a reaction with a target substrate, ozone is consumed and thus inactivated.

Studies employing oxygen-18-labelled ozone have revealed that lung lining fluid takes up proportionally more ozone than either the lung lining fluid cell fraction or

lung tissue.[29] These data, combined with a range of in vitro studies demonstrating interactions between antioxidants and ozone, have led to the general belief that antioxidants present in lung lining fluid protect the lung from oxidative challenge. When ozone reacts with non-antioxidant substrates in lung lining fluid, such as protein or lipid, secondary oxidation products arise that may transmit toxic signals to the underlying epithelium.

NITROGEN DIOXIDE

Nitrogen dioxide is a nitrogen-centred free radical with limited solubility in aqueous solutions. High concentrations of nitrogen dioxide can damage the lung in animal studies, while cell culture experiments indicate that exposure increases cell permeability and injury. Controlled laboratory exposures of humans to high (parts per million range) concentrations of nitrogen dioxide result in a time-dependent inflammatory response in the lung.[30] Like ozone, it reacts with substrates present in the lung lining fluid compartment, and it is therefore unlikely to interact directly with the pulmonary epithelium.[31] Instead, it is the oxidized species arising from a reaction between nitrogen dioxide and the lung lining fluid compartment that are responsible for initiating the signalling cascade that brings inflammatory cells into the lung.

Oxidative potential of particles

It has been argued that as exposure to a broad spectrum of particle types (e.g. vehicle emissions, cigarette and wood smoke) also elicits neutrophilic inflammation,[32] reduced inspiratory capacity[33] and heightened bronchial reactivity,[34] they may act through a common mechanism. Although the epidemiological evidence for particle-induced health effects is extremely strong, major questions remain concerning the mechanisms by which these compositionally heterogeneous species elicit their toxic actions. Indeed, the mechanisms underlying ambient particulate toxicity are more complicated than those for oxidant gases.

Particulate matter is a complex mixture of chemical components in terms of their chemical composition, dependent on the emission source and, in combustion scenarios, the type of fuel being burnt (see Chapter 7). For example, ultrafine particles from sources of combustion generally comprise a carbonaceous core with absorbed substances condensed onto the surface, including organic and elemental carbon, polycyclic aromatic hydrocarbons (PAHs), metals (both redox active and non-redox active), biological compounds such as bacterial endotoxin, as well as sulphate, nitrate, chloride and ammonium.

The composition dictates the surface reactivity of the particles – an important factor in determining particle toxicity[35] and their adverse health effects. Whether these particulate components result in substantial oxidative damage, inflammation and injury depends on their initial

Table 9.3 Responses to particles exposure observed in animal studies

Particle type	Response
Residual oil fly ash or isolated components	Neutrophil influx
	Oedema
	Bronchial reactivity
	Increased infection
	Increased glutathione concentration in the lung
Diesel exhaust	Generation of proinflammatory cytokines, catalase or organic extracts
	Nuclear factor κB activation
	Inflammation
Quinones	Generation of reactive oxygen species
	Inflammation

interactions with these antioxidant defences. It is useful to grade the response of the lung to particle-induced oxidative stress (Table 9.3), with low-level oxidative stress resulting in an upregulation of endogenous extra- and intracellular responses prior to the induction of substantial toxicity.[36]

The interaction of particles with metals to potentiate pulmonary toxicity appears to be important. For example, in the rat lung, ultrafine carbon black induced a significant neutrophil influx, and this inflammatory effect is positively enhanced by the addition of iron salts.[37] However, much of the experimental work examining the contribution of metals to particulate matter toxicity has made use of residual oil fly ash (ROFA), which contains about 10 per cent by weight of water-soluble iron, nickel and vanadium.

The instillation of high concentrations of ROFA into rat airways has been shown to induce neutrophilia, oedema, bronchial hyperreactivity and increased susceptibility to infection in these animals.[38] Equivalent responses have been observed in these studies using only the water-soluble components of these samples.[39] The instillation of ROFA into mice lungs significantly increases the total glutathione concentration of lung lining fluid, whereas this response is attenuated in transgenic mice overexpressing extracellular superoxide dismutase.[40] Furthermore, elevated lung extracellular GSH concentrations following particulate matter challenge is due to an increased activity of c-glutamylcysteine synthase.[41]

Urate concentrations are also increased in the lung lining fluid of rats following the instillation of metal-rich particulates, in association with an increased expression of xanthine oxidase, suggesting that the production of uric acid is directly regulated by iron via regulation of the expression or activity of its enzymatic source.[42]

Consistent with this concept, diesel exhaust particles have been shown to generate free radicals in bronchial and nasal epithelial cells, as well as their organic extracts.[43]

Further evidence for a key role of oxidative stress in the upregulation of proinflammatory cytokines has been demonstrated by the capacity of antioxidants to reduce both nuclear factor κB activation and cytokine release from cells challenged in vitro with diesel exhaust particles or their extracts.[44]

Evidence is also accumulating to suggest that organic components carried on the particle surface play an important role in mediating a toxic effect. Ambient particles have been shown to contain stable organic radicals that have been tentatively identified as quinones,[45] which again are highly redox active molecules that can generate reactive oxygen species.[46] For example, a semiquinone radical, $QH\bullet$, can reduce oxygen to form superoxide, which can undergo dismutation to hydrogen peroxide and finally form the hydroxyl radical in the presence of 'free' iron. Biological reductants such as ascorbate, NAD(P)H and glutathione are then able to reduce the oxidized quinoid back to the reduced state ($QH\bullet$ and the hydroquinone), enabling the reaction to cycle again. This illustrates once more that the interactions between particle constituents and lung lining fluid antioxidants are not always necessarily protective.

The organic fraction of particulate matter, particularly the fine fraction, can also include semi-volatile PAHs. These compounds can induce oxidative stress indirectly through biotransformation by cytochrome P450 and dihydrodiol dehydrogenase to generate the redox active quinones. PAHs and their derivatives are formed during the incomplete combustion and pyrolysis of organic material, and can thus be released into the atmosphere from natural sources (e.g. volcanic eruptions and forest fires) and anthropogenic emissions.[47]

The role of particle size and surface area versus composition as determinants of toxicity

Oxidizing species such as transition metals and the organic compounds described above interact with and deplete lung lining fluid antioxidants in the same manner as gaseous pollutants. Of course, as a consequence, these particles will arrive at the lung surface in a less active form. However, surface reactivity is not the only aspect of particle toxicity. A number of groups have produced evidence indicating that particle size is an important determinant of reactivity. The mechanism by which a large number of particles or a large surface area leads to increased biological activity is not known, but surface area does appear to be the metric that drives the inflammation in vivo caused by low toxicity particles.[23]

Redox balance at the lung surface

The rules that govern the balance between beneficial and detrimental interactions in the lung lining fluid compartment are not well established, but these may contribute in part to the sensitivity of individuals to air pollution.[25] A simplistic viewpoint would be that the greater the range and concentration of antioxidant defences on the lung surface, the better the level of protection from oxidant air pollutants. If this were the case, however, subgroups of the population recognized to be susceptible to air pollution should have decreased lung lining fluid antioxidant defences. This was indeed found in asthmatic individuals, a susceptible subgroup in that they have markedly decreased concentrations of ascorbic acid in lung lining fluid compared with healthy control subjects.[26] However, the same was not found to be true of those healthy subjects who happen to show the largest decrease in lung function following ozone challenge.[48]

It is not yet clear to what extent lung lining fluid antioxidants perform a critical role in reducing the toxic consequences of oxidant challenges to the lung. Ozone elicits a broad spectrum of airway antioxidant responses, with initial losses of vitamin C and urate followed by a phase of augmentation of low molecular weight antioxidant concentrations at the air–lung interface; this suggests that these defences play an important role in this respect. The temporal association between increased lung fluid glutathione concentration following ozone exposure and the loss of this thiol from macrophages implies its mobilization to the lung surface is part of an acute protective adaptation to ozone.[49] Furthermore, given that lung fluid ascorbate can be augmented only transiently by oral vitamin C supplementation, it suggests that the antioxidant status at the lung surface is tightly regulated,[50] for as yet unknown reasons.

CONCLUSION

The lung is exquisitely designed to undertake its primary task – gaseous exchange. Ambient air is sucked down through a labyrinth of branching airways to flaccid alveolar sacs that permit gaseous transfer along defined concentration gradients. Gases other than oxygen and particles small enough to also make their way into the lung are dealt with by an elaborate series of physical, immunological and biochemical defences.

Exposure to a broad spectrum of gases (ozone and nitrogen dioxide) and particle types (e.g. vehicle emissions and cigarette and wood smoke) elicits similar acute responses in the lung, namely neutrophilic inflammation. It is thus possible that these opportunistic visitors to the lung act through common mechanisms, one of which may relate to an ability to cause damaging oxidation reactions or 'oxidative stress'. The precise nature of the mechanisms involved and the tissue responses that occur are a major research focus as acute and chronic respiratory disorders continue to make a major contribution to the public health agenda.

REFERENCES

● = Key primary paper
◆ = Major review article

1. Stinson SF, Loosli CG. Ultrastructural evidence concerning the mode of secretion of electron-dense granules by Clara cells. *J Anat* 1978; **127**(Pt 2): 291–8.
2. Serabjit-Singh CJ, Wolf CR, Philpot RM, Plopper CG. Cytochrome p-450: localization in rabbit lung. *Science* 1980; **207**: 1469–70.
3. Giangreco A, Reynolds SD, Stripp BR. Terminal bronchioles harbor a unique airway stem cell population that localizes to the bronchoalveolar duct junction. *Am J Pathol* 2002; **161**: 173–82.
4. Green FHY, Schürch S, Gehr P, Lee MR. The role of surfactant in disease associated with particle exposure. In: Gehr P, Heyder J (eds) *Particle–Lung Interactions*. New York: Marcel Dekker, 2000: 533–76.
5. Bazzoni G, Dejana E. Endothelial cell-to-cell junctions: molecular organization and role in vascular homeostasis. *Physiol Rev* 2004; **84**: 869–901.
6. Guo M, Breslin JW, Wu MH, Cara J, Gottardi C, Yuan SY. VE-cadherin and β-catenin binding dynamics during histamine-induced endothelial hyperpermeability. *Am J Physiol Cell Physiol* 2008; **294**:977–84.
◆7. Pearlstein DP, Ali MH, Mungai PT, Hynes KL, Gewertz BL, Schumacker PT. Role of mitochondrial oxidant generation in endothelial cell responses to hypoxia. *Arterioscler Thromb Vasc Biol* 2002; **22**: 566–73.
8. Richardson JB. Nerve supply to the lungs. *Am Rev Respir Dis* 1979; **119**: 785–802.
◆9. Belvisi MG. Overview of the innervation of the lung. *Curr Opin Pharmacol* 2002; **2**: 211–15.
10. International Commission on Radiological Protection. Human respiratory tract model for radiological protection. ICRP Publication No. 66. *Ann ICRP* 1994; **24**(1–3): 1–482.
11. Bailey MR, Ansoborio E, Guilmette RA, Paquet F. Updating the ICRP human respiratory tract model. *Radiat Prot Dosimetry* 2007; **127**: 31–34.
12. Bannenberg G, Atzori L, Xue J et al. Sulfur dioxide and sodium metabisulfite induce bronchoconstriction in the isolated perfused and ventilated guinea pig lung via stimulation of capsaicin-sensitive sensory nerves. *Respiration* 1994; **61**: 130–7.
13. Valentine R, Kennedy GL. Inhalation toxicology, fibers. In: Hayes AW (ed.) *Principles and Methods of Toxicology*, 5th edn. Philadelphia: Taylor & Francis, 2007: 1417–21.
14. Matsui H, Randell SH, Peretti SW, Davis CW, Boucher RC. Coordinated clearance of periciliary liquid and mucus from airway surfaces. *J Clin Invest* 1998; **102**: 1125–31.
15. Smith DJ, Gaffney EA, Blake JR. Modelling mucociliary clearance. *Respir Physiol Neurobiol* 2008; **163**: 178–88.
◆16. Davis CW, Lazarowski E. Coupling of airway ciliary activity and mucin secretion to mechanical stresses by purinergic signaling. *Respir Physiol Neurobiol* 2008; **163**(1–3): 208–13.

17. Kreyling WG, Scheuch G. Clearance of particles deposited in the lungs. In: Gehr P, Heyder J (eds) *Particle–Lung Interactions*. New York: Marcel Dekker, 2000: 323–76.

18. Geiser M, Rothen-Rutishauser B, Kapp N *et al.* Ultrafine particles cross cellular membranes by nonphagocytic mechanisms in lungs and in cultured cell. *Environ Health Perspect* 2005; 113: 1555–60.

19. Churg A. Particle uptake by epithelial cells. In: Gehr P, Heyder J (eds) *Particle–Lung Interactions*. New York: Marcel Dekker, 2000: 401–35.

◆20. Moller W, Felten K, Sommerer K *et al.* Deposition, retention, and translocation of ultrafine particles from the central airways and lung periphery. *Am J Respir Crit Care Med* 2008; 177: 426–32.

21. Dreher KL, Jaskot RH, Lehmann JR *et al.* Soluble transition metals mediate residual oil fly ash induced acute lung injury. *J Toxicol Environ Health* 1997; 50: 285–305.

22. Rylander R, Haglind P, Lundholm M. Endotoxin in cotton dust and respiratory function decrement among cotton workers in an experimental cardroom. *Am Rev Respir Dis* 1985; 131: 209–13.

23. Duffin R, Tran CL, Clouter A *et al.* The importance of surface area and specific reactivity in the acute pulmonary inflammatory response to particles. *Ann Occup Hyg* 2002; 46: 242–45.

24. Cross CE, van der Vleit LS, Thiele JJ, Halliwell B. Oxidative stress and antioxidants at biosurfaces: plants, skin and respiratory tract surfaces. *Environ Health Perspect* 1998; 106: 1241–51.

25. Kelly FJ, Mudway IS, Krishna MT, Holgate ST. The free radical basis of air pollution: focus on ozone. *Respir Med* 1995; 89: 647–56.

●26. Kelly FJ, Mudway I, Blomberg A, Frew A, Sandstrom T. Altered lung antioxidant status in patients with mild asthma. *Lancet* 1999; 354: 482–3.

◆27. Mudway IS, Kelly FJ. Ozone and the lung: a sensitivity issue. *Mol Aspects Med* 2000; 21: 1–48.

28. Langford SD, Bidani A, Postlethwait EM. Ozone-reactive absorption by pulmonary epithelial lining fluid constituents. *Toxicol Appl Pharmacol* 1995; 132: 122–30.

29. Hatch GE, Slade R, Harris LP *et al.* Ozone dose and effect in humans and rats. A comparison using oxygen-18 labeling and bronchoalveolar lavage. *Am J Respir Crit Care Med* 1994; 150: 676–83.

30. Sandstrom T, Stjernberg N, Eklund A *et al.* Inflammatory cell response in bronchoalveolar lavage fluid after nitrogen dioxide exposure of healthy subjects: a dose–response study. *Eur Respir J* 1991; 4: 332–9.

31. Kelly FJ, Tetley T. Nitrogen dioxide depletes uric acid and ascorbic acid but not glutathione from lung lining fluid. *Biochem J* 1997; 325: 95–9.

32. Ghio AJ, Kim C, Devlin RB. Concentrated ambient air particles induce mild pulmonary inflammation in healthy human volunteers. *Am J Respir Crit Care Med* 2000; 162: 981–8.

33. Chen R, Tunstall-Pedoe H, Tavendale, R. Environmental tobacco smoke and lung function in employees who never smoked: the Scottish MONICA study. *Occup Environ Med* 2001; 58, 563–8.

34. Nordenhall C, Pourazar J, Blomberg A, Levin JO, Sandstrom T, Adelroth E. Airway inflammation following exposure to diesel exhaust: a study of time kinetics using induced sputum. *Eur Respir J* 2000; 15: 1046–51.

35. Fubini B. Surface reactivity in the pathogenic response to particulates. *Environ Health Perspect* 1997; 105: 1013–20.

36. Li N. Use of a stratified oxidative stress model to study the biological effects of ambient concentrated and diesel exhaust particulate matter. *Inhal Toxicol* 2002; 14: 459–66.

37. Wilson MR, Lightbody JH, Donaldson K, Sales J, Stone V. Interactions between ultrafine particles and transition metals in vivo and in vitro. *Toxicol Appl Pharmacol* 2002; 184: 172–9.

38. Gavett SH, Madison SL, Dreher KL, Winsett DW, McGee JK, Costa DL. Metal and sulfate composition of residual oil fly ash determines airway hyperreactivity and lung injury in rats. *Environ Res* 1997; 72: 162–72.

●39. Dreher KL, Jaskot RH, Lehmann JR *et al.* Soluble transition metals mediate residual oil fly ash induced acute lung injury. *J Toxicol Environ Health* 1997; 50: 285–305.

40. Ghio AJ, Suliman HB, Carter JD, Abushamaa AM, Folz RJ. Overexpression of extracellular superoxide dismutase decreases lung injury after exposure to oil fly ash. *Am J Physiol* 2002; 283: L211–18.

41. Rahman I, Morrison D, Dondaldson K, McNee W. Systemic oxidative stress in asthma, COPD and smokers. *Am J Respir Crit Care Med* 1996; 154: 1055–60.

●42. Ghio, AJ, Kennedy TP, Stonehuerner J *et al.* Iron regulates xanthine oxidase activity in the lung. *Am J Physiol* 2002; 283: L563–72.

43. Sagai M, Saito H, Ichinose T, Kodama M, Mori Y. Biological effects of diesel exhaust particles. I: In vitro production of superoxide and in vivo toxicity in mouse. *Free Rad Biol Med* 1993; 14: 37–47.

44. Hashimoto S, Gon Y, Takeshita I *et al.* Diesel exhaust particles activate p38 MAP kinase to produce interleukin 8 and RANTES by human bronchial epithelial cells and N-acetylcysteine attenuates p38 MAP kinase activation. *Am J Respir Crit Care* 2000; 161: 280–5.

45. Squadrito GL, Dellinger B, Pryor WA. Quinoid redox cycling as a mechanism for sustained free radical generation by inhaled airborne particulate matter. *Free Rad Biol Med* 2001; 31: 1132–8.

46. Bolton JL, Trush MA, Penning TM, Dryhurst G, Monks TJ. Role of quinones in toxicology. *Chem Res Toxicol* 2000; 13: 135–60.

47. Manoli E, Kouras A, Samara C. Profile analysis of ambient and source emitted particle-bound polycyclic aromatic hydrocarbons from three sites in northern Greece. *Chemosphere* 2004; 56: 867–78.

48. Mudway IS, Stenfors N, Blomberg A *et al.* Differences in basal airway antioxidant concentrations are not predictive

of individual responsiveness to ozone: a comparison of
healthy and mild asthmatic subjects. *Free Rad Biol Med*
2001; **31**: 962–74.

49. Behndig A, Blomberg A, Helleday R, Kelly FJ, Mudway IS.
Augmentation of respiratory tract lining fluid ascorbate
concentrations through supplementation with vitamin C.
Inhal Toxicol 2009; **21**: 250–58.

50. Behndig A, Blomberg A, Helleday R, Duggan S, Kelly FJ,
Mudway IS. Antioxidant responses to ozone in healthy
human airway. *Inhal Toxicol* 2009; **21**: 933–42.

10

Health effects of air pollution: acute and chronic

IAN LITCHFIELD, DOUGLAS W. DOCKERY, JON G. AYRES

INTRODUCTION

It took the London smog of 1952 to demonstrate the risk to human health of breathing polluted air in the industrialized cities of the 1940s and 50s.[1] At least 4000 (and probably many more) deaths resulted from cardiac and respiratory disease during that episode. The effects of the London smog should have come as no surprise: earlier incidents in the Meuse Valley in 1930 and in Donora, Pennsylvania in 1948 had shown that high concentrations of industrially generated air pollutants could have a serious effect on health. At the time, scientific opinion believed that the impact on health was a result of the combination of particles and sulphur dioxide, and while a later re-examination of the historical data supported a role for the acidity of the aerosol in contributing to the observed mortality,[2] this hypothesis has since been questioned, highlighting the difficulty of identifying causal pathways in this whole area.

This episode led to the Clean Air Act of 1956, which was introduced to prevent a repeat of these events, and measures such as heightening chimneys, relocating power stations and introducing smoke-free zones all led to a reduction in black smoke levels in the urban environment. By 1970, as the air became measurably cleaner, some evidence of health benefits emerged, with symptoms of chronic bronchitis no longer being so closely influenced by fluctuations in daily pollutant levels.[3] As time passed, however, road traffic increased, and it was realized from work in the USA that pollutants associated with the internal combustion engine had begun to impact on human health.

POLLUTANTS, SOURCES AND EXPOSURES

The sources and factors governing emissions of the major air pollutants and their control are described in Chapter 7. For the purposes of this chapter, UK, European Community and World Health Organization air quality standards are shown in Table 10.1 and define levels of population exposure above which the risk of adverse health effects might occur. Some confusion has arisen regarding the World Health Organization Air Quality Guidelines: these define exposures in terms of concentrations and durations of exposure, and state that, at guideline levels, the majority of the population is unlikely to experience adverse effects as a result of exposure. A common error is to assume that immediately the guideline has been exceeded, most people will experience such effects; however, this is not so, and most guidelines include a margin of safety that will prevent widespread effects until the guideline has been significantly exceeded.

Exposure to air pollution is dependent on the type of source of those pollutants, the strength of the source(s) and the behaviour of the individual(s) potentially exposed. As personal monitoring of pollutant exposures in large numbers of individuals has to date been impossible, the estimation of population exposures has relied on the use of sentinel monitoring sites, despite offering only a crude measure of individual exposure. This problem is discussed in depth in Chapter 5, but it nevertheless remains true that much of the community epidemiology on air pollution is based on sentinel site data, yet has been shown to be robust and repeatable across a wide range of countries and scenarios.

Table 10.1   Air quality standards for criterion air pollutants for the UK, the European Community (EC) and the World Health Organization (WHO)

	Air quality standards		
	WHO (2005 revision)	EC	UK
Sulphur dioxide			
10 minutes	500 µg/m³		
15 minutes	–		100 ppb (286 µg/m³)
24 hours	125 µg/m³ (Interim Target 1) 20 µg/m³ (AQS)		
Annual	Now not needed as adherence to the 24 hour standard will control annual exposures	48.8 ppb if smoke >60 µg/m³ 67.5 ppb if smoke <60 µg/m³	
Nitrogen dioxide			
1 hour	200 µg/m³	70.6 ppb (133 µg/m³)*	150 ppb (282 µg/m³)
Annual	40 µg/m³	26.2 ppb (49 µg/m³)†	
Ozone			
8 hour moving average	100 µg/m³	55 ppb (110 µg/m³)	50 ppb (100 µg/m³)
Particles			
24 hour mean	PM₁₀ 50 µg/m³ PM₂.₅ 25 µg/m³	PM₁₀ 80 µg/m³	PM₁₀ (>50 µg/m³)‡
Annual mean	PM₁₀ 20 µg/m³ PM₂.₅ 10 µg/m³		

AQS, Air Quality Standards; PM, particulate matter; ppb, parts per billion.
*98% centile.
† 50th centile.
‡ Currently under revision to a PM₂.₅ standard.

ASSESSING THE HEALTH EFFECTS OF AIR POLLUTANTS

Health effects of air pollution can result from acute exposure leading to mild short-term impacts such as irritation to the eyes, nose and throat, or more serious effects such as exacerbations of respiratory and cardiovascular diseases resulting in hospital admission or death.[4–6] Effects mostly occur on the day of exposure or the succeeding day, but in some conditions lagged effects are seen over days or even weeks. Chronic exposure over months or years can contribute to both the initiation and the progressive worsening of, in particular, cardiorespiratory disease[6] and can affect lung growth in children.[7]

The relationship between exposure and pollutant exposure for most end points is linear with no evidence for a threshold (i.e. a level below which no effects occur) (Figure 10.1). The question of the existence of a threshold is critical (as has been questioned for ozone) because, if true, this would materially affect calculations of health

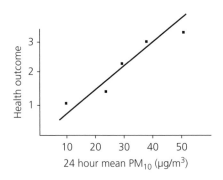

Figure 10.1   Hypothetical exposure response plot for an undefined health outcome (e.g. hospital admissions per day) against 24 hour mean particle exposure. The linearity of the slope allows calculation of an effect size by computing the change in health outcome per unit change in PM exposure.

burden from air pollution. However, for general purposes, non-threshold relationships should be regarded as the norm.

Exposure–response plots such as that shown in Figure 10.1 allow effect size coefficients to be calculated. These are usually expressed as a percentage change in effect (or increase in risk) per unit change in exposure, although different denominators have been used in different studies, which can make direct comparisons less easy. Expressing these exposure–response coefficients in terms of a common metric of exposure facilitates comparisons across studies. Although the term 'exposure–response coefficients' has been used here, few epidemiological studies actually measure personal exposure to air pollutants, the majority instead relating effects to ambient concentrations.

Methods of assessment of health effects

There are a number of ways of measuring the health effects resulting from exposure to air pollution:

- *Epidemiological studies*: Time series studies of routinely collected data and panel studies of potentially susceptible groups such as schoolchildren are used to estimate the effects of short-term exposures. Longitudinal cohort studies provide estimates of the effects of long-term exposures, and to a lesser extent, cross-sectional studies also provide estimates of the effects of long-term exposure. Populations sampled in these natural exposure studies include the most sensitive individuals.
- *Experimental studies on human subjects*: The controlled laboratory exposure of volunteers allows measurements of the physiological or biochemical responses to exposure to one or a combination of pollutants. These studies are usually of healthy, and do not include the most sensitive, individuals.
- *Experimental studies on animals*: Controlled laboratory exposures of animals with known characteristics can include detailed physiological and pathological evaluations of the response. Animal models of susceptible human subgroups have also been evaluated. Multiday or extended exposures that would not be feasible with human subjects can also be undertaken.
- *Experimental in vitro work on cells*: Cells obtained from nasal or bronchoalveolar lavage or cultured in monolayers can be exposed to pollutants, providing mechanistic information.

In addition to a direct measurement of health impacts, a prediction of effects can be made using computer modelling. This requires the use of valid exposure data for the pollutant or pollutants under investigation, incorporating co-exposures such as meteorological variables and individual characteristics. This capacity has been enhanced by the use of geographical information systems (GISs; see box on page 109), which allow the relationships between a range of pollutants and other environmental factors to be explored within an increasingly refined geographical scale.

Effects of short-term exposure to air pollution

The effects of short-term (1–3 day) exposures to air pollutants have been demonstrated for all ranges of severity from physiological responses to symptoms to hospitalizations and to mortality. This was not considered surprising for respiratory disease, but the fact that all-cause (non-trauma) mortality was associated with particle exposure suggested that air pollutants might affect individuals with cardiac disease. This suggestion has subsequently been confirmed, raising questions of potential mechanisms that are discussed below.

ASTHMA: SYMPTOMS AND ADMISSIONS

A number of panel studies of children, usually children with asthma, have demonstrated a link between nitrogen dioxide, ozone and particle exposure, and health end points. Inhaler use and symptoms have been reported to increase by 3 per cent for every $10\,\mu g/m^3$ rise in particulate matter with a diameter of $10\,\mu m$ or less (PM_{10}). Lung function effects tend to be less marked, with peak flow falls of less than 1 per cent for the same increment.[8] However, these North American findings have not in general been replicated in Europe, most notably by the Pediatric Asthma Control Evaluation (PEACE) studies,[9,10] perhaps suggesting that particle size and/or content may be important or that the pollutant mix might be important. Some studies have shown a more marked effect when considering fine particles ($PM_{2.5}$),[11] particularly traffic-related $PM_{2.5}$.[12] Factors specific to the subjects under study are also important: where effects were observed in the North American studies, they were more likely to be seen in children who were either atopic or had pre-existing symptoms, or both.[13]

Apparently in conflict with the variable evidence from panel studies, there is a clear relationship between day-to-day exposure to air pollution and hospital admission.[14,15] Although there are many triggers for asthma attacks (e.g. aeroallergens) that are more important,[16] this does not mean that air pollution is unimportant.

Sulphur dioxide is a potent bronchoconstrictor with a much greater effect, dose for dose, in individuals with asthma compared with healthy individuals. Now that low-sulphur motor vehicle fuels are used in many countries, sulphur from diesel fuels has been become a small contributor to ambient concentrations of sulphur dioxide. The main source of exposure to this gas is from industrial point sources or coal-fired power stations, although high concentrations of sulphur dioxide were historically due to the widespread use of coal for domestic heating. Nevertheless, the Air Pollution and Health, a European Approach (APHEA) studies have consistently shown a link between sulphur dioxide level and hospital admission in Europe. A Canadian study investigated the impact of short-term exposure to emissions from a petrol refinery on children between 2 and 4 years of age living up to 7.5 km from the refinery and showed a relationship between emergency department visits/hospitalizations and modelled same-day peak levels of sulphur dioxide.[17]

One innovative attempt to match personal exposure to pollutants and lung function and inflammatory responses was undertaken in a cross-over study of 60 adults with mild-to-moderate asthma in London, UK.[46] On separate occasions, the subjects were studied while walking along a busy, central road (Oxford Street) and through the less polluted Hyde Park.[18] Oxford Street exposure was associated with worse lung function and increases in neutrophilic inflammation and airway acidification compared with Hyde Park exposure, effects being greater in those with more severe asthma and linked closely with personal $PM_{2.5}$ exposure.

Ozone, particles and sulphur dioxide exposure are thus associated with severe attacks of asthma requiring hospital admission but have variable effects when considering lesser levels of morbidity. However, short-term exposure to city pollution can worsen airway inflammation in asthmatic subjects.

Asthma mortality

Death from asthma is rare, and although it is plausible that air pollution contributes to asthma deaths, there are no historical[1,19,20] or modern data to suggest that air pollution does so. There are, however, case reports of individuals suffering fatal asthma attacks following accidental exposure to high sulphur dioxide concentrations.[21]

CHRONIC OBSTRUCTIVE PULMONARY DISEASE: SYMPTOMS AND ADMISSIONS

A number of studies have demonstrated a relationship between exposure to air pollution and hospital admissions for chronic obstructive pulmonary disease (COPD), showing an increase in hospitalizations of between 1 and 3 per cent for a $10 \mu g/m^3$ rise in PM_{10} in the USA[8] and of around 1 per cent in the APHEA study from Europe.[22,23] The majority of studies point to particles being the more important pollutant, although in some ozone may also play a part, particularly in the summer months.[24] In cities where sulphur dioxide emissions are still significant, this gas is still associated with COPD admissions. For instance, in Sao Paulo, Brazil, the daily number of COPD emergency room visits was related to both PM_{10} and sulphur dioxide with immediate and lagged effects.[25] Associations have also been shown for nitrogen dioxide. In the UK, one study of rural COPD admissions showed a 22 per cent increased risk of admission for a $10 \mu g/m^3$ increase in nitrogen dioxide, which might reflect an association with another unmeasured pollutant such as particle number given that levels of nitrogen dioxide were very low.[26]

Chronic obstructive pulmonary disease mortality

Day-to-day changes in exposure to air pollution are associated with changes in deaths from COPD, most strongly

2–3 days following exposure.[8] In the USA, COPD deaths increased by about 3.4 per cent for each $10 \mu g/m^3$ rise in PM_{10}.[8] In Europe, however, sulphur dioxide still plays a role (even at levels much lower than those seen in past decades), particularly where long-term PM levels are higher.[15,27]

CARDIOVASCULAR DISEASE

Although inhaling polluted air can logically be expected to adversely affect subjects with respiratory disease, it might not seem immediately obvious why such exposures would affect patients with cardiovascular disease.[28] Nevertheless, the evidence that this occurs is overwhelming. The initial finding that all-cause mortality is associated with particle exposure led to a realization that cardiovascular effects were likely and has also led to studies of a wide range of acute cardiovascular events (ranging from myocardial infarction to arrhythmias) and risk factor predictors of these events such as heart rate variability (HRV).

Cardiovascular mortality

In the 1990s, the first clear evidence that air pollution was associated with cardiovascular mortality appeared,[29] and subsequent studies have confirmed this association. A summary estimate was provided by the UK's Committee on Medical Effects of Air Pollutants (COMEAP) report[30] (Figure 10.2) showing that, for a $10 \mu g/m^3$ rise in 24 hour mean PM_{10}, cardiovascular deaths increased by 0.5 per cent.

Effect size varies by diagnosis within the general rubric of 'cardiovascular disease', which will reflect both true differences in actual diagnosis as well as differences in diagnostic practice across countries. For instance, a study from the Netherlands over 8 years observed significant effects for total cardiovascular mortality (relative risk mortality: 1.2 per cent for an $80 \mu g/m^3$ increase in 7 day mean PM_{10}, 2.9 per cent for $40 \mu g/m^3$ 7 day mean sulphur dioxide, 5.5 per cent for $150 \mu g/m^3$ 8 hour mean ozone), lesser effects for myocardial infarction and other ischaemic heart disease deaths (relative risk mortality 0.5 per cent for PM_{10}, 1.5 per cent for sulphur dioxide, 2.6 per cent for ozone), and effects that were most pronounced (three times higher for all pollutants except ozone) for deaths from heart failure and arrhythmia.[31] This also highlights the marked differences in effect across different pollutants even though heterogeneity is also present for other pollutants (Figure 10.2). There is a consistent effect of ozone on cardiovascular deaths even in areas with relatively low exposures.

Particles are a heterogeneous mixture of materials. One source of the heterogeneity may be differences in composition of the particles themselves. A Californian study examined associations of daily cardiovascular mortality with the constituents of $PM_{2.5}$[32] and showed that daily mortality was associated with specific constituents, namely elemental and organic carbon, nitrates, sulphates, copper and potassium, the most marked effect being for organic carbon, nitrates and iron.

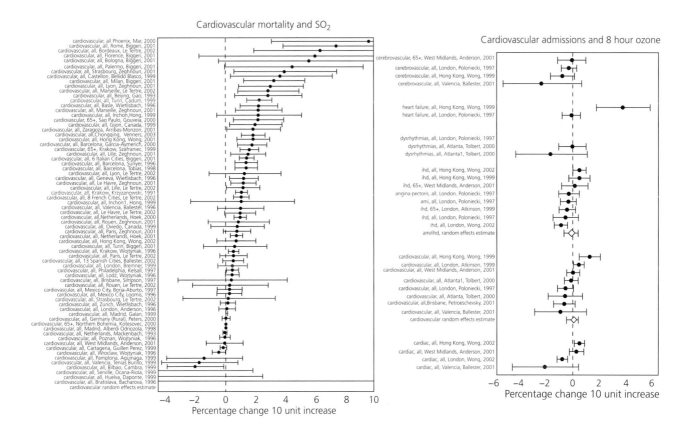

Figure 10.2   Forest plots showing heterogeneity of effect sizes for cardiovascular mortality and sulphur dioxide exposure and cardiovascular admissions and 8 hour ozone from time series studies. Each row represents one published paper for which a mean effect size and 95% confidence intervals are plotted. Reproduced from ref. 30 with permission.

Cardiovascular admissions

Admissions for cardiac disease can be difficult to assess because of differences in diagnostic coding. Where there is a clear diagnosis such as myocardial infarction,[5] there can be more confidence about a clear association with air pollution than, for instance, when the admission diagnosis is a more general diagnosis such as chest pain. Nevertheless, there is a consistent association between admissions for cardiovascular disease and exposure to particles. One meta-analysis showed that a $10\,\mu g/m^3$ reduction in 24 hour average PM_{10} concentration was associated with a 0.8 per cent reduction in cardiovascular admissions.[33] This effect is seen more with increasing age.[34]

These effects can be seen at particle levels within the general air quality standards. For instance, the Determinants of Myocardial Infarction Onset Study showed that a $2.5\,\mu g/m^3$ increase in hourly $PM_{2.5}$ within current air quality standards was associated with around a 5 per cent increased risk of myocardial infarction within 1–2 hours. Furthermore, high 24 hour concentrations of fine particles 1 day before the onset of symptoms were also associated with an elevated risk.[35] The results for the two separate time periods were independent and additive, suggesting the possibility of two, potentially independent mechanisms.

Cardiovascular mortality, but not number of admissions, is associated with ozone exposure. This difference between cardiovascular responses to ozone compared with particles may indicate that ozone is proarrhythmic, resulting in out-of-hospital cardiac death.

Arrhythmias

While the main underlying cause of cardiac deaths is coronary artery disease, the final cause of death is usually a disorder of rhythm. However, not all arrhythmias are due to underlying coronary artery disease. In the West German smog episode of 1985, admissions for arrhythmia increased by some 50 per cent in comparison to the period before and after the event,[19] suggesting that air pollution has a separate effect on the induction of arrhythmias.

This is supported by a panel study investigating episodes of defibrillation in relation to ambient air quality among 100 patients with implantable cardioverter defibrillators in Boston, USA.[36] The frequency of defibrillator discharges showed a significant correlation with increased levels of PM_{10} and $PM_{2.5}$, with a lag time of 2 days and an association with nitrogen dioxide levels on the previous day. In a subgroup of patients who had had at least 10 interventions to treat ventricular arrhythmia, the odds of a discharge tripled, with an increase in nitrogen dioxide from the fifth to the 95th percentile, and increased by 60 per cent for the equivalent rise in $PM_{2.5}$. The 2 day lead time between particle exposure and arrhythmia onset might suggest that particle exposure establishes a milieu that increases susceptibility to subsequent proarrhythmic triggers. However, recent evidence for arrhythmias is not entirely consistent with this.[37]

Effects of long-term exposure to air pollution

Long-term exposure to air pollution may have a greater overall impact on public health than acute exposures,[8] and may have a clear impact on mortality.[38–40] The main effects are seen in COPD and cardiac disease, but there remains uncertainty over whether such an effect is seen in asthma.

ASTHMA

There are persuasive mechanistic arguments to support the assertion that long-term exposure to air pollutants is associated with an increased risk of developing asthma *ab initio* based on immunological, inflammatory and morphogenetic considerations. These factors could act interactively such that exposure to air pollutants could modify the way in which the airways respond to injury, could affect an underlying genetic predisposition to raise immunoglobulin E production or could produce an exaggerated airway response either to endogenous bronchoconstrictor agents or through neural reflexes. As reviewed above, there is substantial epidemiological evidence that exposure to air pollution can trigger attacks and generally exacerbate asthma in patients with this condition, but the epidemiological evidence of an association between long-term air pollution exposure and increased rates of asthma is much more limited.

Traffic studies

Cross-sectional studies of proximity to roads and levels of traffic have suggested associations with the prevalence of asthma. The use of newer technologies such as GIS (see box on page 109) to obtain estimates of pollutant exposure provides new opportunities for improving exposure–response relationships. For instance, a cross-sectional study from Sweden used GIS to link residential address to road traffic and emissions of various nitrogen oxides and found that living within 100 m of a road with more than 10 cars a minute was associated with a diagnosis of asthma (odds ratio [OR] 1.40, 95 per cent confidence interval [CI] 1.04–1.89).[41]

Longitudinal studies

The Seventh Day Adventists study (AHSMOG) suggested that exposure to different components of the pollutant mix (notable particles and ozone) could in turn lead to an increased incidence of asthma,[14] although effects were limited to males. Although this population is helpful in

that smoking is not a confounder, extrapolation to other populations needs be done with caution. The Southern California Children's Health Study suggests that there may be an association of new-onset asthma in relation to exposure to traffic, but the balance of evidence is unconvincing at present.[42]

CHRONIC OBSTRUCTIVE PULMONARY DISEASE

Chronic obstructive pulmonary disease is a disease largely caused by cigarette smoking, and other factors such as occupation or outdoor air pollution have consequently received less attention. Nevertheless, studies from the 1950s in the UK found a higher prevalence of COPD in postmen working in more polluted areas, an association independent of smoking.[43] A further study on postmen found reduced lung function in those who worked in polluted cities compared with less polluted areas.[44] Subsequent research on both sides of the Atlantic has produced similar findings in the general population.[45,46] Raised levels of gaseous and particulate pollution are associated with increased respiratory morbidity,[47] and though evidence exists supporting the worsening of COPD symptoms,[21] there is little in the literature yet to demonstrate a link with new cases.[48]

CARDIOVASCULAR DISEASE

Throughout the Western world, ischaemic heart disease is the leading cause of mortality in men aged over 45 and women over 65. A number of time series investigations have considered the effect of air pollution on respiratory and cardiovascular deaths.[49,50,28] Survival analyses of cohort studies have provided evidence of risk of cardiovascular mortality associated with air pollution.[51] The American Cancer Society study of over half a million people followed since 1982 has been the most influential in this area.[39] Considering fine particles ($PM_{2.5}$), it found a 17 per cent increased risk of death (any non-trauma cause) and a 30 per cent increased risk of cardiopulmonary death in this population in the most compared with the least polluted areas. More recently, long-term exposures have been associated with mortality attributable to ischaemic heart disease, dysrhythmias, heart failure and cardiac arrest. For these causes of death, a $10\,\mu g/m^3$ elevation in fine PM was associated with an 8–18 per cent increase in mortality risk.[52,53] Importantly, these effects were robust to the addition of gaseous pollutants in the models, which appeared in general not to have an impact on chronic disease states.

Intervention studies have also contributed to knowledge in this area. Following the cessation of sales of coal in Dublin in the 1990s, black smoke levels fell by 70 per cent, with an associated fall in annual cardiovascular death rates of 10.3 per cent.[54] In Hong Kong, where legislation meant that ambient sulphur dioxide levels dropped sharply, there was a decline in cardiovascular death rates of 2.0 per cent.[55]

A number of studies have suggested that low socioeconomic status groups are more susceptible to the negative impact of long-term traffic pollution. A recent study explored this relationship further, studying associations between coronary artery calcification and high levels of traffic. Residential exposure to traffic was defined as proximity to major roads using GIS. High traffic and low socioeconomic status were both associated with higher amounts of calcification, but participants with low socioeconomic status and exposure to high traffic volume had the highest levels. Although high traffic levels were associated with high levels of coronary artery calcification in all groups, existing inequalities could be further shaped by traffic exposure.[56]

A recent study followed over 65 800 women in 36 US metropolitan areas for some 6 years in order to explore the role of long-term exposure to fine PM air pollution on cardiovascular disease in postmenopausal females. They found that each increase of $10\,\mu g/m^3$ in $PM_{2.5}$ was associated with an increased OR of 1.24 (95 per cent CI 1.09–1.41) for the onset of a cardiovascular event.[57]

In another study in the USA, some 132 000 adults aged over 30 who participated in the National Health Interview Survey for 6 years, beginning in 1999, were linked to annual $PM_{2.5}$ data from monitors within 20 km of their residence. It was found that a $10\,\mu g/m^3$ increase in exposure was associated with a 5 per cent increased risk of hypertension (OR 1.05, 95 per cent CI 1.00–1.10) and an 8 per cent increased risk of heart disease (OR 1.08, 95 per cent CI 1.00–1.16). Hypertension was found in white, non-Hispanic individuals but not in non-Hispanic black or Hispanic individuals.[58]

A meta-analysis of three large cross-sectional surveys in the UK, undertaken on a population in excess of 19 000 adults older than 45, also examined the relationship between self-reported doctor-diagnosed cardiovascular disease and outdoor air pollutants. Using multilevel regression analysis, the combined estimates showed that an increase of $1\,\mu g/m^3$ in PM_{10} was associated with a 2.9 per cent increased prevalence of heart disease in men and a 1.6 per cent greater prevalence for women. No consistent associations with gaseous pollutants could be established and, taken individually, no association was present in the years 1994 and 1998, although there was a strong association in 2003.[59]

MECHANISMS OF THE EFFECTS OF AIR POLLUTANTS

Particles

A number of mechanisms have been implicated in the health outcomes observed following exposure to PM dependent upon the size, composition and concentration of the PM.

Toxicology

It is likely that inhaled particles act through oxidant stress, largely through the generation of free radicals causing pro-inflammatory effects in the nose, lung and cardiovascular system.[60] High levels of reactive oxygen species change the redox status of the cell and its environment, triggering an inflammatory cascade and, at higher concentrations, apoptosis.[61,62] $PM_{2.5}$ samples taken from kerbsides have shown a greater potential to produce free radicals than those collected from an urban background environment, suggesting that newly generated particles may have more potential for oxidant stress.[63] This could lead to worsening of airway inflammation in COPD[64,65] and also to a worsening instability of atherosclerotic plaques. This is supported by animal studies in which particles promote oxidative lung damage, causing both alveolar and systemic inflammatory responses.[66,67]

This concept is supported by human challenge studies. Diesel exhaust exposure in individuals with coronary artery disease showed enhanced ST depression and an inhibition of tissue plasminogen activator, suggesting that diesel exhaust may have an immediate effect on coronary artery flow while increasing the likelihood of thrombosis.[68] Epidemiologically, carotid intima–media thickness, a measure of subclinical atherosclerosis, is related to mean annual $PM_{2.5}$, with a $10\,\mu g/m^3$ increase in particles being associated with around a 6 per cent increase in carotid intima–media thickness.[69] This suggests that particle exposure is associated with both acute, day-to-day effects and the effects of long-term exposure potentially via similar mechanisms. However, the situation is likely to be more complex than one simple, oxidative stress-mediated pathway.

Altered cardiac autonomic function

The ability of the heart to respond to changes in physiological demands by changing rate (HRV) is of fundamental importance as one factor involved in cardiovascular mortality. Reduced HRV is associated with a greater risk of cardiac arrhythmia and cardiac death,[70–72] and there is consistent evidence from animal studies,[73] human challenge studies[74] and epidemiology[75–77] that air pollutants affect HRV. Effects on blood pressure might also be mediated through changes in HRV.[78] However, many regular activities, including modest exertion and slight changes in ambient temperature, can affect HRV. In particular, respiratory rate affects heart rate via autonomic reflexes (the explanation for so-called sinus arrhythmia in adolescents), and these influences have largely not been dealt with in epidemiological studies. Consequently, clarification of the relationship between air pollutant exposure and HRV needs to be addressed by studies incorporating personal exposure studies that capture information on these interacting influences.

Changes in vascular responsiveness

Both PM and ozone exposure have been shown to induce brachial artery vasoconstriction in healthy adults in laboratory challenge studies.[79] As coronary and brachial artery reactivity are strongly correlated, such changes could promote ischaemia in individuals with underlying coronary artery disease. An enhancement of the endothelial response is associated with atherogenesis, so this mechanism may again be associated with the cardiovascular effects of both short- and long-term exposure.

These four mechanistic hypotheses (inflammation, thrombosis, autonomic influence and arterial reactivity) might each independently, or more likely in combination, explain the observed association between air pollution and both cardiovascular morbidity and mortality. For example, in a susceptible individual with coronary artery disease, exposure to pollution might cause systemic inflammation, increasing the likelihood of plaque rupture. In addition, any adverse influence on cardiac autonomic control, particularly in this individual in whom it is already impaired, would then increase the vulnerability of the acutely ischaemic or failing myocardium to lethal ventricular arrhythmia. Short-term increases in morbidity and mortality from heart failure might also be explained by a combination of arrhythmic deaths, repeated ischaemic insults or impaired cardiac autonomic control leading to tachycardia and hence worsening ventricular function.[51,54]

Away from the cardiorespiratory effects, there is some evidence that particle exposure is cytotoxic, an effect that increases with smaller particle size[80] and with transition metal content.[81] Particles are also mutagenic, with smaller-sized particles having the most marked effect,[82] similar to the pattern for induced DNA breakages.[83,84] Diesel exhaust is regarded by the International Agency for Research on Cancer as a class 1 carcinogen, and this could explain the epidemiological associations of PM with an increased risk of lung cancer.

Gases

The sources of pollutant gases are described in Chapter 7.

SULPHUR DIOXIDE

Sulphur dioxide is a highly irritant gas that is rapidly absorbed by the respiratory tract, making it a potent bronchoconstrictor in asthma. However, the variability in the stimulus required to produce a response is large, between 500 parts per billion (ppb) and in excess of 1500 ppb.[85] In normal subjects, the minimum level for an observed effect is 4 parts per million. It is likely that sulphur dioxide acts on the rapidly adapting receptors in the upper airways and the larger intrathoracic airways, leading directly to bronchoconstriction.[86] At rest, the doses inhaled by individuals with asthma can alter autonomic

balance, leading to the possibility that the gas initially activates neurogenic inflammation and, via a vagally mediated reflex, results in an autonomic response different from that of subjects without the condition.[87] Sulphur dioxide exposure is not classically pro-oxidant.

NITROGEN DIOXIDE

An oxidant gas, nitrogen dioxide can cause acute pulmonary oedema, but effects at ambient levels (15–30 ppb) are harder to discern. Although some changes in spirometric function and bronchial hyperresponsiveness have been observed in asthma sufferers at higher concentrations (1000–3000 ppb) in laboratory studies, the effect size is modest,[88] and there is limited evidence that higher concentrations result in inflammation.[89,90] However, at exposures of 400 ppb, nitrogen dioxide has been shown to exacerbate the bronchoconstrictive response to house dust mite allergen in those sensitized to it.[91,92]

OZONE

The highly reactive oxidative gas ozone can cause bronchoconstriction in normal and asthmatic subjects[93] and also increase, in a dose-related manner, non-specific airway responsiveness in healthy individuals and those with asthma. However, following daily exposure, the response in asthmatic subjects attenuates, suggesting tolerance.[94] It also enhances the bronchoconstrictor effect of allergen in asthma, either alone[95] or in conjunction with nitrogen dioxide.[96]

The inflammatory response to ozone is variable. The majority of studies have shown an increase in neutrophils in bronchoalveolar lavage fluid, with some showing an increase in the levels of certain adhesion molecules.[95,97] There remain, however, marked differences between individuals, and there is no corresponding alteration in air flow with changes in inflammatory markers. There is limited albeit unconfirmed evidence that people with COPD exposed to ozone show decreased lung function and lower oxygen saturations.[98,99]

SUMMARY

On a day-to-day basis, outdoor air pollution is a statistically significant but small contributor to both respiratory and cardiovascular deaths worldwide, and has also been implicated in neonatal deaths. The major causal factors are particles and ozone and, in countries where high-sulphur fuels are still in use, sulphur dioxide. However, longer term exposure is associated with an even greater burden on society, populations with higher exposures suffering shorter life expectancy and, in all probability, more severe cardiopulmonary disease. Air pollution exposure is associated with exacerbations of asthma, but there is as yet no convincing evidence to support a causal role in the primary initiation of the condition even though, mechanistically, this seems attractive. It has been argued that traffic-related air pollution could be causally implicated in the development of asthma.

The most likely mechanistic route by which air pollution exerts its effects is through oxidative stress, whether through components of the particulate fraction (mostly residing in the sub-2.5 µm fraction) or through oxidant gases such as ozone. Whether nitrogen dioxide at current urban background levels has a deleterious effect is debatable, the epidemiological associations potentially being explicable by the gas simply being a marker of traffic and thus acting as a surrogate for another pollutant, most likely a component within the ultrafine particle fraction.

REFERENCES

1. Ministry of Health. *Mortality and Morbidity During the London Fog of December 1952*. Report No. 95. London HMSO, 1954.

2. Lipmann M, Ito K. Separating the effects of temperature and season on daily mortality from those of air pollution in London: 1965–1972. *Inhal Toxicol* 1995; **7**: 85–97.

3. Lawther PJ, Waller RE, Henderson M. Air pollution and exacerbations of bronchitis. *Thorax* 1970; **25**: 525–39.

4. Poloniecki JD, Atkinson RW, Ponce de Leon A, Anderson HR. Daily time series for cardiovascular hospital admissions and previous day's air pollution in London. *Occup Environ Med* 1997; **54**: 534–40.

5. Halonen JI, Lanki T, Yli-Tuomi T, Tiittanen P, Kulmala M, Pekkanen J. Particulate air pollution and acute cardiorespiratory hospital admissions and mortality among the elderly. *Epidemiology* 2009; **20**: 143–53.

6. Peng RD, Chang HH, Bell ML *et al*. Coarse particulate matter air pollution and hospital admissions for cardiovascular and respiratory diseases among Medicare patients. *JAMA* 2008; **299**: 2172–9.

7. Gauderman WJ, Vora H, McConnell R *et al*. Effect of exposure to traffic on lung development from 10 to 18 years of age: A cohort study. *Lancet* 2007; **369**: 571–7.

8. Dockery DW, Pope CA III. Acute respiratory effects of particulate air pollution. *Ann Rev Public Health* 1994; **15**: 107–32.

9. Roemer W, Hoek G, Brunekeef B, Haluszka J, Kalandidi A, Pekkanen J. Daily variations in air pollution and respiratory health in a multicentre study: The PEACE project. *Eur Respir J* 1998; **12**: 1354–61.

10. Roemer W, Hoek G, Brunekeef B *et al*. The PEACE project: General discussion. *Eur Respir Rev* 1998; **8**: 125–30.

11. Dales R, Chen L, Frescura AM, Liu L, Villeneuve PJ. Acute effects of outdoor air pollution on forced expiratory volume in 1 s: a panel study of schoolchildren with asthma. *Eur Respir J* 2009; **34**: 316–323.

12. Gent JF, Koutrakis P, Belanger K, Triche E, Holford TR, *et al*. Symptoms and medication use in children with asthma and traffic-related sources of fine particle pollution. *Environ Health Perspect* 2009; **117**(7): 1168–1174.

13. Brunekreef B, Kinney PL, Ware JH *et al*. Sensitive subgroups and normal variation in pulmonary function response to air pollution episodes. *Environ Health Perspect* 1991; **90**: 189–93.

14. Walter S, Griffiths RK, Ayres JG. Temporal association between hospital admissions for asthma in Birmingham and ambient levels of sulphur dioxide and smoke. *Thorax* 1994; **49**: 133–40.

15. Sunyer J, Spix C, Quenel P *et al*. Urban air pollution and emergency admissions for asthma in four European cities: The APHEA project. *Thorax* 1997; **52**: 760–5.

16. Atkinson RW, Strachan DP, Anderson HR, Hajat S, Emberlin J. Temporal associations between daily counts of fungal spores and asthma exacerbations. *Occup Environ Med* 2006; **63**: 580–90.

17. Kim JJ; American Academy of Pediatrics Committee on Environmental Health. Ambient air pollution: Health hazards to children. *Pediatrics* 2004; **114**: 1699–707.

18. McCreanor J, Culinan P, Nieuwenhuijsen MJ *et al*. Respiratory effects of exposure to diesel traffic in persons with asthma. *N Engl J Med* 2007; **357**: 2348–58.

19. Wichmann HE, Mueller W, Allhof P *et al*. Health effects during a smog episode in West Germany in 1985. *Environ Health Perspec* 1989; **79**: 88–99.

20. Anderson HR, Limb ES, Bland JM, Ponce de Leon A, Strachan DP, Bower JS. Urban air pollution and emergency admissions for asthma in four European cities: The APHEA project. *Thorax* 1995; **50**: 1188–93.

21. Huber AL, Loving TJ. Fatal asthma attack after inhaling sulfur fumes. *JAMA* 1991; **266**: 2225.

22. Spix C, Anderson HR, Schwartz J. Short-term effects of air pollution on hospital admissions of respiratory diseases in Europe: A quantitative summary of APHEA study results. Air Pollution and Health: A European Approach. *Arch Environ Health* 1998; **53**: 54–64.

23. Anderson HR, Cook DG. Passive smoking and sudden infant death syndrome: Review of the epidemiological evidence. *Thorax* 1997; **52**: 1003–9.

24. Ponce de Leon A, Anderson HR, Bland JM, Strachan DP, Bower J. Effects of air pollution on daily hospital admissions for respiratory disease in London between 1987–88 and 1991–92. *Epidemiol Comm Health* 1996; **50**(Suppl. 1): S76–80.

25. Arbex MA, Margarete G, Cendron SP *et al*. Urban air pollution and COPD-related emergency room visits. *J Epidemiol Community Health* 2009; Online. (DOI: 10.1136/jech.2008.078360)

26. Sauerzapf V, Jones AP, Cross J. Environmental factors and hospitalisation for chronic obstructive pulmonary disease in a rural county of England. *J Epidemiol Commun Health* 2009; **63**: 324–8.

27. Katsouyanni K, Touloumi G, Spix C *et al*. Short term effects of ambient sulphur dioxide and particulate matter on mortality in 12 European cities: Results from time series data from the APHEA project. *Br Med J* 1997; **314**: 1663.

28. Dockery DW. Epidemiologic evidence of cardiovascular effects of particulate air pollution. *Environ Health Perspec* 2001; **64**: 36–52.

29. Schwartz J. Air pollution and hospital admissions for respiratory disease. *Epidemiology* 1996; **7**: 20–8.

30. Committee on the Medical Effects of Air Pollutants. 2009. (Chair: JG Ayres.) *Long-term exposure to air pollution: Effect on mortality.* London: Health Protection Agency.

31. Hoek G, Brunekreef B, Fischer P, van Wijnen J. The association between air pollution and heart failure, arrhythmia, embolism, thrombosis, and other cardiovascular causes of death in a time series study. *Epidemiology* 2001; **12**: 357.

32. Ostro BD, Feng W-Y, Broadwin R, Malig BJ, Green RS, Lipsett MJ. The impact of components of fine particulate matter on cardiovascular mortality in susceptible subpopulations. *Occup Environ Med* 2008; **65**: 750–6.

33. Anderson HA, Atkinson RW. *Association between Ambient Particles and Daily Admissions for Cardiovascular Diseases.* London: Department of Health, 2001.

34. Le Tertre A, Medina S, Samoli E *et al.* Short-term effects of particulate air pollution on cardiovascular diseases in eight European cities. *J Epidemiol Commun Health* 2002; **56**: 773–779.

35. Peters A, Dockery DW, Muller JE, Mittleman MA. Increased particulate air pollution and the triggering of myocardial infarction. *Circulation* 2001; **103**: 2810–15.

36. Peters A, Liu E, Verrier RL *et al.* Air pollution and incidence of cardiac arrhythmia. *Epidemiology* 2000; **11** (1): 11–17.

37. Link MS, Dockery DW. Air pollution and the triggering of cardiac arrhythmias. *Curr Opin Cardiol* 2010; **25**: 16–22.

38. Dockery DW, Pope CA III, Xu X *et al.* An association between air pollution and mortality in six US cities. *N Engl J Med* 1993; **329**: 1753–9.

39. Pope CA III, Thun MJ, Nambadoori MM *et al.* Particulate air pollution as a predictor of mortality in a prospective study of US adults. *Am J Respir Crit Care Med* 1995; **151**: 669–74.

40. Beelen R, Hoek G, van den Brandt R *et al.* long-term effects of traffic related air pollution on mortality in a Dutch cohort (NLCS-AIR study). *Environ Health Perspec* 2008; **116**: 196–202.

41. Lindgren A, Stroh E, Montnemery P, Nihlen U, Jakobsson K, Axmon A. Traffic-related air pollution associated with prevalence of asthma and COPD/chronic bronchitis. A cross-sectional study in Southern Sweden. *Int J Health Geograph* 2009; **8**. Online. DOI: 10.1186/1476–072X-8-2.

42. Gauderman WJ, Avol E, Lurmann F *et al.* Childhood asthma and exposure to traffic and nitrogen dioxide. *Epidemiology* 2005; **16**: 737–43.

43. Fairbairn AS, Reid DD. Air pollution and other local factors in respiratory disease. *Br J Prev Soc Med* 1958; **12**: 94–103.

44. Holland WW, Reid D. The urban factor in chronic bronchitis. *Lancet* 1965; **i**: 448.

45. Lambert PM, Reid DD. Smoking, air pollution and bronchitis in Britain. *Lancet* 1970; **295**: 853–7.

46. Burrows B, Kellogg AL, Buskey J. Relationship of symptoms of chronic bronchitis and emphysema to weather and air pollution. *Arch Environ Health* 1968; **16**: 406–13.

47. Sunyer J, Jarvis D, Gotschi T *et al.* Chronic bronchitis and urban air pollution in an international study. *Occup Environ Med* 2001; **63**: 836–43.

48. Salvi SS, Barnes PJ. Chronic obstructive pulmonary disease in non-smokers. *Lancet* 2009; **374**: 733–43.

49. Roemer WH, van Wijnen JH. Daily mortality and air pollution along busy streets in Amsterdam, 1987–1998. *Epidemiology* 2002; **13**: 491.

50. Kwon HJ, Cho SH, Nyberg F, Pershagen G. Effects of ambient air pollution on daily mortality in a cohort of patients with congestive heart failure. *Epidemiology* 2001; **12**: 413–19.

51. Committee on the Medical Effects of Air Pollutants. 2006 (Chair: JG Ayres) *Cardiovascular Disease and Air Pollution.* London: Department of Health.

52. Dockery D, Pope CA III, Spiezer FE, Thun MJ. Comments on the reanalysis project. *J Toxicol Environ Health A* 2003; **66**: 1689–96.

53. Pope CA III, Burnett RT, Thurston GD *et al.* Cardiovascular mortality and long-term exposure to particulate air pollution. *Circulation* 2004; **109**: 71–7.

54. Clancy L, Goodman P, Sinclair H, Dockery DW. Effect of air-pollution control on death rates in Dublin, Ireland: An intervention study. *Lancet* 2002; **360**: 1210–14.

55. Hedley AJ, Wong CM, Thach TQ, Ma S, Lam TH, Anderson HR. Cardiorespiratory and all-cause mortality after restrictions on sulphur content of fuel in Hong Kong: An intervention study. *Lancet* 2002; **360**: 1646–52.

56. Dragano N, Hoffmann B, Moebus S *et al.* Traffic exposure and subclinical cardiovascular disease: Is the association modified by socioeconomic characteristics of individuals and neighbourhoods? Results from a multilevel study in an urban region. *Occup Environ Med* 2009; **66**: 628–35.

57. Miller K, Siscovick D, Sheppard L *et al.* Long-term exposure to air pollution and incidence of cardiovascular events in women. *New Engl J Med* 2007; **356**: 447–58.

58. Johnson D, Parker JD. Air pollution exposure and self-reported cardiovascular disease. *Environ Res* 2009; **109**: 582–9.

59. Forbes L, Patel MD, Rudnicka AR *et al.* Chronic exposure to outdoor air pollution and diagnosed cardiovascular disease: Meta-analysis of three large cross-sectional surveys. *Environmental Health* 2009; **8**: 30.

60. Ayres JG, Borm P, Cassee F *et al.* Evaluating the toxicity of airborne particulate matter and nanoparticles by measuring oxidative stress potential – a workshop report and consensus statement. *Inhal Toxicol* 2008; **20**: 75–99.

61. Xiao GG, Wang M, Li N, Loo JA, Nel AE. Use of proteomics to demonstrate a hierarchical oxidative stress response to diesel exhaust particles in a macrophage cell line. *J Biol Chem* 2003; **278**: 50781–90.

62. Li N, Kim S, Wang M, Froines J, Sioutas C, Nel A. Use of a stratified oxidative stress model to study the biological

effects of ambient concentrated and diesel exhaust particulate matter. *Inhal Toxicol* 2002; **14**: 101–28.

63. de Kok TM, Hogervorst JG, Briede MH *et al.* Genotoxicity and physiochemical characteristics of traffic related ambient particulate matter. *Environ Mol Mutagen* 2005; **46**: 71–80.

64. MacNee W, Donaldson K. Exacerbations of COPD: Environmental mechanisms. *Chest* 2000; **117**: 390S–397S.

65. MacNee W, Donaldson K. Mechanisms of lung injury caused by PM10 and Ultrafine particles. *Eur Respir J* 2003; **21**:47s–51s.

66. Van Eeden SF, Tan WC, Suwa T *et al.* Cytokines involved in the systemic inflammatory response induced by exposure to particulate matter air pollutants. *Am J Respir Crit Care Med* 2001; **164**: 826–30.

67. Goto Y, Hogg J, Shih C, Ishii H, Vincent R, van Eeden S. Exposure to ambient particles accelerates monocyte release from the bone marrow in atherosclerotic rabbits. *Am J Physiol Lung Cell Mol Physiol* 2004; **287**: 79–85.

68. Mills NL, Tornquist H, Gonzalez MC *et al.* Ischemic and thrombotic effects of dilute diesel-exhaust inhalation in men with coronary heart disease. *N Engl J Med* 2007; **357**: 1075–82.

69. Kunzli N, Jerrett M, Mack WJ *et al.* Ambient air pollution and atherosclerosis in Los Angeles. *Environ Health Perspec* 2004; **113**(2): 201–206.

70. Dyer AR, Persky V, Stamler J *et al.* Heart rate as a prognostic factor for coronary heart disease and mortality: Findings in three Chicago epidemiologic studies. *Am J Epidemiol* 1980; **112**: 736–49.

71. Hjalmarson AG, Kjekshus EA, Schieman J, Nicod G, Henning P, Ross H. Influence of heart rate on mortality after acute myocardial infarction. *Am J Cardiol* 1990; **65**: 547–53.

72. Nemec J, Hammill SC, Shen WK. Increase in heart rate precedes episodes of ventricular tachycardia and ventricular fibrillation in patients with implantable cardioverter defibrillators: Analysis of spontaneous ventricular tachycardia database. *Pacing Clin Electrophysiol* 1999; **22**: 1729–38.

73. Lipmann M, Ito K, Hwang JS, Maciejczyk P, Chen LC. Cardiovascular effects of nickel in ambient air. *Environ Health Perspec* 2006; **114**(11): 1662–1669.

74. Tunnicliffe WS, Mark D, Harrison RM, Ayres JG. Effect of particle and sulphur dioxide challenge on heart rate variability in normal and asthmatic subjects. *Eur Respir J* 2001; **17**: 604–8.

75. Romieu L, Tellez-Rojo MM, Lazo M *et al.* Omega-3 fatty acid prevents heart rate variability reductions associated with particulate matter. *Am J Respir Crit Care Med* 2005; **172**: 1534–40.

76. Chuang K-J, Chan C-C, Chen NT *et al.* Effects of particle size fractions on reducing heart rate variability in cardiac and hypertensive patients. *Environ Health Perspec* 2005; **113**: 1693–7.

77. Folino AF, Scapatello ML, Canova C *et al.* Individual exposure to particulate matter and the short-term arrhythmic and autonomic profiles in patients with myocardial infarction. *Eur Heart J* 2009. **30**(13): 1614–1620.

78. Brook RD, Urch B, Dvonch T *et al.* Insights into the mechanisms and mediators of the effects of air pollution exposure on blood pressure and vascular function in healthy humans. *Hypertension* 2009; **54**: 659–67.

79. Brook RD, Brook JR, Urch B *et al.* Inhalation of fine particles air pollution and ozone causes acute arterial vasoconstriction in healthy adults. *Circulation* 2002; **105**: 1534–6.

80. Massolo L, Muller A, Tueros M *et al.* Assessment of mutagenicity and toxicity of different sized fractions of air particulates from LaPlata, Argentina and Liepzig Germany. *Environ Toxicol* 2002; **17**: 219–31.

81. Tong S, Colditz P. Air pollution and sudden infant death syndrome: A literature review. *Paediatr Perinat Epidimiol* 2004; **18** (5): 327–35.

82. Vargas VM. Mutagenic activity as a parameter to assess ambient air quality for protection of the environment and human health. *Mutat Res* 2003; **544**: 313–19.

83. Dellinger B, Pryor WA, Cueto GL *et al.* Role of free radicals in the toxicity of airborne fine particulate matter. *Chem Res Toxicol* 2001; **14**:1371–1377.

84. Healey K, Lingard JJ, Tomlin AS *et al.* Genotoxicty of size fractioned samples of urban particulate matter. *Environ Mol Mutagen* 2005; **47**: 199–211.

85. Sheppard D, Saisho A, Nadel JA, Boushey HA. Exercise increases sulfur dioxide-induced bronchoconstriction in asthmatic subjects. *Am Rev Respir Dis* 1981; **123**: 486–91.

86. Atzori L, Bannenberg G, Corriga AM *et al.* Sulfur dioxide-induced bronchoconstriction via ruthenium red-sensitive activation of sensory nerves. *Respiration* 1992; **59**: 272–78.

87. Tunnicliffe WS, Mark D, Harrison RM, Ayres JG. Effect of particle and sulphur dioxide challenge on heart rate variability in normal and asthmatic subjects. *Eur Respir J* 2001; **17**: 604–08.

88. Folinsbee L. Does nitrogen dioxide exposure increase airways responsiveness? *Toxicol Ind Health* 1992; **8** (5): 273–83.

89. Blomberg A, Krishna MT, Bocchino V *et al.* The inflammatory effects of 2 ppm NO_2 on the airways of healthy subjects. *Am J Respir Crit Care Med* 1997; **156**: 418–24.

90. Blomberg A. Airway inflammatory and antioxidant responses to oxidative and particulate air pollutants – experimental exposure studies in humans. *Clin Exp Allergy* 2000; **30**: 310–17.

91. Tunnicliffe WS, Burge PS, Ayres JG. Effect of domestic concentrations in nitrogen dioxide on airway responses to inhaled allergen in asthmatic patients. *Lancet* 1994; **344**: 1733–6.

92. Strand V, Svartengren M, Rak S, Barck C, Bylin G. Repeated exposure to an ambient level of NO_2 enhances asthmatic response to a non-symptomatic allergen dose. *Eur Respir J* 1998; **12**: 6–12.

93. Hazucha MJ. Relationship between ozone exposure and pulmonary function changes. *Physiol* 1987; **62**: 1671–80.

94. Horstmann DH, Folinsbee LJ, Ives PJ, Abdul-Saleem S, McDonnell WF. Ozone concentration and pulmonary response relationships for 6.6 hour exposures with five hours of moderate exercise to 0.08, 0.10 and 0.12 ppm. *Am Rev Respir Dis* 2009; **142**: 1158–63.

95. Jorres R, Nowak D, Magnussen H. The effect of ozone exposure on allergen responsiveness in subjects with asthma or rhinitis. *Am J Respir Crit Care Med* 1996; **153**: 56–64.

96. Jenkins HS, Devalia JL, Mister RL, Bevan AM, Rusznak C, Davies RJ. The effect of exposure to ozone and nitrogen dioxide on the airway response of atopic asthmatics to inhaled allergen. *Am J Respir Crit Care Med* 1999; **160**: 33–9.

97. Holz O, Jorres R, Timm P *et al*. Ozone-induced airway inflammatory changes differ between individuals and are reproducible. *Am J Respir Crit Care Med* 1999; **159**: 776–84.

98. Solic JJ, Hazucha MJ, Bromberg PA. The acute effects of 0.2 ppm ozone in patients with chronic obstructive pulmonary disease. *Am Rev Respir Dis* 1982; **125**: 664–9.

99. Kehrl HR, Hazucha MJ, Solic JJ, Bromberg PA. Responses of subjects with chronic obstructive pulmonary disease after exposure to 0.3 ppm ozone. *Am Rev Respir Dis* 1985; **131**: 719–24.

11

Point sources

JOSEP M. ANTÓ

A DEFINITION OF A HEALTH-RELATED POINT SOURCE

In the context of epidemiology and public health, a point source is a single identifiable localized source of pollution that may affect the health of the surrounding population. This may include point sources of air and water pollution. Examples of point-source emissions, as considered in this chapter, can be specific, such as combustion furnace flue gas stacks, or more general, such as industrial sites and areas.

Similar to point sources, other types of air pollution sources are line sources, area sources and volume sources. A point source has no geometric dimensions, in contrast to line sources, which are one-dimensional, or area sources, which are two-dimensional. A volume source is a three-dimensional source of diffuse air pollutant emissions, for example emissions from a petrochemical plant. In some circumstances, however, area or volume sources are approached as point sources. In contrast to point sources, diffuse sources of pollution are referred to as non-point sources.

ANTECEDENTS

The formal use of the term 'point source' in modern epidemiology can be traced back to the work done by Knox in the late 1950s and early 60s with respect to the geographical clustering of rare diseases. In a seminal paper titled 'Epidemics of rare diseases', he noted that although epidemics were at that time – as they are now – 'defined on a time basis, the concept of spread in space was implicit'.[1]

In this paper, Knox generalized the concept of the propagation of cases across space and distinguished between 'point features (like asbestos factories), linear features (roads, railways, canals, rivers) and closed areas (contours, woods, urban boundaries, polluted areas)'. Knox went even further in envisioning the future role of geographical information systems, stating that: 'distances from "point features", nearest distances from linear features and closed boundaries, and, for the latter, distinction between "inside" and "outside" are all capable of formal solution by programming methods'. Today, the generalized use of geographical information systems together with registers of contaminating sources facilitates the systematic investigation of health effects due to point sources as Knox formulated.

Among the many examples of point-source episodes that have received wide attention in the scientific literature, the London cholera outbreak described by John Snow continues to be a key historical landmark. This and other more recent examples are considered below.

A poisoning pump in Broad Street, London, UK

This famous cholera outbreak started in London in late August 1854 and reached a peak of mortality on September 2nd. Snow noted that many of the cases occurred near the Broad Street pump or among those who had travelled to the area to obtain water from the pump. He also noted that rates of cholera were much lower in the neighbourhood workhouse, where residents drank from their own pump, and among the employees of a local brewery, many of whom did not drink water at all.

Being convinced that water from the Broad Street pump was at fault, Dr Snow spoke on September 7th to the Board of Guardians, the political group responsible for maintaining the safety and welfare of the area. They listened to his concerns, noted his findings, and on September 8 authorized the removal of the pump handle.[2] What is relevant here for the understanding of epidemiological research of point sources is how the proximity of living near to the Broad Street pump was examined in relation to that individual being affected by cholera.

A polluting steel mill in Utah Valley, USA

The Utah Valley provided a unique opportunity to evaluate the health effects of particulate matter in humans. The area was intermittently exposed to high particle levels with the principal source being a steel mill. Due to a labour dispute, the mill was shut down for some months. The closure and reopening of the steel mill allowed an examination of the relationship between emissions and potential harmful effects on the health of the surrounding populations.

Epidemiological investigations demonstrated an association between both the closure of the steel mill and the reduction in exposure to air pollution particles and changes in morbidity and mortality. The apparent health effects of elevated pollution with particulate matter less than $10\,\mu m$ in diameter observed in the Utah Valley included decreased lung function, an increased incidence of respiratory symptoms, increased school absenteeism, an increase in respiratory hospital admissions, increased mortality, especially respiratory and cardiovascular mortality, and possibly increased rates of lung cancer.

The Utah Valley provided a unique opportunity to evaluate the health effects of respirable particulate pollution in a single homogeneous population because of the concurrence of several unusual circumstances. These included the fact that, during low-level temperature inversion episodes, local emissions become trapped in a stagnant air mass near the valley floor, resulting in highly elevated concentrations of particulate matter less than $10\,\mu m$ in diameter, and that other sources of air pollution such as sulphur dioxide and ozone were relatively low.[3] Crucially, in the case of the Utah Valley, there were appropriate local facilities that allowed an assessment of the temporal relationship between the contaminating steel mill and the health of the surrounding population. So here the time–activity pattern of the point source rather than physical proximity to the point source was the relevant exposure measurement.

A contaminating silo in Barcelona harbour, Spain

During the early 1980s, several asthma outbreaks were reported in Barcelona, Spain, with high fatality rates. An epidemiological monitoring of these outbreaks revealed striking geographical and time clustering, strongly suggesting that the outbreak was a point-source epidemic. The industrial harbour area adjacent to the neighbourhood in which the epidemic occurred was considered to be a probable source of the cause of the outbreak.[4] Subsequent epidemiological investigations revealed that these outbreaks were caused by the inhalation of soybean dust released during the unloading of soybeans at the city harbour.[5] An assessment of those involved in the outbreaks revealed that soybean epidemic asthma was mediated by an immunoglobulin E-mediated allergic reaction.[6]

Following these studies, the unloading of soybeans was stopped until appropriate filters had been installed in the top of the causative silo. The effectiveness of the filters was tested in a before-and-after study that showed a cessation of asthma outbreaks as well as a striking reduction in the rate of severe life-threatening asthma in Barcelona.[7] Following the studies in Barcelona, asthma outbreaks in New Orleans, USA, which had been investigated in the 1960s and 70s, were retrospectively linked to soybean handling in the city harbour.[8]

The investigation of the asthma outbreaks in Barcelona combined the features of both the Broad Street pump outbreak and the Utah Valley steel mill incident. First, the proximity of the affected population to a large industrial harbour pointed to the harbour as the more likely origin, and second, the time–activity pattern of the silo (i.e. unloading versus non-unloading days) was used as both an indicator and a measure of exposure.

Although these historical episodes of disease due to contaminating point sources are classic examples of successful epidemiological research, they illustrate only part of a problem that can be solved. Unfortunately, most of the time, health effects due to putative point sources are very difficult to assess and continue to pose complex challenges to public health services and researchers. In the following sections, the different types of health effect due to contaminating point sources will be described, together with the several methodological issues that are relevant to their investigation. Finally, the different approaches available for the surveillance and control of these events will be reviewed.

TYPES OF POINT-SOURCE EPIDEMIOLOGICAL STUDY

Outbreaks or epidemics known to be due to point-source emissions

There are several diseases that present in epidemic form in the general population and are known to be caused by point-source emissions. One of the best examples is provided by Legionnaires' disease, while asthma outbreaks can also be included in this category. Both types of outbreak provide the same lesson, namely that establishing for the first time that a point source is the cause of a specific health effect can be challenging. However, proving that a point source is the origin of a given epidemic disease facilitates its subsequent identification and control, both at the original place and in future settings.

LEGIONNAIRES' DISEASE, PHILADELPHIA, USA

An explosive, common-source outbreak of pneumonia caused by a previously unrecognized bacterium primarily affected persons attending an American Legion convention in Philadelphia in July, 1976. Twenty-nine of 182 cases were fatal, and the disease was considered to be a bacterial infection. Despite an intense effort, the source of the bacterium was not found, but epidemiological analysis suggested an airborne exposure in the lobby of the headquarters hotel or in the area immediately surrounding the hotel. Person-to-person spread seemed not to have occurred.[9]

To identify the aetiological agent underlying the outbreak, by this time called Legionnaires' disease, patients' serum and tissue specimens were examined in a search for toxins, bacteria, fungi, Chlamydiae, Rickettsiae and viruses. A Gram-negative bacillus was isolated from the lungs of four patients. When compared with controls, patients meeting the clinical criteria of Legionnaires' disease showed diagnostic increases in antibody titres. Diagnostic increases were also found in sporadic cases of severe pneumonia and in stored serum from two other previously unsolved outbreaks of respiratory disease. It was then evident that Legionnaires' disease was caused by a Gram-negative bacterium that was likely to be responsible for local outbreaks.[10]

The discovery of the bacterial origin of Legionnaires' disease (*Legionella pneumophila*) facilitated the development of methods for the relatively easy identification and typing of this group of organisms in pneumonia outbreaks. It was soon evident that most of the institutional and community outbreaks of Legionnaires' disease were due to cooling towers or water reservoirs contaminated by *L. pneumophila*, the identification of these point sources being a necessary step to control the outbreaks.

Although the concept is simple, the identification of the causative source of *Legionella* may be very time-consuming. The type of study necessary to identify a point source is exemplified by the investigation and control of a community outbreak of Legionnaires' disease in Hereford, UK. The outbreak investigation consisted of an epidemiological survey, an identification and environmental investigation of potential sources, a microbiological analysis of clinical and environmental samples, and a mapping of the location of potential sources and the movement and residence of cases.

Each potential source was allocated a 'composite score' based on different zones of exposure and wind direction. All together, 28 cases were identified, with an overall case fatality rate of 7 per cent. All cases had epidemiological links to Hereford city centre. The 'composite score' identified a cluster of cooling towers as being the most likely source of the outbreak. Environmental samples from one of the cooling towers in the cluster and clinical samples from two patients were positive for *L. pneumophila* serogroup 1 and were indistinguishable by molecular subtyping.[11]

In a similar way to that of the first Legionnaires' disease outbreaks, the finding that asthma outbreaks in Barcelona were due to the inhalation of soybean dust released from a silo in the city harbour prompted the identification of similar episodes in Valencia and Tarragona, Spain, Naples, Italy and New Orleans, USA. The latter was a remarkable finding taking into account the fact that asthma outbreaks in New Orleans had been intensively investigated during the 1960s and 70s without finding an origin.[8]

Sporadic cases of otherwise epidemic diseases related to point-source emissions

When considering entities such as Legionnaires' disease or soybean asthma, it is also relevant to consider to what extent sporadic cases can be due to point-source emissions. The origin of non-epidemic cases of Legionnaires' disease in Glasgow, UK, particularly the role of cooling towers, was investigated by comparing the locations of patients' homes in relation to the location of cooling towers. The study population included patients with non-epidemic Legionnaires' disease during 1978–86 and patients with lung cancer during the same period.

Using the locations of patients' homes and cooling towers as defined by postcodes, which provided map grid references accurate to 10 m, the authors estimated the number of expected and observed cases of Legionnaires' disease in census enumeration districts and the distance of the enumeration districts from the nearest cooling tower as defined by five distance categories. There was an inverse association between the distance of residence from any cooling tower and the risk of infection, the population living within 0.5 km of any tower having a relative risk of infection over three times that of people living more than 1 km away. In contrast, there was no such association with respect to travel-related Legionnaires' disease, and for lung cancer the association was weak. The study provides an interesting example of multiple point sources and how the methods to investigate point sources can be applied to sporadic cases of Legionnaires' disease.[12]

In a similar way, the occurrence of non-epidemic cases of asthma in the vicinity of soybean operating harbours was investigated in Valencia and A Coruña, Spain. Asthma admissions were retrospectively identified for the period 1993–95, and harbour activities were investigated in each location showing the absence of epidemic asthma days during the study period. Two approaches were used to assess the association between sporadic cases of asthma and soybean unloading:

- the use of unusual asthma days (days with an unusually high number of emergency room asthma visits) as an effect measure;
- an estimation of the relative increase in the daily number of emergency room visits.

No association between unusual asthma days and soya unloading was observed in either Valencia or A Coruña, except for one particular dock in Valencia. When the association between unloaded products and the daily number of emergency asthma visits was studied, a weak statistically significant association was observed for the unloading of soybeans in A Coruña. These findings suggested that, in the absence of asthma outbreaks, the population living in the vicinity of harbours with soybean unloading could have been at risk of non-epidemic soybean asthma.[13]

Disease clusters with a point source as a matter of concern

A cluster is a localized increased in the occurrence of a disease that is not explicable in terms of the size and distribution of the population and is not due to chance. It is well accepted that the definition and identification of disease clusters is challenging, and because false positives are common, the aetiological investigation of a cluster should only be undertaken when there is enough evidence that the cluster is a true event. The latter requirement means that the first step of a cluster investigation involves only the analysis of the cluster itself irrespective of any potential relationship to a putative point source. If the cluster is confirmed, and the evidence on its nature is consistent enough, testing the relationship between the disease status and exposure to a suspected point source may then become an issue.

NUCLEAR INSTALLATIONS AND CANCER

The complex interplay between the study of a cluster and a point source study is well illustrated by the seminal studies of the cluster of leukaemia in Sellafield, Cumbria, UK, which contributed to the development of methods for cluster investigation.[14]

Following the initial studies in Sellafield, the identification of a local excess of cancer cases in populations living in the vicinity of nuclear installations has received intensive attention, with a number of one-site studies reporting significant increases in leukaemia in children around the reprocessing plants at Sellafield and Dounreay, Caithness (UK), La Hague (France) and Krümmel (Germany).[15] Although these studies showed an increased risk of childhood leukaemia, the reasons for the increase could not be established with sufficient certainty, and several methodological limitations, typical of small-area studies, were considered as alternative explanations.

Among these limitations, the ones that have received most consideration are:

- the lack of a specific a priori hypothesis;
- the small number of cases and low statistical power;
- the presence of reporting, diagnostic or classification bias;
- the possibility that conventional statistical tests may be inappropriate if the underlying spatial distribution of the disease is not random.[16]

Some of these limitations were thoroughly approached in a study conducted to assess the relationship between the risk of childhood leukaemia and non-Hodgkin's lymphoma and proximity of residence to nuclear installations in England and Wales. The study population included children below the age of 15 living in electoral wards within 25 km of 23 nuclear installations and six control sites that had been investigated for suitability for generating stations but had never been used.

One analytical approach was the use of incidence ratios of observed to expected cases. In addition, the authors used what was at that time a new statistical test called the linear risk score test, based on ranks and designed to be sensitive to an excess incidence in close proximity to a putative source of risk. In none of the 25 km circles around the installations was the incidence ratio significantly greater than 1.0. The only significant results for the linear risk score test were for Sellafield, Sizewell (Suffolk, UK) and one of the control sites.[17] A similar, large multisite geographical study assessing the incidence of leukaemia in children aged 0–15 years (1980–90), particularly in reference to the locations of nuclear power facilities, was conducted in Sweden. The study did not find any significant clusters.[18]

An exploration of the aetiology and mechanisms of local clusters near to nuclear sites in places like Sellafield or La Hague, where the available data have suggested the possibility of a genuine causal effect, has been undertaken using case–control studies and has allowed the assessment of potentially relevant exposures. In Sellafield, a case–control study including 52 cases of leukaemia and 1001 controls did show an increased risk for leukaemia and non-Hodgkin's lymphoma in children born near Sellafield and in the children of fathers employed at the plant, particularly those with high radiation dose recordings before their child's conception. The latter suggested that the occupational exposure of male workers to ionizing radiation might be leukaemogenic in their offspring.[19] Unfortunately, the pre-conception occupational exposure hypothesis has proved hard to test.

A case–control study including 27 cases of leukaemia and 192 controls conducted in La Hague, France, did not find an association with occupational radiation exposure in the parents. In contrast, increased significant risks were found for the use of local beaches by mothers and children and the consumption of local fish and shellfish, suggesting that such exposures could partially explain the association between living in the vicinity of the nuclear plant and the increased risk of leukaemia.[20]

Overall, the accumulated evidence suggests that in several places, including Sellafield and La Hague, clusters of leukaemia in children living in the sites' vicinity are likely be due to exposures that are directly or indirectly (via population-mixing) related to the nuclear facilities.[21] Such clusters seem to reflect the effect of local circumstances since systematic multisite studies have not identified clusters in other nuclear facilities.

From point source to disease: point sources potentially harmful for the health of the population

In contrast to the investigation of the outbreaks alluded to above, for which the starting point was the disease, the opposite situation – where emissions from a given point source are considered as potentially harmful to health – is becoming increasingly common. Here, the question usually arises in a reactive context when concerns about safety are raised by the exposed population to the public health authorities.

Studies about the consequences of exposure to single point sources in particular locations (the local approach) are seriously hampered by several limitations such as insufficient sample size, recall bias and confounding by socioeconomic status or deprivation. In contrast, the question of how much harm is to be attributed to a putative point source could be better approached by conducting a study large enough to include many similar point sources (the systematic approach), as has been previously shown by the studies around nuclear installations. Both the local and the systematic approaches are described below.

THE LOCAL APPROACH

Health authorities should always formulate a response to people's concerns about the potential toxicity of emissions released from a suspect point source (e.g. a landfill site or an industrial site). There is no general rule for what an appropriate response should be, but the approach should consider both risk assessment criteria and the local context. In some cases, an ad hoc study may be considered necessary.

Solid-waste incinerator, Mataró, Spain

In Mataró, Spain, concern was raised by residents about the safety levels of a municipal solid-waste incinerator planned for placement in the proximity of an inhabited area, leading the local authorities to commission an epidemiological study. In a biomonitoring study,[22] 104 subjects who lived near (i.e. within 0.5–1.5 km of) the incinerator were compared with 97 subjects living a distance away (i.e. within 3.5–4.0 km) both before the incinerator started functioning in 1995, and 2 years later;

17 workers employed at the incinerator were also included. Dioxins, furans and polychlorinated biphenyls were studied in pooled blood samples, and individual blood and urine samples were analysed for the detection of lead, chromium, cadmium and mercury.

In 1995, blood dioxin levels were similar among both those living close to the incinerator and those living further away (both groups having a mean of about 13 ng international dioxin toxic equivalents/kg fat). In 1997, dioxin and polychlorinated biphenyl levels had increased in both groups of residents by approximately 25 per cent and 12 per cent, respectively. Regarding other contaminants, blood lead levels decreased, but no difference was observed for chromium, cadmium and mercury. Minimal changes were seen among workers. Given the low dioxin stack emissions from this plant (the mean for each of the two stacks over a 30 month period being 2.5 and 0.98 ng international dioxin toxic equivalents/m^3 respectively) and the fact that the blood dioxin levels did not depend on the distance from the residence to the incinerator, the authors considered it unlikely that the small increase in dioxin blood levels resulted from the incinerator's emissions; instead, an increase in serum dioxin levels resulting from dietary intake was considered a more likely explanation.[23]

Industrial sites in the UK

Although petrochemical industries have proliferated all over the world and are commonly located in close proximity to very large urban populations, studies in this area are scarce and mostly restricted to reactive studies in single sites. One of the first studies assessed the incidence and mortality of leukaemia, cancer of the larynx and other cancers near the petrochemical plant at Baglan Bay, South Wales, UK, in response to local concerns of an alleged cluster of cancers. The study population comprised 115 721 people living within 7.5 km of the plant.

There was no excess of mortality, but there was an 8 per cent excess incidence of all cancers within 7.5 km, and a 24 per cent excess of cancer of the larynx with no apparent decline in incidence with distance from the plant. There was no evidence of a decline in leukaemia incidence or mortality with distance, at all ages or in children. Among the other causes included in the mortality study, there was an excess of multiple myeloma within 7.5 km, especially among women, although there was no overall excess of mortality within 7.5 km, and the overall pattern was judged to be consistent with a general excess in the area possibly related to patterns of cancer registration in Wales.[24]

Another study examined the incidence and mortality of cancer near the Pan Britannica Industries factory in Waltham Abbey, Essex, UK, after reports of a possible cluster of all cancers and brain cancer in the vicinity. The study concluded that there was limited and inconsistent evidence for a localized excess of cancer in the vicinity of the Pan Britannica Industries plant and recommended a continued surveillance of mortality and cancer incidence in the locality.[25]

A similar study was conducted in Runcorn, Cheshire, UK, a site of chemical industry activity for over a century where, over time, tons of toxic chemicals have been released into the air and water. Excess kidney disease mortality (nephritis, nephrotic syndrome and nephrosis) was found in the population living within 2 km of the industrial plants (standardized mortality ratio in males 131, with a 95 per cent confidence interval [CI] of 90–185, and in females 161, with a 95 per cent CI of 118–214) compared with a reference population (north-west England). The risk of hospital admissions for kidney disease was also increased, and the area was judged to require further investigation.[26]

Local studies conducted to assess the health impact of living in the vicinity of single point sources are affected by several important limitations. These limitations are sometimes related to the study design:

- before-and-after studies that do not include an appropriate control area;
- a limited sample size, when the size of the study population is not enough to provide risk estimates with sufficient precision;
- migration patterns that may have distorted the study base in a way that cannot be controlled for in the analysis;
- a lack of individual exposure measurements other than distance of the residence to the point source;
- confounding by socioeconomic status.

For these reasons, the approach to local studies should be carefully considered and balanced as both positive and negative results may require further attention.

THE SYSTEMATIC APPROACH

One way to overcome the difficulties involved in single-site studies is to conduct a systematic study including as many sites as possible similar to the one of interest, as described earlier with the study of nuclear sites in Britain. One of the fields where the systematic approach has been widely considered is the investigation of possible harmful effects in populations living in the vicinity of landfill sites.

Landfill sites, Europe

The EUROHAZCON study collected data from seven regional registers of congenital anomalies in five countries including 1089 live births, stillbirths and terminations of pregnancy with non-chromosomal congenital anomalies and 2366 control births without malformation. The mothers were living within 7 km of a landfill site, and 21 sites were included. A zone within a 3 km radius of each site was defined as the 'proximate zone' of most likely exposure to teratogens.[27]

Residence within 3 km of a landfill site was associated with a significantly raised risk of congenital anomaly with a combined odds ratio of 1.33 (95 per cent CI 1.11–1.59) after adjusting for maternal age and socioeconomic status. There was a fairly consistent decrease in risk with distance away from the sites. A significantly raised odds ratio for residence within 3 km of a landfill site was found only for neural tube defects, malformations of the cardiac septa and anomalies of the great arteries and veins.

Although the systematic studies including multiple sites provide a test sufficiently powered to identify a weak combined effect, power to test heterogeneity across sites may be difficult to achieve. In the EUROHAZCON study, there was little evidence of differences in risk between landfill sites, but the power to detect such differences was low because of the relatively small number of people living near each site. In addition, the lack of personal exposure measurements and detailed characterization of the toxicants emitted from the sites were important limitations in the EUROHAZCON study.[27]

The results of the EUROHAZCON study are consistent with a similar study conducted in the UK that used geographical information systems to develop an index of density of waste sites within 2 km of births. The study included 8804 landfill sites, 607 of which were handling hazardous waste, and 10 million births (136 821 with congenital anomalies) during the period 1983–98. An association between density of sites and congenital anomalies was found only for sites handling hazardous wastes in relation to all anomalies combined, cardiovascular defects and hypospadias and epispadias.[28] This study also provided information about chromosomal anomalies, showing a higher risk of such anomalies in people who lived close to sites and the increase being independent of maternal age and socioeconomic status.[29] In contrast, no evidence about an increased risk of low birth weight was found either in a study of the 10 English hazardous waste landfill sites included in the EUROHAZCON study[30] or in another study including 61 Scottish special (hazardous) waste landfill sites.[31]

The same approach has been adopted to investigate the risk patterns of several cancers in the population living near to landfill sites in Great Britain.[32] This study included people living within 2 km of 9565 (from a total of 19 196) landfill sites that were operational at some time from 1982 to 1997, and compared them with those living more than 2 km from a landfill. The study included 89 786 cases of bladder cancer, 36 802 cases of brain cancer, 21 773 cases of hepatobiliary cancer, 37 812 cases of adult leukaemia and 3973 cases of childhood leukaemia. The results showed no excess risks of cancers of the bladder and brain, hepatobiliary cancer or leukaemia in populations living within 2 km of a landfill site. The results were similar if the analysis was restricted to landfill sites licensed to carry special (hazardous) waste.

As important as they are, systematic studies conducted in populations living in the vicinity of waste sites are affected by a number of relevant limitations, the main ones being:

- a lack of detailed information about the contaminants released from the sites – with a consequent lack of direct exposure measurement;
- a restriction of studies to populations living in close vicinity to the sites – so little is known about low-level exposures in the general population;
- the fact that migration patterns in these populations are difficult to capture.

Unfortunately, these problems have no easy solutions, although better exposure measurements, including the use of biomarkers and environmental monitoring data, to define individual exposure offer promising alternatives.[33,34]

Coke works, UK

Another type of point source that has been the subject of systematic studies is the coke works, a major source of smoke and sulphur dioxide. An early study showed that, for several indicators of respiratory health, including cough, sinus trouble, glue ear and wheeze (but not for asthma and chronic bronchitis), there was a gradient of self-reported ill-health, with the highest prevalence in areas closest to the works.[35] A subsequent study conducted in Great Britain included a larger population and showed an excess of all-cause mortality of 3 per cent in those living within less than 2 km of coke works, and a significant decline in mortality with distance from coke works. The increased mortality was larger for cardiovascular causes, especially ischaemic heart disease, and for respiratory deaths, with significant declines in risk with distance for all these causes.[36]

In contrast, a study that included the populations aged 65 years or over and under 5 years living within 7.5 km of four coke works, and used distance from residence to the coke work source as a measure of exposure, did not find an increased risk of emergency hospital admissions with a primary diagnosis of coronary heart disease, stroke, all respiratory diseases, chronic obstructive pulmonary disease or asthma. There was, however, evidence of significant heterogeneity in risk estimates between coke work groups, and for one of the coke works in north-east England there was an increased risk of both respiratory disease and asthma.[37] Regarding other outcomes, one study reported no evidence of an increased risk of low birth weight, stillbirth, neonatal mortality or post-neonatal mortality near coke works.[38]

The studies of coke works are to a large extent subject to the same limitations as those of landfill studies, and in particular there have been indications that deprivation of the population living around coke works may not have been effectively controlled for in analyses.[36]

METHODOLOGICAL ISSUES IN EPIDEMIOLOGICAL STUDIES AROUND POINT SOURCES

The investigation of health effects around point sources is a particular situation in which standard epidemiological designs can rarely be applied. The complexity of studying health patterns in relation to emissions from a contaminant point source is due to several inter-related issues. First, the type of design adopted in most point-source studies does not correspond to the classical epidemiological design. Second, the measurement of exposure usually consists of a rough indirect measure such as the distance from the residence to the point source. Third, area-related confounders such as other environmental exposures and socioeconomic status are difficult to control. Finally, the type of statistical method to be used in these studies differs from those used in the classical epidemiological research.

Point-source studies can most of the time be considered as a particular form of small-area study, both belonging to the broad field of spatial or geographical epidemiology. As mentioned earlier, studies of this type use secondary data for both the exposure and the outcome. Although these studies have provided an individual measure of risk, the limitations of data on exposures and outcomes, together with the lack of information about confounders, place these studies somewhere between ecological and individual studies. The latter is an important issue since ecological biases are very difficult to control, and their influence on risk estimates is very difficult to predict.

Some authors have considered how ecological designs can be improved by the use of individual-level data.[39,40] In some cases, however, it is possible to use the case–control design, as was the case in the Sellafield studies. In other instances, the time–activity patterns of the point source are exploited with time rather than space leading the choice of design, as was the case in the before-and-after studies conducted to investigate the effects of the steel mill of Utah Valley,[3] the incinerator at Mataró[22] and the soybean silo in Barcelona.[7] Although before-and-after studies can also be seen as a type of ecological study, the fact that they are based on groups (time periods) that are compared with themselves, in different periods of time, makes ecological bias unlikely. However, in these studies, background time trends in exposure and/or disease may also bias the risk estimates, the inclusion of control areas being a useful option.

Exposure estimation

The price to pay for point-source studies aiming to provide individual-based estimates is that indirect measures of exposure have to be used. As shown in earlier sections of this chapter, most studies have used different indices of distance from the residence to the point source as an individual measure of exposure. The distance from the residence to the point source is a very crude measure that does not take into account the characteristics of exposure, such as the route of contaminant exposure (ingested or dermal instead of airborne), the time spent in the area or relevant indoor exposures. Consequently, the majority of point-source studies are affected by a substantial degree of exposure misclassification.

Alternatives to alleviate this problem are the use of modelling methods that may provide improved estimates of exposure. In point-source studies, modelling exposure will involve modelling point-source emissions.[41] Whereas modelling of exposure is being increasingly applied to situations such as air pollution, its use in point-source studies is still uncommon.[26] Another approach to improve exposure measurement in this situation is the use of biomarkers. The rationale and applicability of using biomarkers was shown in a transitional study conducted in an industrial metropolitan area of Belgium.[42]

Specific statistical approaches

One important particularity of point-source studies is the need to use special statistical methods. Stone proposed a method of testing the increased risk of a disease around a point source.[43] Stone's test is appropriate to data consisting of counts of the number of cases, which can be ordered in increasing distance from a point source. The test assumes that the number of cases is a mutually independent Poisson co-variate, the expected number of cases being obtained from standardized national or regional incidence rates. The null hypothesis, that the risk is constant, is then tested against the alternative that risk increases monotonically with distance from the source. The Stone method has subsequently been modified to deal with several limitations by allowing for adjustments for socioeconomic confounding and for generally elevated risks near the source, to pooled data around a number of point sources[44] and to allow for co-variate adjustment via a log-linear model.[45]

A more powerful test, the linear risk score, was developed by Bithell in a study of the distribution of childhood leukaemia around nuclear installations in Britain.[46] More recently, in the context of a study regarding an excess risk of perinatal undesirable outcomes near municipal solid-waste incinerators in Japan, Tango considered extensions of score tests in order to allow selection of the best among several prespecified parametric exposure functions. The latter is useful to avoid multiple testing problems and to be applied to a possible situation where the hazardous substance levels have a peak at some distance from a point source.[47]

The opportunity to use Bayesian statistics as an appropriate framework for geographical analysis and disease mapping has been recognized for more than a decade.[48] Bayesian mapping can be used to assess whether there is an excess of disease risk close to a prespecified point

source and allows the frequently encountered extra-Poisson variability to be accommodated through random effects. A random-effects approach may be used for diagnostic purposes, in particular to assess the appropriateness of the distance–risk model.[49]

The many methodological intricacies of geographical epidemiological studies have been thoroughly reviewed, and, when applied appropriately, such methods offer a valuable alternative for point-source studies where classical epidemiological methods cannot be applied.[50]

PUBLIC HEALTH APPROACHES

In the final analysis, protecting the health of a population living in the vicinity of potentially harmful point sources is the main objective, often a challenging one. Owing to the local nature, the concerns of residents about the potential health effects of contaminating point sources are frequently presented to the local public health services. The main issues are then to clarify the nature of the concerns, to assess the types of health problem giving rise to concern and to decide whether or not an ad hoc study is required. Providing scientifically clear answers to such questions is, however, often not possible. Some general recommendations for local public health services and a review of some of the approaches reported in the literature follow in the next section.

Unfortunately, there are no available guidelines specifically addressing the response of the public health services when such concerns are raised. For some of the relevant issues involved in the investigation of a point source, the Centers for Disease Control guidelines for the investigation of clusters can be applied.[51] These guidelines, specifically designed for the investigation of clusters, provide a useful stepwise approach:

1 In general, when facing the investigation of a point source, the first broad step should come from initial contacts with both residents and point-source managers to form estimations of risk. The Small Area Health Statistics Unit (SAHSU) in the UK has developed a suitable model for this initial step.
2 If this step does not provide sufficient information, a more detailed study should be considered. As described earlier, however, local studies are commonly limited by several intrinsic characteristics, including the limited size of the exposed population.
3 Therefore, the possibility of undertaking a well-designed systematic study should be considered as a further option.

The availability of information about the location and emissions of point sources is of crucial importance in facilitating geographical studies covering wide populations. The availability of this type of information obviously varies from country to country. For instance, at the

European level, an important step has been the development of the European Pollutant Emission Register (EPER).[52] The EPER was established in 2000 and results have been reported for the years 2001 and 2004. In 2007, the EPER was replaced by the European Pollutant Release and Transfer Register (European PRTR).

The EPER is a register of industrial plants covering a limited number of activities whenever the amount of eligible emission is beyond a threshold. The threshold values have been chosen in order to include about 90 per cent of the emissions of the industrial facilities looked at. The EPER contains data on the main pollutant emissions to air and water reported by about 10 000 large and medium-sized industrial facilities, covering 50 pollutants and providing descriptions of each of the substances, their uses, their major emission sources and their impacts on human health and the environment. Emissions from the transport sector and from most agricultural sources are not included.

To improve the quality of data, the EPER uses several internal processes including a validation tool covering the types of pollutant, the codes for industrial sectors and the types of geographical coordinate. However, external validation, like the one recently conducted in Spain, could contribute to a more exhaustive ascertainment of data quality.[53]

SAHSU in the UK has developed a Rapid Inquiry Facility able to provide an estimated relative risk for any given condition for the population within defined areas around a point source, relative to the population in a local reference region. The facility uses routinely collected morbidity, mortality and population data on a small-area scale, together with the computing facilities and expertise necessary to run such analyses quickly and efficiently.[54] Currently, other facilities following the SAHSU approach are being developed in other countries. One example is the National Centre for Epidemiology in Spain, which has conducted several geographical studies assessing the increases in morbidity and mortality around point sources.[55]

Assessment of control measures

In some situations, controlling the activity of the contaminating point sources may be a difficult task and may involve the need to develop specific monitoring systems. Although the installation of bag filters in the silo that caused the soybean asthma outbreaks in Barcelona was an effective measure, there was evidence of sporadic relatively high levels of soybean allergens in the city's air. Therefore, other strict protective measures in the unloading process were established to avoid the release of soybean dust into the atmosphere, with allergen emissions showing a very important decrease to levels 95–98 per cent lower; this showed that, with a systematic control programme, industrial soybean operations could function near urban centres without public health risks.[56] A key element of the

approach developed in Barcelona was the environmental monitoring of soybean allergens in the city's air, which provides updated evidence that despite higher levels of soybean allergens on unloading days, there is no association between these levels and the number of emergency room admissions for asthma.[57]

For some other types of point source, specific regulations have been developed to minimize the health effects in exposed populations. Wet cooling systems are often associated with large outbreaks of Legionnaires' disease, and several European countries have legislation for registering such systems. Information about the level of development of such systems was obtained by means of a survey of 39 European countries and regions. Nine countries stated having legislation for the registration of wet cooling systems. Separate legislation was reported to exist at a regional level for two regions in Belgium and three regions in the UK, giving a total of 12 countries/regions with legislation. In nine of these countries/regions, the legislation had been introduced since 2001. All of these countries/regions require periodic microbiological monitoring, and in nine the legislation requires periodic inspection of the systems. Regulations for the registration of wet cooling systems should be required by public health authorities. During an outbreak of legionellosis, a register of wet cooling systems can considerably speed up the investigation process.[58]

Conclusion

Unfortunately, the availability of resources like the ones alluded to above is the exception rather than the rule, and public health services are commonly faced with strikingly limited resources to address the health problems related to contaminating point sources. Although the available knowledge and methods, as reviewed in this chapter, provide a range of useful strategies when facing point-source health-related problems, there is an urgent need for large-scale developments in this field, including the extension of inventories of point sources such as the EPER, the implementation of risk assessment facilities like SAHSU, and the development of more robust environmental monitoring systems. Improving the current risk management standards is a key aspect of any attempt to protect the health of the populations living in the vicinity of contaminating point sources.

REFERENCES

● = Key primary paper
◆ = Major review article

1. Knox G. Epidemics of rare diseases. *Br Med Bull* 1971; **27**: 43–7.
2. Fredrichs RR. History, maps and the internet: UCL's John Snow Site. *SoC Bull* 2001; **34**: 3–7.

●3. Pope CA III. Particulate pollution and health: A review of the Utah valley experience. *J Expo Anal Environ Epidemiol* 1996; **6**: 23–34.

4. Antó JM, Sunyer J. A point-source asthma outbreak. *Lancet* 1986; **1**: 900–3.

●5. Antó JM, Sunyer J, Rodriguez-Roisin R, Suarez-Cervera M, Vazquez L. Community outbreaks of asthma associated with inhalation of soybean dust. Toxicoepidemiological Committee. *N Engl J Med* 1989; **320**: 1097–102.

6. Sunyer J, Antó JM, Rodrigo MJ, Morell F. Case-control study of serum immunoglobulin-E antibodies reactive with soybean in epidemic asthma. *Lancet* 1989; **1**: 179–82.

●7. Antó JM, Sunyer J, Reed CE *et al.* Preventing asthma epidemics due to soybeans by dust-control measures. *N Engl J Med* 1993; **329**: 1760–3.

8. White MC, Etzel RA, Olson DR, Goldstein IF. Reexamination of epidemic asthma in New Orleans, Louisiana, in relation to the presence of soy at the harbor. *Am J Epidemiol* 1997; **145**: 432–8.

●9. Fraser DW, Tsai TR, Orenstein W *et al.* Legionnaires' disease: Description of an epidemic of pneumonia. *N Engl J Med* 1977; **297**: 1189–97.

●10. McDade JE, Shepard CC, Fraser DW, Tsai TR, Redus MA, Dowdle WR. Legionnaires' disease: Isolation of a bacterium and demonstration of its role in other respiratory disease. *N Engl J Med* 1977; **297**: 1197–203.

11. Kirrage D, Reynolds G, Smith GE, Olowokure B; Hereford Legionnaires Outbreak Control Team. Investigation of an outbreak of Legionnaires' disease: Hereford, UK 2003. *Respir Med* 2007; **101**: 1639–44.

12. Bhopal RS, Fallon RJ, Buist EC, Black RJ, Urquhart JD. Proximity of the home to a cooling tower and risk of non-outbreak Legionnaires' disease. *BMJ* 1991; **302**: 378–83.

13. Ballester F, Soriano JB, Otero I *et al.* Asthma visits to emergency rooms and soybean unloading in the harbors of Valencia and A Coruña, Spain. *Am J Epidemiol* 1999; **149**: 315–22.

14. Gardner, MJ. Childhood leukaemia around the Sellafield nuclear plant. In: Elliott P, Cuzick J, English D, Stern R (eds) *Geographical and Environmental Epidemiology: Methods for Small-area Studies.* Oxford: Oxford University Press, 1992.

15. Laurier D, Grosche B, Hall P. Risk of childhood leukaemia in the vicinity of nuclear installations – findings and recent controversies. *Acta Oncol* 2002; **41**: 14–24.

◆16. Beral V. Childhood leukemia near nuclear plants in the United Kingdom: The evolution of a systematic approach to studying rare disease in small geographic areas. *Am J Epidemiol* 1990; **132**: S63–8.

◆17. Bithell JF, Dutton SJ, Draper GJ, Neary NM. Distribution of childhood leukaemias and non-Hodgkin's lymphomas near nuclear installations in England and Wales. *BMJ* 1994; **309**: 501–5.

18. Waller LA, Turnbull BW, Gustafsson G, Hjalmars U, Andersson B. Detection and assessment of clusters of disease: An application to nuclear power plant facilities and childhood leukaemia in Sweden. *Stat Med* 1995; **14**: 3–16.

●19. Gardner MJ, Snee MP, Hall AJ, Powell CA, Downes S, Terrell JD. Results of case-control study of leukaemia and lymphoma among young people near Sellafield nuclear plant in West Cumbria. *BMJ* 1990; **300**: 423–9. [Erratum in: *BMJ* 1992; **305**: 715.]

20. Pobel D, Viel JF. Case-control study of leukaemia among young people near La Hague nuclear reprocessing plant: The environmental hypothesis revisited. *BMJ* 1997; **314**: 101–6.

21. Boutou O, Guizard AV, Slama R, Pottier D, Spira A. Population mixing and leukaemia in young people around the La Hague nuclear waste reprocessing plant. *Br J Cancer* 2002; **87**: 740–5.

22. González CA, Kogevinas M, Gadea E *et al.* Biomonitoring study of people living near or working at a municipal solid-waste incinerator before and after two years of operation. *Arch Environ Health* 2000; **55**: 259–67.

23. González CA, Kogevinas M, Gadea E, Pera G, Päpke O. Increase of dioxin blood levels over the last 4 years in the general population in Spain. *Epidemiology* 2001; **12**: 365.

24. Sans S, Elliott P, Kleinschmidt I *et al.* Cancer incidence and mortality near the Baglan Bay petrochemical works, South Wales. *Occup Environ Med* 1995; **52**: 217–24.

25. Wilkinson P, Thakrar B, Shaddick G *et al.* Cancer incidence and mortality around the Pan Britannica Industries pesticide factory, Waltham Abbey. *Occup Environ Med* 1997; **54**: 101–7. [Erratum in *Occup Environ Med* 1997; **54**: 216.]

26. Hodgson S, Nieuwenhuijsen MJ, Hansell A *et al.* Excess risk of kidney disease in a population living near industrial plants. *Occup Environ Med* 2004; **61**: 717–19.

●27. Vrijheid M, Armstrong B, Abramsky L *et al.* Risk of congenital anomalies near hazardous-waste landfill sites in Europe: The EUROHAZCON study. *Lancet* 1998; **352**: 423–7.

28. Elliott P, Richardson S, Abellan JJ *et al.* Geographic density of landfill sites and risk of congenital anomalies in England. *Occup Environ Med* 2009; **66**: 81–9.

29. Vrijheid M, Dolk H, Armstrong B *et al.* Chromosomal congenital anomalies and residence near hazardous waste landfill sites. *Lancet* 2002; **359**: 320–2.

30. Morgan OW, Vrijheid M, Dolk H. Risk of low birth weight near EUROHAZCON hazardous waste landfill sites in England. *Arch Environ Health* 2004; **59**: 149–51.

31. Morris SE, Thomson AO, Jarup L, de Hoogh C, Briggs DJ, Elliott P. No excess risk of adverse birth outcomes in populations living near special waste landfill sites in Scotland. *Scott Med J* 2003; **48**: 105–7.

32. Jarup L, Briggs D, de Hoogh C *et al.* Cancer risks in populations living near landfill sites in Great Britain. *Br J Cancer* 2002; **86**: 1732–6.

◆33. Vrijheid M. Health effects of residence near hazardous waste landfill sites: A review of epidemiologic literature. *Environ Health Perspect* 2000; **108** (Suppl. 1): 101–12.

◆34. Linzalone N, Bianchi F. [Studying risks of waste landfill sites on human health: Updates and perspectives] [Article in Italian]. *Epidemiol Prev* 2005; **29**: 51–3.

35. Bhopal RS, Phillimore P, Moffatt S, Foy C. Is living near a coking works harmful to health? A study of industrial air pollution. *J Epidemiol Community Health* 1994; **48**: 237–47.

36. Dolk H, Thakrar B, Walls P *et al*. Mortality among residents near cokeworks in Great Britain. *Occup Environ Med* 1999; **56**: 34–40.

37. Aylin P, Bottle A, Wakefield J, Jarup L, Elliott P. Proximity to coke works and hospital admissions for respiratory and cardiovascular disease in England and Wales. *Thorax* 2001; **56**: 228–33.

38. Dolk H, Pattenden S, Vrijheid M, Thakrar B, Armstrong B. Perinatal and infant mortality and low birth weight among residents near cokeworks in Great Britain. *Arch Environ Health* 2000; **55**: 26–30.

39. Jackson C, Best N, Richardson S. Improving ecological inference using individual-level data. *Stat Med* 2006; **25**: 2136–59.

40. Haneuse SJ, Wakefield JC. Hierarchical models for combining ecological and case-control data. *Biometrics* 2007; **63**: 128–36.

41. Nieuwenhuijsen MJ. Environmental exposure assessment. In: Baker D (ed.) *Environmental Epidemiology*, 3rd edn. New York: Oxford University Press, 2008: pp. 41–73.

♦42. Staessen JA, Nawrot T, Hond ED *et al*. Renal function, cytogenetic measurements, and sexual development in adolescents in relation to environmental pollutants: A feasibility study of biomarkers. *Lancet* 2001; **357**: 1660–9.

43. Stone RA. Investigations of excess environmental risks around putative sources: Statistical problems and a proposed test. *Stat Med* 1988; **7**: 649–60.

44. Shaddick G, Elliott P. Use of Stone's method in studies of disease risk around point sources of environmental pollution. *Stat Med* 1996; **15**: 1927–34.

45. Morton-Jones T, Diggle P, Elliott P. Investigation of excess environmental risk around putative sources: Stone's test with covariate adjustment. *Stat Med* 1999; **18**: 189–97.

46. Bithell JF. The choice of test for detecting raised disease risk near a point source. *Stat Med* 1995; **14**: 2309–22.

47. Tango T. Score tests for detecting excess risks around putative sources. *Stat Med* 2002; **21**: 497–514.

48. Elliott P, Martuzzi M, Shaddick G. Spatial statistical methods in environmental epidemiology: A critique. *Stat Methods Med Res* 1995; **4**: 137–59.

49. Wakefield JC, Morris SE. The Bayesian modelling of disease risk in relation to a point source. *J Am Stat Assoc* 2001; **96**: 77–91.

♦50. Elliott P, Savitz DA. Design issues in small-area studies of environment and health. *Environ Health Perspect* 2008; **116**: 1098–104.

51. Centers for Disease Control. Guidelines for investigating clusters for health events. *MMWR* 1990; **39**: 1–23.

52. European Pollutant Emission Register 2009. Available from: http://eper.ec.europa.eu/eper/ (accessed January 5, 2010).

53. García-Pérez J, Boldo E, Ramis R *et al*. Validation of the geographic position of EPER-Spain industries. *Int J Health Geogr* 2008; **7**: 1.

●54. Aylin P, Maheswaran R, Wakefield J *et al*. A national facility for small area disease mapping and rapid initial assessment of apparent disease clusters around a point source: The UK Small Area Health Statistics Unit. *J Public Health Med* 1999; **21**: 289–98.

55. García-Pérez J, Pollán M, Boldo E *et al*. Mortality due to lung, laryngeal and bladder cancer in towns lying in the vicinity of combustion installations. *Sci Total Environ* 2009; **407**: 2593–602.

56. Villalbí JR, Plasencia A, Manzanera R, Armengol R, Antó JM; Collaborative and Technical Support Groups for the study of soybean asthma in Barcelona. Epidemic soybean asthma and public health: New control systems and initial evaluation in Barcelona, 1996–98. *J Epidemiol Community Health* 2004; **58**: 461–5.

57. Rodrigo MJ, Cruz MJ, García MD, Antó JM, Genover T, Morell F. Epidemic asthma in Barcelona: An evaluation of new strategies for the control of soybean dust emission. *Int Arch Allergy Immunol* 2004; **134**: 158–64.

58. Ricketts KD, Joseph C, Lee J, Wewalka G; European Working Group for Legionella Infections. Survey on legislation regarding wet cooling systems in European countries. *Euro Surveill* 2008; **13**: pii, 18982.

Volcanoes

PETER J. BAXTER

The greatest source of influence in Charles Darwin's formulation of the evolutionary theory was Charles Lyell's grand work, *The Principles of Geology*, the first volume of which was published in 1830 just before Darwin embarked on the voyage of the *Beagle*.[1] For the first time, stratigraphical observations from geology and palaeontology were explaining earth history and the role of volcanic and earthquake action: it was on the young, volcanic Galapagos islands where Darwin came across the evidence for the theory of natural selection.

Another scientific revolution occurred in the 1960s, when plate tectonic theory radically changed perceptions of the forces underlying the oceans and continents and their geochemical cycles.[1] Today, with the quadrupling of the world's population in the twentieth century and environmental impacts such as climate change, there is a new sense of urgency behind understanding the forces that shape the earth and its atmosphere, in which volcanoes have an important part.

WHAT IS A VOLCANO?

Most volcanoes form where the dozen or so tectonic plates that make up the shell of the Earth – the crust and lithosphere – are pulling apart at rifts and long mid-ocean ridges, or converging at subduction zones, an ancient and massive geological recycling process between the inner Earth and its surface of minerals and volatile elements such as water, carbon dioxide and sulphur.

At volcanoes, the molten rock (or magma) below the Earth's crust and associated gases are extruded onto the Earth's surface or into the atmosphere. Low-silica magmas have a low viscosity and produce fluid lava flows, but volcanoes with more viscous magmas have a higher gas (or volatile) content and can erupt explosively, producing fluxes of energy and matter that can take the form of natural hazards. Eruptions are driven by the energy from heat trapped in the Earth since its formation 4.5 billion years ago and from the decay of naturally occurring uranium, potassium, thorium and other radionuclides present deep in the Earth.[2]

IMPACTS OF VOLCANIC ERUPTIONS

The Earth's early atmosphere was formed by volcanic gases. The constancy of the atmosphere today is the outcome of a climate system that is fully coupled to the cycles of plate tectonics, weathering, erosion and biological activity. The connection between volcanic eruptions and climate finally became firmly established after the 1991 eruption of Mount Pinatubo, Philippines, and debate continues on the effect that massive releases of magmatic volatiles could have on long-term climate trends.[3]

The large eruptions of Tambora (1815) and Krakatoa (1883), in Indonesia, each killed tens of thousands of people in their vicinity, but they were also responsible for vivid sunsets that inspired artists like J.M.W. Turner and William Ascroft on the other side of the globe. The sulphate aerosols in the stratosphere that scattered the sun's rays to create this effect from Tambora also caused sufficient global cooling for harvests to fail and trigger famine in many countries in 1816 (the 'year without a summer'),[4] and for Krakatoa this effect slowed sea level rise and ocean warming into the following century.[3]

Eruptions on the scale of Tambora could occur with sufficient frequency to warrant concerted global mitigation planning, but for scientists the forecasting of such events remains an elusive goal.

CHEMISTRY OF VOLCANIC EMISSIONS

The gaseous and ash emissions from active volcanoes can cause pollution of air, soils and water over long distances. Volcanoes like Mount Etna, Sicily, the largest and most active in Europe, are in a state of continuous copious degassing that is only occasionally punctuated by eruptions of fluid lava or basaltic explosive activity with moderate ash fall, whereas others like Masaya, Nicaragua, can go through cycles of degassing lasting years at a time. Whereas the effects of a tall volcano like Etna (altitude 3340 m) on the local environment may not be very apparent while degassing up to 20 000 tonnes of sulphur dioxide per day, the low-altitude crater of Masaya enables the gas plume to fumigate the land downwind, which, together with the rain made acid from mixing with the plume, destroys vegetation and alters soil composition over a wide, populated area.[5]

Water vapour and carbon dioxide are the most abundant gases in plumes. Sulphur dioxide is the most important gas for respiratory health as it can trigger asthma attacks in concentrations as low as 400 parts per billion in asthma sufferers, levels that can be found kilometers downwind of an active vent. Estimates indicate that total volcanic emissions constitute 10–35 per cent of the present-day global sulphur dioxide source to the atmosphere, and the total sulphate aerosol burden in the troposphere could be as high as 40 per cent.[6] Sulphate veils in the stratosphere after eruptions also induce ozone loss.

But it is the halogens (fluorine, chlorine, bromine and iodine) and their gases that can have the most profound effects on the atmosphere and hydrosphere, perturbing the tropospheric and stratospheric ozone budgets, and contributing towards the formation of acid rains, volcanogenic air pollution and the acidification of soils and surface waters.[7]

The emission of volatile heavy metals has so far only been poorly quantified, and estimates are at best in orders of magnitude: Etna's emissions are strongly enriched with bismuth, copper, cadmium, tin and zinc, and the volcano is also likely to be a major source of natural mercury for the Mediterranean and Europe, like other volcanoes known to be significant sulphur dioxide emitters on a regional scale.[8]

ERUPTIONS

There are about 700 land volcanoes in the world, about 200 of which are active. Rare super-eruptions can unleash the greatest forces on earth, but fortunately, compared with floods, wind storms and earthquakes, volcanic eruptions occur much less frequently, averaging in recent decades only two to four fatal events world wide every year.[9]

Modern volcanology can be said to have begun in 1980 with the eruption of Mount St Helens in the USA, when, for the first time, the scale and impact of a major explosive eruption could be captured by the media and scientists alike. The lateral blast-driven pyroclastic surge destroyed within minutes a 180 degree swathe of forest as far as 28 km from the crater. The eruption had occurred without any warning, despite the volcano having been under close monitoring by scientists for the 2 months since the start of its unrest.[10] Only 58 people in the wilderness area, which had been mostly evacuated, were killed, but the event showed the enormity of the threat that a similar volcano would present in a heavily populated area.[11]

An estimated 10 per cent of the world's population have settled in areas of active volcanism,[12] and large populations now occupy cities and islands without any regard to the hazard of volcanoes that may have been dormant for decades or centuries. This is the single most important reason for the rapidly growing vulnerability of human populations to volcanic eruptions.

Pyroclastic flows and surges, like the one at Mount St Helens, are among the deadliest eruptive phenomena, being typically fast-moving clouds of ash and gas whose intense heat and high lateral pressures flatten and ignite almost everything in their path. The worst volcanic disaster of the twentieth century occurred in 1902 when 28 000 people died in a fireball after the city of St Pierre on Martinique was struck by a surge from Mont Pelée volcano.[13] The surge hazard was unknown at the time, but scientists saw that the destruction resembled the ruins of Pompeii and Herculaneum, the towns destroyed in the AD 79 eruption of Vesuvius. It was only after study of the eruption of Mount St Helens that scientists finally pieced together the repeated flows and surges generated by collapses in the eruption column of Vesuvius that had swept so devastatingly around the volcano.[14] The largest eruption of the last millennium at Vesuvius was in 1631, but this was followed by centuries of milder eruptions, the last in 1944. Since then, the population in the shadow of Vesuvius has grown by hundreds of thousands.

The most common scenario is for signs of volcanic activity to appear suddenly at a volcano that has been in repose for decades at least and where the population at risk has little idea what to do or expect. The state of unrest may typically continue for months or even years before the volcano erupts or the activity eventually stops. Monitoring volcanoes by scientific teams is essential for attempting to forecast their behaviour and for advising officials and populations on the decisions to take to safeguard life and property.

Unfortunately, predicting the timing, size and type of an eruption is not usually possible in most of these crises, which can become very fraught, and the uncertainty involved can lead to false alarms, leading to unnecessary but economically costly evacuations or false reassurances, which can be disastrous. In such a crisis in 1985, 23 000 inhabitants of Armero, Colombia, perished in a mudflow (lahar) triggered by an eruption of the Nevado del Ruiz volcano when a small summit eruption melted part of its glacier and sent a wall of flood water and mud into the populated valley below.[15] A warning system and evacuation plan would have prevented this disaster – a lesson in disaster vulnerability that was heeded in leading the United Nations to declare the 1990s as the International Decade for Natural Disaster Reduction.

One of the largest eruptions of the twentieth century was at Pinatubo, Philippines, in 1991. After 2 months of unrest, the volcano's activity began to increase sharply, and just before the climactic eruption, volcanologists persuaded the authorities to evacuate tens of thousands of people who would otherwise have died in pyroclastic flows. Yet the ash fall-out from the eruption, which lasted many hours, was responsible for over 300 deaths among those who sheltered inside buildings as the roofs collapsed on top of them under the weight of the accumulated ash.[16] This hazard and the wide range of impacts of volcanic fall-out on transport (air, rail and road) and vital infrastructure in modern cities and conurbations also require very specific mitigation measures.

RISKS FROM VOLCANIC EMISSIONS

Tephra is the mixture of glassy, mineralic or rock fragments emitted in volcanic eruptions. Ash is defined as the fragments 2 mm or less in diameter. The inhalable fraction 10 µm or less in diameter (PM) can constitute about 10–20 per cent by weight of ash deposits in explosive eruptions.[17] In consequence, people in ash-fall areas can be exposed to elevated mean levels of volcanic PM_{10} (about 200–400 µg/m³) for weeks or even months after eruptions, especially those in outdoor occupations. Public perception in affected areas is that volcanic ash is very harmful to the lungs, and this fear is an important reason why people temporarily or even permanently abandon areas if eruptions go on for long periods and there is repeated exposure to ash resuspended by winds and traffic.

Before the Mount St Helens eruption, little was known about the health risks of inhaling volcanic ash, and although our knowledge has improved, there is much more yet to learn about the effects of ashes emitted from different types of volcano. The fine particles ($PM_{2.5}$) do irritate the airways of susceptible people, and acute bronchitis, asthma and an exacerbation of chronic lung diseases can occur in some but not all eruptions with widespread ash fall-out.[17] In certain types of lava dome-forming eruptions, the amount of respirable crystalline silica in the form of cristobalite is substantially increased,[18] and in eruptions lasting years, protective measures against silicosis may be needed, as were instituted in the population to protect mainly children and outdoor workers on

Montserrat, West Indies, in the eruption of the Soufrière Hills volcano that began in 1995.[17]

Fluoride-coated ash has been an important toxicant to sheep and other grazing animals in certain eruptions in Iceland and less commonly elsewhere in the world. Ash should always be tested for volatile substances adsorbed in the erupted plume, including sulphur, halogen and metal species, which can be leached, potentially releasing heavy loadings to soils and water bodies.[19] About 10 per cent of active volcanoes have crater lakes, and some are hyperacid due to volcanic gases discharging through the waters, which become concentrated with elements from dissolved rock, including fluoride; this can then pollute rivers used to irrigate crops and provide water for human and animal consumption. Studies of the Kawah Ijen crater lake in Java have shown effects on soil chemical processes and plant uptake of nutrients, whereas dental fluorosis is widespread in humans in the irrigated areas.[20]

Rarely, crater lakes and deep lakes in volcanic areas, such as Lake Kivu in East Africa, can store huge amounts of carbon dioxide in solution under hydrostatic pressure in their deep layers. In 1986, an overturning of Lake Nyos produced a gas burst in the form of a huge cloud of carbon dioxide that asphyxiated about 1700 people living in the remote valleys below.[21] Magmatic carbon dioxide and radon (from the radioactive decay of uranium) are common soil gases in volcanic areas, and these can become hazardous to human health if they collect inside houses built on top of degassing soils.[22,23] Radon daughters are human lung carcinogens.

MANAGEMENT OF VOLCANIC ACTIVITY

The awareness of the hazards of volcanoes and the wider environmental and planetary consequences of eruptions and degassing volcanoes is only quite recent, but scientists now have a growing understanding of hazardous eruptive phenomena and the key factors that contribute to human, building and economic vulnerability. The main problem is the uncertainty in forecasting major explosive eruptions and the high stakes involved if the area is heavily populated. Just as the evolutionary and tectonic theories provided science with new language and rules, so a new probabilistic framework to constrain the uncertainty and complexity of Earth processes is needed.[24]

At the emergency planning level, the quantification of volcanic risk using Bayesian decision analysis and formal probabilistic reasoning was successfully applied to support decision-making on the delineation of high-risk areas and the need for evacuation in Montserrat it has been developed further in conjunction with major advances in three-dimensional numerical simulation modelling of eruptive phenomena for a future crisis at Vesuvius.[25] Similar work is urgently needed at other dangerous volcanoes around the world.

REFERENCES

◆ = Major review article

◆1. Fortey R. *The Earth: An Intimate History*. London: HarperCollins, 2004.

◆2. Sigurdsson H. Introduction. In: Sigurdsson H, Houghton BF, McNutt SR, Rymer H, Stix J (eds) *Encyclopedia of Volcanoes*. San Diego: Academic Press, 2000: 1–13.

3. Scaillet B. Are volcanic gases serial killers? *Science* 2008; **319**: 1628–9.

4. Oppenheimer C. Climatic, environmental and human consequences of the largest known historic eruption: Tambora volcano (Indonesia) 1815. *Prog Phys Geogr* 2003; **27**: 230–59.

5. Delmelle P, Stix J, Baxter PJ, Garcia-Alvarez, Barquero J. Atmospheric dispersion, environmental effects and potential health hazard associated with the low-altitude gas plume of Masaya volcano, Nicaragua. *Bull Volcanol* 2002; **64**: 423–34.

6. Stevenson DS, Johnson CE, Collins WJ, Derwent RG. The tropospheric sulphur cycle and the role of volcanic SO_2. In: Oppenheimer C, Pyle DM, Barclay J (eds) *Volcanic Degassing*. Special Publication No. 213. London: Geological Society, 2005: 295–305.

7. Pyle DM, Mather TA. Halogens in igneous processes and their fluxes to the atmosphere and oceans from volcanic activity: A review. *Chem Geol* 2009; **263**: 110–21.

8. Pyle DM, Mather TA. The importance of volcanic emissions for the global atmospheric mercury cycle. *Atmos Environ* 2003; **37**: 5115–24.

9. Simkim T, Siebert S, Blong R. Volcano fatalities – lessons from the historical record. *Science* 2001; **291**: 255.

10. Newhall CG, Punongbayan RS. The narrow margin of successful volcanic risk mitigation. In: Scarpa R, Tilling RI (eds) *Monitoring and Mitigation of Volcano Hazards*. Berlin: Springer, 1996: 809–38.

11. Baxter PJ. Medical effects of volcanoes. 1: Main causes of death and injury. *Bull Volcanol* 1990; **52**: 532–44.

12. Small C, Naumann T. Holocene volcanism and the global distribution of human population. *Environ Hazards* 2001; **3**: 93–109.

13. Baxter PJ, Boyle R, Cole P, Neri A, Spence R, Zuccaro G. The impacts of pyroclastic surges on buildings at the eruption of the Soufrière Hills volcano, Montserrat. *Bull Volcanol* 2005; **67**: 292–313.

14. De Carolis E, Patricelli G. *Vesuvius A.D. 79: The Destruction of Pompeii and Herculaneum*. Los Angeles: Getty Publications, 2003.

15. Voight B. The management of volcanic emergencies: Nevado del Ruiz. In: Scarpa R, Tilling RI (eds) *Monitoring and Mitigation of Volcano Hazards*. Berlin: Springer, 1996: 719–69.

16. Spence RJS, Pomonis A, Baxter PJ, Coburn AW, White M, Dayrit M. Building damage caused by the Mount Pinatubo eruption of June 15, 1991. In: Newhall CG, Punongbayan RS (eds) *Fire and Mud: Eruptions and Lahars at Mount Pinatubo, Philippines*. Seattle: University of Washington Press, 1996: 1055–61.

◆17. Horwell CJ, Baxter PJ. The respiratory health hazards of volcanic ash: A review for volcanic risk mitigation. *Bull Volcanol* 2006; **69**: 1–24.

18. Baxter PJ, Bonadonna C, Dupree R *et al*. Cristobalite in volcanic ash of the Soufrière Hills volcano, Montserrat, British West Indies. *Science* 1999; **283**: 1142–5.

19. Witham CS, Oppenheimer C, Horwell CJ. Volcanic ash-leachates: A review and recommendations for sampling methods. *J Volcanol Geotherm Res* 2005; **141**: 299–326.

20. van Rotterdam-Los AMD, Heikens A, Vriend SP, van Bergen MJ, van Gaans PFM. Impact of acid effluent from Kawah Ijen crater lake on irrigated agricultural soils: Soil chemical processes and plant uptake. *J Volcanol Geotherm Res* 2008; **178**: 287–96.

21. Baxter PJ, Kapila M, Mfonfu D. Lake Nyos disaster, Cameroon, 1986: The medical effects of large scale emission of carbon dioxide? *BMJ* 1989; **298**: 1437–41.

22. Baxter PJ, Baubron J-C, Coutinho R. Health hazards and disaster potential of ground gas emissions at Furnas volcano, Sao Miguel, Azores. *J Volcanol Geotherm Res* 1999; **92**: 95–106.

23. Carapezza ML, Badalamenti B, Cavarra L, Scalzo A. Gas hazard assessment in a densely inhabited area of Colli Albani Volcano (Cava dei Selci, Roma). *J Volcanol Geotherm Res* 2003; **123**: 81–94.

◆24. Neri A, Baxter PJ, Blong R (eds). Evaluating explosive eruption risk at European volcanoes. Special Issue. *J Volcanol Geotherm Res* 2008; **178**: 1–591.

25. Baxter PJ, Aspinall WP, Neri A *et al*. Emergency planning and mitigation at Vesuvius: a new evidence based approach. *J Volcanol Geotherm Res* 2008; **178**: 454–73.

OTHER RESOURCES

International Volcanic Health Hazard Network. http://www.ivhhn. org

Marti J, Ernst GGJ (eds). *Volcanoes and the Environment*. Cambridge: Cambridge University Press, 2005.

Oppenheimer C, Francis P. *Volcanoes*, 2nd edn. Cambridge: Cambridge University Press, 2004.

Sigurdsson H, Houghton BF, McNutt SR, Rymer H, Stix J (eds). *Encyclopedia of Volcanoes*. San Diego: Academic Press, 2000.

Smithsonian Global Volcanic Program. http://www.volcano.si.edu

US Geological Survey Cascades Volcano Observatory. http://vulcan. wr.usgs.gov

13

Environmental allergens

MOISÉS A. CALDERÓN, PABLO RODRÍGUEZ DEL RÍO, NARA T. ORBAN

Worldwide changes in the environment can potentially be associated with the remarkably increased rate of allergic diseases, particularly in countries with a Western lifestyle, that has been seen over the last two to three decades. This chapter considers allergic rhino-conjunctivitis and summer-type hypersensitivity in relation to exposure to environmental aero-allergens, taking into consideration epidemiological and basic research data, such as those related to air pollution and environmental tobacco smoke (ETS).

DEFINITION AND CLASSIFICATION

Allergic rhinitis (AR) is defined as 'inflammation of the lining of the nose, characterized by nasal congestion, rhinorrhoea, sneezing and itching.' Most pollen-allergic patients suffer from rhino-conjunctivitis.[1]

Rhinitis can be classified into different groups according to its aetiology (Table 13.1). The traditional seasonal/perennial classification of AR has recently been questioned, and a revised version based on the severity and duration of symptoms has been proposed in the 'Allergic Rhinitis and its Impact on Asthma' guidelines.[1] Intermittent AR is defined by a symptom duration of less than 4 days per week or less than 4 weeks' duration, whereas persistent AR is defined by the presence of symptoms for more than 4 days per week and for at least 4 weeks. The severity of symptoms is divided into mild or moderate/severe according to whether or not the symptoms impact significantly on quality of life.[1]

The impact of hay fever on factors such as performance at work or school can be significant. A British case–control analysis of 1834 students (age 15–17 years, 50 per cent

Table 13.1 Classification of rhinitis

Group	Aetiology
Allergic rhinitis	Intermittent
	Persistent
	Seasonal
	Perennial
Infectious	Viral
	Bacterial
	Acute
	Chronic
Drug related	Aspirin
	Other medications
Occupational	Intermittent
	Persistent
Hormonal	
Other	NARES
	Irritants
	Food
	Emotional
	Atrophic
	Gastro-oesophageal reflux
Idiopathic	

girls) sitting for national examinations showed that current symptomatic AR and use of rhinitis medication were associated with a significantly increased risk of unexpectedly dropping a grade in summer examinations. This is the first time that the relationship between symptomatic AR and poor examination performance has been demonstrated, which has significant implications for clinical practice.[2]

EPIDEMIOLOGY

Allergic rhinitis is a chronic disease of modern times and is considered to be a global health problem,[3] affecting as many as 23 per cent of the population in Western countries[4] and between 10 per cent and 25 per cent of the world population.[5] Half of all sufferers have not been formally diagnosed, yet 80 per cent would benefit from treatment.[4]

Data from the first phase of the International Study of Asthma and Allergies in Childhood (ISAAC) suggested a prevalence of rhino-conjunctivitis symptoms among children 6–7 years of age and 13–14 years of age of 0.8–14.9 per cent and 1.4–39.7 per cent, respectively, across all participants.[6] When the study was repeated several years later, the prevalence had further increased slightly, but with a wide variation between countries and centres. In the younger group, the increase was more remarkable in the Asia-Pacific and Eastern Mediterranean regions, Latin America, North America and Western Europe.[7] In the 13–14-year age group, an increased prevalence was found mostly in Africa, Asia-Pacific, India and Northern and Eastern Europe. These data show how the prevalence of rhino-conjunctivitis is increasing in young children and even more in the youngest group.

The European Community Respiratory Health Survey (ECRHS)[8] was conducted in adults. ECRHS I (1991–1993) shows a median prevalence of hay fever in Europe of 20.9 per cent (range 9.5–40.9 per cent; ECRHS 1996), with a geographical distribution that varies but runs parallel with atopic sensitization, suggesting that this geographical variation is at least in part due to environmental factors.[9] Large families, shared bedrooms, male siblings and dogs were related to less atopy and fewer allergic diseases, supporting an inverse relation between infectious diseases and atopy as described in many other publications.[10,11]

In opposition to the theory of an overall increase in Western Europe, data provided by the Swiss Study of Childhood Allergy and Respiratory Symptoms with respect to Air Pollution and Climate (SCARPOL, 1992–2001) show that the increase in asthma and hay fever among Swiss children has reached a plateau.[12,13]

ALLERGENS AND ENVIRONMENTAL FACTORS

Seasonal upper respiratory symptoms can be caused by pollen grains, especially from grass, trees and weeds. Grass

species are distributed worldwide, and the most common allergies are caused by reactions to grass pollen released in the late spring and early summer. The distribution of different aero-allergens varies between countries and climates. The increased geographical pollen mobility caused by new and different plants being grown in different areas and grains of pollen travelling further may contribute to a great inconsistency in the duration and severity of allergic symptoms.

Pollen grains contain pores through which their associated proteins can be rapidly distributed on the human nasal mucosa and upper airways. The allergenic proteins produced in the pollen of each plant are very specific, accounting for the high degree of variability among humans in their sensitivity to different pollens. It is important to consider that many patients are polysensitized and polyallergic so in such cases, seasonal exposure to several allergens will extend the duration of the symptoms, leading to persistent nasal complaints.

Westernized lifestyles, including rapid urbanization and high levels of vehicle emissions, are epidemiologically correlated to an increase in the frequency of pollen-induced respiratory allergy.[14,15] The prevalence of AR is increased in urban areas.[16–19] It is also thought that meteorological factors such as temperature, wind speed and humidity can affect both the biological and chemical components of this interaction.

In urban areas with high levels of vehicle traffic, the most abundant air pollutants are respirable particulate matter, nitrogen dioxide, ozone and diesel exhaust particles. All these air pollutants are associated with oxidative stress, the activation of several mitogen-activated protein kinases and transcription factors, and disturbances in cell function.[20, 21] These components of air pollution can ordinarily interact with pollen grains or plant-derived submicronic components, and may enhance the risk of both atopic sensitization and exacerbation of symptoms in sensitized subjects.[14,22] In addition, airway mucosal damage and impaired mucociliary clearance induced by air pollution may facilitate the access of inhaled allergens to the cells of the immune system.[14,23,24] Thus, the interaction between natural vegetation, air pollutants and environmental conditions influences plant allergenicity.

Experimental exposure to ETS has been shown to promote the production of allergen-specific immunoglobulin E (IgE) and to increase levels of nasal histamine in individuals with AR caused by short ragweed. Levels of histamine after ETS/ragweed exposure were on average up to 16.6 times higher than after exposure to clean air/ragweed challenge. Moreover, ETS promotes the induction of a T helper cell type 2 (Th2) cytokine nasal milieu (increased interleukin-4 [IL-4], IL-5 and IL-13 and decreased interferon gamma (IFN-γ) production, which is typical of an active allergic response.[25]

Occupational rhinitis can mimic AR symptoms. It is caused by either inhaled low molecular weight compounds (e.g. acid anhydrides used in epoxy resins)[26] or high molecular weight compounds (e.g. flour and animal proteins)[27–29] in the workplace. Patients with occupational rhinitis are symptomatic mainly in the workplace or during the evening after work (late responses) and improve during weekends away from work and during vacations.[30] There is always a period of exposure prior to sensitization. A proportion of those sensitized will develop true occupational allergy with symptoms on exposure to the offending agent, generally months or 1–3 years following first exposure. If exposure is prolonged, symptoms may persist long term, even in the absence of exposure, highlighting the need for the early recognition and avoidance of provoking occupational allergens. Occupational exposures may provoke both allergic and/or irritant rhinitis symptoms. For greater detail, the reader is referred to Hunter's *Diseases of Occupation*.

MECHANISMS

Features of allergic inflammation include an IgE-dependent activation of mast cells and tissue eosinophilia. Following nasal allergen provocation in sensitive subjects, an 'early allergic response' occurs. Clinically this manifests as itching and/or sneezing within seconds or minutes, followed by nasal discharge and congestion that is maximal at 15–30 minutes and resolves within 1–3 hours. About 50–60 per cent of subjects go on to develop a 'late-phase response' that is maximal at 6–12 hours and resolves within 24 hours. The late nasal responses are characterized by nasal

obstruction due to the recruitment, activation and persistence of eosinophils, basophils and activated T-cells at the sites of allergen exposure (Figure 13.1).

Mediators of hypersensitivity

IMMUNOGLOBULIN E

High serum levels of allergen-specific IgE are a feature of AR, while total IgE levels may remain within the normal range. IgE binds to high-affinity receptors (FcεRI) on mast cells and basophils.[31] FcεRI is present on dendritic cells (DCs) in atopic individuals. IgE also binds to the low-affinity IgE receptor FcεRII (CD23) that is present on monocytes/macrophages and on B lymphocytes.

Cross-linking of the adjacent IgE molecules on the mast cell surface by allergen results in mast cell degranulation and the release of mediators of hypersensitivity that include histamine, tryptase and leukotrienes C_4, D_4 and E_4. Histamine stimulates H_1 receptors on sensory nerves and causes vascular dilatation and increased permeability, which contribute to nasal congestion. Tryptase has potent enzymatic activity and breaks down kininogen, leading to the formation of potent vasoactive and inflammatory kinins, including bradykinin. Leukotrienes increase the vascular permeability and induce mucus secretion from the nasal glands. Prostaglandin D_2 is a potent chemotactic factor for T-cells and may induce the release of cytokines. In addition to the release of preformed and lipid-derived mediators following IgE-dependent activation, mast cells

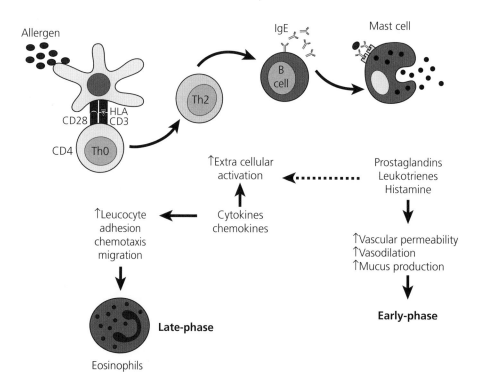

Figure 13.1   Summary of nasal allergic response.

and basophils are known to produce IL-4 and other cytokines that may contribute to the induction of late-phase responses (Figure 13.1).

Effector cells

MAST CELLS

Mast cells are tissue-based inflammatory cells derived from cKIT + CD34 + pluripotent bone marrow stem cells. Mast cells are classified as mucosal (predominantly tryptase-only positive) and connective tissue (both tryptase and chymase positive) types by the use of specific immunostaining. Tryptase-only positive mast cells are predominant in the nasal epithelium of patients with hay fever.

BASOPHILS

Basophils are granulocytes that share many common features with mast cells, including the expression of FcεR1, metachromatic staining and the synthesis and release of histamine and IL-4.[31] Basophils are increased in the nasal epithelium during grass pollen exposure.[32]

EOSINOPHILS

Blood and tissue eosinophilia is the hallmark of allergy.[31] Eosinophils have bilobed nuclei and multiple intracellular granules that contain highly basic proteins including major basic protein and eosinophil cationic protein. Eosinophils are present in allergic tissue sites and increase in number following allergen provocation[33] and during natural seasonal exposure. Eosinophils produce lipid mediators, including leukotriene C_4, platelet activating factor, granulocyte–macrophage colony-stimulating factor (GM-CSF) and cytokines, including IL-4, IL-5 and Eosinophils have many IL surface receptors (IL-3R, IL-5R and GM-CSFR), Ig receptors (FcγRII [CD32] and FcαRI [secretory IgA]), complement receptors (C3aR and C5aR) and chemokine receptors (CCR3).

Eosinophils also selectively express the adhesion molecule VLA-4, the ligand for the eosinophil-selective vascular cell adhesion molecule-1, which is important for the selective recruitment of eosinophils at allergic tissue sites including the nasal mucosa.[33,34]

T-LYMPHOCYTES

T-lymphocytes are pivotal in the pathogenesis of allergic diseases, as the only cells capable of recognizing antigenic material after processing by antigen-presenting cells. Cytokines produced by T-cells play a major role in orchestrating allergic inflammation. Type 1 T helper (Th1) cells produce IFN-γ and IL-2 but not IL-4 or IL-5 after activation. Th2 cells produce mainly IL-4, IL-13 and IL-5 but not IL-2 or IFN-γ. Th2 cells characterize human allergic responses and are present at the mucosal surfaces during the late but not the immediate response to allergen exposure. Th2 cells can also be expanded from the peripheral blood of allergic patients by stimulation with specific allergen in vitro.[35,36]

The evolution of either Th1 responses or Th2 responses, or both, may be determined by the route and dose of antigen as well as the nature of the antigen-presenting cell. For example, high doses of allergen preferentially favour the induction of Th1-type responses.[37]

DENDRITIC CELLS

Dendritic cells are professional antigen-presenting cells that are abundant within the epithelium and submucosa of the upper and lower respiratory tract in patients with allergic diseases.[38] Dendritic cells are highly efficient at capturing, processing and presenting antigen to T-cells. It has been suggested that so-called DC1 cells produce high levels of IL-12 and favour Th1 T-cell development, whereas DC2 cells are low IL-12 producers and support preferential Th2 T-lymphocyte differentiation. Differential functions may depend on their location, their degree of maturation and the local cytokine milieu.[37]

Nasal hyperresponsiveness

Patients with rhinitis, particularly those with AR, tend to show increased sensitivity to multiple environmental triggers such as tobacco smoke, strong perfumes and exhaust fumes. This reaction is called 'nasal hyperresponsiveness' and is thought to be neurally mediated. An exaggerated centrally mediated neural response may be a feature of repetitive allergen or irritant stimulation. A disrupted autonomic response may result in hyperresponsiveness that is clinically manifest as a primarily secretory (parasympathetic) or vascular (sympathetic) response.[39]

CO-MORBIDITY

Rhinitis is often accompanied by sinusitis, collectively termed 'rhino-sinusitis'. Sinusitis can be a common complicating feature of AR, mainly due to the oedema that accompanies AR, which may impact on sinus drainage. Although not due to allergy, nasal polyps may exist on a background of AR.[40,41] A considerable proportion of those with AR also have middle ear symptoms and otitis media with effusion. This is partly due to a disturbance of the normal function of the Eustachian tube.[42,43]

During seasonal exposure to allergens, cough thresholds are decreased. The association of AR with cough may possibly be amplified by the presence of posterior nasal discharge.[44] Gastro-oesophageal reflux, which is known to trigger laryngeal symptoms, has also been implicated as a possible cause of inflammation of the nasopharynx, with associated rhinitis symptoms.[45]

The impact of AR on asthma is now well recognized, and a stepwise approach in the management of both conditions is recommended.[46] Allergic rhinitis in children may be a precursor for the development of asthma. Deterioration of nasal symptoms negatively impacts on bronchial responsiveness and, conversely, the adequate management of rhinitis improves asthmatic symptoms.[47] The diagnosis and adequate treatment of AR is fundamental in asthma management.

DIAGNOSIS

The diagnosis of AR is based on a medical history, physical examination and demonstration of specific IgE to aero-allergens.

Nasal symptoms associated with AR include nasal itching, sneezing, blockage and watery discharge. Symptoms are generally bilateral and may vary between patients. Most patients complain of ocular symptoms, such as watery, red and itchy eyes. It is important to establish the most troublesome symptom and its variability throughout the year. Unilateral symptoms may be due to structural problems such as a deviated nasal septum or malignancy.[48] Increasing unilateral nasal obstruction, blood-stained or purulent nasal discharge, or facial pain requires urgent evaluation in a specialist rhinological setting.

A clinical correlation between the onset and duration of symptoms and exposure to possible allergens is pivotal in diagnosis. Seasonal symptoms are expected in specific pollen allergy, whereas perennial symptoms are commonly the result of exposure to house dust mite, cockroaches, mould and domestic pets.

Nasal medical examination can be easily performed in an outpatient setting using a head mirror and a nasal speculum. A rigid naso-endoscope is an invaluable tool, providing clear views of the interior of the nose. A large, swollen, oedematous inferior or middle turbinate is typical in AR. However, this can be easily confused with a polyp, although nasal polyps are insensitive to touch (in contrast to nasal turbinates), typically pale grey and translucent in appearance and mobile.

Skin-prick tests are easy to perform, inexpensive, and provide helpful information to identify aero-allergens. When negative, skin-testing largely excludes IgE-mediated disease. Skin-testing may be further supported by blood total and allergen-specific IgE concentrations, determined by a radio-allergosorbent test or enzyme-linked immunosorbent test.

Exhaled nasal nitric oxide is a sensitive marker of inflammation. Nitric oxide levels are raised in patients with AR[49] and decreased in sinusitis,[50] severe nasal obstruction and primary ciliary dyskinesia.[51]

Nasal airway measurements using nasal inspiratory peak flow, rhinomanometry and acoustic rhinometry are rarely used in routine allergy practice.

MANAGEMENT

Treatment options include allergen avoidance, pharmacotherapy and allergen-specific immunotherapy (SIT) for patients whose symptoms remain uncontrolled despite pharmacological treatment (Table 13.2).

Allergen avoidance

Complete allergen avoidance for seasonal pollen exposure is not practical and not realistically possible; pharmacotherapy and SIT play a crucial role in symptom control. In occupational settings (latex allergy in particular),[52,53] avoidance is effective.

Pharmacological treatment

This includes topical and oral antihistamines, corticosteroids, decongestants, plus chromones, leukotriene receptor antagonists, topical antimuscarinics and anti-IgE drugs.

ANTIHISTAMINES

Antihistamines can be used for both intermittent and persistent disease regardless of severity. Type H1 antihistamines relieve nasal itching, sneezing, rhinorrhoea and congestion; conjunctival itching, watering and redness; and itching of the palate, throat and ears.

First-generation H1 antihistamines bind to H1 receptors and block the neurotransmitter effect of histamine in the central nervous system (CNS). They penetrate the blood–brain barrier due to their lipophilicity, relatively low molecular weight and lack of recognition by the P-glycoprotein efflux pump that is expressed on the luminal surfaces of non-fenestrated endothelial cells in the vasculature of the CNS. Second-generation H1 antihistamines are specific for H1 receptors and penetrate the CNS poorly, owing to their lipophobicity and affinity for P-glycoprotein that is expressed on vascular endothelial cells in the CNS.[54, 55] Some antihistamines are metabolized via the p450 hepatic system and therefore have potential drug interactions, for example with macrolide antibiotics and antifungal agents. Rarely, but importantly, antihistamines can be arrhythmogenic and therefore potentially fatal.

CORTICOSTEROIDS

Intranasal corticosteroids are the single most effective therapy for AR. Their efficacy is superior to that of antihistamines[56,57] and leukotriene antagonists[58] either

Table 13.2 Management and treatment of allergic rhinitis (AR)

Treatment	Mechanism	Advantages/strengths	Disadvantages/weaknesses	Side-effects	Route
Allergen avoidance	Suppression of surface IgE production	No drug intake	Complete avoidance realistically impossible	None	–
Antihistamines	Block H1 receptors Some antiallergic effect	Highly effective in itching, sneezing and watery rhinorrhoea Rapid effect Second generation compounds have long-lasting effect with no sedation Once-a-day use	Poor relief of blockage	Sedation (mainly first generation drugs) Arrhythmogenic action Polaramine and cetirizine in pregnancy	Oral Ocular Nasal Intravenous Intramuscular
INCSs	Potent suppression of the inflammatory cascade in several steps	Are the single most effective drugs in AR Highly effective in blockage	Days until maximum effect is achieved	Local: dryness, epistaxis Systemic: very rare	Nasal
Systemic corticosteroids		Are the single most effective drugs in AR	Higher chance and increased frequency of side-effects	Suppression of hypothalamic-pituitary-adrenal axis	Oral Intravenous Intramuscular
Chromones	Inhibition of mast cell degranulation	Excellent safety profile Effective for itchiness, sneezing and watery discharge	Lower efficacy than anti-H1 compounds or INCSs Low effect on blockage Need to be taken every 4–6 hours	Minor local effects	Nasal Ocular
Decongestants	Vasoconstriction activating α-adrenergic receptors	Rapid relief of blockage	No effect on itching, sneezing or rhinorrhoea Never use more than 2 weeks	Rhinitis medicamentosa Tachycardia, hypertension Not to be used in pregnancy	Nasal Oral
Leukotriene antagonists	Blockage of cysteinyl leukotriene receptors	Effective for all symptoms	Modest efficacy versus cost	Good safety profile Not to be used in pregnancy	Oral
Ipratropium bromhydrate	Blockage of muscarinic receptors	Highly effective in watery rhinorrhoea	No efficacy for blockage, itching, sneezing or eye symptoms	Local and rare Dryness, irritation and burning	Nasal
Specific allergen immunotherapy	Systemic effect through modulation of cell and humoral immune response	Effective for all nasal symptoms Long-term efficacy	Variable efficacy Continued treatment Subcutaneous injections should be given only in hospitals or clinics fully equipped with anaphylactic emergency equipment	Depending on the route, from local effects to anaphylaxis	Sublingual Subcutaneous

INCS, intranasal corticosteroids.

separately or in combination.[59] Intranasal corticosteroids should form the basis of treatment of AR unless symptoms are mild and intermittent. In moderate-to-severe intermittent AR, it is recommended that treatment is started prior to seasonal exposure and that therapy is maintained throughout the season for maximum symptom control. Preparations are available as aerosols, aqueous suspensions and, in Scandinavia, as dry powder devices. Local side-effects include crusting and dryness without nasal mucosal atrophy. Occasional epistaxis may occur. Topical therapy has virtually no effect on the hypothalamic-pituitary-adrenal axis[60] with the exception of beclomethasone, which has the highest systemic bioavailability.[61]

Oral systemic corticosteroids for AR should be reserved for short courses in severe persistent disease unresponsive to usual therapy; 20–30 mg prednisolone for 5–7 days is recommended.

Intramuscular systemic corticosteroids are not recommended for the treatment of AR.

DECONGESTANTS

These are vasoconstrictor catecholamines that act on alpha-adrenergic capacitance vessels in the nose, thereby decreasing blood flow and mucosal oedema, and resulting in reduced nasal congestion.[62] Topical intranasal preparations have a rapid onset of action that may last up to 12 hours. Oral preparations are active within 30 minutes and may last up to 24 hours. Decongestants are not effective for other symptoms such as sneezing and rhinorrhoea.

Topical intranasal decongestants can burn, sting and cause dryness and occasionally bleeding. If they are used continuously for more than 2–3 weeks, they can produce 'rhinitis medicamentosa',[63] which is an increased dependence on medication with attenuation of the benefit. This situation can be treated by complete withdrawal of the decongestant, possibly with intranasal corticosteroid cover. The side-effects of both topical and oral administration include irritability, tachycardia, dizziness, insomnia, headaches, anxiety and tremors. The use of decongestants is not recommended during pregnancy, in elderly people or for those with hypertension or psychiatric disorders. The role of decongestants should be reserved for the alleviation of an acute deterioration in symptoms, such as during the common cold, or to 'open up' the nose during the introduction of intranasal steroid therapy.

CHROMONES

Sodium cromoglicate and sodium nedocromil are chromones that act through mast cell stabilization. They are particularly recommended for topical intraocular treatment. Intranasal chromones are no more effective than antihistamines or intranasal corticosteroids. Their systemic absorption is poor, so chromones have an excellent safety profile and are commonly used in children[64] and during pregnancy.[65] A drawback is the need for frequent (3–4 times daily) administration.

LEUKOTRIENE RECEPTOR ANTAGONISTS

These block the effect of potent inflammatory mediators of the cysteinyl leukotriene cascade. Montelukast reduces symptoms of nasal congestion as well as rhinorrhoea and sneezing in AR. However, their effects are modest and less predictable than for intranasal corticosteroids or antihistamines.[66] Montelukast may be used in children and is generally well tolerated. The use of montelukast for AR has the potential to improve both nasal and bronchial symptoms.[67]

IPATROPIUM BROMIDE

This is an antimuscarinic compound that reduces watery anterior rhinorrhoea by blocking the parasympathetic function of secretory glands within the nasal mucosa. It is recommended when rhinorrhoea is the main symptom and there is no success with other therapeutic drugs. Concomitant therapy is needed when other nasal symptoms are present.[68]

ANTI–IMMUNOGLOBULIN E

Omalizumab is a recombinant humanized monoclonal anti-IgE antibody that binds to the constant region of the IgE molecule, blocking the interaction of the antibody with mast cells and basophils. Omalizumab has been shown to be effective in AR,[69,70] but the cost of this treatment precludes its routine use in the absence of severe associated allergic asthma.

Allergen-specific immunotherapy

SIT involves giving gradually increasing doses of allergen. Allergen-specific immunotherapy interferes with the basic mechanism of allergy and alters the natural course of allergic diseases.[47,71] It inhibits both early and late responses to allergen exposure. Allergen-specific immunotherapy increases allergen-specific IgG, particularly the IgG4 isotype, which blocks not only IgE-dependent histamine release from basophils but also IgE-mediated antigen presentation to T-cells.[37] It also acts on T-cells to modify peripheral and mucosal Th2 responses to allergen in favour of Th1 responses, and increases IL-10 production in peripheral blood and on mucosal surfaces.[72]

Allergen-specific immunotherapy is indicated in severe AR unresponsive to usual pharmacotherapy or in patients whom pharmacotherapy causes undesirable side-effects. It is more effective when there is a single dominant allergen.

Specific immunotherapy is effective in reducing symptoms and the need for rescue medication.[73,74] It can produce improvement in hay fever symptoms over and above that which can be achieved by pharmacotherapy alone. In addition, unlike pharmacotherapy, SIT provides long-term clinical benefits such as long-term disease remission, the prevention of new atopic sensitizations and reduction in disease progression from rhinitis to asthma.[75]

Traditionally, SIT has been administered as a course of subcutaneous injections (SCIT). Although efficacious, SCIT has the potential risk of systemic reactions, hence the requirement that treatment is given only in hospitals or clinics fully equipped with anaphylactic emergency equipment. Moreover, the inconvenience of frequent hospital/clinic visits and the discomfort associated with injections can reduce patient compliance.

Sublingual immunotherapy (SLIT) is considered an efficacious and very safe alternative to SCIT.[76–78] It has been widely used in many countries in Central Europe, where more than 50 per cent of the current population of patients receiving specific immunotherapy are on SLIT.[3] The favourable safety profile of SLIT makes this treatment suitable for home administration, giving the opportunity to offer it to a wider population. More studies are needed to confirm the optimal dosage and the long-term efficacy of SLIT.

CONCLUSION

The prevalence of allergic rhino-conjunctivitis and summer-type hypersensitivity due to environmental aeroallergens has increased dramatically over the last three decades. Environmental factors, such as air pollution and ETS, may contribute to or exacerbate this global problem. A better understanding of this chronic health problem and adequate management of the disease, including SIT where appropriate, will contribute to the improvement of symptoms and patients' quality of life.

REFERENCES

1. Bousquet J, Van Cauwenberge P, Khaltaev N; Aria Workshop Group; World Health Organization. Allergic rhinitis and its impact on asthma. *J Allergy Clin Immunol.* 2001; **108**(5 Suppl.): S147–334.
2. Walker S, Khan-Wasti S, Fletcher M *et al.* Seasonal allergic rhinitis is associated with a detrimental effect on examination performance in United Kingdom teenagers: case-control study. *J Allergy Clin Immunol* 2007; **120**: 381–7.
3. Bousquet J, Demoly P. Specific immunotherapy – an optimistic future. *Allergy* 2006; **61**: 1155–8.
4. Bauchau V, Durham SR. Prevalence and rate of diagnosis of allergic rhinitis in Europe. *Eur Respir J* 2004; **24**: 758–64.
5. Salib RJ, Harries PG, Nair SB, Howarth PH. Mechanisms and mediators of nasal symptoms in non-allergic rhinitis. *Clin Exp Allergy* 2008; **38**: 393–404.
6. Strachan D, Sibbald B, Weiland S *et al.* Worldwide variations in prevalence of symptoms of allergic rhinoconjunctivitis in children: The International Study of Asthma and Allergies in Childhood (ISAAC). *Pediatr Allergy Immunol* 1997; **8**: 161–76.
7. Asher MI, Montefort S, Björkstén B *et al.* Worldwide time trends in the prevalence of symptoms of asthma, allergic rhinoconjunctivitis, and eczema in childhood: ISAAC Phases One and Three repeat multicountry cross-sectional surveys. *Lancet* 2006; **368**: 733–43.
8. European Community Respiratory Health Survey. Variations in the prevalence of respiratory symptoms, self-reported asthma attacks, and use of asthma medication in the European Community Respiratory Health Survey (ECRHS). *Eur Respir J* 1996; **6**: 687–95.
9. Janson C, Anto J, Burney P *et al.* The European Community Respiratory Health Survey: What are the main results so far? *Eur Respir J.* 2001; **18**: 598–611.
10. Matricardi PM, RosminiF, Riondino S *et al.* Exposure to foodborne and orofecal microbes versus airborne viruses in relation to atopy and allergic asthma: Epidemiological study. *BMJ* 2000; **320**: 412–17.
11. Stelmach I, Smejda K, Jerzynska J *et al.* Decreased markers of atopy in children with presumed early exposure to allergens, unhygienic conditions, and infections. *Ann Allergy Asthma Immunol* 2007; **99**: 170–7.
12. Grize L, Gassner M, Wülthrich B *et al.* Trends in prevalence of asthma, allergic rhinitis and atopic dermatitis in 5–7 year old Swiss children from 1992 to 2001. *Allergy* 2006; **61**: 556–62.
13. Braun-Fahrlander C, Gassner M, Grize L *et al.* No further increase in asthma, hay fever and atopic sensitization in adolescents living in Switzerland. *Eur Respir J* 2004; **23**: 407–13.
14. D'Amato G, Cecchi L, Bonini S *et al.* Allergenic pollen and pollen allergy in Europe. *Allergy* 2007; **62**: 976–90.
15. Saxon A, Diaz-Sanchez D. Air pollution and allergy: you are what you breathe. *Nat Immunol* 2005; **6**: 223–6.
16. Ishizaki T, Koizumi K, Ikemori R, Ishiyama Y, Kushibiki E. Studies of prevalence of Japanese cedar pollinosis among the residents in a densely cultivated area. *Ann Allergy* 1987; **58**: 265–70.
17. Braun-Fahrlander C, Gassner M, Grize L *et al.* Prevalence of hay fever and allergic sensitization in farmer's children and their peers living in the same rural community: SCARPOL team: Swiss study on Childhood Allergy and Respiratory Symptoms with Respect to Air Pollution. *Clin Exp Allergy* 1999; **29**: 28–34.
18. Von Ehrenstein OS, Von Mutius E, Illi S *et al.* Reduced risk of hay fever and asthma among children and farmers. *Clin Exp Allergy* 2000; **30**: 87–93.
19. Riedler J, Eder W, Oberfeld G, Schreuer M. Austrian children living on a farm have less hay fever, asthma and allergic sensitization. *Clin Exp Allergy* 2000; **30**: 194–200.

20. Kelly FJ. Dietary antioxidants and environmental stress. *Proc Nutr Soc* 2004; **63**: 579–85.

21. Pourazar J, Mudway IS, Samet JM *et al.* Diesel exhaust activates redox-sensitive transcription factors and kinases in human airways. *Am J Physiol Lung Cell Mol Physiol* 2005; **289**: L724–30.

22. Knox RB, Suphioglu C, Taylor P *et al.* Major grass pollen allergen Lol p 1 binds to diesel exhaust particles: Implications of asthma and air pollution. *Clin Exp Allergy* 1997; **27**: 246–51.

23. D'Amato G, Liccardi G, D'Amato M, Holgate S. Environmental risk factors and allergic bronchial asthma. *Clin Exp Allergy* 2005; **35**: 1113–24.

24. Nordenhäll C, Pourazar J, Ledin MC *et al.* Diesel exhaust enhances airway responsiveness in asthmatic subjects. *Eur Respir J* 2001; **17**: 909–15.

25. Enomoto M, Tierney WJ, Nozaki K. Risk of human health by particulate matter as a source of air pollution – comparison with tobacco smoking. *J Toxicol Sci* 2008; **33**: 251–67.

26. Nielsen J, Welinder H, Bensryd I, Rylander L, Skerfving S. Ocular and airway symptoms related to organic acid anhydride exposure – a prospective study. *Allergy* 2006; **61**: 743–9.

27. Brisman J, Järvholm B, Lillienberg L. Exposure–response relations for self reported asthma and rhinitis in bakers. *Occup Environ Med* 2000; **57**: 335–40.

28. Campbell CP, Jackson AS, Johnson AR, Thomas PS, Yates DH. Occupational sensitization to lupin in the workplace: occupational asthma, rhinitis, and work-aggravated asthma. *J Allergy Clin Immunol* 2007; **119**: 1133–9.

29. Draper A, Newman Taylor A, Cullinan T, Cullinan P. Estimating the incidence of occupational asthma and rhinitis from laboratory animal allergens in the UK, 1999–2000. *Occup Environ Med* 2003; **60**: 604–5.

30. Hellgren J. Occupational rhinosinusitis. *Curr Allergy Asthma Rep* 2008; **8**: 234–9.

31. Prussin C, Griffith DT, Boesel KM, Lin H, Foster B, Casale TB. Omalizumab treatment downregulates dendritic cell FcepsilonRI expression. *J Allergy Clin Immunol* 2003; **112**: 1132–8.

32. Wilson DR, Irani AM, Walker SM *et al.* Grass pollen immunotherapy: symptomatic improvement correlates with reductions in eosinophils and IL-5 mRNA expression in the nasal mucosa during the pollen season. *J Allergy Clin Immunol* 2001; **107**: 971–6.

33. Rajakulasingam K, Durham SR, O'Brien F *et al.* Enhanced expression of high-affinity IgE receptor (Fc epsilon RI) alpha chain in human allergen-induced rhinitis with co-localization to mast cells, macrophages, eosinophils, and dendritic cells. *J Allergy Clin Immunol* 1997; **100**: 78–86.

34. Gangur V, Oppenheim JJ. Are chemokines essential or secondary participants in allergic responses? *Ann Allergy Asthma Immunol* 2000; **84**: 569–79.

35. Romagnani S. Immunologic influences on allergy and the TH1/TH2 balance. *J Allergy Clin Immunol* 2004; **113**: 395–400.

36. Larché M, Akdis CA, Valenta R. Immunological mechanisms of allergen-specific immunotherapy. *Nature* 2006; **6**: 761–71.

37. Till SJ, Francis JN, Nouri-Aria K, Durham SR. Mechanisms of immunotherapy. *J Allergy Clin Immunol* 2004; **113**: 1025–34.

38. Holt PG, Upham JW. The role of dendritic cells in asthma. *Curr Opin Allergy Clin Immunol* 2004; **4**: 39–44.

39. Sarin S, Undem B, Sanico A, Togias A. The role of the nervous system in rhinitis. *J Allergy Clin Immunol* 2006; **118**: 999–1016.

40. Spector SL. The role of allergy in sinusitis in adults. *J Allergy Clin Immunol* 1992; **90**: 518–20.

41. Baroody M. Allergic rhinitis: Broader disease effects and implications for management. *Otolaryngol Head Neck Surg* 2003; **128**: 616–31.

42. Luong A, Roland PS. The link between allergic rhinitis and chronic otitis media with effusion in atopic patients. *Otolaryngol Clin North Am* 2008; **41**: 311–23.

43. Nguyen LH, Manoukian JJ, Tewfik TL *et al.* Evidence of allergic inflammation in the middle ear and nasopharynx in atopic children with otitis media with effusion. *J Otolaryngol* 2004; **33**: 345–51.

44. Niimi A. Geography and cough aetiology. *Pulm Pharmacol Ther* 2007; **20**: 383–7.

45. Loehrl TA, Smith TL, Darling RJ *et al.* Autonomic dysfunction, vasomotor rhinitis, and extraesophageal manifestations of gastroesophageal reflux. *Otolaryngol Head Neck Surg* 2002; **126**: 382–7.

46. Ryan MW. Asthma and rhinitis: Comorbidities. *Otolaryngol Clin North Am* 2008; **41**: 283–95.

47. Bousquet J, Khaltaev N, Cruz AA *et al.* Allergic Rhinitis and its Impact on Asthma (ARIA) 2008 update (in collaboration with the World Health Organization, GA(2)LEN and AllerGen). *Allergy* 2008; **63**(Suppl. 86): 8–160.

48. Benoit MM, Bhattacharyya N, Faquin W, Cunningham M. Cancer of the nasal cavity in the pediatric population. *Pediatrics* 2008; **121**: e141–5.

49. Boot JD, de Kam ML, Mascelli MA *et al.* Nasal nitric oxide: Longitudinal reproducibility and the effects of a nasal allergen challenge in patients with allergic rhinitis. *Allergy* 2007; **62**: 378–84.

50. Deja M, Busch T, Bachmann S *et al.* Reduced nitric oxide in sinus epithelium of patients with radiologic maxillary sinusitis and sepsis. *Am J Respir Crit Care Med* 2003; **168**: 281–6.

51. Lundberg JO, Weitzberg E, Nordvall SL, Kuylenstierna R, Lundberg JM, Alving K. Primarily nasal origin of exhaled nitric oxide and absence in Kartagener's syndrome. *Eur Respir J* 1994; **7**: 1501–4.

52. Taylor JS, Erkek E. Latex allergy: Diagnosis and management. *Dermatol Ther* 2004; **17**: 289–301.

53. Brown RH, Taenkhum K, Buckley TJ, Hamilton RG. Different latex aeroallergen size distributions between powdered surgical and examination gloves: Significance for environmental avoidance. *J Allergy Clin Immunol* 2004; **114**: 358–63.

54. Simons FE. Advances in H1-antihistamines. *N Engl J Med* 2004; **351**: 2203–17.

55. Simons FE, Silver NA, Gu X, Simons KJ. Skin concentrations of H1-receptor antagonists. *J Allergy Clin Immunol* 2001; **107**: 526–30.

56. Weiner JM, Abramson MJ, Puy RM. Intranasal corticosteroids versus oral H1 receptor antagonists in allergic rhinitis: Systematic review of randomised controlled trials. *BMJ* 1998; **317**: 1624–9.

57. Yáñez A, Rodrigo GJ. Intranasal corticosteroids versus topical H1 receptor antagonists for the treatment of allergic rhinitis: A systematic review with meta-analysis. *Ann Allergy Asthma Immunol* 2002; **89**: 479–84.

58. Nathan RA. Leukotriene receptor antagonists are not as effective as intranasal corticosteroids for managing nighttime symptoms of allergic rhinitis. *J Allergy Clin Immunol* 2005; **116**: 463–4.

59. Pullerits T, Praks L, Ristioja V, Lötvall J. Comparison of a nasal glucocorticoid, antileukotriene, and a combination of antileukotriene and antihistamine in the treatment of seasonal allergic rhinitis. *J Allergy Clin Immunol* 2002; **109**: 949–55.

60. Wilson AM, McFarlane LC, Lipworth BJ. Effects of repeated once daily dosing of three intranasal corticosteroids on basal and dynamic measures of hypothalamic-pituitary-adrenal-axis activity. *J Allergy Clin Immunol* 1998; **101**(4 Pt 1): 470–4.

61. Skoner DP, Rachelefsky GS, Meltzer EO *et al.* Detection of growth suppression in children during treatment with intranasal beclomethasone dipropionate. *Pediatrics* 2000; **105**: E23.

62. Passàli D, Salerni L, Passàli GC, Passàli FM, Bellussi L. Nasal decongestants in the treatment of chronic nasal obstruction: efficacy and safety of use. *Expert Opin Drug Saf* 2006; **5**: 783–90.

63. Ramey JT, Bailen E, Lockey RF. Rhinitis medicamentosa. *J Investig Allergol Clin Immunol* 2006; **16**: 148–55.

64. Baena-Cagnani CE. Safety and tolerability of treatments for allergic rhinitis in children. *Drug Saf* 2004; **27**: 883–98.

65. Keleş N. Treatment of allergic rhinitis during pregnancy. *Am J Rhinol* 2004; **18**: 23–8.

66. Wilson AM, O'Byrne PM, Parameswaran K. Leukotriene receptor antagonists for allergic rhinitis: A systematic review and meta-analysis. *Am J Med* 2004; **116**: 338–44.

67. Philip G, Nayak AS, Berger WE *et al.* The effect of montelukast on rhinitis symptoms in patients with asthma and seasonal allergic rhinitis. *Curr Med Res Opin* 2004; **20**: 1549–58.

68. Dockhorn R, Aaronson D, Bronsky E *et al.* Ipratropium bromide nasal spray 0.03% and beclomethasone nasal spray alone and in combination for the treatment of rhinorrhea in perennial rhinitis. *Ann Allergy Asthma Immunol* 1999; **82**: 349–59.

69. Casale TB. Anti-immunoglobulin E (omalizumab) therapy in seasonal allergic rhinitis. *Am J Respir Crit Care Med* 2001; **164**(8 Pt 2): S18–21.

70. Chervinsky P, Casale T, Townley R *et al.* Omalizumab, an anti-IgE antibody, in the treatment of adults and adolescents with perennial allergic rhinitis. *Ann Allergy Asthma Immunol* 2003; **91**: 160–7.

71. Bousquet J, Lockey R, Malling HJ. Allergen immunotherapy: Therapeutic vaccines for allergic diseases. A WHO Position Paper. *J Allergy Clin Immunol* 1998; **102**: 558–562.

72. Francis JN, Till SJ, Durham SR. Induction of IL-10 + CD4$^+$CD25$^+$ T cells by grass pollen immunotherapy. *J Allergy Clin Immunol* 2003; **111**: 1255–61.

73. Calderon M, Alves B, Jacobson M *et al.* Allergen injection immunotherapy for seasonal allergic rhinitis. *Cochrane Database Syst Rev* 2007; (1): CD001936.

74. Wilson DR, Torres LM, Durham SR. Sublingual immunotherapy for allergic rhinitis: Systematic review and meta-analysis. *Allergy* 2005; **60**: 4–12.

75. James LK, Durham SR. Update on mechanisms of allergen injection immunotherapy. *Clin Exp Allergy* 2008; **38**: 1074–88.

76. Durham SR, Yang WH, Pedersen MR, Johansen N, Rak S. Sublingual once-daily grass-pollen immunotherapy: A randomised controlled trial in seasonal allergic rhinoconjunctivitis. *J Allergy Clin Immunol* 2006; **117**: 802–9.

77. Dahl R, Kapp A, Colombo G *et al.* Sublingual grass allergen tablet immunotherapy provides sustained clinical benefit with progressive immunologic changes over 2 years. *J Allergy Clin Immunol* 2008; **121**: 512–18.

78. Didier A, Malling HJ, Worm M *et al.* Optimal dose, efficacy, and safety of once-daily sublingual immunotherapy with a 5-grass pollen tablet for seasonal allergic rhinitis. *J Allergy Clin Immunol* 2007; **120**: 1338–45.

SUMMER HYPERSENSITIVITY PNEUMONITIS/ALVEOLITIS

LISA HILL, JON G. AYRES

Summer hypersensitivity pneumonitis (SHP) is the most prevalent form of hypersensitivity pneumonitis in Japan.[1] Sensitization to repeated inhalation of antigen leads to this immunologically mediated lung disease, the most common offending antigens being *Trichosporon asahii* and *Trichosporon mucoides.*[2] These fungi are found in temperate and subtropical areas including most Western countries, where they are also a cause of SHP. This is a true environmental condition and has no occupational causal links. The incidence of the disease remains undetermined but in Japan is estimated to be several hundred cases a year and is twice as common in women than in men. This is thought to be due to a greater exposure to the offending antigens among female home-makers.[3]

CLINICAL FEATURES

The condition is characterized by repeated, consecutive summertime episodes of cough, fever and dyspnoea with resolution in the autumn. There is a familial pattern with symptoms provoked by patients' home environments. Investigation reveals a blood neutrophilic leukocytosis, a negative skin test to tuberculin with no clear association with atopy. Antibodies to *Trichosporon* are found in both serum and bronchoalveolar lavage fluid. Serodiagnosis can be made by assaying for anti-Trichosporon antibodies using a commercially available kit.[4] While symptomatic, patients show a moderately decreased ventilatory capacity, often a markedly decreased arterial partial pressure of oxygen, and diffuse nodular shadows on chest X-ray. Histologically, appearances are consistent with an alveolitis and/or pneumonitis with interstitial epithelioid cell granulomas without central necrosis in 63 per cent of cases.[5]

Patients respond positively to treatment with corticosteroids. In addition, disinfection of the colonized location to remove *Trichosporon* prevents recurrence of the disease and is the key management approach, particularly in prevention of progression to pulmonary fibrosis.[1] Without intervention, recurrence rate the following year is approximately 40 per cent.[3]

PROGNOSIS

As with other forms of hypersensitivity pneumonitis, pulmonary fibrosis can develop in those with chronic SHP and the diagnosis is often missed in patients with apparent idiopathic pulmonary fibrosis, largely due to an inadequate history being taken. Chronic, untreated SHP may also lead to emphysema, spontaneous pneumothorax, cor pulmonale, respiratory failure and death. A high index of suspicion is required to correctly diagnose SHP as, with appropriate treatment, progression to pulmonary fibrosis can be prevented.

MECHANISMS

Initiation and progression of the disease involve immune complex and T-cell mediation. Host factors have been shown to play a role in SHP with an increase in frequency of the gene suppressor HLA-DQw3 on chromosome 6 being identified in patients. It has been suggested that cigarette-smoking has a protective effect on the incidence of SHP[3] but this may be partly due to false-negative diagnoses in smokers.

References

● = Key primary paper
◆ = Major review article

●1. Ando M, Arima K, Yoneda R, Tamura M. Japanese summer-type hypersensitivity pneumonitis. Geographic distribution, home environment, and clinical characteristics of 621 cases. *Am Rev Respir Dis* 1991; **144**: 765–9.

2. Ohtani Y, Ochi J, Mitaka K *et al.* Chronic summer-type hypersensitivity pneumonitis initially misdiagnosed as idiopathic interstitial pneumonia. *Intern Med* 2008; **47**: 857–62.

◆3. Ando M, Suga M, Nishiura Y, Miyajima M. Summer-type hypersensitivity pneumonitis. *Intern Med* 1995; **34**: 707–12.

4. Ando M. Pathogenesis of summer-type hypersensitivity pneumonitis. *Jap J Med Mycol* 2000; **41**: 137–41.

5. Kawai T, Tamura M, Murao M. Summer-type hypersensitivity pneumonitis. A unique disease in Japan. *Chest* 1984; **85**: 311–17.

EXPOSURE TO COMPOSTING EMISSIONS AND HEALTH

PETER SYKES

Composting is a common process, and occupational exposure to emissions is well recognized. However, a significant number of individuals live near to commercial composting sites, and concern has been expressed by such individuals that emissions from these sites are a cause of ill-health.

THE COMPOSTING PROCESS

Composting operations rely on the decomposition of organic materials through promoting the action of microorganisms. The composting process has been described in three phases,[1] in which different organisms thrive at different stages, their growth and survival being influenced by temperature, moisture content, oxygen content and the material being composted.

Phase One – high-rate composting (4–40 days)

Simple carbohydrates and proteins are readily degraded first by mesophiles and then by thermophilic species as the temperature rises above 45 °C.

Phase Two – stabilization (20–60 days)

Thermophilic temperatures (<50 °C) are attained. Thermophilic organisms such as thermophilic actinomycetes, *Bacillus* spp. and *Thermus* spp., have been shown to dominate, whereas thermotolerant fungi such as *Aspergillus* and *Penicillium* have been widely reported. These organisms readily break down cellulose.

Phase Three – maturation (variable)

This is characterized by a reduction in temperature as metabolic activity decreases. Mesophilic *Actinomycetes* and fungi predominate and are thought to be responsible for degrading and converting lignins.

During composting operations, these microorganisms become airborne, forming a 'bioaerosol'. Bioaerosols liberated from composting operations may contain varying quantities of actinomycetes, thermophilic bacteria, fungal spores, Gram-positive bacteria, Gram-negative bacteria, endotoxins, mycotoxins, glucans and volatile organic compounds.[2]

HEALTH EFFECTS – OCCUPATIONAL EXPOSURES

The effects of exposure to bioaerosols on respiratory health have been described in numerous occupational studies. Reported conditions include aspergillosis in immunocompromised individuals,[3] allergic rhinitis and asthma, possibly chronic obstructive pulmonary disease, extrinsic allergic alveolitis (farmer's lung) when prolonged (usually occupational) exposure occurs, toxic pneumonitis and upper airway irritation.[2,4] It is thus entirely plausible that emissions might affect the health of the population living near commercial composting activities.

HEALTH EFFECTS – ENVIRONMENTAL EXPOSURES

Although many measurements of airborne concentrations of organisms have been made within and in the vicinity of composting plants, which give ample evidence for the existence of a hazard especially to composting workers, there have been very few studies of health effects from which any quantitative indication of risk can be derived for members of the public.

Significant increases in off-site concentrations of viable bacteria, viable fungi and endotoxins during periods of site activity have been reported.[5] Concentrations of thermophilic actinomycetes, moulds and total bacteria in excess of 10^5 colony-forming units/m^3 at 200 m from the composting facilities have been described.[6] Wheeler et al.[7] suggest that emissions from composting facilities decline with distance from the source, and concentrations measured at distances of 100–150 m were mostly close to zero. A reduction in bioaerosol concentrations to background levels has been reported at distances of anywhere between 200 and 500 m from the source.[2,8,9]

There has been relatively little investigation of the effects of community exposure to bioaerosols. There is evidence of an increased reporting of skin rashes and irritative airways complaints in residents living in close proximity to composting facilities,[9] but further work is needed to characterize the true risks to the public's health from composting activities.

References

1. Gilbert EJ, Riggle DS, Holland FD. *Large-Scale Composting – a Practical Manual for the UK*. Wellingborough, Northamptonshire: Composting Association, 2001.
2. Swan JR, Crook B, Gilbert EJ. Microbial emissions from composting sites. In: Harrison R (ed.) *Environmental and Health Impact of Solid Waste Management Activities*. Issues in Environmental Science and Technology, No. 18. London: Royal Society of Chemistry, 2002: 73–101.
3. Millner P. Bioaerosols and composting. *BioCycle* 1995; **36**: 48–54.

4. Bunger J, Schlappler-Scheele B, Hilgers R, Hallier EA. 5-year follow-up study on respiratory disorders and lung function in workers exposed to organic dust from composting plants. *Int Arch Occup Environ Health* 2007; **80**: 306–12.
5. Hryhorczuk D, Curtis L, Scheff P *et al.* Bioaerosol emissions from a suburban yard waste composting facility. *Ann Agric Environ Med* 2001; **8**: 177–85.
6. Herr CEW, zur Nieden A, Jankofsky M, Stilianakis NI, Boedeker R-H, Eikmann TF. Effects of bioaerosol polluted outdoor air on airways of residents: a cross sectional study. *Occup Environ Med* 2003; **60**: 336–42.
7. Wheeler PA, Stewart I, Dumitrean P, Donovan B. *Health Effects of Composting – a Study of Three Compost Sites and Review of Past Data.* R&D Technical Report P1-315/TR. Bristol: Environment Agency, 2001.
8. Herr CE, Nieden Az A, Stilianakis NI, Eikmann TF. Health effects associated with exposure to residential organic dust. *Am J Ind Med* 2004; **46**: 381–5.
9. Recer GM, Browne ML, Horn E, Hill K, Boehler W. Ambient air levels of *Aspergillus fumigatus* and thermophilic actinomycetes in a residential neighbourhood near a yard waste composting facility. *Aerobiologia* 2001; **17**: 99–108.

14

Indoor air pollution in developed countries

ISABELLA MYERS, ROBERT L. MAYNARD

INTRODUCTION

Developed countries are those with a high level of economic achievement and extensive industrialization – they are, in comparative terms, rich. Such countries tend to have addressed many of the environmental problems that damage health in poorer, developing countries, and tend to have high standards for such essentials as air quality, water quality and drainage. At the same time, housing has been improved, and one could expect, perhaps wrongly, that the indoor environment would be conducive to good health. This is broadly true, but problems still exist – and not only in the poorer parts of developed countries. The poorer members of developed countries continue to live in poor conditions. Houses may be damp and cold, and overcrowding remains a problem. In addition, smoking is more common among the poor than the rich, and childhood exposure to second-hand tobacco smoke continues to damage health. A solution to this problem has yet to be found. The inappropriate use of cooking appliances for space-heating is also commonplace. These present further risks to health.

Economic development and a concern to reduce emissions of carbon dioxide have led to newly built houses being better insulated. This reduces the need for space-heating but, if coupled with reduced ventilation, brings further problems. Damp is a consequence of poor ventilation, and damp leads to mould growth and the multiplication of house mites. Enthusiastic attempts to insulate houses and a lack of attention to ventilation is thought by some to have led to an increase in allergic diseases in Nordic countries and, consequently, to the focus on indoor air pollution by research workers.

Insulation can bring problems of its own: the release of formaldehyde (HCHO) gas from cavity wall insulation during the immediate post-installation period provides one example. Whether this causes significant damage to health is arguable, even though formaldehyde is a class 1 carcinogen, and concentrations in semi-permanent structures can exceed the current World Health Organization (WHO) *Air Quality Guidelines* of 0.1 mg/m^3 as a 30 minute average (which was set prior to the reclassification of formaldehyde in 2004).[1] Furniture and fittings can give off organic air pollutants (from glues), and artificial boarding (e.g. chipboard) can give off, again, formaldehyde. Concerns that indoor exposure to volatile organic compounds can cause sick building syndrome have been raised.

Indoor air pollution is often regarded as a problem of homes. This may be because the other great indoor environment – the workplace – tends to be better regulated. In the UK, the Health and Safety Work at Work Act applies to workplaces but not to homes. The Act is sometimes seen as applying more to industrial premises than to offices, hospitals and schools. This is incorrect – the Act applies to all these locations. However, standards set for workplaces are seldom as demanding as those insisted upon for ambient (outdoor) air, and this leads to confusion about the levels of air pollutants to which people may be comparatively safely exposed. Some people of course work at home, and it may be asked, who regulates their working environment? The answer is, they do – but they may then need advice to help them do this.

The regulation of outdoor air by the control of sources of air pollutants is a feature of developed countries. The air in the home is not subject to such regulation, and reliance is placed on product safety standards and industry-incentivized reductions in emitted pollutants from appliances and materials. Regulation, in the outdoor sense, implies standards and monitoring with all the necessary attendant criteria for the location of monitors and methods of reporting and quality assurance of the data produced.

This has not been seen as possible (or acceptable) in the home, even though such an approach is taken in the workplace. As soon as standard-setting for indoor air (in the home) is attempted, serious difficulties arise. These range from questions of how standards could be enforced and conditions monitored, to those difficult issues of personal freedom to act as we please in our own homes. This has led to the approach being broadly restricted to building and product safety standards and the provision of guidance and advice. Going further than this has been very difficult indeed.

But it is far from clear how large an effect indoor air pollution has on health in developed countries, largely because the detection of small increases in risks to health requires large studies with substantial statistical power. It is thought that risks at an individual level are likely to be small because indoor concentrations of the common air pollutants are low – lower that is than those producing an obvious risk to health. The key word here is 'obvious'. That such risks can and do occur due to accidents and the poor maintenance of, for example, heating devices is clear: people die as a result of at-home exposure to carbon monoxide every year in developed countries. But whether the levels of air pollutants found in well-managed homes damage health is less easy to demonstrate. This is odd: similar levels found outdoors have been widely accepted as damaging health, and it is increasingly accepted that concepts of safe levels and thresholds of effect are misleading.

The reason for this disparity of evidence is that the epidemiological methods applied with great success to discovering the effects on health of outdoor air pollutants have been found to be difficult or impossible to apply to indoor air pollutants. For example, time series methodology that has revolutionized our understanding of the effects of outdoor air pollutants depends on the day-to-day variation in outdoor levels of pollutants produced, largely, by varying meteorological conditions. Meteorological conditions have, as far as is known, a lesser effect on indoor pollution levels. In the indoor air field, we cannot rely on central monitoring sites to reflect average exposure[2] – homes vary from one to another. Research workers have focused on studies of panels of people living in homes with, for example, different heating sources.[3] Panels tend to be small in comparison with the hundreds of thousands and sometimes millions of people studied by time series methods. Detecting small or perhaps modest effects by methods applicable indoors is, simply, difficult.

In developing countries, where indoor levels of air pollutants may be high in comparison with conditions in developed countries, the problem is less difficult and effects have been shown (see Chapter 15). Extrapolating from the effects seen on high-level exposure to the effects that may or may not occur at much lower level exposure is difficult and may require assumptions to be made. Such assumptions certainly can be made, but they are difficult, or perhaps impossible, to test.

SOURCES OF INDOOR AIR POLLUTANTS IN DEVELOPED COUNTRIES

In this chapter, we focus on chemical air pollutants of non-biological origin. Thus, antigens produced by mites and moulds are not discussed. Pollutants found in indoor air come from a variety of sources, as described below.

From outdoors

Depending on the level of ventilation, the indoor environment equilibrates with the outdoor environment at varying speeds. Outdoor sources of air pollutants, for example traffic, power generation and chemical reactions taking place in the atmosphere, are larger than indoor sources that deliver their products into the indoor air. Of course, indoor sources such as coal fires and gas heaters with outdoor venting affect outdoor levels of air pollutants. In the coal-burning period of domestic heating in the UK and in other urban areas of the world, space-heating with coal fires was a major cause of outdoor air pollution and coal smoke smog.

Outdoor air pollution largely enters houses via ventilation. Thus, close to busy roads, nitrogen dioxide produced by traffic will enter houses, and indoor levels are likely to exceed those in houses further from the road. Ozone is a pollutant produced outdoors as a result of the photochemical breakdown of nitrogen dioxide. Ozone will infiltrate from outdoors to indoors, but indoor levels remain low as a result of rapid reactions between ozone and furniture and fittings indoors. Similarly, particles produced outdoors pass indoors, and indoor concentrations of particulate matter with a diameter less than $2.5\,\mu m$ ($PM_{2.5}$) can, in the absence of indoor sources, approach 60 per cent of those outdoors.[4]

Infiltration increases in summer when windows and doors tend to be left open, although nearer the equator such seasonal differences in infiltration are less marked. That infiltration can lead to very high concentrations of pollutants indoors is unlikely in developed countries with well-regulated outdoor concentrations; infiltration can, however, certainly add to the effects of indoor sources of air pollutants.

From heating and cooking using fossil fuels indoors

Indoor heating and cooking devices can be divided into those which vent to the outdoor air and those which do not. The latter are less common than the former in developed countries, although badly maintained propane space-heaters and mobile gas fires are potential sources of indoor air pollution. Paraffin (kerosene) heaters used to be a problem in the UK; such devices tended to be poorly maintained and were put into use only in cold weather – a time when windows and doors were likely to be firmly closed. Gas water heaters, especially when used in poorly ventilated bathrooms, have also given rise to dangerously high levels of carbon monoxide but are now less common than in the past.

Gas cookers, on the other hand, are very common, and although current building regulations call for good ventilation in kitchens, this is by no means always present. Poorly maintained grills are a particularly potent source of nitrogen dioxide. Using an open oven as a means of warming a kitchen or living room is a potential danger. Of course, all these devices are safe if used appropriately and if well maintained. This is more likely to be the case in the homes of the well-off than in those of the poor, even in developed countries.

Devices that vent to the outdoor air are common in developed countries. Gas fires and boilers and oil-powered and coke-powered boilers are all commonplace and if adequately maintained and properly used cause few problems. If, however, the venting to the outdoor air is inadequate or blocked, or if the burners in gas- and oil-fired devices are old or poorly adjusted, dangerous concentrations of carbon monoxide can build up indoors. This should be well known, but accidents continue to occur and foolish actions such as venting a gas fire into the cavity of a wall, leading to the poisoning of a person upstairs or in the adjacent property, are not unknown. That this is a real problem is shown by the accidental deaths that occur each year in the UK and USA as a result of carbon monoxide poisoning.

In England, there are approximately 50 deaths a year from unintentional carbon monoxide poisoning,[5] and in the USA there are around 500.[6] Deaths may well represent the tip of the 'effects-iceberg': many more people are likely to be exposed to sublethal concentrations. In recent years, attention has focused on exposure to subsymptomatic concentrations of carbon monoxide that can lead to neurological effects. 'Carbon monoxide flu' is sometimes used as a term to describe such effects.[7,8] A difficulty in accepting such effects is caused by the tendency to equate the effects of exposure to carbon monoxide with levels of carboxyhaemoglobin. This is certainly a guide to the effects of higher levels of exposure but is perhaps less useful at low levels. It is known that carbon monoxide is a signalling molecule, and it may be that the unexplained effects of exposure to carbon monoxide may depend upon its function as such, rather than on a reduction in oxygen supply to the tissues.

Gas flames generate ultrafine particles.[9] The luminosity of flames is caused by the presence of very hot, incandescent, carbon particles emitting heat and light. A luminous flame also generates carbon monoxide and is a sign of a badly adjusted gas jet. A deposition of carbon (lamp black) on walls and china-clay radiants is a further sign of malfunctioning gas-burning devices.

From fittings, insulation and furnishings

As noted above, glues and solvents give off volatile organic compounds. Formaldehyde is a gas that is released when chipboard, for example, is sawn. Such compounds are produced by new fittings (e.g. a new carpet with some form of rubberized backing) and from upholstery. It is less easy to say whether these sources present a significant risk to health, and this is discussed further below.

From people and their activities

Smoking is injurious to health – this is widely accepted as far as active smoking is concerned and, increasingly so, as regards passive smoking. A recent study in Scotland showed that the ban on smoking in public places, including bars, has a significant effect on symptoms in non-smokers and, remarkably, smokers working in such places.[10] Exposure to cigarette smoke damages the health of children: symptoms of asthma and glue ear are typically more common in children growing up in houses with smokers present,[1] and there is a dose–response effect – symptoms are fewest where no parents smoke, worse where the father alone smokes, worse still where the mother alone smokes and worst of all where both parents smoke. Smoking is likely to be the major source of particles and nitrogen dioxide in homes in which smokers live. This is remarkable – indoor air conditions are very seriously and adversely affected by smoking, and it cannot be doubted that this affects health.

People also generate indoor pollutants as a result of hobby activities: any work involving organic solvents (painting and decorating, model-building, repairing pieces of furniture, etc.) is likely to release pollutants indoors. It is unlikely that occasional exposure to such sources has a significant effect on health, although effects in the occupational setting have been clearly described among painters.[11–13]

One common source of indoor air pollutants is the integral garage: petrol vapour and organic pollutants from oil spills and from stored solvents and paints may spread from the garage (workshop) into the house. Demonstrating effects on health is again difficult, but it is clear that a hazard exists.

EXPOSURE TO CHEMICAL AIR POLLUTANTS INDOORS

Nitrogen dioxide

People living in developed countries spend, on average, perhaps 90 per cent of their lives indoors. This includes the time spent indoors at work and indoors at home. Young children and old people may spend more than 90 per cent of their time in the home. Exposure to nitrogen dioxide in the home will vary from room to room: one might expect concentrations of pollutants generated by gas cookers to be higher in the kitchen than in the bedrooms, and this is indeed the case. However, concentrations in bedrooms in houses in which gas cookers were used were shown in 1993 by Lambert *et al.* to be significantly higher than those in homes where electric cookers were used (Table 14.1),[14] and it is likely that these findings reflect current conditions.

Sources such as gas cookers are used for only comparatively short periods, although it will be noted that the data shown in the Table 14.1 report two weekly average concentrations. A study by Ross in 1994 reported peak hourly average concentrations in addition to weekly averages (Table 14.2).[15]

High hourly average concentrations of nitrogen dioxide occurred in the kitchen, but, more surprisingly, high concentrations were also recorded in the bedroom and living room. This suggests that air pollutants produced in one room spread readily throughout the house. The

difference in concentrations recorded in 'gas-cooking homes' and in 'electric-cooking homes' is striking. It will also be noted that peak hourly concentrations in kitchens exceed the current short-term WHO guideline for nitrogen dioxide: $200\,\mu g/m^3$ (1 hour average). The WHO *Air Quality Guidelines* report that 'Animal and human experimental toxicology indicates that nitrogen dioxide is itself – in short-term concentrations exceeding $200\,\mu g/m^3$ – a toxic gas with significant health effects.'[1] The inclusion of the words 'in itself' is intended to separate the effects considered here from those of lower concentrations outdoors where the possibility of nitrogen dioxide acting as a surrogate for other pollutants (especially particles) arises.

Interestingly, the WHO *Air Quality Guidelines* for long-term exposure to nitrogen dioxide (annual average concentration $40\,\mu g/m^3$) are based on studies of the effects of indoor exposure to nitrogen dioxide on respiratory infections in young children.[1] This work was first used as a basis for standard- or guideline-setting in a report on

Table 14.1 Indoor nitrogen dioxide (NO_2) concentrations in $\mu g/m^3$ (parts per billion) during 1998–91 in the homes of 1205 infants living in Albuquerque, New Mexico

Cooker type	Summer NO₂ bedroom	Winter NO₂ bedroom	Winter NO₂ living room	Winter NO₂ kitchen
Gas	26.3 SD = 18.8 (14 SD = 10) 5% > 58.3 (31)	39.5 SD = 41.4 (21 SD = 22) 5% > 94 (50)	54.5 SD = 90.2 (29 SD = 48) 5% > 124.1 (66)	63.9 SD = 62.0 (32 SD = 33) 5% > 152.3 (81)
Electric	13.2 SD = 11.3 (7 SD = 6) 5% > 26.3 (14)	13.2 SD = 11.3 (7 SD = 6) 5% > 30 (16)		

The data shown in the table report two weekly average concentrations.
SD, standard deviation.
Reproduced from Lambert *et al.*,[14] with permission.

Table 14.2 Continuous and passive sampling of nitrogen dioxide in $\mu g/m^3$ (parts per billion) in 12 UK homes

Location	Cooking appliance	Number of readings	Maximum 1 hour average ± SD, range		Weekly average ± SD, range	
Kitchen	Gas	10	438 ± 270 100–1115	(233 ± 144) (53–593)	45 ± 15 24–71	(24 ± 8) (13–38)
	Electric	2	55 ± 28 26–83	(29 ± 15) (14–44)	15 ± 9.4 (5.6–22.6)	(8 ± 5) (3–12)
Living room	Gas	9	212 ± 147 70–555	(113 ± 78) (37–295)	26 ± 7 17–47	(14 ± 4) (9–25)
	Electric	1	9.4	(5)	0	
Bedroom	Gas	8	248 ± 186 30–573	(132 ± 99) (16–305)	23 ± 11.3 38–34	(12 ± 6) (2–18)
	Electric	2	45 ± 9.4 36–53	(24 ± 5) (19–28)	43 ± 5.6 5.6–15	(6 ± 3) (3–8)

SD, standard deviation.
Reproduced from Ross,[15] with permission.

nitrogen dioxide from the International Programme on Chemical Safety.[16] This is an unusual occurrence: evidence of the effects of a pollutant indoors being used to set an outdoor air quality guideline.

Evidence of the effects on health of outdoor exposure to low concentrations of nitrogen dioxide is confounded by the possible effects of the ambient fine particulate aerosol. Concentrations of fine particles ($PM_{2.5}$) and concentrations of nitrogen dioxide tend to be closely correlated in urban areas, making separation as regards effects on health difficult or impossible.[17,18] That nitrogen dioxide can affect the capacity of the lung to deal with infectious organisms has been shown in both in vitro[18] and in vivo (animal)[19,20] studies. These findings support the case for the association between indoor concentrations and the prevalence of respiratory infections in children being causal. Whether this is the case outdoors is a subject of debate.

Carbon monoxide

Time-series studies have reported associations between outdoor, low concentrations of carbon monoxide in urban areas and acute episodes of cardiovascular disease, notably myocardial infarction,[21,22] although it is debatable whether this association is causal. Like nitrogen dioxide, outdoor concentrations of carbon monoxide are correlated with the concentrations of fine particles. This is unsurprising as these three pollutants share the same source: traffic. Indoor exposure to high concentrations of carbon monoxide can kill, and this, as stated above, is the cause of many accidental deaths in the UK and the USA.

It has been generally accepted that the mechanism of effect of carbon monoxide is explained by its avidity for binding to haemoglobin, leading to a reduction in oxygen carriage and a left shift of the oxyhaemoglobin dissociation curve. Tissues such as the heart and brain are acutely dependent on a normal supply of oxygen and suffer damage if this is impaired. In recent years, post-anoxic damage by free radicals formed on reperfusion has been identified as a further mechanism of neuronal injury. This mechanism operates during recovery from carbon monoxide poisoning and amplifies the initial injury caused by carbon monoxide inhalation.[23]

This may explain some of the delayed (post-exposure) effects of carbon monoxide on the brain. Damage tends to be greatest in the basal ganglia – perhaps because the globus pallidus lies at the periphery of two arterial supplies. Acute exposure to low concentrations of carbon monoxide in healthy subjects is not generally thought to be dangerous, but less is known of the effects of chronic exposure from malfunctioning heating devices burning gas or other fossil fuels, particularly among vulnerable groups.

Cigarette smoke is also a potent source of indoor carbon monoxide.[24] In many developed countries, including the UK, carbon monoxide alarms are advised as a means of providing a warning if carbon monoxide concentrations increase. This is clearly helpful but should not be seen as a cheap alternative to the proper fitting, use and maintenance of fossil fuel-burning appliances. The use of substandard devices, especially in poorly ventilated bedrooms, mobile homes or caravans, is potentially very dangerous.

Volatile organic compounds

A large number of organic compounds can be identified in indoor air. Fabrics, carpets, furniture, glues, deodorants, pesticides and perfumes all contribute to the complex mixture. Among these chemicals are many regarded as harmless to health (or about which little is known), as well as recognized carcinogens such as benzene. Once again, smoking is an important source of these compounds in some homes. Low concentrations of some organic compounds can be detected by their distinctive odour. Polishes and cleaning products produce such compounds – this is sometimes deliberate, and lemon-smelling compounds are often added to, for example, washing-up liquids.

Monitoring all the organic compounds found in indoor air is a large task, and, for many of them, concentrations are likely to be too low to be interpreted using standard toxicological data. One approach to the problem has been to measure total volatile organic compounds (TVOC) and try to relate TVOC levels to effects on health. A great deal of work has been done in this area, and a detailed account has been provided in the Institute for Environment and Health (IEH) report on indoor quality in the home.[25] Table 14.3 shows the results of a detailed analysis of volatile organic compounds from two apartments in Copenhagen.

Occupancy affects the concentrations of a number of the compounds analysed. It will also be noted that some compounds, for example benzene, are carcinogenic, and whereas acute exposure to low concentrations is unlikely to be associated with a significant risk to health, long-term exposure will contribute to the risk of cancer – in the case of benzene, to the risk of leukaemia. This risk can be calculated by use of the unit risk factor for benzene derived in the WHO *Air Quality Guidelines*: 'The geometric mean of the range of estimates of the excess lifetime risk of leukaemia at an air concentration of $1\,\mu g/m^3$ is 6×10^{-6}.' This can also be presented as 'lifetime exposure to $17\,\mu g/m^3$ benzene is associated with an excess lifetime risk of 1 in 10 000'. The basis of the calculation is set out in the WHO *Air Quality Guidelines*.

The IEH report recorded that the average indoor concentration of benzene in urban homes tended to be about 2.5 parts per billion (ppb), or $8\,\mu g/m^3$. This is lower than the original outdoor air standard set in the UK in 1994 for benzene (5 ppb or $16.2\,\mu g/m^3$) but above outdoor concentrations in the UK – about $2\,\mu g/m^3$ – and above the current UK Air Quality Standard of 1 ppb ($3.2\,\mu g/m^3$).

Table 14.3   Mean, maximum and minimum concentrations in $\mu g/m^3$ of 21 volatile organic compound (VOC) samples on diffusive samplers in two apartments in Copenhagen, Denmark

VOC	Vacant			Occupied		
	Mean	Minimum	Maximum	Mean	Minimum	Maximum
Decane	16	<2	44	50	10	167
Undecane	21	5	64	25	10	52
Dodecane	6	<2	31	50	<2	214
α-Pinene	156	42	278	137	45	230
β-Pinene	23	2	55	18	<1	49
3-Carene	78	17	151	83	27	151
Limonene	7	<2	21	20	<2	133
Benzene	3.2	1.3	7.2	23.3	1.6	131
Benzene (outdoor)	3.0	1.8	5.3	–	–	–
Toluene	16	5	51	84	15	392
Toluene (outdoor)	7	4	12	–	–	–
Ethylbenzene	5	<2	15	13	<2	55
Ethanol	–	<5	<5	229	<5	1326
Butanol	104	22	254	83	28	199
Ethylacetate	30	3	77	29	0	83
Butylacetate	68	8	161	62	17	195
Texanol*	754	<10	4009	487	<10	2800
Formaldehyde	208	63	384	135	14	276
Pentanal	25	<2	60	18	<2	36
Hexanal	61	7	149	44	9	119
Benzaldehyde	16	<2	48	15	<2	37
Acetone	32	7	63	40	16	148
Butanone	2	<1	9	6	<1	20

*2,4,4-trimethyl-1,3-pentanediol monoisobutyrates.
Reproduced from Institute for Environment and Health,[25] with permission.

If we exclude carcinogens, it is difficult to accept that low concentrations of mixed organic compounds present a significant risk to health, based on conventional toxicological testing. However, the detection of odour and other effects including eye irritation have been found to be linked with symptoms, or at least a loss of 'comfort', indoors.

There is no doubt that strong and unpleasant odours can trigger significant effects including headaches and vomiting; that mild odours can do this seems unlikely – at least in most people. Some people, however, appear to be remarkably sensitive to low concentrations of odoriferous organic compounds, and this takes us into the vexed issue of multiple chemical sensitivity. For some this is a well-accepted syndrome, whereas for others it cannot be well defined with sufficient precision to allow meaningful studies. The latter view was taken in the UK by the Department of Health Advisory Committee on Toxicity of Chemicals in Food, Consumer Products and the Environment.[26] This area is further complicated by assertions that exposure to organic chemicals can trigger or enhance allergen responses, which has led to the growing but ill-defined field of psycho-immuno-neuroendocrine toxicology. Some guidance can, however, be provided with

respect to volatile organic compounds, the IEH report[25] concluding:

> Based on chamber studies, TVOC concentrations greater than 25 mg/m³ (note mg not μg) may cause acute irritancy and other transient effects. Such concentrations are unlikely to be encountered under normal domestic conditions but could occur during painting or excessive solvent usage.

Formaldehyde

Formaldehyde is an irritant gas that has been classified by the International Agency for Research on Cancer as a human carcinogen (Group 1).[27] It occurs indoors at, generally, low concentrations, but in premises with new furnishings, furniture and fittings made from various artificial boards (e.g. particle board/chipboard) or premises that are cavity-insulated with urea formaldehyde foam insulation, concentrations can rise to well above average levels. Extensive studies of concentrations in homes have been undertaken in the USA and the UK.[25] In a larger

Table 14.4 Average concentration of formaldehyde in mg/m³ in various atmospheric environments

Source	Estimated formaldehyde concentration	Range of formaldehyde exposure (mg/day)*
Outdoor air (10%) of time)	0.01	0.02
Indoor air		
Home (65% of time)		
Conventional	0.04–0.15	0.5–2.0
Prefabricated (chipboard)	0.08–0.90	1.0–10.0
Workplace (25% of time)		
Without occupational		
exposure	0.04–0.16	0.2–0.8
With 1 mg/m³		
occupational exposure	1.0	5.0
Environmental tobacco smoke	0.02–0.20	0.1–1.0
Smoking (20 cigarettes/day)		1.0

*Assuming a respiratory volume of 20 m³ per day.
Reproduced from Institute for Environment and Health,[25] with permission.

UK study, concentrations of 0.020–0.025 mg/m³ were found (Table 14.4).

Formaldehyde has a characteristic odour, the odour threshold being between 0.06 and 1.2 mg/m³.[28] Interestingly, this range overlaps with that for throat and eye irritation, 0.01–3.0 mg/m³, with the eyes being most sensitive. Concentrations in mobile homes can exceed these figures. In 1991, Liu *et al.* reported a study of US mobile homes where weekly average exposures were reported as 11.8 mg/m³ hours and where individuals complained of burning eyes, cough, fatigue and dizziness.[29] Other work has reported asthma and bronchitis to be more common among children living in homes in which formaldehyde concentrations exceed 0.7 mg/m³.[30] Chamber studies report no effects on indices of lung function in adults exposed to 2.4 and 3.6 mg/m³ for 40 and 180 minutes, respectively.[31,32] Interestingly, patients with a history of asthma and hyper-reactivity of the airways showed no response to concentrations of 0.85 mg/m³ formaldehyde during a 90 minute exposure.[33]

Guidelines for formaldehyde have been recommended by the WHO: to prevent significant sensory inhalation in the general population, the recommended ceiling is 0.1 mg/m³ (for a short-term exposure – 30 minute average concentration). When this guideline was set in 2000, it was felt that it would also protect against more than a negligible risk of upper respiratory tract cancer. It should be noted that some individuals will be able to detect the odour of formaldehyde at concentrations below the WHO guideline value.

SETTING GUIDELINES FOR DOMESTIC INDOOR AIR QUALITY

Air quality guidelines for outdoor air have been recommended by the WHO.[1,35,36] Standards are available in developed countries for workplaces (see the websites of the American Conference of Governmental Industrial Hygienists and the UK Health and Safety Executives; weblinks at the end of the chapter). In the European Community, the WHO *Air Quality Guidelines* are used as basis for limit values for outdoor air pollutants,[34] and in the USA, the Environmental Protection Agency sets the National Ambient Air Quality Standards. Despite this, guidelines or standards for domestic air quality are generally not available.

It would, however, be inaccurate to say that the WHO has not considered this problem: chapters dealing with indoor air pollution appear in both the 2000 (second edition) of the WHO *Air Quality Guidelines* for Europe and in the later *Air Quality Guidelines Global Update*.[1,36] These chapters provide a useful background to the problem. The WHO is, however, at the time of writing, in the process of producing its first series of guidelines specific to indoor air quality: dampness and mould, (selected) chemicals and products of combustion. But the lack of a quantitative health-based guideline published in the first book of the series prompts the question: 'What obstacles stand in the way of setting such guidelines?'

It is generally accepted that standards imply some capacity for enforcement and that enforcement implies monitoring to ensure the observance of standards. These requirements are clearly impossible, or at least very difficult, to achieve when considering people's homes, and this has been a major stumbling block to setting indoor air quality standards. Although the WHO has been unable to provide or recommend a quantitative health-based guideline value or threshold of contamination for dampness and mould growth,[37] it does provide recommended measures, formulated from rigorous reviews of the available scientific literature, to enable occupants and built environment professionals to prevent and reduce damp and mould growth. Although few would doubt that people should be free to do as they wish in their own homes, such guidance can be of help. In rented accommodation, the landlord bears the responsibility for ensuring that the tenants are not exposed to unacceptable risk, and such risks could be assessed against standards. Given this, standards or guidelines would be useful.

A second and more difficult objection arises from a commonly asked question: 'If indoor mixes with outdoor air and there are standards and guidelines for outdoor air, why not simply apply these indoors?' At first glance, this seems sensible, but we should consider the evidence on which outdoor standards and guidelines are based. In the case of some pollutants, chamber studies provide the evidence, and there is no reason to assume that such standards would be less applicable (or suitable) indoors than outdoors. Chamber studies and toxicological studies have the great advantage that exposure tends to be measurable, although ill-health in the context of indoor air is invariably related to the effects of long-term exposure on chronic diseases or persistent symptoms rather than acute exposures, which relate better to chamber studies. In toxicological studies involving laboratory animals, some allowance for interspecies differences in sensitivity needs to be made, but this is common problem in all toxicological work.

Epidemiological studies present less tractable problems. Consider time series studies. Here, the unit of analysis is 'the day'. We know, usually from a central outdoor monitoring site, how concentrations of pollutants vary from day to day, and we relate this to variations in counts of health-related (or ill-health-related) end points such as deaths and hospital admissions. This leads to coefficients linking daily average concentrations and risks to health. But exposure is not measured – all we tend to know is that average exposure correlates well with concentration,[38] although, when inhaled, not necessarily with lung dose. It should be recalled that these studies reflect only a comparatively short duration of exposure outdoors each day: perhaps 10 per cent of an individual's day. To use such studies to predict the effects of indoor exposure for the other 90 per cent of the day seems unwise.

Studies using a cohort design are of even less use in the indoor environment. These studies are designed to look at areas or cities and to compare these in terms of long-term outdoor average concentrations of air pollutants and risk of death at any age.[39,40] The results of one large and rightly highly regarded study[40] might be expressed in the following terms: if you live in a city in which the long-term average concentration of fine particles (particulate matter with a diameter less than $2.5\,\mu m$) is $10\,\mu g/m^3$ greater than in a second city, your risk of death from cardiovascular disease is increased (in comparison with what it would be if you lived in the second city) by an average 6 per cent at any adult age.

Such findings allow calculations of loss of life expectancy in populations. But nothing is said of exposure, and this is important. The following question, for example, cannot be answered: 'If I live in a house in which the concentration of fine particles is 50 per cent of that of my neighbour, how much lower will my risk be?' The studies tell us about cities (or areas). This is the unit of analysis, just as the day is the unit of analysis in time series studies. To predict the effects of varying indoor or outdoor exposure to pollutants on individuals, we would need a study design in which the unit of analysis was the individual. Such studies are expensive to undertake and thus tend to be limited in size. Small studies lack the statistical power necessary to detect small increases in risk. Air pollution at ordinary indoor and outdoor concentrations is associated with small increases in risk.

Yet more difficult is the failure of studies of the effects of outdoor air pollutants (or of associations between outdoor concentrations and risks to health) to detect a clear threshold of effect even for non-cancer end points such as deaths from heart disease and admissions to hospital for respiratory disease. This 'failure' to detect a threshold may be due to an averaging of exposures and also to the perhaps wide distribution of sensitivity to air pollutants in the general population. A move away from outdoor air quality standards expressed in terms of concentrations and averaging periods has begun in some countries, including the UK. Standards are being replaced by policies of progressive, cost–benefit tested reductions in concentrations with defined interim targets. This seems sensible and in line with the epidemiological findings but is clearly a poor basis for setting traditional indoor air quality standards.

The problem of providing guidance on indoor air quality has been considered in the UK by the Department of Health Advisory Committee on the Medical Effects of Air Pollutants.[41] In general, it was considered that when outdoor air quality standards were based on chamber studies (e.g. sulphur dioxide or carbon monoxide) or on occupational studies (e.g. benzene), these standards could be applied indoors with acceptable confidence. For particles, an important air pollutant, both indoor and outdoors, no such advice could be given.

If concentrations of pollutants indoors (in the home) are not regulated – as they are not in the UK – can anything be done to ensure acceptable indoor air quality? The answer to this question is, yes. The following measures are recommended:

- the provision of advice on how to keep down levels of pollutants indoors; this includes advice on the use and maintenance of fossil-fuelled devices such as gas fires and cookers;
- advice to install both a smoke alarm and a carbon monoxide alarm; these devices should be of an acceptable International Organization for Standardization standard;
- building regulations to ensure adequate ventilation;
- product safety information to provide advice on the use of paints and solvents;
- advice on suitable insulation techniques;
- the banning of dangerous products such as asbestos;
- advice against smoking.

CONCLUSION

Indoor air pollution is a neglected area of public health. In developed countries, indoor air tends not to be seen as a risk to health – but this is incorrect. Potentially dangerous sources of air pollutants occur indoors and cause deaths and serious injury every year in developed countries such as the UK and the USA. Regulating indoor air quality is difficult, but good advice can be provided. If this advice is followed, the risks posed to health by indoor air pollution can be reduced.

REFERENCES

● = Key primary paper
◆ = Major review article

◆ 1. World Health Organization. *Air Quality Guidelines for Europe*, 2nd edn. WHO Regional Publications, European Series, No. 91. Copenhagen: WHO, 2000.

2. Hoek G, Kos G, Harrison R *et al.* Indoor–outdoor relationships of particle number and mass in four European cities. *Atmos Environ* 2008; **42**: 156–69.

3. Hasselblad V, Eddy DM, Kotchmar DJ. Synthesis of environmental evidence: Nitrogen dioxide in epidemiological studies. *J Air Waste Manage Assoc* 1992; **42**: 662–71.

◆ 4. Dockery DW, Spengler JD. Indoor–outdoor relationships of sulphates and particles. *Atmos Environ* 1981; **15**: 335–43.

5. Department of Health. Recognising Carbon Monoxide Poisoning – 'Think CO'. Available from: http://www.dh.gov.uk/cmo (accessed September 12, 2009).

6. Centers for Disease Control and Prevention. Unintentional non-fire-related carbon monoxide exposures United States, 2001–2003. *MMWR* 2005; **54**: 36–9.

7. Townsend CL, Maynard RL. Changing views on carbon monoxide. *Clin Exp Allergy* 2002; **32**: 172–4.

8. Townsend CL, Maynard RL. Effects on health of prolonged exposure to low concentrations of carbon monoxide. *Occup Env Med* 2002; **59**: 708–11.

9. Dennekamp M, Howarth S, Dick SA, Cherrie JW, Donaldson K, Seaton A. Ultrafine particles and nitrogen oxides generated by gas and electric cooking. *Occup Env Med* 2001; **58**: 511–16.

● 10. Ayres JG, Semple S, MacCalman L *et al.* Bar workers' health and environmental tobacco smoke exposure (BHETSE): Symptomatic improvement in bar staff following smoke-free legislation in Scotland. *Occup Environ Med* 2009; **66**: 339–46.

11. Dick F, Semple S, Soutar A, Osborne A, Cherrie JW, Seaton A. Is colour vision impairment associated with cognitive impairment in solvent exposed workers? *Occup Environ Med* 2004; **61**: 76–8.

12. Dick F, Semple S, Osborne A *et al.* Organic solvent exposure, genes, and risk of neuropsychological impairment. *QJM* 2002; **95**: 379–87.

13. Chen R, Semple S, Dick F, Seaton A. Nasal, eye, and skin irritation in dockyard painters. *Occup Environ Med* 2001; **58**: 542–3.

14. Lambert WE, Samet JM, Hunt WC, Skipper BJ, Schwab M, Spengler JD. *Nitrogen Dioxide and Respiratory Illness in Children*. Part II: *Assessment of Exposure to Nitrogen Dioxide*. Health Effects Institute Research Report No. 58. Cambridge, MA: Health Effects Institute, 1993.

◆ 15. Ross D. *Continuous and Passive Monitoring of Nitrogen Dioxide in UK Homes*. (BRE) Note B109/94. Watford: Building Research Establishment, 1994.

16. International Programme on Chemical Safety. *Nitrogen Oxides*, 2nd edn. Environmental Health Criteria No. 188. Geneva: World Health Organization, 1997.

◆ 17. Gauderman WJ, Avol E, Lurmann F *et al.* Childhood asthma and exposure to traffic and nitrogen dioxide. *Epidemiology* 2005; **6**: 737–43.

18. Frampton MW, Smeglin AM, Roberts NJ, Finkelstein JN, Morrow PE, Utell MJ. Nitrogen dioxide exposure in vivo and human alveolar macrophage inactivation of influenza virus in vitro. *Environ Res* 1989; **48**: 179–92.

19. Ehrlich R, Henry MC. Chronic toxicity of nitrogen dioxide. I: Effect on resistance to bacterial pneumonia. *Arch Environ Health* 1968; **17**: 860–5.

20. McGrath JJ, Oyervides J. Effects of nitrogen dioxide on resistance to *Klebsiella pneumoniae* in mice. *J Am Coll Toxicol* 1985; **4**: 227–31.

21. Morris RD, Naumova EN, Munesinghe RL. Ambient air pollution and hospitalization for congestive heart failure among elderly people in seven large US cities. *Am J Public Health* 1995; **85**: 1361–5.

● 22. Morris RD, Naumova EN. Carbon monoxide and hospital admissions for congestive heart failure: Evidence of an increased effect at low temperatures. *Environ Health Perspect* 1998; **106**: 649–53.

● 23. Thom SR. Dehydrogenase conversion to oxidase and lipid peroxidation in brain after carbon monoxide poisoning. *J Appl Physiol* 1992; **73**: 1584–9.

24. Institute for Environment and Health. *IEH Assessment on Indoor Air Quality in the Home (2): Carbon Monoxide*. Assessment A5. Available from: http://www.cranfield.ac.uk/health/researchareas/environmenthealth/ieh/ieh%20publications/a5.pdf (accessed November 26, 2009).

25. Institute for Environment and Health. *IEH Assessment on Indoor Air Quality in the Home: Nitrogen Dioxide, Formaldehyde, Volatile Organic Compounds, House Dust Mites, Fungi and Bacteria*. Assessment A2. Leicester: University of Leicester, Institute for Environment and Health, 1996.

26. Department of Health, Food Standards Agency. Committee on the Toxicity of Chemicals in Food, Consumer Products and the Environment. Annual Report 2000. Available from: http://cot.food.gov.uk/pdfs/cotcomcocrep_cot.pdf (accessed November 26, 2009).

27. International Agency for Research on Cancer. *IARC Monographs on the Evaluation of Carcinogenic Risks to Humans*. Volume 88: *Formaldehyde, 2-Butoxyethanol and 1-tert-Butoxypropan-2-ol*. Lyon: IARC, 2006.

28. Samet JM, Marbury MC, Spengler JD. Health effects and sources of indoor air pollution. Part II. *Am Rev Respir Dis* 1988; **137**: 221–42.

◆ 29. Liu KS, Huang FY, Hayward JF, Brugere J, Goldberg M. Irritant effects of formaldehyde-exposure in mobile homes. *Environ Health Perspect* 1991; **94**: 91–4.

30. Krzyzanowski M, Quackenboss JJ, Lebowitz MD. Chronic respiratory effects of indoor formaldehyde-exposure. *Environ Res* 1990; **52**: 117–25.

31. Schachter EN, Witck TJ, Tosun T, Beck GE. A study of respiratory effects from exposure to 2 ppm formaldehyde in healthy subjects. *Arch Environ Health* 1986; **41**: 229–39.

32. Sauder LR, Green DJ, Chatham MD, Kulle TJ. Acute
pulmonary response to formaldehyde exposure in healthy
nonsmokers. *J Occup Med* 1986; **28**: 420–4.

33. Harving H, Korsgaard J, Pedersen OF, Mølhave I, Dahl R.
Pulmonary function and bronchial reactivity in asthmatics
during low-level formaldehyde exposure. *Lung* 1990; **168**:
15–21.

34. European Commission. Legislation. Ambient Air Quality.
http://ec.europa.eu/environment/air/legis.htm (accessed
November 27, 2009).

◆35. World Health Organization. *Air Quality Guidelines for
Europe*. WHO Regional Publications, European Series,
No. 23. Copenhagen: WHO, 1987.

36. World Health Organization. (2006) *Air Quality Guidelines.
Global Update 2005. Particulate Matter, Ozone,
Nitrogen Dioxide and Sulfur Dioxide*. Available from:
http://www.euro.who.int/Document/E90038.pdf (accessed
November 26, 2009).

37. World Health Organization. WHO Guidelines for Indoor
Air Quality: Dampness and Mould. Available from:
http://www.euro.who.int/document/E92645.pdf (accessed
September 12, 2009).

38. Mage DT, Buckley TJ. The relationship between personal
exposures and ambient concentrations of particulate

matter. Paper No 95-MP18.01, 88th Annual Meeting of the
Air and Waste Management Association, San Antonio,
18–23 June, 1995.

●39. Dockery DW, Pope CA III, Xu X *et al*. An association
between air pollution and mortality in six U.S. cities. *NEJM*
1993; **329**: 1753–9.

40. Pope CA III, Burnett RT, Thun MJ *et al*. Lung cancer,
cardiopulmonary mortality, and long-term exposure
to fine particulate air pollution. *JAMA* 2002; **287**:
1132–41.

41. Department of Health, Committee on the Medical
Effects of Air Pollutants. Guidance on the Effects on
Health of Indoor Air Pollutants. Available from:
http://www.advisorybodies.doh.gov.uk/comeap/PDFS/
guidanceindoorairqualitydec04.pdf (accessed November 26,
2009).

FURTHER RESOURCES

American Conference of Governmental Industrial Hygienists:
  http://www.acgih.org
Environmental Protection Agency: http://www.epa.gov
Health and Safety Executive: http://www.hse.gov.uk

15

Indoor air pollution in developing countries

OM P. KURMI, JON G. AYRES

Most people spend approximately 90 per cent of their time indoors, more in the case of elderly and sick people. The indoor environment can thus influence health through exposure to emissions from cooking and heating, environmental tobacco smoke, the inflow of polluted outdoor air and various biological exposures such as house dust mites, fungi and bacteria. The effects of the indoor environment in developed countries have been covered in Chapter 14; we address here the problems associated with the indoor environment in the less economically developed countries (LEDCs) where indoor air quality is dominated by emissions from dirty fuels such as unprocessed biomass, coal and dung cake for cooking and heating, placing women and children in particular at risk of both acute and long-term ill-health.

HOUSEHOLD ENERGY IN LEDCS

More than 3 billion people, around half the world's population, use unprocessed biomass to meet their basic household energy demands.[1] In many areas of Africa, Central America and Asia, over 90 per cent of rural homes use solid fuel as the primary cooking and/or heating fuel (Figure 15.1).[2] The world's total energy consumption from biomass decreased from 50 per cent in 1900 to around 14 per cent in the early 2000s,[3] wood providing around 15 per cent of energy needs in LEDCs overall, rising to 75 per cent in tropical Africa. However, rises in the prices of kerosene and bottled gas have increased the use of biomass fuels and slowed the transition to cleaner fuels. In LEDCs, the varying use of different types of fuel will result in differential exposures. For instance, people in remote areas lacking electricity use kerosene or wood as a fuel and are thus exposed to mixtures of pollutants, different from their urban counterparts.

Kitchen type (Figure 15.2) and the design of living areas in houses in LEDCs can increase exposure to air pollutants by several fold through inadequate ventilation and lack of flues, the rate of clearance of indoor air pollutants generated from cooking thus being determined in most cases by natural ventilation. Exposure to indoor air pollutants during the winter is several times higher than in the other seasons as people sit around fires to protect themselves from the cold. Residential biomass smoke also contributes to outdoor pollutant concentrations during the winter season when wood is burnt for heating purposes.

COMPOSITION OF BIOMASS SMOKE

One of the main components of biomass smoke is carbon (5–20 per cent of wood smoke as particulate mass), which is found in the particulate fraction of the smoke and is present across a range of particle sizes. Biomass smoke also contains more than 250 organic compounds, varying mainly by the type of fuel burnt and the combustion conditions.[4] Smoke from the incomplete and inefficient combustion of biomass contains different, partially oxidized chemicals compared with smoke from efficiently burning fires as well as organic derivatives such as endotoxin. The partial oxidation of carbon produces carbon monoxide instead of carbon dioxide; nitrogen-containing materials can yield hydrogen cyanide, ammonia and nitrogen oxides; and chlorine (e.g. in polyvinyl chloride) or other halogens may lead to the production of

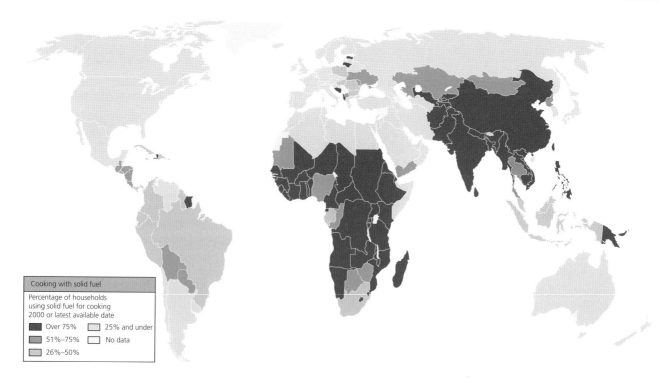

Figure 15.1 Worldwide estimates of solid fuel use. (Reproduced from Mackay *et al.*,[2] with permission.)

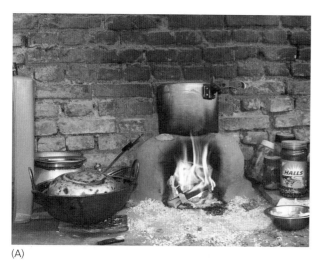

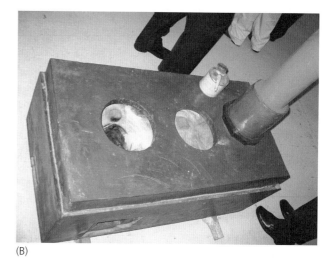

(A)

(B)

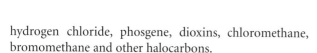

Figure 15.2 Traditional stove (A) and improved stove (B).

hydrogen chloride, phosgene, dioxins, chloromethane, bromomethane and other halocarbons.

An assessment of exposure to biomass can be made either simply on the basis of history (exposed/non-exposed) or by the measurement of airborne particles or carbon monoxide levels.

MEASUREMENT OF EXPOSURE TO BIOMASS SMOKE

Particulate matter (PM) present in biomass smoke is classified on the basis of aerodynamic diameter, which

takes into account particle size, mass and shape. It is important to quantify PM exposure and make sure that the methods used for assessing levels of exposure are accurate. Currently, two main techniques, one gravimetric and the other photometric, are used for this purpose.

Gravimetric techniques have been widely used to measure the mass concentration of particles deposited on filters in both indoor and outdoor environments. They provide a measure of the integrated sample and time-averaged concentrations over a given period, and are generally regarded as the primary method in the measurement of airborne PM. Gravimetric methodology cannot provide real-time measurements and requires long sampling periods, usually hours, so that sufficient mass can be collected on the filter for analysis, although the sampling time will depend on the reason for sampling (measurement of mass or analysis of content) and the likely level of exposure, higher levels requiring shorter sampling times.

However, photometric methods are widely used to measure the micrometre and submicrometre range of airborne particles in both indoor and outdoor environments, providing real-time measurements in a continuous and repeated manner. They have been widely used to measure aerosol concentrations in occupational and environmental settings. This approach is satisfactory provided that there is a consistent relationship with results obtained from gravimetric dust samplers as the light-scattering devices rely on indirect sensing techniques that require more frequent calibration.

Photometric devices are simpler to use and are less labour intensive than gravimetric methods, where filters need to be weighed on a high-precision balance before and after sampling in well-defined environmental conditions. Photometric devices, especially when measuring combustion-derived particulates, over-read levels compared with gravimetric measures.[5] Photometric devices thus need to be calibrated regularly depending on the source in use and the environmental conditions under study.

TOXICOLOGY OF BIOMASS SMOKE

Overall, relatively little is known about the toxicology of biomass smoke, with limited information on the effects of wood smoke but none for other biomass fuels such as dung or crop residues (Table 15.1).

The lung

Particulate matter deposits differentially in the lung, depending largely on particle size but with other factors playing a role (see Chapter 9).

ANIMAL STUDIES

Rats exposed subchronically to wood smoke at concentrations of 1–10 mg/m^3 over weeks showed reduced carbon monoxide-diffusing capacity and increased airway resistance along with mild chronic inflammation and squamous metaplasia in the larynx, alveolar macrophage hyperplasia and slight thickening of the alveolar septae.[6] While these changes are perhaps unsurprising, a number of other acute and subchronic effects have been reported (Table 15.2).

HUMAN STUDIES

Acute exposure to sulphur dioxide increases bronchial reactivity in normal subjects and can cause bronchoconstriction in asthmatic individuals at levels of around 100 parts per billion. For nitrogen dioxide, acute effects are only seen at high concentrations (over 1 part per million), but lower concentrations can enhance bronchial responses to allergens.[7] Longer-term exposure may increase susceptibility to viral lung infections. Dung-generated particles appear to have high oxidative potential, depleting physiologically relevant antioxidants such as ascorbate, urate and glutathione.[8]

Immune system

There is some evidence that wood smoke exposure can impair macrophage function and be mutagenic in animal studies,[4] while human studies have shown that wood smoke causes greater levels of DNA damage in lymphocytes than does exposure to liquefied petroleum gas combustion products.[9]

The eye

Wood smoke condensates damage the lens in rats, causing discoloration and opacities, probably through oxidation by polycyclic aromatic compounds and metal ions.[10] More commonly, chemicals such as aldehydes and acrolein can cause eye irritation and sometimes conjunctivitis.

Blood

Carbon monoxide released from biomass burning binds with haemoglobin, producing carboxyhaemoglobin. Potentially, this can reduce oxygen transport to key organs and the developing fetus, which may result in low birth weight and perinatal death.[11] In chronically biomass smoke-exposed Indian women, activation of circulating platelets, neutrophils and monocytes has been reported, with higher levels of leukocyte–platelet aggregates.[12] As a number of studies on ambient air pollution suggest that particulate pollutants increase fibrinogen levels, thus enhancing blood coagulation,[13] it is plausible that biomass smoke exposure could be a risk factor for cardiovascular events.

There have been very few controlled exposure studies[14] of human exposure to biomass smoke, but there is a suggestion that exposure at levels of around 250 μg/m^3 is associated with an increase in circulating factor VIII and serum amyloid A, both of which confer a cardiovascular risk.

HEALTH EFFECTS OF BIOMASS SMOKE EXPOSURE

Whereas clues to the direct health effects of biomass smoke can be derived from epidemiological studies of

Table 15.1 Major health-damaging pollutants from biomass combustion

	Examples*	Source	Notes	Mode of toxicity
Particulate matter	Fine particles (PM$_{2.5}$)	Condensation of combustion gases; incomplete combustion	Transported over long distances; primary and secondary production[†]	Inflammation and oxidative stress; may be allergenic
	Respirable particles	Condensation of combustion gases; incomplete combustion	For biomass smoke, approximately equal to fine particles	
	Inhalable particles (PM$_{10}$)	Condensation of combustion gases; incomplete combustion; entrainment of vegetation and ash fragments	Coarse[†] + fine particles. Coarse particles are not transported far and contain mostly soil and ash	Inflammation and oxidative stress; may be allergenic
Inorganic gases	Carbon monoxide	Incomplete combustion	Transported over distances	Asphyxiant
	Ozone	Secondary reaction product of nitrogen dioxide and hydrocarbons	Only present downwind of fire; transported over long distances	Irritant
	Nitrogen dioxide	High-temperature oxidation of nitrogen in air; some contribution from fuel nitrogen	Reactive	Irritant
Hydrocarbons	Many hundreds Unsaturated: 40+, e.g. *1,3-butadiene*	Incomplete combustion	Some transport; also react to form organic aerosols. Species vary with biomass and combustion conditions	Irritant, carcinogenic, mutagenic
	Saturated: 25+, e.g. n-*hexane*			Irritant, neurotoxic
	Polycyclic aromatic: 20+, e.g. *benzo[a]pyrene*			Mutagenic, carcinogenic
	Monoaromatics: 28+, e.g. *benzene, styrene*			Carcinogenic, mutagenic
Oxygenated organics	Hundreds Aldehydes: 20+, e.g. *acrolein, formaldehyde*	Incomplete combustion	Some transport; also react to form organic aerosols. Species vary with biomass and combustion conditions	Irritant, carcinogenic, mutagenic
	Organic alcohols and acids: e.g. *methanol, acetic acid*			Irritant, teratogenic
	Phenols: 33+, e.g. catechol, cresol (methylphenols)			Irritant, carcinogenic, mutagenic, teratogenic
	Quinones: hydroquinone, fluorenone, anthraquinone			Irritant, allergenic, redox active, oxidative stress and inflammation, possibly carcinogenic
Chlorinated organics	Methylene chloride, methyl chloride, dioxin	Requires chlorine in biomass		Central nervous system depressant (methylene chloride), possibly carcinogenic
Free radicals	Semiquinone-type radicals	Little is known about their formation		Redox active, cause oxidative stress and inflammatory response, possibly carcinogenic

PM, particulate matter.
*Compounds in italics are either criteria air pollutants or hazardous air pollutants under Section 112 of the US Clean Air Act.
[†]Particles are created directly during the combustion process and also formed later from emitted gases through condensation and atmospheric chemical reactions.
[†]Coarse particles are defined as those between 2.5 and 10 μm in size.
Adapted from Naeher *et al*,[4] with permission.

ambient air pollution in the developed world, studies investigating the adverse affects of solid fuel smoke on health are fewer.

Nevertheless, there is good evidence that an increased risk of acute lower respiratory tract infections and the development of chronic obstructive pulmonary disease (COPD) and lung cancer (the latter from coal use) are associated with the prolonged use of solid fuels. Studies have also linked exposure to biomass smoke to asthma, cataracts, tuberculosis, adverse pregnancy outcomes (in particular low birth weight), ischaemic heart disease, interstitial lung disease and nasopharyngeal and laryngeal cancers.

Table 15.2 Toxicological effects of acute and subchronic wood exposure in animal studies

Acute: single exposures	Subchronic: repeated exposure
Necrotizing tracheobronchial epithelial cell injury	Desquamation of airway epithelial lining
Acute tracheobronchial and bronchiolar inflammatory response	Pulmonary oedema
Acute mucociliary dysfunction	Neutrophilic peribronchiolar and perivascular infiltration
Alveolar macrophage dysfunction	Bronchiolitis
Airway hyperresponsiveness	Lymphoid follicle hyperplasia
Lung compliance reduction	Late eosinophilia
Reduction in ventilatory response	Bacterial clearance reduction
	Mild emphysema
	Lung cancer

Respiratory effects

CHRONIC OBSTRUCTIVE PULMONARY DISEASE

The term COPD was developed in the 1980s, replacing multiple previously used terms such as chronic bronchitis and emphysema. Chronic obstructive pulmonary disease is now defined in terms of lung function and symptoms, although symptoms known to be associated with chronic bronchial inflammation can occur in the presence of normal lung function. The definition and classification used at present is that formulated by the Global Initiative for Obstructive Lung Disease (Table 15.3).[15]

Chronic obstructive pulmonary disease is recognized as a major chronic disease of developed countries and is increasingly being recognized as being very prevalent, especially in the poor, in LEDCs.[2] The main contributory factors are cigarette smoke, occupational exposures and exposure to biomass smoke. Lower socioeconomic status increases the risk of developing COPD, although which component factors (e.g. poor housing, poor nutrition, low income or no/poor education) are the most important in influencing COPD and to what extent is unclear.

The prevalence of active cigarette-smoking varies by both country and gender within a country, so will affect different populations differently. Passive smoking may also be a risk factor for COPD as maternal smoking during pregnancy poses a risk to the fetus by affecting lung growth and development in utero.[16] Chronic obstructive pulmonary disease is related to a number of occupations that are of relevance as co-exposures when considering the effects of biomass smoke on lung function in the developing world. These include coal-mining, hard-rock-mining and tunnel-working among others.[17] Occupational dust exposures have been estimated to account for approximately 15 per cent of the morbidity from COPD.[18]

Table 15.3 Spirometric classification of chronic obstructive pulmonary disease (COPD) severity based on post-bronchodilator forced expiratory volume in 1 second (FEV_1)

COPD stages	Spirometric classification	Respiratory symptoms
I: Mild	$FEV_1/FVC < 0.70$ and $FEV_1 \geq 80\%$ predicted	May produce chronic cough and sputum, but not always
II: Moderate	$FEV_1/FVC < 0.70$ and $50\% \leq FEV_1 < 80\%$ predicted	Shortness of breath typically developing on exertion, and cough, sometimes with sputum production
III: Severe	$FEV_1/FVC < 0.70$ and $30\% \leq FEV_1 < 50\%$ predicted	Greater shortness of breath, reduced exercise capacity, fatigue and repeated exacerbations
IV: Very severe	$FEV_1/FVC < 0.70$ and $FEV_1 < 30\%$ predicted or $FEV_1 < 50\%$ predicted plus chronic respiratory failure	Chronic respiratory failure (arterial $PaO_2 < 8.0\,kPa$ (60 mmHg), with or without arterial $PaCO_2 > 6.7\,kPa$ (50 mmHg))

FVC, forced vital capacity; $PaCO_2$, partial pressure of carbon dioxide; PaO_2, partial pressure of oxygen.
Adapted from Global Initiative for Obstructive Lung Disease,[15] with permission.

Outdoor air pollution not only contributes to day-to-day changes in hospital admissions and mortality for COPD, but is also associated with an increased prevalence of the disease (see Chapter 10 for a fuller account). In the developing world, major cities have extremely high levels of outdoor air pollution, but city-dwellers in these countries often use biomass fuel less than those living in rural areas, where ambient levels are low (although contributions to ambient levels from indoor biomass burning can be significant).

A number of studies have shown associations between biomass smoke from different fuels and the prevalence of COPD,[19,20] chronic bronchitis[21] and changes in lung function.[22] Many of these studies have methodological weaknesses (no control group, no direct measurement of exposure or inadequate allowance for confounders), but the overall associations are reasonably robust, although there is a level of heterogeneity in reported effect sizes (Figure 15.3).

The most important co-factors when considering the development of COPD in relation to biomass smoke exposure are gender (females), smoking status, occupational dust exposure and socioeconomic status. However, allowing for these, there is a near threefold risk of developing COPD, defined using lung function testing, in populations exposed in the long term to biomass smoke (Figure 15.3).

Some studies, rather than considering the prevalence of defined COPD, have looked at lung function differences between exposed and unexposed populations. In one study,[23] although both exposed men and women had worse lung function, the decrement was significantly more in women who did the cooking, especially in those using wood as fuel. Lung function loss seems to relate to increasing age and duration of cooking times.[24] Work from Nepal has also shown a deleterious effect of biomass smoke exposure on lung function in young adults, suggesting that there may be an effect of biomass smoke on lung growth.[25]

CHRONIC BRONCHITIS

When using reported symptoms as an index of chronic lung disease, it is likely that the reported risks will be lower as the production of phlegm, minor degrees of cough and mild breathlessness are common in rural areas. Rural dwellers perceive these symptoms as 'normal' and thus not requiring medical treatment, which may be a source of reporting bias. While this is important when considering health burden, it is also important in terms of prognosis as people from rural areas often lack proper medical facilities locally and have to travel quite long distances to get treatment, thus allowing COPD to remain undiagnosed until late.

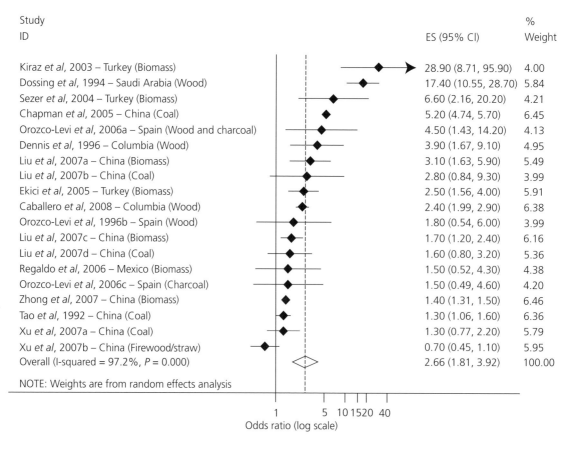

Figure 15.3 Summary of studies reporting chronic obstructive pulmonary disease due to exposure to solid fuels. CI, confidence interval; ES, effect size.

The major cause of chronic bronchitis, as defined using combinations of symptoms, notably cough and phlegm production,[26] is cigarette-smoking in the developed world, but it remains important in biomass-exposed populations.[2,4] However, trying to apportion the relative contribution of smoking and biomass exposure to the development of COPD in these populations is difficult because of the problems in determining cumulative exposures over time.

The prevalence of chronic bronchitis varies considerably in a range of countries (Figure 15.4), with a greater than doubling in risk of chronic bronchitis in those exposed: time exposed daily to smoke is a main driver of response, and cooking with biomass outside is associated with a lower prevalence compared with cooking indoors.[21] However, in some studies, the differences in prevalence are not as marked. For instance, a cross-sectional study from India reported a significantly higher prevalence of chronic bronchitis in women using biomass fuel (2.9 per cent) compared with liquefied petroleum gas (LPG) (2.5 per cent), kerosene (1.3 per cent) or mixed fuels (1.2 per cent).[27]

PATHOLOGY OF CHRONIC LUNG DISEASE

The pathology of chronic lung disease due to biomass exposure is poorly understood, although one study of non-

smoking women reported severely reduced lung function, with high-resolution computed tomography scan findings showing increased lung volumes, generalized or focal emphysema and thickening of the interlobular septae.[28] Only one other study has attempted to identify emphysema as an outcome from biomass smoke exposure[29] in a study in a hilly region of Nepal, reporting a prevalence of 3.1 per cent using World Health Organization radiological criteria.

INTERSTITIAL LUNG DISEASE

There are some anecdotal reports and short case-studies from LEDCs that have linked exposure to biomass smoke with interstitial lung disease, mostly referred to as 'hut lung', while studies from India suggest that populations exposed to biomass smoke are at risk of developing non-occupational, environment-related pneumoconiosis.[30] However, the effect of other potential causal exposures, notably organic dusts, is very likely to play a role, and whether biomass smoke does lead to interstitial lung disease must remain uncertain at present.

ACUTE RESPIRATORY INFECTIONS

Acute lower respiratory tract infections result in over 4 million deaths per year worldwide, over two-thirds

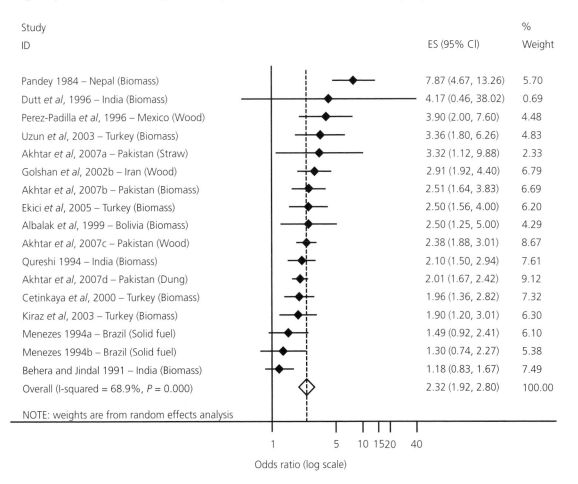

Figure 15.4 Summary studies reporting chronic bronchitis due to exposure to solid fuels. CI, confidence interval; ES, effect size.

occurring in LEDCs.[31] Globally, they form the second most common cause of death in children under the age of 5 in the world after neonatal deaths (17 per cent and 37 per cent respectively), and they lead the list when calculating the impact as total disability-adjusted life–years.[32] Deaths due to respiratory diseases are highest in African countries followed by eastern Mediterranean and south-east Asian countries,[31] where most of the people have low socioeconomic status and are poor.

Evidence for acute respiratory infection being caused by solid fuel smoke exposure

As with COPD, factors such as age, nutritional status, environmental tobacco smoke exposure, location of cooking and crowding all contribute to the risk of acute lower respiratory tract infection, but biomass exposure is a major factor. Overall, young children exposed to solid fuel smoke have two to three times more risk of serious acute respiratory infection than unexposed children.[33] A longitudinal study in Nepalese children under 2 years of age showed a doubling in lower respiratory tract infection with biomass smoke exposure reported by the mother, with a suggestion of a dose–response relationship. Similarly, a longitudinal study in rural Kenya in children under the age of 5 found a more obvious exposure–response relationship with evidence of a plateau with daily PM_{10} exposures above 2000 $\mu g/m^3$ (Figure 15.5).[34]

The same effect is seen in slightly older children (up to the age of 5): one study from Zimbabwe showed a greater than doubling risk of suffering from acute respiratory infection compared with children from households using clean fuel. A 1 year cohort study of 500 Gambian children under 5 years old looking at risk factors for lower respiratory tract infection found a six times higher risk in girls than boys, perhaps due to the fact that girls are carried on their mother's back more often than boys while cooking and are thus exposed more to biomass smoke.[35] The

mechanisms are unknown but may be by adversely affecting the specific and non-specific defences of the respiratory tract against pathogens.[36]

ASTHMA

There is a wide variation in the prevalence of asthma worldwide, especially in children, the reasons for which are not entirely clear: some studies in LEDCs have considered possible associations with biomass/solid fuel pollutant exposure. A study of 11–17-year-old school children in Nepal suggested that the risk of asthma in children increased with use of biomass fuels,[37] as did similar studies from Kenya, India and Guatemala. Overall, exposure to indoor air pollution increases the risk of developing asthma by around 65 per cent.

CARCINOGENIC EFFECTS

Emissions from combustion of coal for domestic purposes have been classified as a group 1 (definite) carcinogen by International Agency for Research on Cancer, while emissions from combustion of biomass for domestic purposes are probably carcinogenic to man (group 2a), implying that differences in the content of different solid fuels are important causal factors.[38]

Exposure to coal smoke is associated with an increased risk of lung cancer, most of the information coming from China.[39] Other studies have shown that a potential confounding factor, cooking fumes, was also causally related to lung cancer,[40] but whether these two factors act independently or additively is not known. Overall, the relative risk estimated from random effects models is around 1.55 for women and 1.20 for men.

For non-coal solid fuel smoke exposures, the evidence is less strong. A hospital-based case–control study in non-smoking women from Osaka, Japan, reported that

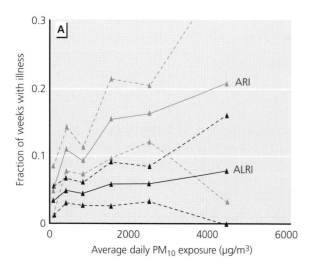
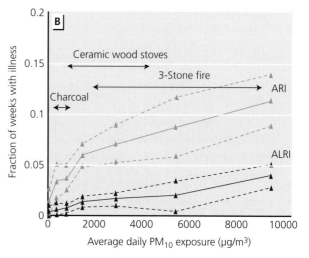

Figure 15.5 Exposure–response relationship for acute respiratory infection (ARI) and acute lower respiratory infection (ALRI). PM, particulate matter. (Reproduced from Ezzati *et al.*,[34] with permission.)

wood- or straw-burning increased the risk of lung cancer,[41] while non-smoking women in rural Mexico who were exposed to wood smoke for at least 50 years had a greater risk of lung cancer after adjusting for age, education, socioeconomic status and environmental tobacco smoke exposure,[42] findings similar to those seen in a Canadian study.[43] The overall effect size for non-coal smoke was 2.5 for women and 0.7 for men.

PULMONARY TUBERCULOSIS

The evidence to suggest that exposure to biomass smoke increases the risk of tuberculosis is inconsistent, with both positive[44] and negative[45] studies. There are theoretical reasons why biomass smoke exposure could increase this risk. Other particulate exposures such as cigarette-smoking also increase the risk by suppression of local immunity in the lung. Biomass exposure interferes with the mucociliary defences of the lungs and decreases several antibacterial properties of lung macrophages, such as adherence and phagocytosis.[46]

Cardiovascular effects

A number of epidemiological studies in developed countries have shown that ambient air pollution is associated with an increased risk of hospital admission for cardiovascular disease.[47] Pope *et al.* have reported that fine particulate air pollution is a risk factor for cause-specific cardiovascular disease mortality via mechanisms that probably include pulmonary and systemic inflammation, accelerated atherosclerosis and altered cardiac autonomic function.[47]

Currently, however, there is only one published study from Guatemala related to the cardiovascular effects of biomass smoke. The study from Guatemala was a stove intervention study that showed a small effect in reducing blood pressure (3–4 mmHg) as smoke exposure fell.[48] The change in exposure in that study was substantial.

Low birth weight and infant mortality

Exposure to ambient particles has been associated with adverse pregnancy and perinatal effects.[49] Some studies from the developing world suggest that indoor air pollution is associated with adverse birth outcomes independent of child's sex, birth order, mother's nutritional status, pregnancy care, mother's education, household living standards and other factors.

LOW BIRTH WEIGHT

A cohort study from a semi-rural area of Pakistan reported that cooking with wood during pregnancy was significantly associated with low birth weight,[50] with a prevalence of low birth weight of 22.7 per cent among wood users and 15 per cent among natural gas users. There was also a possible effect on mean birth weight, infants born to wood users

being 82 g lighter than those born to natural gas users. A more marked effect on birth weight was found in Zimbabwe, where babies born to mothers using biomass fuel were on average 175 g lighter compared with babies born to mothers using LPG, natural gas or electricity.[51] Similar work from Guatemala on over 1700 women and newborn children found a prevalence of low birth weight of 19.9 per cent in open wood fire users compared with 16.8 per cent in those whose homes had chimneys on their stoves, and 16.0 per cent in 365 electricity and gas users, independent of key maternal, social and economic factors.[52]

A large Chinese study of nearly 75 000 primiparous live births with a gestational age of 37–44 weeks reported a significant exposure–response relationship between maternal exposure to ambient sulphur dioxide and total suspended particles and infant birth weight.[53] The study reported adjusted odds ratios for low birth weight of 1.11 and 1.10 for each $100 \, \mu g/m^3$ increase in sulphur dioxide and total suspended particles respectively, and also estimated a 7.3 and 6.9 g reduction in birth weight for each $100 \, \mu g/m^3$ increase in sulphur dioxide and total suspended particles, respectively.

There is some evidence for biomass smoke exposure being associated with infant mortality.[54]

The mechanisms for these perinatal effects are likely to be multifactorial and may include changes in placental blood flow or oxygen delivery, although there is no direct evidence to support these suggestions.

Cataract

Long-term exposure to biomass smoke might damage the eye. Exposure can result in eye irritation, with similar effect sizes for different fuels. More importantly, biomass smoke exposure is associated with a high risk of cataract, with increased risks of over threefold compared with non-biomass-exposed individuals. A study of the 1992–93 National Family Health Survey in India in over 170 000 people over the age of 30 showed an 18 per cent prevalence of blindness in biomass fuel users, with biomass users experiencing a 30 per cent increased risk for both men and women.[55] The association was significant for both men and women separately. Similar findings have been found in a second study from India and in Nepal.

MANAGEMENT OF EXPOSURE TO BIOMASS SMOKE

The main approach to reducing biomass exposure indoors is either to provide flued stoves, which reduce (although tend not to remove completely) smoke exposure, or to provide more efficiently burning stoves.

Work in Guatemala found that women using traditional stoves (three-stone open fires) reported significantly more morning cough, daytime cough and daytime phlegm than those using improved cook stoves (Plancha) (see Figure 15.2

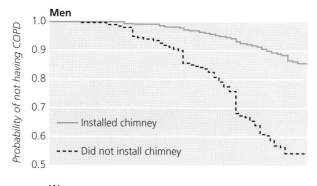

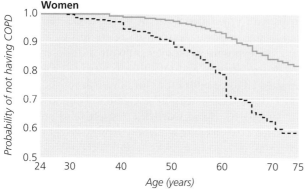

Figure 15.6 Product limit survival plots showing the probability of not having chronic obstructive pulmonary disease (COPD) by age in years in men and women according to whether they had a chimney. (Adapted from Chapman et al.,[20] with permission.)

above). In China, a longitudinal study followed the prevalence of COPD in dwellings with open fires compared with the incidence in dwellings where flued stoves were installed,[20] revealing a remarkable reduction in COPD associated with the intervention, although the benefit did not really start to be noticeable until about 10 years.

SUMMARY

In summary, there is sufficient evidence to show that exposure to biomass/solid fuel causes respiratory problems (acute lower respiratory tract infection, COPD and possibly worsening asthma). Coal smoke causes lung cancer, although whether smoke from other biomass fuels is carcinogenic is unclear. Evidence is also good for a causal relationship between biomass smoke and cataract, but less so for tuberculosis. Some studies suggest that exposure to biomass smoke may lead to premature birth or low birth weight. Exposure to biomass smoke appears to increase blood pressure but, although theoretically plausible, no association has been shown with coronary artery disease.

Intervention studies should focus on providing communities with the capability to reduce biomass smoke exposure rather than simply providing them with more

efficient stoves to enable a sustainable approach to the problem. It should also be borne in mind that biomass smoke makes a considerable contribution to climate change (see Chapter 48), so further approaches to alternatives to biomass fuels need to be sought while accepting that, for most individuals, the 'best' fuel is that which is readily available and cheap. The immediate way forward is the provision of more efficient stoves, but approaches to alternative fuels need to be strongly considered.

REFERENCES

● = Key primary paper

◆ = Major review article

1. World Health Organization. Fuel for Life – Household Energy and Health. Available from: http://www.who.int/indoorair/publications/fuelforlife.pdf (accessed September 14, 2009).
2. Mackay R, Rehfuess E, Gordon B. *Inheriting the World: The Atlas of Children's Health and the Environment.* Geneva: World Health Organization, 2004.
3. Bruce N, Perez-Padilla R, Albalak R. The Health Effects of Indoor Air Pollution Exposure in Developing Countries. WHO/SDE/OEH/02.05. Available from: http://whqlibdoc.who.int/hq/2002/WHO_SDE_OEH_02.05.pdf (accessed September 14, 2009).
4. Naeher LP, Brauer M, Lipsett M et al. Woodsmoke health effects: a review. *Inhal Toxicol* 2007; **19**: 67–106.
5. Kurmi OP, Semple S, Steiner M, Henderson GD, Ayres JG. Particulate matter exposure during domestic work in Nepal. *Ann Occup Hygiene* 2008; **52**: 509–17.
6. Tesfaigzi Y, Singh SP, Foster JE et al. Health effects of subchronic exposure to low levels of wood smoke in rats. *Toxicol Sci* 2002; **65**: 115–25.
7. Tunnicliffe WS, Burge PS, Ayres JG. Effect of domestic concentrations of nitrogen dioxide on airway responses to inhaled allergen in asthmatic patients. *Lancet* 1994; **344**: 1733–6.
◆8. Mudway I, Duggan S, Venkataraman C, Habib G, Kelly F, Grigg J. Combustion of dried animal dung as biofuel results in the generation of highly redox active fine particulates. *Part Fibre Toxicol* 2005; **2**: 6.
9. Pandey AK, Bajpayee M, Parmar D et al. DNA damage in lymphocytes of rural Indian women exposed to biomass fuel smoke as assessed by the Comet assay. *Environ Mol Mutagen* 2005; **45**: 435–41.
10. Rao CM, Qin C, Robison WG Jr, Zigler JS Jr. Effect of smoke condensate on the physiological integrity and morphology of organ cultured rat lenses. *Curr Eye Res* 1995; **14**: 295–301.
11. Torres-Duque C, Maldonado D, Perez-Padilla R, Ezzati M, Viegi G. Biomass fuels and respiratory diseases: a review of the evidence. *Proc Am Thorac Soc* 2008; **5**: 577–90.
12. Ray MR, Mukherjee S, Roychoudhury S et al. Platelet activation, upregulation of CD11b/CD18 expression on

leukocytes and increase in circulating leukocyte-platelet aggregates in Indian women chronically exposed to biomass smoke. *Hum Exp Toxicol* 2006; **25**: 627–35.

13. Chuang KJ, Chan CC, Su TC, Lee CT, Tang CS. The effect of urban air pollution on inflammation, oxidative stress, coagulation, and autonomic dysfunction in young adults. *Am J Respir Crit Care Med* 2007; **176**: 370–6.

◆14. Barregard L, Sallsten G, Gustafson P *et al.* Experimental exposure to wood-smoke particles in healthy humans: effects on markers of inflammation, coagulation, and lipid peroxidation. *Inhal Toxicol* 2006; **18**: 845–53.

15. Global Initiative for Obstructive Lung Disease. Executive Summary: Global Strategy for the Diagnosis, Management, and Prevention of Chronic Obstructive Pulmonary Disease. Available from: http://www.goldcopd.org/Guidelineitem. asp?l1=2&l2=1&intId=996 (accessed September 14, 2009).

16. Tager IB, Ngo L, Hanrahan JP. Maternal smoking during pregnancy. Effects on lung function during the first 18 months of life. *Am J Respir Crit Care Med* 1995; **152**: 977–83.

17. Hnizdo E, Baskind E, Sluis-Cremer GK. Combined effect of silica dust exposure and tobacco smoking on the prevalence of respiratory impairments among gold miners. *Scand J Work Environ Health* 1990; **16**: 411–22.

18. Balmes J, Becklake M, Blanc P *et al.* American Thoracic Society Statement: Occupational contribution to the burden of airway disease. *Am J Respir Crit Care Med* 2003; **167**: 787–97.

●19. Zhong N, Wang C, Yao W *et al.* Prevalence of chronic obstructive pulmonary disease in China: a large, population-based survey. *Am J Respir Crit Care Med* 2007; **176**: 753–60.

●20. Chapman RS, He X, Blair AE, Lan Q. Improvement in household stoves and risk of chronic obstructive pulmonary disease in Xuanwei, China: retrospective cohort study. *BMJ* 2005; **331**: 1050.

◆ 21. Albalak R, Frisancho AR, Keeler GJ. Domestic biomass fuel combustion and chronic bronchitis in two rural Bolivian villages. *Thorax* 1999; **54**: 1004–8.

22. Behera D, Jindal SK, Malhotra HS. Ventilatory function in nonsmoking rural Indian women using different cooking fuels. *Respiration* 1994; **61**: 89–92.

23. Saha A, Rao NM, Kulkarni PK, Majumdar PK, Saiyed HN. Pulmonary function and fuel use: a population survey. *Respir Res* 2005; **6**: 127.

24. Sumer H, Turaclar UT, Onarlioglu T, Ozdemir L, Zwahlen M. The association of biomass fuel combustion on pulmonary function tests in the adult population of Mid-Anatolia. *Soz Praventivmed* 2004; **49**: 247–53.

25. Kurmi OP, Sean S, Steiner M, Simkhada PP, Ayres JG. Relationship between biomass fuel smoke and lung function in Nepal. Presented at American Thoracic Society Conference, Toronto, Canada, 17–21 May, 2008.

26. Medical Research Council's Committee on the Aetiology of Chronic Bronchitis. Standardized Questionnaires on Respiratory Symptoms. *Br Med J* 1960; **2**: 1665.

◆27. Behera D, Jindal SK. Respiratory symptoms in Indian women using domestic cooking fuels. *Chest* 1991; **100**: 385–8.

28. Ozbay B, Uzun K, Arslan H, Zehir I. Functional and radiological impairment in women highly exposed to indoor biomass fuels. *Respirology* 2001; **6**: 255–8.

◆29. Pandey MR. Prevalence of chronic bronchitis in a rural community of the Hill Region of Nepal. *Thorax* 1984; **39**: 331–6.

30. Saiyed HN, Sharma YK, Sadhu HG *et al.* Non-occupational pneumoconiosis at high altitude villages in central Ladakh. *Br J Ind Med* 1991; **48**: 825–9.

31. World Health Organization. *Global Burden of Disease – 2004 Update.* Geneva: World Health Organization, 2008.

32. World Health Organization Statistical Information System. Available from: http://www.who.int/whosis/data/Search.jsp (accessed September 14, 2009).

◆33. Smith KR, Samet JM, Romieu I, Bruce N. Indoor air pollution in developing countries and acute lower respiratory infections in children. *Thorax* 2000; **55**: 518–32.

◆34. Ezzati M, Kammen DM. Quantifying the effects of exposure to indoor air pollution from biomass combustion on acute respiratory infections in developing countries. *Environ Health Perspect* 2001; **109**: 481–8.

35. Armstrong JR, Campbell H. Indoor air pollution exposure and lower respiratory infections in young Gambian children. *Int J Epidemiol* 1991; **20**: 424–9.

36. Reynolds HY. Defense mechanisms against infections. *Curr Opin Pulm Med* 1999; **5**: 136–42.

37. Melsom T, Brinch L, Hessen JO *et al.* Asthma and indoor environment in Nepal. *Thorax* 2001; **56**: 477–81.

38. Straif K, Baan R, Grosse Y, Secretan B, El Ghissassi F, Cogliano V. Carcinogenicity of household solid fuel combustion and of high-temperature frying. *Lancet Oncol* 2006; **7**: 977–8.

39. Du YX, Cha Q, Chen XW *et al.* An epidemiological study of risk factors for lung cancer in Guangzhou, China. *Lung Cancer* 1996; **14**(Suppl.1): S9–37.

◆40. Ko YC, Cheng LS, Lee CH *et al.* Chinese food cooking and lung cancer in women nonsmokers. *Am J Epidemiol* 2000; **151**: 140–7.

41. Sobue T. Association of indoor air pollution and lifestyle with lung cancer in Osaka, Japan. *Int J Epidemiol* 1990; **19**(Suppl.1): S62–6.

42. Hernandez-Garduno E, Brauer M, Perez-Neria J, Vedal S. Wood smoke exposure and lung adenocarcinoma in non-smoking Mexican women. *Int J Tuberc Lung Dis* 2004; **8**: 377–83.

43. Ramanakumar AV, Parent ME, Menzies D, Siemiatycki J. Risk of lung cancer following nonmalignant respiratory conditions: evidence from two case-control studies in Montreal, Canada. *Lung Cancer* 2006; **53**: 5–12.

44. Perez-Padilla R, Perez-Guzman C, Baez-Saldana R, Torres-Cruz A. Cooking with biomass stoves and tuberculosis: a case control study. *Int J Tuberc Lung Dis* 2001; **5**: 441–7.

45. Shetty N, Shemko M, Vaz M, D'Souza G. An epidemiological evaluation of risk factors for tuberculosis in South India: a matched case control study. *Int J Tuberc Lung Dis* 2006; **10**: 80–6.

46. Fick RB Jr, Paul ES, Merrill WW, Reynolds HY, Loke JS. Alterations in the antibacterial properties of rabbit pulmonary macrophages exposed to wood smoke. *Am Rev Respir Dis* 1984; **129**: 76–81.

47. Pope CA 3rd, Burnett RT, Thurston GD *et al*. Cardiovascular mortality and long-term exposure to particulate air pollution: epidemiological evidence of general pathophysiological pathways of disease. *Circulation* 2004; **109**: 71–7.

◆48. McCracken JP, Smith KR, Diaz A, Mittleman MA, Schwartz J. Chimney stove intervention to reduce long-term wood smoke exposure lowers blood pressure among Guatemalan women. *Environ Health Perspect* 2007; **115**: 996–1001.

49. Bobak M. Outdoor air pollution, low birth weight, and prematurity. *Environ Health Perspect* 2000; **108**: 173–6.

50. Siddiqui AR, Gold EB, Yang X, Lee K, Brown KH, Bhutta ZA. Prenatal exposure to wood fuel smoke and low birth weight. *Environ Health Perspect* 2008; **116**: 543–9.

51. Mishra V, Dai X, Smith KR, Mika L. Maternal exposure to biomass smoke and reduced birth weight in Zimbabwe. *Ann Epidemiol* 2004; **14**: 740–7.

52. Boy E, Bruce N, Delgado H. Birth weight and exposure to kitchen wood smoke during pregnancy in rural Guatemala. *Environ Health Perspect* 2002; **110**: 109–14.

53. Wang X, Ding H, Ryan L, Xu X. Association between air pollution and low birth weight: a community-based study. *Environ Health Perspect* 1997; **105**: 514–20.

54. Rinne ST, Rodas EJ, Rinne ML, Simpson JM, Glickman LT. Use of biomass fuel is associated with infant mortality and child health in trend analysis. *Am J Trop Med Hyg* 2007; **76**: 585–91.

55. Mishra VK, Retherford RD, Smith KR. Biomass cooking fuels and prevalence of blindness in India. *J Environ Med* 1999; **1**: 189–99.

Respiratory diseases from infectious agents

16

Nosocomial transmission and control of SARS

BENJAMIN J. COWLING, STEVEN RILEY, WING HONG SETO, GABRIEL M. LEUNG

INTRODUCTION

Severe acute respiratory syndrome (SARS) originated as a zoonotic disease but rapidly became primarily a nosocomial disease. Sustained epidemics have not recurred in humans following the original outbreak. Subclinical or asymptomatic infection was very rare, and the peak infectivity was usually at least 1 week after the onset of symptoms, by which time, with a high clinical index of suspicion, the patient would have already been hospitalized; transmissibility of the pathogen is relatively low except in special circumstances such as during clinical procedures. Empirical experience during the 2002–03 global epidemic confirmed the dominance of a within-hospital spread of the virus, particularly in the context of superspreading events; in addition, the wide heterogeneity of within-hospital transmission correlated with the intensity and stringency of infection control procedures in apparently similar settings.

In late 2002, the SARS coronavirus emerged in humans in southern China and caused a global outbreak that had a severe impact on public health, international travel and trade. A common feature of the various SARS outbreaks worldwide was the role of hospitals in initiating and maintaining the epidemic. Out of 8096 probable cases of SARS by the end of the global epidemic, 1706 (21 per cent) were infections of healthcare workers.[1] In Singapore and Canada, more than 40 per cent of the cases were among healthcare workers, and 57 per cent of the Vietnamese cases were in healthcare workers (Table 16.1).

Importantly, transmission within heathcare settings affected other groups in addition to healthcare workers. In the largest hospital outbreak, at the Prince of Wales Hospital in Hong Kong, almost one-third of the cases were among other patients (admitted prior to infection with SARS) and hospital visitors.[2] Similar trends were observed in other large hospital outbreaks (Table 16.2).[2–12]

The first recorded human case of SARS infection was identified on November 16th, 2002 in the city of Foshan in Guangdong Province, China.[13] In February 2003, an infected doctor travelled from Guangdong to Hong Kong, transmitting the disease to 12 guests staying at his hotel and then also to multiple healthcare workers and patients

Table 16.1 Number of probable cases of severe acute respiratory syndrome (SARS) by region, proportion of cases among healthcare workers and number of imported cases

Region	Total number of probable SARS cases	Number (%) of SARS cases among healthcare workers	
China	5327	1002	(19%)
Hong Kong	1755	86	(22%)
Taiwan	346	68	(20%)
Canada	251	109	(43%)
Singapore	238	97	(41%)
Vietnam	63	36	(57%)
Other regions*	116	8	(7%)
Total	8096	1706	(21%)

* Other regions including Australia, Macau SAR, France, Germany, India, Indonesia, Italy, Kuwait, Malaysia, Mongolia, New Zealand, Philippines, Republic of Ireland, Republic of Korea, Romania, Russian Federation, South Africa, Spain, Sweden, Switzerland, Thailand, United Kingdom, and USA.

Adapted from World Health Organization,[1] with permission.

Table 16.2   Features of large severe acute respiratory syndrome (SARS) outbreaks in hospitals

Hospital	Location	Date of admission of first case (2003)	Number of hospital infections				
			Total	Healthcare workers	Visitors	Other patients	Superspreaders
Hanoi French Hospital[3]	Hanoi, Vietnam	February 26	56	36	18	16	0
Chang Guang Memorial Hospital[4]	Kaohsiung, Taiwan	April 26	33	17	0	16	0
Tan Tock Seng Hospital[5–7]	Singapore	March 1	105	60	32	13	3
Prince of Wales Hospital[2,8]	Hong Kong, China	March 4	259	175	19	65	1
Scarborough Grace Hospital[9]	Toronto, Canada	March 7	84	50	18	18	0
National University Hospital[7,10]	Singapore	March 23*	9	3	n/a	n/a	1
Singapore General Hospital[7,10]	Singapore	March 24	59	40	n/a	n/a	1
First Hospital of Peking University[11]	Beijing, China	March 24	n/a	18	n/a	n/a	0
Pingjin Hospital[12]	Tianjin, China	April 15	n/a	111	n/a	n/a	0

n/a, data not available.
*The case that initiated the large outbreak was admitted on April 8.

at a local hospital after admission.[14] With an average time from infection to onset of symptoms of around 5 days,[15] many of the guests infected in 'hotel M' had left Hong Kong by the time they became ill, seeding outbreaks in Vietnam, Singapore and Toronto.[14]

One guest travelled to Vietnam on February 26th, 2003 and was admitted to the Hanoi French Hospital. Nine secondary cases were suspected by March 4th,[16] and in total there were 62 SARS cases among staff, patients, visitors and their close contacts, including 56 staff or visitors.[3] The outbreak in Singapore began when another 'hotel M' guest was admitted to Tan Tock Seng Hospital upon her return from Hong Kong on March 1st, 2003. Nosocomial transmission ensued shortly after her hospitalization, and when infected patients sought medical advice from other hospitals, an interhospital outbreak, and consequently a SARS epidemic, was underway.[6,10]

The Canadian outbreak began when yet another 'hotel M' guest returned to Toronto on February 23rd, 2003.[9] The patient became ill upon arrival, and transmission to a family member who was later admitted to a community hospital led to a large nosocomial outbreak.[9] Hospital transmission played a significant role in initiating and sustaining this outbreak, accounting for 72 per cent of cases in Toronto.[17]

CLINICAL AND EPIDEMIOLOGICAL CHARACTERISTICS OF SARS

SARS infection was characterized by severe lower respiratory tract infection.[18] The most common symptoms at presentation included fever, dyspnoea, non-productive cough, chills or rigors, myalgias and malaise.[19–21] Approximately 10 per cent of patients died,[1] and the greatest predictors for the risk of mortality included older age, the presence of co-morbid conditions, male sex, haziness or infiltrates on chest radiography, less than 95 per cent oxygen saturation on room air, a high lactate dehydrogenase level, and high neutrophil and low platelet counts.[22] The mean time from onset of fever to an abnormal radiograph was around 5 days,[23] while viral shedding typically peaked at 12–14 days after the onset of the first symptoms.[24,25]

Detailed studies of exposures to potential infection have determined that the time from infection to onset of symptoms averaged around 5 days, while 95 per cent of infected subjects developed symptoms within 10–14 days.[15,26,27] Early in the epidemic, it was typical for patients to be admitted 5–7 days after symptom onset, by which time their condition had become quite severe.[28] However, a measure of success in public health control was seen by the reduction in average times from onset to admission to 1–2 days.[27,29] Rapid admission and the isolation of suspected cases was important because it reduced the opportunity for community transmission before later-stage infection had been firmly established. On average, patients spent 3–4 weeks in hospital before either succumbing to the disease or recovering sufficiently to be discharged.[27]

A distinguishing feature of the epidemiology of SARS infections that made it primarily nosocomial was the lack of asymptomatic or subclinical infections. During and subsequent to the epidemic, a series of seroprevalence surveys were conducted in most of the affected areas in various subgroups including healthcare workers at affected hospitals, close contacts of SARS patients, other inpatients and members of the general community. A systematic review of these surveys found that around 15 per cent of wild animal handlers in southern China had seroconverted with asymptomatic or subclinical infections, perhaps due to frequent zoonotic challenges, but among other subgroups (even the close contacts of confirmed cases) the average seropositivity rate was 0.10 per cent in more than 20 000 individuals tested.[30]

MODES OF TRANSMISSION

Understanding how SARS spread from person to person is important in designing adequate infection control strategies. Since hospital transmission played a major role in the epidemic, within-hospital infection control measures were essential in containing the outbreak. SARS appeared to be spread most commonly via direct close contact. Healthcare workers who performed direct patient care duties often had the highest attack rates, highlighting the increased exposure risk associated with direct contact.[3,31] Contact precautions were also shown to be effective in preventing transmission.[32]

Although there is substantial evidence to support the key role of transmission through droplet and direct contact, there is relatively little evidence to support the hypothesis that SARS could be transmitted by the airborne route.[33] One modelling study of the spread of illness in the Amoy Gardens housing estate in Hong Kong, outside the hospital setting, suggests that airborne spread played a role.[34] However, given that other data reported a lack of airborne transmission despite unprotected extended exposures in healthcare settings,[35–37] the World Health Organization classified SARS as a disease with 'opportunistic airborne' transmission, to indicate that the disease naturally spreads by non-airborne routes but under special environmental conditions may spread by the airborne route.[38,39] Diseases that are spread by opportunistic airborne transmission do not require special airborne infection isolation measures, for example negative-pressure isolation rooms, but special precautions are recommended for high-risk procedures.

Yet another mode of transmission may be via fomites – inanimate objects capable of transmitting infectious organisms from one individual to another, such as linens.[40] The SARS coronavirus was capable of surviving on dried, inert surfaces and was found on hospital surfaces.[41] The documentation of SARS cases among non-medical support staff implied possible transmission via fomites, droplets and airborne particles.[42] The array of possible transmission modes indicates the challenges that public health authorities faced in devising effective infection control strategies.

TRANSMISSIBILITY OF SARS

The basic reproductive number R_0 is a central concept of infectious disease epidemiology and has been used extensively to help describe key features of the epidemiology of SARS. It is defined as the average number of secondary infections resulting from one typically infectious index case in a susceptible population.[43] If the reproductive number exceeds 1, an outbreak can be sustained. Therefore, the aim of any public health intervention during the outbreak phase of emergence of a novel pathogen must be to reduce the effective reproductive number below 1 so that the outbreak will peter out. The basic reproductive number of SARS has been estimated to be between 2 and 3,[44,45] meaning that an infected case will on average infect two or three other people. In these terms, SARS was considerably less transmissible than other respiratory disease such as measles, but more transmissible than human immunodeficiency virus.[46,47]

Although it is often useful to think only of the total transmissibility of a pathogen, the basic reproductive number can also be allocated to different risk groups, infection stages or settings. For example, by considering the following two factors, we can use R_0 to define SARS as primarily a nosocomial infection. First, infection led to severe disease requiring hospitalization, with very few subclinical or asymptomatic infections.[48,49] Therefore, almost all transmission occurred from individuals who were admitted to hospital at some point. Second, viral loads in infected individuals, probably correlated with infectiousness,[25,50] typically increased after the onset of first symptoms, peaking around a week later,[25] by which time the cases had typically been hospitalized, especially as the causative pathogen had been identified and the index of clinical suspicion was heightened following community outbreaks.[27] Therefore, because the vast majority of infected individuals were admitted to hospital and peak infectiousness occurred well after admission in most cases, a large proportion of R_0 can be attributed to that setting.

The main modes of transmission for SARS appear to have been droplet spread, which often occurred during high-risk medical procedures, or through common inanimate vectors such as shared equipment or surfaces, or more seriously perhaps through clinical personnel. Apart from a large community outbreak at the Amoy Gardens housing estate in Hong Kong,[34] ongoing hospital transmission seems to have been responsible for sustaining the outbreaks in most affected regions. Therefore, the eventual control of the epidemic can be attributed to intensive efforts to control nosocomial transmission.

SUPERSPREADERS AND NOSOCOMIAL TRANSMISSION

In addition to nosocomial infection, one of the most notable features of the SARS epidemic was the role of superspreaders in amplifying the epidemic. For example, in Singapore, the index case infected in Hong Kong's 'hotel M' was directly associated with 172 subsequent infections through chains of transmission. One hundred and eighteen (69 per cent) of these cases were recorded as secondary cases of the initial index case and just four other superspreaders who may each have infected 10 or more other individuals (Figure 16.1).[51] However, some care is required when interpreting the case-tracing data gathered at the time of the outbreak.

The outbreak at The Prince of Wales Hospital provides an ideal opportunity to tease apart the potential contribution of superspreading events and nosocomial transmission because both certainly featured to some extent.[2] It has been shown, using a mathematical model of transmission, that the superspreading event may have contributed fewer direct infections than was first thought.[8] Some care should be taken when defining the number of secondary infections arising from a superspreader. For the purposes of infection control and to help understand the relative importance of alternative routes of transmission, one should only count directly infected patients as members of a superspreading cluster; therefore, in the Prince of Wales Hospital, only those infected by the index case should be considered to be members of the superspreading cluster.

This strict definition of superspreaders ensures that potentially effective infection control measures are not overlooked. For example, it seems likely that, at the Prince of Wales Hospital, a significant number of staff members who may have initially been assigned as infectees of the

superspreader were, in fact, infected by other members of staff.[8] Therefore, in any future similar outbreak, due attention should be given to reducing the effective levels of contact between staff as well as between patients and staff.

INFECTION CONTROL

A common feature described by case reports of hospital outbreaks is the speed at which outbreaks developed under initially lax infection control measures contrasted with the almost immediate control of outbreaks once stringent measures were implemented.[6,10,12,31,52–56] There are also reports that when good basic infection control measures are in place, there is effective control of transmission.[57] In Taiwan, the control of the initial outbreak in March and April led to complacency, and a lapse in hospital infection control procedures in treating an unidentified SARS patient triggered a series of nosocomial outbreaks in seven hospitals.[53] In Toronto, enhanced infection control practices appeared to have ended the outbreak, but an outbreak initially among nursing staff led to a second wave of infections.[54]

Hospitals in heavily affected regions employed a variety of infection control measures to successfully contain this SARS outbreak and subsequently the local epidemics.[6,55,58,59] These interventions can be grouped into the categories of engineering controls, administrative and work practice

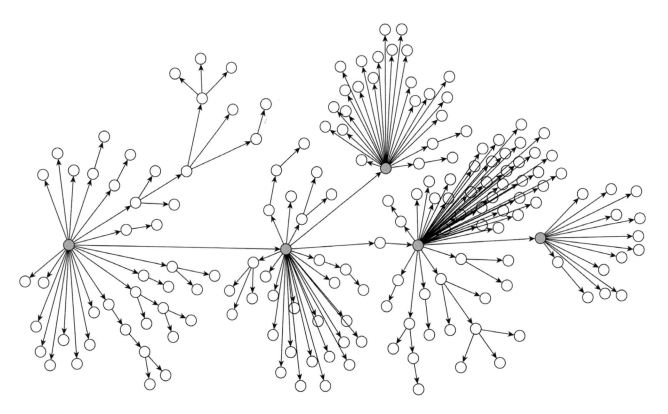

Figure 16.1   Contact tracing of a outbreak of severe acute respiratory syndrome (SARS) in a hospital in Singapore.[51] One hundred and eighteen (69 per cent) of the 172 cases were recorded as secondary cases from just five 'superspreaders' (shaded).

controls, and personal protection equipment.[60] Delayed isolation and admission to a non-isolation facility may also have been factors associated with increased transmission,[4,5] and engineering controls such as negative-pressure isolation rooms, anterooms, local ventilation and the physical isolation of SARS cases may have been important in reducing possible transmission.[17,60]

The use of personal protective equipment such as gloves, gowns, surgical masks or N95 respirators had differing degrees of effectiveness, but their simultaneous and proper use lowered exposure risks.[32,37,61,62] Gowns and masks effectively prevented SARS contraction among healthcare workers during the Vietnamese and Hong Kong outbreaks.[16,32] However, the use of surgical masks versus N95 respirators was a subject of controversy during the SARS epidemic,[32,63,64] especially important during times of supply shortage. The use of surgical masks appeared to be effective in the Vietnamese experience, when N95 respirators were unavailable early in the outbreak.[16] An important factor contributing to the lower patient-to-healthcare worker transmission rate was the proper use of personal protective equipment, which required training and fit-testing. Proper fit-testing and the consistent proper use of personal protective equipment were important factors in reducing the contraction risk.[65,66]

A wide range of administrative and work practice controls were used in conjunction with personal protective equipment to reduce the risk of exposure of healthcare workers. Hospital interventions included patient triaging, the quarantine of exposed individuals, the prevention of interfacility patient and staff transfer, the establishment of a dedicated SARS team, visitor restrictions, and temperature monitoring of workers, among other infection control measures.[4,10,67] The early identification of probable SARS cases was essential in preventing and containing outbreaks.[5,7] Temperature-monitoring enabled the early detection of SARS in healthcare workers in some settings, while the establishment of a SARS team limited staff-to-patient transmission risks. Dedicating a local hospital to SARS and closing down emergency departments were among several larger-scale interventions used.[10] Due to the difficulty and inconsistency in the implementation of infection control measures within emergency departments, dedicating an entire SARS facility may be more practical and efficient, especially in the future, when large-scale outbreaks that would overwhelm the capacity of a dedicated facility appear unlikely.[68–70]

Despite the importance of infection control strategies in containing the SARS epidemic, there were individuals hospitalized with SARS who did not cause nosocomial outbreaks in the absence of infection control measures.[37] Evidence suggested that patient factors also played a role in determining the intensity of transmission. For example, more severe disease, proxied by lactate dehydrogenase levels,[22,27] was associated with a higher risk of transmission.[5]

FUTURE EPIDEMICS

SARS-like coronaviruses isolated from bats are thought to be the ancestors of the SARS coronavirus,[71,72] while similar viruses have also been isolated from civet cats,[73] a potential animal reservoir and the likely route into humans via live animal markets; many of the early cases were among butchers and chefs working with exotic meats. Re-emergence of the virus into humans remains possible, and the trading of civet cats in animal markets continues in Guangdong province despite its official ban.[74] However if SARS were to re-emerge in the immediate future, it is unlikely that large-scale outbreaks would result provided that the initial cases were handled with appropriate caution.

The SARS outbreak was in many ways a lucky escape.[75] Fundamentally, the virus does not possess the epidemiological properties that would allow it to spread more easily (i.e. a low basic reproductive number, especially subject to social distancing and nosocomial infection control interventions) or more quickly (i.e. a relatively longer generation or doubling time, compared, for example, with influenza). However, precisely because of this reason and subject to the SARS coronavirus not mutating into something more sinister from a public health viewpoint, the incentive to develop and mass-produce a vaccine appears a distant possibility. There is as yet no effective therapy to treat those infected. If a SARS-like virus were to emerge in 20 or 30 years' time, it is entirely possible that the collective knowledge and memory of the healthcare profession in the region in which SARS emerged might have waned substantially. If that is the case, initial clusters would not be recognized with sufficient speed and another global outbreak would become more likely.

Therefore lessons learned from the 2002–03 outbreak must be heeded, and corrective action followed through and institutionalized as standard infection control processes in healthcare facilities, much like bloodborne and gastrointestinal universal precautions against human immunodeficiency virus/hepatitis or *Clostridium difficile* infection.[76–79] Moreover, another respiratory pathogen sharing many similar features with SARS coronavirus, pandemic influenza or even interpandemic disease might be much more difficult to control, the three influenza pandemics of the twentieth century having resulted in unprecedented morbidity and mortality over only a few months each time.[80] Now is the time to develop, trial, implement and evaluate universal respiratory precautions in the design of hospitals and clinical operations.[76–79]

ACKNOWLEDGMENTS

We gratefully acknowledge research funding from the Research Fund for the Control of Infectious Diseases of the Government of the Hong Kong SAR. We thank Trevor Yuen for invaluable assistance with this literature review, as well as Vicky Fang for assistance in drawing the figure.

REFERENCES

● = Key primary paper

◆ = Major review article

1. World Health Organization. Summary of Probable SARS Cases with Onset of Illness from 1 November 2002 to 31 July 2003. Available from: http://www.who.int/csr/sars/country/table2004_04_21/en/index.html (accessed September 21, 2009).

2. Wong TW, Lee CK, Tam W et al. Cluster of SARS among medical students exposed to single patient, Hong Kong. Emerg Infect Dis 2004; 10: 269–76.

3. Reynolds MG, Anh BH, Thu VH et al. Factors associated with nosocomial SARS-CoV transmission among healthcare workers in Hanoi, Vietnam, 2003. BMC Public Health 2006; 6: 207.

4. Liu JW, Lu SN, Chen SS et al. Epidemiologic study and containment of a nosocomial outbreak of severe acute respiratory syndrome in a medical center in Kaohsiung, Taiwan. Infect Control Hosp Epidemiol 2006; 27: 466–72.

5. Chen MI, Chow AL, Earnest A et al. Clinical and epidemiological predictors of transmission in severe acute respiratory syndrome (SARS). BMC Infect Dis 2006; 6: 151.

6. Chen MI, Leo YS, Ang BS et al. The outbreak of SARS at Tan Tock Seng Hospital – relating epidemiology to control. Ann Acad Med Singapore 2006; 35: 317–25.

7. Chen MI, Loon SC, Leong HN, Leo YS. Understanding the super-spreading events of SARS in Singapore. Ann Acad Med Singapore 2006; 35: 390–4.

8. Kwok KO, Leung GM, Lam WY, Riley S. Using models to identify routes of nosocomial infection: a large hospital outbreak of SARS in Hong Kong. Proc Biol Sci 2007; 274: 611–17.

9. Varia M, Wilson S, Sarwal S et al. Investigation of a nosocomial outbreak of severe acute respiratory syndrome (SARS) in Toronto, Canada. CMAJ 2003; 169: 285–92.

10. Gopalakrishna G, Choo P, Leo YS et al. SARS transmission and hospital containment. Emerg Infect Dis 2004; 10: 395–400.

11. Li L, Cheng S, Gu J. SARS infection among health care workers in Beijing, China. JAMA 2003; 290: 2662–3.

12. Wang SX, Li YM, Sun BC et al. The SARS outbreak in a general hospital in Tianjin, China – the case of super-spreader. Epidemiol Infect 2006; 134: 786–91.

●13. Zhong NS, Zheng BJ, Li YM et al. Epidemiology and cause of severe acute respiratory syndrome (SARS) in Guangdong, People's Republic of China, in February, 2003. Lancet 2003; 362: 1353–8.

14. Update: Outbreak of Severe Acute Respiratory Syndrome - Worldwide, 2003. Morb Mortal Wkly Rep 2003; 52: 241–8.

15. Cowling BJ, Muller MP, Wong IO et al. Alternative methods of estimating an incubation distribution: examples from severe acute respiratory syndrome. Epidemiology 2007; 18: 253–9.

16. Nishiura H, Kuratsuji T, Quy T et al. Rapid awareness and transmission of severe acute respiratory syndrome in Hanoi French Hospital, Vietnam. Am J Trop Med Hyg 2005; 73: 17–25.

17. McDonald LC, Simor AE, Su IJ et al. SARS in healthcare facilities, Toronto and Taiwan. Emerg Infect Dis 2004; 10: 777–81.

18. Gu J, Korteweg C. Pathology and pathogenesis of severe acute respiratory syndrome. Am J Pathol 2007; 170: 1136–47.

19. Poutanen SM, Low DE, Henry B et al. Identification of severe acute respiratory syndrome in Canada. N Engl J Med 2003; 348: 1995–2005.

20. Tsang KW, Ho PL, Ooi GC et al. A cluster of cases of severe acute respiratory syndrome in Hong Kong. N Engl J Med 2003; 348: 1977–85.

21. Lee N, Hui D, Wu A et al. A major outbreak of severe acute respiratory syndrome in Hong Kong. N Engl J Med 2003; 348: 1986–94.

22. Cowling BJ, Muller MP, Wong IO et al. Clinical prognostic rules for severe acute respiratory syndrome in low- and high-resource settings. Arch Intern Med 2006; 166: 1505–11.

23. Grinblat L, Shulman H, Glickman A et al. Severe acute respiratory syndrome: radiographic review of 40 probable cases in Toronto, Canada. Radiology 2003; 228: 802–9.

24. Cheng PK, Wong DA, Tong LK et al. Viral shedding patterns of coronavirus in patients with probable severe acute respiratory syndrome. Lancet 2004; 363: 1699–700.

●25. Peiris JS, Chu CM, Cheng VC et al. Clinical progression and viral load in a community outbreak of coronavirus-associated SARS pneumonia: a prospective study. Lancet 2003; 361: 1767–72.

26. Cai QC, Xu QF, Xu JM et al. Refined estimate of the incubation period of severe acute respiratory syndrome and related influencing factors. Am J Epidemiol 2006; 163: 211–16.

27. Leung GM, Hedley AJ, Ho LM et al. The epidemiology of severe acute respiratory syndrome in the 2003 Hong Kong epidemic: an analysis of all 1755 patients. Ann Intern Med 2004; 141: 662–73.

28. Donnelly CA, Ghani AC, Leung GM et al. Epidemiological determinants of spread of causal agent of severe acute respiratory syndrome in Hong Kong. Lancet 2003; 361: 1761–6.

29. Liang WN, Liu M, Chen Q et al. Assessment of impacts of public health interventions on the SARS epidemic in Beijing in terms of the intervals between its symptom onset, hospital admission, and notification. Biomed Environ Sci 2005; 18: 153–8.

30. Leung GM, Lim WW, Ho LM et al. Seroprevalence of IgG antibodies to SARS-coronavirus in asymptomatic or subclinical population groups. Epidemiol Infect 2006; 134: 211–21.

31. Ho AS, Sung JJ, Chan-Yeung M. An outbreak of severe acute respiratory syndrome among hospital workers in a community hospital in Hong Kong. Ann Intern Med 2003; 139: 564–7.

●32. Seto WH, Tsang D, Yung RW et al. Effectiveness of precautions against droplets and contact in prevention of nosocomial transmission of severe acute respiratory syndrome (SARS). Lancet 2003; 361: 1519–20.

◆33. Li Y, Leung GM, Tang JW et al. Role of ventilation in airborne transmission of infectious agents in the built environment – a multidisciplinary systematic review. Indoor Air 2007; 17: 2–18.

34. Yu IT, Li Y, Wong TW et al. Evidence of airborne transmission of the severe acute respiratory syndrome virus. N Engl J Med 2004; 350: 1731–9.

35. Park BJ, Peck AJ, Kuehnert MJ et al. Lack of SARS transmission among healthcare workers, United States. Emerg Infect Dis 2004; 10: 244–8.

36. Peck AJ, Newbern EC, Feikin DR et al. Lack of SARS transmission and US SARS case-patient. Emerg Infect Dis 2004; 10: 217–24.

37. Chen YC, Chen PJ, Chang SC et al. Infection control and SARS transmission among healthcare workers, Taiwan. Emerg Infect Dis 2004; 10: 895–8.

38. Weinstein RA. Planning for epidemics – the lessons of SARS. N Engl J Med 2004; 350: 2332–4.

39. Roy CJ, Milton DK. Airborne transmission of communicable infection – the elusive pathway. N Engl J Med 2004; 350: 1710–12.

40. Yu IT, Sung JJ. The epidemiology of the outbreak of severe acute respiratory syndrome (SARS) in Hong Kong – what we do know and what we don't. Epidemiol Infect 2004; 132: 781–6.

41. Dowell SF, Simmerman JM, Erdman DD et al. Severe acute respiratory syndrome coronavirus on hospital surfaces. Clin Infect Dis 2004; 39: 652–7.

42. Lau JT, Tsui H, Lau M, Yang X. SARS transmission, risk factors, and prevention in Hong Kong. Emerg Infect Dis 2004; 10: 587–92.

43. Anderson RM, May RM. Infectious Diseases of Humans: Dynamics and Control. Oxford: Oxford University Press, 1991.

44. Lipsitch M, Cohen T, Cooper B et al. Transmission dynamics and control of severe acute respiratory syndrome. Science 2003; 300: 1966–70.

45. Riley S, Fraser C, Donnelly CA et al. Transmission dynamics of the etiological agent of SARS in Hong Kong: impact of public health interventions. Science 2003; 300: 1961–6.

46. Fraser C, Riley S, Anderson RM, Ferguson NM. Factors that make an infectious disease outbreak controllable. Proc Natl Acad Sci USA 2004; 101: 6146–51.

●47. Lloyd-Smith JO, Schreiber SJ, Kopp PE, Getz WM. Superspreading and the effect of individual variation on disease emergence. Nature 2005; 438: 355–9.

48. Leung GM, Chung PH, Tsang T et al. SARS-CoV antibody prevalence in all Hong Kong patient contacts. [erratum appears in Emerg Infect Dis 2004 Oct; 10(10): 1890]. Emerg Infect Dis 2004; 10: 1653–6.

◆49. Leung GM, Lim WW, Ho LM et al. Seroprevalence of IgG antibodies to SARS-coronavirus in asymptomatic or subclinical population groups. Epidemiol Infect 2003; 134: 211–21.

50. Pitzer VE, Leung GM, Lipsitch M. Estimating variability in the transmission of severe acute respiratory syndrome to household contacts in Hong Kong, China. Am J Epidemiol 2007; 166: 355–63.

51. Severe acute respiratory syndrome – Singapore, 2003. Morb Mortal Wkly Rep 2003; 52: 405–11.

52. Wilder-Smith A, Teleman MD, Heng BH et al. Asymptomatic SARS coronavirus infection among healthcare workers, Singapore. Emerg Infect Dis 2005; 11: 1142–5.

53. Ho MS, Su IJ. Preparing to prevent severe acute respiratory syndrome and other respiratory infections. Lancet Infect Dis 2004; 4: 684–9.

54. Ofner-Agostini M, Wallington T, Henry B et al. Investigation of the second wave (phase 2) of severe acute respiratory syndrome (SARS) in Toronto, Canada. What happened? Can Commun Dis Rep 2008; 34: 1–11.

55. Dwosh HA, Hong HH, Austgarden D et al. Identification and containment of an outbreak of SARS in a community hospital. CMAJ 2003; 168: 1415–20.

56. Lee N, Sung JJ. Nosocomial transmission of SARS. Curr Infect Dis Rep 2003; 5: 473–6.

57. Seto WH, Ching TY, Ho PL. Understanding and ensuring that infection control of SARS is achievable in the hospital. In: Chan JCK, Wong VCW (eds) Challenges of Severe Acute Respiratory Syndrome. Oxford: Elsevier, 2006: Chapter 10.

58. Yen MY, Lin YE, Su IJ et al. Using an integrated infection control strategy during outbreak control to minimize nosocomial infection of severe acute respiratory syndrome among healthcare workers. J Hosp Infect 2006; 62: 195–9.

59. Tsai MC, Arnold JL, Chuang CC et al. Impact of an outbreak of severe acute respiratory syndrome on a hospital in Taiwan, ROC. Emerg Med J 2004; 21: 311–16.

60. Thorne CD, Khozin S, McDiarmid MA. Using the hierarchy of control technologies to improve healthcare facility infection control: lessons from severe acute respiratory syndrome. J Occup Environ Med 2004; 46: 613–22.

61. Chia SE, Koh D, Fones C et al. Appropriate use of personal protective equipment among healthcare workers in public sector hospitals and primary healthcare polyclinics during the SARS outbreak in Singapore. Occup Environ Med 2005; 62: 473–7.

62. Gomersall CD, Joynt GM, Ho OM et al. Transmission of SARS to healthcare workers. The experience of a Hong Kong ICU. Intensive Care Med 2006; 32: 564–9.

◆63. Gamage B, Moore D, Copes R et al. Protecting health care workers from SARS and other respiratory pathogens: a review of the infection control literature. Am J Infect Control 2005; 33: 114–21.

64. Loeb M, McGeer A, Henry B et al. SARS among critical care nurses, Toronto. Emerg Infect Dis 2004; 10: 251–5.

65. Ofner-Agostini M, Gravel D, McDonald LC et al. Cluster of cases of severe acute respiratory syndrome among Toronto healthcare workers after implementation of infection control precautions: a case series. Infect Control Hosp Epidemiol 2006; 27: 473–8.

66. Lau JT, Fung KS, Wong TW et al. SARS transmission among hospital workers in Hong Kong. *Emerg Infect Dis* 2004; **10**: 280–6.

67. Ho PL, Tang XP, Seto WH. SARS: hospital infection control and admission strategies. *Respirology* 2003; **8**(Suppl.): S41–5.

68. Chang WT, Kao CL, Chung MY et al. SARS exposure and emergency department workers. *Emerg Infect Dis* 2004; **10**: 1117–19.

69. Chen WK, Cheng YC, Chung YT, Lin CC. The impact of the SARS outbreak on an urban emergency department in Taiwan. *Med Care* 2005; **43**: 168–72.

70. Chen WK, Wu HD, Lin CC, Cheng YC. Emergency department response to SARS, Taiwan. *Emerg Infect Dis* 2005; **11**: 1067–73.

71. Chu DK, Poon LL, Chan KH et al. Coronaviruses in bent-winged bats (*Miniopterus* spp.). *J Gen Virol* 2006; **87**: 2461–6.

72. Li W, Shi Z, Yu M et al. Bats are natural reservoirs of SARS-like coronaviruses. *Science* 2005; **310**: 676–9.

73. Wang M, Yan M, Xu H et al. SARS-CoV infection in a restaurant from palm civet. *Emerg Infect Dis* 2005; **11**: 1860–5.

74. Chen H. Civet Cats Found at Restaurants Again. *China Daily*, February 14, 2007. Available from: http://www. chinadaily.com.cn/china/2007–02/14/content_808890.htm (accessed September 21, 2009).

75. Wallinga J, Teunis P. Different epidemic curves for severe acute respiratory syndrome reveal similar impacts of control measures. *Am J Epidemiol* 2004; **160**: 509–16.

76. Onodera N, Sakurai S, Kobayashi S. [Effectiveness of newly applied infection control policies to suppress the number of cases with hospital-acquired influenza infection at Iwate Medical University Hospital – comparison of the 2004/5 and 2005/6 seasons]. *Kansenshogaku Zasshi* 2007; **81**: 681–8.

77. Gagneur A, Vallet S, Talbot PJ et al. Outbreaks of human coronavirus in a paediatric and neonatal intensive care unit. *Eur J Pediatr* 2008; **167**: 1427–34.

78. Leekha S, Zitterkopf NL, Espy MJ et al. Duration of influenza A virus shedding in hospitalized patients and implications for infection control. *Infect Control Hosp Epidemiol* 2007; **28**: 1071–6.

79. Salgado CD, Giannetta ET, Hayden FG, Farr BM. Preventing nosocomial influenza by improving the vaccine acceptance rate of clinicians. *Infect Control Hosp Epidemiol* 2004; **25**: 923–8.

80. Morens DM, Fauci AS. The 1918 influenza pandemic: insights for the 21st century. *J Infect Dis* 2007; **195**: 1018–28.

17

Epidemic and pandemic influenza

JONATHAN S. NGUYEN-VAN-TAM

Of all the respiratory virus infections that affect humans, influenza stands out as by far the most important. Through a combination of regular (winter) seasonal epidemics and occasional pandemics, the total morbidity and mortality inflicted by the virus is immense. In recent years, even greater attention has been refocused on influenza due to the threat to human health posed by avian influenza viruses, most notably influenza A/H5N1 and A/H7N7. Although the timing of a pandemic is always unpredictable, many experts considered that the next one was overdue; few, however, perceived the most likely source to be an A/H1N1 virus, or Mexico to be the most obvious epicentre. This most recent turn of events in the history of human influenza proves above all else that the disease remains highly unpredictable.

CLINICAL PRESENTATION

Human influenza presents as an acute illness characterized predominantly by cough, malaise and feverishness (each of these occurring in over 80 per cent of adult cases), typically of rapid onset. Other additional symptoms (in order of frequency) are: (50–79 per cent of cases) chills, headache, anorexia, coryza, myalgia and sore throat; (less than 50 per cent) new or changed sputum, dizziness, hoarseness, chest pain; (below 10 per cent) vomiting and diarrhoea.[1] A typical illness lasts up to 5 days.

In most individuals, influenza is self-limiting; however, a severe and often fatal primary viral pneumonia is occasionally described. A range of secondary complications may also occur, including acute bronchitis, pneumonia, otitis media (in children), myocarditis, pericarditis and neurological sequelae (febrile convulsions and Reye's syndrome in children; encephalitis).[1] Although the most common complication is acute bronchitis, the most significant is bacterial pneumonia, for which the common organisms described are *Streptococcus pneumoniae*, *Staphylococcus aureus* and *Haemophilus influenzae*.[2] Across the three influenza pandemics of the twentieth century, the incidence of bacterial pneumonia complicating influenza was estimated to be in the range of 15–20 per cent.[3,4]

In some patients, recovery from influenza is followed by a period of fatigue and lethargy lasting up to several weeks. Influenza is associated with more severe outcomes in the following groups: neonates and children under 2 years of age; the elderly, especially those over 75 years; and persons with underlying co-morbidities (e.g. asthma, diabetes, chronic obstructive pulmonary disease and cardiac failure) in whom the acute infection may destabilize the underlying condition.[5]

VIROLOGY, CLASSIFICATION AND ANIMAL RESERVOIRS

Influenza viruses are negative-strand RNA viruses from the family *Orthomyxoviridae* and are classified into three subtypes, denoted A, B and C. Influenza A and B are associated with the classical syndromic picture of influenza in humans, described above, and are considered to be of major public health importance. In contrast, influenza C causes a mild respiratory illness and is considered to be a rarer cause of the milder 'common cold' syndrome and, on its own, of relatively low public health significance.[6]

Influenza A is further classified into subtypes denoted by the combination of haemagglutinin and neuraminidase antigens expressed on the surface of the virus. In total there are 16 haemagglutinins, the most recent of these described in 2005,[7] and nine neuraminidases. This explains the notation A/H5N1, A/H3N2, etc. In contrast, influenza B is much less antigenically heterogeneous and is therefore not classified into subtypes. Nevertheless, both influenza A and B viruses exhibit the high error rate during replication typical of RNA viruses, and therefore mutate frequently into new antigenically distinct strains (*antigenic drift*), especially influenza A. This antigenic variability explains the need to incorporate new strains into seasonal influenza vaccines on an almost annual basis. New strains are classified according to the date and location in which they were first described, for example A/Solomon Island/3/2006; B/Malaysia/2506/2004.

In addition to the phenomenon of antigenic drift, influenza A viruses have the unique potential for variability by a second more dramatic means. Influenza A viruses may acquire novel haemagglutinin or neuraminidase antigens from the pool of available antigens in the environment, which are different from those currently established in humans. This is believed to occur through a process of genetic reassortment brought about through co-infection of a susceptible species (e.g. the pig) with an animal (avian) influenza virus and a human influenza virus.[8,9] This process is known as *antigenic shift* and believed to have been responsible for some, such as the 1957 (A/H1N1) and 1968 (A/H3N2), but not all of the human pandemics of the twentieth century.[10,11]

It is important to note that although surface antigens may be fully substituted during antigenic shift, not all the internal genetic material is bound to change. For example, influenza A/H1N1 was replaced in human circulation in 1957 by a new pandemic virus with entirely different surface antigens (A/H2N2), but although four new genes were acquired, the remainder were preserved from the previous human A/H1N1 virus.[11] Until recently, the classical understanding was that antigenic shift was the means by which a new human pandemic virus emerged. However the re-emergence of influenza A/H1N1 in 1977, after its previous disappearance in 1956, was not associated with a pandemic.[12,13] There is now evidence that the virus that produced the greatest ever human pandemic in 1918 (A/H1N1) originated from an avian virus but was definitely mammalian by 1918, suggesting that it may have been adapting in humans for some time before the pandemic began, through a process of gradual genetic change rather than abrupt reassortment.[14]

The realization that human influenza pandemics may occur as a result of *genetic adaptation* as well as antigenic shift has heightened concern about the pandemic threat posed by the current zoonotic spread of A/H5N1 in birds and its rare incursion into humans and possible early signs of adaptation (see box p. 221). However, the recent emergence of a novel A/H1N1 virus has rechallenged many previous assumptions about the emergence of pandemic influenza. Although the new pandemic virus is a genuine reassortment,[15] it is of the same subtype as the A/H1N1 viruses that have circulated constantly since 1977. It is therefore the first known occasion on which a human pandemic virus has emerged from the same subtype as a virus currently in circulation (see box p. 221). Nevertheless, human pandemics have only ever been described due to influenza A viruses, and it is believed that only they, and not influenza B viruses, have pandemic potential.

Influenza B is considered to be a human pathogen with a human reservoir. In contrast, influenza A is considered to have an extensive environmental reservoir in birds, notably wild aquatic shore birds, although a fairly wide variety of mammalian species can also be infected, including pigs,[16] horses,[17] seals,[18] mink[19] and whales.[20] The emergence of A/H5N1 in humans in 1997,[21] and its rapid re-emergence in 2003, prompting concerns about a pandemic, have also led to important observational and experimental findings demonstrating inherent susceptibility and transmissibility within other species, notably felids such as tigers,[22,23] leopards,[23] and domestic cats.[24,25]

THE HISTORY OF EPIDEMICS AND PANDEMICS

Although the influenza virus was first identified in 1933,[26] accounts of 'epidemic fevers' in historical texts reveal possible influenza epidemics and pandemics as far back as the mid-sixteenth century.[27] Although virological confirmation is impossible, these past events are described as explosive outbreaks of febrile respiratory illness associated with rapid community spread and often excess mortality; they are therefore most likely to have been due to influenza. The origin of the word 'influenza' is unknown, but it may be derived from the Latin language, in which the occurrence of the disease was commonly attributed to the influence of adverse astrological events. In time, this may have led to a modified expression *influenza del freddo*, meaning 'influence of the cold'. The word influenza is believed to have first been used in English in 1743, when it was adopted, with an anglicized pronunciation, during an outbreak of the disease in Europe. It is suggested that an average of three or four human pandemics occur each century, giving a roughly 3–4 per cent annual risk.[28]

There is sero-archaeological evidence linking influenza to human pandemics since the late nineteenth century. It is almost certain that a human pandemic occurred in 1889,[27] and that the A/H2 and A/H3 subtypes circulated in humans between 1889 and the emergence of A/H1N1 in 1918.[29] In the twentieth century, pandemics occurred due to A/H1N1 in 1918 ('Spanish flu'), A/H2N2 in 1957 ('Asian flu') and A/H3N2 in 1968 ('Hong Kong flu'). In 1976 in Fort Dix, New Jersey, USA, an outbreak of influenza A/H1N1 ('swine flu') occurred in a closed military institution but failed to spread into the wider community, although it prompted widespread fears of a further pandemic like the one in 1918,[30] and triggered a mass vaccination programme across the USA. One year later, influenza A/H1N1 did re-emerge in humans, but did not displace A/H3N2 or produce a human pandemic, the reasons for which are unknown. However, the 1977 virus was most closely related to one that circulated in 1946, and not to the 1918 virus.[12,13]

Besides the occurrence of pandemic influenza, influenza occurs seasonally, producing regular epidemics. These tend to be larger and more severe in the years soon after a pandemic, and to become smaller in impact after a subtype has been in circulation for several decades. This phenomenon has been observed in the UK over the last two decades, where the last sizeable epidemic was in 1989[31] but activity has been exceptionally low since the millennium winter of 1999/2000 (Figure 17.1).[32] Nevertheless, it has been suggested that cumulative morbidity and mortality of seasonal influenza both exceed that of the rarer pandemic variety;[33] it should therefore not be underestimated as a major public health issue.

EPIDEMIOLOGY OF SEASONAL INFLUENZA

The epidemiology of seasonal influenza is characterized by winter epidemics of variable size in the temperate zones of the world, each one typically lasting 8–10 weeks. Usually, one influenza A subtype (H3N2 or H1N1) or influenza B will dominate during the epidemic period, but this is far from always the case and 'mixed epidemics' are possible. Over the remainder of the winter period (November to March in the northern hemisphere), influenza continues to circulate at much lower levels, and A/H3N2, A/H1N1 and B are all usually recognized. Although not much

diagnosed clinically by medical practitioners during the warmer summer months, influenza outbreaks are well described,[34,35] suggesting that virus circulates all year round. In tropical and subtropical zones, the seasonality of influenza is much less polarized – indeed, some regions regularly experience two separate peaks per annum, corresponding with the rainy seasons.[36,37]

Many theories abound for why influenza seasonality occurs, including the influence of solar radiation (ultraviolet light),[38] the effects of temperature and humidity on virus survival,[39,40] and also social theories relating to human overcrowding, indoor living and reduced home ventilation during the winter.[41,42] No single theory has been proven, and although the hypothesis based on patterns of human interaction during the colder winter months seems very intuitive, the issue is almost certainly multifactorial. Longitudinal studies of respiratory virus infection in families that took place in the late 1960s and 1970s in the USA have established that seasonal influenza is characterized by a high annual attack rate in children and teenagers, which declines markedly with age.[43,44] This is especially true for influenza B, which affects adults much less frequently.[45]

In contrast, although attack rates in the elderly are lowest, infection in this group is undoubtedly associated with the highest levels of morbidity, mortality and consequential effects on health services. Excess mortality in the elderly clearly distinguishes influenza from other respiratory viruses, except perhaps respiratory syncytial virus (RSV). It is now well recognized that, when a severe epidemic occurs, influenza produces a surplus of deaths in the elderly over and above those which would have occurred anyway in the winter.[33] Similarly, at all ages, the rate of secondary complications due to influenza infection are higher in persons with underlying co-morbidities, for

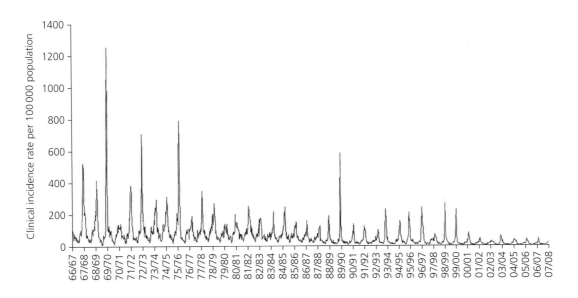

Figure 17.1 Clinical incidence of influenza-like illness in England and Wales per 100 000 population, 1967–2007. (Data kindly supplied by the Royal College of General Practitioners Sentinel Primary Care Network – Weekly Returns Service.)

example asthma, chronic obstructive pulmonary disease and diabetes, compared with those who are 'healthy'.[5] This explains why influenza vaccines should be targeted at the elderly and those with chronic illness.

Subclinical (asymptomatic) infections are well described in the large sero-epidemiological surveys, and typically account for about 50 per cent of all serologically detectable infections.[45,46] This illustrates that although influenza is described classically as a severe respiratory illness, it often also presents in milder forms that, without the use of sensitive diagnostic techniques such as the polymerase chain reaction, are difficult to distinguish from the host of other common acute respiratory virus infections that occur each winter. Thus, epidemiological and vaccine effectiveness studies are particularly challenging to perform.

Although influenza in children is widely recognized, and in most cases is non-serious, there is a recent growing awareness that the number of hospitalizations of children associated with influenza is higher than was initially recognized.[47] These studies are gradually changing the evidence base in favour of more widespread vaccination of children, although it has long been asserted that vaccinating children might have a favourable effect on household transmission, thereby reducing the incidence in adults,[48] a finding that is now supported by new modelling data in a pandemic context.[49]

INFLUENZA TRANSMISSION AND SURVIVAL

Surprisingly little is known about influenza transmission. Although it is assumed that the virus is transmitted predominantly by the respiratory route, i.e. through coughing and sneezing, the relative contributions of large particles (droplets over 5 μm in size), which travel short distances and settle quickly, small particles and droplet nuclei, both with the potential to stay suspended for far longer and travel further, and contact transmission (direct from person to person, and indirect via fomites) are not adequately understood.[50] The role of aerosol transmission is particularly hotly debated.[51] Most epidemiological studies and the descriptions from nosocomial outbreaks point to short-range transmission that occurs principally via large particles (droplets),[52] except in certain healthcare settings where known aerosol-generating procedures (e.g. endotracheal intubation) are being performed. But definitive research in this area is badly needed.

Infected individuals shed influenza virus in proportion to the severity of their symptoms and the level of their fever,[53] so it can be inferred that they are most infectious to others very soon after the onset of symptoms. An adult is likely to remain infectious to others for 3–5 days after the onset of symptoms, by which time virus shedding is usually very low.[54,55] However, it is known that children and the immunocompromised may excrete virus for much longer periods and that virus titres in young children tend to be higher than in adults.[53,56–59] The role of asymptomatic

persons in transmission is not adequately known but is likely to be substantially lower, although still rarely described.[60,61]

Influenza virus survival is also incompletely understood. Data that are almost 30 years old, generated by Bean et al., suggest that human influenza viruses survive on hard, non-porous surfaces, in quantities that are transferable to hands, for up to 24 hours, but only for up to 2 hours on soft porous surfaces.[62] However, these data do not assist in understanding the deposition of viruses from naturally coughing and sneezing patients, or the true extent to which detectability on surfaces equates with the potential to infect others. It is known that avian influenza viruses can survive on experimentally contaminated surfaces for at least 6 days at 37 °C,[63] but survival is prolonged, for at least 1 month, in cold agricultural and aquatic environments.

Although these data may assist in the conduct of environmental disinfection following avian influenza outbreaks in poultry premises, they do not assist in our understanding of influenza transmission from person to person. The influenza virus is not robust, and hand-washing with soap and water will inactivate the virus in human settings, as will alcohol-based cleansers.[64] A better understanding of human influenza transmission and environmental survival would help towards making clearer recommendations for seasonal and pandemic infection control procedures in healthcare settings and in the home, especially regarding the roles of environmental cleaning and respiratory personal protective equipment.

EPIDEMIOLOGY OF PANDEMIC INFLUENZA

An influenza pandemic occurs when a novel influenza virus emerges in humans that is antigenically unrelated to its immediate predecessors (those influenza A viruses in current circulation), i.e. there is little or no population immunity or cross-protection. In addition, the new virus must be capable of causing clinically significant illness and must spread efficiently from person to person. In the case of the novel influenza A/H1N1 pandemic virus, all of these conditions have been fulfilled, even though the virus is of the same subtype as one of the currently circulating interpandemic viruses (seasonal A/H1N1).

The pandemic of 1918, caused by influenza A/H1N1, was the most devastating in human history.[65] It is conservatively estimated that about 40 million persons died worldwide. The pandemic occurred in three distinct waves in the northern hemisphere: the first in spring/summer 1918, which was relatively small in size and intensity; the second in autumn 1918, which was the most severe wave; and the third in early 1919, which was of moderate intensity.[66] It is notable that the severe second wave and the moderate third wave both occurred during winter in the northern hemisphere, suggesting that pandemic influenza also has a winter seasonal predilection. After the emergence of the 1918 virus, the pattern of age-specific mortality changed dramatically from being highest in the elderly to highest in young adults of working age.[66] A similar change, if repeated in a future pandemic, will have major implications for critical national infrastructures and business continuity. Overall in 1918/19, the case fatality rate due to pandemic influenza was 2.5 per cent.

The subsequent pandemics of 1957 and 1968 were comparatively mild. Case fatality rates were in the order of 0.4–0.5 per cent and it is estimated that around 1 million persons died in each.[66] It is also hypothesized that the difference in severity between 1918 on the one hand and 1957 and 1968 on the other might relate to the fact that the former probably emerged by genetic adaptation,[14] whereas the latter two emerged by genetic reassortment.[10,11] Nevertheless, in all three pandemics of the twentieth century there are remarkable similarities in population clinical attack rates, which all lie in the narrow range of 33–45 per cent.

PANDEMIC PREPAREDNESS

Because of the serious potential impact of a future pandemic,[67,68] many governments have been involved in detailed preparedness planning. Rapid globalization since the last pandemic in 1968 means that spread will be extremely rapid when the next one occurs,[69] as has already proved to be the case with the novel A/H1N1 pandemic virus. Although influenza A/H5N1 ('avian flu') may well have been regarded by many as the most likely current threat, and has certainly provided the stimulus for action to many nations, it was by no means certain that the next pandemic would emerge from an H5 progenitor virus.

While it would be unlikely that a true pandemic vaccine would ever be available until at least 6 months after the next pandemic virus emerged, far more can now be done to prepare than was possible in 1968. Neuraminidase inhibitors offer a therapeutic approach to pandemic influenza that is not subtype specific,[70] although there are certain risks inherent in stockpiling associated with the possible emergence of resistance,[71,72] and logistic challenges regarding rapid population access. Strategies based on treatment alone may have far less impact than those based on treatment and household post-exposure prophylaxis, but the amount of drugs needed for each strategy varies dramatically as well.[49] Governments should also consider the role to be played by antibiotics in the treatment of secondary bacterial pneumonia, and these also warrant consideration of stockpiling.[2] Finally, biomathematical modelling has confirmed the potential importance of public health countermeasures such as school closures,[49] and the likely futility of others such as international travel restrictions and entry screening at ports.[69,73]

In addition, the first human A/H5N1 vaccine is now available in Europe for pre-pandemic use, and several more are reaching licensure. Some governments may decide to acquire these as an additional safeguard against a future H5 pandemic. The available data already suggest that these vaccines will be highly immunogenic (two doses usually being required) and offer marked cross-protection between virus clades of the same subtype.[74–76] Even a poorly matched A/H5N1 vaccine given to a large proportion of the population in advance of a pandemic (of the same subtype) will be likely to have marked public health benefit.[49] The same technologies used to develop human H5N1 vaccines are now being applied very rapidly to the development of vaccines against the novel A/H1N1 pandemic virus, but the occurrence of an A/H1N1 pandemic in 2009 does not imply that the threat from A/H5N1 has suddenly receded.

CONCLUSION

Influenza continues to pose a major public health threat in both its epidemic and pandemic forms. Although the epidemiology of influenza in humans is well described, relatively little is still known about its transmission from person to person and its survival in the environment. In addition, the burden of disease in children may be underrecognized. Because of rapid globalization, the threat posed by a pandemic is considerable. However, neuraminidase inhibitors and novel vaccines are now available to supplement public health countermeasures.

REFERENCES

● = Key primary paper
◆ = Major review article

◆1. Nicholson KG. Human influenza. In: Nicholson KG, Webster RG, Hay AJ (eds) *Textbook of Influenza*. Oxford: Blackwell Science, 1998: 219–64.

◆2. Gupta RK, George R, Nguyen-Van-Tam JS. Bacterial pneumonia and pandemic influenza planning. *Emerg Infect Dis* 2008; **14**: 1187–92.

◆3. Brundage JF. Interactions between influenza and bacterial respiratory pathogens: Implications for pandemic preparedness. *Lancet Infect Dis* 2006; **6**: 303–12.

4. Soper GA. The pandemic in the army camps. *JAMA* 1918; **71**: 1899–909.

◆5. Nguyen-Van-Tam JS. Epidemiology of influenza. In: Nicholson KG, Webster RG, Hay AJ (eds) *Textbook of Influenza*. Oxford: Blackwell Science, 1998: 181–206.

6. Daly JM, Wood JM, Robertson JS. Cocirculation and divergence of human influenza viruses. In: Nicholson KG, Webster RG, Hay AJ (eds) *Textbook of Influenza*. Oxford: Blackwell Science, 1998: 168–77.

7. Fouchier RA, Munster V, Wallensten A *et al.* Characterization of a novel influenza A virus hemagglutinin subtype (H16) obtained from black-headed gulls. *J Virol* 2005; **79**: 2814–22.

8. Scholtissek C. Pigs as 'mixing vessels' for the creation of new pandemic influenza A viruses. *Med Principles Pract* 1990; **2**: 65–71.

9. Castrucci MR, Donatelli I, Sidoli L, Barigazzi G, Kawaoka Y, Webster RG. Genetic reassortment between avian and human influenza A viruses in Italian pigs. *Virology* 1993; **193**:503–6.

10. Kawaoka Y, Krauss S, Webster RG. Avian-to-human transmission of the PB1 gene of influenza A viruses in the 1957 and 1968 pandemics. *J Virol* 1989; **63**: 4603–8.

●11. Scholtissek C, Rohde W, von Hoyningen V, Rott R. On the origin of the human influenza virus subtypes H2N2 and H3N2. *Virology* 1978; **87**: 13–20.

12. Kung HC, Jen KF, Yuan WC, Tien SF, Chu CM. Influenza in China in 1977: recurrence of influenza virus A subtype H1N1. *Bull WHO* 1978; **56**: 913–18.

13. Scholtissek C, von Hoyningen V, Rott R. Genetic relatedness between the new 1977 epidemic strains (H1N1) of influenza and human influenza strains isolated between 1947 and 1957. *Virology* 1978; **89**: 613–17.

◆14. Reid AH, Taubenberger JK. The origin of the 1918 pandemic influenza virus: A continuing enigma. *J Gen Virol* 2003; **84**: 2285–92.

●15. Dawood FS, Jain S, Finelli L *et al.* Emergence of a novel swine-origin influenza A (H1N1) virus in humans. *New Engl J Med* 2009; **360**: 2605–15.

●16. Shope RE. Swine influenza. III: Filtration experiments and aetiology. *J Exp Med* 1931; **54**: 373–85.

17. Sovinova O, Tumova B, Pouska F, Nemec J. Isolation of a virus causing respiratory diseases in horses. *Acta Virol* 1958; **1**: 52–61.

18. Webster RG, Hinshaw VS, Bean WJ *et al.* Characterization of an influenza A virus from seals. *Virology* 1981; **113**: 712–24.

19. Yagyu K, Yanagawa R, Matsuura Y, Fukushi H, Kida H, Noda H. Serological survey of influenza A virus infection in mink. *Jpn J Vet Sci* 1982; **44**: 691–3.

20. Hinshaw VS, Bean WJ, Geraci JR, Fiorelli P, Early G, Webster RG. Characterization of two influenza A viruses from a pilot whale. *J Virol* 1986; **58**: 655–6.

◆21. Tam JS. Influenza A (H5N1) in Hong Kong: An overview. *Vaccine* 2002; **20**(Suppl. 2): S77–81.

●22. Keawcharoen J, Oraveerakul K, Kuiken T *et al.* Avian influenza H5N1 in tigers and leopards. *Emerg Infect Dis* 2004; **10**: 2189–91.

●23. Thanawongnuwech R, Amonsin A, Tantilertcharoen R *et al.* Probable tiger-to-tiger transmission of avian influenza H5N1. *Emerg Infect Dis* 2005; **11**: 699–701.

24. Songsermn T, Amonsin A, Jam-on R *et al.* Avian influenza H5N1 in naturally infected domestic cat. *Emerg Infect Dis* 2006; **12**: 681–3.

●25. Rimelzwaan GF, van Riel D, Baars M *et al.* Influenza A virus (H5N1) infection in cats causes systemic disease with potential novel routes of virus spread between hosts. *Am J Pathol* 2006; **168**: 176–83.

●26. Smith W, Andrewes CH, Laidlaw PP. A virus obtained from influenza patients. *Lancet* 1933; **ii**: 66–8.

27. Creighton C. Influenzas and epidemic agues. In: Creighton C (ed.) *A History of Epidemics in Britain*, 2nd edn. London: Frank Cass, 1965: 300–433.

◆28. Potter CW. Chronicle of influenza pandemics. In: Nicholson KG, Webster RG, Hay AJ (eds) *Textbook of Influenza*. Oxford: Blackwell Science, 1998: 3–18.

29. Masurel N, Marine WM. Recycling of Asian and Hong Kong influenza A virus hemagglutinins in man. *Am J Epidemiol* 1973; **97**: 44–9.

●30. Goldfield M, Bartley JD, Pizzuti W, Black HC, Altman R, Halperin WE. Influenza in New Jersey in 1976: Isolations of influenza A/New Jersey/76 virus at Fort Dix. *J Infect Dis* 1977; **136**(Suppl): S347–55.

31. Ashley J, Smith T, Dunnell K. Deaths in Great Britain associated with the influenza epidemic of 1989/90. *Popul Trends* 1991; **65**: 16–20.

32. Fleming DM, Elliot AJ. Lessons from 40 years' surveillance of influenza in England and Wales. *Epidemiol Infect* 2008; **136**: 866–75.

33. Simonsen L, Clarke MJ, Williamson GD, Stroup DF, Arden NH, Schonberger LB. The impact of influenza epidemics on mortality: introducing a severity index. *Am J Public Health* 1997; **87**: 1944–50.

34. Young LC, Dwyer DE, Harris M *et al.* Summer outbreak of respiratory disease in an Australian prison due to an influenza A/Fujian/411/2002(H3N2)-like virus. *Epidemiol Infect* 2005; **133**: 107–12.

35. Kohn MA, Farley TA, Sundin D, Tapia R, McFarland LM, Arden NH. Three summertime outbreaks of influenza type A. *J Infect Dis* 1995; **172**: 246–9.

36. Alonso WJ, Viboud C, Simonsen L, Hirano EW, Daufenbach LZ, Miller MA. Seasonality of influenza in Brazil: A travelling wave from the Amazon to the subtropics. *Am J Epidemiol* 2007; **165**: 1434–42.

37. Chew FT, Doraisingham S, Ling AE, Kumarasinghe G, Lee BW. Seasonal trends of viral respiratory tract infections in the tropics. *Epidemiol Infect* 1998; **121**: 121–8.

●38. Hope-Simpson RE. The role of season in the epidemiology of influenza. *J Hyg Camb* 1981; **86**: 35–47.

39. Hemmes JH, Winkler KC, Kool SM. Virus survival as a seasonal factor in influenza and poliomyelitis. *Nature* 1960; **188**: 430–1.

40. Schaffer FL, Soergel ME, Straube DC. Survival of airborne influenza virus: Effects of propagating host, relative humidity, and composition of spray fluids. *Arch Virol* 1976; **51**: 263–73.

41. Jordan WS Jr. The mechanism of spread of Asian influenza. *Am Rev Resp Dis* 1961; **2**: 29–40.

42. Thacker SB. The persistence of influenza A in human populations. *Epidemiol Rev* 1986; **8**: 129–41.

●43. Monto AS, Kiouhmehr F. The Tecumseh study of respiratory illness. IX: Occurrence of influenza in the community, 1966–1971. *Am J Epidemiol* 1975; **102**: 553–63.

●44. Hall CE, Cooney MK, Fox JP. The Seattle Virus Watch. IV: Comparative epidemiologic observations of infections with influenza A and B viruses, 1965–69, in families with young children. *Am J Epidemiol* 1973; **98**: 365–80.

45. Davis LE, Caldwell GG, Lynch RE, Bailey RE, Chin DY. Hong Kong influenza: The epidemiologic features of a high

school family study analysed and compared with a similar study during the 1957 Asian influenza epidemic. *Am J Epidemiol* 1970; **92**: 240–7.

●46. Fox JP, Cooney MK, Hall CE, Foy MF. Influenza virus infections in Seattle families, 1975–79. II: Pattern of infection in invaded households and relation of age and prior antibody to occurrence of infection and related illness. *Am J Epidemiol* 1982; **116**: 228–42.

47. Teo SS, Nguyen-Van-Tam JS, Booy R. Influenza burden of illness, diagnosis, treatment and prevention: What is the evidence in children and where are the gaps? *Arch Dis Child* 2005; **90**: 532–6.

◆48. Reichert TA, Sugaya N, Fedson DS, Glezen WP, Simonsen L, Tashiro M. The Japanese experience with vaccinating schoolchildren against influenza. *N Engl J Med* 2001; **344**: 889–96.

●49. Ferguson NM, Cummings DA, Fraser C, Cajka JC, Cooley PC, Burke DS. Strategies for mitigating an influenza pandemic. *Nature* 2006; **442**: 448–52.

◆50. Brankston G, Gitterman L, Hirji Z, Lemieux C, Gardam M. Transmission of influenza A in human beings. *Lancet Infect Dis* 2007; **7**: 257–65.

51. Tellier R. Review of aerosol transmission of influenza A virus. *Emerg Infect Dis* 2006; **12**: 1657–62.

◆52. Bridges CB, Kuehnert MJ, Hall CB. Transmission of influenza: Implications for control in hospital settings. *Clin Infect Dis* 2003; **37**: 1094–1101.

53. Hall CB, Douglas RG, Geiman JM, Meagher MP. Viral shedding patterns of children with influenza B infection. *J Infect Dis* 1979; **140**: 610–13.

54. Morris JA, Kasel JA, Saglam M, Knight V, Loda F. Immunity to influenza as related to antibody levels. *N Engl J Med* 1966; **274**: 527–35.

55. Murphy BR, Chahlub EG, Nusinoff SR, Kasel J, Chanock RM. Temperature-sensitive mutants of influenza virus. 3: Further characterisation of the ts-1 (E) influenza A recombinant (H3N2) in man. *J Infect Dis* 1973; **128**: 479–87.

56. Hall CB, Douglas RG. Nosocomial influenza infection as a cause of intercurrent fever in infants. *Paediatrics* 1975; **55**: 673–7.

57. Munoz FM, Campbell JR, Atmar RL *et al.* Influenza A virus outbreak in a neonatal intensive care unit. *Pediatr Infect Dis J* 1999; **18**: 811–15.

58. Englund JA, Champlin RE, Wyde PR *et al.* Common emergence of amantadine- and rimantadine-resistant influenza A viruses in symptomatic immunocompromised adults. *Clin Infect Dis* 1998; **26**: 1418–24.

59. Evans KD, Kline MW. Prolonged influenza A infection responsive to rimantadine therapy in a human immunodeficiency virus-infected child. *Pediatr Infect Dis J* 1995; **14**: 332–4.

60. Sheat K. An investigation into an explosive outbreak of influenza – New Plymouth. *Commun Dis N Z* 1992; **92**: 18–19.

61. Frank AL, Taber LH, Wells CR, Wells JM, Glezen WP, Paredes A. Patterns of shedding of myxoviruses and paramyxoviruses in children. *J Infect Dis* 1981; **144**: 433–41.

●62. Bean B, Moore BM, Sterner B, Petersen LR, Gerding DN, Balfour HH Jr. Survival of influenza viruses on environmental surfaces. *J Infect Dis* 1982; **146**: 47–51.

63. Tiwari A, Patnayak DP, Chander Y, Parsad M, Goyal SM. Survival of two avian respiratory viruses on porous and nonporous surfaces. *Avian Dis* 2006; **50**: 284–7.

64. Schurmann W, Eggers HJ. Antiviral activity of an alcoholic hand disinfectant: Comparison of the in vitro suspension test with in vivo experiments on hands, and on individual fingertips. *Antiviral Res* 1983; **3**: 25–41.

65. Crosby AW. *America's Forgotten Pandemic: The Influenza of 1918*. Cambridge: Cambridge University Press, 1989.

◆66. Nguyen-Van-Tam JS, Hampson AW. The epidemiology and clinical impact of pandemic influenza. *Vaccine* 2003; **21**: 1762–8.

67. Meltzer MI, Cox NJ, Fukuda K. The economic impact of pandemic influenza in the United States: Priorities for intervention. *Emerg Infect Dis* 1999; **5**: 659–71.

68. Hak E, Meijboom MJ, Buskens E. Modelling the health-economic impact of the next influenza pandemic in the Netherlands. *Vaccine* 2006; **24**: 6756–60.

●69. Cooper BS, Pitman RJ, Edmunds WJ, Gay NJ. Delaying the international spread of pandemic influenza. *PLoS Med* 2006; **3**: e212.

◆70. Ward P, Small I, Smith J, Suter P, Dutkowski R. Oseltamivir (Tamiflu) and its potential for use in the event of an influenza pandemic. *J Antimicrob Chemother* 2005; **55**(Suppl. 1): i5–21.

●71. de Jong MD, Tran TT, Truong HK *et al.* Oseltamivir resistance during treatment of influenza A (H5N1) infection. *N Engl J Med* 2005; **353**: 2667–72.

72. Pandemic (H1N1) 2009 briefing note 1. Viruses resistant to oseltamivir (Tamiflu) identified. *Wkly Epidemiol Rec* 2009; **84**: 299.

●73. Pitman RJ, Cooper BS, Trotter CL, Gay NJ, Edmunds WJ. Entry screening for severe acute respiratory syndrome (SARS) or influenza: Policy evaluation. *BMJ* 2005; **331**:1242–3.

●74. Leroux-Roels I, Borkowski A, Vanwolleghem T *et al.* Antigen sparing and cross-reactive immunity with an adjuvanted rH5N1 prototype pandemic influenza vaccine: A randomised controlled trial. *Lancet* 2007; **370**: 580–9.

●75. Leroux-Roels I, Bernhard R, Gérard P, Dramé M, Hanon E, Leroux-Roels G. Broad clade 2 cross-reactive immunity induced by an adjuvanted clade 1 rH5N1 pandemic influenza vaccine. *PLoS ONE* 2008; **3**: e1665.

●76. Ehrlich HJ, Müller M, Oh HM *et al.* A clinical trial of a whole-virus H5N1 vaccine derived from cell culture. *N Engl J Med* 2008; **358**: 2573–84.

AVIAN INFLUENZA

JONATHAN S. NGUYEN-VAN-TAM

Avian influenza (AI) has been recognized in poultry for over a century but was first attributed to the influenza A virus in 1955. Feral ducks form the natural reservoir; virus replicates preferentially in the gastrointestinal tract and is excreted in extremely high concentration in the faeces. The duration of infection is typically 1 month.

These features, together with mass congregation prior to seasonal migration, produce ideal environmental conditions for the transmission and mixing of AI virus subtypes and the maintenance of a potent animal reservoir. Because feral ducks remain healthy yet excrete the virus copiously, clear opportunities exist for spread to other feral and poultry birds, as migrating flocks land in search of food and contaminate the local environment of other birds.[1] AI viruses have been isolated from the free-living birds of at least 18 families, especially wild aquatic shore birds.

AI produces symptomatic illness in poultry. This is usually mild and consists of ruffled feathers, mild respiratory symptoms, depression and lowered egg production. These symptoms are attributable to low-pathogenic viruses (LPAIs). LPAIs occur in outbreaks, and only A/H9N2 could be considered endemic in certain regions, notably the Middle East. LPAIs have the capacity to mutate into variants that are highly pathogenic in poultry (HPAIs). This has so far been described with viruses of the H5 and H7 subtypes, and was first recorded in Scotland in 1959. The symptoms of HPAI in poultry are severe, including egg drop, severe respiratory symptoms, cyanosis, diarrhoea, haemorrhage and facial oedema. Within a poultry house or unit, contagion is rapid, and mortality often exceeds 90 per cent within 48 hours.

Large outbreaks of HPAI have been described in many parts of the world from 1983 onwards, including the USA, Mexico, Pakistan, Hong Kong SAR, Italy, The Netherlands, Canada, South Africa and the UK.[2] HPAI A/H5N1 is now entrenched in poultry in many parts of Asia, Africa and the Middle East, and the movement of poultry and people (contaminated shoes and clothing), contaminated vehicles, equipment, feed and cages may well contribute significantly.

Human infections with AI are well documented for subtypes H5N1, H7N2, H7N3, H7N7 and H9N2, but not all of these viruses have been highly pathogenic variants. With two major exceptions, these have been sporadic cases, associated with close contact with infected birds and no human-to-human transmission. However, the outbreak of HPAI A/H7N7 in the Netherlands in 2003 and human HPAI A/H5N1 infections since 1997 have given rise to the greatest public health concern.

In the Netherlands in 2003, a large outbreak of HPAI A/H7N7 in poultry resulted in 453 health complaints (mainly conjunctivitis, but also some influenza-like illnesses) in poultry workers and farmers and their immediate families, 89 of whom were confirmed to have H7N7 infection. There was evidence of limited human-to-human transmission, and one veterinarian died.[3]

In 1997, 18 cases of HPAI A/H5N1 occurred in Hong Kong residents coinciding with an outbreak in local live poultry markets; six cases were fatal. H5N1 re-emerged in humans in 2003 in Hong Kong SAR, and in the period 2003-07, 351 cases were reported to the World Health Organization, of which 217 (62 per cent) proved fatal. These cases were spread across 14 countries in Asia, Africa and parts of the Middle East. The infection in humans produces a severe illness characterized by fever, dyspnoea, cough and pneumonia (in over 80 per cent of cases) often progressing rapidly to acute respiratory distress syndrome. Diarrhoea is also reported more frequently than with seasonal influenza, and leukopenia, thrombocytopenia and disordered liver function are relatively common findings.[4]

It should be borne in mind that large proportions of the human population in Asia, Africa and many parts of the Middle East are exposed to poultry on a widespread, almost daily basis, through small-scale 'backyard' husbandry. In spite of this, human infections with H5N1 remain rare, although the pandemic threat remains considerable. The most potent route of transmission is from avian to human, through the handling of sick or dead H5N1-infected poultry. The most risk-prone activities are slaughtering, de-feathering, evisceration, play (young children) and cock fighting.

However, at least one-quarter of all cases cannot be explained by avian-to-human contact, and environment-to-human transmission is most likely implicated. Plausible routes include walking through live bird markets (exposure to faecal dust), the ingestion of raw poultry products, contact with fomites and fertilizer containing poultry faeces, and swimming or bathing in heavily virus-contaminated water courses. Human-to-human transmission has been recorded during very close contact with severely ill patients; however, so far, these events have proved extremely rare, and the chains of transmission have been extremely short (two or three people) and non-sustained. There is no convincing evidence to date of widespread mild or asymptomatic infections occurring.[4,5]

References

● = Key primary paper
◆ = Major review article

◆1. Ito T, Kawaoka Y. Avian influenza. In: Nicholson KG, Webster RG, Hay AJ. (eds) *Textbook of Influenza*. Oxford: Blackwell Science, 1998: 126–36.

◆2. World Health Organization. Avian Influenza: Assessing the Pandemic Threat. Available from: http://www.who.int/csr/disease/influenza/WHO_CDS_2005_29/en/index.html (accessed August 4, 2009)

●3. Koopmans M, Wilbrink B, Conyn M *et al.* Transmission of H7N7 avian influenza A virus to human beings during a large outbreak in commercial poultry farms in the Netherlands. *Lancet* 2004; **363**: 587–93.

◆4. Writing Committee of the Second World Health Organization Consultation on clinical aspects of human infection with avian influenza A (H5N1) virus. Update on avian influenza A (H5N1) virus infection in humans. *N Engl J Med* 2008; **358**: 261–73.

◆5. Writing Committee of the World Health Organization Consultation on human influenza A/H5. (H5N1) virus. Avian influenza A (H5N1) infection in humans. *N Engl J Med* 2005; **353**: 1374–85 [Erratum in *N Engl J Med* 2006; **354**: 884.]

2009 PANDEMIC INFLUENZA A/H1N1

JONATHAN S. NGUYEN-VAN-TAM

Influenza A/H1N1 has a long association with humans. An influenza A/H1N1 virus was responsible for the first and most severe pandemic of the twentieth century in 1918, and remained in continuous circulation until 1956. A/H1N1 then re-emerged in 1977 and has remained in global circulation alongside A/H3N2 viruses and influenza B until the present day; however, a pandemic was not declared in 1977, and a significant impact of the virus was only ever described in children and young adults. It is less well remembered that a different A/H1N1 of swine origin had in fact brought the world to the brink of a pandemic one year earlier in 1976. This outbreak of 'swine flu' in Fort Dix, USA, is covered in Chapter 17 but is the first documented occasion on which an influenza virus of swine origin has caused widespread human disease.

In March 2009, Mexico experienced an extensive outbreak of acute respiratory illness whose aetiology was unknown at the time. Some cases were reported to be severe, and attention was drawn to the occurrence of severe pneumonia and a number of fatalities in young adults. The epidemic curve in Mexico had begun to accelerate dramatically by mid-April. On April 23rd, 2009, in the process of routinely characterizing clinical isolates of influenza reported to the Centers for Communicable Disease, the USA identified a small number of non subtypable human influenza A infections from its southern states, mainly those bordering Mexico. These viruses were investigated further and characterized to be a novel reassortant A/H1N1, containing six genes from a currently circulating North American swine flu virus and two new ones from a Eurasian swine influenza virus. At least some of the most recent Mexican cases were then subsequently identified to be due to the same virus, suggesting that international spread was already underway.

Mexico subsequently declared a Public Health Emergency of International Concern (PHEIC) to the World Health Organization (WHO) on April 25th, 2009. The rapid assessment of a spreading novel influenza virus prompted the declaration of WHO Pandemic Alert Phase 4 on April 27th, followed by Phase 5 on April 29th, 2009. Although considered to be of swine origin, the virus represented a new reassortant that had never previously been identified in a species other than man, and was highly antigenically dissimilar to recent A/H1N1 seasonal viruses. However, its precise route of emergence has not yet been defined.

Clinical descriptions of the infections from Mexico initially suggested a disease with a broad spectrum of clinical severity from mild to fatal. Although the clinical attack rate was highest in children and lowest in the elderly (consistent with an increasing prevalence of cross-reactive antibodies with advancing age), the burden of hospitalization and deaths appeared to be associated with younger adults of working age (20–49 years), but the case fatality rate increased markedly with age. Although the precise numerical values for these indicators were not certain at this stage due to significant problems in defining appropriate denominators, the overall trends described above have now been reflected in every affected country of the world.

During May and June 2009, sustained community transmission of the virus developed in the USA and

Canada, initially driven by cases in urban areas and large outbreaks centred on schools. In addition, rapid introduction of the virus to many other countries, especially the UK and Spain, occurred via returning travellers. After seeding of the virus by returning travellers, the pattern of community activity seen in USA and Canada (school and urban outbreaks) was repeated in most affected countries. By late May 2009, it was becoming clear that community transmission was well established in several WHO Regions, fulfilling the requirements for declaration of a pandemic (WHO Alert Phase 6), which was formally made on June 11th.

Like previous influenza viruses, the new pandemic variant has demonstrated its propensity for seasonality. In the southern hemisphere winter period (June–August 2009) very substantial pandemic influenza activity has been observed, whereas in most places in Europe (except in the UK) the late spring wave was small, and activity declined dramatically over the summer across the whole of the northern hemisphere. It is uncertain whether the reason for the summer decline in Europe was entirely due to reduced seasonal transmission, or at least in part due to social distancing in children and teenagers produced as a consequence of planned school closures during the vacation period. Pandemic influenza activity re-established itself in early autumn 2009 in the northern hemisphere, soon after the schools reopened. In sharp contrast to 1918, however, the autumn wave has not been as large as many experts predicted, and the virulence of the virus has not appreciably altered. As this book goes to print in early 2010, pandemic activity has peaked or is declining all across the northern hemisphere.

A clearer clinical picture of the pandemic virus has now emerged. The 2009 pandemic can be considered to have been mild, and even less severe than those in 1957 and 1968, with a very high rate of asymptomatic illness. The case fatality rate lies in the range of 0.1–0.02 per cent (compared with 2.5 per cent in 1918), and most cases are self-limiting. Estimates of the reproductive number of the virus have tended to fall within the range 1.4–1.6, indicating moderate transmissibility. Notwithstanding, the rate of hospitalization in clinically apparent cases is probably 1 per cent or less in most healthcare systems, although some individual estimates are higher. Compared with seasonal influenza, these hospitalized cases remain unusual because of the overrepresentation of young adults of working age and children, and the very unusual requirement for assisted ventilation in 10–20 per cent of those admitted, although bacterial complications are less common than was anticipated. Although a very clear signal has already emerged in relation to underlying chronic conditions (including asthma and other pulmonary conditions, pregnancy and morbid obesity) as strong risk factors for hospitalization and death, at least one half of those admitted to hospital and about 20 per cent of those who

died due to confirmed pandemic influenza in the UK did not have underlying illnesses.

By the end of 2009, the pandemic had caused none of the widespread societal disruption that might have been expected during a severe pandemic (e.g. A/H5N1), but intensive care services in most locations experienced considerable and sustained pressure for several months, caring primarily for young adults and children with viral pneumonia and respiratory distress. To date, the virus has shown remarkably little genetic variation, regardless of where it has been isolated, and in general terms it has remained sensitive to both licensed neuraminidase inhibitors, although resistant to adamantanes from the outset. Nevertheless, oseltamivir-resistant viruses (with the H275Y mutation) have been reported in small numbers. Although this situation will require careful future monitoring, there is no obvious suggestion that the emergence of resistance is being driven by selection pressure from the widespread use of antiviral drugs. A pandemic vaccine became generally available in late September 2009, and vaccination programmes are well underway in many parts of the world.

The biggest remaining questions relate to what will happen in the future. It already seems clear that seasonal influenza A/H1N1 has been replaced by the pandemic variant. It is not yet clear whether the previously dominant pre-pandemic A/H3N2 subtype will decline in importance or even disappear. It is most likely that the pandemic influenza A/H1N1 virus will continue to cause illness in younger age groups for the next few years, but the timing and intensity of human influenza remain as unpredictable as ever.

Further reading

ANZIC Influenza Investigators. Critical care services and 2009 H1N1 influenza in Australia and New Zealand. *N Engl J Med* 2009; **361**: 1925–34.

Donaldson LJ, Rutter PD, Ellis BM *et al.* Mortality from pandemic A/H1N1 2009 influenza in England: Public health surveillance study. *BMJ* 2009; **339**: b5213. doi: 10.1136/bmj.b5213 [Epub 2009 Dec 10].

European Centre for Disease Prevention and Control. *The Influenza H1N1 2009 Pandemic Experiences from the Southern Hemisphere*. Eurosurveillance Special Edition. Stockholm: European Centre for Disease Prevention and Control, 2010.

European Centre for Disease Prevention and Control. *Tracking the Influenza H1N1 2009 Pandemic May–October 2009*. Eurosurveillance Special Edition. Stockholm: European Centre for Disease Prevention and Control, 2010.

Garten RJ, Davis CT, Russell CA *et al.* Antigenic and genetic characteristics of swine-origin 2009 A(H1N1) influenza viruses circulating in humans. *Science* 2009; **325**: 197–201.

Hancock K, Veguilla V, Lu X *et al.* Cross-reactive antibody responses to the 2009 pandemic H1N1 influenza virus. *N Engl J Med* 2009; **361**: 1945–52.

Itoh Y, Shinya K, Kiso M *et al.* In vitro and in vivo characterisation of new swine-origin H1N1 influenza viruses. *Nature* 2009; **460**: 1021–5.

Jain S, Kamimoto L, Bramley AM *et al.* Hospitalized patients with 2009 H1N1 influenza in the United States, April–June 2009. *N Engl J Med* 2009; **361**; 1935–44.

Jamieson DJ, Honein MA, Rasmussen SA *et al.* H1N1 2009 influenza virus infection during pregnancy in the USA. *Lancet* 2009; **374**: 451–8.

Louie JK, Acosta M, Winter K *et al.* Factors associated with death or hospitalization due to pandemic 2009 influenza A (H1N1) infection in California. *JAMA* 2009; **302**: 1896–902.

Miller E, Hoschler K, Hardelid P *et al.* Incidence of 2009 pandemic influenza A H1N1 infection in England: A cross-sectional serological study. *Lancet* 2010. doi: 10.1016/S0140-6736(09)62126-7 [Epub 2010 Jan 21].

Novel Swine-Origin Influenza A (H1N1) Virus Investigation Team; Dawood FS, Jain S, Finelli L *et al.* Emergence of a novel swine-origin influenza A (H1N1) virus in humans. *N Engl J Med* 2009; **360**: 2605–15. [Erratum in *N Engl J Med* 2009; **361**: 102.]

Perez-Padilla R, de la Rosa-Zamboni D, Ponce de Leon S *et al.* Pneumonia and respiratory failure from swine-origin influenza A(H1N1) in Mexico. *N Engl J Med* 2009; **361**: 680–9.

Van-Tam J, Sellwood C (eds). *Introduction to Pandemic Influenza*. Wallingford: CAB International, 2010.

18

Legionnaires' disease

JOHN V. LEE, GORDON L. NICHOLS

FIRST RECOGNIZED OUTBREAK

Legionnaires' disease was first recognized following an outbreak of disease among a convention of US army veterans being held in a hotel in Philadelphia in July 1976. Out of 4400 people, 76 were affected, of whom 29 died. The outbreak of pneumonia took 6 months to pin down to a specific organism using animal inoculation and the eventual demonstration of a novel bacterium,[1] eventually termed *Legionella pneumophila*. Legionnaires' disease is an important community-acquired pneumonia.[2,3] The organisms responsible are derived from water environments that are mostly manmade, but the organism is transmitted through the air as aerosols.

Travel-related infection occurs associated with hotels, and a European Working Group for *Legionella* Infections has developed a surveillance system for *Legionella* infections that can trace cases occurring in different countries back to an individual resort hotel.[4] Outbreaks have been associated with various sorts of cooling tower, hotel and hospital hot and cold water systems, and a variety of other devices using water such as misters for food display cabinets. *Legionella* spp. have been responsible for outbreaks of legionellosis in spa pools on cruise ships, in hotels and leisure centres and in holiday homes, with large outbreaks associated with spa pools on display. The only natural sources of human infection that have been reported are natural hot springs.

CHARACTERISTICS OF LEGIONNAIRES' DISEASE

Compared with other pneumonias, Legionnaires' disease has few particular distinguishing clinical features, but patients are more frequently smokers, aged over 40, male (3:1 male:female ratio) and present with neurological signs, evidence of multisystem involvement and diarrhoea. Infection is more common in those who are immunocompromised or immunosuppressed, such as patients following organ transplant.[5–11] The attack rate in community outbreaks is usually rather low (less than 1 per cent). Although the mortality can be 4–6 per cent in travel-associated cases,[4] the mortality in hospital-acquired Legionnaires' disease can be up to 20 per cent.

The disease can be severe, leading to life-threatening acute lobar or bronchopneumonia that progresses to extrapulmonary symptoms and multisystem failure. Non-respiratory symptoms include headache, weakness, myalgia, fever and rigors, while cough is usually non-productive with or without haemoptysis. Liver enzymes (transaminases, alkaline phosphatase and bilirubin) may be raised, elevated creatinine phosphokinase and aldolase can sometimes occur, while proteinuria, haematuria and renal insufficiency are infrequent. When patients die, it is mostly as a result of respiratory insufficiency. Legionnaires' disease is acquired by the inhalation of aerosols containing

Legionella either separately or within amoebae or amoebal vesicles. There is no evidence that the infection can be passed from person to person by coughing.

The incidence can vary from 0 to 34 per million population per year. Within the UK, it is estimated that about 2–5 per cent of individuals with pneumonia who require admission to hospital have Legionnaires' disease, although only about 10 per cent of these are detected. There is substantial underascertainment of infection resulting from a lack of appreciation of the disease and the limitations of diagnosis. The use of urinary antigen testing has greatly improved diagnosis across Europe and led to improvements in ascertainment. Treatment is usually with a fluoroquinolone, a beta-lactam and a macrolide, alone or in combination.[12–14]

PONTIAC FEVER

Pontiac fever is an acute flu-like illness without any pneumonic manifestations and was recognized as a specific entity some years before the causal organism was identified. The attack rate can be high, affecting both young and old alike. Pontiac fever has been caused by a respiratory hypersensitivity to *L. pneumophila*, *L. anisa*, *L. feeleii* and *L. micdadei*, although the organism is not normally cultured from affected patients. 'Legionellosis' refers to both Legionnaires' disease and Pontiac fever.

LEGIONELLA SPP.

There are 54 described species of the genus *Legionella* and over 70 serogroups (Table 18.1). Only a small percentage of these have been detected in patients with disease.[15] The genus lies within the gamma subgroup of the class Proteobacteria. Although 19 *Legionella* species are able to cause human disease the majority of cases around the world are due to *L. pneumophila* serogroup 1, while *L. longbeachae* is an important cause of community-acquired pneumonia in Australia that has been traced to potting composts (cases linked to potting compost having also occurred in other countries).

A number of schemes have been developed for typing *L. pneumophila*. An internationally developed method based on the sequencing of parts of seven genes is now being widely applied.[16,17] Some sequence types (ST) of *L. pneumophila* serogroup 1 (e.g. ST 47) are more associated with human disease than others although rarely isolated from the environment in the absence of cases.[18]

Legionella spp. usually grow in association with other organisms. Many *Legionella* species can be isolated using agar culture media containing specific growth factors (cysteine and iron), and the organisms are intracellular through much of their life-cycle, within a range of protozoa including *Acanthamoeba*, *Echinamoeba*, *Tetrahymena*, *Hartmannella*, *Naegleria*, *Vahlkampfia* and *Cyclidium* as

Table 18.1 Recognized species of *Legionella*

Species	Human disease	Reference
Legionella adelaidensis	Unknown	64
Legionella anisa	Yes	65
Legionella beliardensis	Unknown	66
Legionella birminghamensis	Yes	67
Legionella bozemanii	Yes	68
Legionella brunensis	Unknown	69
Legionella busanensis	Unknown	70
Legionella cherrii	Unknown	71
Legionella cincinnatiensis	Yes	72
Legionella donaldsonii	Unknown	73
Legionella drancourtii	Unknown	74
Legionella dresdenensis	Unknown	100
Legionella drozanskii	Unknown	75
Legionella dumoffii	Yes	68
Legionella erythra	Yes	71
Legionella fairfieldensis	Unknown	76
Legionella fallonii	Unknown	75
Legionella feeleii	Yes	77
Legionella geestiana	Unknown	78
Legionella gormanii	Yes	79
Legionella gratiana	Unknown	80
Legionella gresilensis	Unknown	66
Legionella hackeliae	Yes	81
Legionella impletisoli	Unknown	82
Legionella israelensis	Unknown	83
Legionella jamestowniensis	Unknown	82
'Candidatus *Legionella jeonii*'	Unknown	84
Legionella jordanis	Yes	85
Legionella lansingensis	Yes	86
Legionella londiniensis	Unknown	78
Legionella longbeachae	Yes	87
Legionella lytica	Unknown	88
Legionella maceachernii	Yes	89
Legionella micdadei	Yes	68
Legionella moravica	Unknown	69
Legionella nautarum	Unknown	78
Legionella oakridgensis	Yes	90
Legionella parisiensis	Yes	91
Legionella pneumophila	Yes	92
Legionella quateirensis	Unknown	78
Legionella quinlivanii	Unknown	93
Legionella rowbothamii	Unknown	75
Legionella rubrilucens	Unknown	94
Legionella sainthelensi	Yes	95
Legionella santicrucis	Unknown	96
Legionella shakespearei	Unknown	97
Legionella spiritensis	Unknown	94
Legionella steigerwaltii	Unknown	71
Legionella taurinensis	Unknown	94
Legionella tucsonensis	Yes	98
Legionella wadsworthii	Yes	99
Legionella waltersii	Unknown	93
Legionella worsleiensis	Unknown	78
Legionella yabuuchiae	Unknown	82

well as within the macrophages of people's lungs. The amoebal associations are thought to be important in disease transmission by allowing many individual bacteria within an amoeba to survive better and to enter the lungs in an infective dose in either amoebal cysts or vesicles.

DIAGNOSIS

Legionnaires' disease and Pontiac fever are diagnosed by the detection of antigen in urine, polymerase chain reaction (PCR) and culture. Antibody testing and culture were commonly used, but the widespread use of urinary antigen testing has allowed much better ascertainment of the disease in many European countries. However, these screening systems are specifically focused on *L. pneumophila*, and there is probably an underestimation of disease caused by other species. Culture from patients uses selective culture media with activated carbon, iron and cysteine both with and without acid pre-treatment. The urinary antigen test is effective in diagnosing the acute phase of infection (80 per cent sensitive), but is less so later in the disease. The British Thoracic Society has produced guidelines for the clinical diagnosis of severe community pneumonias.

LEGIONELLOSIS IN DEVELOPING COUNTRIES

The occurrence of infections caused by *Legionella* spp. in developing countries is poorly understood. The common occurrence of these organisms in most warm aqueous environments suggests that infection should be common. However, diagnosis is generally poor and identified outbreaks uncommon.

SOURCES OF *LEGIONELLA* SPP. CAUSING HUMAN DISEASE

Legionella species are ubiquitous in freshwater habitats worldwide and have been isolated from streams, rivers, lakes, hydrothermal waters, groundwater sediments and mud, particularly in warm waters. They are not found naturally in seawater (as they will not grow in seawater) but can be in run-off from land. They can be transmitted through wet cooling systems (cooling towers and evaporative condensers),[19–27] air scrubbers,[28–30] spa pools,[31,32] including those on display,[33–38] taps,[8,39] parts of distribution systems,[40] showers,[41–45] distribution systems on ships (particularly cruise ships),[46–48] indoor (but not outdoor) decorative fountains,[49–51] food misting,[52,53] car washes, the commissioning of water systems, dental water and ice. There is also some evidence for transmission through contaminated drinking water in hospitals as a result of aspiration by patients[43] and possible transmission

to neonates by birthing pools.[54] Transmission has occurred from naturally infected hot springs and has been reported in association with the use of water alone in windscreen washers. The seasonal increase in sporadic legionellosis in the summer months appears to be related to humidity and temperature, although the sources of infection remain unclear.[55]

Legionella usually grow in warm aquatic environments in association with other organisms in biofilm. A risk of infection will arise when the legionellae released from the biofilm into the water are subsequently aerosolized, for example by a spray in a cooling tower, a shower, turning on a tap or bubbles rising through the water in a spa pool. They can grow at between 20°C and 40°C and are phagocytosed by a variety of free-living protozoa, where they can remain relatively protected from extremes of temperature, osmolarity and pH.

OUTBREAK INVESTIGATION

Cases in the community can be difficult to investigate. Where there is more than one case linked in space and time, an investigation should search for common risk factors. Outbreak investigation is multidisciplinary, requiring, for example, input from epidemiologists, health and safety inspectors, environmental health officers, clinical and environmental microbiologists, engineers and water treatment specialists. Considerable resources may be required. In all investigations, it is important to identify potential sources as quickly as possible, sample them and then render them safe by a precautionary disinfection or other means. The investigation of outbreaks is discussed in detail by Bartram *et al.*[15]

Where cases are linked to recent travel, they are reported to the European Surveillance Scheme for Travel Associated Legionnaires' Disease (EWGLINET). This was run in the UK from 1993 but passed to European Centre for Disease Prevention and Control (ECDC) in 2010. Any cases where the patient has stayed in a hotel during the presumed incubation period are reported centrally. The scheme organizer collates the reports, and if two or more cases have stayed in the same hotel within a 2 year period, this is reported as a potential cluster and investigations are initiated in the Member State.

PUBLIC HEALTH AND CONTROL MEASURES

Control of Legionnaires' disease has been through trying to identify the main sources of contamination for humans and acting to reduce these.[56] The control of outbreaks and sporadic disease has focused on the water safety plan approach used in the World Health Organization (WHO) framework for safe drinking water. The key components in this approach include system assessment, monitoring and

Table 18.2 Examples of the assessment of local systems for *Legionella* control following the World Health Organization Water Safety Plan approach

	Steps	Examples
System assessment	Survey and describe the system Hazard analysis to identify factors encouraging amplification, points where amplification may occur or points of heightened exposure	Identify key components, tanks valves, water heaters, outlets, etc. *Growth factors* Quality of the incoming water Overall cleanliness of the system Temperature Disinfectant residues
		Design and construction of the system Use of appropriate construction materials Maintenance of water flow and turnover Adequacy of insulation Ease of access for maintenance and cleaning
		Susceptibility of population exposed Renal or other organ transplant wards Haematology wards
Monitoring	Identify control measures	Improve insulation Increase flow Improver control to avoid water temperature of 25–45 °C Remove unused outlets and pipes Replace unsuitable materials Introduce supplementary disinfection
	Define limits of acceptable performance	Hot water reaches >50 °C at the tap Cold remains below 20 °C Chlorine >0.2 mg/L in cold systems *Legionella pneumophila* count <100/L
	Establish procedures to verify that the control measures are working and will meet targets	Procedures detailing frequency of monitoring temperature, disinfectant residuals, and sampling for *Legionella*
Management and communication	Develop supporting programmes	Staff training Verification of suppliers, e.g. laboratory accreditation Research programme to improve control technologies
	Prepare management procedures	Written scheme of control Actions to be taken in response to monitoring failures/incidents/ emergency situations
	Establish documentation and communication procedures	Written risk assessment Identification of monitoring points and schedule of monitoring Identification of key personnel and responsibilities Periodic meeting of infection control team to review monitoring data Audit and review of records and results of operational monitoring

management and communication, and examples of its application are shown in Table 18.2.

In some countries, standard methods have been developed to test the ability of materials to support microbial growth. This has led to the selection of more suitable materials for tap washers, piping and other components that are less supportive of biofilm growth (which supports the growth of *Legionella* spp.) and has helped in reducing the contamination of tap washers[45] and

other components used within distribution.[57,58] *Legionella* spp. can be reduced in distribution systems through the control of water temperature, with hot water distributed at close to 60 °C so that it reaches the outlets at hotter than 50 °C, and cold water below 20 °C. Unfortunately, conflicts can arise between the recommendations for energy conservation and the prevention of scalding and the control of *Legionella*. Within the UK, failsafe thermostatic mixer valves have been widely fitted in hospitals, and it is then very difficult to maintain control downstream of the thermostatic mixer valves.

Evidence from the USA indicates that the disinfectant chosen for treatment and as a residual within mains water distribution systems can play a role in preventing the colonization of buildings, and thereby outbreaks. Monochloramine is thought to be more protective than chlorine, probably because it is more persistent in the distribution system such that sufficient residual remains up to the point of entry into the building.[59–62] Control of *Legionella* in domestic water systems is usually through the control of temperature and supplementary disinfection, coupled with good design and maintenance.

Control of the contamination of cooling towers requires good housekeeping to minimize the accumulation of dirt and deposits within them and the associated cooling system. This is combined with the control of scale and corrosion by appropriate chemical inhibitors, and the limitation of biofilm formation using biocides. Spa pool operation can present problems, and good management, regular washing and disinfection are important in preventing outbreaks of infection.[63] Warm industrial water use can lead to outbreaks. Large outbreaks are luckily relatively uncommon, but environmental health vigilance is required in this area to ensure that standards of maintenance are ensured. When a heavily contaminated cooling tower is producing plumes containing *Legionella*, these have caused infections up to 6 km away. It is important that the potential risks associated with individual cases are investigated in a timely way so that the number of outbreaks can be reduced.

The detection of *Legionella* spp. by culture and/or PCR is increasingly being undertaken as an audit of control. Some countries require wet cooling systems to be monitored on a regular basis (e.g. 2–4 times per year). Healthcare premises should be regularly monitored. In a hot or cold water system, the greater proportion of outlets that are positive, the greater the risk. Higher counts (e.g. over 1000/L) represent an increased risk, but where high-risk immunocompromised patients are being treated, the presence of any detectable *Legionella* may be deemed an unacceptable risk. In some countries, spa pools are also monitored.

Any water system in which the water can be warm and there are opportunities for aerosolization of the water may cause a problem. It may take several years before types of equipment perceived as potential sources of *Legionella* spp. are confirmed to be associated with human cases, as occurred with air scrubbers and vehicle washes. Contributory factors in outbreaks include bad management, the interruption or lack of biocidal controls, temperature, design, construction and maintenance.

REFERENCES

1. McDade JE, Shepard CC, Fraser DW, Tsai TR, Redus MA, Dowdle WR. Legionnaires' disease: Isolation of a bacterium and demonstration of its role in other respiratory disease. *N Engl J Med* 1977; **297**: 1197–203.

2. Hirani NA, Macfarlane JT. Impact of management guidelines on the outcome of severe community acquired pneumonia. *Thorax* 1997; **52**: 17–21.

3. Neill AM, Martin IR, Weir R et al. Community acquired pneumonia: Aetiology and usefulness of severity criteria on admission. *Thorax* 1996; **51**: 1010–6.

4. Ricketts K, McNaught B, Joseph C. Travel-associated legionnaires disease in Europe: 2005. *Euro Surveill* 2007; 12.

5. Oren I, Zuckerman T, Avivi I, Finkelstein R, Yigla M, Rowe JM. Nosocomial outbreak of *Legionella pneumophila* serogroup 3 pneumonia in a new bone marrow transplant unit: Evaluation, treatment and control. *Bone Marrow Transplant* 2002; **30**: 175–9.

6. Knirsch CA, Jakob K, Schoonmaker D et al. An outbreak of *Legionella micdadei* pneumonia in transplant patients: Evaluation, molecular epidemiology, and control. *Am J Med* 2000; **108**: 290–5.

7. Kool JL, Fiore AE, Kioski CM et al. More than 10 years of unrecognized nosocomial transmission of legionnaires' disease among transplant patients. *Infect Control Hosp Epidemiol* 1998; **19**: 898–904.

8. Levin AS, Caiaffa Filho HH, Sinto SI, Sabbaga E, Barone AA, Mendes CM. An outbreak of nosocomial Legionnaires' disease in a renal transplant unit in Sao Paulo, Brazil. Legionellosis Study Team. *J Hosp Infect* 1991; **18**: 243–8.

9. Ampel NM, Wing EJ. *Legionella* infection in transplant patients. *Semin Respir Infect* 1990; **5**: 30–7.

10. Dowling JN, Pasculle AW, Frola FN, Zaphyr MK, Yee RB. Infections caused by *Legionella micdadei* and *Legionella pneumophila* among renal transplant recipients. *J Infect Dis* 1984; **149**: 703–13.

11. Goldstein JD, Keller JL, Winn WC Jr, Myerowitz RL. Sporadic Legionellaceae pneumonia in renal transplant recipients. A survey of 70 autopsies, 1964 to 1979. *Arch Pathol Lab Med* 1982; **106**: 108–11.

12. Martinez D, Alvarez R, V, Ortiz de Zarate MM et al. Management in the emergency room of patients requiring hospital treatment of community-acquired pneumonia. *Rev Esp Quimioter* 2009; **22**: 4–9.

13. Pedro-Botet ML, Yu VL. Treatment strategies for *Legionella* infection. *Expert Opin Pharmacother* 2009; **10**: 1109–21.

14. Kakeya H, Ehara N, Fukushima K et al. Severe Legionnaires' disease successfully treated using a combination of fluoroquinolone, erythromycin, corticosteroid, and sivelestat. *Intern Med* 2008; **47**: 773–7.

15. Bartram J, Chartier Y, Lee JV, Pond K, Surman-Lee JV. *Legionella and the Prevention of Legionellosis*. Geneva: World Health Organization, 2007.

16. Gaia V, Fry NK, Afshar B et al. Consensus sequence-based scheme for epidemiological typing of clinical and environmental isolates of *Legionella pneumophila*. *J Clin Microbiol* 2005; **43**: 2047–52.

17. Ratzow S, Gaia V, Helbig JH, Fry NK, Luck PC. Addition of neuA, the gene encoding N-acylneuraminate cytidylyl transferase, increases the discriminatory ability of the

consensus sequence-based scheme for typing *Legionella pneumophila* serogroup 1 strains. *J Clin Microbiol* 2007; **45**: 1965–8.

18. Harrison TG, Afshar B, Doshi N, Fry NK, Lee JV. Distribution of *Legionella pneumophila* serogroups, monoclonal antibody subgroups and DNA sequence types in recent clinical and environmental isolates from England and Wales (2000–2008). *Eur J Clin Microbiol Infect Dis* 2009; **28**: 781–91.

19. Ferre MR, Arias C, Oliva JM *et al*. A community outbreak of Legionnaires' disease associated with a cooling tower in Vic and Gurb, Catalonia (Spain) in 2005. *Eur J Clin Microbiol Infect Dis* 2009; **28**: 153–9.

20. Mouchtouri VA, Goutziana G, Kremastinou J, Hadjichristodoulou C. *Legionella* species colonization in cooling towers: Risk factors and assessment of control measures. *Am J Infect Control* 2010 **38** (1): 50–5.

21. Carducci A, Verani M, Battistini R. *Legionella* in industrial cooling towers: Monitoring and control strategies. *Lett Appl Microbiol* 2010 **50** (1): 24–9.

22. de Olalla PG, Gracia J, Rius C *et al*. [Community outbreak of pneumonia due to *Legionella pneumophila*: Importance of monitoring hospital cooling towers.] *Enferm Infecc Microbiol Clin* 2008; **26**: 15–22.

23. Castilla J, Barricarte A, Aldaz J *et al*. A large Legionnaires' disease outbreak in Pamplona, Spain: Early detection, rapid control and no case fatality. *Epidemiol Infect* 2008; **136**: 823–32.

24. Sonder GJ, van den Hoek JA, Bovee LP *et al*. Changes in prevention and outbreak management of Legionnaires disease in the Netherlands between two large outbreaks in 1999 and 2006. *Euro Surveill* 2008; **13**.

25. Hugosson A, Hjorth M, Bernander S *et al*. A community outbreak of Legionnaires' disease from an industrial cooling tower: Assessment of clinical features and diagnostic procedures. *Scand J Infect Dis* 2007; **39**: 217–24.

26. Morton S, Bartlett CL, Bibby LF, Hutchinson DN, Dyer JV, Dennis PJ. Outbreak of legionnaires' disease from a cooling water system in a power station. *Br J Ind Med* 1986; **43**: 630–5.

27. Dondero TJ Jr, Rendtorff RC, Mallison GF *et al*. An outbreak of Legionnaires' disease associated with a contaminated air-conditioning cooling tower. *N Engl J Med* 1980; **302**: 365–70.

28. Wedege E, Bergdal T, Bolstad K *et al*. Seroepidemiological study after a long-distance industrial outbreak of legionnaires' disease. *Clin Vaccine Immunol* 2009; **16**: 528–34.

29. Nygard K, Werner-Johansen O, Ronsen S *et al*. An outbreak of legionnaires disease caused by long-distance spread from an industrial air scrubber in Sarpsborg, Norway. *Clin Infect Dis* 2008; **46**: 61–9.

30. Nygard K. Update: Outbreak of legionnaires disease in Norway traced to air scrubber. *Euro Surveill* 2005; **10**: E050609.

31. Beyrer K, Lai S, Dreesman J *et al*. Legionnaires' disease outbreak associated with a cruise liner, August 2003: Epidemiological and microbiological findings. *Epidemiol Infect* 2007; **135**: 802–10.

32. Foster K, Gorton R, Waller J. Outbreak of legionellosis associated with a spa pool, United Kingdom. *Euro Surveill* 2006; **11**: E060921.

33. Alsibai S, Bilo dB, Janin C, Che D, Lee JV. Outbreak of legionellosis suspected to be related to a whirlpool spa display, September 2006, Lorquin, France. *Euro Surveill* 2006; **11**: E061012.

34. Ruscoe Q, Hill S, Blackmore T, McLean M. An outbreak of *Legionella pneumophila* suspected to be associated with spa pools on display at a retail store in New Zealand. *N Z Med J* 2006; **119**: U2253.

35. Boshuizen HC, Neppelenbroek SE, Van Vliet H *et al*. Subclinical *Legionella* infection in workers near the source of a large outbreak of Legionnaires disease. *J Infect Dis* 2001; **184**: 515–18.

36. Benkel DH, McClure EM, Woolard D *et al*. Outbreak of Legionnaires disease associated with a display whirlpool spa. *Int J Epidemiol* 2000; **29**: 1092–8.

37. McEvoy M, Batchelor N, Hamilton G *et al*. A cluster of cases of legionnaires' disease associated with exposure to a spa pool on display. *Commun Dis Public Health* 2000; **3**: 43–5.

38. Legionnaires disease associated with a whirlpool spa display – Virginia, September–October, 1996. *Morb Mortal Wkly Rep* 1997; **46**: 83–6.

39. Ott M, Bender L, Marre R, Hacker J. Pulsed field electrophoresis of genomic restriction fragments for the detection of nosocomial *Legionella pneumophila* in hospital water supplies. *J Clin Microbiol* 1991; **29**: 813–15.

40. Memish ZA, Oxley C, Contant J, Garber GE. Plumbing system shock absorbers as a source of *Legionella pneumophila*. *Am J Infect Control* 1992; **20**: 305–9.

41. Tossa P, Deloge-Abarkan M, Zmirou-Navier D, Hartemann P, Mathieu L. Pontiac fever: An operational definition for epidemiological studies. *BMC Public Health* 2006; **6**: 112.

42. Darelid J, Bengtsson L, Gastrin B *et al*. An outbreak of Legionnaires' disease in a Swedish hospital. *Scand J Infect Dis* 1994; **26**: 417–25.

43. Blatt SP, Parkinson MD, Pace E *et al*. Nosocomial Legionnaires' disease: Aspiration as a primary mode of disease acquisition. *Am J Med* 1993; **95**: 16–22.

44. Hanrahan JP, Morse DL, Scharf VB *et al*. A community hospital outbreak of legionellosis. Transmission by potable hot water. *Am J Epidemiol* 1987; **125**: 639–49.

45. Colbourne JS, Pratt DJ, Smith MG, Fisher-Hoch SP, Harper D. Water fittings as sources of *Legionella pneumophila* in a hospital plumbing system. *Lancet* 1984; **1**: 210–13.

46. Sedgwick J, Joseph C, Chandrakumar M, Harrison T, Lee J, de Jong B. Outbreak of respiratory infection on a cruise ship. *Euro Surveill* 2007; **12**: E070809.

47. Regan CM, McCann B, Syed Q *et al*. Outbreak of Legionnaires' disease on a cruise ship: Lessons for

international surveillance and control. *Commun Dis Public Health* 2003; **6**: 152–6.

48. Cayla JA, Maldonado R, Gonzalez J *et al.* A small outbreak of Legionnaires' disease in a cargo ship under repair. *Eur Respir J* 2001; **17**: 1322–7.

49. Palmore TN, Stock F, White M *et al.* A cluster of cases of nosocomial legionnaires disease linked to a contaminated hospital decorative water fountain. *Infect Control Hosp Epidemiol* 2009; **30**: 764–8.

50. O'Loughlin RE, Kightlinger L, Werpy MC *et al.* Restaurant outbreak of Legionnaires' disease associated with a decorative fountain: An environmental and case-control study. *BMC Infect Dis* 2007; **7**: 93.

51. Hlady WG, Mullen RC, Mintz CS, Shelton BG, Hopkins RS, Daikos GL. Outbreak of Legionnaires' disease linked to a decorative fountain by molecular epidemiology. *Am J Epidemiol* 1993; **138**: 555–62.

52. Anon. Legionnaires' disease. Outbreak associated with a mist machine in a retail food store. *Wkly Epidemiol Rec* 1990; **65**: 69–70.

53. Mahoney FJ, Hoge CW, Farley TA *et al.* Communitywide outbreak of Legionnaires' disease associated with a grocery store mist machine. *J Infect Dis 1992*; **165**: 736–9.

54. Franzin L, Cabodi D, Scolfaro C, Gioannini P. Microbiological investigations on a nosocomial case of *Legionella pneumophila* pneumonia associated with water birth and review of neonatal cases. *Infez Med* 2004; **12**: 69–75.

55. Ricketts KD, Charlett A, Gelb D, Lane C, Lee JV, Joseph CA. Weather patterns and Legionnaires' disease: a meteorological study. *Epidemiol Infect* 2009; **137**: 1003–12.

56. Health and Safety Commission. *Legionnaires' Disease: The control of* Legionella *Bacteria in Water Systems.* Approved Code of Practice and Guidance L8. London: HSC, 2000.

57. Rogers J, Dowsett AB, Dennis PJ, Lee JV, Keevil CW. Influence of plumbing materials on biofilm formation and growth of *Legionella pneumophila* in potable water systems. *Appl Environ Microbiol* 1994; **60**: 1842–51.

58. Anon. *Water Supply (Water Fittings) Regulations 1999.* Statutory Instrument SI **1999**:1148.

59 Moore MR, Pryor M, Fields B, Lucas C, Phelan M, Besser RE. Introduction of monochloramine into a municipal water system: Impact on colonization of buildings by *Legionella* spp. *Appl Environ Microbiol* 2006; **72**: 378–83.

60. Kool JL, Carpenter JC, Fields BS. Effect of monochloramine disinfection of municipal drinking water on risk of nosocomial Legionnaires' disease. *Lancet* 1999; **353**: 272–7.

61. Kool JL, Bergmire-Sweat D, Butler JC *et al.* Hospital characteristics associated with colonization of water systems by *Legionella* and risk of nosocomial legionnaires' disease: A cohort study of 15 hospitals. *Infect Control Hosp Epidemiol* 1999; **20**: 798–805.

62. Heffelfinger JD, Kool JL, Fridkin S *et al.* Risk of hospital-acquired legionnaires' disease in cities using monochloramine versus other water disinfectants. *Infect Control Hosp Epidemiol* 2003; **24**: 569–74.

63. Newbold J, Copping S, Deans J *et al. Management of Spa pools – Controlling the risks of infection.* London: HPA/HSE, 2006.

64. Benson RF, Thacker WL, Lanser JA, Sangster N, Mayberry WR, Brenner DJ. *Legionella adelaidensis*, a new species isolated from cooling tower water. *J Clin Microbiol* 1991; **29**: 1004–6.

65. Gorman GW, Feeley JC, Steigerwalt A, Edelstein PH, Moss CW, Brenner DJ. *Legionella anisa*: A new species of *Legionella* isolated from potable waters and a cooling tower. *Appl Environ Microbiol* 1985; **49**: 305–9.

66. Lo PF, Riffard S, Meugnier H *et al. Legionella gresilensis* sp. nov. and *Legionella beliardensis* sp. nov., isolated from water in France. *Int J Syst Evol Microbiol* 2001; **51 (Pt 6)**:1949–57.

67. Wilkinson HW, Thacker WL, Benson RF *et al. Legionella birminghamensis* sp. nov. isolated from a cardiac transplant recipient. *J Clin Microbiol* 1987; **25**: 2120–2.

68. Wilkinson HW, Fikes BJ. Detection of cell-associated or soluble antigens of *Legionella pneumophila* serogroups 1 to 6, *Legionella bozemanii, Legionella dumoffii, Legionella gormanii,* and *Legionella micdadei* by staphylococcal coagglutination tests. *J Clin Microbiol* 1981; **14**: 322–5.

69. Wilkinson HW, Drasar V, Thacker WL *et al. Legionella moravica* sp. nov. and *Legionella brunensis* sp. nov. isolated from cooling-tower water. *Ann Inst Pasteur Microbiol* 1988; **139**: 393–402.

70. Park MY, Ko KS, Lee HK, Park MS, Kook YH. *Legionella busanensis* sp. nov., isolated from cooling tower water in Korea. *Int J Syst Evol Microbiol* 2003; **53**(Pt 1):77–80.

71. Edelstein PH, Edelstein MA. Evaluation of the Merifluor-Legionella immunofluorescent reagent for identifying and detecting 21 *Legionella* species. *J Clin Microbiol* 1989; **27**: 2455–8.

72. Thacker WL, Benson RF, Staneck JL *et al. Legionella cincinnatiensis* sp. nov. isolated from a patient with pneumonia. *J Clin Microbiol* 1988; **26**: 418–20.

73. Huang SW, Hsu BM, Ma PH, Chien KT. *Legionella* prevalence in wastewater treatment plants of Taiwan. *Water Sci Technol* 2009; **60**: 1303–10.

74. La Scola B, Birtles RJ, Greub G, Harrison TJ, Ratcliff RM, Raoult D. *Legionella drancourtii* sp. nov., a strictly intracellular amoebal pathogen. *Int J Syst Evol Microbiol* 2004; **54**(Pt 3): 699–703.

75. Adeleke AA, Fields BS, Benson RF *et al. Legionella drozanskii* sp. nov., *Legionella rowbothamii* sp. nov. and Legionella *fallonii* sp. nov.: Three unusual new *Legionella* species. *Int J Syst Evol Microbiol* 2001; **51**(Pt 3): 1151–60.

76. Thacker WL, Benson RF, Hawes L *et al. Legionella fairfieldensis* sp. nov. isolated from cooling tower waters in Australia. *J Clin Microbiol* 1991; **29**: 475–8.

77. Moss CW, Bibb WF, Karr DE, Guerrant GO, Lambert MA. Cellular fatty acid composition and ubiquinone content of *Legionella feeleii* sp. nov. *J Clin Microbiol* 1983; **18**: 917–19.

78. Dennis PJ, Brenner DJ, Thacker WL *et al*. Five new *Legionella* species isolated from water. *Int J Syst Bacteriol* 1993; **43**: 329–37.

79. Morris GK, Steigerwalt A, Feeley JC *et al. Legionella gormanii* sp. nov. *J Clin Microbiol* 1980; **12**: 718–21.

80. Bornstein N, Marmet D, Surgot M *et al. Legionella gratiana* sp. nov. isolated from French spa water. *Res Microbiol* 1989; **140**: 541–52.

81. Wilkinson HW, Thacker WL, Steigerwalt AG, Brenner DJ, Ampel NM, Wing EJ. Second serogroup of *Legionella hackeliae* isolated from a patient with pneumonia. *J Clin Microbiol* 1985; **22**: 488–9.

82. Kuroki H, Miyamoto H, Fukuda K *et al. Legionella impletisoli* sp. nov. and *Legionella yabuuchiae* sp. nov., isolated from soils contaminated with industrial wastes in Japan. *Syst Appl Microbiol* 2007; **30**: 273–9.

83. Bercovier H, Fattal B, Shuval H. Seasonal distribution of legionellae isolated from various types of water in Israel. *Isr J Med Sci* 1986; **22**: 644–6.

84. Park M, Yun ST, Kim MS, Chun J, Ahn TI. Phylogenetic characterization of Legionella-like endosymbiotic X-bacteria in *Amoeba proteus*: A proposal for 'Candidatus *Legionella jeonii*' sp. nov. *Environ Microbiol* 2004; **6**: 1252–63.

85. Cherry WB, Gorman GW, Orrison LH *et al. Legionella jordanis*: A new species of *Legionella* isolated from water and sewage. *J Clin Microbiol* 1982; **15**: 290–7.

86. Thacker WL, Dyke JW, Benson RF *et al. Legionella lansingensis* sp. nov. isolated from a patient with pneumonia and underlying chronic lymphocytic leukemia. *J Clin Microbiol* 1992; **30**: 2398–401.

87. Moss CW, Karr DE, Dees SB. Cellular fatty acid composition of *Legionella longbeachae* sp. nov. *J Clin Microbiol* 1981; **14**: 692–4.

88. Palusinska-Szysz M, Choma A, Russa R, Drozanski WJ. Cellular fatty acid composition from *Sarcobium lyticum* (*Legionella lytica* comb. nov.) – an intracellular bacterial pathogen of amoebae. *Syst Appl Microbiol* 2001; **24**: 507–9.

89. Fox A, Rogers JC, Fox KF *et al*. Chemotaxonomic differentiation of legionellae by detection and characterization of aminodideoxyhexoses and other unique sugars using gas chromatography-mass spectrometry. *J Clin Microbiol* 1990; **28**: 546–52.

90. Qu PH, Yin YB, Hu ZH *et al*. [Research on the procedure for recovery and species identification of *Legionella* from surface environmental water.] *Zhonghua Yu Fang Yi Xue Za Zhi* 2008; **42**: 653–7.

91. O'Connell WA, Dhand L, Cianciotto NP. Infection of macrophage-like cells by *Legionella* species that have not been associated with disease. *Infect Immun* 1996; **64**: 4381–4.

92. Fraser DW, Deubner DC, Hill DL, Gilliam DK. Nonpneumonic, short-incubation-period Legionellosis (Pontiac fever) in men who cleaned a steam turbine condenser. *Science* 1979; **205**: 690–1.

93. Benson RF, Thacker WL, Daneshvar MI, Brenner DJ. *Legionella waltersii* sp. nov. and an unnamed *Legionella* genomospecies isolated from water in Australia. *Int J Syst Bacteriol* 1996; **46**: 631–4.

94. Lo PF, Riffard S, Meugnier H *et al. Legionella taurinensis* sp. nov., a new species antigenically similar to *Legionella spiritensis*. *Int J Syst Bacteriol* 1999; **49**(Pt 2): 397–403.

95. Campbell J, Bibb WF, Lambert MA *et al. Legionella sainthelensi*: A new species of *Legionella* isolated from water near Mt. St. Helens. *Appl Environ Microbiol* 1984; **47**: 369–73.

96. Benson RF, Thacker WL, Fang FC, Kanter B, Mayberry WR, Brenner DJ. *Legionella sainthelensi* serogroup 2 isolated from patients with pneumonia. *Res Microbiol* 1990; **141**: 453–63.

97. Verma UK, Brenner DJ, Thacker WL, Benson RF, Vesey G, Kurtz JB *et al. Legionella shakespearei* sp. nov., isolated from cooling tower water. *Int J Syst Bacteriol* 1992; **42**: 404–7.

98. Thacker WL, Benson RF, Schifman RB *et al. Legionella tucsonensis* sp. nov. isolated from a renal transplant recipient. *J Clin Microbiol* 1989; **27**: 1831–4.

99. Edelstein PH, Brenner DJ, Moss CW, Steigerwalt AG, Francis EM, George WL. *Legionella wadsworthii* species nova: A cause of human pneumonia. *Ann Intern Med* 1982; **97**: 809–13.

100. Lück CP, Jacobs E, Röske I, Schröter-Bobsin U, Dumke R, Gronow S. *Legionella dresdenensis* sp. nov. isolated from the river Elbe near Dresden in Germany. *Int J Syst Evol Microbiol* [Epub ahead of print].

OTHER RESOURCES

- The British Thoracic Society guidelines for the diagnosis of community pneumonias are available from: http://www.brit-thoracic.org.uk/Portals/0/Clinical%20Information/Pneumonia/Guidelines/CAPGuideline-full.pdf

BURKHOLDERIA SPECIES AND THE RHIZOSPHERE

T.L. PITT

The genus *Burkholderia* is named after the American microbiologist Walter Burkholder, who first coined the species epithet *cepacia* (from the Latin *cepa*, meaning onion) for *Pseudomonas* organisms causing slippery skin rot in onions. The species *Pseudomonas cepacia*, along with six other species belonging to the *Pseudomonas* ribosomal RNA group II, were transferred to the new genus *Burkholderia* by Yabuuchi *et al.* in 1992.[1] To date, there are over 40 species within the genus, characterized by high biochemical versatility and distributed in an array of ecological niches. These range from traditional plant pathogens such as *B. gladioli*, to opportunist agents associated with respiratory infection in people with cystic fibrosis (*B. cepacia* complex), and highly pathogenic species for man and animals such as *B. mallei* and *B. pseudomallei*.

Burkholderia are natural residents of the rhizosphere and are components of a complex microbial community (e.g. *Rhizobium*, *Sphingomonas*, *Pseudomonas* and *Actinomycetes*), but have been shown to be the dominant culturable population in maize, peanut and rice plants.[2] This predominance may be explained by the production of plant defence degrading compounds, the ability to fix atmospheric nitrogen, the expression of high-affinity siderophores to chelate iron from the environment, and the synthesis of, as well as resistance to, antibiotics.

Some *Burkholderia* species play a role in plant and leaf nodulation by a symbiotic interaction with another microbe, while others have been identified growing in conjunction with fungal endomycorrhizae. These endosymbionts are characterized by a relatively small genome (1.4 Mb compared with 7.5 Mb in other species) and possess genes important for the colonization of eukaryotic cells.[3] More exotically, *Burkholderia* colonizes the midgut of Heteropterae, which feed on rice and soybean plants and are also present in ant species that cultivate symbiotic fungus gardens; these gardens may also contain *Burkholderia* that produce an antibiotic which protects both the fungus and the ants.[4] The phytopathogenic *Burkholderia* elaborate a variety of extracellular factors to obtain nutrition from the host plant tissues or induce vascular dysfunction through wounding that leads to wilting. The classic picture of macerated onion tissue associated with *B. cepacia* is caused by a single endo-polygalacturonase active at low pH.

These varied properties of the genus have been widely exploited by industry for biocontrol, bioremediation and plant growth promotion.

Members of the *B. cepacia* complex have received special attention as they are often associated with opportunistic infection in humans. They are frequent contaminants of water supplies, and, owing to their intrinsic resistance to many antibacterial compounds, numerous outbreaks in hospitals have been documented involving the contamination of antiseptics, infusion fluids and tubing for irrigation. People with cystic fibrosis are susceptible to infection with these bacteria, and some species, such as *B. cenocepacia*, can have a significant impact on life expectancy and quality of life in these individuals.[5]

Burkholderia pseudomallei is common in water and soil in parts of South East Asia and Northern Australia, and infections can be acquired from these sources. It causes the disease melioidosis, which commonly presents as acute pulmonary infection with septicaemia or local wound infection. Mortality is high if the condition is untreated, and relapse is common. Diabetes and renal insufficiency are predisposing risk factors for infection. Chronic infection is characterized by the formation of multiple abscesses in organs, particularly the spleen and liver. Disease in Western countries is usually associated with travel to endemic areas, but sporadic cases from other tropical areas are reported.[6] *Burkholderia mallei* is the cause of glanders in equines, and human infection is rare.

References

● = Key primary paper

◆ = Major review article

●1. Yabuuchi E, Kosako Y, Oyaizu H *et al.* Proposal of *Burkholderia* gen. nov.; and transfer of seven species of the *Pseudomonas* homology group II to the new genus, with the type species *Burkholderia cepacia* (Palleroni and Holmes 1981) comb.nov. *Microbiol Immunol* 1992; **36**: 1251–75.

◆2. Balandreau J, Mavingui P. Beneficial interactions of *Burkholderia* spp. with plants. In: Coeyne T, Vandamme P (eds) Burkholderia, *Molecular Biology and Genomics*. Norfolk, UK: Horizon Bioscience, 2007: 129–51.

●3. Ruiz Lozano JM, Bonfante P. A *Burkholderia* strain living inside the arbuscular mycorrhizal fungus *Gigaspora margarita* possesses the *vac*B gene, which is involved in host cell colonization by bacteria. *Microb Ecol* 2000; **39**: 137–44.

●4. Valmir Santos A, Dillon RJ, Dillon VM, Reynolds SE, Samuels RI. Occurrence of the antibiotic producing bacterium *Burkholderia* spp. in colonies of the leaf cutting ant *Atta sexdens rubropilosa*. *FEMS Microbiol Lett* 2004; **239**: 319–23.

◆5. Govan JRW. *Burkholderia cepacia* complex and *Stenotrophomonas maltophilia*. In: Bush A, Alton EWFW, Davies JC, Griesenbach U (eds) *Cystic Fibrosis in the 21st Century*. Progress in Respiratory Research Vol. 34. Basel: Karger, 2006: 145–52.

◆6. Pitt T, Simpson AJH. *Pseudomonas* and *Burkholderia* spp. In: Gillespie SH, Hawkey PM (eds) *Principles and Practice of Clinical Bacteriology*, 2nd edn. London: Wiley, 2005: 427–43.

Q-FEVER

JON G. AYRES

Q (query)-fever is caused by the rickettsia-like, spore-bearing organism *Coxiella burnettii*, a cause of endemic abortion in sheep and cattle.[1] The organism is widespread worldwide, and many other animals are known to act as reservoirs. Infection is by the inhaled route, the incubation period being variable and partly related to the infecting dose, averaging about 21 days.[1] Fewer than 10 organisms can cause a clinical infection, and because of its potency, *Coxiella burnettii* has in the past been considered as a germ warfare weapon. The highest human exposures are seen in at-risk occupations in rural areas, notably farmers and abattoir workers.

Non-occupational disease has been documented following windborne outbreaks[2-4] usually associated with specific meteorological conditions, notably high winds, often at the time of lambing or calving. Other outbreaks have been attributed to a range of non-occupational sources, although the exact cause of an outbreak is often not clearly identified.

ACUTE Q-FEVER

Acute Q-fever is a pneumonic illness with a high swinging fever, profuse sweating and often profound weight loss. Neurological symptoms or transient complications (ranging from headache to paresis) are common, but recovery is usual and death in the acute illness is rare.[5] Patients are usually treated with broad-spectrum antibiotics before a specific diagnosis is made. It has often been recommended that tetracycline or a macrolide should be used, although there is no clinical trial evidence to support this. The best antibiotic identified by in vitro studies is rifampicin.

CHRONIC Q-FEVER

Chronic Q-fever occurs insidiously, usually presenting as chronic endocarditis (the aortic or mitral valve being most commonly affected) but more rarely as granulomatous hepatitis or osteomyelitis, and even more rarely with bone marrow involvement.[1] Treatment for chronic Q-fever is unsatisfactory although doxycycline and hydroxyquinoline have been recommended, albeit on limited evidence. Cardiac valve replacement is often needed. A history of preceding acute Q-fever is relatively uncommon in this condition.

Q-FEVER FATIGUE SYNDROME

Q-fever fatigue syndrome (QFS) has recently been recognized as a specific form of post-infection fatigue.[6]

This has been reported following both occupational and environmental exposure. The spectrum of symptoms is very similar to that of classical chronic fatigue syndrome (CFS) although in the occupational setting, where repeated exposure to the organism can occur (which would be unusual where exposure occurred non-occupationally), symptoms can occur with severe apparent exacerbations. Recurrent episodes of painful lymphadenopathy have been recognized in abattoir workers. There is no specific treatment for QFS, but approaches along the lines of graduated exercises, as is the case with chronic fatigue syndrome, may be appropriate.

DIAGNOSIS AND PATHOGENESIS

The initial diagnosis of acute Q-fever is made with complement-fixing antibodies or through immunofluorescence. Phase 2 immunoglobulin G antibodies rise acutely and settle back to lower levels by about 9 months. If there is a rise in titre of phase 1 antibodies, the risk of developing chronic Q-fever is increased, perhaps representing an altered immune response resulting from persistence of the antigen.[7]

The *Coxiella* genome has been detected in bone marrow many years after the initial infection, which may be important in Q-fever reactivation (sometimes seen in pregnancy), Q-fever endocarditis and QFS.[8] It has been postulated that persistent genomic fragments cause differential cytokine dysregulation in susceptible individuals, thus permitting these different clinical patterns to become manifest. A vaccination programme in Australia has proved effective at reducing disease in those working in contact with animals.[9]

References

1. Sawyer LA, Fishbein DB, McDade JE. Q fever: current concepts. *Rev Infect Dis* 1987; **9**: 935–46.
2. Hawker JI, Ayres JG, Blair I *et al.* (Q Fever Group). A large Q fever outbreak in the West Midlands: windborne spread into a metropolitan area? *Commun Dis Pub Health* 1998; **1**: 180–7.
3. Lyytikainen O, Zlese T, Schwartlander B *et al.* Outbreak of Q fever in Lohra-Rollshausen, Germany, Spring 1996. *Eurosurveillance* 1997; **2**: 9–11.
4. Armengaud A, Kessalis N, Desenclos JC *et al.* Urban outbreak of Q fever, Briancon, France, March to June 1996. *Eurosurveillance* 1997; **2**: 12–13.
5. Smith DL, Ayres JG, Blair I *et al.* (Q Fever Group). A large Q fever epidemic in the West Midlands: clinical features. *Respir Med* 1993; **87**: 509–16.

6. Wildman M, Smith EG, Groves J, Ayres JG. Chronic fatigue syndrome following acute Q fever: 10 year follow up of the 1989 outbreak cohort. *QJM* 2002; **95**: 527–38.

7. Marmion BP, Storm PA, Ayres J, Semendric L, Harris RJ. Long term persistence of *Coxiella burnetii* after acute primary Q fever: a cooperative study of persistent markers of infection in Q fever patients in the Birmingham (UK) outbreak

and in sporadic cases in Australia. *QJM* 2005; **98**: 7–20.

8. Helbig K, Harris R, Ayres J *et al.* Variation in immune response genes in the post Q-fever fatigue syndrome, Q fever endocarditis and uncomplicated acute primary Q fever. *QJM* 2005; **98**: 565–74.

9. Gidding HF, Wallace C, Lawrence GL, McIntyre PB. Australia's national Q fever vaccination program. *Vaccine* 2009; **27**: 2037–41.

PSITTACOSIS (CAPTIVE BIRDS)

ROBERT M. SMITH

In the UK in recent years, there has been an increasing trend for pet birds to be sold through large chain stores in addition to being available from more conventional high-street pet shops. This may encourage the purchase of birds – and other animals – without adequate preparation or planning. Many of the birds sold in this way originate from a relatively small number of suppliers.

Chlamydophila psittaci is a bacterium in the family Chlamydiaceae that can be transmitted from pet birds to humans; the resulting infection is colloquially known as 'psittacosis', 'parrot fever' or 'ornithosis'. Psittacosis in humans presents as a generalized acute chlamydial disease with an incubation period of 1–4 weeks. The clinical presentation may be variable with fever, headache, myalgia and either upper or lower respiratory tract symptoms that are often disproportionately mild when compared with the extensive pneumonia that may be demonstrated radiologically.

Although human disease may range from mild to moderate, it can be severe, especially when untreated as well as in the elderly. Mortality is, however, less than 1 per cent. Treatment is by conventional antibiotics, although doxycycline is the antibiotic of choice where the diagnosis is suspected.

Apparently healthy birds may shed *Chlamydophila* that can then infect other birds or humans. Psittacines

are physiologically able to cope adequately with the infection, unlike other orders of birds, which may show a history of disease, such as sneezing, or may have obvious discharges in or around the nares or beak, which may be evidence of respiratory infection. The signs of chlamydiosis in birds vary with the species of bird, the virulence of the chlamydial strain, the stresses on the bird and the route of exposure; there are no pathognomonic signs or lesions.

Chlamydiosis is a systemic disease with signs that include lethargy, ruffled feathers and anorexia and a serous or purulent ocular and/or nasal discharge. Diarrhoea, if it occurs, may be greenish-yellow. Psittacines may only develop signs of the disease when severely stressed, with the organism being excreted in the faeces and/or nasal discharges of infected birds. In some cases, the first sign of illness is sudden death. Shedding may be intermittent and is exacerbated by stress from transportation, crowding, chilling or even breeding.

The organism is resistant to desiccation and can remain infectious for some months. Infected birds can excrete high concentrations of organisms in their faeces and, if untreated, pose a hazard not only to other birds, but also to humans. Pet psittacines in pet shops, aviaries and homes are most likely to infect humans.

19

Aspergillosis, mucormycosis, cryptococcosis, coccidioidomycosis and histoplasmosis

ELIZABETH M. JOHNSON

Members of the kingdom Fungi are eukaryotic organisms that lack chlorophyll and must therefore obtain their nutrients from external sources. There are several important classes of fungal infection that are acquired primarily by the respiratory route, and many moulds may also cause infection of wounds or by accidental subcutaneous inoculation. The organisms that cause these opportunistic infections are saprobes living on dead, decaying organic matter, are recognized plant and animal pathogens that are acquired from the environment or are constituents of the faecal flora of animals and birds.

These fungi share a means of aerial dispersal that involves the production of large numbers of spores that are in many cases small enough to penetrate to the alveoli following inhalation. Infections are therefore usually initially acquired via the respiratory tract and are often primarily pulmonary, although following sinus or lung infection all have the capacity to cause life-threatening infection by haematogenous dissemination to other organs. The propensity to spread depends largely on the host's underlying immune status.

ASPERGILLOSIS

The spectrum of disease caused by *Aspergillus* species ranges from allergic reactions following the inhalation of spores by atopic individuals or those encountering repeated or overwhelming exposure, through to frequently fatal disseminated disease encountered predominantly in severely immunocompromised patients. Spores trapped in the mucous secretions of patients with cystic fibrosis can lead to

acute bronchopulmonary aspergillosis.[1] Sinus infection, keratitis, otomycosis and wound infections are seen in otherwise healthy individuals. Aspergilloma occurs when pre-existing lung cavities are colonized,[2,3] and a more severe form is chronic cavitating aspergillosis.[4] The progressively more invasive chronic necrotizing aspergillosis is encountered in debilitated patients, and invasive aspergillosis in immunocompromised patients.[5-7]

Many *Aspergillus* species also produce powerful mycotoxins. The repeated ingestion of aflatoxin, produced primarily by *Aspergillus flavus*, and other mycotoxins can cause hepatitis, cirrhosis and liver cancer. Clusters of cases have been identified particularly in children when populations have eaten grains stored under poor conditions.[8-10]

Aspergilllus species epidemiology

Spores of the genus *Aspergillus* are ubiquitous in the environment and have been found on every continent. This genus is characterized by the production of large numbers of dry spores suited for air dispersal, and in studies of environmental air sampling this genus is one of the predominant organisms. The most abundant production of spores is associated with growth on straw, hay, leaf litter and grass compost with a high moisture content.[11,12]

The dose necessary for establishing invasive disease is unknown, but it is clear that individuals with normal pulmonary function and an intact immune system can usually withstand extensive exposure without contracting infection, whereas those who are severely immunocompromised are vulnerable to much lower inocula.[13] Inhalation of conidia is the usual mechanism of infection, and it has been shown that the alveolar macrophages form a first-line cellular defence against inhaled *Aspergillus* conidia and that the neutrophils are an important defence against conidia that have germinated to form hyphae. Thus, a reduction in the number or function of these cells is a major predisposing factor leading to invasive disease.[14]

Members of the *Aspergillus fumigatus* species complex are those most frequently implicated in disease, with at least 66 per cent of invasive infection being due to this species,[7] although in some superficial infections such as otomycosis, *A. niger* appears to predominate.[15] *Aspergillus* spp. have traditionally been identified phenotypically by the distinctive appearance of their colonial and microscopic morphology (Figure 19.1). However, molecular identification techniques have revealed that most *Aspergillus* species are really complexes that contain a large number of cryptic species. These cannot readily be distinguished by morphology visible under the light microscope, and some distinctions are only possible at the molecular level as several genetically distinct species often exist within a single morphospecies.[16] Currently, the *Aspergillus* section *Fumigati* comprises in excess of 29 species of *Neosartorya* and 14 species of *Aspergillus*.

INVASIVE ASPERGILLOSIS

Invasive aspergillosis is a devastating infection, often nosocomial, that occurs most frequently in those suffering severe immunosuppression due to disease or treatment for it. Prolonged neutropenia ($<0.5 \times 10^9$ neutrophils/L) of typically more than 12 days, corticosteroid use and acquired immune deficiency syndrome (AIDS) are major factors predisposing to invasive disease, with the majority of infections seen in patients with haematological malignancy.[6,7,17,18] In all patients, invasive aspergillosis is usually respiratory in origin, most often infecting the lungs but occasionally manifesting as a sinus infection.

Haematogenous dissemination from the primary site, especially to the brain, is associated with high mortality.[19] The highest-risk group for acquiring invasive pulmonary infection includes those undergoing bone marrow transplantation, particularly allogeneic transplant requiring powerful immunosuppressive regimes. This is often associated with the need for high-dose corticosteroids to manage graft-versus-host disease, which can lead to invasive infection several months after the transplant.[7,20,21] In patients undergoing a solid organ transplant, the highest risk is associated with lung transplantation.[22]

The source of infection can be difficult to determine but may stem from high airborne spore counts resulting from construction work or plant decomposition. In order to protect patients from the risk of inhaling *Aspergillus* spores, standards of air quality involving the use of high-efficiency particulate air filtration have been recommended for units housing bone marrow transplant recipients, especially during phases of profound neutropenia.[22]

Diagnosis and treatment

The early diagnosis of invasive aspergillosis is critical to a favourable outcome, and clinical diagnosis is improved by the use of high-resolution computed tomography scans of the chest early in the course of infection to look for the presence of a halo sign. Although not pathognomonic for invasive fungal disease, this is a useful adjunct to diagnosis in high-risk patient groups.[23]

Laboratory diagnosis is by means of direct microscopy of respiratory secretions, bronchoalveolar lavage fluids or tissues for the presence of hyaline, branching, septate hyphae; this is often enhanced by staining with a fluorescent brightener followed by culture on glucose–peptone agar and incubation at 37 and 42 °C.[24]

Blood culture is often negative even in disseminated disease, and although it is helpful to look for a raised titre of immunoglobulin (Ig) G antibody in immunocompetent patients with aspergilloma and IgE antibody in patients with allergic symptoms, antibodies are often not detected in those with invasive disease. In such cases, other markers of infection have been sought, and galactomannan antigen detection, beta-D-glucan detection and molecular methods such as the polymerase chain reaction (PCR) have been widely investigated.[24–27] However, only the first two have been accepted by the European Organization for Research and Treatment of Cancer as diagnostic criteria for helping to establish 'proven', 'probable' and 'possible' invasive fungal disease.[28]

Treatment modalities have improved greatly in recent years, although invasive disease is still associated with a high morbidity and mortality. Owing to difficulties in making an early diagnosis, empirical treatment is still often employed, although there is a move towards more targeted

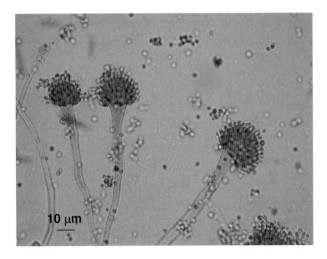

Figure 19.1   Sporing heads of *Aspergillus fumigatus*.

treatment. Large trials of empirical therapy have shown caspofungin to be as effective as liposomal amphotericin B, with fewer side-effects.[29] Trials for the treatment of invasive aspergillosis have established voriconazole and liposomal amphotericin B as effective first-line agents,[30,31] and there have been successful salvage therapy trials with caspofungin and posaconazole.[32,33] There is also good evidence for the use of itraconazole and posaconazole in prophylaxis for high-risk patients.[34,35] All these agents are reviewed in the Infectious Diseases Society of America's clinical practice guidelines for the treatment of invasive aspergillosis.[36]

MUCORMYCOSIS (ZYGOMYCOSIS)

Zygomycete fungi are common food spoilage organisms. Several genera can cause infection, and these are characterized by an ability to grow at 37 °C. Those species most often implicated in human disease are members of the order Mucorales: *Rhizopus arrhizus*, *Rhizopus microsporus* group, *Rhizo rhizopodiformis*, *Rhizomucor pusillus*, *Mucor circinelloides* and *Lichtheimia corymbifera* (previously *Absidia corymbifera*).[37]

The predominance of the order Mucorales in infection led to the term 'mucormycosis', but the term 'zygomycosis' was considered to be more comprehensive, also encompassing the less common infections caused by the Entomophthorales: *Conidiobolus coronatus* and *Basidiobolus ranarum*. However, it has long been recognized that the phylum Zygomycota is polyphyletic, and since molecular analyses have been possible, the taxonomy of this phylum has been in a considerable state of flux, the majority of human pathogens now being included in a new subphylum Mucoromycotina.[38]

Although infection can follow the deposition of spores onto the susceptible tissue of burns or other open wounds, leading to a rapidly invasive infection with marked necrosis, the most common presentation is as rhinocerebral zygomycosis following the inhalation of spores.[37] The zygomycete fungi are characterized by having broad, almost aseptate hyphae. These fungi are angioinvasive, targeting and growing along blood vessels, which means they can spread very rapidly within and between contiguous tissues. The physical mass of the fungus occludes the blood vessels, causing ischaemia and localized necrosis, which, if visible externally, may be the first clinical sign of disease. If not recognized early, the fungus can rapidly spread from the nasal sinus to the orbit and the brain, hence the term 'rhinocerebral zygomycosis'. Spores that are inhaled more deeply into the lungs in a susceptible patient result in pulmonary zygomycosis, which mimics invasive aspergillosis and is hard to diagnose. Infection of the gastrointestinal tract is also difficult to diagnose.

Patients with uncontrolled diabetes with ketoacidosis and individuals with neutropenia are most vulnerable to infection with mucoraceous moulds due to a reduction in cell-mediated immunity. High-dose corticosteroid use and high iron levels are other predisposing factors, whereas an infection of wounds can follow the deposition of spores.[37] Neonatal infection can be particularly rapidly progressive and devastating as neonatal skin is delicate and friable and presents no physical barrier to the invasion of hyphae.[39] Although infection is usually sporadic involving individual cases, there have been occasional outbreaks associated with contaminated fomites such as sticking plaster, wound dressings and wooden tongue depressors, which were in the past used for holding intravenous lines and monitoring equipment in situ.[40]

Diagnosis and treatment

It is important that zygomycete infections are distinguished from invasive aspergillosis and other mould infections as only a few of the systemically active antifungal agents are effective against the former.[41] Early diagnosis is essential to a successful outcome owing to the rapid progression of infection. Direct microscopy of tissue is the fastest way to make a diagnosis, based on the appearance of broad, ribbon-like, thin-walled, almost aseptate hyphae; a fluorescent brightener can help to reveal the hyphae. Pan-fungal PCR followed by sequencing may be used to identify the fungus but has been used mainly on tissue samples as it lacks the sensitivity for use as a diagnostic test on blood samples. There are currently no antigen tests available to detect this group of fungi, and the detection of beta-D-glucan is ineffective as this is not a major cell wall component in this group.

Treatment focuses on rectifying the underlying predisposing factor, surgical debridement and the administration of lipid amphotericin products, often at higher doses than those used for invasive aspergillosis; new approaches also include the use of hyperbaric oxygen and cytokine therapy.[41] More recently, there have been publications supporting the use of the extended-spectrum triazole posaconazole as salvage therapy.[42]

CRYPTOCOCCOSIS

Several species of the yeast *Cryptococcus* have been implicated in human infection, and different species are thought to differ in their pathogenicity. Although there are 19 species in the genus *Cryptococcus*, few are capable of growth at 37 °C and therefore able to cause disease in warm-blooded animals. Within the species *Cryptococcus neoformans* are several varieties classified as serotypes A, B, C, D and AD.[43] Types A, D and AD were traditionally recognized as being *Cryptococcus neoformans* var. *neoformans*, and types B and C as *Cryptococcus neoformans* var. *gattii*. It has since become apparent that serotype A, which is the most common in Europe, is sufficiently different to be classified as a variety in its own right: *Cryptococcus neoformans* var. *grubii*.[44–46] Reports of infections with the less pathogenic species *Cryptococcus albidus* and *Cryptococcus laurentii* and others are, although rare, increasing in incidence.[47–49]

Infection is acquired by inhalation, and in an immunocompetent host this may result in a mild flu-like illness, which resolves spontaneously. Studies suggest high exposure rates to *Cryptococcus neoformans* in children living in urban areas, with the majority of children above the age of 2 years living in the Bronx, New York, demonstrating antibodies reactive with *Cryptococcus neoformans* proteins.[50]

In the immunocompromised individual, the yeast appears to have a predilection for the central nervous system (CNS), resulting in life-threatening cryptococcal meningitis. There is a steady incidence of cryptococcal meningitis in patients not infected with human immunodeficiency virus (HIV) who have decreased cell-mediated immunity, for example those taking steroids for sarcoidosis, systemic lupus erythematosus or solid organ transplantation, and those with a haematological malignancy.[51–53] Occasionally, no underlying abnormality can be found.

Cryptococcosis is, however, now predominantly a disease of HIV-infected individuals, is recognized as the most common CNS fungal infection associated with HIV infection[54] and is classified as an AIDS-defining illness.[55–57] The widespread use of highly active antiretroviral therapy to control HIV infection has resulted in a reduction in incidence of cryptococcosis in countries where such therapy is readily available. There are, however, many areas, such as Africa and South-East Asia, where the AIDS epidemic is less controlled and cryptococcosis has emerged as the second most prevalent opportunistic infection in this group after tuberculosis.

Cryptococcus is an encapsulated yeast 4–6 μm in diameter that reproduces by budding. The capsule, together with melanin production, is thought to be a virulence factor protecting the cells from the killing mechanisms of phagocytic cells.[58] The sexual form (teleomorph) is the mould *Filobasidiella neoformans* or *Filobasidiella bacillispora* depending on the anamorph variety, a basidiomycete that produces multiple basidiospores. These are smaller than the yeast form (1–3 μm in diameter) and potentially a better candidate for aerial dispersal, although the sexual form has not been isolated from patients or the environment so the role of basidiospores in disease acquisition remains unknown.

There is a strong environmental association between *Cryptococcus neoformans* var. *neoformans* and var. *grubii* and soil contaminated with pigeon or other bird guano, and they are geographically widespread.[59,60] The yeasts replicate in the gut with no ill effects to the birds, possibly due to their higher body temperature than humans.[59] When excreted, however, the pigeon guano acts as a natural selective medium due to the presence of low molecular weight nitrogenous compounds. The yeast form can withstand desiccation and exposure to ultraviolet light, and can therefore survive for long periods as the guano dries out and

is dispersed by air currents. It is believed that the smaller desiccated yeast cells are then inhaled and that this can result in pulmonary infection. In the immunocompromised patient, lung infection can progress to haematogenous dissemination and spread to the CNS, resulting in life-threatening cryptococcal meningitis and sometimes cutaneous cryptococcosis or osteomyelitis. In males, the prostate has been implicated as a sanctuary site in recurrent disease.[61]

The variety *gattii* is geographically more restricted to tropical and subtropical areas, and in Australia and Africa there is a strong association with *Eucalyptus camaldulensis*.[62] This variety has more recently been found causing an outbreak in immunocompetent humans and animals on Vancouver Island in Canada, where there is also a tentative association with *Eucalyptus* plants.[63–65] Infections with var. *gattii* are more often found in individuals without recognized underlying predisposing factors and tend to be more aggressive and harder to treat than those caused by var. *neoformans* or var. *grubii*.[66,67]

Diagnosis and treatment

A drop of cerebrospinal fluid (CSF) from a patient with cryptococcal meningitis placed in a drop of Indian ink reveals budding yeasts surrounded by the thick polysaccharide capsule, which displaces the ink (Figure 19.2).[68] The detection of capsular material by a latex agglutination test is another sensitive method by which the diagnosis can be confirmed using samples of either serum or CSF.[69] Culture of respiratory secretions or CSF may yield a more or less mucoid colony depending on the size of the capsule. Such isolates can often be identified by commercial sugar assimilation methods or by amplification of the ITS1 and ITS2 regions of the large ribosomal subunit followed by sequencing and comparison with Internet-based databases.

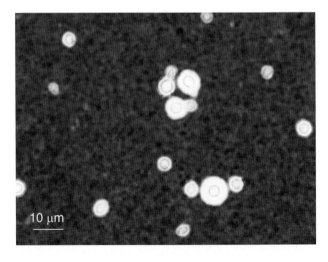

Figure 19.2 Indian ink stain of *Cryptococcus neoformans*, revealing the polysaccharide capsule.

Before the advent of amphotericin B, disseminated cryptococcal disease was uniformly fatal with an average duration of 6 weeks. The treatment of choice for cryptococcal meningitis still hinges on a combination of amphotericin B and flucytosine for the first 14 days as this rapidly sterilizes the CSF. Following this, oral fluconazole is used as maintenance therapy; fluconazole can also be used as primary therapy in disease not affecting the CNS.[70] At one time, life-long maintenance was required following infection in HIV-infected patients, but with advances in antiretroviral therapy, it has been found that maintenance can be stopped after the prolonged stabilization of CD4 counts.[71,72]

COCCIDIOIDOMYCOSIS

Coccidioidomycosis is a pulmonary infection acquired by the inhalation of arthrospores of the dimorphic fungus *Coccidioides immitis* or the more recently described *Coccidioides posadasii*.[73] Infection occurs in very restricted geographical locations in the south-western USA, Mexico and small areas of Central and South America, although the areas of endemicity are increasing, as evidenced by the presence of infection in small rodents from adjacent areas. Diagnoses made outside these areas have been in travellers returning from endemic areas or have occasionally been due to the exposure of individuals to dust or vegetation from endemic areas.[74–76]

The fungus is thermally dimorphic and grows as a mycelial form in the environment that readily breaks into unicellular arthroconidia by a process known as rhexolysis. This procedure results in the production of numerous spores with small amounts of cell wall material left on them, which markedly enhances their aerodynamic properties, allowing them to travel readily on air currents. Following inhalation, the arthroconidia reach the alveoli where they convert to spherules, the in vivo growth form, at 37 °C. Each spherule is a thick-walled structure that swells, matures and differentiates to produce multiple endospores. Rupture of the mature spherules to release the endospores starts the cycle again and leads to pulmonary coccidioidomycosis.

The resulting respiratory infection is mostly a mild febrile illness known as 'valley fever' and widely suffered by those resident in endemic areas, as evidenced by skin test positivity to coccidin antigen.[74] Endospores occasionally spread haematogenously to cause life-threatening disseminated disease; this happens most frequently in immunocompromised individuals, but pregnant women and certain racial groups, notably those from the Philippines, are also at increased risk.

An 'outbreak' of coccidioidomycosis was observed from 1991 to 1994. There had been an 11-fold increase in the mean number of cases from 1955 to 1990, and Fisher and colleagues investigated whether or not this was a point source outbreak associated with a shift to increased pathogenicity of a particular strain of *Coccidioides*.[77]

Molecular analysis of the isolates involved revealed that there was considerable genetic diversity; however, it was found that the principle factors governing the epidemic were not genetic but environmental, linked to cyclical periods of rain and drought, which led to a great increase in population size of the fungus. Isolates from patients in New York had multilocus genotypes similar to those found in Arizona, suggesting that infections had been acquired in the known area of endemicity.

Diagnosis and treatment

All clinical samples should be handled under a hood, and in Europe this should be housed in a hazard containment level 3 facility as *Coccidioides* is classified as a hazard group 3 organism. In the USA, it is classified as biosafety level 2, but propagation requires level 3 facilities. It is known that the infective dose is small and may be as low as 10 fungal spores; before protective handling facilities were introduced, there were frequent infections resulting from laboratory exposure.[62]

Diagnosis is by microscopic examination of sputum, bronchoalveolar lavage or other body fluids or tissues for the presence of fungal spherules containing endospores, which comprise the growth form encountered in vivo. These samples should then be incubated at 30 °C to encourage growth of the mould form of the fungus as it is very difficult to obtain spherule production in vivo. Once there is a white, floccose mould growth, microscopic examination will reveal the presence of arthrospore production in which the spores are separated by empty cells that split by a process known as rhexolysis (Figure 19.3). Identification of the fungus is by means of its microscopic morphology and exoantigen production and, if necessary,

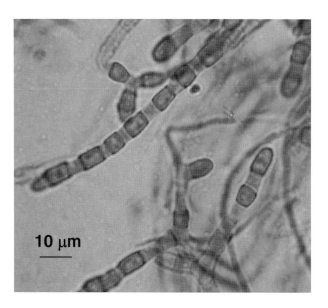

Figure 19.3 Arthrospores of *Coccidioides immitis*.

PCR amplification and sequencing of its DNA. Non-culture methods include the detection of antibodies by immunodiffusion and complement fixation tests.[62]

Many patients with pulmonary infection do not require treatment, but in immunocompromised patients or those showing signs of dissemination, the initial treatment of choice is amphotericin B followed by oral itraconazole or fluconazole, although there are fewer relapses with the former. If there is meningeal involvement, the latter is preferred.[78]

HISTOPLASMOSIS

Histoplasmosis is the most common endemic mycosis in the USA and is also the most common systemic mycosis imported into Europe.[79] The dimorphic moulds *Histoplasma capsulatum* var. *capsulatum* and *Histoplasma capsulatum* var. *duboisii* are the two causative agents of histoplasmosis in humans, whereas *Histoplasmosis capsulatum* var. *farciminosum* causes infection in horses. In Europe, these are classified as hazard group 3 organisms.

These moulds exhibit thermal dimorphism, which means that they have two different growth forms: in the environment and at temperatures of 30°C they grow as filamentous moulds, but at 37°C or *in vivo* they grow as budding yeasts. The in vitro mould forms of the two varieties affecting humans are indistinguishable as both produce multiple teardrop-shaped microconidia and larger tuberculate macroconidia that have distinctive surface projections. However, the yeast forms are readily differentiated due to their size: that of var. *capsulatum* resembles *Candida glabrata* in shape and size (2–4 μm diameter) and is often found within phagocytic cells, whereas that of var. *duboisii* is about 10 times as large and is often seen forming short chains.

The major endemic area for *Histoplasma capsulatum* var. *capsulatum* follows the Mississippi river delta in Eastern North America, although cases have been reported from many other areas, including South-East Asia and Africa as well as some European countries. Individuals resident in these areas are infected in childhood. The endemic area for var. *duboisii* is more restricted, being found mainly between the tropics of Cancer and Capricorn on the African continent.[80]

With both forms, infection follows the inhalation of spores from the mould form growing in the environment, and histoplasmosis is thus primarily a pulmonary infection; it is asymptomatic or only mildly symptomatic in most people. High concentrations are found in bird and bat guano, and infection often follows occupational exposure due to construction and environmental clean-up work or exposure as a result of recreational activities such as spelunking (caving).

Histoplasma has quite specific growth requirements, and the presence of high concentrations of guano, especially under blackbird roosts and around chicken coops, provides the right humidity, acidity and presence of nitrogenous compounds to lead to profuse mycelial growth.[80,81] Although, in contrast to bats, birds themselves are not infected, it is believed that they may contribute to the environmental spread of the organism on their feet and feathers, while bats excrete the organism in their faeces.[82]

Although many individuals are exposed on a daily basis and may merely suffer a mild respiratory infection, dissemination occurs in some individuals, and the disease can become life-threatening. Most cases are sporadic, but there have been reports of large-scale outbreaks involving numerous individuals. Histoplasmosis is an AIDS-defining illness and has emerged as an important opportunistic pathogen in HIV-infected individuals residing in endemic areas.[80] A presentation of the disease – acute septic histoplasmosis – has been recognized in this group of patients.

Diagnosis and treatment

The diagnosis of *Histoplasma capsulatum* var. *capsulatum* is by the observation of small (2–3 μm diameter), budding yeast cells often seen within macrophages either in respiratory or tissue samples, in particular Giemsa-stained bone marrow smears. The yeast form of the var. *duboisii* can be differentiated by its larger diameter (8–15 μm). Growth at 37°C on slopes of blood or bone heart infusion agar will encourage the growth of the yeast form, whereas the mould form will grow at 30°C. Mould colonies are white to beige and spreading, with a powdery surface. Microscopic examination of the mould form will reveal multiple small microconidia formed along the sides of hyphae and distinctive large, tuberculate macroconidia (Figure 19.4).[82]

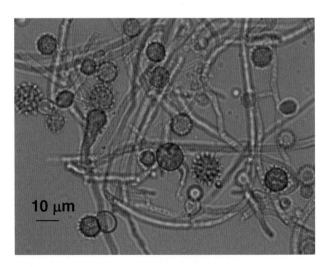

Figure 19.4   Tuberculate macroconidia of *Histoplasma capsulatum*.

Non-culture methods include the detection of antibodies by immunodiffusion or complement fixation tests, and an antigen test currently available in the USA is helpful in HIV-infected patients, who may not mount an antibody response.[83]

Many patients with pulmonary infection will not require treatment. HIV-infected patients and those with disseminated disease should, however, initially be treated with lipid forms of amphotericin B followed by itraconazole.[84]

REFERENCES

● = Key primary paper
◆ = Major review article

1. Rosenberg M, Patterson R, Mintzer R et al. Clinical and immunological criteria for the diagnosis of bronchopulmonary aspergillosis. Ann Intern Med 1977; 86: 405–14.
◆2. Aslam P, Eastridge C, Hughes F. Aspergillosis of the lung – an 18 year experience. Chest 1971; 59: 28–32.
3. Kauffman CA. Quandary about treatment of aspergillomas persists. Lancet 1996; 347: 1640.
◆4. Denning DW, Riniotis K, Dobrashian R et al. Chronic cavitary and fibrosing pulmonary and pleural aspergillosis: Case series, proposed nomenclature change and review. Clin Infect Dis 2003; 37(Suppl. 3): S265–80.
5. Austwick PKC. Pathogenicity. In: Raper KB, Fennel DI (eds) The Genus Aspergillus. Baltimore: Williams & Wilkins, 1965: 82–126.
◆6. Denning DW. Invasive aspergillosis. Clin Infect Dis 1998; 26: 781–803.
◆7. Patterson TF, Kirkpatrick WR, White M et al. Invasive aspergillosis. Disease spectrum, treatment practices, and outcomes. 13 Aspergillus Study Group. Medicine 2000; 79: 250–60.
8. Dhatt PS, Parida NK, Das Chaudhury PK et al. Aflatoxins and Indian childhood cirrhosis. Indian J Paediatr 1982; 19: 407–8.
9. Denning DW. Aflatoxin and human disease. A review. Adverse Drug React Acute Poisoning Rev 1987; 4: 175–209.
10. Hedayati MT, Pasqualotto AC, Warn PA et al. Aspergillus flavus: Human pathogen, allergen and mycotoxins producer. Microbiology 2007; 153: 1677–92.
11. Emmons CW. The Jekyll–Hydes of mycology. Mycopathologia 1960; 52: 669–80.
12. Eastwood DJ. The fungus flora of composts. Brit Med Soc Trans 1952; 35: 215–20.
◆13. Patterson TF. Aspergillosis. In: Dismukes WE, Pappas PG, Sobel JD (eds) Clinical Mycology. Oxford: Oxford University Press, 2003: 221–40.
◆14. Kauffman HF, Tomee JF. Defence mechanisms of the airways against Aspergillus fumigatus: Role in invasive aspergillosis. Chem Immunol 2002; 81: 94–113.
15. Loh KS, Tan KK, Kumarasinghe G et al. Otitis externa – the clinical pattern in a tertiary institution in Singapore. Ann Acad Med Singapore 1998; 27: 215–18.
16. Balajee SA, Houbraken J, Verweij PE et al. Aspergillus species identification in the clinical setting. Stud Mycol 2007; 59: 39–46.
17. Walsh TJ, Dixon DM. Nosocomial aspergillosis: Environmental microbiology, hospital epidemiology, diagnosis and treatment. Eur J Epidemiol 1989; 5: 131–42.
18. Denning DW, Follansbee SE, Scolaro M et al. Pulmonary aspergillosis in the acquired immunodeficiency syndrome. N Engl J Med 1991; 324: 654–62.
◆19. Lin SJ, Schranz J, Teutsch SM. Aspergillosis case-fatality rate: Systematic review of the literature. Clin Infect Dis 2001; 32: 358–66.
20. Wald A, Leisenring W, van Burik J-A et al. Epidemiology of Aspergillus infections in a large cohort of patients undergoing bone marrow transplantation. J Infect Dis 1997; 175: 1459–66.
●21. Marr KA, Carter RA, Crippa F et al. Epidemiology and outcome of mould infections in hematopoetic stem cell transplant recipients. Clin Infect Dis 2002; 34: 909–17.
22. Patterson JE, Peters J, Calhoon JH et al. Investigation and control of aspergillosis and other filamentous fungal infections in solid organ transplant recipients. Transpl Infect Dis 2000; 2: 22–8.
●23. Greene RE, Sclamm HT, Oestmann JW et al. Imaging findings in acute invasive pulmonary aspergillosis: Clinical significance of the halo sign. Clin Infect Dis 2007; 44: 373–9.
◆24. Hope WW, Walsh TJ, Denning DW. Laboratory diagnosis of invasive aspergillosis. Lancet Infect Dis 2005; 5: 609–22.
25. Odabasi Z, Marttiuzzi G, Estey E et al. β-D-Glucan as a diagnostic adjunct for invasive fungal infections: Validation, cutoff development, and performance in patients with acute myelogenous leukaemia and myelodysplastic syndrome. Clin Infect Dis 2004; 39: 199–205.
◆26. White PL, Barnes RA. Aspergillus PCR: Platforms, strengths and weaknesses. Med Mycol 2006; 44: S191–8.
●27. Otrosky-Zeichner L, Alexander BD, Kett DH et al. Multicentre clinical evaluation of the (1–3) β-D-glucan assay as an aid to diagnosis of fungal infection in humans. Clin Infect Dis 2005; 41: 654–9.
●28. De Pauw B, Walsh TJ, Donnelly JP et al. Revised definitions of invasive fungal disease from the European Organization for Research and Treatment of Cancer/Invasive Fungal Infections Cooperative Group and the National Institute of Allergy and Infectious Diseases Mycoses Study Group (EORTC/MSG) consensus group. Clin Infect Dis 2008; 46: 1813–21.
29. Walsh TJ, Teppler H, Donowitz GR et al. Caspofungin versus liposomal amphotericin B for empirical antifungal therapy in patients with persistent fever and neutropenia. N Engl J Med 2004; 351: 1391–402.
●30. Herbrecht R, Denning DW, Patterson TF et al. Voriconazole versus amphotericin B for primary therapy of invasive aspergillosis. N Engl J Med 2002; 347: 408–15.

31. Cornely OA, Maertens J, Bresnik M *et al.* Liposomal amphotericin B, an initial therapy for invasive mold infection: A randomized trial comparing a high-loading dose regimen with standard dosing (AmBiLoad trial). *Clin Infect Dis* 2007; **44**: 1289–97.

32. Maertens J, Raad I, Petrikkos G *et al.* Efficacy and safety of caspofungin for treatment of invasive aspergillosis in patients refractory to or intolerant of conventional therapy. *Clin Infect Dis* 2004; **39**; 1563–71.

33. Walsh TJ, Raad I, Patterson TF *et al.* Treatment of invasive aspergillosis with posaconazole in patients refractory to or intolerant of conventional therapy: An externally controlled trial. *Clin Infect Dis* 2007; **44**: 2–12.

♦34. Prentice AG, Glasmacher A, Hobson RP *et al.*, for the British Committee for Standards in Haematology. Guidelines on the Management of Invasive Fungal Infection During Therapy for Haematological Malignancy. Available from: http://www.bcshguidelines.com/pdf/IFI-therapy.pdf (accessed January 6, 2009).

35. Cornely OA, Maertens J, Winston DJ *et al.* Posaconazole vs fluconazole or itraconazole prophylaxis in patients with neutropenia. *N Engl J Med* 2007; **356**: 348–59.

♦36. Walsh TJ, Anaissie EJ, Denning DW *et al.* Treatment of aspergillosis: Clinical practice guidelines of the Infectious Diseases Society of America. *Clin Infect Dis* 2008; **46**: 327–60.

♦37. Ellis DH. Systemic zygomycosis. In: Merz WG, Hay RJ (eds) *Topley and Wilson's Microbiology and Microbial Infections*, 10th edn. London: Hodder Arnold, 2005: 659–87.

●38. Hibbett DS, Binder M, Bischoff JF. A higher-level phylogenetic classification of the Fungi. *Mycol Res* 2007; **111**: 509–47.

39. Linder N, Keller N, Huri C. Primary cutaneous mucormycosis in a premature infant: Case report and review of the literature. *Am J Perinatol* 1998; **15**: 35–8.

40. Mitchell SJ, Gray J, Morgan ME *et al.* Nosocomial infection with *Rhizopus microsporus* in pre-term infants: Association with wooden tongue depressors. *Lancet* 1996; **348**: 441–3.

♦41. Rogers TR. Treatment of zygomycosis: Current and new options. *J Antimicrob Chemother* 2008; **61**(Suppl. 1): i35–9.

●42. Greenberg RN, Mullane K, van Burik J-AH *et al.* Posaconazole as salvage therapy for zygomycosis. *Antimicrob Agents Chemother* 2006; **50**: 126–33.

43. Kwon-Chung KJ, Bennett JE, Theodore TS. *Cryptococcus bacillispora* sp. nov.: Serotype B-C of *Cryptococcus neoformans. Int J System Bacteriol* 1978; **28**: 616–20.

44. Franzot SP, Salkin IF, Casadevall A. *Cryptococcus neoformans* var. *grubii*: Separate varietal status for *Cryptococcus neoformans* serotype A isolates. *J Clin Microbiol* 1999; **37**: 838–40.

45. Kwong-Chung KJ, Varma A. Do major species concepts support one, two or more species within *Cryptococcus neoformans? FEMS Yeast Res* 2006; **6**: 574–87.

46. Lin X, Heitman J. The biology of the *Cryptococcus neoformans* species complex. *Ann Rev Microbiol* 2006; **60**: 69–105.

47. Johnson LB, Bradley SF, Kauffman CA. Fungaemia due to *Cryptococcus laurentii* and a review of non-neoformans cryptococcaemia. *Mycoses* 1998; **4**: 227–80.

48. McCurdy LH, Morrow JD. Infections due to non-*neoformans* cryptococcal species. *Compr Ther* 2003; **29**: 95–101.

49. Khawcharoeporn T, Apisarnthanarak A, Mundy LM. Non-*neoformans* cryptococcal infections: A systematic review. *Infection* 2007; **35**: 51–8.

50. Goldman DL, Khine H, Abadi J *et al.* Serologic evidence for *Cryptococcus neoformans* infection in early childhood. *Paediatrics* 2001; **107**: e66.

51. Vichez RA, Fung J, Kusne S. Cryptococcosis in organ transplant recipients: An overview. *Am J Transplant* 2002; **2**: 575–80.

52. Marik PE. Fungal infections in solid organ transplantation. *Expert Opin Pharmacother* 2006; **7**: 297–305.

53. Warnatz K. Cryptococcosis in HIV-negative immunodeficiency. *Clin Adv Hematol Oncol* 2008; **6**: 448–62.

54. Currie BP, Casadevall A. Estimation of the prevalence of cryptococcal infection among HIV-infected individuals in New York City. *Clin Infect Dis* 1994; **19**: 1029–33.

55. Sugar AM. Overview: Cryptococcosis in the patient with AIDS. *Mycopathologia* 1991; **114**: 153–7.

56. Mitchell TG, Perfect JR. Cryptococcosis in the era of AIDS 100 years after the discovery of *Cryptococcus neoformans. Clin Microbiol Rev* 1995; **8**: 515–48.

♦57. Waters L, Nelson M. Cryptococcal disease and HIV infection. *Expert Opin Pharmacother* 2005; **6**: 2633–44.

58. Steenbergen JN, Nosanchuk JD. 'Ready made' virulence and 'dual use' virulence factors in pathogenic environmental fungi – the *Cryptococcus neoformans* paradigm. *Curr Opin Microbiol* 2003; **6**: 332–7.

59. Emmons CW. Saprophytic sources of *Cryptococcus neoformans* associated with the pigeon (*Columbia livia*). *Am J Hyg* 1955; **62**: 227–32.

60. Kwong-Chung KJ, Bennett JE. Epidemiologic differences between the two varieties of *Cryptococcus neoformans. Am J Epidemiol* 1984; **120**: 123–30.

61. Larsen RA, Bozzette SA, McCutchan A, Chiu J, Leal MAE, Richman DD. Persistent *Cryptococcus neoformans* infection of the prostate after successful treatment of meningitis. *Ann Intern Med* 1989; **111**: 125–8.

♦62. Kwong-Chung KJ, Bennett JE. *Medical Mycology.* London: Lea & Febiger, 1992.

63. Upton A, Fraser JA, Kidd SE *et al.* First contemporary case of human infection with *Cryptococcus gattii* in Puget Sound: Evidence for spread of the Vancouver Island outbreak. *J Clin Microbiol* 2007; **45**: 3086–8.

64. McDougall L, Kidd SE, Galanis E *et al.* Spread of *Cryptococcus gattii* in British Columbia, Canada and detection in the Pacific Northwest, USA. *Emerg Infect Dis* 2007; **13**: 42–50.

65. Bartlett KH, Kidd SE, Kronstad JW. The emergence of *Cryptococcus gattii* in British Columbia and the Pacific Northwest. *Curr Infect Dis Rep.* 2008; **10**: 58–65.

66. Sorrell TC. *Cryptococcus neoformans* variety *gattii. Med Mycol* 2001; **39**: 155–68.

67. Nicol AM, Hurrell C, McDowell W *et al.* Communicating the risks of a new, emerging pathogen: The case of *Cryptococcus gattii. Risk Anal* 2008; **28**: 373–86.

68. Zerpa R, Huicho L, Guillen A. Modified India ink preparation for *Cryptococcus neoformans* in cerebrospinal fluid specimens. *J Clin Microbiol* 1996; **34**: 2290–1.

69. Goodman JS, Kaufman L, Koenig MG *et al*. Diagnosis of cryptococcal meningitis: Value of immunological detection of cryptococcal antigen. *N Engl J Med* 1971; **285**: 434–6.

♦70. Saag MS, Graybill RJ, Larsen RA *et al*. Practice guidelines for the management of cryptococcal disease. *Clin Infect Dis* 2000; **30**: 710–18.

71. Martinez E, Garcia-Viejo MA, Marcos MA. Discontinuation of secondary prophylaxis for cryptococcal meningitis in HIV-infected patients responding to highly active anti-retroviral agents. *AIDS* 2000; **14**: 2615.

72. Vibhagool A, Sungkanuparph S, Mootsikapun P *et al*. Discontinuation of secondary prophylaxis of cryptococcal meningitis in human immunodeficiency virus-infected patients treated with highly active antiretroviral therapy: A prospective, multicenter randomized study. *Clin Infect Dis* 2003; **36**: 1329–31.

●73. Fischer MC, Koenig GL, White TJ *et al*. Molecular and phenotypic description of *Coccidioides posadasii* sp. nov., previously recognized as the non-Californian population of *Coccidioides immitis. Mycologia* 2002; **94**: 73–84.

♦74. Pappagianis D. Coccidioidomycosis. In: Merz WG, Hay RJ (eds) *Topley and Wilson's Microbiology and Microbial Infections,* 10th edn. London: Hodder Arnold, 2005: 502–18.

♦75. Stevens DA. Coccidioidomycosis. *N Engl J Med* 1995; **322**: 1077–82.

76. Schneider E, Hajjeh RA, Speigel RA *et al*. A coccidioidomycosis outbreak following the Northridge, California, earthquake. *JAMA* 1997; **277**: 904–8.

77. Fisher MC, Koenig GL, White TJ *et al*. Pathogenic clones versus environmentally driven population increase: Analysis of an epidemic of the human fungal pathogen *Coccidioides immitis. J Clin Microbiol* 2000; **38**: 807–13.

♦78. Galgiani JN, Ampel MN, Blair JE. IDSA guidelines: Coccidioidomycosis. *Clin Infect Dis* 2005; **41**: 1217–23.

79. Panackal AA, Hajjeh RA, Cetron MS *et al*. Fungal infections among returning travelers. *Clin Infect Dis* 2002; **35**: 1088–95.

♦80. Cano M, Hajjeh RA. The epidemiology of histoplasmosis: A review. *Semin Respir Infect* 2001; **16**: 109–18.

81. Chick EW, Compton SB, Pass T *et al*. Hitchcock's birds, or the increased rate of exposure to *Histoplasma* from blackbird roost sites. *Chest* 1981; **80**: 434–8.

♦82. Shwartz J. *Histoplasmosis.* New York: Praeger, 1981.

♦83. Wheat LJ. Improvements in diagnosis of histoplasmosis. *Exp Opin Biol Ther* 2006; **6**: 1207–21.

♦84. Wheat LJ, Friefeld AG, Kleiman MB. Clinical practice guidelines for the management of patients with histoplasmosis: 2007 update by the Infectious Diseases Society of America. *Clin Infect Dis* 2007; **46**: 807–25.

20

Diseases of air travel

DAVID L. HAGEN

INTRODUCTION

Every year, airlines carry more than 2 billion passengers worldwide.[1] With the cost of travel decreasing in real terms, what was once considered the realm of the more affluent in society is now more widely accessible than ever.[2] This profound change in our leisure and business life has led to increasing concerns about the effects of spending long periods of time in close proximity to others, in what would be considered an unnatural environment. The World Tourism Organization has predicted that international arrivals are expected to reach nearly 1.6 billion by the year 2020, with East Asia and the Pacific, Asia, the Middle East and Africa forecasted to record growth rates of over 5 per cent per year, compared with the world average of 4.1 per cent.[3] This provides opportunities for hitherto distant threats arising from infectious disease and other environmental agents to be transmitted to not only holiday-makers, but also to those in their home countries upon their return.

Although the public perception is that travelling by air is hazardous, evidence suggests that passengers' health is not at increased risk and that the transmission of infectious disease is not facilitated by the cabin environment any more than it would be by any other mode of transport. It has been suggested that the opportunity for infection to spread is greater in airport terminals, where passengers from various points of origin and destinations are gathered together to eat, rest and utilize toilet facilities.[4]

THE CABIN ENVIRONMENT

Air supply to cabins

Prior to the introduction of the modern generation of aircraft in the 1970s and 80s, cabins were ventilated largely with fresh air that was compressed, humidified and cooled by the engines in a rather inefficient process. In part to increase fuel economy and reduce operating costs, aircraft manufacturers designed ventilation systems that recirculated cabin air.[5] This recirculation of air resulted in a higher relative humidity as frequent renewal of the moister cabin air mixes with outside air. Most modern aircraft now recirculate up to 50 per cent of the already pressurized cabin air in the ventilation systems.[6]

High-efficiency particulate air filters

Modern aircraft use high-efficiency particulate air (HEPA) filters, which reduce the number of microscopic particles from the recirculated air before mixing it with external, sterile air and allowing it to re-enter the passenger cabin. These filters can remove more than 99 per cent of particles between 0.1 and 0.3 μm in diameter, which is the standard used as this size is the most difficult to block and hence provides the gold standard for filtration, with virtually all particles below 0.1 μm being blocked in the filtration dynamics (C. Thibeault, Medical Advisor, International Air

Transport Association, personal communication, June 2008). Most airborne particles, including bacteria and fungi, are larger than this and are therefore effectively filtered as long as proper aircraft maintenance is carried out.[7] Although viruses can be smaller than 0.3 μm, they usually form colonies or clumps larger than 0.3 μm that cannot pass through HEPA filters.

Humidity

The cabin of a modern aircraft has a low humidity, with a range of between 5 and 20 per cent, compared with the average humidity in buildings of approximately 30–50 per cent. Contrary to popular belief, the humidity is lower in first and business class sections than it is in economy owing to the closer proximity of individuals giving off moisture. Although this level of humidity may give rise to ocular and nasal symptoms due to decreased tear film stability and nasal patency,[8] recent studies have suggested that the health effects are minimal, particularly related to deep vein thrombosis,[9] which would seem to be more related to immobilization.

Air flow

In older aircraft, the general flow of circulating air was from the front of the aircraft to the rear. In modern aircraft, however, the airflow is circular, coming from the ceiling vents downwards towards the floor. Here the flow is vented and either exhausted out of the cabin or filtered and recirculated.[4] This circular pattern hinders the flow of air lengthwise in the cabin and is important in limiting the airborne spread of particles, and hence infections, to those passengers in the same or adjacent rows of the aircraft.

Air is completely changed at least 20 times per hour, compared with 12 air exchanges per hour in a typical office building and 5 exchanges per hour in most homes, further reducing the likelihood of transmission of airborne particles.[5,10] An often-quoted study sites an outbreak of influenza in 1979 among passengers when the air circulation system was switched off for a 3-hour period on the ground,[11] implying the importance of air flow.

Cabin pressure

Commercial aircraft typically maintain a cruising altitude of 35 000–40 000 feet (10 500–12 000 m)[9] above sea level, and air pressure inside the cabin is equivalent to an altitude of 5000–8000 feet (1500–2400 m).[12] At this altitude, the reduced barometric pressure and thus partial pressure of oxygen is approximately 120 mmHg (16.0 kPa^2), which is 75 per cent of its sea level value of around 160 mmHg (21.3 kPa). Although this will lead to a fall in arterial oxygen tension from 95 mmHg (12.7 kPa) to 53–64 mmHg

(7.0–8.5 kPa), it will, owing to the shape of the oxygen dissociation curve, only lead to a fall in oxygen saturation from 97 per cent to approximately 90 per cent. This fall is compensated by the normal physiological response and is well tolerated by healthy individuals. However, this decrease in oxygen saturation needs to be taken into account for those with severe cardiac or pulmonary conditions or anaemia.[12]

Ozone

Aircraft flying at the upper operational range of altitude and those flying in or near significant storms may encounter higher levels of outside ozone. Although most ozone is converted to oxygen by the high temperature and pressure in the compression stages of the aircraft engine prior to being circulated in the cabin, a University of California study has found instances of ozone levels in the cabin higher than limits set by the US Federal Aviation Administration.[13] Modern commercial aircraft have catalytic/ozone converters, which should maintain not more than 0.1 parts per million of ozone for 3 hours, with a maximum of 0.25 parts per million at any time.[2]

Cosmic radiation

Cosmic radiation exposure on aircraft is a function of altitude, latitude, solar activity and cumulative time spent flying. Exposure is many times greater at commercial aircraft altitudes than at ground level since the atmosphere provides considerable protection from this source. An additional factor is due to the earth's magnetic field, which deflects some of the cosmic radiation away. This shielding is more effective over the equator and least effective at the poles, a common transcontinental route. The final factor is the sun, whose magnetic field causes a variation in the amount reaching the earth according to the 11 year solar cycle. The sun also emits solar flares that consist of energetic particles such as photons; these are, however, thought to contribute very little to the overall exposure.[14]

Both ozone and cosmic radiation exposure are felt to be insignificant for ordinary travellers but relevant as occupational exposure, especially for pregnant women.[6] Canada recommends that pregnant women who expect to fly more than 200 hours over the course of their pregnancy should seek advice.[14]

DISEASES AND AIR TRAVEL

Infectious disease

The World Health Organization (WHO) issued its first set of regulations intended to prevent the spread of diseases in 1951. They concentrated only on six 'quarantinable' diseases: cholera, plague, relapsing fever, smallpox, typhus and yellow fever. These regulations were called the International Sanitary Regulations and were renamed the International Health Regulations in 1969.[15] Since that time, other issues have appeared as international concerns. To account for this, three fundamental principles have been incorporated into the latest version:

1. replacing the list of specific diseases with more generic illness;
2. including chemical, biological and radiological agents as well as infectious ones;
3. making some incidents notifiable within 24 hours to the WHO if they fulfil the criteria to constitute a Public Health Emergency of International Concern.

Public Health Emergencies of International Concern are reported through a newly established National Focal Point for each country. In addition, the emphasis for member states has changed from control at borders to containment at source for international threats.

The stated intention of the International Health Regulations is to 'prevent, protect against, control and provide a public health response to the international spread of disease in ways that are commensurate with and restricted to public health risks, and which avoid unnecessary interference with international traffic and trade'.[15]

International organizations

There are three primary organizations which advise the international air travel industry on public health and other issues:

1. the International Civil Aviation Organization (ICAO), which represents its contracting countries and whose responsibilities are at country level;
2. the Airports Council International, which represents its individual airports;
3. the International Air Transport Association (IATA), which is a trade association representing the airline industry worldwide.

Each has developed plans and guidelines for their respective areas of responsibility, most of which are available on the Internet.

Misconceptions of risk

There is a mistaken belief amongst the travelling public, often reinforced by public health officials, that if one person on board an aircraft has suffered from an infectious disease, all the rest of the passengers are at high risk of acquiring that infection. There is little evidence to support this supposition and, in addition, clear guidelines to follow

in the event of incidents of infectious disease on aircraft among the crew or passengers, to mitigate any such incident.

Transmission of infection

There are three main routes by which respiratory infections can be transmitted on an aircraft: droplet spread, contact transmission and airborne particles. Droplet spread involves large particles which contain organisms that settle relatively rapidly. These droplets are produced by coughing, sneezing or talking and are assumed to be limited to less than 1 m of spread.

Direct contact transmission occurs when there is skin-to-skin contact and the transfer of live organisms either directly from the index case to another person or indirectly when a surface is contaminated and organisms are transferred by touch to a mucous membrane.

Airborne transmission involves relatively small suspensions of microorganisms, produced by coughing and sneezing, which may disperse more widely and are usually inhaled by the recipient host.

Foodborne disease may be caused by bacterial or viral contamination of food or water, or may be caused by intoxication through chemical contaminants such as toxins of biological origin or chemicals.

TUBERCULOSIS

Tuberculosis is usually transmitted via droplets from the throat or lungs of people with active respiratory disease but may also spread by direct airborne transmission. The Centers for Disease Control and Prevention in the USA uncovered some evidence that tuberculosis may be transmitted on long flights by symptomatic individuals by looking at incidents between 1993 and 1995 (see also Box 20.1). In these events, 2600 passengers and crew on 191 flights were investigated in six separate incidents. Only two of the six produced evidence of possible transmission, and no individuals developed active tuberculosis.[5] Three factors were identified as contributing to possible transmission: sitting within two rows of the index case, having a long duration of flight, and a high relative infectiveness of the index case. This formed the basis of the first guidelines issued by the WHO in 1998, which recommended that in the event that a passenger with sputum-positive tuberculosis had travelled on a commercial flight of more than 8 hours in the previous 3 months, the airline should inform those seated in the same row plus two rows in front and two rows behind that they were at risk, albeit a low one.[16]

Multiple drug-resistant tuberculosis, although more difficult to treat than drug-sensitive disease, seems to not be more transmissible[17] and hence is less significant in dealing with air travel incidents than recent publicity would suggest. Two subsequent revisions of the WHO guidance have been made with minor changes, mainly involving the responsibilities of airlines and public health agencies.[16]

In 2007, despite being advised otherwise, a man from the USA travelled to Europe, within Europe and returned to North America suffering from drug-resistant tuberculosis. Subsequent studies found no other passengers were infected despite widespread publicity and hence enhanced case ascertainment.[18,19] In December 2007, a woman flew from India to the USA while infected with drug-resistant tuberculosis, and although a second case was subsequently found, it is not known whether he acquired the disease in India unrelated to the index case.[19] It is estimated that 10 per cent of the worldwide population carries latent tuberculosis infection, and therefore the subsequent screening of passengers must be performed in such a way as to minimize false-positive results and undue anxiety among the travelling public.[17,20]

SEVERE ACUTE RESPIRATORY SYNDROME

The severe acute respiratory syndrome (SARS) coronavirus is predominantly spread in droplets from the respiratory tract of the index case.[21] Faecal or airborne transmission is less frequent but was suggested as a mechanism in an analysis of computational fluid dynamics predicting the detailed airflow pattern in the air shafts of a housing complex that was affected in Hong Kong.[22]

SARS is an interesting disease with regard to air travel due to several factors:

- it was a newly emerging global threat first recognized in 2003;

- it spread rapidly to more than two dozen countries in North America, South America, Europe and Asia before the outbreak was contained;
- it was spread readily by close contact;
- it was amenable to proactive efforts due to the fact that it was not felt to be infectious until symptoms presented,[23] it has a relatively long incubation period (3–10 days[24]) and general infection control precautions are the suggested actions.[23,25,26]

SARS made its first appearance in November 2002 in the Guangdong province of southern China and appeared to spread when a treating physician fell ill and travelled to Hong Kong via air, leading to further cases in the province.[25] Recommendations were given by the WHO and other public health authorities throughout the world and included:

- issuing travel alerts that provided information about the disease and risks;
- issuing travel advisories that recommended against non-essential travel to the affected area(s);
- issuing advice to airline staff and national airport authorities on managing suspected cases on aircraft;
- issuing advice to households where a SARS contact resided;
- issuing advice to healthcare facilities when a suspected case was admitted;
- issuing general control of infection advice for public facilities including hotels.[26]

The SARS outbreak presented one of the first severe new diseases to spread rapidly through air travel and provided important lessons that would subsequently be drawn upon in planning for pandemic influenza.[27,28] Given the scale of air travel in the modern world, experience here may prove more useful for this sector than those of the influenza pandemics of 1918, 1957 and 1968.[29,30] Much attention was given to exit screening, by both medical questionnaire and thermal imaging, in affected countries, but this proved disruptive and costly, requiring individual and public health action for febrile persons.[30]

According to flight schedule provider OAG, the number of scheduled flights worldwide fell by 3 per cent – equivalent to 2.5 million seats – in mid-June 2003 compared with the year before. Flights to and from China showed a drop in passenger numbers of 45 per cent,[31] and the outbreak cost the world's airlines and travel-related industries an estimated US$40 billion. In addition, it altered the public's perception of risk of in-flight transmission of disease.[32,33]

PANDEMIC INFLUENZA

As discussed in Chapter 17, a worldwide outbreak of influenza occurs when a novel influenza virus subtype emerges and infects people, causing serious illness and spreading easily and sustainably among humans. There will be little or no immunity to the new virus, and hence it will cause higher attack rates and more severe illness than those caused by pre-existing influenza viruses. In contrast to the entirely reactive response to the SARS outbreak previously outlined, the response to the threat of an influenza pandemic has been proactive and facilitated by the implementation of the International Health Regulations (2005).[1]

As we discovered earlier, preparedness planning for influenza is primarily based on its transmission through droplets, although the efficiency of other routes of transmission such as aerosol or contact with contaminated surfaces remains unclear. The mean incubation time is thought to be 2 days but can vary from 1 to 7 days, and transmission during the asymptomatic period is assumed to be negligible; however, this may not be correct for a small group of 'superspreader' cases and children.[34,35]

Widely accepted modelling suggests that a 90 per cent restriction on European air travel would delay the peak of the pandemic by only 1–2 weeks. Restrictions on travel from specific locations, for instance south-east Asia, would also be ineffective given the indirect flows of people from Asia to the rest of the world as well as flows of people who would rapidly become infected in outbreaks in other countries.[36,37] However, there is a view in a recent study indicating that restricting air travel to the USA might have some effect.[38]

A WHO technical consultation was held in Geneva in 2004, attended by more than 100 experts from 33 countries, and has stated:

> providing information to domestic and international travellers (risks to avoid, symptoms to look for, when to seek care) is better use of health resources than formal screening. Entry screening of travellers at international borders will incur considerable expense with a disproportionately small impact on international spread, although exit screening should be considered in some situations.[29]

The layered approach

North America, the UK, and many other countries have adopted what is termed a 'layered approach' whereby several levels of response overlap and complement each other. This approach is necessary in pandemic influenza as it is likely that: (1) the causes of influenza-like illness in passengers will be varied; (2) asymptomatic infected individuals will not be detected by screening; and (3) travellers who are incubating the illness at the beginning of a long-haul flight and are asymptomatic may develop symptoms en route. The layered approach divides the actions into those at pre-embarkation, en route and upon arrival at the destination airport.[39]

Pre-embarkation measures may include:

- medical assessment of fitness to fly (see below);
- a self-administered medical questionnaire with assessment;
- the questioning of passengers by trained staff;
- thermal imaging;
- screening by check-in or gate staff supported by airline contracted ground-based medical support (which is routine at present).

Generic communicable disease control applied to pandemic influenza

En route generic measures include enforcing existing IATA guidelines on dealing with suspected communicable diseases,[40] which will facilitate appropriate action in recognizing and dealing with any passenger fulfilling the criteria stated. Implementing these guidelines should give cabin crew the confidence to avoid such situations as occurred when a 16-year-old girl flying from Hawaii to New York on a school trip was removed from her flight due to an acute episode of coughing.[41]

The guidelines indicate that cabin crew should obtain contact details from all travellers seated in the same row, two rows in front and two rows behind the sick traveller utilizing Passenger Locator Cards.[42] These cards were developed by the WHO to obtain public health contact tracing information and have been adapted for use by airlines and public health authorities internationally. Obtaining passenger data through airline manifest information continues to be problematic due to the nature of the details held by airlines, which are for financial purposes, and due to confidentiality issues.[43] These measures have been supplemented by the ICAO's introduction in July 2007 of a system to increase the window for mounting a public health response by reporting suspected cases of communicable disease via air traffic control services[44] rather than relying on last-minute contact with the destination airport.

Despite evidence from the SARS response, *arrival* measures may include a consideration of thermal screening utilizing newer-generation equipment, or having public health staff perform assessments on self-administered questionnaires completed upon landing or en route.[45] Current generic arrival measures rely on *isolation*, which is the separation and restriction of movement of ill and potentially infectious individuals. *Quarantine*, which is the separation and restriction of the movement of persons who, while not yet ill, have been potentially exposed to a communicable disease, would require a large investment in resources (to staff, accommodate and supply basic day-to-day needs in a secure area). In addition, this would require each country to pass legislation to ensure compliance and enforcement; it would also require a policy to be put in place for the removal of quarantine measures through near-patient or rapid testing, or via an evidence-based clinical assessment.

NOROVIRUS

Noroviruses, also known as small round structured viruses or Norwalk-like viruses, are the most common cause of gastroenteritis in the developed world and therefore a significant problem to the airline industry, where there are shared toilet facilities and a constant turnover of new and susceptible travellers and staff.

Generally causing a mild illness, transmission on board an aircraft can be through the same mechanism as on land:

- infected food handlers on the ground or in the air who may contaminate food eaten raw or post-cooking/heating;
- food contaminated from water containing sewage;
- person-to-person spread via the faeco-oral route either from environmental surfaces or aerosol transmission during vomiting;
- contaminated drinking water supplied to aircraft or contaminated in holding tanks or hoses.[46]

There are IATA guidelines for cabin crew (Box 20.2)[40] and for cleaning crew[47] in the event of this frequent occurrence, and each country's public health authority will have protocols in place for staff at ports of entry to assess and document the incident. Although acquisition of the infection will almost always be prior to boarding (incubation usually being 24–48 hours[24]), it is important to find the source and treat those passengers in need of healthcare.

Aircraft disinfection following an incident can be difficult, not only due to the rapid turnover of aircraft, but also due to the cabin materials and electronics on board. Aircraft manufacturers have advised the WHO in producing guidance on substances that may be used. A working group is currently revising the guidelines on aircraft disinfection.[48]

ASSESSING FITNESS TO FLY

The global increase in air travel has brought with it a wider range of individuals than previously have flown. Travellers include the elderly and those with a wide range of pre-existing medical conditions, and therefore physicians need to be aware of the physiological stresses of flight in order to properly advise their patients, not only for the welfare of the individual, but also to avoid costly and inconvenient diversions of aircraft.[49] Conditions that warrant consideration include, in part:

- cardiovascular disease – including angina, coronary artery bypass grafting, valvular heart disease and recent cerebrovascular accident;
- respiratory disease – including asthma, chronic obstructive pulmonary disease, bronchiectasis and cystic fibrosis, respiratory infection and the presence of a pneumothorax;
- pregnancy;

> **BOX 20.2: Suspected communicable disease – International Air Transport Association guidelines for cabin crew**
>
> Fever of 38°C/100°F or greater associated with one or more of the following:
>
> - Appearing obviously unwell
> - Persistent coughing
> - Impaired breathing
> - Persistent diarrhoea
> - Persistent vomiting
> - Skin rash
> - Bruising or bleeding without previous injury
> - Confusion of recent onset

- recent surgical conditions – including day surgery, neurosurgical or ophthalmological procedures involving trapped gases or increased oxygen consumption;
- diabetes;
- haematological disorders;
- trauma/orthopaedic procedures;
- deep vein thrombosis.[12]

There is a plethora of information available for medical professionals and passengers to access, and most major airlines and government agencies concerned with health and air travel have also published useful documents.

FUME EVENTS

Recently, there have been anecdotal reports of adverse health consequences from the release of harmful compounds into the cabin air environment.[50] Specific types of aircraft have been implicated, and the compounds concerned include volatile organic compounds, semi-volatile organic compounds and tricresyl phosphate. It is alleged that these events occur due to engine oil or fuel leaks from badly designed or faulty seals and overfilling, which cause the toxic substances to be drawn from the engines via bleed air, as explained earlier in the section on the cabin environment.[51] It is also alleged that events such as this may occur in up to 1 in 2000 flights, but evidence is lacking.

The subject was brought to the UK House of Lords Select Committee on Science and Technology in 2000,[6] who commented that they had seen no evidence that cabin air was monitored or sampled routinely or during incidents. The topic was revisited again in the updated House of Lords session in 2007,[51] and is the subject of an ongoing study at Cranfield University in the UK where the sampling of cabin air will be performed to capture and analyse compounds present routinely and during such an event.

AIRCRAFT DISINSECTION

Since the beginnings of international air travel, there has been concern that mosquito vectors and the diseases they transmit might be introduced by aircraft into non-indigenous countries. Many countries insist that arriving aircraft be disinsected when they have come from areas where insect vector-borne diseases are endemic. Accepted proof of disinsection may be either a certificate of residual disinsection or evidence of used aerosol insecticide cans presented to the country's public health inspectors. If not satisfied, the public health authority may choose to spray the cabin of the aircraft.[50]

Compiling the list of airports and other areas that are currently considered endemic is the responsibility of the WHO according to Annex 5 of the International Health Regulations,[15] but at the time of writing the only list available is for the purpose of fulfilling vaccination requirements and advising on prophylaxis. This list is based on areas where malaria is endemic and does not account for other common insect-borne diseases such as dengue fever and Chikungunya virus, and these may need to be considered. In addition, some individual countries' airports lie at different altitudes and within different environments, and each requires a separate risk assessment. Concern has been expressed about the possible adverse effects on passengers and crew of the application of pyrethroid aerosol sprays,[52,53] commonly used as the agents for disinsection.

The most direct evidence of transmission of disease by mosquitoes on aircraft is termed 'airport malaria', which is cases of malaria in or near international airports, among people who have not travelled to areas where it is endemic or who have not recently received blood or human tissue products.

REFERENCES

● = Key primary paper
◆ = Major review article

◆1. World Health Organization. The World Health Report 2007: A Safer Future: Global Public Health Security in the 21st Century. Available from: http://www.who.int/whr/2007/en (accessed August 2009).

2. British Medical Association. The Impact of Flying on Passenger Health: A Guide for Healthcare Professionals. Available from: http://www.bma.org.uk/health_promotion_ethics/transport/Flying.jsp (accessed August 2009).

3. World Tourism Organization. Tourism 2020 Vision. Available from: http://www.unwto.org/facts/pub.html (accessed August 2009).

4. Australian Transport Safety Bureau. Passenger Health – the Risk Posed by Infectious Disease in the Aircraft Cabin. 2008. Available from: http://www.atsb.gov.au/publications/2008/ar2007050.aspx (accessed August 2009).

●5. Leder K, Newman D. Review: Respiratory infections during air travel. *Intern Med J* 2005; **35**: 50–5.

6. House of Lords Science and Technology Committee. Fifth Report: Air Travel and Health. Available from: http://www.publications.parliament.uk/pa/ld199900/ldselect/ldsctech/121/12101.htm (accessed August 2009).

7. Australian Medical Association Council of Scientific Affairs. Report 10: Airborne Infections on Commercial Flights. Available from: http://www.ama-assn.org/ama/no-index/about-ama/13598.shtml (accessed August 2009).

8. Norback D, Lindgren T, Wieslander G. Changes in ocular and nasal signs and symptoms among air crew in relation to air humidification on intercontinental flights. *Scand J Work Environ* 2006; **32**: 138–44.

9. Schreijer AJM, Cannegieter SC, Caramella M *et al.* Fluid loss does not explain coagulation activation during air travel. *Thromb Haemost* 2008; **99**: 985–6.

10. Hunt EH, Space DR. (1994). The Airplane Cabin Environment. Issues Pertaining to Flight Attendant Comfort. Available from: http://www.boeing.com/commercial/cabinair/ventilation.pdf (accessed August 2009).

11. Moser MR, Bender TR, Margolis HS, Noble GR, Kendal AP, Ritter DG. An outbreak of influenza aboard a commercial airliner. *Am J Epidemiol* 1979; **110**: 1–6.

12. Civil Aviation Authority. Assessing Fitness to Fly: Guidelines for Medical Professionals from the Aviation Health Unit, UK Civil Aviation Authority. Available from: http://www.caa.co.uk/docs/923/FitnessToFlyPDF_FitnesstoFlyPDF%20Feb%2009.pdf (accessed August 2009).

13. Demerjian D. That Airplane Air You're Breathing Might Be a Little Heavy on the Ozone. 8 May 2008. Available from: http://www.wired.com/autopia/2008/05/study-finds-ill/ (accessed August 2009).

14. Health Canada. Cosmic Radiation Exposure and Air Travel. Available from: http://www.hc-sc.gc.ca/ewh-semt/radiation/comsic-cosmique-eng.php (accessed August 2009).

●15. World Health Organization. The International Health Regulations (2005). Available from: http://www.who.int/ihr/en (accessed August 2009).

◆16. World Health Organization. *Tuberculosis and Air Travel: Guidelines for Prevention and Control*, 3rd edn. Geneva: World Health Organization, 2008.

17. Department of Health. *The Interdepartmental Working Group on Tuberculosis: Prevention and Control of Tuberculosis in the United Kingdom*. London: DoH, 1998.

18. Block I. Air travellers test clean in TB scare. *Montreal Gazette*, 21 September 2007 Available from: http://www.canada.com/story_print.html?id=a731f6ad-4d56-476c-bd86-dd2c80a5f0a2&sponsor= (accessed August 2009).

19. Swift M. Second TB case on India flight. *San Jose Mercury News*, April 18, 2008.

●20. National Institute for Health and Clinical Excellence. *Tuberculosis: Clinical Diagnosis and Management of Tuberculosis, and Measures for its Prevention and Control*. London: NICE, 2006.

◆21. Kamps B, Hoffmann C (eds). *SARS Reference: Transmission*. Flying Publisher. Available from: http://www.sarsreference.com (accessed August 2009).

22. Yu I, Li Y, Wong TW *et al.* Evidence of airborne transmission of the severe acute respiratory syndrome virus. *N Eng J Med* 2004; **350**: 1731–9.

23. Chow JY, Anderson SR, Delpech V *et al.* SARS: UK public health response – past, present and future. *Commun Dis Public Health* 2003; **6**: 209–15.

24. Heymann D (ed.). *Control of Communicable Diseases Manual*, 18th edn. Washington, DC: American Public Health Association, 2004.

•25. Pickles H. Screening international travellers in China for SARS. *Commun Dis Public Health* 2003; **6**: 216–20.

26. Centers for Disease Control and Prevention. Public Health Guidance for Community-Level Preparedness and Response to Severe Acute Respiratory Syndrome (SARS) Version 3. Available from: http://www.cdc.gov/ncidod/sars/guidance (accessed August 2009).

27. Macnair T. Health Conditions – Severe Acute Respiratory Syndrome (SARS). Available from: www.bbc.co.uk/health/conditions/sars1.shtml (accessed August 2009).

28. World Health Organization. WHO Guidelines for the Global Surveillance of Severe Acute Respiratory Syndrome. Updated Recommendations, October 2004. Available from: http://www.who.int/csr/resources/publications/WHO_CDS_CSR_ARO_2004_1/en (accessed August 2009).

29. World Health Organization. *WHO Consultation on Priority Public Health Interventions Before and During an Influenza Pandemic, Geneva 16–18 March 2004.* Geneva: WHO, 2004.

30. World Health Organization Writing Group. Nonpharmaceutical Interventions for Pandemic Influenza, International Measures. *Emerg Infect Dis* [serial on the Internet]. 2005. Available from: http://www.wpro.who.int/NR/rdonlyres/3B18284F-4443-47A8-8548- B630CF3FDA76/0/EID_2006_ Nonpharmaceu-ticalinterventionsforpandemicfluinternationalmeasures.pdf (accessed August 2009).

31. BBC News. SARS Hits Airlines 'More Than War'. Available from: http://news.bbc.co.uk/1/hi/business/2986612.stm (accessed August 2009).

32. Olsen SJ, Chang H, Cheung TY *et al.* Transmission of the severe acute respiratory syndrome on aircraft. *N Engl J Med* 2003; **349**: 2416–22.

33. Bowen JT Jr, Laroe C. Airline networks and the international diffusion of severe acute respiratory syndrome (SARS). *Geogr J* 2006; **172**: 130–44.

34. Carrat F, Vergu E, Ferguson NM *et al.* Time lines of infection and disease in human influenza: a review of volunteer challenge studies. *Am J Epidemiol* 2008; **167**: 775–85.

35. Lloyd-Smith JO, Schreiber SJ, Kopp PE, Getz WM. Superspreading and the effect of individual variation on disease emergence. *Nature* 2005; **439**: 355–9.

36. World Health Organization. WHO Strategic Action Plan for Pandemic Influenza, 2006. Available from: http://www.who.int/csr/resources/publications/influenza/WHO_CDS_EPR_GIP_2006_2/en (accessed August 2009).

37. Department of Health. *Pandemic influenza: Modelling Summary, Pandemic Influenza Scientific Advisory Group; Subgroup on Modelling, November 2007.* London: DoH.

38. Brownstein JS, Wolfe CJ, Mandl KD. Empirical evidence for the effect of airline travel on inter-regional influenza spread in the United States. *PLoS Medicine* 2006; **3**: e401. Available from: http://www.plosmedicine.org/article/info%3Adoi%2F10.1371%2Fjournal.pmed.0030401 (accessed August 2009).

39. Security and Prosperity Partnership of North America. *North American Plan For Avian & Pandemic Influenza.* Available from: http://www.spp-psp.gc.ca/eic/site/spp-psp.nsf/eng/00092.html (accessed August 2009).

40. International Air Transport Association. Suspected Communicable Disease: General Guidelines for Cabin Crew. Available from: http://www.iata.org/NR/rdonlyres/DD29D97F-0E8C-4CBD-B575-1F5067174941/0/Guidelines_cabin_crew_May2009.pdf (accessed August 2009).

41. Associated Press. Coughing Fit Gets Girl Kicked off Flight. Available from: http://www.msnbc.msn.com/id/17859629 (accessed August 2009).

42. World Health Association. Public Health Passenger Locator Card. Available from: http://www.who.int/ihr/PLC.pdf (accessed August 2009).

43. McKenna M. Tracing Air Travellers at Risk for Disease Still Tough. Available from: http://www.cidrap.umn.edu/cidrap/content/influenza/panflu/news/jun1008airline.html (accessed August 2009).

44. International Civil Aviation Association. Communication ref: AN 5/22 - 07/55, 2007.

45. Roos R. Hawaii Begins Testing Some Arriving Travellers for Flu. Available from: http://www.cidrap.umn.edu/cidrap/content/influenza/panflu/news/jun0608screening.html (accessed August 2009).

46. Hawker J, Begg N, Blair I, Reintjes R, Weinberg J. *Communicable Disease Control Handbook*, 2nd edn. Oxford: Blackwell Publishing, 2005.

47. International Air Transport Association. Suspected Communicable Disease: General Guidelines for Cleaning Crew. Available from: http://www.iata.org/NR/rdonlyres/23EA32B7-EC3E-4EED-B4FA-EFD7C07B58BC/0/Guidelines_cleaning_crew_Dec2008.pdf (accessed August 2009).

•48. World Health Organization. Guide to Hygiene and Sanitation in Aviation, 3rd edn, advance copy. Available from: http://www.who.int/water_sanitation_health/hygiene/ships/guide_hygiene_sanitation_aviation_3_edition.pdf (accessed August 2009).

♦49. Aerospace Medical Association. Medical Guidelines for Airline Travel, 2nd edn. *Aviat Space Environ Med* **74**(Suppl.): A1–20.

50. Starmer-Smith C. Is Cabin Air Making Us Sick? Available from: http://www.telegraph.co.uk/travel/travelnews/759562/Is-cabin-air-making-us-sick.html (accessed August 2009).

51. House of Lords Science and Technology Committee. Air Travel and Health: An Update. 2007. London: Science and Technology Committee.

52. Gratz N, Steffen R, Cocksedge W. Why aircraft disinsection? *Bull World Health Organ* 2000; **78**: 995–1004.

53. Sutton PM, Vergara X, Beckman BS, Nicas M, Das R. Pesticide illness among flight attendants due to aircraft disinsection. *Am J Ind Med* 2007; **50**: 345–6.

21

Environmental mycobacteria

JOSEPH O. FALKINHAM III

A substantial proportion of the more than 100 reported species of *Mycobacterium* are environmental opportunists that cause disease in humans and animals.[1,2] The environmental opportunistic mycobacteria are normal inhabitants of natural water, engineered water systems (e.g. household plumbing) and soils. They persist and grow on their own in those habitats, unlike *Legionella*, which need other microorganisms.

Because of this ability to grow in water and soils, humans are surrounded by the environmental opportunistic mycobacteria, and disease follows from the overlap of human and mycobacterial habitats. For example, mycobacteria such as *Mycobacterium avium* and *Mycobacterium intracellulare* are normal inhabitants of drinking water distribution systems[3] and household plumbing,[4] both of which are shared with humans. Engineered systems, such as drinking water distribution systems and household plumbing, select for mycobacterial proliferation and persistence because they provide an environment that is ideal for mycobacteria.

ENVIRONMENTAL OPPORTUNISTIC PATHOGENIC MYCOBACTERIA

Table 21.1 lists the major species of environmental *Mycobacterium* infecting humans. In the USA, the most commonly reported species associated with infection are *M. avium* and *M. intracellulare*.[1] However, other species are recovered, and there are noteworthy geographical differences. For example, *Mycobacterium simiae* appears more commonly in Texas and the surrounding states than in other parts of

the USA,[5] and *Mycobacterium malmoense* is more frequently recovered in Europe than the USA.[6] Disease caused by *Mycobacterium xenopi* appears sporadically and is usually associated with localized outbreaks.[7] Both slowly growing (colony formation in greater than 7 days) and rapidly growing (colony formation in less than 7 days) species are associated with disease. Skin and soft tissue infections can be caused by both slowly[8] and rapidly[9] growing mycobacteria. Many cases of nosocomial mycobacteria infection are caused by the rapidly growing mycobacteria.[10] Two species are regularly reported as animal disease agents: *Mycobacterium marinum* in fish and *Mycobacterium avium* subspecies *paratuberculosis*, the causative agent of Johne's disease in cattle. It has also been proposed that *M. avium* subspecies *paratuberculosis* causes Crohn's disease in humans.

The structure and composition of the mycobacterial envelope is the major determinant of their ecology and virulence (Table 21.2). Mycobacteria have a thick, lipid-rich

Table 21.1 Environmental opportunistic mycobacteria

Slowly growing mycobacteria (colony formation ≥ 7 days)	Rapidly growing mycobacteria (colony formation 3–7 days)
Mycobacterium avium	*Mycobacterium abscessus*
Mycobacterium intracellulare	*Mycobacterium chelonae*
Mycobacterium kansasii	*Mycobacterium fortuitum*
Mycobacterium marinum	*Mycobacterium immunogenum*
Mycobacterium malmoense	
Mycobacterium simiae	

Table 21.2 Factors influencing distribution of mycobacteria in natural and human engineered environments

Factor	Impacts in habitats	
	Natural habitats	**Engineered habitats**
Hydrophobicity	Attach to particulates	Attach to surfaces
	Biofilm formation	Biofilm formation
	Concentration at air–water interfaces	
	Antimicrobial resistance	Antimicrobial resistance
	Hydrocarbon utilization	Hydrocarbon utilization
Growth at low pH	High numbers in acidic, brown-water swamps and boreal (peat) soils	
Humic and fulvic acid	High numbers in acidic, brown-water	Growth in drinking water distribution
Growth stimulation	swamps and boreal (peat) soils	systems and household plumbing
Temperature resistance		Survive in buildings and home hot water systems

true outer membrane that makes cells hydrophobic and impermeable.[11–13] Impermeability to hydrophilic compounds is likely to contribute to their slow growth and to antibiotic and disinfectant resistance. Hydrophobicity drives the preferential attachment to surfaces and concentration in aerosol droplets.[14] The environmental opportunistic mycobacteria can grow in natural waters with greater than 50 μg carbon per litre.[15]

DISEASES CAUSED BY ENVIRONMENTAL MYCOBACTERIA

The incidence of infections (principally pulmonary disease) caused by the environmental mycobacteria appears to be increasing, from 1–2 per 100 000 in 1990 to 8–10 per 100 000 in 2005.[16] In the USA, that translates to 30 000 active cases. Disease presentations include pulmonary disease,[1,17] cervical lymphadenitis,[18] skin infections,[17] furunculosis[19] and disseminated disease in individuals with acquired immune deficiency syndrome or those who are immunosuppressed due to cancer, chemotherapy, or coincident with transplantation.[1,20]

Risk factors for mycobacterial pulmonary disease among immunocompetent individuals include lung damage, such as pneumoconiosis, black lung, smoking or alcoholism.[17] Patients with cystic fibrosis can be infected

with the rapidly growing mycobacterium *Mycobacterium abscessus* acquired from their environment.[21] Individuals with gastro-oesphageal reflux disease are also at higher risk of pulmonary disease caused by the environmental mycobacteria.[22,23] Furthermore, there has been a new presentation of mycobacterial pulmonary disease in slender, elderly men and women who lack any of the classic risk factors.[24–26] One study of such elderly patients identified that some had mutations in the chloride membrane transport protein CFTR.[27]

Two species of environmental mycobacteria have been associated with skin infections: *M. marinum* and *M. haemophilum*.[8] It is not surprising that both species have a growth temperature optimum of 30 °C and cannot be recovered on laboratory medium if incubated at 37 °C. An important risk factor for the acquisition of *M. marinum* infection is superficial cuts and exposure to infected fish.[17] Thus, fishermen and individuals keeping aquaria are at risk of infection. *Mycobacterium haemophilum* skin infections are found in immunosuppressed individuals and have been associated with kidney dialysis.[8]

There is a long association between mycobacterial exposure and hypersensitivity pneumonitis. Hypersensitivity pneumonitis is produced in rabbits exposed to cell envelope fractions,[28] and mycobacterial cells can elicit hypersensitivity reactions in macrophage cells.[29] Recently, the inhalation of mycobacteria-containing aerosols generated from hot tubs was linked to hypersensitivity pneumonitis.[30,31] It has been hypothesized that an exposure to aerosols of metal recovery fluids in the automobile industry is responsible for outbreaks of hypersensitivity pneumonitis. Mycobacteria, including a novel species *Mycobacterium immunogenum*, have been isolated from metal recovery fluids linked to hypersensitivity pneumonitis.[32] Mycobacteria are probably introduced during mixing the 100 per cent metal recovery fluid with water to produce the emulsion used to cool the working surfaces of cutting and grinding tools and carry off particulates. Mycobacteria can metabolize many of the hydrocarbon constituents of metal recovery fluid[33] and survive the addition of disinfectant used to inhibit microbial growth. Thus, like drinking water distribution systems and household plumbing, this engineered environment selects for mycobacterial persistence and growth.

TREATMENT OF MYCOBACTERIAL DISEASE

The American Thoracic Society has published recommended diagnostic criteria and treatment guidelines for mycobacterial disease.[34] A combination of antibiotics is usually required, in some instances for quite a long time. Attendant with multiple drug therapy is the potential problem of multiple side-effects and drug–drug interactions. The treatment guidelines are suggested regimens, because there have not been sufficient large-scale drug treatment trials to compare different regimens. If a patient can tolerate the multiple drug regimens, disease symptoms disappear. However, it is understood that patients may never be 'cured' of mycobacteria, because mycobacteria can enter a dormant stage and reappear to cause disease later in life.[35]

ENVIRONMENTAL COMPARTMENTS INHABITED BY MYCOBACTERIA

A wide variety of environmental compartments are inhabited by mycobacteria (Box 21.1) as part of the normal microbial flora. Once they colonize a habitat, they grow, persist and are almost impossible to eradicate. Natural waters,[36,37] drinking water and drinking water distribution systems,[3,38,39] as well as building[40] household water and plumbing systems,[4,41] all yield mycobacteria, especially *M. avium* and *M. intracellulare*, in significant numbers (over 1000 colony-forming units per millilitre). Aerosols collected above natural waters[42] or generated by bubbling[14] have high numbers of mycobacteria. In fact, the hydrophobic mycobacteria are concentrated on air bubbles in water leading to a concentration of mycobacteria on the bubble surface; this, when it bursts at the water surface, leads to the formation of an ejected droplet highly concentrated (1000–10 000-fold) in mycobacterial numbers.[14]

The environmental mycobacteria readily form biofilms.[43–45] It is likely that biofilm formation is responsible for the persistence of environmental mycobacteria in drinking water distribution systems and household plumbing, attachment preventing the loss of these slow-growing bacteria through washout. Hydrophobicity drives the attachment of mycobacteria to surfaces, in particular to pipes in drinking water distribution systems[3] and household plumbing.[4] Environmental mycobacteria in biofilms are more resistant to disinfectants[45] and antibiotics.[46]

Natural soils,[47] particularly peats and boreal forest soils,[48] and packaged potting soils[49] harbour high numbers of mycobacteria (over 10^6 colony-forming units per gram). Thus, it is not surprising that mycobacteria can be isolated from dusts generated by disturbing soil.[49] The hydrophobicity of mycobacteria is likely to promote the binding of mycobacteria to soil particulate matter. This hypothesis is supported by the observation that the number of mycobacteria entering water treatment facilities has been shown to be proportional to the turbidity.[3]

OVERLAP OF HUMAN AND MYCOBACTERIAL HABITATS IS CHARACTERISTIC OF INFECTION

Mycobacterial disease is a consequence of exposure in habitats occupied by both mycobacteria and humans. A number of such habitats where infection has been traced to mycobacteria in the environment include drinking water,[50] showers,[4] hot tubs and spas,[51] footbaths[19] and peat and potting soils.[49] In those studies, mycobacteria of the same species and sharing the same DNA fingerprint as the patient's isolate were isolated from the patient's environment. The overlap of the habitats is not the only factor influencing infection, because infection requires pre-existing host conditions.

MYCOBACTERIAL TRANSMISSION AND INFECTION ROUTES

Routes of mycobacterial transmission include droplet aerosols generated above natural waters and as a consequence of splashing (e.g. showers) or bubbling (e.g. hot tubs and spas).[14] The measurement of aerosol droplets ejected from water has shown that a proportion are small enough to enter human alveoli (less than 5 μm in diameter).[14,42] Dusts generated by dropping potting soils contain mycobacteria of the same species and sharing the same DNA fingerprint as the patients providing the soil,[49] supporting the hypothesis that mycobacterial infection as a consequence of soil exposure is via the inhalation of dusts. For children with cervical lymphadenitis, the likely route of infection is swallowing water.[18]

WHY ARE MYCOBACTERIA IN THE ENVIRONMENT?

A number of physiological traits support the survival, growth and persistence of mycobacteria in the environment. Cell surface hydrophobicity is the major trait because it promotes attachment to surfaces so that slow-growing mycobacteria are not washed out of habitats. Furthermore, it is a determinant of the concentration of mycobacteria in air bubbles and their ejection into the air in droplets.[14] The hydrophobic surface layers reduce transport[11] but also protect against antimicrobial agents.[45,46] Resistance to the disinfectants used in water treatment (e.g. chlorine) promotes mycobacterial growth and persistence in drinking water distribution systems and household plumbing. Antibiotic resistance is due, in part, to the impermeable surface of mycobacterial cells. Finally, the environmental mycobacteria are oligotrophs, able to grow in water with very low levels of organic carbon (i.e. over 50 μg assimilable

---

BOX 21.1: Habitats of environmental opportunistic mycobacteria

- Natural waters
- Drinking water distribution systems
- Household plumbing
- Hot tubs, spas and therapy pools
- Natural and household/building aerosols
- Soils, especially boreal forest soils and peats
- Metal working fluid systems
- Aquaria

organic carbon per litre).[15] This collection of traits supports the notion that engineered habitats such as drinking water distribution systems and household plumbing select for mycobacterial persistence and proliferation.

REFERENCES

● = Key primary paper
◆ = Major review article

◆1. Wayne LG, Sramek HA. Agents of newly recognized or infrequently encountered mycobacterial diseases. *Clin Microbiol Rev* 1992; **5**: 1–25.

◆2. Tortoli E. Impact of genotypic studies on mycobacterial taxonomy: the new mycobacteria of the 1990s. *Clin Microbiol Rev* 2003; **16**: 319–54.

3. Falkinham JO III, Norton CD, LeChevallier MW. Factors influencing numbers of *Mycobacterium avium*, *Mycobacterium intracellulare*, and other mycobacteria in drinking water distribution systems. *Appl Environ Microbiol* 2001; **67**: 1225–31.

●4. Falkinham JO III, Iseman MD, de Haas P, van Soolingen D. *Mycobacterium avium* in a shower linked to pulmonary disease. *J Water Health* 2008; **6**: 209–13.

5. Conger NG, O'Connell RJ, Laurel VL *et al*. *Mycobacterium simiae* outbreak associated with a hospital water supply. *Infect Control Hosp Epidemiol* 2004; **25**: 1050–5.

6. Zaugg M, Salfinger M, Opravil M, Luthy R. Extrapulmonary and disseminated infections due to *Mycobacterium malmoense*: case report and review. *Clin Infect Dis* 1993; **16**: 540–9.

7. Costrini AM, Mahler DA, Gross WM, Hawkins JE, Yesner R, D'Esopo ND. Clinical and roentgenographic features of nosocomial pulmonary disease due to *Mycobacterium xenopi*. *Am Rev Respir Dis* 1981; **123**: 104–9.

8. Dobos KM, Quinn FD, Ashford DA, Horsburgh RC, King CH. Emergence of a unique group of necrotizing mycobacterial diseases. *Emerg Infect Dis* 1999; **5**: 367–78.

9. Uslan DZ, Kowalski TJ, Wengemack NL, Virk A, Wilson JW. Skin and soft tissue infections due to rapidly growing mycobacteria. *Arch Dermatol* 2006; **142**: 1287–92.

◆10. Wallace RJ Jr, Brown BA, Griffith DE. Nosocomial outbreaks/pseudo-outbreaks caused by nontuberculous mycobacteria. *Annu Rev Microbiol* 1998; **52**: 453–90.

◆11. Brennan PJ, Nikaido H. The envelope of mycobacteria. *Annu Rev Biochem* 1995; **64**: 29–63.

◆12. Daffe M, Draper P. The envelope layers of mycobacteria with reference to their pathogenicity. *Adv Microbiol Physiol* 1998; **39**: 131–203.

●13. Hoffman CA, Leis M, Niederweis M, Plizko JM, Engelhardt H. Disclosure of the mycobacterial outer membrane: cryo-electron tomography and vitreous sections reveal the lipid bilayer structure. *Proc Natl Acad Sci USA* 2008; **105**: 3963–7.

●14. Parker BC, Ford MA, Gruft H, Falkinham JO III. Epidemiology of infection by nontuberculous mycobacteria. IV: Preferential aerosolization of *Mycobacterium intracellulare* from natural waters. *Am Rev Respir Dis* 1983; **128**: 652–6.

15. Norton CD, LeChevallier MW, Falkinham JO III. Survival of *Mycobacterium avium* in a model distribution system. *Water Res* 2004; **38**: 1457–66.

◆16. Marras TK, Chedore P, Ying AM, Jamieson F. Isolation prevalence of pulmonary non-tuberculous mycobacteria in Ontario, 1997–2003. *Thorax* 2007; **62**: 661–6.

◆17. Wolinsky E. Nontuberculous mycobacteria and associated diseases. *Am Rev Respir Dis* 1979; **119**: 107–59.

●18. Wolinsky E. Mycobacterial lymphadenitis in children: a prospective study of 105 nontuberculous cases with long-term follow up. *Clin Infect Dis* 1995; **20**: 954–63.

19. Winthrop KL, Abrams M, Yakrus M *et al*. An outbreak of mycobacterial furunculosis associated with footbaths at a nail salon. *N Engl J Med* 2002; **346**: 1366–71.

◆20. Falkinham JO III. Epidemiology of infection by nontuberculous mycobacteria. *Clin Microbiol Rev* 1996; **9**: 177–215.

21. Jonsson BE, Gilljam M, Lindblad A, Ridell M, Wold AW, Welinder-Olsson C. Molecular epidemiology of *Mycobacterium abscessus*, with focus on cystic fibrosis. *J Clin Microbiol* 2007; **45**: 1497–504.

22. Thomson RM, Armstrong JG, Looke DF. Gastroesophageal reflux disease, acid suppression, and *Mycobacterium avium* complex pulmonary disease. *Chest* 2007; **131**: 1166–72.

23. Koh WJ, Lee JH, Kwon YS *et al*. Prevalence of gastroesophageal reflux disease in patients with nontuberculous mycobacterial disease. *Chest* 2007; **131**: 1825–30.

●24. Prince DS, Peterson DD, Steiner RM *et al*. Infection with *Mycobacterium avium* complex in patients with predisposing conditions. *N Engl J Med* 1989; **321**: 863–8.

25. Reich JM, Johnson RE. *Mycobacterium avium* complex pulmonary disease. Incidence, presentation, and response to therapy in a community setting. *Am Rev Respir Dis* 1991; **143**: 1381–5.

26. Kennedy TP, Weber DJ. Nontuberculous mycobacteria. An underappreciated cause of geriatric lung disease. *Am J Respir Crit Care Med* 1994; **149**: 1654–8.

●27. Kim JS, Tanaka N, Newell JD *et al*. Nontuberculous mycobacterial infection. CT scan findings, genotype, and treatment responsiveness. *Chest* 2005; **128**: 3863–9.

28. Richerson HB, Suelzer MT, Swanson PA, Butler JE, Koop WC, Rose EF. Chronic hypersensitivity pneumonitis produced in the rabbit by the adjuvant effect of inhaled muramyl dipeptide (MDP). *Am J Pathol* 1982; **106**: 409–20.

29. Huttunen K, Ruotsalainen M, Iivanainen E, Torkko P, Katila M-L, Hirvonen M-R. Inflammatory responses in RAW264.7 macrophages caused by mycobacteria isolated from moldy houses. *Environ Toxicol Pharmacol* 2000; **8**: 237–44.

30. Rickman OB, Ryu JH, Fidler ME, Kalra S. Hypersensitivity pneumonitis associated with *Mycobacterium avium* complex and hot tub use. *Mayo Clin Proc* 2002; **77**: 1233–7.

31. Marras TK, Wallace RJ Jr, Koth LL, Stulbarg MS, Cowl CT, Daley CL. Hypersensitivity pneumonitis reaction to

Mycobacterium avium in household water. *Chest* 2005;
127: 664–71.

32. Moore JS, Christensen M, Wilson RW *et al.* Mycobacterial
    contamination of metalworking fluids: involvement of a
    possible new taxon of rapidly growing mycobacteria.
    Am Ind Hyg Assoc J 2000; **61**: 205–13.

33. Krulwich TA, Pelliccione NJ. Catabolic pathways of
    coryneforms, nocardias, and mycobacteria. *Annu Rev
    Microbiol* 1979; **33**: 95–111.

◆34. Griffith DE, Aksamit T, Brown-Elliott BA *et al.* An official
     ATS/IDSA statement: diagnosis, treatment, and prevention
     of nontuberculous mycobacteria diseases. *Am J Respir Crit
     Care Med* 2007; **175**: 367–416.

35. Wayne LG, Hayes LG. An *in vitro* model for the sequential
    study of shiftdown of *Mycobacterium tuberculosis* through
    two stages of nonreplicating persistence. *Infect Immun*
    1996; **64**: 2062–9.

●36. Falkinham JO III, Parker BC, Gruft H. Epidemiology of
     infection by nontuberculous mycobacteria. I: Geographic
     distribution in the eastern United States. *Am Rev Respir Dis*
     1980; **121**: 931–7.

37. von Reyn CF, Waddell RD, Eaton T *et al.* Isolation of
    Mycobacterium avium complex from water in the United
    States, Finland, Zaire, and Kenya. *J Clin Microbiol* 1993; **31**:
    3227–30.

●38. duMoulin GC, Stottmeier KD. Waterborne mycobacteria: an
     increasing threat to health. *ASM News* 1986; **52**: 525–9.

39. Covert TC, Rodgers MR, Reyes AL, Stelma GN Jr. Occurrence
    of nontuberculous mycobacteria in environmental samples.
    Appl Environ Microbiol 1999; **65**: 2492–6.

●40. duMoulin GC, Stottmeier KD, Pelletier PA, Tsang AY,
     Hedley-Whyte J. Concentration of *Mycobacterium avium*
     by hospital hot water systems. *J Am Med Assoc* 1988; **260**:
     1599–601.

41. Nishiuchi Y, Maekura R, Kitada S *et al.* The recovery of
    Mycobacterium avium-intracellulare complex (MAC) from

the residential bathrooms of patients with pulmonary
MAC. *Clin Infect Dis* 2007; **45**: 347–51.

●42. Wendt SL, George KL, Parker BC, Gruft H, Falkinham JO III.
     Epidemiology of infection by nontuberculous mycobacteria.
     III: Isolation of potentially pathogenic mycobacteria from
     aerosols. *Am Rev Resp Dis* 1980; **122**: 259–63.

43. Schulze-Röbbecke R, Fischeder R. Mycobacteria in biofilms.
    Zentbl Hyg Umweltmed 1989; **188**: 385–90.

44. Torvinen E, Suomalainen S, Lehtola MJ *et al.* Mycobacteria in
    water and loose deposits of drinking water distribution systems
    in Finland. *Appl Environ Microbiol* 2004; **70**: 1973–81.

45. Steed KA, Falkinham JO III. Effect of growth in biofilms on
    chlorine susceptibility of *Mycobacterium avium* and
    Mycobacterium intracellulare. Appl Environ Microbiol
    2006; **72**: 4007–100.

46. Falkinham JO III. Growth in catheter biofilms and antibiotic
    resistance of *Mycobacterium avium. J Med Microbiol* 2007;
    56: 250–4.

47. Brooks RW, Parker BC, Gruft H, Falkinham JO III. Epidemiology
    of infection by nontuberculous mycobacteria. V: Numbers in
    eastern United States soils and correlation with soil
    characteristics. *Am Rev Respir Dis* 1984; **130**: 630–3.

48. Iivanainen EK, Martikainen PJ, Raisanen ML, Katila M-J.
    Mycobacteria in boreal coniferous forest soils. *FEMS
    Microbiol Ecol* 1997; **23**: 325–32.

●49. De Groote MA, Pace NR, Fulton K, Falkinham JO III.
     Relationship between *Mycobacterium* isolates from
     patients with pulmonary mycobacterial infection and
     potting soils. *Appl Environ Microbiol* 2006; **72**: 7602–6.

●50. von Reyn CF, Maslow JN, Barber TW, Falkinham JO III,
     Arbeit RD. Persistent colonisation of potable water as a
     source of *Mycobacterium avium* infection in AIDS. *Lancet*
     1994; **343**: 1137–41.

51. Mangione EJ, Huitt G, Lenaway D *et al.* Nontuberculous
    mycobacterial disease following hot tub exposure. *Emerg
    Infect Dis* 2001; **7**: 1039–42.

SECTION C

Diseases related to exposure to non-infectious material

22

Chemical transmission through the food chain

JANET A.M. KYLE, GERALDINE McNEILL

The safety of the food supply has been an area of major public concern since early times. 'Food scares' can have a rapid and long-lasting impact on the population's consumption patterns and on the economic viability of affected food producers. Enforcement of legislation to reduce the risk of contamination of the food supply is an important function of national and international bodies. However, information on the possible toxic effects of different contaminants and on the levels of exposure from diet is often incomplete, leaving opportunity for consumer concern about the possible health effects of the food supply. Food contamination incidents are often widely reported, and public concern about the implications of novel processes for the safety of foods is high.

Although the level of exposure of better-known food contaminants is generally decreasing in higher income countries, international trade and the increasing complexity of food-processing mean that opportunities for contamination still occur in all parts of the world. Population groups who are particularly vulnerable to high levels of exposure are the very young, those with unusual diets and those reliant on a small number of foods or food sources.

This chapter covers the routes by which chemicals can be introduced into the food chain, which are summarized in Table 22.1. Specific examples, such as pesticides and acrylamide, are used to illustrate general aspects of the chemical contamination of foods, as, for many of the examples in the table, the health effects are less well understood. Contamination from microorganisms and their products, such as mycotoxins (e.g. aflatoxin), are covered in other chapters of this book. Estimating dietary intake and exposure to chemicals in the food chain is an integral, albeit challenging, part of monitoring their presence and health risks; consequently, a section of this chapter will outline the most frequently used methods mentioned in earlier sections.

CONTAMINATION DURING FOOD PRODUCTION

In both crop and animal food production, chemical contamination can occur as a result of contaminants in the environment in which the plants or animals are produced, or from the excessive application of chemicals designed to promote production, such as pesticides, fertilizers and other growth promoters.

Table 22.1 Sources of contaminants in the food chain

Link in food chain	Type of potential contaminants
Production	Pesticide residues, environmental toxicants, e.g. heavy metals, veterinary medicines, fertilizers and chemicals in animal feedstuffs
Processing	Pesticide residues, foreign bodies, additives e.g. nitrites, and food contact materials
Packaging	Food contact materials, microbial hazards and additives
Storage	Pesticide residues, foreign bodies, dioxins, microbial hazards, mycotoxins and fumigants
Home preparation	Food contact materials, chemicals from preparation and cooking and microbial hazards

Environmental contaminants

Toxins in the air, water or soil can enter the food chain through plants cultivated on the contaminated land and through animals reared in the contaminated environment. Bioaccumulation, whereby contaminants reach higher concentrations in species higher up the food chain, for example marine predators and livestock, may occur, particularly for contaminants that are persistent within animal tissues, such as heavy metals or lipophilic organic compounds.

Dioxin-like compounds (DLCs) include dioxins, furans and polychlorinated biphenyls (PCBs) with dioxin-like activity. Dioxins and furans are by-products of the combustion of organic matter so are produced, for example, through the burning of tropical forest or the incineration of household waste. PCBs, a group of 209 congeners used in the manufacture of electrical goods, have been prohibited in industrial countries since the late 1980s, but levels in the environment have decreased relatively slowly due to their high persistence.[1] The toxic and chemical effects of these compounds are wide ranging and include carcinogenic, hepatic, endocrine, immune and neurological effects.[2,3]

Based on these adverse health effects, tolerable daily intakes (TDIs) of 2 pg and 1–4 pg total toxic equivalents (TEQs) per kilogram body weight per day (for definitions of these, see Table 22.2) were derived for dioxins and PCBs by the European Commission and World Health Organization (WHO), respectively.[4] Intakes of DLCs and PCBs are normally expressed as TEQs as there are many mixtures of these compounds with different toxicity factors, which are multiplied to give a TEQ value.[5]

Although DLCs can enter the human body through air and water, the major source of DLCs in man is through the food chain. Due to bioaccumulation, levels of these lipophilic compounds are particularly high in animal products, with milk, meat and oily fish being major sources.[2] One of the more common routes to dioxin and PCB food contamination tracks back to contaminated animal feed used to feed, for example, fish, pigs, cows and poultry. This has resulted in raised dioxin levels in meat, milk and egg products, leading to their withdrawal from the human food supply as levels were above set legal limits.[6,7]

A number of studies have assessed the level of DCLs and PCBs in foodstuffs and then estimated dietary intake, showing that levels in several populations from developed and industrialized countries might exceed set exposure limits.[2,8] In the UK, average levels of dietary exposure to dioxins and DLCs have fallen since the early 1980s,[4] with average dietary intakes by adults and schoolchildren tending to be below the TDIs, even though the upper levels

Table 22.2 Terms used in the regulation of contaminants in the food chain

Term	Definition
Maximum residue level (MRL)	The maximum concentration of chemical residue (expressed as milligrams of residue per kilogram of food) legally permitted in or on foods or feedstuffs
No observed adverse effect level (NOAEL)	The highest dose of active chemical in a toxicological investigation that does not cause ill-effects
Toxic equivalency factor (TEF)	A measure of the relative toxicological potency of a chemical compared with a well-characterized reference compound. TEFs can be used to sum the toxicological potency of a mixture of chemicals that are all members of the same chemical class, having common structural, toxicological and biochemical properties
Total toxic equivalent (TEQ)	A method of comparing the total relative toxicological potency within a sample. It is calculated as the sum of the product of the concentration of each congener multiplied by its toxic equivalency factor (TEF)
Acceptable daily intake (ADI)	An estimate of the amount of a substance in food or drink, expressed on a body weight basis (e.g. mg/kg body weight), that can be ingested daily over a lifetime by humans without appreciable health risk
Acute reference dose (ARfD)	An estimate of the amount of a substance in food or drink, expressed on a body weight basis, that can be ingested in a period of 24 hours or less without appreciable health risk
Tolerable daily intake (TDI)	An estimate of the amount of contaminant, expressed on a body weight basis (e.g. mg/kg body weight), that can be ingested daily over a lifetime without appreciable health risk
Provisional tolerable daily intake (PTDI)	A reference value indicating the safe level of intake of a contaminant, calculated on a daily basis for contaminants that do not accumulate in the human body. It is a primary health standard applying to total exposure (i.e. both food and non-food sources)
Provisional tolerable weekly intake (PTWI)	The reference value used to indicate the safe level of intake of a contaminant. The PTWI is calculated on a weekly basis for contaminants that may accumulate in the human body over time, in order to minimize the significance of daily variations in intake. It is a primary health standard that applies to total exposure (i.e. both food and non-food sources)

of dietary intake (the 97.5th centile of intake; for a definition, see later) seem to be slightly above the European Union (EU) TDI. However, for younger children (toddlers), estimates of average exposure tend to exceed the EU TDI by around 2-fold.[4] Despite this, similar findings have been reported across Europe.[9] 'Biomarker of exposure' studies support the dietary exposure studies with PCB and DLC concentrations in human milk, blood and serum being monitored.[10–12] The consumption of oily fish and shellfish appears to be an important predictor of exposure,[13,14] with fish-eating populations tending to consume high levels of dioxins and PCBs.[8] Levels of the persistent DLCs are essentially falling but are still close to established safe levels; governments globally are thus developing strategies for further reducing exposure to the toxic contaminants.

Heavy metals may also enter the food chain from the industrial contamination of land or water. Mercury from industrial processes such as coal-fired power stations, mining and the combustion of waste containing mercury may enter rivers and hence the sea. In water, mercury is converted to methyl mercury, which can cross the blood–brain barrier and placenta and exerts toxic effects on the developing nervous system.[15] Mercury poisoning can also occur in adults exposed to high intakes, and results in disturbed sensation and lack of coordination.

Dietary exposure safety limits indicate the provisional tolerable weekly intake (PTWI; see Table 22.2 for a definition) for methyl mercury is 1.6 μg/kg body weight per week. Larger fish such as shark, swordfish and marlin have higher concentrations, and hence pregnant women are advised to avoid or to limit their intake of these fish, whereas other adults are advised to have no more than one portion per week. Tuna, which contains intermediate levels, is recommended for consumption in moderation by pregnant women.[16] Interestingly, selenium in fish may counteract the toxic effects of mercury at moderate concentrations by selenoproteins acting as mercury-chelating agents.[17] Pan-European dietary intake assessment indicates that, in Europe, typical levels of exposure do not exceed the PTWI, but communities eating high quantities of fish are at risk of exceeding the safe limits of mercury exposure.[2]

Another metal that enters the food chain via water is arsenic from industrial waste. In the inorganic form, arsenic is known to cause cancers such as skin and bladder tumours. Historically, fish and shellfish have been the main dietary source of this metal. In some areas, however, groundwater contains elevated levels of arsenic: in Bangladesh, high levels are found due to drinking water wells being sunk to levels at which high arsenic concentrations are found.

Rice grown in paddy fields is particularly efficient in taking up arsenic from soils, and in areas with high arsenic levels in water, the concentrations in rice may reach higher health risk levels. Rice is the staple food for many people in South-East Asia but is also consumed in other parts of the world and used to make breakfast cereals, crackers, milk and infant foods.[18] Rice is also cultivated in other parts of the

world, often on flood plains that may suffer from industrial contamination. A survey of the arsenic content of rice from different areas found the highest levels in rice from the USA (Michigan) and France (Camargue) and the lowest levels in rice from Egypt, although due to a variation in speciation and in average rice consumption, populations in Bangladesh are likely to be at highest risk of elevated inorganic arsenic intake.[19] As this is a relatively recent area of research, studies of inorganic arsenic intake among frequent consumers of rice-based foods (babies, ethnic minorities, vegans and individuals with coeliac disease) may be needed to determine whether this poses a significant risk to human health.

In summary, environmental contaminants including dioxins, PCB and heavy metals are present in the food chain and have the potential to exert adverse health effects on the population. There are several other environmental contaminants found in the foodstuffs but not investigated here that also pose a risk to health; these include other heavy metals such as lead and cadmium, brominated flame retardants and radionuclides. Further reading on these contaminants is available in the book on food safety edited by D'Mello.[20]

Pesticides and pesticide residues

Pesticide control in food production dates back to the beginnings of agriculture circa 8000 BC. The Ancient Sumarians reportedly applied sulphur to crops to control mites and insects around 2500 BC, while the Chinese employed biocontrol measures circa 324 BC by introducing ants to citrus groves to control caterpillars.[21] Essentially, with the exception of various mixtures of natural repellents and poisons, primarily inorganic compounds including arsenic, ash (burnt plant residue), copper and mercury and later petroleum products and extracts, pesticide use was limited, frequently resulting in crop failure, famine and mass emigration. One of the best known examples was the Irish potato famine of 1845, where the fungal disease 'blight' repeatedly destroyed potato crops over a 6 year period, resulting in around 1 000 000 deaths. This, combined with other crop failures such as the destruction of French vineyards by mildew (1882), resulted in more systematic research and the development of initially complex mixtures of minerals and natural plant extracts.

The synthesis of dichlorodiphenyltrichloroethane (DDT) in 1939, a potent and highly toxic insecticide and the first organic pesticide to be commercially marketed in the late 1940s, led the way. Intense research and development, fuelled by the need to feed devastated post-war populations, resulted in a revolution in pest and weed control in food production and a major shift from their application on high-value, small-acreage crops, such as soft fruits, to major crops including corn, potatoes and grains, and to the routine application of pesticides. This widespread usage was facilitated by the development, mass production and routine application of new synthetic pesticides, herbicides and growth regulators. By the end of the twentieth century, around 1300 pesticide products were marketed for application on food crops and animal feeds.[22]

The modern term 'pesticide' encompasses all chemical natural and synthetic substances (Table 22.3), known as insecticides, fungicides and herbicides and plant growth regulators. Despite the global expenditure on pesticides almost tripling between 1995 and 2001 to $31.8 billion, annual usage fell slightly by 0.3 billion kg to 2.3 billion kg.[23] The application of pesticides is clearly an important part of modern agriculture, enabling more efficient food production through a reduction of losses due to crop infestations and diseases through the control of insects, fungi, rodents and weeds. Yet pesticides are biologically active chemical substances with potential acute and long-term health implications, with reported links to cancer, congenital malformations, reproductive effects and neurotoxicity, as well as actions on the central nervous system, an aspect covered more extensively in Chapter 25.

Consequently, since the 1960s, strict regulations and controls on safe usage have gradually been introduced to which the agricultural and food industries across the globe must adhere. A number of international and national regulatory bodies now ensure the safety of pesticides in the food chain. Within the EU, there are currently around 850 pesticides approved for agricultural use, although individual countries approve and ban different numbers and types. For example, the UK has approximately 350 approved pesticides that are closely regulated, monitored and controlled by the Chemicals Regulation Directorate (CRD).[24] Pesticides are authorized for use on specific crops, at set concentrations, with a maximum number of applications and fixed treatment methods, and at specific times or stages of production, all designed to minimize the risk of pesticide residues being present on food items when they are ready for consumption. Residues do, however, continue to be found on foods.[25]

The most frequently detected pesticide residues in the diet are insecticides, fungicides and plant growth regulators (Table 22.4), and the remainder of this section will focus on these types of pesticide.

INSECTICIDES

Numerous different classes of insecticide have been designed for food crops and animal feeds, the largest groups of which can be classified by their chemical structure to include organochlorine compounds, organophosphorus compounds, pyrethroids and carbamates (see Table 22.3). Increasingly, however, a wide range of new classes of 'reduced-risk' insecticide are being developed,

Table 22.3 Types of pesticide found in the food chain[25–27]

Group of pesticide	Common examples of pesticide residues found in foods			
Insecticides				
Organochlorines	DDT	Endosulphan	Dieldrin	Lindane (γ-HCH)
Organophosphates	Chlorpyrifos	Dimethoate	Malathion	Diazinon
Carbamates	Carbendazim	Thiophanate-methyl	Benomyl group	Carbaryl
Pyrethroids/pyrethrins	Cypermethrin	Deltamethrin	Permethrin	
Fungicides	Maneb group	Methiocarb and carbaryl	Cypermethrin	Bitertanol
Herbicides	Glyphosate	Diquat	2,4-D	Thiocarbamates
Plant growth regulators	Chlormequat	Maleic hydrazide	Carbaryl	Ethoxyquin
Fumigants	Bromide	Hydrogen phosphide (phosphine)		

Table 22.4 Residues most frequently found in the US Total Diet Study[27]

Pesticide	Type	% of samples containing residue	Detection range (mg/kg)	MRL (mg/kg food)
DDT	Insecticide, OC	25%	0.0001–0.109	1
Endosulphan	Insecticide, OC	16%	0.0001–0.0756	15
Malathion	Insecticide, OP	16%	0.0002–0.069	100
Chlorpyrifos methyl	Insecticide, OP	15%	0.0001–0.028	
Dieldrin	Insecticide, OC	13%	0.0001–0.022	–
Chlorpyrifos	Insecticide, OP	7%	0.0001–0.044	–
Permethrin	Insecticide, pyrethroid	7%	0.0003–1.796	100
Chlorpropham	Herbicide and PGR	6%	0.0005–1.513	
Thiabendazole	Fungicide	5%	0.001–0.508	40
Carbaryl	Insecticide and PGR	5%	0.001–0.217	200

MRL, maximum residue level; OC, organochlorine; OP, organophosphate; PGR, plant growth regulator.

such as oxadiazines and nicotinoids. Comprehensive lists of the many different types of pesticide are available from the CRD[24] pesticides register and the US Environmental Protection Agency pesticides fact sheets.[28]

Organochlorines are persistent insecticides that include the well-known compound DDT, widely used in crop and food production during the 1950s through to the 1970s before a global ban came into force in the 1980s and it was replaced with less persistent alternatives such as organophosphates. Acute oral exposures to organochlorine compounds are classified as either 'highly hazardous' or 'moderately hazardous' to health.[29] However, in regions where vector-borne diseases including malaria are prevalent, DDT continues to be applied.

Despite restricted agricultural use, around 90 per cent of organochlorines, such as DDT and its metabolites (total DDT), detected in human tissues are thought to be of dietary origin and continue to be detected in food items, particularly animal and fish products.[30] Several organochlorines persist in the environment for several years, DDT having a half-life of 4–5 years in soil[31] and around 15 years in sea water[32] before degrading to the less toxic metabolites dichlorodiphenyldichloroethane (DDD) and dichlorodiphenyldichloroethylene (DDE). The persistent nature of these lipophilic compounds is reflected in their ability to bioaccumulate in body fats, which is one reason for their continued detection in animal and fish products.

Organochlorine residues (mainly DDT metabolites and dieldrin) are most frequently identified in oily fish. Residue-monitoring programmes show that, despite the continued detection of these residues in oily fish, levels in the UK fell 10-fold between 2000 and 2008,[25] and residues rarely occur in low-fat white fish or shellfish. Detection rates in animal products are around 20 per cent of samples analysed in the UK and USA, but levels are also diminishing.[25,33] In plant-based foods, organochlorine residues, such as endosulphan, are occasionally detected (<3 per cent of food samples analysed) across Europe.[26] This rate is increased in developing countries, areas where the organochlorine ban was implemented more recently, areas where DDT is employed to control malaria and areas where infringements of the ban may occur.[34] In summary, organochlorine residues detected in foods across Europe rarely exceed the maximum residue levels (MRL; for a definition, see Table 22.2) for foods.[25,26]

Assessing the dietary intake of organochlorine residues, the established levels of acceptable daily intake (ADI; for a definition, see Table 22.2) are now very rarely exceeded. For example, the ADI for DDT and its metabolites (total DDT) is 20 μg/kg body weight per day,[35] the estimated intake by a mainly fish-eating Inuit community from Greenland was 0.0185 μg/kg body weight per day in 2004, almost a tenth of the 0.125 μg total DDT per kilogram body weight per day intake calculated in 1976.[36] This trend is mirrored in developed Western countries where a more mixed diet of fish-, meat- and plant-based foods is consumed. The average dietary intake of total DDT has been estimated to be less than 2 μg per day for the average

adult[37] and child.[9,38,39] Essentially, several dietary intake studies show levels of total DDT intake to be well within the ADI, typically below 0.2 per cent.[27,40]

However, the intake in developing countries tends to be higher, but still below the set ADIs. For example, the total DDT intake from Indian vegetarian diets ranged from 0.8 to 17.9 μg/kg body weight per day.[34] This Indian study also found higher levels of intake of lindane (γ-HCH) and endosulphan compared with European and American populations; both are known to be the least persistent of the organochlorine insecticides.[22] A similar difference has been observed between Western and former Soviet States of Eastern Europe. Dietary intake levels of DDE were reported to be 3–4 times higher in a Polish population than one from West Germany.[41] The ban for using these insecticides in Eastern Europe did not come into effect until around 10 years after Western Europe, and furthermore the stockpiling of old pesticides has led to contamination of the surrounding soils. Biomonitoring of organochlorine pesticides supports these regional differences[41] and highlights the persistence of the organochlorines, as well as the falling concentrations of these insecticides over time in human breast milk,[10,42] adipose tissue, serum and blood.[43]

Organophosphates are a large class of compounds with a range of chemical structures, properties and applications. Used mainly as insecticides, the active compounds include chlorpyrifos and malathion (see Table 22.3). These highly toxic compounds are powerful and effective insecticides that rapidly degrade, do not accumulate in the environment and initially became one of the main replacements for the organochlorines.[22] In the UK, currently authorized organophosphates[24] are typically classified as 'moderately hazardous' or 'slightly hazardous' to health.[29] Note, as with all pesticides, that different organophosphates have different uses for different crops.

One of the more commonly detected organophosphates, chlorpyrifos, is mainly used on a wide range of fruit, vegetables and cereal crops. Between 2004 and 2006, over 92 per cent of foods analysed for pesticide residues in Europe did not contain chlorpyrifos residues, while less than 0.2 per cent of samples contained residues at or above the compound's MRL. Fruit, namely oranges, apples and grapes, most frequently contained chlorpyrifos residues.[26] Note that when analysing the food items, the products are not washed or peeled; for example, the whole orange with its rind is examined, although the rind is not typically eaten.

Organophosphate compounds can be highly toxic with acute exposure to high doses, and previous reports have suggested that the diet is the main route of exposure to organophosphates.[44] This observation was supported by recent studies feeding children an organic diet free of organophosphate pesticide residues, in which the urinary excretion of these compounds diminished significantly, that of chlorpyrifos to non-detectable levels.[45,46]

The Australian Total Diet Study[40] estimated dietary exposure to chlorpyrifos residues for the highest risk group toddlers to be less than 0.6 per cent of the 0.01 mg/kg body weight per day ADI. Total-diet studies and duplicate diet trials (see below for a description) have repeatedly reported low dietary exposure to the most frequently detected organophosphate residues, normally well below the ADI values for adults and high-risk group children.[27,34,40,47] For example, the typical US adult intakes of chlorpyrifos and malathion were 0.3 and 5.5 µg per adult per day, respectively, the ADIs being 10 and 20 µg/kg body weight per day.[48] However, exceedences of the acute reference dose (ARfD; for a definition, see Table 22.2) have been reported for fruit and vegetables,[25,26] highlighting the existence of the potential for exposure to organophosphate residues, particularly on the part of adults or children frequently eating high quantities of fruit and vegetables.

In the UK, pyrethroids, the most frequently applied group of insecticides,[49] are synthetic forms of the light-sensitive natural pesticide pyrethrin. Replacing organophosphates in agriculture, pyrethroid manufacturers employed stereochemistry to minimize the actual dosage of compounds required to treat crops effectively.[22] The combination of lower levels of application and the non-persistent nature of this pesticide has meant that the most frequently applied type of pesticide is one of the least often detected pesticide residues in plant foods.[26] However, these compounds have been found to be toxic at high doses and are classed as 'moderately hazardous' or 'slightly hazardous' to health.[29]

In comparison to organochlorines and organophosphates, relatively few pyrethroid intake and exposure studies have been conducted. In the UK between 2000 and 2007, assessments of the risk to consumer health of any pyrethroid residues detected in food items above their MRL have consistently found residue levels to be below their ADI.[25] ARfDs have occasionally been exceeded, particularly when assessing the exposure risk in younger children,[25,26] highlighting a need for further research into the potential risk to health. This is reinforced by biomarker assessment that shows non-occupationally pesticide-exposed populations excrete urinary pyrethoid metabolites.[50] It is important to note that other routes of exposure – dermal and inhalational – contribute to the excretion of these metabolites. However, dietary exposure has recently been linked to the urinary excretion of pyrethroid metabolites.[51,52]

Carbamates, in a similar way to pyrethroids, have superseded organophosphates in terms of rate of usage in the UK.[49] They are mainly biodegradable and tend not to accumulate in the food crops. Residues identified in foods include carbendazim and carbaryl (see Table 22.3). These compounds range in toxicity in acute doses from 'moderately hazardous' to 'unlikely to present acute hazard in normal use' to health.[29] In a similar way to pyrethyroids, assessment of dietary exposure is relatively limited. The limited studies indicate that short-term carbamate intake estimates tend to be below the ADI,[53–55] although assessment of ARfDs after the detection of residues as part of monitoring programmes has found

exceedences.[25–27] Further information on dietary intake and risk assessment can be found on the UK CRD website.[24]

FUNGICIDES AND HERBICIDES

Representing 80 per cent of pesticides used in UK agriculture,[49] fungicides and herbicides are a structurally very diverse groups of compounds; examples include carbaryl and glyphosate respectively (see Table 22.3). Fungicides and herbicides currently authorized in the UK[24] tend to be classified as 'slightly hazardous' to health or 'unlikely to present acute hazard in normal use'.[29]

UK-approved fungicides generally have low toxicity, are non-persistent and are used to control fungal growth mainly on fruit, vegetable and cereal crops pre and post harvest. There are two main types of fungicides – 'protectant' and 'eradicant' – protecting plants against fungal disease and treating crops already exhibiting a fungal infection, respectively. It has, however, been suggested that high doses of fungicides have demonstrated the potential to be carcinogenic or endocrine disruptors.[56,57] The US Environmental Protection Agency, for example, when assessing the compound boscalid, acknowledged a 'suggestive carcinogenic potential' but concluded that the evidence was not sufficient to assess its human carcinogenic potential.[28]

In Europe, the most frequently detected residues in plant foods tend to be of the lower toxicity risk category.[26] The most frequently detected fungicide residues include the maneb group of compounds and bitertanol. Degradation products of dithiocarbamate fungicides such as the maneb group are often found in raw unwashed fruit and vegetables,[25,26] but have also been detected in processed fruit-based soft drinks[58] and ready meals.[59] This is a reflection of the post-harvest application of fungicides to extend the life and quality of fresh produce.

Herbicides play an important role in weed control, with widespread application on main crops including cereals, rice and soybeans. Herbicides tend to be applied to the soil when, or soon after, crops are planted, before the edible parts – fruits, vegetables and cereals – have developed, thus reducing the risk of residue contamination in ready-to-eat foodstuffs.[22] This is reflected by the relatively infrequent detection of herbicides in EU pesticide residue-monitoring programmes. Low-level concentrations of residues have, however, occasionally been detected,[25,26] but rarely above set safety limits. Further reading on fungicide and herbicide residues in foods is available in the book by Watson.[60]

Dietary intake, total-diet and duplicate diet assessment of fungicide and herbicide residues are more limited than those of the extensively investigated organochlorines and organophosphates. Total-diet studies have reported fungicide and herbicide residue exposure being well below the ADI and ARfD values for adults and the high-risk group of children,[27,40] while the UK Pesticides Residue Committee rarely reports any exceedence of herbicide ARfDs.[25]

PLANT GROWTH REGULATORS

Altering the ageing process, growth and development of food crops, the use of plant growth regulators enhances yield, rate of growth and ripening during production and storage. This class of compounds is not persistent in the environment but is relatively frequently found in food products such as cereals, cereal products, fruit and vegetables.[25] Some early plant growth regulators, including ethylene, were used to improve the ripening of fruit such as bananas.[61] Today, there are several classes of plant growth regulator, some of which are also herbicides and insecticides; for example, the insecticide carbaryl is also used as a growth regulator to thin apples from trees. Other examples of plant growth regulators include chlormequat and maleic hydrazide, with toxicity classifications of 'slightly hazardous' and 'unlikely to present acute hazard in normal use' respectively.[29] A review of published literature highlights the limited research into plant growth regulators and any potential health effects.

A relatively commonly applied and detected growth regulator residue is chlorpropham; one of its permitted uses is to inhibit potato sprouting, and it has a temporary ADI of 0.1 mg/kg body weight, which has rarely been exceeded. Chlormequat residue is one of the more frequently detected forms of growth regulator; levels have previously been monitored in cereals and cereal products such as bread, mushrooms and various fruit and vegetables (Pesticides Residue Committee and EU residue-monitoring programmes).[25,26]

A recent review of the 1998–2002 UK pesticide residue-monitoring programmes found that cereals, in particular oats, frequently contained chlormequat residues. Products containing the outer husk of cereal grains were more likely to contain residues; for example, fewer white than wholemeal or brown bread samples contained the contaminant.[62] This observation was reflected in other cereal products containing less refined cereal flours and husks, such as bran flakes and cereal bars. It should be noted that MRLs were again rarely exceeded.[25,26] Reynolds and colleagues[62] found ARfD, daily and long-term daily intakes to be well within ARfD and ADI values for chlormequat across all consumer groups from infants to the elderly.

MONITORING PROGRAMMES FOR PESTICIDE RESIDUES IN FOODS

Within the EU, the number of reported cases, with potentially serious risks to health, of pesticide contaminants in foods mainly of plant origin doubled between 2006 and 2007 to 180 cases.[6] National and international rolling programmes monitoring pesticide residues in foodstuffs consistently show fruit, vegetables, starchy foods and grains as the food groups most likely to contain pesticides residues in detectable levels. Within the EU, as part of a rolling food residue-monitoring programme,[26] over 65 000 samples of fruit, vegetables, cereals and processed products were analysed during 2006 for over 769 different pesticide residues. Of these, 54 per cent of samples contained no detectable pesticide residues, whereas 6.6 per cent were above European Union MRLs. Fruit and vegetables most commonly contained residues (Figure 22.1). Figure 22.1 indicates that foods for the most vulnerable age group – 'infants' – are the least likely to contain detectable levels of residues, a pattern repeated across the globe.[27,40]

In the UK, one of the government's dietary recommendations is to eat at least five portions of fruit and vegetables per day. To encourage this, all schoolchildren in England aged between 4 and 6 years are given fruit and vegetables as part of the Department of Health's 'school fruit and vegetable scheme'.[63] The CRD routinely collects a small number of fruit and vegetable samples from the scheme's produce

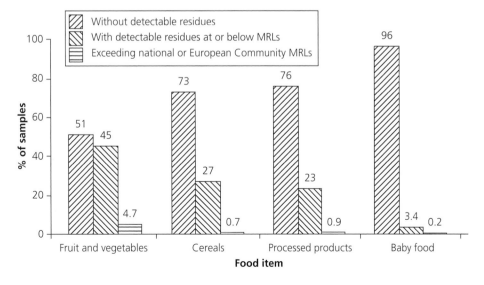

Figure 22.1   Monitoring results for food of plant origin from the European Union surveillance program, 2006. MRL, maximum residual level. (Data from EUROPA Food and Veterinary Office.[26])

suppliers for pesticides residues analysis to ensure that residue levels are within MRLs. Out of 470 unwashed or peeled fruit and vegetable samples analysed, 77 per cent contained residues within legal margins, while 55 per cent of samples contained multiple residues.[25] It is important to emphasize that 98 per cent of detected residues were within permissible limits, that the number of samples analysed was not statistically representative of the over 350 million pieces of fruit and vegetables distributed to schools, and that the produce would be washed before distribution to the children.

Interestingly, a review of residues detected between 1996 and 2005 in the EU indicates that the percentage of fruit, vegetable and cereal samples not containing pesticide residues fell from 60 per cent in 1996 to 52 per cent in 2005, whereas the level of detected residues within the legally permitted concentration margins (below the MRL), increased by 6 per cent to 43 per cent of contaminated samples in 2005. This may reflect improvements in laboratory measurement techniques and a lowering of the assays' lower limits of detection of residues, which increasingly reflect a pesticide's MRL.[26] Alternatively, it may reflect the recent expansion of the EU and subsequent enlargement of the rolling pesticide programme.

Multiple pesticide residues are increasingly being detected in food samples, for example 28 per cent of samples analysed in the EU during 2006. Two or three different residues are most frequently found, although up to eight residues have been detected.[26] It is also important to note there may be several different food sources contributing to the daily intake of a range of residues as the human diet typically encompasses numerous food groups including cereal products, starchy foods (potatoes, rice and pasta), fruit and vegetables, nuts and seeds, fish and meat, dairy products, and beverages such as coffee and fruit juices. A review of the risk of multiple residues suggests that low-level risks of exposure, as potential adverse health effects, are unsubstantiated.[64] Robust risk assessment methods to assess the cumulative and synergistic effects of multiple residues on health are currently being developed.[65]

In summary, humans are exposed to low levels of pesticide residues directly by eating plant-based products and indirectly after consuming animal products, including milk products and eggs where the animals have been fed contaminated feedstuffs. Consequently, when assessing pesticide residue exposure, it is important to consider the different potential foodstuffs in which residues may occur and the potential accumulative effect of the intake of multiple food residues, highlighting the importance of duplicate and total-diet studies (see below for a more in-depth description of dietary intake methods).

Veterinary medicine residues

Foods of animal origin can potentially contain toxic residues of veterinary drugs such as antibiotics, antimicrobial agents, fungicides and growth regulators.

Consequently, veterinary medicines, like pesticides, are strictly controlled by regulatory bodies legislating approval of their use and adherence to dosage and animal treatment guidelines, and evaluating toxicity risks of residues, setting, for example, MRLs and ADIs.[66] A strict regulation of drug use has ensured that less than 0.3 per cent of 38 759 samples analysed in the UK during 2007 exceeded statutory limits or reference points.[67]

Veterinary residues found in foods in Europe during 2007 include the banned antibiotics the nitrofurans and chloramphenicol detected in fish, meat and poultry products.[6] Nitrofuran antibiotic drugs, such as furazolidone and nitrofurazone, were previously widely used in food animal production. Today, the most common countries of origin of contaminated foods are Asian countries where 'nitrofuran' food scares occurred in the early 2000s. Nitrofurans are rapidly metabolized but produce persistent potentially carcinogenic and mutagenic metabolites in animal tissues.[68] These metabolites are also resistant to conventional cooking methods and cold storage.[69]

There is evidence that antibiotic resistance in food-borne infection in humans can be linked to the use of, for example, antimicrobial drugs in food-producing animals, which leads to the emergence of resistant bacteria, including *Campylobacter* and *Salmonella*, not pathogenic to the animal but potentially pathogenic to humans.[70] Other banned and potentially toxic veterinary contaminants detected in the UK are malachite and leucomalachite green fungicidal and parasiticide dyes in fish and shellfish, antimicrobial and heavy metal residues in meat products, and naphthalene in honey.[67] Further reading on veterinary medicine residues is available in the review by Paige and Tollefson.[70]

Fertilizers

Improving plant growth and yield, both organic and inorganic fertilizers are commonly used in food production. The main components of inorganic fertilizers are nitrogen, phosphorus and potassium, with additional elements including calcium, magnesium and sulphur as well as trace metals. Phosphorus fertilizers are known to contain cadmium and fluorine contaminants.[71] Cadmium exposure may have adverse health effects, especially nephrotoxicity, renal disease and increased cancer risk,[72] although dietary exposure assessment has repeatedly indicated intake levels within estimated safe limits.[73–75]

Nitrogen fertilizers have previously been linked with negative health effects but are subject to mixed findings. One reason for this is that they are rich in non-toxic nitrates, which can be metabolized to produce more toxic nitrites and *N*-nitroso compounds.[76,77] Nitrate residues from fertilizers can also add to naturally occurring nitrates in foods, particularly vegetables, and in drinking water.[78] They are also found in high levels in processed meats such as bacon, to which sodium nitrite is added as a preservative.

Bacterial action on nitrates, either before consumption or in the gastrointestinal tract, results in the formation of nitrites, which in large doses can lead to cases of 'blue baby syndrome', i.e. the cyanosis of young infants due to the formation of methaemoglobin.[79,80] In the acid conditions of the stomach, nitrites can be converted to *N*-nitroso compounds, which are carcinogenic in animal models, although human evidence is equivocal.[81] The dietary source of the nitrates may be important: in human populations, fruit and vegetable (and hence nitrate) consumption is generally associated with a lower risk of gastrointestinal cancer, which may be a result of the inhibitory effect of vitamin C on *N*-nitroso compound formation.[82] For a recent review of the food sources of nitrates and their potential impact on health, refer to Hord and colleagues.[83]

CONTAMINATION INTRODUCED DURING FOOD PROCESSING

In the food chain, there are many steps between food cultivation and food consumption. Even in traditional rural economies, the extraction of human foodstuffs from plants such as sugar from cane, oil from seeds or refined flour from cereal grains may involve extensive processing. Animal products such as milk, meat and fish are mostly perishable so often require processing for preservation, particularly where refrigeration is not available. In industrialized societies, the controls on the processing of raw foodstuffs are greater, but the degree of processing typically involves many different stages, each of which may be a possible entry point for contaminants.

Industrial processing of foods

Processed foods form a large proportion of the Western diet, a side-effect of this being the application and use of industrial treatments to modify food flavour, texture and shelf life. Processing techniques include industrially produced ingredients such as hydrogenated vegetable oil and preservation techniques such as canning, drying and pasteurization.

TREATMENT TO ENHANCE TASTE OR TEXTURE

An example of this is hydrolysed vegetable protein, i.e. protein treated to release individual amino acids, which include glutamic acid, better known as monosodium glutamate (MSG), a flavour enhancer. MSG produced by the hydrolysis of vegetable protein does not need to be declared as an additive on the label. If the hydrolysis is carried out using acid, by-products such as the chloropropanols, 3-monochloropropane 1,2 diol or 3-MCPD, which is known to be carcinogenic and mutagenic in rodents,[84,85] are also formed. Consequently, controls on

permitted levels of 3-MCPD in foods and dietary intake have been introduced.[86] The highest recorded levels have been found in non-traditionally brewed soy sauces, but some other, more common food products in the UK, such as sliced bread, crackers, beef-burgers and processed cheese, have also been found to contain high levels.[87–89] The dietary intake of 3-MCPD by a Spanish population was recently determined to be less than 0.01 per cent of the maximum TDI (2 mg/kg body weight per day).[90] Alternative methods for hydrolysing protein, which take longer and therefore increase the cost of production, do not lead to the formation of 3-MCPD.

TREATMENT FOR PRESERVATION

High-temperature heat treatment, such as may occur during canning or bottling, may lead to the formation of furan from the breakdown of amino acids or polyunsaturated fatty acids; this can also be formed by the degradation of pentose sugars, typically found in non-digestible carbohydrates such as bran or maize cobs.[91] Furan and its metabolite, cis-2-butene-1,4-dial, have been classified by the International Agency for Research in Cancer as 'possibly carcinogenic in man',[92] with cytotoxicity and carcinogenic activity indicated in laboratory models.[93,94] High furan levels have been found in roasted coffee beans and contribute to the aroma of freshly roasted coffee, but the furan is volatile so that brewed coffee contains lower levels than coffee beans.[95] Other common foods found to contain furan include potato crisps and canned and jarred foods including baby foods.[96–98] Exposure assessment for furan in humans is limited, although recent dietary intake estimates indicate that adults in the EU may consume around 0.78 µg/kg body weight per day, obtained mainly from coffee, while infants may ingest 0.27–1.01 µg/kg body weight per day.[99] A marker for liver damage, gamma-glutamyltranspeptidase, has also recently been found to be strongly correlated with urinary furan excretion in humans.[100] Experts have advised that levels of furan in food should be 'as low as reasonably practicable'.[94]

Another group of carcinogens that can be formed during heat treatment are polycyclic aromatic hydrocarbons (PAHs) such as benzo(a)pyrene, which is carcinogenic and mutagenic,[101,102] and is formed in oil heated to high temperatures. The highest levels are usually found in smoked and barbecued foods, particularly those with a high intrinsic fat content or foods cooked with added fat, from which fat can drip onto the heat source below and produce fumes containing PAHs, which rise onto the food above. Levels can be reduced by using processes in which the heat is applied from above, so that oils do not drip onto the heat source, or by using leaner meat or fish and adding little or no oil in the cooking process.

PAHs are also produced in other industrial processes that involve the burning of organic matter, and may enter the food chain through the contamination of air, soil and water, leading to detectable levels in cereals, vegetables and fish. Oils and fats themselves may also contain PAHs that are produced during treatment of the oil seeds at high temperatures. Among non-smokers, over 70 per cent of the non-occupational exposure to PAHs is attributable to diet.[103] Modification of processing has led to relatively low levels of PAH contamination of foods, although higher levels have been found in food supplements and smoked and canned fish.[104] This is reflected by dietary exposure in the UK diminishing 2–5-fold between 1979 and 2000.[105] Due to their toxicity, it is not, however, possible to define a level of PAH intake that is without possible risk.[105]

More recently, it has been recognized that foods containing starch that are heated to high temperatures, such as potato chips, crisps, bread and bakery products, may contain high levels of acrylamide.[106] Other studies have confirmed this finding and reported high levels in other foods that contain carbohydrate, such as chocolate and meat products.[107] Long-term dietary exposure estimates range from 0.3 to 0.8 μg/kg body weight per day.[108,109] Acrylamide, with its active metabolite glycidamine, has been classified by the International Agency for Research on Cancer as 'probably carcinogenic to humans'.[110]

Studies of acrylamide intake in case–control and longitudinal studies of cancer are in progress, with recent studies finding no link.[111,112] These may have been hampered by variable levels and a lack of information on acrylamide in foods, which has led to the exploration and development of biomarkers of intake. One study using haemoglobin adducts suggested that both diet and cigarette smoke contributed to acrylamide exposure,[113] while another of the urinary excretion of acrylamide suggested that children might be more at risk of high exposure to acrylamide than adults.[114]

USE OF ADDITIVES

Additives are common in processed foods, not only to enhance colour and flavour and to improve preservation, but also to meet statutory or other demands. For example, the addition of calcium, usually as calcium chloride, to mineral water is required by law in many countries. The additives are often produced by industrial processes, and the quality control of those added to foods should be paramount. However, on one occasion in the UK, the calcium added to mineral water accidentally contained higher levels of calcium bromide than usual, and when ozone was added to the water during production, the levels of bromate, a known carcinogen, reached twice the legal limit, leading to large numbers of bottles of water being withdrawn.[115]

Another example is the use of toxic illegal food colourants such as the use of the chemical colourant Sudan 1 (1-phenylazo-2-naphthol) to give an orange–red colour to chilli powder.[116] Although this is illegal in many countries due to the carcinogenic nature of Sudan 1, in 2005 a batch

of Worcester sauce that was used in the production of other common foods such as pizzas and ready meals was found to contain the colourant, leading to a food scare in which more than 350 products were removed from UK supermarket shelves. Legally approved artificial food colours in the diet of young children have recently been linked with hyperactivity,[117] leading EU regulatory bodies to recommend the need for further research.

DELIBERATE ADULTERATION

The adulteration of foods for economic gain has a long history. The practice of adding colouring agents, water or other lower cost ingredients to commercial foods was widespread before the twentieth century, when legislation to control these practices was first introduced. The contamination of foods may still, however, occur as a deliberate act designed to increase the value of the food.

An example of this is the addition of melamine to food to increase the nitrogen content for tests that use nitrogen as an index of protein content. Melamine ingestion can lead to the formation of kidney stones and ultimately renal failure. An outbreak of kidney stones in cats and dogs in North America was traced to the melamine contamination of pet food.[118] More recently, the addition of melamine to milk by Chinese farmers in an attempt to increase the protein content to meet local trade requirements led to a global health scare. Dried milk with high melamine levels was fed to infants, resulting in kidney stones and other complications, including several deaths.[119] This has led to calls for a greater regulation of the melamine content of foods.[120] The contamination of foods as a deliberate act of sabotage is also a possibility, and the threat of 'food terrorism' is taken seriously at international level.[121] The contamination of baby foods with pieces of glass is also periodically reported, although the deliberate sabotaging of products is rarely demonstrated.

Food storage and packaging

During food-processing, food comes into contact with a wide range of materials, such as metals in the implements and machinery used to gather or process foods and the containers used to store or wrap processed foods. Canned foods may become contaminated from the metals of the cans or the coating materials. Tin plate used in many canned foods consists of steel coated in tin, which may enter the food, although this is limited if the internal surface of the can is lacquered.[122] Lead from the solder used in canning can also migrate into the food, although welding is now rather more common than soldering and leads to lower lead levels in food.[123]

The use of plastic packages, including bottles, trays and wraps, is now commonplace for processed foods. The plastics contain a range of chemicals that are added to alter the durability, appearance, heat or cold tolerance or other qualities of the packaging. Some of these compounds can migrate into foods, the amount depending on a range of factors such as the surface area of food in contact with the plastic, the fat content of the food and the temperature and duration of storage.[122,124]

Food preparation within the home

Even home cooking at high temperatures by grilling or deep frying can lead to the formation of acrylamide and PAHs, as described above. The removal of surface contaminants, for example pesticides and fungicides, may be influenced by washing practices: one survey of the impact of different domestic processes on pesticide residues on plant products suggested that the reduction in residues on fruits and vegetables from boiling or washing was variable, whereas the cooking of rice was associated with the virtual removal of pesticides in the husk.[125] Peeling fruits and vegetables was also said to result in an almost complete removal of residues as they show little penetration into the flesh.[126] However, veterinary residues, such as nitrofuran and malachite green, tend to persist after cooking.[69,127] Similarly, processing contaminants 3-MCPD and furan (see above) also remain in varying levels after cooking.[128,129]

Metals can enter food prepared in the home from cooking vessels, for example iron, nickel and chromium from stainless steel (iron alloy) saucepans, particularly during the cooking of acidic foods, and particularly with oxalic acid found in plant products such as rhubarb, spinach, chocolate and nuts. Nickel can be released under mildly acidic conditions at boiling temperatures, raising the possibility of nickel-induced dermatitis in people sensitive to nickel,[130] although one report suggests that the release of nickel after the first use of a vessel is minimal.[131] Iron and chromium are more likely to have health benefits rather than do harm in the doses released, and the provision of stainless steel cookware has been suggested as a method of reducing the prevalence of iron deficiency anaemia in vulnerable populations;[132] a recent trial did not, however, find any evidence of benefit.[133] Aluminium from saucepans used to cook acid foods was at one time suggested as a risk factor for the development of Alzheimer's disease, since high levels of aluminium are found in the characteristic beta-amyloid plaques in the brain tissue of patients, but subsequent research focused on the role of aluminium from drinking water rather than from the diet.[134]

Another material used in tableware, particularly children's tableware and picnicware, which can lead to contamination of foods, is melamine. Melamine-ware also contains formaldehyde, which was found to migrate at levels above those recommended when the vessels were exposed to fruit juice or mild acetic acid at 70 °C for 2 hours.[135]

Tableware can also be contaminated, for example with cleaning agents such as detergent. 'Milton', a preparation of sodium hypochlorite (bleach) and sodium chloride, is widely used as a disinfectant for bottles for infant formula but if prepared in high concentration may lead to a high intake of sodium.[136]

ESTIMATING DIETARY INTAKE AND EXPOSURE TO CONTAMINANTS

Monitoring the concentration of contaminants in the food chain is carried out by several international and national bodies. Since 1961, the Codex Alimentarius Commission of the Food and Agriculture Organization (FAO) and the WHO[137] has been used to standardize food safety codes for international trade and consumer protection. It currently involves 176 countries and defines MRLs for a number of residues such as pesticides in foods.

In 1976, the WHO established the Global Environment Monitoring System Food Contamination Monitoring and Assessment Program (GEMS/Food)[138] in cooperation with partner organizations in over 70 countries. This programme facilitates the monitoring of a wide range of contaminants, where possible through the use of total-diet studies. These studies involve collecting samples of foodstuffs as eaten from a representative range of outlets and preparation of a pooled sample that contains each food or food group in proportion to the average amount consumed by an individual within the population, as derived from dietary surveys of individuals. The pooled sample can then be analysed for the concentration of any contaminant. A more flexible approach is for separate samples to be prepared for major food groups (e.g. fruits, dairy foods and meats) and the analysis of contaminants to be carried out in each sample; this can then be used, in conjunction with dietary intake data, to estimate the intake of the average but also the highest consumers of these foods (typically those at the 97.5th centile of the intake distribution).

The Joint FAO/WHO Expert Committee on Food Additives[139] (JECFA) has been meeting since 1956 to consider the safety of food contaminants and to establish safe levels. To date, JECFA has evaluated the safety of over 1500 food additives, approximately 40 food contaminants and naturally occurring toxins and around 90 veterinary medicine residues. The parallel Joint FAO/WHO Meeting on Pesticide Residues[140] carries out similar activities for pesticide residues in foods.

In the UK, the Food Standards Agency oversees a total-diet study in which food samples for 20 major food groups are prepared each year. The contribution of individual foods to these groups is based on purchasing data from the annual Expenditure and Food Survey.[141] Food samples are purchased from 24 randomly selected towns and are prepared in accordance with usual consumer practice. The food groups are chosen to separate foods that are common sources of contaminants (e.g. offal is separate from carcase meat) and to provide information on food groups that make a major contribution to the average UK diet (e.g.

bread and milk). Estimates of average and 97.5th centile intake are derived for children aged 1.5–4.5 years, children aged 4–18 years and adults from ad hoc population-based surveys carried out as part of the National Diet and Nutrition Survey programme. Estimates of exposure to contaminants per kilogram body weight in these age groups is then calculated and compared with health-based guidance values such as JECFA estimate of the PTWI.

An analysis of the intake of 24 metals, including arsenic, mercury and lead, in the 2006 total-diet survey concluded that the population exposure to most metals was at low levels compared with health-based guidance values and was similar to or lower than that in 2000 apart from aluminium, barium and manganese.[141] The data from the total-diet study also highlight how exposure to chemicals in food, when calculated on a per kilogram body weight basis, is considerably higher in smaller children than adults. As an example, the mean exposure to methyl mercury in 2006 (using upper bound concentrations) was 52 per cent of the JECFA PTWI in children aged 1.5–4.5 years compared with 22 per cent in adults weighing 60 kg.

Data from total-diet studies are invaluable in providing information on average exposure and trends, but are dependent on up-to-date purchasing and consumption data in a representative sample of the population. Alternatively, dietary exposure estimates can be modelled or simulated by combining contaminant residue data from monitoring programmes, such as the pesticide and veterinary residue and national food and dietary surveillance programmes; this is the favoured approach employed by the European Union. These programmes adopt random or targeted approaches to residue monitoring and then model acute and chronic exposure risk assessments, based on complex statistical modelling techniques.[65] Until recently, the modelling of risk was based on combinations of maximum single contaminant levels and the maximum intake of individual food items; newer modelling techniques assessing the cumulative effects of ingesting combinations of several different contaminants from combinations of different food items are now being developed.[65,142]

In the case of more specific investigations, ad hoc surveys of exposure to contaminants in individuals or population subgroups may be required. Unfortunately, for ad hoc surveys, information on individual or subpopulation dietary intakes of different foods, along with chemical analysis of specific food items consumed over the period of interest, would be required, and this information is rarely available. Although the national consumption statistics of each food group can be used along with national analyses of the contaminant levels in these groups from a total-diet study, this assumes that the individual or population consumes foods with the same concentration of contaminants as the samples analysed in the total-diet study.

An alternative approach that takes into account individual variation and the concentration of the contaminants in all the food consumed is to collect a 'duplicate diet', i.e. a second sample of each food consumed over a period of, for example, a week by the individual. This sample can be homogenized and analysed for the contaminants of interest. The approach is simple in principle but poses many practical challenges, not least the storage of food samples, which is likely to explain why it is infrequently used.

An alternative approach for assessing the exposure of individuals that avoids the need for duplicate diet collection is to measure the concentration of the contaminant or a metabolite or 'biomarker' in a biological tissue. The suitability of different tissues varies according to the absorption, metabolism and excretion of the contaminant of interest, and not all contaminants can be investigated using this approach. The urinary excretion of heavy metals or pesticide residues, ideally from a 24 hour collection as opposed to a spot sample, has, however, been used in a number of studies. Other tissues that may be used to estimate exposure to heavy metals include hair (if free of cosmetics) and nails; bone mineral content and milk tooth enamel have also been investigated. Biological samples often carry the advantage that they reflect the exposure over months or years, as opposed to dietary samples, which are more likely to reflect exposure over a week at most. This is particularly important for contaminants that may vary between food samples (e.g. different varieties or foods from different producers, or with preparation methods, e.g. the washing and peeling of fruit). Unfortunately, the concentration of contaminants in the tissues is often very low in absolute terms, which poses technical challenges for their accurate measurement. Measures of biomarker exposure do not, however, distinguish between different sources of exposure. For example, the urinary excretion of some pesticide metabolites such as pyrethoids may be the result of occupational or household exposure.[46,142]

In summary, the monitoring of exposure to food contaminants at the national level requires a range of information from high-quality surveys on food purchase, individual dietary intake and food chemical analysis. Obtaining information on the exposure of individuals or population subgroups is more challenging due to variations in the intake of foods and food preparation methods between individuals, and differences in the concentration of contaminants in food between samples and over time.

SUMMARY

Chemical contaminants in the food chain are wide ranging, often entering and remaining on foods until ingestion by the human population. It is important to note that an estimated 30 per cent of food crops worldwide are lost during production, while a further 20 per cent are ruined post harvest. This highlights the need for a balance between a need for chemicals such as pesticides and preservatives to prevent food shortages, malnutrition and famine, and the risks associated with dietary exposure to toxic compounds. This chapter has outlined some of the main transmission routes of chemicals in the food chain, and concludes that, unless intentionally added, chemicals are usually present at low levels. However, the long-term risk of chronic low-level exposure to complex mixtures of toxic compounds is little understood, and it is therefore important to fully develop our understanding of their health implications.

REFERENCES

◆ = Major review article

◆1. European Food Safety Authority. Opinion of the Scientific Panel on Contaminants in the Food Chain on a request from the Commission related to the presence of non-dioxin-like polychlorinated biphenyls (PCB) in feed and food. *EFSA J* 2005; **284**: 1–137.

2. Commission of the European Communities. Food Contaminants – Dioxins and PCBs. Communication from the Commission to the Council, the European Parliament and the European Economic and Social Committee: Community Strategy for Dioxins, Furans and Polychlorinated Biphenyls COM (2001) 593 final. Available from: http://www.ec.europa.eu/food/food/chemicalsafety/contaminants/dioxins_en.htm (accessed November 20, 2009).

3. World Health Organization/International Agency on Research in Cancer. *Polychlorinated Dibenzo-para-Dioxins and Polychlorinated Dibenzofurans.* IARC Monograph on the Evaluation of Carcinogenic Risks to Humans, Vol. 69. Lyon: IARC, 1997.

4. Committee on Toxicity of Chemicals in Food, Consumer Products and the Environment. Statement on the tolerable daily intake for dioxins and dioxin like polychlorinated biphenyls. Available from: http://cot.food.gov.uk/pdfs/cot-diox-full.pdf (accessed November 27, 2009).

5. Van den Berg M, Birnbaum LS, Denison M *et al.* The 2005 World Health Organization reevaluation of human and mammalian toxic equivalency factors for dioxins and dioxin-like compounds. *Toxicol Sci* 2006; **93**: 223–41.

6. European Food Safety Authority. The Rapid Alert System for Food and Feed (RASFF) Annual Report 2007. Available from: http://www.ec.europa.eu/food/food/rapidalert/report2007_en.pdf (accessed November 20, 2009).

7. Bernard A, Broeckaert F, De Poorter G *et al.* The Belgian PCB/dioxin incident: Analysis of the food chain contamination and health risk evaluation. *Environ Res* 2002; **88**: 1–18.

◆8. Domingo JL, Bocio A. Levels of PCDD/PCDFs and PCBs in edible marine species and human intake: A literature review. *Environ Int* 2007; **33**: 397–405.

9. Wilhelm M, Schrey P, Wittsiepe J, Heinzow B. Dietary intake of persistent organic pollutants (POPs) by German children using duplicate portion sampling. *Int J Hyg Environ Health* 2002; **204**(5–6): 359–62.

10. Polder A, Skaare JU, Skjerve E *et al.* Levels of chlorinated pesticides and polychlorinated biphenyls in Norwegian breast milk (2002–2006), and factors that may predict the level of contamination. *Sci Total Environ* 2009; **407**: 4584–90.

11. Agudo A, Goñi F, Etxeandia A *et al.* Polychlorinated biphenyls in Spanish adults: Determinants of serum concentrations. *Environ Res* 2009; **109**: 620–8.

12. Bilau M, De Henauw S, Schroijen C *et al.* The relation between the estimated dietary intake of PCDD/Fs and levels in blood in a Flemish population (50–65 years). *Environ Int* 2009; **35**: 9–13.

13. Arisawa K, Uemura H, Hiyoshi M *et al.* Dietary intake of PCDDs/PCDFs and coplanar PCBs among the Japanese population estimated by duplicate portion analysis: a low proportion of adults exceed the tolerable daily intake. *Environ Res* 2008; **108**: 252–9.

14. Rylander C, Sandanger TM, Brustad M. Associations between marine food consumption and plasma concentrations of POPs in a Norwegian coastal population. *J Environ Monit* 2009; **11**: 370–6.

15. Castoldi AF, Johansson C, Onishchenko N *et al.* Human developmental neurotoxicity of methylmercury: Impact of variables and risk modifiers. *Regul Toxicol Pharmacol* 2008; **51**: 201–14.

16. Committee on Toxicity of Chemicals in Food, Consumer Products and the Environment. Science Advisory Committee on Nutrition. *Advice on Fish Consumption Benefits and Risks.* London: Stationery Office, 2004.

17. Peterson SA, Ralston SV, Peck DV *et al.* How might selenium moderate the toxic effects of mercury in stream fish of the Western US? *Environ Sci Technol* 2009; **43**: 3919–25.

18. Sun GX, Williams PN, Zhu YG *et al.* Survey of arsenic and its speciation in rice products such as breakfast cereals, rice crackers and Japanese rice condiments. *Environ Int* 2009; **35**: 473–5.

19. Meharg AA, Williams PN, Adomako E *et al.* Geographical variation in total and inorganic arsenic in polished (white) rice. *Environ Sci Technol* 2009; **43**: 1612–7.

◆20. D'Mello JPF (ed.) *Food Safety: Contaminants and Toxins.* Oxford: CABI, 2003.

21. Van Emden HF. *Pest and Vector Control.* New York: Cambridge University Press, 2004.

22. Cabras P. Pesticides: toxicology and residues in food. In: D'Mello JPF (ed.) *Food Safety: Contaminants and Toxins* (pp. 91–124). Oxford: CABI, 2003.

23. Fishel FM. *Pesticide Use Trends in the U.S.: Global Comparison.* pp. 1–143. Gainsville, FL: University of Florida, Pesticide Information Office, 2007.

24. UK Chemicals Regulation Directorate, Health and Safety Executive. CRD (Pesticides) Databases. Available from: http://www.pesticides.gov.uk/databases.asp (accessed November 20, 2009).

25. Pesticide Residues Committee. Pesticides Residues Committee Annual Reports 2000–2008. Available from: http://www.pesticides.gov.uk/prc.asp?id=959 (accessed November 20, 2009).

26. EUROPA Food and Veterinary Office – Special Reports: Pesticides Monitoring Reports 1996–2007. Available from: http://www.ec.europa.eu/food/fvo/specialreports/pesticides_index_en.htm (accessed November 20, 2009).

27. US Food and Drugs Administration. Residue Monitoring Reports: FDA Pesticide Program Residue Monitoring: 1993–2007. Available from: http://www.fda.gov/Food/FoodSafety/FoodContaminantsAdulteration/Pesticides/ResidueMonitoringReports/default.htm (accessed November 20, 2009).

28. United States Office of Prevention, Pesticides Environmental Protection and Toxic Substances Agency (7501C). Pesticide Fact Sheet: Boscalid. Available from: http://www.epa.gov/opprd001/factsheets/boscalid.pdf (accessed November 20, 2009).

♦29. World Health Organization. The WHO Recommended Classification of Pesticides by Hazard and Guidelines to Classification. Geneva: WHO/IPCS, 2005.

30. World Health Organization. DDT and its Derivatives in Drinking Water. WHO/SDE/WSH/03.04/89. Geneva: WHO, 2004.

31. Woodwell GM, Craig PP, Johnson HA. DDT in the biosphere: Where does it go? Science 1971; 174: 1101.

32. Edwards CA. Persistent Pesticides in the Environment. Boca Raton, FL: CRC Press, 1973.

33. Schafer KS, Kegley SE. Persistent toxic chemicals in the US food supply. J Epidemiol Community Health 2002; 56: 813–17.

34. Kumari B, Kathpal TS. Monitoring of pesticide residues in vegetarian diet. Environ Monit Assess 2009; 151(1–4): 19–26.

35. World Health Organization. Pesticide Residues in Food – 2000. Evaluation-2000. Part II: Toxicology. Joint FAO/WHO Meeting on Pesticide Residues. WHO/PCS/01.3. Geneva: WHO, 2001.

36. Deutch B, Dyerberg J, Pedersen HS et al. Dietary composition and contaminants in north Greenland, in the 1970s and 2004. Sci Total Environ 2006; 370(2–3): 372–81.

37. Galal-Gorchev H. Dietary intake of pesticide residues: Cadmium, mercury, and lead. Food Addit Contam 1991; 8: 793–806.

38. Chung SW, Kwong KP, Yau JC. Dietary exposure to DDT of secondary school students in Hong Kong. Chemosphere 2008; 73: 65–9.

39. Darnerud PO, Atuma S, Bjerselius AR, Petersson Grawe GK, Becker W. Dietary intake estimations of organohalogen contaminants (dioxins, PCB, PBDE and chlorinated pesticides, e.g. DDT) based on Swedish market basket. Food Chem Toxic 2006; 44: 1597–606.

40. Australian Food Standards Agency 20th Australian Total Diet Survey. Available from: http://www.foodstandards.gov.au/_srcfiles/Final_20th_Total_Diet_Survey.pdf (accessed November 20, 2009).

41. Galassi S, Bettinetti R, Neri MC et al. pp'DDE contamination of the blood and diet in central European populations. Sci Total Environ 2008; 390: 45–52.

42. Konishi Y, Kuwabara K, Hori S. Continuous surveillance of organochlorine compounds in human breast milk from 1972 to 1998 in Osaka, Japan. Arch Environ Contam Toxicol 2001; 40: 571–8.

43. Nakata H, Kawazoe M, Arizono K et al. Organochlorine pesticides and polychlorinated biphenyl residues in foodstuffs and human tissues from China: Status of contamination, historical trend, and human dietary exposure. Arch Environ Contam Toxicol 2002; 43: 473–80.

44. Clayton CA, Pellizzari ED, Whitmore RW et al. Distributions, associations, and partial aggregate exposure of pesticides and polynuclear aromatic hydrocarbons in the Minnesota Children's Pesticide Exposure Study (MNCPES). J Expo Anal Environ Epidemiol 2003; 13: 100–11.

♦45. Lu C, Barr DB, Pearson MA et al. Dietary intake and its contribution to longitudinal organophosphorus pesticide exposure in urban/suburban children. Environ Health Perspect 2008; 116: 537–42.

46. Lu C, Barr DB, Pearson M et al. A longitudinal approach to assessing urban and suburban children's exposure to pyrethroid pesticides. Environ Health Perspect 2006; 114: 1419–23.

47. Kawahara J, Yoshinaga J, Yanagisawa Y. Dietary exposure to organophosphorus pesticides for young children in Tokyo and neighboring area. Sci Total Environ 2007; 378: 263–8.

48. Gunderson EL. FDA Total Diet Study, July 1986–April 1991: Dietary intakes of pesticides, selected elements, and other chemicals. J AOAC Int 1995; 78: 1353–63.

49. Food and Environment Research Agency. Pesticide Usage Statistics 2006. Available from: http://pusstats.csl.gov.uk/myindex.cfm (accessed November 20, 2009).

50. Heudorf U, Butte W, Schulz C et al. Reference values for metabolites of pyrethroid and organophosphorous insecticides in urine for human biomonitoring in environmental medicine. Int J Hyg Environ Health 2006; 209: 293–9.

51. Schettgen T, Heudorf U, Drexler H et al. Pyrethroid exposure of the general population – is this due to diet? Toxicol Lett 2002; 134(1–3): 141–5.

52. Riederer AM, Bartell SM, Barr DB et al. Diet and nondiet predictors of urinary 3-phenoxybenzoic acid in NHANES 1999–2002. Environ Health Perspect 2008; 116: 1015–22.

53. Rawn DF, Roscoe V, Trelka R et al. N-methyl carbamate pesticide residues in conventional and organic infant foods available on the Canadian retail market, 2001–03. Food Addit Contam 2006; 23: 651–9.

54. Caldas ED, Miranda MC, Conceição MH et al. Dithiocarbamates residues in Brazilian food and the potential risk for consumers. Food Chem Toxicol 2004; 42: 1877–83.

55. Tasioopoulou S, Chiodini AM, Vellere F et al. Results of the monitoring program of pesticide residues in organic food of plant origin in Lombardy (Italy). J Environ Sci Health B 2007; 42: 835–41.

56. Colburn T, Von Saal FS, Soto AM. Developmental effects of endocrine disrupting chemicals in wildlife and humans. Environ Health Perspect 1993; 101: 378–84.

57. Jaga K, Dharmani C. The epidemiology of pesticide exposure and cancer: A review. *Rev Environ Health* 2005; **20**: 15–38.

58. García-Reyes JF, Gilbert-López B, Molina-Díaz A *et al.* Determination of pesticide residues in fruit-based soft drinks. *Anal Chem* 2008; **80**: 8966–74.

59. Lorenzin M. Pesticide residues in Italian ready-meals and dietary intake estimation. *J Environ Sci Health B* 2007; **42**: 823–33.

♦60. Watson D. *Pesticides, Veterinary and Other Residues in Food.* Cambridge: Woodhead Publishing, 2004.

61. Marriott J. Bananas – physiology and biochemistry of storage and ripening for optimum quality. *Crit Rev Food Sci Nutr* 1980; **13**: 41–88.

62. Reynolds SL, Hill AR, Thomas MR *et al.* Occurrence and risks associated with chlormequat residues in a range of foodstuffs in the UK. *Food Addit Contam* 2004; **21**: 457–71.

63. UK Department of Health. 5-a-day general information. School Fruit and Vegetable Scheme. Available from: http://www.dh.gov.uk/en/Publichealth/Healthimprovement/FiveADay/FiveADaygeneralinformation/DH_4002149 (accessed November 20, 2009).

64. Committee on Toxicity of Chemicals in Food, Consumer Products and the Environment. Risk Assessment of Mixtures of Pesticides and Similar Substances. Available from: http://cot.food.gov.uk/pdfs/reportindexed.pdf (accessed November 27, 2009).

♦65. World Health Organization. *Dietary Exposure Assessment of Chemicals in Food: Report of a Joint FAO/WHO Committee.* WHO/WA/701. Geneva: WHO, 2008.

66. Veterinary Medicines Directorate. Available from: http://www.vmd.gov.uk (accessed November 20, 2009).

67. Veterinary Residues Committee. Annual Report 2007. Available from: http://www.vet-residues-committee.gov.uk/Reports/annual.htm (accessed November 20, 2009).

68. Van Koten-Vermeulen JEM, Wouters MFA, Van Leeuwen FXR. *Report of the 40th Meeting of the Joint FAO/WHO Expert Committee on Food Additives (JECFA).* Geneva: WHO, 1993.

69. Cooper KM, Kennedy DG. Stability studies of the metabolites of nitrofuran antibiotics during storage and cooking. *Food Addit Contam* 2007; **24**: 935–42.

70. Paige JC, Tollefson L. Veterinary products: Residues and resistant pathogens. In: D'Mello JPF (ed.) *Food Safety: Contaminants and Toxins* (pp. 293–314). Oxford: CABI, 2003.

71. Loganathan P, Hedley MJ, Grace ND. Pasture soils contaminated with fertilizer-derived cadmium and fluorine: Livestock effects. *Rev Environ Contam Toxicol* 2008; **192**: 29–66.

72. Satarug S, Moore MR. Adverse health effects of chronic exposure to low-level cadmium in foodstuffs and cigarette smoke. *Environ Health Perspect* 2004; **112**: 1099–103.

73. Nasreddine L, Parent-Massin D. Food contamination by metals and pesticides in the European Union. Should we worry? *Toxicol Lett* 2002; **127**(1–3): 29–41.

74. Food Standards Agency. Measurement of the Concentrations of Metals and Other Elements from the 2006 UK Total Diet Study. Available from: http://www.food.gov.uk/multimedia/pdfs/fsis0109metals.pdf (accessed November 20, 2009).

75. Martí-Cid R, Llobet JM, Castell V *et al.* Dietary intake of arsenic, cadmium, mercury, and lead by the population of Catalonia, Spain. *Biol Trace Elem Res* 2008; **125**: 120–32.

76. Santamaria P. Nitrate in vegetables: toxicity, content, intake and EC regulation. *J Sci Food Agric* 2006; **86**: 10–17.

77. Gangolli SD, van den Brandt PA, Feron VJ *et al.* Nitrate, nitrite and N-nitroso compounds. *Eur J Pharmacol* 1994; **292**: 1–38.

78. McMullen SE, Casanova JA, Gross LK *et al.* Ion chromatographic determination of nitrate and nitrite in vegetable and fruit baby foods. *J AOAC Int* 2005; **88**: 1793–6.

79. Savino F, Maccario S, Guidi C *et al.* Methemoglobinemia caused by the ingestion of courgette soup given in order to resolve constipation in two formula-fed infants. *Ann Nutr Metab* 2006; **50**: 368–71.

80. Knobeloch L, Salna B, Hogan A *et al.* Blue babies and nitrate-contaminated well water. *Environ Health Perspect* 2000; **108**: 675–8.

81. European Food Safety Authority. Nitrate in vegetables: Scientific opinion of the panel on contaminants in the food chain. *EFSA J* 2008; **689**: 1–79.

82. Lunn JC, Kuhnle G, Mai V *et al.* The effect of haem in red and processed meat on the endogenous formation of N-nitroso compounds in the upper gastrointestinal tract. *Carcinogenesis* 2007; **28**: 685–90.

83. Hord NG, Tang Y, Bryan NS. Food sources of nitrates and nitrites: The physiologic context for potential health benefits. *Am J Clin Nutr* 2009; **90**: 1–10.

84. Committee on Carcinogenicity of Chemicals in Food, Consumer Products and the Environment (2000). Carcinogenicity of 3-Monochloro propane 1,2-diol (3-MCPD). COC Statement COC/00/S5. Available from: http://www.advisorybodies.doh.gov.uk/mcpd1.htm (accessed November 27, 2009).

85. Committee on Mutagenicity of Chemicals in Food, Consumer Products and the Environment. Mutagenicity of 3-Monochloro propane 1,2-diol (3-MCPD) COC Statement COC/00/S$. Available from: http://www.advisorybodies.doh.gov.uk/com/mcpd2.htm (accessed November 27, 2009).

86. European Commission. Setting Maximum Levels for Certain Contaminants in Foodstuffs. Commission Regulation (EC) No 466/2001 1. *Official Journal of the European Communities*, L77/1. Available from: http://www.eur-lex.europa.eu/JOIndex.do (accessed November 20, 2009).

87. Hamlet CG, Sadd PA, Crews C *et al.* Occurrence of 3-chloro-propane-1,2-diol (3-MCPD) and related compounds in foods: A review. *Food Addit Contam* 2002; **19**: 619–31.

88. Crews C, Hasnip S, Chapman S *et al.* Survey of chloropropanols in soy sauces and related products purchased in the UK in 2000 and 2002. *Food Addit Contam* 2003; **20**: 916–22.

89. Fu WS, Zhao Y, Zhang G *et al.* Occurrence of chloropropanols in soy sauce and other foods in China between 2002 and 2004. *Food Addit Contam* 2007; **24**: 812–19.

90. León N, Yusà V, Pardo O *et al.* Determination of 3-MCPD by GC-MS/MS with PTV-LV injector used for a survey of Spanish foodstuffs. *Talanta* 2008; **75**: 824–31.

91. Maga JA. Furans in foods. *CRC Crit Rev Food Sci Nutr* 1979; **11**: 355–400.

92. International Agency for Research on Cancer. *Dry Cleaning, Some Chlorinated Solvents and Other Industrial Chemicals.* IARC Monographs, Vol. 63. Lyon: IARC, 1995.

93. National Toxicology Program (NTP). *Toxicology and Carcinogenesis Studies of Furan in F-344/N Rats and B6C3F1 Mice.* NTP Technical Report No. 402. Research Triangle Park, NC: US Department of Health and Human Services, Public Health Service, National Institute of Health, 1993.

94. European Food Standards Agency. Report of the Scientific Panel on Contaminants in the Food Chain on provisional findings on furan in food (Question N° EFSA-Q-2004–109). *EFSA J* 2004; **137**: 1–20.

95. Crews C, Castle L. A review of the occurrence, formation and analysis of furan in heat-processed foods. *Trends Food Sci Technol* 2007; **18**: 365–72.

96. Jestoi M, Järvinen T, Järvenpää E *et al.* Furan in the baby-food samples purchased from the Finnish markets – determination with SPME–GC-MS. *Food Chem* 2009; **117**: 522–8.

97. Morehouse KM, Nyman PJ, McNeal TP *et al.* Survey of furan in heat processed foods by headspace gas chromatography/mass spectrometry and estimated adult exposure. *Food Addit Contam Part A* 2008; **25**: 259–64.

98. Food Standards Agency. Survey of Process Contaminants in Retail Foods 2008. Food Survey Information Sheet No. 03/09. Available from http://www.food.gov.uk/multimedia/pdfs/fsis0309acrylamide.pdf (accessed November 20, 2009).

99. European Food Safety Authority. Results on the Monitoring of Furan Levels in Food: A report of the Data Collection and Exposure Unit in Response to a Request from the European Commission. Available from: http://www.efsa.europa.eu/cs/BlobServer/Report/datex_report_furan_en.pdf (accessed November 27, 2009).

100. Jun HJ, Lee KG, Lee YK *et al.* Correlation of urinary furan with plasma gamma-glutamyltranspeptidase levels in healthy men and women. *Food Chem Toxicol* 2008; **46**: 1753–9.

101. Joint FAO/WHO Expert Committee on Food Additives. Sixty-fourth Meeting, Rome, 8–17 February 2005. Summary and conclusions. Available from: http://www.who.int/ipcs/food/jecfa/summaries/summary_report_64_final.pdf (accessed November 20, 2009).

102. Ramesh A, Walker SA, Hood DB *et al.* Bioavailability and risk assessment of orally ingested polycyclic aromatic hydrocarbons. *Int J Toxicol* 2004; **23**: 301–33.

103. Phillips DH. Polycyclic aromatic hydrocarbons in the diet. *Mutat Res* 1999; **443**: 139–47.

104. European Food Safety Authority. Findings of the EFSA Data Collection on Polycyclic Aromatic Hydrocarbons in Food. A Report from the Unit of Data Collection and Exposure on a Request from the European Commission. Available from: http://www.efsa.europa.eu/EFSA/efsa_locale-1178620753812_1211902589337.htm (accessed November 20, 2009).

105. Committee on Toxicity of Chemicals in Food, Consumer Products and the Environment. Polycyclic Aromatic Hydrocarbons in the 2000 Total Diet Study. TOX/2002/26. Available from: http://cot.food.gov.uk/pdfs/TOX-2002-26.PDF (accessed November 27, 2009)

106. Tareke E, Rydberg P, Karlsson P *et al.* Analysis of acrylamide, a carcinogen formed in heated foodstuffs. *J Agric Food Chem* 2002; **50**: 4998–5006.

107. European Food Safety Authority. Results on the Monitoring of Acrylamide Levels in Food. A Report of the Data Collection and Exposure Unit in Response to a Request from the European Commission. Available from: http://www.efsa.europa.eu/cs/BlobServer/Report/datex_report_acrylamide_en.pdf (accessed November 27, 2009).

108. Joint FAO/WHO Expert Committee on Food Additives. Evaluation of Certain Food Contaminants. Sixty-fourth Report of the Joint FAO/WHO Expert Committee on Food Additives. World Health Organization Technical Report Series No. 930. Available from: http://whqlibdoc.who.int/trs/WHO_TRS_930_eng.pdf (accessed November 27, 2009).

109. Mills C, Tlustos C, Evans R *et al.* Dietary acrylamide exposure estimates for the United Kingdom and Ireland: Comparison between semiprobabilistic and probabilistic exposure models. *J Agric Food Chem* 2008; **56**: 6039–45.

110. International Agency for Research on Cancer. *Some Industrial Chemicals.* IARC Monograph, Vol. 60. Lyon: IARC, 1994.

111. Wilson KM, Mucci LA, Cho E *et al.* Dietary acrylamide intake and risk of premenopausal breast cancer. *Am J Epidemiol* 2009; **169**: 954–61.

112. Wilson KM, Bälter K, Adami HO *et al.* Acrylamide exposure measured by food frequency questionnaire and hemoglobin adduct levels and prostate cancer risk in the Cancer of the Prostate in Sweden Study. *Int J Cancer* 2009; **124**: 2384–90.

113. Wirfält E, Paulsson B, Törnqvist M *et al.* Associations between estimated acrylamide intakes and haemoglobin AA adducts in a sample from the Malmö Diet and Cancer cohort. *Eur J Clin Nutr* 2008; **62**: 314–23.

114. Heudorf U, Hartmann E, Angerer J. Acrylamide in children – exposure assessment via urinary acrylamide metabolites as biomarkers. *J Hyg Environ Health* 2008; **212**: 135–41.

115. Food Standards Agency. Product Withdrawal of Dasani Bottled Still Water. Available from: http://www.food.gov.uk/enforcement/alerts/2004/mar/dasani (accessed November 20, 2009).

116. European Food Safety Authority. Opinion of the Scientific Panel on Food Additives, Flavourings, Processing Aids and Materials in Contact with Food on a request from the Commission to review the toxicology of a number of dyes illegally present in food in the EU. *EFSA J* 2005; **263**: 1–71.

117. McCann D, Barrett A, Cooper A *et al.* Food additives and hyperactive behaviour in 3-year-old and 8/9-year-old children in the community: A randomised, double-blinded, placebo-controlled trial. *Lancet* 2007; **370**: 1560–7.

118. Dobson RL, Motlagh S, Quijano M *et al.* Identification and characterization of toxicity of contaminants in pet food leading to an outbreak of renal toxicity in cats and dogs. *Toxicol Sci* 2008; **106**: 251–62.

119. Ingelfinger JR. Melamine and the global implications of food contamination. *N Engl J Med* 2008; **359**: 2745–8.

120. Lancet. Melamine and food safety in China [Editorial]. *Lancet* 2009; **373**: 353.

121. World Health Organization. *Terrorist Threats to Food: Guidelines for Strengthening and Evaluation of Prevention and Response Systems.* Geneva: WHO, 2008.

122. Blunden S, Wallace T. Tin in canned food: An understanding of occurrence and effect. *Food Chem Toxicol*; 2003; **41**: 1651–62.

123. Jorhem L, Slorach S. Lead, chromium, tin, iron and cadmium in food in welded cans. *Food Addit Contam* 1987; **4**: 309–16.

124. Castle LC, Jickells SM. *A Systematic Evaluation of Chemical Migration During Low Temperature Storage of Packaged Foodstuffs.* CSL Report FD 00/61. York: Central Science Laboratory, 2001.

125. Holmes MJ, Hart A, Northing P *et al.* Dietary exposure to chemical migrants from food contact materials: A probabilistic approach. *Food Addit Contam* 2005; **22**: 907–19.

126. International Union of Pure and Applied Chemistry. Effects of storage and processing on pesticide residues in plant products. *Pure Appl Chem* 1994; **66**: 335–56.

127. Mitrowska K, Posyniak A, Zmudzki J. The effects of cooking on residues of malachite green and leucomalachite green in carp muscles. *Anal Chim Acta* 2007; **586**(1–2): 420–5.

128. Crews C, Brereton P, Davies A. The effects of domestic cooking on the levels of 3-monochloropropanediol in foods. *Food Addit Contam* 2001; **18**: 271–80.

129. Roberts D, Crews C, Grundy H, Mills C, Matthews W. Effects of cooking on furan in convenience foods. *Food Addit Contam* 2008; **25**, 25–31.

130. Kuligowski J, Halperin KM. Stainless steel cookware as a significant source of nickel, chromium and iron. *Arch Environ Contam Toxicol* 1992; **23**: 211–15.

131. Flint GN, Packirisamy S. Purity of food cooked in stainless steel utensils. *Food Addit Contam* 1997; **14**: 115–26.

132. Geerligs PD, Brabin BJ, Omari AA. Food prepared in iron cooking pots as an intervention for reducing iron-deficiency anaemia in developing countries: A systematic review. *J Hum Nutr Diet* 2003; **16**: 275–81.

133. Talley L, Woodruff BA, Seal A *et al.* Evaluation of the effectiveness of stainless steel cooking pots in reducing iron-deficiency anaemia in food aid-dependent populations. *Publ Health Nutr* 2009 Apr 1. [Epub ahead of print]

134. Ferreira PC, Piai Kde A, Takayanagui AM. Aluminum as a risk factor for Alzheimer's disease. *Rev Lat Am Enfermagem* 2008; **16**: 151–7.

135. Bradley EL, Boughtflower V, Smith TL *et al.* Survey of the migration of melamine and formaldehyde from melamine food contact articles available on the UK market. *Food Addit Contam* 2005; **22**: 597–606.

136. Lucas A. Hypochlorite sterilising fluid as a source of dietary sodium in gavage-fed infants. *Lancet* 1977; **2**: 144–5.

137. Food and Agriculture Association/World Health Organization Food Standards. Codex Alimentarius. Available from: http://www.codexalimentarius.net/web/index_en.jsp (accessed November 20, 2009).

138. World Health Organization. Global Environment Monitoring System – Food Contamination Monitoring and Assessment Program (GEMS/Food). Available from: http://www.who.int/foodsafety/chem/gems/en (accessed November 20, 2009).

139. Food and Agriculture Association/World Health Organization. Joint FAO/WHO Expert Committee on Food Additives (JECFA). Available from: http://www.who.int/ipcs/food/jecfa/en (accessed November 20, 2009).

140. Food and Agriculture Association/World Health Organization. JMPR: Joint FAO/WHO Meeting on Pesticide Residues. Available from: http://www.who.int/ipcs/food/jmpr/en (accessed November 20, 2009).

141. Defra (2009). Family Food – Report on the Expenditure and Food Survey. Available from: http://statistics.defra.gov.uk/esg/publications/efs/default.asp (accessed November 27, 2009).

♦142. Tran L, Glass R, Ritchie P, Sleeuwenhoek A, MacCalman L, Cherrie JW. Estimation of Human Intake of Pesticides from All Potential Pathways. Institute of Occupational Medicine Research Report TM/08/01. Available from: http://www.foodbase.org.uk//admintools/reportdocuments/281–1–503_T10005.pdf (accessed November 20, 2009).

23

Biotoxins and xenobiotics

SALLY BRADBERRY, ALLISTER VALE

Biotoxins are usually defined as poisons that are produced by or derived from living organisms. These natural poisons include some of the most toxic agents known. Biotoxins that enter the human body do not replicate like pathogens and are not communicable. Interestingly, ricin and saxitoxin are listed in the Chemical Weapons Convention (Schedule 1).

Some organisms contain biotoxins that are derived from other organisms. For example, the dinoflagellate *Gymnodinium breve* is the primary source of brevetoxin (see Table 34.1), which is toxic to fish and humans and causes neurotoxic shellfish poisoning (see below). The dinoflagellate, *Gambierdiscus toxicus*, is responsible for the production of maitotoxins and ciguatoxins. It lives in epiphytic association with various seaweeds and free in coral rubble. The dead coral and marine algae are eaten by herbivorous fish; these fish accumulate and concentrate the toxins produced by *Gambierdiscus toxicus*. The herbivorous fish are eaten by larger carnivorous fish such as barracuda, snapper and grouper. These may then be eaten by humans, and ciguatera fish poisoning may result (see below).

Xenobiotics (from the Greek *xenos* meaning foreigner, stranger; and *bios* meaning life) are chemicals found in an organism which are not produced by or expected to be in the organism. The term is often used in the context of pollutants such as dioxins, dioxin-like chemicals such as polychlorinated biphenyls (PCB), and DDT (bis[4-chlorophenyl]-1,1,1-trichloroethane), which did not exist in nature before their synthesis by man.

The first part of this chapter will review the toxicology of plant, mushroom and marine biotoxins, with particular focus on ricin and abrin. The chapter concludes with a review of the clinical impact of dioxins and DDT.

PLANT BIOTOXINS

Life-threatening poisoning from plant ingestion is rare,[1–3] although many plants contain potentially toxic substances. These include antimuscarinic agents, calcium oxalate crystals, cardiogenic glycosides, pro-convulsants, cyanogenic compounds, mitotic inhibitors, nicotine-like alkaloids, alkylating agent precursors, sodium channel activators and toxic proteins (toxalbumins).[1–3]

Although many plants contain gastrointestinal toxins, these rarely give rise to life-threatening sequelae. In contrast, other botanical poisons may cause specific organ damage,

Table 23.1 Plants containing antimuscarinic agents

Genus and species	Common name	Toxins
Atropa belladonna	Deadly nightshade	Hyoscyamine, atropine
Brugmansia sanguinea	Angel's trumpet	Hyoscyamine, atropine
Datura stramonium	Thorn apple, jimsonweed	Hyoscyamine, atropine
Hyoscyamus niger	Black henbane, stinking nightshade, poison tobacco	Hyoscyamine
Solanum dulcamara	Woody nightshade	Solanum alkaloids, e.g. solanine
Solanum nigrum	Black nightshade	Solanum alkaloids
Solanum pseudocapsicum	Christmas cherry, Jerusalem cherry	Solanum alkaloids
Solanum tuberosum	Potato	Solanum alkaloids

and death may occur from only small ingestions of yew (genus *Taxus*), oleander (*Thevetia peruviana* [yellow oleander] and *Nerium oleander*) and cowbane (genus *Cicuta*).

Antimuscarinic agents

Plants containing antimuscarinic agents belong to the nightshade family, Solanaceae (Table 23.1). The ingestion of species containing hyoscyamine and/or atropine causes a classical antimuscarinic syndrome with tachycardia, dry, warm skin, urinary retention, absent bowel sounds, delirium, hallucinations and possibly convulsions.[4,5] Central nervous system (CNS) effects are generally less common following the ingestion of solanum species that predominantly cause gastrointestinal upset. Features may persist for hours to days. Management is supportive.

Calcium oxalate crystals

Some plants contain needle-shaped crystals of calcium oxalate (Table 23.2), which can be released by mechanical stimulation. These crystals can penetrate mucous membranes and induce histamine release. Pain and irritation follow skin or eye contact. Following ingestion, inflammation may be sufficiently severe to cause oropharyngeal oedema. Systemic toxicity with hypocalcaemia does not occur since the crystals are insoluble. The management of skin and eye exposures involves decontamination by irrigation with adequate analgesia. Protecting the patency of the airway is the priority following ingestion, and assessment of damage by endoscopic examination may be required.

Cardiotoxic steroids

Several plants contain cardiotoxic steroids that fall structurally into two main groups: cardenolides and bufadienolides (Table 23.3). The best known examples are the foxglove (*Digitalis purpurea*) and yellow oleander (*Thevetia peruviana*), which contain cardenolide cardiac glycosides that inhibit Na^+/K^+ ATP-ase. Ingestion causes a similar syndrome to digoxin poisoning. Arrhythmias and

Table 23.2 Plants containing calcium oxalate crystals

Genus and species	Common name
Caladium bicolor	Angel wings, caladium
Caryota mitis	Fishtail palm
Colocasia esculenta	Elephant's ear
Dieffenbachia picta	Dumb cane
Epipremnum aureum	Amarillo, devil's ivy
Monstera deliciosa	Swiss cheese plant
Philodendron selloum	Sweetheart vine
Spathiphyllum species	Peace lily

hyperkalaemia can be rapidly and safely reversed by the administration of digoxin-specific antibody fragments.[6,7]

Pro-convulsants

Plants containing pro-convulsants are listed in Table 23.4. There is a wide variation in the convulsant potency of these toxins; for example, cicutoxin is a far stronger convulsant than ranunculin. The precise mechanism of seizure

Table 23.3 Plants containing cardiotoxic steroids

Genus and species	Common name	Toxins
Adonis vernalis	Yellow pheasant's eye	Adonitoxin (cardenolide)
Convallaria majalis	Lily-of-the-valley	Convallatoxin (cardenolide)
Digitalis purpurea	Foxglove	Digitoxin (cardenolide)
Helleborus niger	Christmas rose	Hellebrin (bufadienolide)
Hyacinthoides non-scripta	Bluebell	Scillarin (bufadienolide)
Nerium oleander	Oleander	Adynerin (cardenolide)
Ornithogalum umbellatum	Star-of-Bethlehem	Convallatoxin (cardenolide)
Thevetia peruviana	Yellow oleander	Peruvoside (cardenolide)
Urginea maritima	Squill, Red squill	Scillarin (bufadienolide)

Table 23.4 Plants containing pro-convulsants

Genus and species	Common name	Toxins
Aethusa cynapium	Fool's parsley	Aethusin
Anemone coronaria	Anemone	Ranunculin
Blighia sapida	Ackee fruit plant	Hypoglycin
Caltha palustris	Marsh marigold	Protoanemonin
Caulophyllum thalictroides	Blue cohosh	Methylcytisine
Cicuta virosa	Cowbane, water hemlock	Cicutoxin
Clematis vitalba	Wild clematis, old man's beard	Ranunculin
Conium maculatum	Hemlock	Coniine
Coriaria myrtifolia	Myrtle-leaved sumach	Coriamyrtin
Laburnum anagyroides	Laburnum	Cytisine
Nicotiana tabacum	Tobacco plant	Nicotine
Oenanthe crocata	Hemlock water dropwort	Oenanthotoxin
Ranunculus acris	Buttercup	Ranunculin
Strychnos nux-vomica	Strychnine	Strychnine

induction has not been elucidated for all toxins but includes gamma-aminobutyric acid antagonism, excitatory amino acid mimicry, an imbalance of acetylcholine homeostasis, hypoglycaemia and sodium channel disruption. The seizures produced by cicutoxin are usually generalized tonic-clonic in nature.[8] Strychnine antagonizes the postsynaptic inhibitory amino acid glycine at the spinal cord motor neurone, causing muscle hyperactivity without loss of consciousness.[9] Management is supportive, with a judicious use of benzodiazepines, although these may not be effective.

Cyanogenic compounds

With the exception of *Sambucus nigra*, all the species listed in Table 23.5 belong to the rose family, Rosaceae. These plants contain two principal cyanogenic glycosides: prunasin in the vegetative organs, and amygdalin exclusively in the seeds. Plants containing these compounds typically do so in only very small amounts such that cyanide poisoning is only likely after massive ingestions of vegetation or chewing multiple seeds. In these cases, cyanide release requires hydrolysis in the gastrointestinal tract so features of cyanide poisoning are delayed for up to a few hours. Nausea, vomiting, epigastric pain, diarrhoea, salivation, a flushed face, headache and shivering may occur with hypotension, convulsions, metabolic acidosis, coma and respiratory paralysis in severe cases. Fatalities have occurred.[10]

Mitotic inhibitors

Some plants contain mitotic inhibitors (Table 23.6) that interfere with the polymerization of microtubules necessary for spindle formation during cell division. Effects are most apparent in rapidly dividing cells, including those of the gastrointestinal and haematological systems. Ingestion causes nausea and vomiting, which may progress to gastrointestinal mucosal ulceration and necrosis. Features of CNS toxicity include headache, ataxia, seizures and encephalopathy. Multisystem organ failure ensues in

the most severe cases, and fatalities have occurred.[11] Bone marrow failure has also been reported. Management is supportive, including the conventional treatment of bone marrow failure if required.

Nicotine–like alkaloids

The ingestion of plants containing nicotine-like alkaloids causes a stimulation of nicotinic cholinergic receptors resulting in hypertension, tachycardia, sweating, hypersalivation, vomiting, muscle fasciculations and weakness. Depolarizing neuromuscular blockade, seizures and death may occur in severe cases.[12] Plants in this category (Table 23.7) also feature in Table 23.4 due to the pro-convulsant effects of nicotine-like alkaloids. Management is supportive.

Alkylating agent precursors

The pyrrolizidine alkaloids in these plants (Table 23.8) are metabolized to pyrroles, which damage hepatic sinusoidal and pulmonary endothelial cells. Endothelial repair and

Table 23.5   Plants containing cyanogenic compounds

Genus and species	Common name	Toxins
Cotoneaster horizontalis	Wall cotoneaster	Prunasin, amygdalin
Malus sylvestris	Crab apple	Prunasin, amygdalin
Prunus armeniaca	Apricot	Prunasin, amygdalin
Prunus domestica	Plum	Prunasin, amygdalin
Prunus dulcis var. amara	Bitter almond	Prunasin, amygdalin
Prunus laurocerasus	Cherry laurel	Prunasin, amygdalin
Sambucus nigra	Elder	Prunasin

Table 23.6   Plants containing mitotic inhibitors

Genus and species	Common name	Toxins
Catharanthus roseus	Madagascar periwinkle	Vincamine, vincristine
Colchicum autumnale	Autumn crocus, meadow saffron	Colchicine
Gloriosa superba	Glory lily	Colchicine
Podophyllum peltatum	Mayapple	Podophyllotoxin
Vinca minor	Lesser periwinkle	Vincamine, vincristine

Table 23.7   Plants containing nicotine-like alkaloids

Genus and species	Common name	Toxins
Caulophyllum thalictroides	Blue cohosh	Methylcytisine
Conium maculatum	Hemlock	Coniine
Laburnum anagyroides	Laburnum	Cytisine
Nicotiana tabacum	Tobacco plant	Nicotine

Table 23.8   Plants containing alkylating agent precursors

Genus and species	Common name	Toxins
Echium plantagineum	Purple viper's bugloss	Echimidine
Senecio jacobaea	Ragwort	Jacobine, senecionine

hypertrophy result in veno-occlusive disease. Symptoms are gradual in onset, with non-specific anorexia and abdominal pain progressing to hepatic cirrhosis. Human poisonings have occurred from the chronic ingestion of herbal teas[13] and from the ingestion of grain contaminated with the seeds of plants containing these alkaloids.

Sodium channel activators

Plants containing these agents (Table 23.9) cause persistent sodium influx at neuronal and cardiac membranes by stabilizing the open configuration of voltage-gated sodium channels. Membrane depolarization is prolonged, leading to seizures and arrhythmias. Other features include vomiting, colicky diarrhoea, paraesthesiae, muscle fasciculations, weakness and paralysis.[14,15] Management is supportive. No specific therapy for arrhythmias has proven superior, although based on the mechanism of toxicity, sodium channel blocking drugs such as lidocaine, flecainide or amiodarone may be useful. Intravenous magnesium has also successfully terminated ventricular tachycardia induced by these plants.[16]

Toxic proteins (Toxalbumins)

Plants containing these toxins (Table 23.10) inhibit protein synthesis. Chief among these are ricin and abrin, which are described in greater detail in the next section.

Table 23.9   Plants containing sodium channel activators

Genus and species	Common name	Toxins
Aconitum napellus	Monkshood	Aconitine
Kalmia angustifolia	Sheep laurel	Grayanotoxin
Pieris formosa	Pieris	Grayanotoxin
Rhododendron ponticum	Rhododendron	Grayanotoxin
Veratrum album	False hellebore	Protovrine
Zigadenus paniculatus	Death camas	Zigadenine

Table 23.10   Plants containing toxic proteins

Genus and species	Common name	Toxins
Abrus precatorius	Jequirity bean	Abrin
Hura crepitans	Sandbox tree	Huratoxin
Jatropha cathartica	Jicamilla	Curcin
Momordica charantia	Bitter gourd	Momordin
Phoradendron tomentosum	American mistletoe	Phoratoxin
Ricinus communis	Castor oil plant	Ricin
Robinia pseudoacacia	False acacia, black locust	Robin

RICIN AND ABRIN

Ricin and abrin are globular glycoproteins with a similar chemical composition, although they are derived from genetically unrelated plants. Ricin makes up 1–5 per cent by weight of the beans of the castor oil plant *Ricinus communis*, whereas abrin is obtained from the seeds of *Abrus precatorius* (common names jequirity bean or rosary pea). The oil obtained from castor beans by cold-pressing is used as a purgative and laxative, while hot-pressing followed by solvent extraction is used to produce specialist oils and lubricants. The residue is used as a cattle feed or as a fertilizer, after ricin has been destroyed by heating. Ricin can be extracted easily from the waste mash generated by castor oil production or from whole castor beans. The resulting product is a soluble white powder that is stable under ambient conditions but can be detoxified by heating for 10 minutes at 80 °C or for 1 hour at 50 °C.[17]

In recent times, ricin and abrin have been recognized as potential chemical weapons. They are certainly highly toxic to mammalian cells, abrin being even more toxic than ricin in in vitro studies.[18] However, the use of either toxin to cause mass casualties would require either aerosolization by means of a dispersal device or its addition to food or beverages as a contaminant. Both toxins are approximately 1000-fold less toxic by ingestion compared with injection or inhalation, and neither is absorbed through intact skin. The lethal dose of ricin by inhalation or injection is about 5–10 μg/kg.[19]

Mechanisms of toxicity

Ricin and abrin comprise an A chain and a B chain, linked by a single disulphide bond. The A chain confers cellular toxicity, while the B chain is essential for cell binding. Ricin and abrin bind to cell surface carbohydrates, cells of the reticuloendothelial system being particularly susceptible. Once internalized, the A chain attacks the ribosomes, thereby inhibiting protein synthesis.[20] This cessation of protein synthesis triggers programmed cell death (apoptosis) and involves mitochondrial membrane damage and the production of reactive oxygen species.[21–23] Many of the features seen in poisoning can be explained by toxin-induced endothelial cell damage, which leads to fluid and protein leakage and tissue oedema, causing so-called 'vascular leak syndrome'.

Clinical features

Ricin and abrin are toxic via all routes, although the features of poisoning and severity of toxicity vary markedly with the dose and route of exposure. Most documented cases involve eating castor beans. Beans swallowed whole may pass through the gastrointestinal tract intact, whereas chewing facilitates ricin release. Vomiting, diarrhoea and abdominal pain ensue. Gastrointestinal fluid and electrolyte loss may be substantial and complicated by haematemesis or melaena, hypovolaemic shock and multiorgan failure. Non-human primates exposed to ricin by inhalation develop a fibrinopurulent necrotizing pneumonia, typically after a dose-dependent delay of 8–24 hours. Non-pulmonary effects do not occur.[24]

Among the handful of reports of parenteral administration, the most well known is the assassination of the Bulgarian refugee Georgi Markov, who died 3 days after being stabbed with an umbrella believed to be loaded with a ricin-containing pellet. Fatigue, nausea, vomiting and fever developed over 24 hours, followed by necrotic lymphadenopathy at the injection site. Pre-terminal complications included gastrointestinal haemorrhage, hypovolaemic shock and renal failure.[25]

Diagnosis and management

Ricin and abrin can be detected by immunoabsorbent assay for up to 48 hours after exposure.[26,27] The detection of antitoxin antibodies could aid diagnosis in those who survive for 2–3 weeks, but they would not be detected in those who died soon after exposure. Management is primarily symptomatic and supportive, although prophylaxis by immunization with inactivated toxoid or genetically engineered A chain, or treatment with antitoxin antibody (or antibody fragments), is a realistic future therapeutic option.[28]

MUSHROOM BIOTOXINS

Poisoning due to higher fungi (mushrooms) is usually accidental, although the ingestion of hallucinogenic ('magic') mushrooms is invariably intentional. Accidental poisoning with cytotoxic and neurotoxic mushrooms is rare in the UK but more common in Scandinavia and other parts of Europe. In the USA, it has been estimated that there are some 50 cases per year. Hallucinogenic mushrooms may be picked deliberately for their effects or purchased from shops that sell botanical products. Mushrooms may contain cytotoxic agents (e.g. amatoxins and orellanin) and neurotoxic agents (muscarine, psilocybin, isoxazoles and gyromitrin), whereas other species cause gastroenteritis only.

Cytotoxic mushroom poisoning

Cytotoxic mushroom poisoning is caused by amatoxins and orellanin.[29]

AMATOXIN POISONING

Amatoxins are found in *Amanita phalloides*, *Amanita virosa* and *Amanita verna*, and in some *Galerina* and *Lepiota* spp.

Amatoxins are cyclic octapeptides that inhibit transcription from DNA to mRNA by blocking nuclear RNA polymerase II; this results in impaired protein synthesis and cell death.[29] Alternative proposed mechanisms include the induction of apoptosis, the formation of oxygen free radicals and the depletion of hepatic glutathione.[29] Amatoxins are rapidly absorbed and distributed, and uptake is particularly high in the parenchymal cells of the liver, in the kidneys and in the intestinal mucosa. Excretion is mainly renal, but significant amounts are also excreted in bile and faeces.

Clinical features and management

Intense watery diarrhoea starts 8–24 hours after ingestion and persists for 24 hours or longer. Patients often become severely dehydrated. Signs of liver damage appear during the second day, and hepatic failure may ensue. Impaired kidney function is often seen both because of fluid loss and as a result of direct renal damage.

In all patients, fluid, electrolyte and acid–base disturbances should be corrected and renal and hepatic function supported. The value of silibinin and benzylpenicillin is not proven. Silibinin prevents the uptake through hepatocyte membranes of alpha-amanitin and inhibits the effects of tumour necrosis factor-alpha, which exacerbates lipid peroxidation. Benzylpenicillin may also interfere with alpha-amanitin uptake, but it more likely acts through effects on eukaryotic DNA replication. Silibilin 5 mg/kg intravenously over 1 hour followed by 20 mg/kg per 24 hours for 3 days should be considered in those presenting after eating a substantial number of mushrooms. Benzylpenicillin 300 mg/kg per 24 hours has been used as an alternative. Some recent experimental and clinical data suggest that acetylcysteine might also be of value. Liver transplantation is occasionally necessary.

ORELLANIN POISONING

Orellanin is a potent nephrotoxin found in, for example, *Cortinarius orellanus* and *Cortinarius speciosissimus*. Orellanin has a bipyridyl structure, and its metabolite inhibits protein synthesis in the kidneys. Histopathological changes are interstitial nephritis with oedema and leukocyte infiltration, tubular necrosis, basal membrane rupture and eventually fibrosis.

Clinical features and management

Symptoms are typically delayed for 2–4 days (up to 14 days in some cases). Some patients suffer a mild gastrointestinal disturbance before developing signs of renal impairment, headache, fatigue, intense thirst, chills, muscular discomfort and abdominal, lumbar and flank pain. Transient polyuria with proteinuria, haematuria and, characteristically, leukocyturia is followed by oliguria and then anuria. Renal function may recover only partially; end-stage renal failure is reported in about 10–40 per cent of cases.

Management involves careful monitoring and haemodialysis/haemofiltration if renal failure supervenes. Renal transplantation may be required.

Neurotoxic mushroom poisoning

Muscarine is found in, for example, *Inocybe* spp., *Clitocybe* spp. and *Mycena pura*. Muscarine stimulates cholinergic receptors in the autonomic nervous system and produces clinical patterns similar to those seen in muscarinic plant poisoning (see above).

Clinical features and management

Diarrhoea, abdominal pain, diaphoresis, salivation, lachrymation, miosis, bronchorrhoea, bronchospasm, bradycardia and hypotension occur. Atropine 1–2 mg intravenously (children 0.02–0.05 mg/kg) should be given to manage the cholinergic syndrome.

Isoxazole poisoning

Isoxazoles (e.g. ibotenic acid, muscimol and muscazone) occur in *Amanita muscaria* and *Amanita pantherina* and act as gamma-aminobutyric acid agonists.

Clinical features and management

Nausea, vomiting, inebriation, euphoria, confusion, anxiety, visual disturbances and hallucinations occur often within 30 minutes. Severe agitation and violent behaviour are occasionally seen. Other features include myoclonic jerks, muscle fasciculation, seizures (particularly in children) and coma. Peripheral anticholinergic and, by exception, cholinergic symptoms may also occur (trace amounts of muscarine being occasionally found also in these fungi).

Symptomatic and supportive care should be given as necessary. Diazepam 5–10 mg (children 0.1–0.2 mg/kg), repeated as required, should be administered for anxiety, agitation and seizures. Chlorpromazine or haloperidol may be added if necessary.

Gyromitrin poisoning

Gyromitrin is found in *Gyromitra* species, including in particular the false morel (*Gyromitra esculenta*) and *Cudonia circinans*. Gyromitrin decomposes in the stomach to form hydrazines that reduce pyridoxine in the CNS, and hence the gamma-aminobutyric acid synthesis causes glutathione depletion in red blood cells and may form free oxygen radicals that bind to hepatic macromolecules.

Clinical features and management

Vapours from the mushrooms are irritating to the eyes and respiratory tract. Gastrointestinal symptoms appear 5–8 hours after exposure. Vertigo, sweating, diplopia, headache, dysarthria, incoordination and ataxia may follow. Rarely, seizures, coma, haemolysis, methaemoglobinaemia, hypoglycaemia and hepatic damage have been observed.

Symptomatic and supportive care is required, and it is wise to administer a glucose infusion to prevent hypoglycaemia. Pyridoxine 25 mg/kg, as an infusion over 30 minutes, should be given after substantial ingestion and in cases of severe CNS toxicity. Repeat doses may be required. When seizures are not cured by this measure, diazepam should be given.

Hallucinogenic mushroom poisoning

Psilocybin is found in, for example, *Psilocybe* and *Panaeolus* spp. These mushrooms are usually ingested intentionally for their hallucinogenic effects. Psilocybin is a potent hallucinogen producing pharmacological effects similar to those of lysergic acid diethylamide (LSD; stimulation of the central serotonin receptors and blockade of the peripheral serotonin receptors). Phenylethylamine has also been found in some species and may be responsible for the sympathomimetic effects.

Clinical features and management

Symptoms occur within 20–60 minutes. Effects include an altered sense of time and space, depersonalization, hallucinations (sometimes extremely bizarre), derealization and euphoria, and symptoms such as vertigo, anxiety, agitation, headache, nausea, tachycardia, mydriasis, flushing, fever and seizures (rare). Fever and seizures have been seen in children. Symptoms are usually maximal within 2 hours and disappear within 4–6 hours, although 'flashbacks' may recur after weeks or months.

Rest, reassurance and observation in a quiet environment are beneficial. If there is severe anxiety and agitation, diazepam, 5–10 mg initially (children 0.1–0.2 mg/kg), repeated if necessary, is useful. The addition of haloperidol or chlorpromazine is sometimes of value.

Mushroom-induced gastrointestinal disease

Many mushrooms (e.g. *Paxillus*, *Agaricus*, *Entoloma*, *Boletus*, *Hebeloma*, *Tricholoma*, *Russula*, *Lactarius* and *Ramaria*) produce only gastrointestinal upset.

Clinical features and management

Nausea, vomiting, abdominal pain and diarrhoea occur within a few hours after ingestion. Fluid and electrolyte imbalance may ensue. Symptoms are usually mild and resolve within a few hours.

Admission to hospital is seldom necessary. However, if the symptoms are intense, treatment is best undertaken in hospital to ensure adequate rehydration (particularly in children and the elderly).

Antabuse syndrome

'Antabuse syndrome' is caused by *Coprinus atramentarius* and other *Coprinus* spp., *Clitocybe clavipes* and *Boletus luridus*. Coprin (or a metabolite) blocks acetaldehyde dehydrogenase, so the antabuse syndrome results if such mushrooms are ingested with alcohol. The risk persists for about 1 week after ingestion.

Clinical features and management

The clinical features are similar to those of the antabuse syndrome caused by the combination of disulfiram and ethanol (flush, sweating, nausea, headache, anxiety, tachycardia, hypotension, dyspnoea and collapse). Symptomatic and supportive care should be given as required.

Paxillus syndrome

Paxillus syndrome is caused by *Paxillus involutus*. Thermolabile toxins may cause intense gastroenteritis if *Paxillus involutus* is ingested without adequate cooking. Furthermore, this mushroom contains strongly antigenic components, which may after repeated exposure induce a dramatic syndrome of a rapid onset of severe gastroenteritis, haemolysis and subsequent renal failure.

Clinical features and management

Symptomatic and supportive care should be given as necessary.

MARINE BIOTOXINS[30,31]

A number of marine biotoxins (see Chapter 34) represent a significant and expanding threat to human health in many parts of the world. The impact is visible in terms of not only human poisoning following the consumption of contaminated shellfish or fish, but also the killing of large numbers of marine animals and birds. The shellfish syndromes are caused by the human consumption of contaminated shellfish products, whereas ciguatera fish poisoning is caused by the consumption of subtropical and tropical marine carnivorous fish that have accumulated ciguatera toxins through the marine food chain.

Five shellfish poisoning syndromes are recognized:[31]

1. paralytic shellfish poisoning;
2. diarrhoeic shellfish poisoning;
3. amnesic shellfish poisoning;
4. neurotoxic shellfish poisoning;
5. azaspiracid shellfish poisoning.

An alternative categorization to that based on clinical features is also used, and this is based on the toxin. For example, okadaic acid poisoning is responsible for diarrhoeic shellfish poisoning, domoic acid poisoning is responsible for amnesic shellfish poisoning, and saxitoxin poisoning causes paralytic shellfish poisoning.

Paralytic shellfish (saxitoxin) poisoning[32]

This is uncommon and is caused by bivalve molluscs being contaminated with neurotoxins, including saxitoxin, produced by the toxic dinoflagellates belonging to the genus *Alexandrium*, which may occur both in tropical and moderate climate zones. Shellfish grazing on these algae can accumulate the toxins, but the shellfish itself is resistant to their harmful effects. Saxitoxin blocks voltage-gated sodium channels in nerve and muscle cell membranes, thereby blocking nerve signal transmission.

Clinical features and management

Following human ingestion, symptoms develop within 30 minutes. The illness is characterized by paraesthesiae of the mouth, lips, face and extremities and is often accompanied by nausea, vomiting and diarrhoea. In more severe cases, dystonia, dysphagia, muscle weakness, paralysis, ataxia and respiratory depression occur. In one outbreak in 1987 involving 187 cases, there were 26 deaths, fatalities being highest among young children.[33] Management is symptomatic and supportive.

Diarrhoeic shellfish (okadaic) poisoning[34]

Okadaic acid toxins are usually produced by dinoflagellates belonging to the genus *Dinophysis*, although the genus *Prorocentrum* can also produce these toxins. Okadaic acid inhibits the activity of the protein phosphatases 1 and 2a. It has been suggested that okadaic acid may induce diarrhoea by stimulating the phosphorylation of proteins that control sodium secretion by intestinal cells or by enhancing the phosphorylation of cytoskeletal junctional elements, resulting in increased permeability to solutes, which leads to the passive loss of fluids.

Clinical features and management

The predominant symptoms are diarrhoea, nausea, vomiting and abdominal pain. Symptoms tend to occur between 30 minutes and a few hours after shellfish consumption, with patients recovering within 2 or 3 days. Treatment is symptomatic and supportive.

Amnesic shellfish (domoic acid) poisoning[35]

Amnesic shellfish poisoning is caused by domoic acid. The syndrome should be known more accurately as domoic acid poisoning because amnesia is not always present.

Clinical features and management

Symptoms include abdominal cramps, vomiting, disorientation and memory loss, axonal sensorimotor neuropathy, seizures, coma and death. In the first amnesic shellfish poisoning outbreak in 1987 reported from Prince Edward Island in Canada and involving 107 individuals, the first symptoms were experienced between 15 minutes and 38 hours after mussel consumption. The most common symptoms were nausea (77 per cent), vomiting (76 per cent), abdominal cramps (51 per cent), headache (43 per cent), diarrhoea (42 per cent) and memory loss (25 per cent). There was a close correlation between memory loss and age: those under 40 were more likely to have diarrhoea and those over 50 to have memory loss. Memory loss was predominantly short-term.[36]

Neurotoxic shellfish (brevetoxin) poisoning[37]

Neurotoxic shellfish poisoning is caused by brevetoxins produced by the dinoflagellate *Gymnodinium breve*. Brevetoxins open voltage-gated sodium ion channels in the cell membrane. This alters the membrane properties of excitable cell types in ways that enhance the inward flow of sodium ions into the cell. Brevetoxins appear to produce sensory symptoms by transforming fast sodium channels into slower ones, resulting in persistent activation and repetitive firing.

Clinical features and management

The symptoms of neurotoxic shellfish poisoning occur within 30 minutes to 3 hours, last a few days and include nausea, vomiting, diarrhoea, chills, sweats, reversal of temperature, hypotension, arrhythmias, numbness, tingling, paraesthesia of the lips, face and extremities, cramps, bronchoconstriction, paralysis, seizures and coma. Treatment is primarily supportive.

Azaspiracid shellfish poisoning[38,39]

In November 1995, at least eight people in The Netherlands became ill after eating mussels cultivated at Killary Harbour, Ireland.[40] Although the features they developed (nausea, vomiting, diarrhoea and stomach cramps) were similar to those of diarrhoeic shellfish poisoning, concentrations of okadaic acid were very low. Further investigation showed that features were caused by azaspiracid. Azaspiracids are produced by dinoflagellates, and it is known that mussels are the most affected species.

Ciguatera fish poisoning[41]

Over 400 fish species have been reported as ciguatoxic (*Cigua* is Spanish for poisonous snail), although barracuda, red snapper, amberjack and grouper are most commonly implicated. Ciguatera fish contain ciguatoxin, maitotoxin and scaritoxin, which are lipid-soluble, heat-stable compounds that are derived from dinoflagellates such as *Gambierdiscus toxicus*. Ciguatoxin opens voltage-sensitive sodium channels at the neuromuscular junction, and maitotoxin opens calcium channels of the cell plasma membrane.

Clinical features and management

The onset of symptoms may occur from a few minutes to 30 hours after the ingestion of toxic fish. Features typically appear between 1 and 6 hours and include abdominal cramps, nausea, vomiting and watery diarrhoea. In some cases, numbness and paraesthesiae of the lips, tongue and throat occur. Other features described include malaise, dry mouth, a metallic taste, myalgia, arthralgia, blurred vision, photophobia and transient blindness. In more severe cases, hypotension, cranial nerve palsies and respiratory paralysis have been reported. The mortality in severe cases may be as high as 12 per cent. Recovery takes from 48 hours to 1 week in the mild form and from one to several weeks in the severe form.

XENOBIOTICS

Dioxins

Dioxins and dioxin-like chemicals form a large group of chemicals that are structurally related, have a common mechanism of action and are environmentally and biologically persistent (e.g. the half-life of 2,3,7,8-tetrachlorodibenzo-*p*-dioxin [TCDD] in humans has been estimated to be 7–11 years, albeit with wide individual variation[42]). Dioxins exert their effects via high-affinity binding to a specific cellular protein, the aryl hydrocarbon receptor.[43,44] Dioxins did not exist prior to industrialization except in very small amounts due to natural combustion and geological processes.

The group includes polychlorinated dibenzo-*p*-dioxins (PCDDs), pentachlorodibenzofurans (PCDFs) and polychlorinated biphenols (PBCs) (Figure 23.1). The most toxic dioxin, 2,3,7,8-TCDD, was a contaminant of Agent Orange, a herbicide used in the Vietnam War.[45] Dioxins have also been found in Times Beach, Missouri,[46] in Love Canal, Niagara Falls[47] and in Seveso, Italy,[48,49] the latter following an industrial explosion in 1976. Occupational dioxin exposure has also occurred in Amsterdam.[50] Dioxins came to public attention again with the poisoning of President Viktor Yushchenko of Ukraine in 2004.[51]

Transient acute health effects including headache, pruritus, chloracne, fatigue, irritability, inability to have erections or ejaculations, personality changes, abdominal pain, diarrhoea, insomnia, hepatic dysfunction (particularly hepatomegaly and increased alanine transaminase, aspartate transaminase and gamma-glutamyl transpeptidase activities) and respiratory irritation have been reported, particularly following occupational exposure.[52] One individual who was exposed in an unidentified way to TCDD developed chloracne with pruritus; her face and then her body became densely covered with cysts, and she exhibited palmo-plantar keratoderma, epigastric pain,

(a)

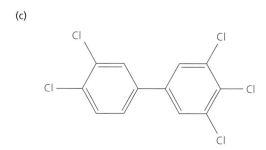

(b)

(c)

Figure 23.1 Dioxins: (a) 2,3,7,8-Tetrachlorodibenzo-*p*-dioxin (2,3,7,8-TCDD); (b) 2,3,4,7,8-Pentachlorodibenzofuran (2,3,4,7,8-PCDF); (c) 3,3',4,4'5-Pentachlorobiphenyl (PCB 126).

nausea and vomiting, anorexia and amenorrhoea.[53] Her TCDD concentration was 144 000 pg/g blood fat, the highest concentration reported to date (equivalent to a body burden of 1.6 mg TCDD).

In humans, longer term exposure to dioxins has been shown to be a risk factor for cancer,[54] immune deficiency[55] and reproductive and developmental abnormalities.[56] Endocrine disruption, including diabetes[57] and thyroid disorders,[58] has also been described. An increased mortality from ischaemic heart disease has been associated with occupational exposure to high concentrations of dioxins.[59,60]

Polychlorinated biphenyls

There are no natural sources of PCBs. They are a synthetic family of molecules that consist of 209 isomers formed by the addition of chlorine atoms to a biphenyl nucleus (Figure 23.1c). The resulting PCBs are either oily non-volatile liquids or solids. There is little information about the individual isomers of PCBs since they were generally produced as mixtures. For example, in the US several mixtures (Aroclor 1016, 1242, 1254, 1260 and 1268) were commercially produced until 1977. Since production ceased in the USA in 1997 (700 000 tonnes of PCBs being produced between 1929 and 1997), PCBs have been placed in landfills, incinerated or exported, or have escaped to the

air, water or soil, if they are no longer in use in electrical equipment.

The toxicological concern regarding PCBs relates primarily to their environmental persistence. Because they do not degrade easily, even at high temperatures, they were frequently used as insulators and coolants. Their oily nature was responsible for their use as heat-resistant lubricants. Because of their resistance to degradation, and hence environmental persistence, the production of PCBs was halted in the USA and in Western Europe in approximately 1977. They continued to be manufactured, however, in Eastern Europe until the 1990s.

As a result of the cessation of most, or all, PCB production, PCBs are often not detectable in biological samples in young people today; this was not, however, true in decades past.[61] In the USA, PCBs have been documented to exist in approximately one-third of major hazardous waste sites identified by the Environmental Protection Agency. They are known to concentrate up the food chain and are found in high concentrations in the fat tissue of fish and aquatic mammals such as seals and whales. However, environmental persistence does not equate to toxicity.

The health effects of PCBs in humans, other than rashes, have been poorly characterized. Furthermore, the interpretation of many of the studies on PCBs is complicated by the almost inevitable contamination of PCBs with PCDFs and PCDDs. Most of the information on the toxicology of PCBs in humans derives from epidemiological studies on chronically exposed populations. There have also been investigations of two major outbreaks of contaminated rice oil: the Yusho Cohort, which occurred in Japan,[62] and the Yu-Cheng Cohort, which occurred in Taiwan in 1979.[63,64] Between these two cohorts, approximately 3700 individuals were affected. All of these populations studied were simultaneously exposed to PCDFs, although the role of these compounds was in many instances either not recognized or not studied.

Although high-dose animal studies have demonstrated renal and hepatic toxicity, these studies appear to have little relevance to any reasonable human environmental exposure. The major concerns regarding the human toxicology of PCBs relate to possible neurobehavioural effects,[65] abnormal thyroid function, immune dysfunction and hepatocellular malignancies.[61] However, there are no convincing studies in humans supporting these associations. The Environmental Protection Agency[66] and International Agency for Research on Cancer (IARC)[67] have designated PCBs as probable human carcinogens. This designation is, however, based primarily on high-dose exposures in rodents and very limited human data.

DDT (see also Chapter 25, p. 297)

DDT was first synthesized in 1874, and its insecticidal properties were described in the late 1930s.[68,69] Its chemical structure is shown in Figure 23.2, and it is the archetypical organochlorine. DDT became widely used in agriculture to control insects but was banned in 1970 in Sweden, in 1972 in the USA (the decision being greatly influenced by the publication of Rachel Carson's book, *Silent Spring*) and in 1986 in the UK, largely on the basis of ecological considerations, including its persistence in the environment and sufficient bioaccumulation and toxic effects to interfere with reproduction in pelagic birds.[70]

Toxic effects in humans did not have a role in bans enacted during the 1970s, although these concerns contributed to the 2001 Stockholm Convention on Persistent Organic Pollutants, which recommended a worldwide ban on a number of organochlorine pesticides. The convention became legally binding on May 17th, 2004, although some countries in Sub-Saharan Africa requested exemption from the ban on DDT. In September 2006, the World Health Organization recommended a wider use of indoor spraying with DDT (and other insecticides) to control malaria, stressing the importance of controlled use to reduce human exposure; hence the availability of DDT is likely to continue.

Technical-grade DDT contains 65–80 per cent p,p'-DDT, 15–21 per cent o,p'-DDT and up to 4 per cent p,p'-DDD (bis[4-chlorophenyl]-1,1-dichloroethane). When sprayed, DDT can drift, sometimes for long distances, and in the soil it can evaporate or attach to wind-blown dust. In the environment, DDT breaks down to p,p'-DDE (bis[4-chlorophenyl]-1,1-dichloroethene),[68] an extremely stable compound that resists further environmental breakdown or metabolism by organisms. The general population is exposed to DDT mainly through food, whereas occupational exposures are mainly through inhalation and dermal contact.[70]

MECHANISMS OF TOXICITY

DDT interferes with sodium channels in the axonal membrane by a mechanism similar to that of pyrethroid insecticides.[71,72] DDT delays the closing of the sodium channels once they have opened, while having little or no effect on closed channels. Thus, although DDT has little or no effect on the resting potential or the rising phase and peak amplitude of the action potential, it greatly prolongs the depolarizing (negative) afterpotential of the action potential, and this produces a period of increased neuronal excitability immediately after the spike phase. This, in turn, enhances the probability of repetitive firing and the insurgence of a 'train' of action potentials. DDT inhibits Ca^{2+}- ATPase, which contributes to membrane instability.[73]

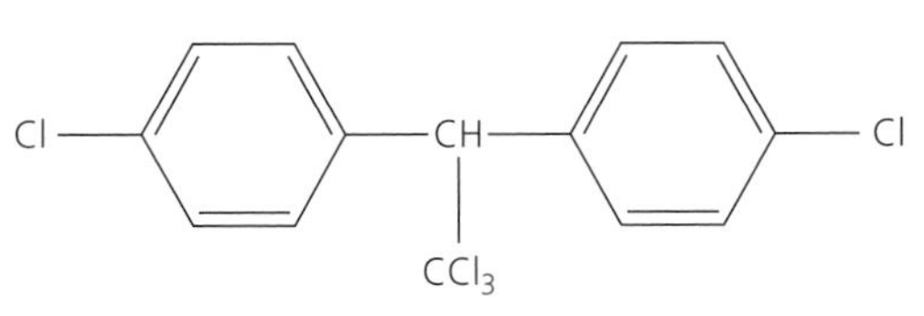

TOXICOKINETICS

The toxicokinetics of DDT have been reviewed elsewhere.[8,74,75] Most DDT dust is of such large particle size ($\geqslant 250$ μm) that any that is inhaled is deposited in the upper respiratory tract and is eventually swallowed.[76] Absorption from the gastrointestinal tract is generally slow. Although the absorption of large doses may be facilitated by fat in food, the absorption of small doses, such as those found in the residues of food, is virtually complete and is also facilitated by the presence of fat in food.[68] Animal studies suggest that the concentration of DDT in serum accurately reflects the concentration in the brain.[68]

In humans, DDT is converted to DDE (1,1'-(2,2-dichlorethenylidene)-bis[4-chlorobenzene]), which is stored in fat even more avidly than the parent compound, and to 1,1-dichloro-2,2-bis(p-chlorophenyl) ethane (DDD). DDE and DDD are then metabolized primarily in the kidney by a variety of steps to 2,2-bis(4-chlorophenyl)-acetic acid (DDA), the main excretory product, at least in occupationally exposed workers. Mean blood concentrations of DDT, DDE and DDD were 0.9 μg/L, 8.0 μg/L and 1.5 μg/L, respectively, in 30 workers exposed to a variety of pesticides for many years.[77] Laws *et al.*[78] found concentrations of DDA of 0.01–2.67 mg/L (mean 0.9 mg/L) in workers exposed occupationally for 11–19 years.

DDT is stored preferentially in fat, although the uptake of DDT by fat is slow; thus, much more is distributed to other tissues following a single, large dose and much more to adipose tissue following many small doses. Following repeated doses, storage in adipose tissue increases rapidly at first and then more gradually until a steady state is reached. The storage of DDT is proportional to the dose.[79,80] In man, the time necessary to reach storage equilibrium is at least 1 year.[80] The steady-state fat concentration at 19–21 months in volunteers administered DDT 3.5 mg and 35 mg each day was a mean of 50 mg/kg and 281 mg/kg.[79]

CLINICAL FEATURES

The use of DDT is generally safe; large populations have been exposed to the compound for 60 years with little acute toxicity apart from a few reports of accidental and intentional poisoning.[81–94]

A number of experimental studies in humans in the 1940s and 50s have shown that individuals administered DDT 6 mg/kg orally generally exhibited no illness, although perspiration, headache and nausea were reported.[95] Convulsions have been reported at doses of 16 mg/kg or higher.[82] Velbinger[96,97] exposed himself and two volunteers to oral doses of DDT 250 mg (3.6 mg/kg), 500 mg (7.1 mg/kg), 750 mg (10.7 mg/kg), 1000 mg (14.3 mg/kg) or 1500 mg (21.4 mg/kg). Increased sensitivity to taste was reported in

Figure 23.2   DDT (bis[4-chlorophenyl]-1,1,1-tricholoroethane).

volunteers exposed to DDT 250 and 500 mg. Six hours after exposure to DDT 750 or 1000 mg, disturbance of sensitivity of the lower part of the face, mild ataxia, nausea, cold clammy skin and hypersensitivity to touch were observed. Paraesthesiae of the tongue and around the mouth and nose, disturbances of equilibrium, dizziness, confusion, tremors, mild ataxia, malaise, headache, fatigue and severe vomiting were observed in volunteers within 10 hours of an oral dose of DDT 1500 mg; complete recovery occurred within 24 hours of exposure.[96,97]

Similar symptoms have been reported after the accidental or intentional ingestion of DDT.[81–94] DDT poisoning usually results in paraesthesiae, dizziness, headache, tremor, confusion and fatigue. Doses as high as 285 mg/kg taken accidentally did not cause death.[93]

Twenty-four volunteers ingested technical or p,p'-DDT at rates up to 35 mg per man per day for 21.5 months.[79] They were then observed for an additional 25.5 months, and 16 were followed up for 5 years. The storage of DDT and DDE and the excretion of DDA were proportional to the dosage. The fat of those receiving technical insecticide at the highest rate contained 105–619 parts per million of DDT when feeding stopped. The average dosage of p,p'-DDT administered in this study was 555 times the average intake of all DDT-related compounds by 19-year-old men in the general population and 1250 times their intake of p,p'-DDT. Since no definite clinical or laboratory evidence of injury by DDT was found in this study, these factors indicate a high degree of safety of DDT for the general population.[79]

In contrast, it has been shown that prolonged occupational exposure to DDT is associated with reduced verbal attention, visuomotor speed and sequencing and with increased neuropsychological and psychiatric symptoms in a dose–response pattern (that is, per year of DDT application) in retired workers aged 55–70 years in Costa Rica.[98]

RISK OF CANCER

Although extensively studied, there is no convincing evidence that DDT or its metabolite DDE increases human cancer risk. Mainly on the basis of animal data, DDT is classified as a possible carcinogen (class 2B) by the IARC[99] and as a reasonably anticipated human carcinogen by the US National Toxicology Program.[100] Breast cancer has been examined most closely for an association with p,p'-DDE. However, large epidemiological studies[101–109] and subsequent pooled meta-analyses[110–112] have failed to confirm the association.

Previous case–control studies have suggested that a history of DDT use was associated with a raised risk of non-Hodgkin's lymphoma,[113,114] but subsequent studies[115] using measurements of total DDT concentrations in serum did not find such an increased risk. The association of DDT with multiple myeloma,[116–118] prostate and testicular cancer,[119,120] endometrial cancer[121–123] and colorectal cancer[124] was sought, but results have been inconclusive or generally do not support an association.

REFERENCES

● = Key primary paper

◆ = Major review article

1. Frohne D, Pfänder HJ. *Poisonous Plants. A Handbook for Doctors, Pharmacists, Toxicologists, Biologists and Veterinarians*, 2nd edn. London: Manson Publishing, 2005.
2. Nelson LS, Shih RD, Balick MJ. *Handbook of Poisonous and Injurious Plants*, 2nd edn. New York: Springer, 2007.
3. Cooper MR, Johnson AW, Dauncey EA. *Poisonous Plants and Fungi: An Illustrated Guide*, 2nd edn. London: TSO, 2003.
4. Soneral SN, Connor NP. Jimson weed intoxication in five adolescents. *Wis Med J* 2005; **104**: 70–2.
5. Şaksen H, Odabas D, Akbayram S *et al*. Deadly nightshade (*Atropa belladonna*) intoxication: An analysis of 49 children. *Hum Exp Toxicol* 2003; **22**: 665–8.
●6. Eddleston M, Rajapakse S, Rajakanthan *et al*. Anti-digoxin Fab fragments in cardiotoxicity induced by ingestion of yellow oleander: A randomised controlled trial. *Lancet* 2000; **355**: 967–71.
◆7. Rajapakse S. Management of yellow oleander poisoning. *Clin Toxicol* 2009; **47**: 206–12.
◆8. Schep LJ, Slaughter RJ, Becket G, Beasley DM. Poisoning due to water hemlock. *Clin Toxicol* 2009; **47**: 270–8.
9. Shadnia S, Moiensadat M, Abdollahi M. A case of acute strychnine poisoning. *Vet Hum Toxicol* 2004; **46**: 76–9.
10. Lasch EE, El Shawa R. Multiple cases of cyanide poisoning by apricot kernels in children from Gaza. *Pediatrics* 1981; **68**: 5–7.
11. Sundov Z, Nincevic Z, Definis-Gojanovic M *et al*. Fatal colchicine poisoning by accidental ingestion of meadow saffron – case report. *Forensic Sci Int* 2005; **149**: 253–6.
12. Heath KB. A fatal case of apparent water hemlock poisoning. *Vet Hum Toxicol* 2001; **43**: 35–6.
13. Kumana CR, Ng M, Lin HJ *et al*. Hepatic veno-occlusive disease due to toxic alkaloid herbal tea. *Lancet* 1983; **2**: 1360–1.
14. Moritz F, Compagnon P, Kaliszczak IG *et al*. Severe acute poisoning with homemade *Aconitum napellus* capsules: Toxicokinetic and clinical data. *Clin Toxicol* 2005; **43**: 873–6.
15. Lin C-C, Chan TYK, Deng J-F. Clinical features and management of herb-induced aconitine poisoning. *Ann Emerg Med* 2004; **43**: 574–9.
16. Travis AD, Gummin DD, McCann P, Knuths JR. Monkshood-induced dysrhythmia treated with magnesium. *J Toxicol Clin Toxicol* 2002; **40**: 646.
17. Burrows WD, Renner SE. Biological warfare agents as threats to potable water. *Environ Health Perspect* 1999; **107**: 975–84.
18. Griffiths GD, Lindsay CD, Upshall DG. Examination of the toxicity of several protein toxins of plant origin using bovine pulmonary endothelial cells. *Toxicology* 1994; **90**: 11–27.
19. Franz DR, Jaax NK. Ricin toxin. In: Zajtchuk R, Bellamy RF (eds) *Medical Aspects of Chemical and Biological Warfare. Textbook of Military Medicine. Part I: Warfare, Weaponry, and the Casualty* (pp. 631–42). Washington DC: Office of the Surgeon General at TMM Publications, 1997.

◆20. Lord MJ, Jolliffe NA, Marsden CJ *et al*. Ricin: Mechanisms of cytotoxicity. *Toxicol Rev* 2003; **22**: 53–64.

21. Qu X, Qing L. Abrin induces HeLa cell apoptosis by cytochrome *c* release and caspase activation. *J Biochem Mol Biol* 2004; **37**: 445–53.

22. Shih S-F, Wu Y-H, Hung C-H, Yang H-Y, Lin J-Y. Abrin triggers cell death by inactivating a thiol-specific antioxidant protein. *J Biol Chem* 2001; **276**: 21870–7.

23. Narayanan S, Surolia A, Karande AA. Ribosome-inactivating protein and apoptosis: Abrin causes cell death via mitochondrial pathway in Jurkat cells. *Biochem J* 2004; **377**: 233–40.

24. Wilhelmsen C, Pitt L. Lesions of acute inhaled lethal ricin intoxication in rhesus monkeys. *Vet Pathol* 1993; **30**: 482.

25. Crompton R, Gall D. Georgi Markov – death in a pellet. *Med Leg J* 1980; **48**: 51–62.

26. Leith AG, Griffiths GD, Green MA. Quantification of ricin toxin using a highly sensitive avidin/biotin enzyme-linked immunosorbent assay. *J Forensic Sci Soc* 1988; **28**: 227–36.

27. Shyu H-F, Chiao D-J, Liu H-W, Tang S-S. Monoclonal antibody-based enzyme immunoassay for detection of ricin. *Hybrid Hybridomics* 2002; **21**: 69–73.

28. Marsden CJ, Smith DC, Roberts LM, Lord JM. Ricin: Current understanding and prospects for an antiricin vaccine. *Expert Rev Vaccines* 2005; **4**: 229–37.

◆29. Karlson-Stiber C, Persson H. Cytotoxic fungi – an overview. *Toxicon* 2003; **42**: 339–49.

◆30. Committee on Toxicity. *COT Statement on Risk Assessment of Marine Biotoxins of the Okadaic Acid, Pectenotoxin, Azaspiracid and Yessotoxin Groups in Support of Human Health*. London: Food Standards Agency COT Secretariat, 2007.

31. Do Nascimento JLM, Oliveira KRM, Crespo-Lopez ME *et al*. Methylmercury neurotoxicity and antioxidant defenses. *Indian J Med Res* 2008; **128**: 373–82.

◆32. FAO. Paralytic shellfish poisoning (PSP). In: *Marine Biotoxins* (pp. 5–52). FAO Food and Nutrition Paper No. 80. Rome: Food and Agriculture Organization of the United Nations, 2004.

33. Rodrigue DC, Etzel RA, Hall S *et al*. Lethal paralytic shellfish poisoning in Guatemala. *Am J Trop Med Hyg* 1990; **42**: 267–71.

◆34. Food and Agriculture Organization. Diarrhoeic shellfish poisoning (DSP). In: *Marine Biotoxins* (pp. 53–95). FAO Food and Nutrition Paper No. 80. Rome: Food and Agriculture Organization of the United Nations, 2004.

◆35. Food and Agriculture Organization. Amnesic shellfish poisoning (ASP). In: *Marine Biotoxins* (pp. 97–136). FAO Food and Nutrition Paper No. 80. Rome: Food and Agriculture Organization of the United Nations, 2004.

◆36. Todd ECD. Domoic acid and amnesic shellfish poisoning – a review. *J Food Prot* 1993; **56**: 69–83.

◆37. Food and Agriculture Organization. Neurologic shellfish poisoning (NSP). In: *Marine Biotoxins* (pp. 137–72). FAO Food and Nutrition Paper No. 80. Rome: Food and Agriculture Organization of the United Nations, 2004.

38. Opinion of the Scientific Panel on Contaminants in the Food Chain on a request from the European Commission on marine biotoxins in shellfish – azaspiracid group. *EFSA J* 2008; **723**: 1–52.

◆39. Food and Agriculture Organization. Azaspiracid shellfish poisoning (AZP). In: *Marine Bbiotoxins* (pp. 173–84). FAO Food and Nutrition Paper No. 80. Rome: Food and Agriculture Organization of the United Nations, 2004.

40. McMahon T, Silke J. Winter toxicity of unknown aetiology in mussels. *Harmful Algae News* 1996; **14**: 2.

◆41. FAO. Ciguatera fish poisoning (CFP). In: *Marine Biotoxins* (pp. 185–218). FAO Food and Nutrition Paper No. 80. Rome: Food and Agriculture Organization of the United Nations, 2004.

42. Pirkle JL, Wolfe WH. Estimates of the half-life of 2,3,7,8-tetrachlorodibenzo-*p*-dioxin in Vietnam veterans of Operation Ranch Hand. *J Toxicol Environ Health* 1989; **27**: 165–71.

◆43. Mandal PK. Dioxin: A review of its environmental effects and its aryl hydrocarbon receptor biology. *J Comp Physiol B* 2005; **175**: 221–30.

◆44. Bradshaw TD, Bell DR. Relevance of the aryl hydrocarbon receptor (AhR) for clinical toxicology. *Clin Toxicol (Phila)* 2009; **47**: 632–42.

◆45 Committee to Review the Health Effects in Vietnam Veterans of Exposure to Herbicides. *Veterans and Agent Orange. Update 2004*, 5th edn. Washington DC: National Academies Press, 2005.

46. Kimbrough RD, Carter CD, Liddle JA, Cline RE. Epidemiology and pathology of a tetrachlorodibenzodioxin poisoning episode. *Arch Environ Health* 1977; **32**: 77–86.

47. Smith RM, O'Keefe PW, Aldous KM, Hilker DR, O'Brien JE. 2,3,7,8-tetrachlorodibenzo-*p*-dioxin in sediment samples from Love Canal storm sewers and creeks. *Environ Sci Technol* 1983; **17**: 6–10.

48. Consonni D, Pesatori AC, Zocchetti C *et al*. Mortality in a population exposed to dioxin after the Seveso, Italy, accident in 1976: 25 years of follow-up. *Am J Epidemiol* 2008; **167**: 847–58.

49. Pesatori AC, Consonni D, Bachetti S *et al*. Short- and long-term morbidity and mortality in the population exposed to dioxin after the "Seveso accident". *Ind Health* 2003; **41**: 127–38.

50. Dalderup LM, Zellenrath D. Dioxin exposure: 20 year follow-up. *Lancet* 1983; **2**: 1134–5.

51. Sorg O, Zennegg M, Schmid P *et al*. 2,3,7,8-Tetrachlorodibenzo-*p*-dioxin (TCDD) poisoning in Victor Yushchenko: Identification and measurement of TCDD metabolites. *Lancet* 2009; **374**: 1179–85.

52. Sweeney MH, Mocarelli P. Human health effects after exposure to 2,3,7,8-TCDD. *Food Addit Contam* 2000; **17**: 303–16.

53. Geusau A, Abraham K, Geissler K *et al*. Severe 2,3,7,8-tetrachlorodibenzo-*p*-dioxin (TCDD) intoxication: Clinical and laboratory effects. *Environ Health Perspect* 2001; **109**: 865–9.

54. Steenland K, Piacitelli L, Deddens J, Fingerhut M, Chang LI. Cancer, heart disease, and diabetes in workers exposed to 2,3,7,8-tetrachlorodibenzo-*p*-dioxin. *J Natl Cancer Inst* 1999; **91**: 779–86.

55. Weisglas-Kuperus N, Patandin S, Berbers GAM *et al*. Immunologic effects of background exposure to polychlorinated biphenyls and dioxins in Dutch preschool children. *Environ Health Perspect* 2000; **108**: 1203–7.

56. Guo YL, Yu ML. The Yucheng rice oil poisoning incident. In: Schecter A, Gasiewicz TA (eds) *Dioxins and Health*, 2nd edn. (pp. 893–920). Hoboken, NJ: Wiley, 2003.

57. Longnecker MP, Michalek JE. Serum dioxin level in relation to diabetes mellitus among Air Force Veterans with background levels of exposure. *Epidemiology* 2000; **11**: 44–8.

58. Pavuk M, Schecter AJ, Akhtar FZ, Michalek JE. Serum 2,3,7,8-tetrachlorodibenzo-p-dioxin (TCDD) levels and thyroid function in Air Force veterans of the Vietnam War. *Ann Epidemiol* 2003; **13**: 335–43.

59. Flesch-Janys D, Berger J, Gurn P *et al.* Exposure to polychlorinated dioxins and furans (PCDD/F) and mortality in a cohort of workers from a herbicide-producing plant in Hamburg, Federal Republic of Germany. *Am J Epidemiol* 1995; **142**: 1165–75.

60. Hooiveld M, Heederik DJJ, Kogevinas M *et al.* Second follow-up of a Dutch cohort occupationally exposed to phenoxy herbicides, chlorophenols, and contaminants. *Am J Epidemiol* 1998; **147**:891–901.

◆61. Kimbrough RD, Krouskas CA. Human exposure to polychlorinated biphenyls and health effects: A critical synopsis. *Toxicol Rev* 2003; **22**: 217–33.

62. Onozuka D, Yoshimura T, Kaneko S, Furue M. Mortality after exposure to polychlorinated biphenyls and polychlorinated dibenzofurans: A 40-year follow-up study of Yusho patients. *Am J Epidemiol* 2009; **169**: 86–95.

63. Hsu ST, Ma CI, Hsu SK *et al.* Discovery and epidemiology of PCB poisoning in Taiwan: A four-year follow-up. *Environ Health Perspect* 1985; **59**: 5–10.

64. Guo YL, Yu M-L, Hsu C-C, Rogan WJ. Chloracne, goiter, arthritis, and anemia after polychlorinated biphenyl poisoning: 14-year follow-up of the Taiwan Yucheng cohort. *Environ Health Perspect* 1999; **107**: 715–19.

◆65. Faroon O, Jones D, de Rosa C. Effects of polychlorinated biphenyls on the nervous system. *Toxicol Ind Health* 2000; **16**: 305–33.

◆66. US EPA. *PCBs: Cancer Dose–Response Assessment and Application to Environmental Mixtures.* EPA/600/P–96/001F. Washington, DC: Environmental Protection Agency, 1996.

67. International Agency for Research on Cancer. Polychlorinated biphenyls and polybrominated biphenyls – summary of data reported and evaluation. *IARC Monogr Eval Carcinog Risks Hum* 1978; **18**: 1–124.

68. International Programme on Chemical Safety. *Environmental Health Criteria 9. DDT and its Derivatives.* Geneva: World Health Organization, 1979.

69. Mellanby K. *The DDT story.* Farnham, Surrey: British Crop Protection Council, 1992.

70. Rogan WJ, Chen A. Health risks and benefits of bis (4-chlorophenyl)-1,1,1-trichloroethane (DDT). *Lancet* 2005; **366**: 763–73.

71. Vijverberg HPM, Zalm JM, Bercken J. Similar mode of action of pyrethroids and DDT on sodium channel gating in myelinated nerves. *Nature* 1982; **295**: 601–2.

72. Narahashi T. The role of ion channels in insecticide action. In: Narahashi T, Chambers JE (eds) *Insecticide Action: From Molecule to Organism* (pp. 55–84). New York: Plenum Press, 1989.

73. Matsumura F, Ghiasuddin SM. Characteristics of DDT-sensitive Ca-ATPase in the axonic membrane. In: Narahashi T (ed.) *Neurotoxicology of Insecticides and Pheromones* (pp. 245–57). New York: Plenum Press, 1979.

74. Smith AG. Chlorinated hydrocarbon insecticides. In: Hayes WJ Jr, Laws ER Jr (eds) *Handbook of Pesticide Toxicology.* Vol. 2 (pp. 731–915). San Diego, CA: Academic Press, 1991.

◆75. Agency for Toxic Substances and Disease Registry. *Toxicological Profile for DDT, DDE and DDD.* ATSDR Toxicological Profiles. Atlanta, GA: ATSDR, US Public Health Service, 2002.

76. Hayes WJ Jr. *Toxicology of Pesticides.* Baltimore, MD: Williams & Wilkins, 1975.

77. Guardino X, Serra C, Obiols J *et al.* Determination of DDT and related compounds in blood samples from agricultural workers. *J Chromatogr A* 1996; **719**: 141–7.

78. Laws ER Jr, Curley A, Biros FJ. Men with intensive occupational exposure to DDT. A clinical and chemical study. *Arch Environ Health* 1967; **15**: 766–75.

79. Hayes WJ Jr, Dale WE, Pirkle CI. Evidence of safety of long-term, high, oral doses of DDT for man. *Arch Environ Health* 1971; **22**: 119–35.

80. Hayes WJ Jr, Durham WF, Cueto C Jr. The effect of known repeated oral doses of chlorophenothane (DDT) in man. *JAMA* 1956; **162**: 890–7.

81. Mülhens K. Uber die Bedeutung der Dichlor-diphenyl-trichlor-methylmethanpräparate als Arthropodengift in der Seuchenbekämpfung unter Berücksichtigung eigener Erfahrungen. *Dtsch Med Wochenschr* 1946; **71**: 164–9.

82. Hsieh HC. DDT intoxication a family of Southern Taiwan. *Arch Ind Health* 1954; **10**: 344–6.

83. Dale WE, Gaines TB, Hayes WJ, Pearce GW. Poisoning by DDT: Relation between clinical signs and concentration in rat brain. *Science* 1963; **142**: 1474–6.

84. Council on Pharmacy and Chemistry. Report to the Council: Pharmacologic and toxicologic aspects of DDT (chlorophenothane USP). *JAMA* 1951; **145**: 728–33.

85. Mackeras IM, West RFK. "DDT" poisoning in man. *Med J Aust* 1946; **1**: 400–1.

86. Cunningham RE, Hill FS. Convulsions and deafness following ingestion of DDT. *Pediatrics* 1952; **9**: 745–7.

87. Hill WR, Damini CR. Death following exposure to DDT. Report of a case. *N Engl J Med* 1946; **235**: 897–9.

88. Reingold IM, Lasky II. Acute fatal poisoning following ingestion of a solution of DDT. *Ann Intern Med* 1947; **26**: 945–7.

89. Campbell AMG. DDT poisoning in man: A suspected case. *Lancet* 1949; **2**: 1178.

90. Biden-Steele K, Stuckey RE. Poisoning by DDT emulsion: Report of a fatal case. *Lancet* 1946; **2**: 235–6.

91. Hill KR, Robinson G. A fatal case of DDT poisoning in a child, with an account of two accidental deaths in dogs. *Br Med J* 1945; **2**: 845–7.

92. Smith NJ. Death following accidental ingestion of DDT. Experimental studies. *JAMA* 1948; **136**: 469–71.

93. Garrett RM. Toxicity of DDT for man. *J Med Assoc State Ala* 1947; **17**: 74–6.

94. Francone MP, Mariani FH, Demare C. Clinica de la intoxicacion por DDT. *Rev Asoc Med Argent* 1952; **66**: 56–9.

95. Hayes WJ Jr. Chlorinated hydrocarbon insecticides. In: *Pesticides Studied in Man* (pp. 172–283). Baltimore, MD: Williams & Wilkins, 1982.

96. Velbinger HH. Beitrag zur Toxikologie des "DDT" – Wirkstoffes Dichlor-diphenyl-trichlormethylmethan. *Pharmazie* 1947; **2**: 268–74.

97. Velbinger HH. Zur Frage der "DDT" – Toxizität für Menschen. *Dtsch Gesundheitsw* 1947; **2**: 355–8.

98. van Wendel de Joode B, Wesseling C, Kromhout H *et al.* Chronic nervous-system effects of long-term occupational exposure to DDT. *Lancet* 2001; **357**: 1014–16.

99. International Agency for Research on Cancer. Occupational exposures in insecticide application, and some pesticides. DDT and associated compounds (group 2B). *IARC Monogr Eval Carcinog Risks Hum* 1991; **53**: 179–250.

100. US Department of Health and Human Services, Public Health Service, National Toxicology Program. Dichlorodiphenyltrichloroethane (DDT). CAS no 50–29-3. In: *Report on Carcinogens (RoC)*. Available from: http:// ehp.niehs.nih.gov/roc/toc11.html#toc (accessed November 23, 2009).

101. Wolff MS, Zeleniuch-Jacquotte A, Dubin N, Toniolo P. Risk of breast cancer and organochlorine exposure. *Cancer Epidemiol Biomarkers Prev* 2000; **9**: 271–7.

102. Van't Veer P, Lobbezoo IE, Martín-Moreno JM *et al.* DDT (dicophane) and postmenopausal breast cancer in Europe: case-control study. *Br Med J* 1997; **315**: 81–5.

103. Helzlsouer KJ, Alberg AJ, Huang HY *et al.* Serum concentrations of organochlorine compounds and the subsequent development of breast cancer. *Cancer Epidemiol Biomarkers Prev* 1999; **8**: 525–32.

104. Demers A, Ayotte P, Brisson J *et al.* Risk and aggressiveness of breast cancer in relation to plasma organochlorine concentrations. *Cancer Epidemiol Biomarkers Prev* 2000; **9**: 161–6.

105. Zheng T, Holford TR, Mayne ST *et al.* Risk of female breast cancer associated with serum polychlorinated biphenyls and 1,1-dichloro-2,2?-bis(*p*-chlorophenyl)ethylene. *Cancer Epidemiol Biomarkers Prev* 2000; **9**: 167–74.

106. Gammon MD, Wolff MS, Neugut AI *et al.* Environmental toxins and breast cancer on Long Island. II: Organochlorine compound levels in blood. *Cancer Epidemiol Biomarkers Prev* 2002; **11**: 686–97.

107. Pavuk M, Cerhan JR, Lynch CF *et al.* Case-control study of PCBs, other organochlorines and breast cancer in Eastern Slovakia. *J Expo Anal Environ Epidemiol* 2003; **13**: 267–75.

108. Hunter DJ, Hankinson SE, Laden F *et al.* Plasma organochlorine levels and the risk of breast cancer. *N Engl J Med* 1997; **337**: 1253–8.

109. Zheng T, Holford TR, Mayne ST *et al.* DDE and DDT in breast adipose tissue and risk of female breast cancer. *Am J Epidemiol* 1999; **150**: 453–8.

110. Laden F, Collman G, Iwamoto K *et al.* 1,1-Dichloro-2,2-bis(*p*-chlorophenyl)ethylene and polychlorinated biphenyls and breast cancer: Combined analysis of five US studies. *J Natl Cancer Inst* 2001; **93**: 768–76.

111. Lopez-Cervantes M, Torres-Sanchez L, Tobias A, Lopez-Carrillo L. Dichlorodiphenyldichloroethane burden and breast cancer risk: A meta-analysis of the epidemiologic evidence. *Environ Health Perspect* 2004; **112**: 207–14.

112. Snedeker SM. Pesticides and breast cancer risk: A review of DDT, DDE, and dieldrin. *Environ Health Perspect* 2001; **109**: 35–47.

113. Cantor KP, Blair A, Everett G *et al.* Pesticides and other agricultural risk factors for non-Hodgkin's lymphoma among men in Iowa and Minnesota. *Cancer Res* 1992; **52**: 2447–55.

114. Woods JS, Polissar L, Severson RK, Heuser LS, Kulander BG. Soft tissue sarcoma and non-Hodgkin's lymphoma in relation to phenoxyherbicide and chlorinated phenol exposure in western Washington. *J Natl Cancer Inst* 1987; **78**: 899–910.

115. Rothman N, Cantor KP, Blair A *et al.* A nested case-control study of non-Hodgkin lymphoma and serum organochlorine residues. *Lancet,* 1997; **350**: 240–4.

116. Cocco P, Blair A, Congia P *et al.* Proportional mortality of dichloro-diphenyl-trichloroethane (DDT) workers: A preliminary report. *Arch Environ Health* 1997; **52**: 299–303.

117. Nanni O, Falcini F, Buiatti E *et al.* Multiple myeloma and work in agriculture: results of a case-control study in Forli, Italy. *Cancer Causes Control* 1998; **9**: 277–83.

118. Cocco P, Kazerouni N, Zahm SH. Cancer mortality and environmental exposure to DDE in the United States. *Environ Health Perspect* 2000; **108**: 1–4.

119. Cocco P, Benichou J. Mortality from cancer of the male reproductive tract and environmental exposure to the anti-androgen *p,p'*- dichlorodiphenyldichloroethylene in the United States. *Oncology* 1998; **55**: 334–9.

120. Ritchie JM, Vial SL, Fuortes LJ *et al.* Organochlorines and risk of prostate cancer. *J Occup Environ Med* 2003; **45**: 692–702.

121. Sturgeon SR, Brock JW, Potischman N *et al.* Serum concentrations of organochlorine compounds and endometrial cancer risk (United States). *Cancer Causes Control* 1998; **9**: 417–24.

122. Weiderpass E, Adami HO, Baron JA *et al.* Organochlorines and endometrial cancer risk. *Cancer Epidemiol Biomarkers Prev* 2000; **9**: 487–93.

123. Hardell L, Van Bavel B, Lindstrom G *et al.* Adipose tissue concentrations of p,p?-DDE and the risk for endometrial cancer. *Gynecol Oncol* 2004; **95**: 706–11.

124. Howsam M, Grimalt JO, Guinó E *et al.* Organochlorine exposure and colorectal cancer risk. *Environ Health Perspect* 2004; **112**: 1460–6.

24

Drinking water safety and standards for drinking water

JOHN FAWELL

Safe drinking water is one of the essentials of life, but drinking water contains many constituents and contaminants that can also threaten well-being. The most important of these are generally microbiological contaminants in the form of pathogens, ranging from viruses through bacteria to parasites, many of which contribute significantly to the death toll from the lack of safe drinking water in so many parts of the world. In addition, some chemicals that can be present in drinking water can also impact on health or the acceptability of drinking water. There is, however, a significant difference between pathogens and chemicals. Pathogens act within a short period of exposure and even very low numbers are capable of causing disease, if only in a small number of individuals, while chemicals generally require long exposure to high concentrations.

There are also substances for which there is little evidence of actual health effects from their presence in drinking water but which it is considered important to control to ensure that they do not cause problems in the future; for others, there is a need to provide reassurance for consumers because of a public fear of their possible effects.

Our knowledge of the contaminants and constituents in drinking water has increased significantly over the past four decades as a consequence of improved methods of analysis for both chemicals and microbiological contaminants. This has resulted in a greater awareness of the presence of trace amounts of many chemicals.

Drinking water is taken from many sources: groundwater, which may or may not be well protected from the surface ingress of pollutants; rivers, lakes and reservoirs, which may be vulnerable to surface contamination and pollution; and small supplies based around wells and springs. Increasingly, large supplies may have more than one source in order to increase the security of supply, while new sources such as desalination are making an increasing contribution.

This chapter provides a brief overview of some of the key contaminants that have some issues for drinking water, and the role of standards and guidelines in assuring drinking water quality.

WATER CONTAMINANTS – OCCURRENCE AND HEALTH ISSUES

Microbiological contaminants

Pathogens are the greatest threat to human health, arising from the discharge of animal faeces and human faeces from sewage or from septic tanks. Pathogens on fields and on urban surfaces can also be washed off following rainfall. Because microorganisms can multiply in the affected host, the infective dose can be very low, sometimes one organism, and a single dose can lead to disease. Drinking water treatment was devised to remove pathogens, and multiple-barrier water treatment is designed to ensure that the barriers are sufficient to prevent contamination by all pathogens. The processes can include settlement in reservoirs, coagulation, sedimentation and filtration, including membranes and activated carbon, often with oxidation by ozone and disinfection with chemical disinfectants such as chlorine and, increasingly, ultraviolet irradiation. Chlorine and chloramine are also used to help to protect distribution systems from contamination subsequent to water treatment.

Surface waters are particularly vulnerable to contamination, and this is reflected in the higher level of treatment usually applied to surface water compared with groundwater, which is often well protected from contamination. Not all groundwater is well protected though, and pathogens can be found as a consequence of surface infiltration or infiltration from leaking sewers and septic tanks. Small supplies and private supplies, particularly in rural areas, are often vulnerable to contamination and remain a significant source of concern in most countries. The issues surrounding waterborne microbial disease are well documented by the World Health Organization (WHO) and are covered in their *Guidelines for Drinking-water Quality*.[1] They are also covered in depth in Chapters 32 and 33 of this volume.

Chemical constituents and contaminants

NATURAL CONSTITUENTS

Water contains traces of many minerals that arise from the rocks and soils through which it passes. Most of these are present in minute concentrations, but some are present at much higher levels, depending on the nature of the geology. Some such as calcium and magnesium are potentially beneficial and, although they may cause scaling, are not considered to pose any hazard to health. Indeed, there is continuing interest in the possible negative association between hard water, including calcium and magnesium, and chronic heart disease. Although there have been many studies, the relationship remains controversial. The WHO has considered the evidence,[2–4] and the data suggest that the replacement of calcium and magnesium removed in treatment by reverse osmosis, but not to naturally soft water, may be appropriate for health reasons.

Some constituents, such as selenium, are essential for human nutrition, but at high intakes, to which water containing high concentrations would contribute, it may give rise to adverse effects, such as on liver protein synthesis. However, affected populations are rare and usually localized.[1] A small number, particularly arsenic and fluoride, are known to cause health effects through the consumption of high concentrations in drinking water.

Fluoride, which can be beneficial at low concentrations, is found in high concentrations in many parts of the world. Where concentrations exceed 2–3 mg/L, and depending on exposure from all sources, dental fluorosis can occur with varying degrees of severity. As concentrations increase and intake is above 6 mg per day, skeletal fluorosis can occur,

which in its most severe form, at intakes of 14 mg per day and above, is crippling and has a major impact on the affected populations (see Chapter 29).[1,5–7]

Arsenic is an important groundwater contaminant in many parts of the world, including the Indian subcontinent, China, South America and northern Europe. In many of these areas, concentrations of arsenic can be sufficient to cause several conditions, including dermal lesions, peripheral neuropathy and cancers of the skin, bladder and lung, with significant morbidity and mortality. Arsenic remains the subject of intense research to determine whether there is a concentration that can be practically achieved but that provides an acceptable risk to health. There remain uncertainties as to the shape of the dose–response curve at low doses for carcinogenicity, and this remains a source of controversy. The WHO guideline value is 10 μg/L based on practical considerations while taking into account health outcomes. However, achieving this concentration in many small rural supplies in developing countries is difficult, and a compromise is required that will reduce the effects on health while still supplying microbiologically safe water.[1]

A constituent that is also found in groundwater is uranium, which is present naturally. As with other such substances, the problem is greatest for small supplies for which resources are limited. The issue for uranium in drinking water is not its radioactivity but its potential for toxicity to the kidney. Data from laboratory animals are unhelpful in identifying a safe intake for man, but data from human populations indicate that it may be less toxic than previously thought. Guidelines and standards currently range from 15 to 30 μg/L, but these may be excessively conservative with regard to kidney toxicity. There is a need for more research on exposed human populations in order to confirm safe concentrations for human consumption.[1,8]

Although there are many possible constituents in drinking water, most have little impact except in a few very special circumstances, such as those encountered in highly mineralized waters. There are, however, those which can impact on the acceptability of drinking water. Iron and manganese fall into this category. Both substances can be found in solution in anaerobic waters, but when oxidized they form insoluble coloured precipitates. The concentrations at which discoloration occurs are well below those that might raise concerns for health, particularly since the bioavailability of the oxide precipitates is lower than that of the dissolved salts. Both have been considered by the WHO.[1]

Surface water sources also contain natural organic substances from the breakdown of plant matter, giving rise to humic and fulvic acids that produce colour in water. In addition, surface waters that are still or slow-flowing can be affected by blooms of algae, the most important of which are the cyanobacteria, or blue–green algae. Although all blooms of algae and diatoms can interfere with treatment, cyanobacteria can also produce the substances geosmin and 2-methylisoborneol that impact on taste at extremely low concentrations of a few nanograms per litre. They can also produce a range of toxins including microcystins and cylindrospermopsin, which are liver toxins and also possible tumour promoters, and saxitoxin and anatoxin a, which are neurotoxins. These substances have caused significant problems in many parts of the world, and it is important that every effort is made to prevent blooms of cyanobacteria in drinking water sources, by a reduction of phosphate as the key nutrient and a management of the sources to disrupt the growth cycle. Presently, there is only a guideline/standard for microcystin LR of 1.0 μg/L, but toxicity data are available for others, and cylindrospermopsin appears to be commonly found in many waters associated with cyanobacterial blooms.[1,9]

Problems are increasingly encountered with the availability of water for drinking water supplies in many parts of the world, either due to a shortage of water in arid regions, such as the middle east, or due to the salination of freshwater supplies through an overexploitation of groundwater in coastal regions or a mobilization of salt from inland salt deposits. As a consequence, there is increasing dependence on desalination. Salt waters frequently contain high levels of bromide and boron, which are more difficult to remove in the desalination process. Bromide is of low toxicity, but there has been concern over the potential reproductive effects of boron. Several authorities agreed that it was appropriate to develop a tolerable daily intake using a reduced uncertainty factor. The standard of 1 mg/L developed by the European Union (EU) was based on an allocation of 10 per cent of the tolerable daily intake to drinking water. However, actual data from overall exposure show that intake from other sources is low and a higher allocation factor, for example 20 per cent, is appropriate.[10–12] A higher standard is of great significance for desalination processes because the removal of boron requires tighter membranes and much higher energy. A new guideline for boron of 24 mg/L has just been published by the WHO (http://www.who.int/water_sanitation_health/dwq/chemicals/boron/en/).

AGRICULTURAL CONTAMINANTS

Agriculture is a potentially significant source of microbial contaminants but it is also a source of chemical contaminants. Nutrients, consisting of phosphate and nitrate, are important. Phosphate can cause blooms of cyanobacteria in water sources but is of no direct concern for drinking water. Nitrate can reach both surface water and groundwater by leaching from soils when there is insufficient plant growth to take up the excess. This can be due to artificial fertilizers, organic manures or autumn ploughing of grassland. Wells can also be contaminated through poorly sited manure stores and badly sited or poorly constructed septic tanks. Nitrate can also be reduced to nitrite in anaerobic waters.

The primary concern for health with nitrate and nitrite in drinking water is the development of methaemoglobinaemia, or blue baby syndrome, in bottle-fed infants. This is now almost unknown in public water supplies, particularly those with adequate pathogen control, since microbial contamination also appears to play an important role. Nitrate can be reduced to nitrite in the gastrointestinal tract of infants, and nitrite can reduce haemoglobin to methaemoglobin. Infants are considered to be at much higher risk because of the high intake of water in relation to body weight, while enzymes for converting methaemoglobin back to haemoglobin are poorly developed. Most cases of methaemoglobinaemia associated with drinking water now are those from the use of small private wells with little or no treatment and high levels of nitrate and microbial contamination.[1,13,14] Because both nitrate and nitrite are important, standards and guidelines usually consider both together by the use of a simple formula:

$$\frac{Conc^n \text{ of nitrate (mg/L)}}{50 \text{ mg/L}} + \frac{Conc^n \text{ of nitrate (mg/L)}}{3 \text{ mg/L}} \leq 1.0$$

Pesticides are other contaminants that are associated with agriculture, including forestry, but they can also arise from their use in controlling weeds on non-crop land. Pesticides, particularly those herbicides that are more water soluble and do not break down rapidly, may reach groundwater, where they can persist. However, many pesticides can reach surface water as a consequence of overspray and run-off following rainfall, including less water-soluble compounds adsorbed to particulate matter. This means that the occurrence and concentrations of pesticides in surface water can vary significantly with time and conditions, and are also dependent on their pattern of use. The concentrations of pesticides are generally extremely low, and many are removed in drinking water treatment; this is certainly true of those which are of low water solubility. Currently, there is little credible evidence that any pesticides cause health effects through drinking water from public supplies, but they retain the potential to be a threat.

INDUSTRIAL CONTAMINANTS

This group includes contaminants from industry and from human settlements. They can be from large industry or small local industries and can potentially cover a very wide range of substances. More information on assessing the contaminants from these and other sources can be found in *Chemical Safety of Drinking-water: Assessing Priorities for Risk Management*.[15] The most commonly occurring contaminants are briefly discussed below.

Oils are used in large quantities and often cause contamination. They are invariably complex mixtures containing a wide range of substance of differing molecular size. The larger molecules are of limited concern for drinking water because of their low solubility and mobility. However, smaller molecules, particularly from the aromatic fractions, are a significant nuisance in drinking water, causing unpleasant taste and odour at low concentrations, usually well below any concentration of direct concern for health. These include the 'BTEX' compounds (benzene, toluene, ethyl benzene and xylene), the alkyl naphthalenes and the petroleum additive methyl tertiary butyl ether.[16,17] They can not only reach drinking water sources, but also penetrate plastic distribution pipes and service lines and have caused major incidents such as the diesel contamination of Burncrooks water treatment works in the west of Scotland.[18]

Solvents, including tri and tetrachloroethene, carbon tetrachloride and 1,1,1-trichloroethane, have been widely used in industry. The handling of such substances was often lax, and disposal on land was common. Such practice is no longer allowed, but there are many sites where past activity has resulted in the contamination of groundwater because of the mobility of these substances. They are also volatile and are lost from surface water to the atmosphere but this is not possible in groundwater, where they are persistent. Although there have been epidemiological studies that claim to show an association between various adverse health effects and low concentrations in drinking water, a causal relationship is not very plausible.[19] However, these substances are of concern, and there are very tight standards for drinking water.

The collection and treatment of domestic sewage has been a major contributor to the fight against the spread of human pathogens from faeces, but a number of issues have arisen regarding substances that may also be present in treated waste water discharges to surface water that are also sources of drinking water. Following the identification of intersex in fish in waters receiving treated sewage effluent, investigation showed the presence of natural and synthetic hormones from humans and, in a number of cases, industrial chemicals from cleaning and other products, although these show very low potency as oestrogens. There is very strong evidence that there is only a small chance of endocrine-disrupting chemicals reaching drinking water intakes, and they are removed in the treatment trains commonly employed for such surface waters.[20]

There has also been concern regarding the presence of pharmaceutical residues, again primarily from human excretion. There is currently little evidence of concentrations of concern reaching drinking water, and there is evidence of removal in treatment.[21] Such issues are often a matter of public perception, but the increasing pressure on water resources and the need to consider the reuse of waste water mean that they are of some significance. The key is to reduce their presence in treated waste water, which means that there is a need for new more sophisticated approaches to treatment. Although it is unlikely that this can be introduced rapidly in view of the massive investment required, and there also remains the problem of small communities with limited resources, it is important that progress in developing new approaches is made.

There are many other threats to drinking water quality from industry and the domestic use of chemicals and materials, many of which result from spills of chemicals, either to sewers, which can result in a disabling of the biological processes in waste water treatment, or directly to water sources. Such events are best addressed by prevention and preparedness, which are considered below under 'Drinking water safety plans'.

CHEMICALS ARISING FROM THE USE OF CHEMICALS AND MATERIALS IN WATER SUPPLY

A number of chemicals are used in the drinking water supply, primarily in the treatment of drinking water. These include coagulants, coagulant aids, oxidants and disinfectants. Although these chemicals should be of a standard to prevent the contribution of unwanted contaminants, it is not always possible to achieve this without creating conditions that will compromise treatment. It is, therefore, important to ensure that treatment processes are optimized to minimize the concentrations of unavoidable contaminants. Examples of such chemicals are aluminium and iron salts used as coagulants where the primary issue is preventing the deposition of discoloured sediment in distribution.

There have been a number of studies suggesting a relation between aluminium in drinking water and Alzheimer's disease. While most scientists in the field do not consider that this is causal, due to the data that show a low absorption of aluminium from drinking water and the uncertainties inherent in the epidemiology, it is appropriate to seek to minimize aluminium residuals to minimize the risk of discolouration and to allay public fears. The epidemiology indicates that even in the studies showing a positive association, this is weak and does not continue below a concentration of about 100 μg/L, which can be achieved by large well-run treatment works.[1] The Joint WHO/Food and Agriculture Organization Expert Committee on Food Additives and Contaminants has considered aluminium intake from all sources and has suggested a Provisional Tolerable Weekly Intake of 1 mg/kg body weight, which would equate to a drinking water value of about 400 μg/L (rounded value) assuming a 10 per cent allocation of the tolerable daily intake to drinking water for a 60 kg adult drinking 2 L of water per day.[22] Although there may be a requirement for investment in treatment to improve the capability of the treatment works, there will be additional benefits associated with improved coagulation.

Oxidants are used in treatment to oxidize organic and inorganic chemicals and to disinfect the final water before it enters distribution. These substances can react with naturally occurring organic matter, humic and fulvic acids, and inorganic substances such as bromide, to form a wide range of unwanted by-products. The best studied of the disinfectants is chlorine, which produces a large number of halogenated by-products, mostly at concentrations of less than 1 μg/L but some at much higher concentrations. The dominant groups of substances are the trihalomethanes, of which chloroform is usually, but not always, present at the highest concentration, depending on the bromide present, and the haloacetic acids, of which the di- and trichloro compounds are present at the highest concentrations.

Although there are data from laboratory animal studies showing that some of these chemicals may cause cancer, it is the epidemiological studies that have gained most attention. A number of studies show a weak association between trihalomethanes or chlorination and some cancers, particularly bladder cancer and to a lesser extent colon cancer. Although some substances have been shown to cause colon cancer in laboratory animals at relatively high doses, dosing in drinking water does not appear to be as potent as dosing by gavage in corn oil. The view remains that the data are insufficient to conclude causality. In addition, there are considerable difficulties with assessing the exposure of subjects as this is subject to significant individual variation and long latent periods, confused by a steady decrease in by-product levels over the past 25 years following the introduction of standards.

In addition to concerns over cancer, some epidemiological studies have shown an association between various adverse birth outcomes and trihalomethanes or haloacetic acids. Although there is a good deal of inconsistency between the studies, associations, when found, are weak, and the laboratory animal data do not provide convincing support for a causal relationship between by-products and adverse birth effects, particularly at the relatively low concentrations that are increasingly prevalent in drinking water.[23,24]

Other by-products such as bromate can arise from ozonation or the electrolytic generation of sodium hypochlorite from brine with high bromide levels. Standards have been set, but bromate is reduced in the gastrointestinal tract and by extracellular glutathione so standards set using mathematical models with linear extrapolation are likely to be excessively conservative.[25] Chlorine dioxide produces fewer organic by-products than chlorine but provides little residual disinfection capacity and breaks down to form chlorite and, to a lesser extent, chlorate. The latter also forms in hypochlorite solution that is stored under the wrong conditions or for too long. There are appropriate standards and guidelines for all of these inorganic substances. Chloramine is being increasingly used to provide residual disinfection in distribution as a means of reducing trihalomethanes, which continue to form.[1]

However, if not controlled properly, nitrite can form in distribution, and low levels of n-nitrosodimethylamine have also recently been found in some systems, although these are well below the WHO guideline value of 100 ng/L and even below 10 ng/L.[26]

Materials and chemicals that are used in contact with drinking water may also be a source of contaminants in drinking water. The use of lead as a plumbing material was eventually identified as a significant source of lead exposure in areas in which the water was acidic. As a consequence, significant efforts have been made to replace lead pipes or to treat the water to reduce the ability of the water to dissolve lead. The WHO has set a health-based guideline value of 10 μg/L, which has been widely adopted around the world.[1] This guideline value is designed to protect the most vulnerable section of the population – bottle-fed infants. Lead still gives rise to problems, but this must be set against the overall decrease in lead exposure from all sources and the fall in blood levels in children and adults.

However, the experience with lead highlighted the issue of materials and the need to control contamination from this source. A number of larger countries operate approval schemes for chemicals and materials used in contact with drinking water so that those approved meet stringent specifications. The WHO has also recommended that member states should ensure that such schemes are in place, even if this means using information from other existing schemes.[1]

GUIDELINES AND STANDARDS FOR DRINKING WATER QUALITY

The most important source of information for drinking water standards is the WHO *Guidelines for Drinking Water Quality*,[1] which are regularly revised and updated. These provide a point of departure for national or regional standards, for example the EU, but should be adapted according to local conditions taking into account geographical circumstances, health priorities, costs and other practical considerations. Guidelines are usually non-enforceable, whereas standards established by states are usually legally enforceable.

There may be several objectives in setting guidelines and standards:

- To protect public health, for example related to microbiology or arsenic.
- To ensure that drinking water is acceptable to consumers, although values are normally only incorporated into national standards, because of local variations in what is acceptable, for example iron.
- To provide reassurance to consumers. This may include political or precautionary standards such as the standard of 0.1 μg/L for pesticides in the EU, which is not scientifically based and is not a health-based standard.

- To provide a benchmark for water supply operations, for example pH.
- To provide a benchmark against which to judge compliance with standards.

However, it is important that, whatever the reason for setting a standard, the basis of the standard is clear. There are two associated reasons for this. The first is so that, in the event of a standard being exceeded, there is no confusion for health authorities regarding appropriate action; the second is so that consumers do not become unnecessarily concerned and lose confidence in the water supply.

It is also important to be aware of the methods used to derive health-based values and the conservatism inherent in them. For example, when a proportion of an acceptable or tolerable daily intake is allocated to drinking water, this is often quite conservative if there is only limited information on exposure from other sources. In addition, when a theoretical mathematical model is used to estimate the risks from carcinogens, the figure taken is usually the upper 95 per cent confidence interval on the calculation with actual risks being much lower and potentially zero. This is particularly the case where the actual shape of the dose–response curve is non-linear. Such considerations are of great importance in determining the benefits of a particular value against the costs of achieving it and also the implications of exceeding that value and the actions that should be taken.

Drinking water safety plans

The standard for microbiological safety is zero *Escherichia coli* in a 100 mL sample. This is not a strictly health-based standard because *E. coli* is used as an indicator of faecal contamination and therefore the potential for pathogens to be present. However, the sample size is very small in relation to the supply, and pathogens may clump or be present as a short peak. It is, therefore, important to assess other operational information to ensure that treatment is operating at its optimum. Reliance on the measurement of individual substances or indicators at the tap has been the traditional approach to assuring the safety and acceptability of drinking water. For chemicals, this is reliant on a lengthening list of parameters that must be monitored, often at high cost with little benefit. However, the approach cannot account for all potential contaminants in a practical manner.

The WHO and the International Drinking Water Community have recognized this problem and have called for a change in approach, which is rapidly being adopted as best practice all over the world.[27] The approach – drinking water safety plans – is built around hazard identification, risk assessment and establishing clear management and control of risks from the source to the tap. The approach uses a broad range of tools that include traditional means of assuring safety but also introduces formal operating

systems for demonstrating that the barriers, from pollution control to treatment, through distribution management to the tap, are working efficiently at all times. Drinking water standards and guidelines are an essential tool for assuring the safety and quality of drinking water, and these have developed in response to increasing knowledge about water quality. For large municipal supplies, the guidelines and standards are the main benchmark against which they will be judged, but there are many small supplies with much fewer resources for which different more pragmatic means of assuring safety are required.

REFERENCES

● = Key primary paper

● 1. World Health Organization Guidelines for Drinking-water Quality. Third Edition Incorporating the Second Addendum 2008. Available at: http://www.who.int/water_sanitation_health/dwq/gdwq3rev/en/index.html (accessed July 19, 2009).
2. World Health Organization. *WHO Meeting of Experts on the Possible Protective Effect of Hard Water Against Cardiovascular Disease*. Washington DC, USA, April 27–28, 2006. WHO/SDE/WSH/06.06. Geneva: WHO, 2006.
3. Morris RW, Walker M, Lennon LT, Shaper AG, Whincup PH. Hard drinking water does not protect against cardiovascular disease: new evidence from the British Regional Heart Study. *Eur J Cardiovasc Prev Rehabil* 2008; **15**: 185–9.
4. Catling L, Abubaker I, Lake I, Swift L, Hunter P. Review of Evidence for Relationship Between Incidence of Cardiovascular Disease and Water Hardness. Final Report for Contract DWI/70/2/176, 2005. Available from: http://www.dwi.gov.uk/research/reports/DWI70_2_176_water_hardness.pdf (accessed July 19, 2009).
5. International Program on Chemical Safety. Fluorides. EHC 227. Available from: http://www.inchem.org/documents/ehc/ehc/ehc227.htm (ac cessed July 19, 2009).
6. Fawell J, Bailey K, Chilton J, Dahi E, Fewtrell L, Magara Y. *Fluoride in Drinking-water*. WHO Drinking-water Quality Series. London: IWA Publishing, 2006.
7. National Research Council. *Fluoride in Drinking Water: A Scientific Review of EPA's Standards*. Washington DC: National Academies Press, 2006.
8. Kurttio P, Harmoinen A, Saha H *et al*. Kidney toxicity of ingested uranium from drinking water. *Am J Kidney Dis* 2006; **47**: 972–82.
9. Chorus I, Bartram J. *Toxic Cyanobacteria in Water. A Guide to their Public Health Consequences, Monitoring and Management*. London: E & FN Spon, published on behalf of WHO, 1999.
10. International Program on Chemical Safety. *Boron*. EHC 204. Geneva: WHO, 1998.
11. Dourson M, Maier A, Meek B, Renwick A, Ohanian E, Poirier K. Boron tolerable intake: re-evaluation of

toxicokinetics for data-derived uncertainty factors. *Biol Trace Elem Res* 1998 **66**(1–3): 453–63.

12. UK Expert Group on Vitamins and Minerals. *Revised Review of Boron*. Food Standards Agency EVM/99/23/P. Revised August 2002. London: Food Standards Agency.

13. Fewtrell L. Drinking-water nitrate, methaemoglobinaemia and global burden of disease: a discussion. *Environ Health Perspect* 2004; **112**: 1371–4.

14. Schmoll O, Howard J, Chilton J, Chorus I. *Protecting Ground Water for Health. Managing the Quality of Drinking-water*. Geneva: WHO, co-published with IWA, UK, 2005.

15. Thompson T, Fawell J, Kunikane S *et al. Chemical Safety of Drinking-water: Assessing Priorities for Risk Management*. Geneva: WHO, 2007.

16. World Health Organization. Petroleum Products in Drinking-water. Background Document for Development of WHO *Guidelines for Drinking-water Quality*. Available from: http://www.who.int/water_sanitation_health/dwq/chemicals/Petroleum%20Productsrev071105.pdf (accessed July 19, 2009).

17. Fawell J. MTBE: WHO guidelines and taste and odour issues for drinking water. In: Barceló, D (ed.) *The Handbook of Environmental Chemistry 5-R Water Pollution, Fuel Oxygenates*. Berlin: Springer, 2007.

18. Fraser R. The Burncrooks Enquiry. Report on the Disruption to Public Water Supplies in the Area Served by Burncrooks Waterworks, December 1997. Scottish Office, 1998. Available from: http://www.scotland.gov.uk/library/documents5/burn-00.htm (accessed July 19, 2009).

19. Watson RE, Jacobsen CE, Williams AL, Howard WB, DeSesso JM. Trichloroethylene-contaminated drinking water and congenital heart defects: a critical analysis of the literature. *Reprod Toxicol* 2006; **21**: 117–47.

20. Wenzel A, Müller J, Ternes T. Study on Endocrine Disrupters in Drinking Water. Final Report ENV.D.1/ETU/2000/0083. Available from: http://www.europa.nl/research/endocrine/pdf/drinking_water_en.pdf (accessed July 19, 2009).

21. Watts C, Maycock D, Crane M, Fawell J, Goslan E. Desk Based Review of Current Knowledge on Pharmaceuticals in Drinking Water and Estimation of Potential Levels. DEFRA Project: CSA 7184/WT02046/DWI70/2/213. Available from: http://www.dwi.gov.uk/research/reports/dwi70-2-213.pdf (accessed July 19, 2009).

22. Joint FAO/WHO Expert Committee on Food Additives. *Safety Evaluation of Certain Food Additives and Contaminants*. Sixty-seventh meeting. WHO Food Additives Series No. 58. Geneva: WHO, 2007.

23. International Programme on Chemical Safety. *Disinfectants and Disinfectant By-products*. EHC 216. Geneva: WHO, 2000.

24. Tardiff RG, Carson ML, Ginevan ME. Updated weight of evidence for an association between adverse reproductive and developmental effects and exposure to disinfection by-products. *Regul Toxicol Pharmacol* 2006; **45**: 185–205.

25. Bull RJ, Cotruvo JA. A research strategy to improve risk estimates for bromate in drinking water. *Toxicology* 2006; **221**: 2–3.

26. World Health Organization. N-Nitrosodimethylamine in Drinking-water. Background Document for Development of WHO *Guidelines for Drinking-water Quality*. Available from: http://www.who.int/water_sanitation_health/dwq/chemicals/ndma2ndadd.pdf (accessed July 19, 2009).

27. UK Drinking Water Inspectorate. A Brief Guide to Drinking Water Safety Plans. Available from: http://www.dwi.gov.uk/guidance/Guide%20to%20wsp.pdf (accessed July 19, 2009).

25

Pesticides: herbicides, insecticides and rodenticides

FINLAY D. DICK

PESTICIDE DEFINITION

Pesticides are a diverse group of agents employed to control living organisms that pose health or economic threats. They may be manmade (synthetic) or naturally occurring (biological) and may be active against a narrow (selective) or wide (broad spectrum) range of pests. Some act on contact, whereas others do so systemically. They are often grouped by the pest they control (e.g. insecticides) but may be categorized by chemical structure. For example, insecticides can be categorized as carbamates, organochlorines and so on. Pesticides can be categorized by their acute toxicity using the World Health Organization's publication *The WHO Recommended Classification of Pesticides by Hazard and Guidelines to Classification.*[1] Herbicides are also classed by mode of action[2,3] to guide weed-killer selection when dealing with herbicide resistance.

PESTICIDE USAGE

The US Environmental Protection Agency estimates that the world usage of pesticides in 2001 was around 2.4 billion kilograms of active ingredient, at a cost of $32 billion.[4] The USA accounted for more than a third of world expenditure on pesticides and 20 per cent of pesticide use. Herbicides were the largest category at 37 per cent, with insecticides at 24 per cent and fungicides at 9 per cent.

Pesticides used have changed over time, reflecting cost, efficacy and legislation. Pesticide application has become increasingly sophisticated, with electrostatic spraying,

ultra low-volume applications, the microencapsulation of active ingredients and adjuvants[5] to increase efficacy. Many of the most hazardous pesticides[1] have been banned by developed nations, but in developing countries, where the regulation of import, manufacture, sale and use is less stringent, they may still be used.[6] The insecticide dichlorodiphenyltrichloroethane (DDT) has been banned in most countries, owing to its impact on wildlife, but remains in use in some nations.[7] Organochlorine insecticides have little acute mammalian toxicity but show biopersistence, concentrating in adipose tissues: humans' body burden of these persistent organic pollutants is declining, at least where their use has been banned.[8–10]

Some organic farming accreditation schemes[11,12] permit a very limited use of some, naturally occurring, pesticides or allow their use, on welfare grounds, for animals. The Soil Association estimates that organic farmers use around 2 per cent of the pesticides used in equivalent non-organic enterprises.[13]

Pesticides may be used at all stages of growing crops. Seed dressings are used to prevent fungal infections or to repel animals and birds. Crops may be treated to prevent or treat pests, to modify growth or to desiccate foliage prior to harvest. Crops in storage may be treated to prevent a range of pests. Governments may require that products are fumigated, for example with methyl bromide, to prevent economically important pests and diseases being imported. Some insecticides are used in veterinary practice for the prevention or treatment of insect infestations on farm and companion animals. In addition, some insecticides are used as human medicines to control pests such as head lice or for the vector control of insects. Fungicides, insecticides and rodenticides are employed in buildings to prevent, or treat, mould, insect and rodent infestations, respectively. Pesticides, especially herbicides, are widely used in the amenity sector in parks and on golf courses.

EXPOSURE ROUTES

Pesticide exposure may occur by inhalation, dermal absorption or ingestion. The route of exposure is influenced by the application method, the agent and its formulation. Pesticides can be applied in several ways including spraying using a knapsack sprayer, a vehicle-mounted boom sprayer or a fixed- or rotary-wing aircraft. Although spraying is the most common application method, other approaches include crop-dusting, fogging, irrigation ('chemigation') and soil injection. In confined spaces, such as greenhouses, smoke bombs or candles may be employed. Insect infestations in buildings may be treated by applying pesticides to the cracks and crevices where insects hide. For those pesticides used on animals, plunge-dipping, showering, drenching (the oral administration of veterinary medicines) or pour-on treatments may be employed.

Inhalation is the primary route of exposure, especially for volatile or semi-volatile agents, but some pesticides show significant dermal absorption: for organophosphorous pesticides, this is the primary route of exposure. Mass poisonings have occurred due to pesticide-contaminated clothing and cosmetics. In 1981, warfarin-contaminated talcum powder caused acute haemorrhages in 741 Vietnamese children, of whom 177 died.[14] The ingestion of pesticides can occur due to hand-to-mouth transfer following dermal exposure, mouthing behaviour in young children, intentional ingestion with suicidal intent and the ingestion of pesticide-contaminated foodstuffs or water.

Suicide by pesticide ingestion is underascertained, but estimates suggest that more than 250 000 people take their own life each year in this way, representing a third of all suicides worldwide.[15] The global pattern of suicide using pesticides does not reflect pesticide usage but rather the proportion of the populace with ready access to them, so it is in the rural areas of developing countries where the problem is greatest. Measures such as banning the most hazardous pesticides[16] and providing secure pesticide storage boxes for farmers can reduce this burden.[17]

Exposure can occur at any stage in the manufacture, transport, distribution, application or disposal of pesticides: occupational groups are generally at greatest risk. Non-occupational exposures typically occur due to dietary intake or the domestic[18] or hobby use of pesticides. However, in addition to these exposure pathways, the public may be exposed to take-home contamination, by-stander/residential exposure from agricultural spraying, environmental contamination around housing, contamination of water, accidental release of pesticides (or precursors) during manufacture, distribution[19] or use.

Pesticide contamination of foodstuffs can occur by four mechanisms:[14]

1. contamination while in storage or transport;
2. the diversion of pesticide-dressed seeds to food;
3. the accidental use of pesticides in foods;
4. the inappropriate or illegal use of pesticides on food crops.[6,14]

Food contamination in storage can occur when pesticides and foodstuffs are stored or transported together. International regulations govern the transport of such hazardous substances, but in developing countries with limited literacy, weak regulation and poor enforcement such events still occur. A survey of 258 farmers in one Chinese region found that 25 per cent had purchased pesticides from food retailers who were not licensed pesticide vendors.[20] Such practices create the potential to contaminate foodstuffs if pesticide containers leak during storage.

Pesticide-treated seeds can result in episodes of mass poisoning where the original seeds were intended for planting or as poison bait, but were diverted for human consumption.[14] One incident in Iraq led to over 5000 hospital admissions and 280 deaths due to methyl mercury poisoning from fungicide-treated wheat.[21] An epidemic of porphyria cutanea tarda occurred in south-eastern Turkey from 1955 to 1957 when wheat treated with the fungicide hexachlorobenzene was diverted to food use, poisoning around 4000 people. Between 1000 and 2000 children died, leading to the loss of a generation of children in some villages.[22]

Direct food contamination may occur due to the incorrect labelling or packing of pesticides as foods, or the inappropriate storage of usually granular or crystalline pesticides, such as barium carbonate (a rodenticide), in kitchens, with subsequent confusion with foods such as salt (see also Chapter 22, p. 259).[14]

Illegal use on food crops

Where pesticide withdrawal periods (the minimum safe intervals between application and harvest) are not observed, residues may remain on crops, in milk or in meat. Poisonings have occurred following unlicensed applications such as spraying aldicarb on water melons, which absorb it into their flesh so poisoning the consumer.[14] Developed countries monitor pesticide residues in foods to ensure that they do not exceed the maximum permissible residue levels, but the situation may be very different in developing countries, with some foods exceeding these limits.[6]

Accidental exposure in the home

Many households use pesticides,[18,23,24] so creating the potential for domestic exposure. If kept in leaking or damaged packages[25] or in inappropriate containers such as lemonade bottles,[26] they may be both accessible and attractive to children. Where pesticides are applied in the home, infants may be preferentially exposed owing to their extended time at home and their behaviour, motor development, activity levels and physiological factors (high respiratory rate and high metabolic rate).[27,28] Toddlers exhibit behaviours such as mouthing,[29] leading to a greater exposure to environmental contaminants than in older children.[30] Children may be exposed to garden pesticides indoors, as well as outdoors, due to the transport indoors of lawn pesticides on shoes and pets: a 'no shoes in the house' policy reduces indoor contamination.[31] Children living in poverty may experience greater exposure owing to poor-quality housing and the frequent use of legal and illegal pesticides.[32]

Take-home contamination

Take-home contamination may lead to occupationally exposed workers contaminating their vehicles[33,34] and homes with pesticides.[35] Several studies have found that the children of agricultural workers have higher pesticide levels than other children.[34,36–38] A study in El Salvador found that living with a farmer who had used methyl parathion (a World Health Organization class IA toxicity pesticide, i.e. extremely hazardous) in the previous fortnight was associated with acute symptoms, independent of whether the individual themselves worked in agriculture. Whether this reflected take-home contamination, environmental contamination around the home, water contamination or multiple exposure pathways was unclear.[39] A study in rural Washington state found that children's urinary organophosphorous metabolites fluctuated with seasonal agricultural spraying independent of parental occupation.[40]

Exposure to spray drift

Children may be exposed to pesticides owing to their use in schools[41] or, less commonly, from spray drift from adjacent farms.[41,42] An analysis of three pesticide surveillance schemes in the USA between 1998 and 2002 found that 2593 people developed acute illnesses following pesticide exposure in schools (including 830 cases due to exposure to disinfectants), with an annual incidence of 7.4 cases per million children.[41] Adults can also be exposed in the same way. This is likely to be an underestimate given the known underreporting to these schemes.

Accidents

The public and workers may be exposed to pesticides following chemical incidents. The worst such disaster happened in Bhopal, Madhya Pradesh, in central India in the early hours of December 3rd, 1984. A pesticides plant, operated by a subsidiary of the Union Carbide Company, released a toxic gas cloud, containing methyl isocyanate, following a run-away exothermic reaction.[43] Between 100 000 and 200 000 people were exposed to the toxic plume, which spread over 40 square kilometres.[44] Estimates of deaths vary,[44,45] but at least 3800 people lost their lives[43] and 15 000 were injured.[44] Studies of long-term health effects have been limited, but survivors suffer eye, throat and chest problems, reproductive difficulties and neurodevelopmental problems.[43]

Another major pesticide release occurred near Mount Shasta, northern California, USA, on the night of July 14th, 1991 when a freight train derailment released 19 000 gallons of the pesticide metam sodium into the Sacramento River.[19] Nearby residents reported respiratory irritation and some developed reactive airways dysfunction syndrome. Fire in pesticide stores, although rare, can affect emergency personnel and residents. On May 31st, 1986, the village of Canning, Nova Scotia,[46] was evacuated after fire destroyed an agricultural store containing pesticides. Water used to control the blaze polluted nearby watercourses with 1.2 million litres of pesticide-contaminated water. Firemen, policemen and a local resident required hospital treatment. The village was evacuated for 6 days, and the site required a month-long decontamination.

Environmental contamination

Environmental contamination from pesticides can occur due to spills during storage or mixing, overspray, spray drift, off-gassing, run-off into watercourses, leaching into groundwaters or inappropriate disposal. Pesticide contamination may thus affect the air,[42,47] water[48–50] and soil,[51] with exchange between these media.

The inappropriate storage of pesticides occurs in both developed[26,52] and developing[6,53–55] countries. In one South African survey,[54] 67 per cent of farm pesticide stores had pesticide contaminated floors. The inappropriate location of stores near wells, streams and ponds or in low-lying areas vulnerable to flooding can threaten water supplies.

During pesticide-mixing, spills can occur if the spray tank is overfilled, thus contaminating soil and groundwater.[56] One measure to reduce environmental contamination from such on-farm sources is the bio-bed: a grass-covered pit filled with straw, peat and soil above a layer of clay with a gravel base. The tractor and sprayer are reversed over the bio-bed, and tank-filling and washing are then carried out. Such pits capture effluent, preventing water contamination.[57] 'Back-siphoning' occurs where the pesticide mixing tank is above the water source, so contaminating the water supply when the water is turned off and the dilute pesticide is drawn back into the water supply. Similar problems may arise during chemical irrigation unless an antisiphon device is employed.

Overspray occurs during aerial spraying when spraying extends beyond the intended spray zone. Spray drift can contaminate the air, fields and nearby habitations: this is one source of diffuse contamination of water courses.[50] A well-maintained sprayer used by an operator who observes guidance on 'no-spray' buffer zones[58] adjacent to field margins, watercourses and habitations and who avoids spraying in windy conditions should minimize such occurrences. Hedges and broad-leaved trees reduce spray drift and run-off entering surface waters. Spray drift can affect human health, although UK data[26] suggest that, unlike in some countries, such events are rarely associated with hospital admissions. Leachate can contaminate groundwater: soil type and underlying geology influence leaching. Factors that increase leaching include a high water table, sandy soil, soil with a low organic content, soil macropores[51] and underlying rock fractures.[59]

Most pesticide sprayed on crops falls on soil or is lost as run-off, with as little as 1 per cent of pesticide reaching the intended site.[5] Pesticide run-off is increased by rain,[50,60] irrigation after spraying or the combination of relatively impermeable soil (evident by a tendency to puddle in heavy rain) and rain flushing pesticides into drains. The contamination of water supplies with pesticides[6,48–50,61] is well described, sometimes exceeding published limits.[6,49]

Volatile pesticides, such as the fumigant methyl bromide, vaporize after application,[47] with sometimes tragic consequences. Methyl bromide vapour can seep into sewers and conduits, fatally poisoning neighbouring residents.[62,63] An alternative soil fumigant, metam sodium, breaks down to methyl isothiocyanate,[64] and although this is less volatile than methyl bromide, off-gassing has poisoned humans.[65] Methyl bromide is to be withdrawn under the Montreal protocol owing to its ozone-depleting effects, although some countries wish to retain it, for example for strawberry-growing in California.[66] Measures to reduce the release of soil fumigants include deep soil injection, covering treated soil with impermeable plastics, soil compaction and water irrigation.[64]

STORAGE AND DISPOSAL OF PESTICIDES

The United Nation's Food and Agriculture Organization estimates that developing nations hold 500 000 tonnes of obsolete pesticides[53] that have passed their expiry date, are now banned or are no longer required. Their disposal is challenging as many stocks are in poor condition, are in leaking containers, and have contaminated surrounding soils.[54,55] Similar issues with obsolete or illegal pesticides stored on farms have been identified in developed countries.[52]

The ill-advised disposal of waste pesticide, for example by burying concentrates on farms, can lead to environmental contamination.[52] Discarded pesticide containers have led to poisoning in developing countries where robust containers are prized and contaminated pesticide containers may be reused for water or foods.[14] The Food and Agriculture Organization has run an obsolete pesticide disposal programme in Africa and the Middle East for a number of years, but by 2006 only 3000 tonnes had been destroyed, mostly by high-temperature incineration in European waste facilities. A cheaper approach is disposal by high-temperature incineration in cement kilns, which exist in many developing countries. Experiments have shown proof of concept, and this seems a promising alternative to specialized waste incinerators.[67]

The environmental fate of pesticide varies depending on both the pesticide's chemistry and the soil to which it is applied. Some pesticides, such as the organochlorines, are biopersistent so have fallen out of favour. In contrast, some pesticides are inactivated on contact with soil, are metabolized by soil microorganisms[59] or degrade on exposure to sunshine, thus reducing their potential for environmental contamination.

HEALTH EFFECTS

Pesticides may produce acute or chronic health effects owing to their active ingredients or to adjuvants. Concerns have been raised regarding the toxicity of adjuvants, which, in some countries, are not declared on pesticide labels.[68] Advice on the recognition and management of pesticide poisoning has been produced by the US Environmental Protection Agency and is available online.[69]

Acute effects

Acute poisoning following environmental exposure to some pesticides is well recognized. There are few established antidotes: hospital fatality rates for organophosphorous poisoning exceed 10 per cent, and over 50 per cent for poisoning with paraquat or the rodenticide aluminium phosphide.[70] Organophosphorous pesticides show acute toxicity, and the management of such poisonings has been reviewed.[71] Organophosphorous pesticides inhibit the enzyme acetylcholinesterase, preventing postsynaptic breakdown of acetylcholine. Acetylcholinesterase reactivation may occur spontaneously or following the early administration of pralidoxime. Over several hours, 'ageing' of the enzyme may occur due to irreversible binding, rendering oximes ineffective.

The signs and symptoms of acute organophosphorous intoxication are due to muscarinic (miosis, lacrimation, salivation, bronchorrhoea, bronchospasm, vomiting, diarrhoea, urinary frequency, bradycardia and hypotension), nicotinic (hypertension, tachycardia, mydriasis, fasciculation and muscle weakness) and central nervous system effects (confusion, seizures and respiratory depression). The diagnosis can be confirmed by measuring plasma butyrylcholinesterase or red cell acetylcholinesterase activity, but this rarely influences acute management.[71] Treatment includes resuscitation, fluids, oxygen, atropine (to reverse the muscarinic effects), pralidoxime and diazepam (for seizures), but optimal therapy has yet to be established.[71]

The intermediate syndrome[72] develops 24–96 hours after exposure to organophosphorous pesticides, giving proximal muscle weakness and cranial nerve palsies: death may occur due to respiratory paralysis. Organophosphorous-induced delayed neuropathy[73] occurs 1–3 weeks after exposure to organophosphorous pesticides, such as tri-ortho-cresyl phosphate, which inhibit neuropathy target esterase. It is characterized by paraesthesia, distal muscle wasting, ataxia and spasticity.

Young children, especially boys under 5 years of age, account for half of non-intentional pesticide poisonings in some case series.[28] An American study found that, in the period 1993–95, 7434 children aged under 6 years were exposed to pesticides: most showed no ill effects, and there were no deaths.[74] Measures to reduce this burden include improved packaging, substitution with less toxic agents and reduced concentrations of the active ingredient.

Chronic effects

Chronic health effects that some have linked to pesticides include neurodevelopmental effects, cancer, reproductive effects, congenital malformations (hypospadias and cryptorchidism), asthma and Parkinson's disease. Studies of such outcomes are difficult, particularly in terms of exposure assessment, as most pesticides lack long-term biomarkers of exposure. Organochlorines are an exception, and researchers have measured organochlorines in serum, adipose tissue, hair, breast milk, umbilical cord serum, umbilical cord and meconium. Organochlorine levels in maternal serum, umbilical cord serum and umbilical cord (without blood) are correlated, but some argue that the most sensitive measure for determining fetal organochlorine exposure is umbilical cord.[75] Lactation and weight loss increase the elimination of organochlorines in adults.[76]

Many studies have retrospectively assessed pesticide exposure, with the risk of recall bias. Weaknesses in exposure estimation are evident, with some inferring exposure on the basis of occupation and others using low-quality exposure metrics. Some have undertaken multiple analyses, thus increasing the likelihood of identifying spurious associations.

NEURODEVELOPMENTAL DELAY

Antenatal or childhood pesticide exposures may have adverse effects on neurodevelopment.[32] One review[77] concluded that there was some evidence of an association between neurodevelopmental problems and exposure to organophosphorous pesticides, although the evidence for organochlorines was less consistent. Some studies of prenatal exposure to organophosphorous pesticides have found an association with abnormal reflexes at birth[78] or neurodevelopmental problems.[79–81] Others have found associations between neurodevelopmental delay and prenatal exposure to DDT or its main metabolite 2,2-bis(p-chlorophenyl)-1,1-dichloroethylene (DDE).[82–84] Impaired social behaviour in children has been linked to hexachlorobenzene exposures in utero.[85] Nonetheless, whatever the DDT level at birth, subsequent breast-feeding is beneficial for children (see also Chapter 23).[83,86]

CANCER

Cancers which have been linked with pesticide exposures include brain cancer, breast cancer, prostate cancer, testicular cancer, leukaemia and lymphoma. Several meta-analyses have explored these effects,[87–90] but most examined heavily exposed occupational groups, although some studied environmentally exposed groups.[91,92] Teitelbaum[93] has reviewed the exposure assessments used in these studies and the many difficulties in retrospective assessment, including information bias, recall bias and exposure misclassification.

BRAIN CANCER

Brain cancer has been linked to farming: the authors of one meta-analysis (33 studies) concluded that, although there was evidence of a positive association between farming and brain cancer, the associations were weak.[94] Whether this association relates to pesticides or other agricultural exposures, such as animal viruses, is unclear. Some studies[92,95–100] suggest that the offspring of exposed parents are at a modestly increased risk of brain tumours,[101] although other studies do not.[102,103] Although there is limited evidence of an association between pesticide exposure and childhood brain tumours, the possibility of recall bias must be borne in mind when interpreting these findings.

BREAST CANCER

The association between pesticide exposure and breast cancer has been extensively studied due to concerns regarding the weak oestrogenic effects of organochlorine pesticides.[104] By the 1990s, several small case–control studies had suggested an association between organochlorine levels and breast cancer. In 1993, a nested case–control study set within the New York University Women's Health study found a significant association between DDE and breast cancer, with a 4-fold increase in relative risk between the 10th and 90th percentile of serum DDE concentration.[105] However, most subsequent studies failed to confirm this association,[106–116] and a meta-analysis[87] concluded that there was no association between DDE and breast cancer risk. Thus, despite early concerns that organochlorine pesticides were associated with breast cancer, the weight of evidence does not support this association.[117]

PROSTATE CANCER

There is some evidence for an association between pesticides and prostate cancer, but it is inconclusive and largely relates to occupational rather than environmental exposure.[118,119]

TESTICULAR CANCER

The incidence of testicular cancer has been rising in Western countries, although the cause is unknown. One case–control study found elevated levels of hexachlorobenzene and chlordanes in the mothers of men with testicular cancer.[120] A case–control study of 754 men with seminoma or teratoma found that p,p'-DDE levels were associated with these tumours.[121] These observations require further study.

LEUKAEMIA, LYMPHOMAS AND MULTIPLE MYELOMA

The incidence of non-Hodgkin's lymphoma increased in the second half of the twentieth century, and some linked this to persistent organic pollutants such as chlorophenols.[89] No association was found between residential herbicide use and non-Hodgkin's lymphoma in one study.[122] However, non-Hodgkin's lymphoma in children has been associated with their mother's domestic pesticide use.[123] The Northern California Childhood Leukaemia Study found that the use of professional pest treatments 1 year before and up to 3 years after birth was associated with childhood leukaemia (odds ratio [OR] 2.8, 95 per cent confidence interval [CI] 1.4–5.7).[124] A French case–control study[125] found that maternal pesticide use was associated with an increased risk of acute leukaemia. A study of children with Down syndrome found that maternal pesticide exposure was significantly associated with acute lymphoblastic leukaemia in the child.[126] Insecticidal shampoos containing pyrethroids have been associated with leukaemia.[125]

A meta-analysis of occupational exposure to pesticides and haematopoietic cancers found significantly increased odds ratios for non-Hodgkin's lymphoma [OR 1.35, 95 per cent CI 1.2–1.5] and non-significantly increased odds for leukaemia [OR 1.35, 95 per cent CI 0.9–2.0] and multiple myeloma [OR 1.16, 95 per cent CI 0.99–1.36].[89] These were case–control studies, and the possibility of recall bias must be considered.[127,128]

REPRODUCTIVE EFFECTS

A systematic review of pesticide effects on human sperm[129] concluded that the evidence suggested an effect on sperm quality. However, methodological weaknesses were identified in some studies, including low-quality exposure assessment, small sample size and a failure to control for confounders. The insecticides fenvalerate (a pyrethroid) and carbaryl (a carbamate) were associated with adverse effects on sperm in five studies.[130] Few studies examined environmentally exposed men, and the evidence for this weak association largely relates to occupational exposures.

Pesticides have been linked to hypospadias and cryptorchidism, but the evidence is inconclusive.[130–135] An American case–control study of hypospadias, cryptorchidism and maternal serum DDT and DDE found no association despite this cohort being recruited during 1959–67 when DDT use was high.[130] A criticism of this study is that breast milk is a better index of infants' exposure to organochlorine pesticides than maternal serum. A Dutch case–control study found that paternal pesticide exposure was associated with hypospadias in sons.[134] A prospective study[132] examined breast milk DDE and cryptorchidism and found a non-significant trend (OR 2.16, 95 per cent CI 0.94–4.98). Similar results were reported in a prospective study which found that 17 of 22 organochlorine pesticides analysed were elevated in the breast milk of mothers whose sons had cryptorchidism when compared with the mothers of healthy boys.[133] A Spanish study found significant associations between placental organochlorines (o,p'-DDT, p,p'-DDT, lindane, mirex and endosulfan alpha) and male urogenital malformations.[135] In contrast, an Italian case–control study found little evidence of an association between parental exposure to endocrine disruptors (including pesticides) and hypospadias or cryptorchidism.[131]

Maternal DDE and its association with time to pregnancy has been studied, with inconsistent results, although on balance they do not support an important association.[136, 137] A retrospective cohort study of women poisoned by the consumption of hexachlorobenzene-treated wheat found an association between serum hexachlorobenzene and an increased risk of spontaneous abortion.[22] A retrospective survey of the risk of stillbirth from occupational and residential exposures, set in California, found an association between women's third-trimester residential pesticide exposure and stillbirth (OR 1.7, 95 per cent CI 1.0–2.9).[138] An Australian study[139] found no association between low-level maternal DDT and DDE and any reproductive outcomes. There is little evidence of adverse effects of pesticides on reproduction except among women heavily exposed to hexachlorobenzene.

RESPIRATORY EFFECTS

Children's exposure to organochlorines, in utero or from breast milk, may be associated with asthma. A German study[140] that examined breast-feeding and serum DDE in 7–8-year-old children found that the protective effect of breast-feeding on asthma was attenuated in children with the highest DDE levels. A Spanish study[141] found that DDE levels in cord serum, among children in the highest quartile of exposure, were significantly associated with wheezing when aged 4 years (relative risk 2.63, 95 per cent CI 1.19–4.69). Although other studies are both negative and positive for asthma or respiratory symptoms, the balance points towards an association with exacerbation of pre-existing disease or possibly initiation.

PARKINSON'S DISEASE

Pesticide exposures have been linked to Parkinson's disease in case–control and cohort studies.[142] A meta-analysis[143] of 19 case–control studies of Parkinson's disease and pesticide exposure found a combined OR of 1.94 with 95 per cent CI of 1.49–2.53. A US cohort study[144] of over 140 000 individuals found an increased relative risk of Parkinson's disease among pesticide-exposed individuals (relative risk 1.7, 95 per cent CI 1.2–2.3). Which pesticides are responsible is not known, but paraquat, organochlorine, organophosphorous and carbamate pesticides have all been implicated.[145] Much of the evidence draws on data from occupational groups, but rural residence and well-water use (factors likely to be surrogates for pesticide exposure) have also been associated with Parkinson's disease.

In summary, acute health effects due to environmental exposure to some pesticides, such as organophosphorous insecticides and soil fumigants, are well established. The evidence that environmental exposure to these and other agents is associated with long-term health effects such as cancer is less consistent. This uncertainty, in part, reflects the many difficulties in undertaking such studies. There is strong evidence that organochlorine insecticides are not associated with breast cancer. There is some evidence suggestive of associations between pesticide use and neurodevelopmental problems, childhood cancers, haematopoietic cancers, hypospadias and cryptorchidism, reduced sperm quality and childhood asthma. These associations are based on limited data, and further studies are required to confirm these observations. The association between pesticides and Parkinson's disease is well established, but which agents are responsible for this association is unknown.

REFERENCES

● = Key primary paper
◆ = Major review article

1. World Health Organization. *The WHO Recommended Classification of Pesticides by Hazard and Guidelines to Classification: 2004.* Geneva: World Health Organization, 2005.
2. Herbicide Resistance Action Committee. Classification of Herbicides According to Mode of Action. Available from: http://www.plantprotection.org/HRAC/ (accessed August 7, 2008).
3. Mallory-Smith CA, Retzinger EJ. Revised classification of herbicides by site of action for weed resistance management strategies. *Weed Technol* 2003; **17**: 605–19.
4. Kiehly T, Donaldson D, Grube A *et al. Pesticide Industry Sales and Usage: 2000 and 2001 Market Estimates.* Washington, DC: US Environmental Protection Agency, 2004.
5. Faers MA, Pontzen R. Factors influencing the association between active ingredient and adjuvant in the leaf deposit of adjuvant-containing suspoemulsion formulations. *Pest Manag Sci* 2008; **64**: 820–33.
6. Tariq MI, Afzal S, Hussain I, Sultana N. Pesticides exposure in Pakistan: a review. *Environ Int* 2007; **33**: 1107–22.
7. Turusov V, Rakitsky V, Tomatis L. Dichlorodiphenyl-trichloroethane (DDT): ubiquity, persistence and risks. *Environ Health Perspect* 2002; **110**: 125–8.
8. Smith D. Worldwide trends in DDT levels in human breast milk. *Int J Epidemiol* 1999; **28**: 179–88.
9. Dallaire F, Dewailly E, Laliberté C *et al.* Temporal trends of organochlorine concentrations in umbilical cord blood of newborns from the lower north shore of the St. Lawrence river (Québec, Canada). *Environ Health Perspect* 2002; **110**: 835–8.
10. Lackmann GM. Neonatal serum *p,p'*-DDE concentrations in Germany: chronological changes during the past 20 years and proposed tolerance level. *Paediatr Perinat Epidemiol* 2005; **19**: 31–5.
11. US Department of Agriculture National Organic Program. National List of Allowed and Prohibited Substances. Available from: http://www.ams.usda.gov/AMSv1.0/getfile?dDocName=STELPRDC5068682&acct=nopgeninfo (accessed December 11, 2008).
12. Soil Association. Soil Association Organic Standards, Revision 16. Available from: http://92.52.112.178/web/sacert/sacertweb.nsf/e8c12cf77637ec6c80256a6900374463/4d7054234b8da20a8025740b0012f83f/$FILE/ATTW3W7S/Soil%20Association%20Organic%20Standards%20for%20Producers%202009.pdf (accessed July 19, 2009).
13. Soil Association. Pesticides and Organic Farming – a Last Resort. Information sheet. Available from: http://92.52.112.178/web/sa/saweb.nsf/89d058cc4dbeb16d80256a73005a2866/cd9bd47fbe5715bc802573100034f97e?OpenDocument (accessed July 19, 2009).
14. Ferrer A, Cabral R. Recent epidemics of poisoning by pesticides. *Toxicol Lett* 1995; **82/83**: 55–63.
◆15. Gunnell D, Eddleston M, Phillips MR, Konradsen F. The global distribution of fatal pesticide self-poisoning: systematic review. *BMC Public Health* 2007; **7**: 357.
16. Eddleston M, Karalliedde L, Buckley N *et al.* Pesticide poisoning in the developing world – a minimum pesticides list. *Lancet* 2002; **360**: 1163–7.

17. Konradsen F, Pieris R, Weerasinghe M et al. Community uptake of safe storage boxes to reduce self-poisoning from pesticides in rural Sri Lanka. BMC Public Health 2007; 7: 13.

18. Berkowitz GS, Obel J, Deych E et al. Exposure to indoor pesticides during pregnancy in a multiethnic, urban cohort. Environ Health Perspect 2003; 111: 79–84.

19. Cone JE, Wugofski L, Balmes JR et al. Persistent respiratory health effects after a metam sodium pesticide spill. Chest 1994; 106: 500–8.

20. Zhang H, Lu Y. End-users' knowledge, attitude, and behaviour towards safe use of pesticides: a case study in the Guanting Reservoir area, China. Environ Geochem Health 2007; 29: 513–20.

21. Damluji SF, Tikriti S. Mercury poisoning from wheat. BMJ 1972; 1: 804.

22. Jarrell J, Gocmen A, Foster W et al. Evaluation of reproductive outcomes in women inadvertently exposed to hexachlorobenzene in southeastern Turkey in the 1950s. Reprod Toxicol 1998; 12: 469–76.

23. Bouvier G, Blanchard O, Momas I, Seta N. Pesticide exposure of non-occupationally exposed subjects compared to some occupational exposure: a French pilot study. Sci Total Environ 2006; 366: 74–91.

24. Grey CN, Nieuwenhuijsen MJ, Golding J; ALSPAC Team. Use and storage of domestic pesticides in the UK. Sci Total Environ 2006; 368: 465–70.

25. Robbins AL, James CF, Nash DF, Ruark HE. Poisoning involving improperly stored parathion. West J Med 1977; 126: 231–3.

26. Leverton K, Cox V, Battershill J, Coggon D. Hospital admission for accidental pesticide poisoning among adults of working age in England, 1998–2003. Clin Toxicol (Phila) 2007; 45: 594–7.

27. Cohen Hubal EA, Sheldon LS, Burke JM et al. Children's exposure assessment: a review of factors influencing children's exposure, and the data available to characterize and assess that exposure. Environ Health Perspect 2000; 108: 475–86.

28. Garry VF. Pesticides and children. Toxicol Appl Pharmacol 2004; 198: 152–63.

29. Tulve NS, Suggs JC, McCurdy T et al. Frequency of mouthing behavior in young children. J Expo Anal Environ Epidemiol 2002; 12: 259–64.

30. Freeman NC, Jimenez M, Reed KJ et al. Quantitative analysis of children's microactivity patterns: the Minnesota Children's Pesticide Exposure Study. J Expo Anal Environ Epidemiol 2001; 11: 501–9.

31. Nishioka MG, Lewis RG, Brinkman MC et al. Distribution of 2,4-D in air and on surfaces inside residences after lawn applications: comparing exposure estimates from various media for young children. Environ Health Perspect 2001; 109: 1185–91.

32. Landrigan PJ, Claudio L, Markowitz SB et al. Pesticides and inner city children: exposures, risks and prevention. Environ Health Perspect 1999; 107(Suppl. 3): 431–7.

33. Curl CL, Fenske RA, Kissel JC et al. Evaluation of take-home organophosphorus pesticide exposure among agricultural workers and their children. Environ Health Perspect 2002; 110: A787–92.

34. Coronado GD, Vigoren EM, Thompson B et al. Organophosphate pesticide exposure and work in pome fruit: evidence for the take-home pesticide pathway. Environ Health Perspect 2006; 114: 999–1006.

35. Curwin BD, Hein MJ, Sanderson WT et al. Pesticide contamination inside farm and nonfarm homes. J Occup Environ Hyg 2005; 2: 357–67.

36. Loewenherz C, Fenske RA, Simcox NJ et al. Biological monitoring of organophosphorus pesticide exposure among children of agricultural workers in central Washington State. Environ Health Perspect 1997; 105: 1344–53.

37. Lu C, Fenske RA, Simcox NJ, Kalman D. Pesticide exposure of children in an agricultural community: evidence of household proximity to farmland and take home exposure pathways. Environ Res 2000; 84: 290–302.

38. Curwin BD, Hein MJ, Sanderson WT et al. Pesticide dose estimates for children of Iowa farmers and non-farmers. Environ Res 2007; 105: 307–15.

39. Azaroff LS, Neas LM. Acute health effects associated with nonoccupational pesticide exposure in rural El Salvador. Environ Res 1999; 80: 158–64.

40. Koch D, Lu C, Fisker-Andersen J et al. Temporal association of children's pesticide exposure and agricultural spraying: report of a longitudinal biological monitoring study. Environ Health Perspect 2002; 110: 829–33.

41. Alarcon WA, Calvert GM, Blondell JM et al. Acute illnesses associated with pesticide exposure at schools. JAMA 2005; 294: 455–65.

42. Kawahara J, Horikoshi R, Yamaguchi T et al. Air pollution and young children's inhalation exposure to organophosphorus pesticide in an agricultural community in Japan. Environ Int 2005; 31: 1123–32.

43. Broughton E. The Bhopal disaster and its aftermath: a review. Environ Health 2005; 4: 6.

44. Bhopal Working Group. The public health implications of the Bhopal disaster. Report to the Program Development Board, American Public Health Association. Am J Public Health 1987; 77: 230–6.

45. Gupta PK. Pesticide exposure – Indian scene. Toxicology 2004; 198: 83–90.

46. Environment Canada. Environmental Emergencies. Pesticide Warehouse Fire. Available from: http://www.ec.gc.ca/ee-ue/default.asp?lang=en&n=532CB16E (accessed December 18, 2008).

47. Lee S, McLaughlin R, Harnly M et al. Community exposures to airborne agricultural pesticides in California: ranking of inhalation risks. Environ Health Perspect 2002; 110: 1175–84.

48. Tariq MI, Afzal S, Hussain I. Pesticides in shallow groundwater of Bahawalnagar, Muzafargarh, D.G. Khan

and Rajan Pur districts of Punjab, Pakistan. *Environ Int* 2004; **30**: 471–9.

49. Leong KH, Tan LLB, Mustafa AM. Contamination levels of selected organochlorine and organophosphate pesticides in the Selangor River, Malaysia between 2002 and 2003. *Chemosphere* 2007; **66**: 1153–9.

50. Donald DB, Cessna AJ, Sverko E, Glozier NE. Pesticides in surface drinking-water supplies of the northern Great Plains. *Environ Health Perspect* 2007; **115**: 1183–91.

51. Kjaer J, Olsen P, Ullum M, Grant R. Leaching of glyphosate and amino-methylphosphonic acid from Danish agricultural field sites. *J Environ Qual* 2005; **34**: 608–20.

52. Slingerland DT, May E, Miles M, Church L. Reclamation of pesticides in New York State. *Am J Ind Med* 2002; (Suppl 2): 43–8.

53. Food and Agriculture Organization. Baseline Study on the Problem of Obsolete Pesticide Stocks. FAP Pesticide Disposal Series N.9. Available from: http://www.fao.org/DOCREP/003/X8639E/x8639e01.htm#P131_1808 (accessed December 18, 2008).

54. Aquiel Davie M, Africa A, London L. Disposal of unwanted pesticides in Stellenbosch, South Africa. *Sci Total Environ* 2006; **361**: 8–17.

55. Haylamicheal ID, Dalvie MA. Disposal of obsolete pesticides, the case of Ethiopia. *Environ Int* 2009; **35**: 667–73.

56. Helweg A, Bay H, Hansen HPB et al. Pollution at and below sites used for mixing and loading of pesticides. *Int J Environ Anal Chem* 2002; **82**: 583–90.

57. Pilar Castillo M del, Torstensson L, Stenström J. Biobeds for environmental protection from pesticide use – a review. *J Agric Food Chem* 2008; **56**: 6206–19.

58. Woods N, Craig IP, Dorr G, Young B. Spray drift of pesticides arising from aerial application in cotton. *J Environ Qual* 2001; **30**: 697–701.

59. Borggaard OK, Gimsing AL. Fate of glyphosate in soil and the possibility of leaching to ground and surface waters: a review. *Pest Manag Sci* 2008; **64**: 441–56.

60. Potter TL, Truman CC, Bosch DD, Bednarz CW. Cotton defoliant runoff as a function of active ingredient and tillage. *J Environ Qual* 2003; **32**: 2180–8.

61. Gao J, Liu L, Liu X et al. The occurrence and spatial distribution of organophosphorous pesticides in Chinese surface water. *Bull Environ Contam Toxicol* 2009; **82**: 223–9.

62. Langård S, Rognum T, Fløtterød O, Skaug V. Fatal accident resulting from methyl bromide poisoning after fumigation of a neighbouring house: leakage through sewage pipes. *J Appl Toxicol* 1996; **16**: 445–8.

63. Horowitz BZ, Albertson TE, O'Malley M, Swenson EJ. An unusual exposure to methyl bromide leading to fatality. *J Toxicol Clin Toxicol* 1998; **36**: 353–7.

64. Li LY, Barry T, Mongar K, Wofford P. Modeling methyl isothiocyanate soil flux and emission ratio from a field following a chemigation of metam-sodium. *J Environ Qual* 2006; **35**: 707–13.

65. O'Malley M, Barry T, Verder-Carlos M, Rubin A. Modeling of methyl isothiocyanate air concentrations associated with community illnesses following a metam-sodium sprinkler application. *Am J Ind Med* 2004; **46**: 1–15.

66. Norman CS. Potential impacts of imposing methyl bromide phaseout on US strawberry growers: a case study of a nomination for a critical use exemption under the Montreal Protocol. *J Environ Manage* 2005; **75**: 167–76.

67. Karstensen KH, Kinh NK, Thang LB et al. Environmentally sound destruction of obsolete pesticides in developing countries using cement kilns. *Environ Sci Policy* 2006; **9**: 577–86.

68. Cox C, Surgan M. Unidentified inert ingredients in pesticides: implications for human and environmental health. *Environ Health Perspect* 2006; **114**: 1803–6.

69. Reigart JR, Roberts JR. *Recognition and Management of Pesticide Poisonings*, 5th edn. Washington, DC: United States Environmental Protection Agency, 1999.

70. Buckley NA, Eddleston M, Dawson AH. The need for translational research on antidotes for pesticide poisoning. *Clin Exp Pharmacol Physiol* 2005; **32**: 999–1005.

●71. Eddleston M, Buckley NA, Eyer P, Dawson AH. Management of acute organophosphorous pesticide poisoning. *Lancet* 2008; **371**: 597–607.

72. Senanayake N, Karalliedde L. Neurotoxic effects of organophosphorus insecticides. An intermediate syndrome. *N Engl J Med* 1987; **316**: 761–3.

73. Senanayake N, Johnson MK. Acute polyneuropathy after poisoning by a new organophosphate insecticide. *N Engl J Med* 1982; **306**: 155–7.

74. Spann MF, Blondell JM, Hunting KL. Acute hazards to young children from residential pesticide exposures. *Am J Public Health* 2000; **90**: 971–3.

75. Fukata H, Omori M, Osada H et al. Necessity to measure PCBs and organochlorine pesticide concentrations in human umbilical cords for fetal exposure assessment. *Environ Health Perspect* 2005; **113**: 297–303.

76. Wolff MS, Britton JA, Teitelbaum SL et al. Improving organochlorine biomarker models for cancer research. *Cancer Epidemiol Biomarkers Prev* 2005; **14**: 2224–36.

77. Jurewicz J, Hanke W. Prenatal and childhood exposure to pesticides and neurobehavioral development: review of epidemiological studies. *Int J Occup Med Environ Health* 2008; **21**: 121–32.

78. Engel SM, Berkowitz GS, Barr DB et al. Prenatal organophosphate metabolite and organochlorine levels and performance on the Brazelton neonatal behavioural assessment scale in a multiethnic pregnancy cohort. *Environ Health Perspect* 2007; **165**: 1397–404.

79. Grandjean P, Harari R, Barr DB, Debes F. Pesticide exposure and stunting as independent predictors of neurobehavioral deficits in Ecuadorian school children. *Pediatrics* 2006; **117**: e546–56.

80. Rauh VA, Garfinkel R, Perera FP et al. Impact of prenatal chlorpyrifos exposure on neurodevelopment in the first

3 years of life among inner city children. *Pediatrics* 2006; **118**: e1845–59.

81. Eskenazi B, Marks AR, Bradman A *et al.* Organophosphate pesticide exposure and neurodevelopment in young Mexican-American children. *Environ Health Perspect* 2007; **115**: 792–8.

82. Ribas-Fitó N, Torrent M, Carrizo D *et al.* In utero exposure to background concentrations of DDT and cognitive functioning among preschoolers. *Am J Epidemiol* 2006; **164**: 955–62.

83. Eskenazi B, Marks AR, Bradman A *et al.* In utero exposure to dichlorodiphenyltrichloroethane (DDT) and dichlorodiphenyldichloroethylene (DDE) and neurodevelopment among young Mexican American children. *Pediatrics* 2006; **118**: 233–41.

84. Torres-Sánchez L, Rothenberg SJ, Schnaas L *et al.* In utero p,p'-DDE exposure and infant neurodevelopment: a perinatal cohort in Mexico. *Environ Health Perspect* 2007; **115**: 435–9.

85. Ribas-Fitó N, Torrent M, Carrizo D *et al.* Exposure to hexachlorobenzene during pregnancy and children's social behavior at 4 years of age. *Environ Health Perspect* 2007; **115**: 447–50.

86. Ribas-Fitó N, Júlvez J, Torrent M *et al.* Beneficial effects of breastfeeding on cognition regardless of DDT concentrations at birth. *Am J Epidemiol* 2007; **166**: 1198–202.

♦87. López-Cervantes M, Torres-Sánchez L, Tobías A, López-Carrillo L. Dichlorodiphenyldichloroethane burden and breast cancer risk: a meta-analysis of the epidemiologic evidence. *Environ Health Perspect* 2004; **112**: 207–14.

88. Basill KL, Vakil C, Sanborn M *et al.* Cancer health effects of pesticides: systematic review. *Can Fam Physician* 2007; **53**: 1704–11.

89. Merhi M, Raynal H, Cahuzac E *et al.* Occupational exposure to pesticides and risk of hematopoietic cancers: meta-analysis of case-control studies. *Cancer Causes Control* 2007; **18**: 1209–26.

90. Van Maele-Fabry G, Duhayon S, Mertens C, Lison D. Risk of leukaemia among pesticide manufacturing workers: a review and meta-analysis of cohort studies. *Environ Res* 2008; **106**: 121–37.

91. Zahm SH, Ward MH. Pesticides and childhood cancer. *Environ Health Perspect* 1998; **106**(Suppl. 3): 893–908.

♦92. Infante-Rivard C, Weichental S. Pesticides and childhood cancer: an update of Zahm and Ward's 1998 review. *J Toxicol Environ Health B* 2007; **10**: 81–9.

93. Teitelbaum SL. Questionnaire assessment of nonoccupational pesticide exposure in epidemiologic studies of cancer. *J Expo Anal Environ Epidemiol* 2002; **12**: 373–80.

94. Khuder SA, Mutgi AB, Schaub EA. Meta-analyses of brain cancer and farming. *Am J Ind Med* 1998; **34**: 252–60.

95. Cordier S, Mandereau L, Preston-Martin S *et al.* Parental occupations and childhood brain tumors: results of an international case-control study. *Cancer Causes Control* 2001; **12**: 865–74.

96. Feychting M, Plato N, Nise G, Ahlbom A. Paternal occupational exposures and childhood cancer. *Environ Health Perspect* 2001; **109**: 193–6.

97. Wijngaarden E van, Stewart PA, Olshan AF *et al.* Parental occupational exposure to pesticides and childhood brain cancer. *Am J Epidemiol* 2003; **157**: 989–97.

98. Efird JT, Holly EA, Preston-Martin S *et al.* Farm-related exposures and childhood brain tumours in seven countries: results from the SEARCH International Brain Tumour Study. *Paediatr Perinat Epidemiol* 2003; **17**: 201–11.

99. Pogoda JM, Preston-Martin S. Household pesticides and risk of pediatric brain tumours. *Environ Health Perspect* 1997; **105**: 1214–20.

100. Rosso AL, Hovinga ME, Rorke-Adams LB *et al.* A case-control study of childhood brain tumours and fathers' hobbies: a Children's Oncology Group study. *Cancer Causes Control* 2008; **19**: 1201–7.

101. Kerr MA, Nasca PC, Mundt KA *et al.* Parental occupational exposures and risk of neuroblastoma: a case-control study (United States). *Cancer Causes and Control* 2000; **11**: 635–43.

102. Howe GR, Burch JD, Chiarelli AM *et al.* An exploratory case-control study of brain tumors in children. *Cancer Research* 1989; **49**: 4349–52.

103. Heacock H, Hertzman C, Demers PA *et al.* Childhood cancer in the offspring of male sawmill workers occupationally exposed to chlorophenate fungicides. *Environ Health Perspect* 2000; **108**: 499–503.

104. Davis DL, Bradlow HL, Wolff M *et al.* Medical hypothesis: xenoestrogens as preventable causes of breast cancer. *Environ Health Perspect* 1993; **101**: 372–7.

•105. Wolff MS, Toniolo PG, Lee EW *et al.* Blood levels of organochlorine residues and risk of breast cancer. *J Natl Cancer Inst* 1993; **85**: 648–52.

106. Krieger N, Wolff MS, Hiatt RA *et al.* Breast cancer and serum organochlorines: a prospective study among white, black, and Asian women. *J Natl Cancer Inst* 1994; **86**: 589–99.

107. Dorgan JF, Brock JW, Rothman N *et al.* Serum organochlorine pesticides and PCBs and breast cancer risk: results from a prospective analysis (USA). *Cancer Causes Control* 1999; **10**: 1–11.

108. Hunter DJ, Hankinson SE, Laden F *et al.* Plasma organochlorine levels and the risk of breast cancer. *N Engl J Med* 1997; **337**: 1253–8.

109. Moysich KB, Ambrosone CB, Vena JE *et al.* Environmental organochlorine exposure and postmenopausal breast cancer risk. *Cancer Epidemiol Biomarkers Prev* 1998; **7**: 181–8.

110. Helzlsouer KJ, Alberg AJ, Huang HY *et al.* Serum concentrations of organochlorine compounds and the subsequent development of breast cancer. *Cancer Epidemiol Biomarkers Prev* 1999; **8**: 525–32.

111. Zheng T, Holford TR, Mayne ST *et al.* Risk of female breast cancer associated with serum polychlorinated biphenyls and 1,1-dichloro-2,2'-bis(*p*-chlorophenyl) ethylene. *Cancer Epidemiol Biomarkers Prev* 2000; **9**: 167–74.

112. Wolff MS, Berkowitz GS, Brower S *et al.* Organochlorine exposures and breast cancer risk in New York City women. *Environ Res* 2000; **84**: 151–61.

113. Laden F, Hankinson SE, Wolff MS *et al.* Plasma organochlorine levels and the risk of breast cancer: an extended follow-up in the Nurses' Health Study. *Int J Cancer* 2001; **91**: 568–74.

•114. Laden F, Collman G, Iwamoto K *et al.* 1,1-Dichloro-2,2-bis(*p*-chlorophenyl)ethylene and polychlorinated biphenyls and breast cancer: combined analysis of five U.S. studies. *J Natl Cancer Inst* 2001; **93**: 768–76.

115. Raaschou-Nielsen O, Pavuk M, Leblanc A *et al.* Adipose organochlorine concentrations and risk of breast cancer among postmenopausal Danish women. *Cancer Epidemiol Biomarkers Prev* 2005; **14**: 67–74.

116. Gatto NM, Longnecker MP, Press MF *et al.* Serum organochlorines and breast cancer: a case-control study among African-American women. *Cancer Causes Control* 2007; **18**: 29–39.

117. Salehi F, Turner MC, Phillips KP *et al.* Review of the etiology of breast cancer with special attention to organochlorines as potential endocrine disruptors. *J Toxicol Environ Health B Crit Rev* 2008; **11**: 276–300.

118. Van Maele-Fabry G, Willems JL. Occupation related pesticide exposure and cancer of the prostate: a meta-analysis. *Occup Environ Med* 2003; **60**: 634–42.

119. Van Maele-Fabry G, Libotte V, Willems J, Lison D. Review and meta-analysis of risk estimates for prostate cancer in pesticide manufacturing workers. *Cancer Causes Control* 2006; **17**: 353–73.

120. Hardell L, van Bavel B, Lindström G *et al.* Increased concentrations of polychlorinated biphenyls, hexachlorobenzene, and chlordanes in mothers of men with testicular cancer. *Environ Health Perspect* 2003; **111**: 930–4.

121. McGlynn KA, Quraishi SM, Graubard BI *et al.* Persistent organochlorine pesticides and risk of testicular germ cell tumors. *J Natl Cancer Inst* 2008; **100**: 663–71.

122. Hartge P, Colt JS, Severson RK *et al.* Residential herbicide use and risk of non-Hodgkin lymphoma. *Cancer Epidemiol Biomarkers Prev* 2005; **14**: 934–7.

123. Buckley JD, Meadows AT, Kadin ME *et al.* Pesticide exposures in children with non-Hodgkin lymphoma. *Cancer* 2000; **89**: 2315–21.

124. Ma X, Buffler PA, Gunier RB *et al.* Critical windows of exposure to household pesticides and risk of childhood leukemia. *Environ Health Perspect* 2002; **110**: 955–60.

125. Menegaux F, Baruchel A, Bertrand Y *et al.* Household exposure to pesticides and risk of childhood acute leukaemia. *Occup Environ Med* 2006; **63**: 131–4.

126. Alderton LE, Spector LG, Blair CK *et al.* Child and maternal household chemical exposure and the risk of acute leukemia in children with Down's syndrome: a report from the Children's Oncology Group. *Am J Epidemiol* 2006; **164**: 212–21.

127. Schüz J, Spector LG, Ross JA. Bias in studies of parental self-reported occupational exposure and childhood cancer. *Am J Epidemiol* 2003; **158**: 710–16.

128. Belson M, Kingsley B, Holmes A. Risk factors for acute leukemia in children: a review. *Environ Health Perspect* 2007; **115**: 138–45.

•129. Perry MJ. Effects of environmental and occupational pesticide exposure on human sperm: a systematic review. *Hum Reprod Update* 2008; **14**: 233–42.

130. Bhatia R, Shiau R, Petreas M *et al.* Organochlorine pesticides and male genital anomalies in the child health and development studies. *Environ Health Perspect* 2005; **113**: 220–4.

131. Carbone P, Giordano F, Nori F *et al.* The possible role of endocrine disrupting chemicals in the aetiology of cryptorchidism and hypospadias: a population-based case-control study in rural Sicily. *Int J Androl* 2007; **30**: 3–13.

132. Brucker-Davis F, Wagner-Mahler K, Delattre I *et al.* Cryptorchidism at birth in Nice area (France) is associated with higher prenatal exposure to PCBs and DDE, as assessed by colostrum concentrations. *Hum Reprod* 2008; **23**: 1708–18.

133. Damgaard IN, Skakkebaek NE, Toppari J *et al.* Persistent pesticides in human breast milk and cryptorchidism. *Environ Health Perspect* 2006; **114**: 1133–8.

134. Pierik FH, Burdorf A, Deddens JA *et al.* Maternal and paternal risk factors for cryptorchidism and hypospadias: a case-control study in newborn boys. *Environ Health Perspect* 2004; **112**: 1570–6.

135. Fernandez MF, Olmos B, Granada A *et al.* Human exposure to endocrine-disrupting chemicals and prenatal risk factors for cryptorchidism and hypospadias: a nested case-control study. *Environ Health Perspect* 2007; **115**(Suppl. 1): 8–14.

136. Law DC, Klebanoff MA, Brock JW *et al.* Maternal serum levels of polychlorinated biphenyls and 1,1-dichloro-2,2-bis(p-chlorophenyl)ethylene (DDE) and time to pregnancy. *Am J Epidemiol* 2005; **162**: 523–32.

137. Axmon A, Thulstrup A-M, Rignell-Hydbom A *et al.* Time to pregnancy as a function of male and female serum concentrations of 2,2′4,4′5,5′-hexachlorobiphenyl (CB-153) and 1,1-dichloro-2,2-bis(*p*-chlorophenyl)-ethylene (*p,p′*-DDE). *Hum Reprod* 2006; **21**: 657–65.

138. Pastore LM, Hertz-Picciotto I, Beaumont JJ. Risk of stillbirth from occupational and residential exposures. *Occup Environ Med* 1997; **54**: 511–18.

139. Khanjani N, Sim MR. Maternal contamination with dichlorodiphenyltrichloroethane and reproductive outcomes in an Australian population. *Environ Res* 2006; **101**: 373–9.

•140. Karmaus W, Davis S, Chen Q *et al.* Atopic manifestations, breast-feeding protection and the adverse effect of DDE. *Paediatr Perinat Epidemiol* 2003; **17**: 212–20.

141. Sunyer J, Torrent M, Muñoz-Ortiz L. Prenatal dichlorodiphenyldichloroethylene (DDE) and asthma in children. *Environ Health Perspect* 2005; **113**: 1787–90.

♦142. Brown TP, Rumsby PC, Capelton AC *et al.* Pesticides and Parkinson's disease – is there a link? *Environ Health Perspect* 2006; **114**: 156–64.

143. Priyadarshi A, Khuder SA, Schaub EA, Shrivastava S. A meta-analysis of Parkinson's disease and exposure to pesticides. *Neurotoxicology* 2000; **21**: 435–40.

144. Ascherio A, Chen H, Weisskopf MC *et al.* Pesticide exposure and risk for Parkinson's disease. *Ann Neurol* 2006; **60**: 197–203.

145. Dick FD. Parkinson's disease and pesticide exposures. *Br Med Bull* 2007; **79–80**: 219–31.

26

Lead

BRIAN L. GULSON

Lead is the most studied of the toxic metals. In spite of a knowledge of its toxicity since Roman times and thousands of articles being written about lead, there are still ongoing cases of lead poisoning, especially in young children and in occupational settings. Furthermore, many clinicians and agencies have minimal familiarity with lead and its various aspects. Lead has no physiological use in living species, including plants.

This chapter can only briefly highlight several aspects of lead, and the interested reader is directed towards excellent review documents produced by, for example, the US Environmental Protection Agency (EPA) in its revised *Air Quality Criteria for Lead* document,[1] the US Centers for Disease Control and Prevention,[2] and the International Agency for Research on Cancer.[3] This chapter will focus on human aspects of lead rather than its effect in the environment or the very important animal research, and will also focus more closely on environmentally rather than occupationally exposed individuals. Furthermore, the reader may detect a slight bias towards the information on lead in bone, but this is because bone is the major repository of lead in the body, lead in blood is dominated from bone lead under equilibrium conditions, lead can be mobilized from the skeleton during times of physiological stress, and devices for measurement of lead in bone are undergoing refinement.

USES OF LEAD

Lead occurs naturally, especially when concentrated into large mineral deposits, which are found in most continents. Human activities have increased levels more than a thousand-fold in the last 300 years, with much of this increase occurring in the second half of the twentieth century with an increased use in motor vehicles. Because of its low melting point and chemistry, lead readily forms alloys with other metals. Some of the major uses of lead are illustrated in Figure 26.1; the overwhelming use is in lead–acid batteries for transportation, and with recent developments in the storage capacity of lead–acid batteries, their use can only increase. The other major past use was as tetra-alkyl lead compounds in gasoline for motor vehicles, a use that is declining internationally. Production figures for lead are illustrated in Figure 26.2.

POTENTIAL EXPOSURE TO LEAD

Humans may be exposed to lead from several sources and via several pathways (Figure 26.3).[1]

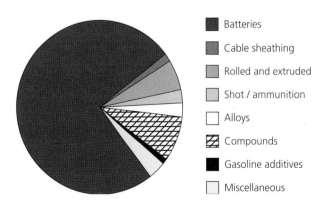

- Batteries
- Cable sheathing
- Rolled and extruded
- Shot / ammunition
- Alloys
- Compounds
- Gasoline additives
- Miscellaneous

Figure 26.1 Lead uses in 2009. (Adapted from the International Lead Association, with permission.)

As reflected in Figure 26.2, lead production and consumption are not diminishing, and hence occupational and industrial exposure is still an important issue. The main industries are mining and smelting, battery manufacture, the recycling of products such as

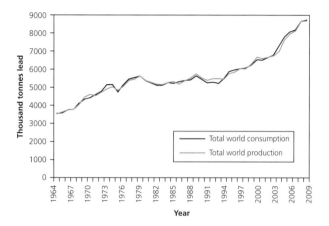

Figure 26.2 World production and consumption of lead. (Adapted from the International Lead Association with permission.)

batteries and electronic waste,[4] and ship repair and demolition.

Activities that can generate lead dust and/or fumes and produce environmental exposure include: the restoration of homes, boats, cars and furniture coated with lead-based paints (probably the most important source of lead exposure in communities that are not industrially exposed); pottery (glazing and firing); soldering (radiators and stained glass); lead-casting (to make ammunition, fishing 'sinkers' and toy soldiers); and the burning of lead-stabilized plastics or materials coated with lead-based paints. Other potential sources of lead include ceramic ware (generally only a problem if it is used for cooking, but especially if it has been improperly fired), toys, some 'traditional' medicines and supplements,[5] some cosmetics and hair dyes, and jewellery.[6]

Although lead from gasoline additives and paint was a major source of direct exposure in the past, these categories cannot be dismissed as they are now indirect sources of exposure. That is, gasoline lead and paint lead from earlier renovations may still be present in soil and house dust and may be resuspended by wind.[8] Houses built prior to the 1970–80s may still contain lead paint in various components, especially the windows and door trims.

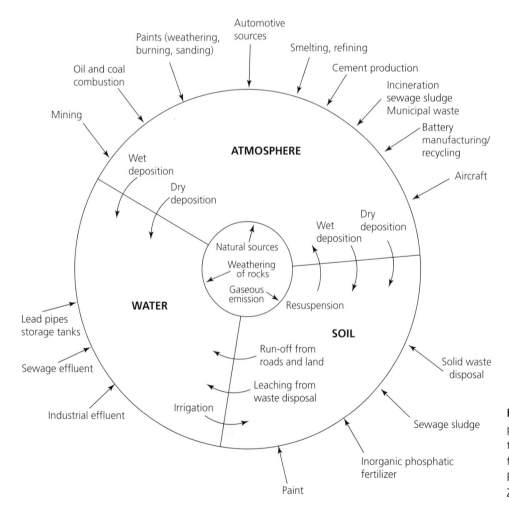

Figure 26.3 Transport pathways for lead in the environment. (Amended from US Environmental Protection Agency[1] and Zabel[7], with permission.)

The elimination of lead solder in canned food has resulted in decreased levels of exposure from this source. For example, the average dietary lead intake in the USA is about 1 μg lead per day per kilogram body weight,[9] and similar levels have been reported in Australia in the first decade of the twenty-first century.[10]

Lead in drinking water is commonly included in dietary intakes but may be a significant contributor of lead by itself. Elevated lead levels may derive from the corrosion of lead pipes, lead-based solder, or brass or bronze fixtures within a residence; the levels also depend on temperature, residence time and amount flushed from the pipes. Lead concentrations are generally low (below the action level of 15 μg/L of the US EPA), but in recent years the increasing use of chloramine in water distribution systems in place of chlorination as a disinfection process has led to notable elevations of lead in tap water in some US communities.[11]

Decreases in mobile sources of lead in the USA, resulting from the phase-out of gasoline lead additives, created a 98 per cent decline in airborne emissions from 1970 to 2003. The phase-out of gasoline lead, the removal of lead from canned foods and increased public awareness of the hazards and health effects of lead has resulted in a decline in blood lead levels in children aged 1–5 years from a geometric mean of approximately 15 μg/dL in 1976–80 to around 1–2 μg/dL in the period 2000–04, as shown by the National Health and Nutrition Examination Surveys (NHANES).[2] Similar declines in blood lead levels have been observed in several countries (India,[12] Taiwan,[13] Chile,[14] China[15] and Sweden[16]).

With decreasing inhalation exposure, the focus has shifted to other sources and pathways of lead. In the 1990s, soil lead was targeted, one major study being the Three City Lead Study in Boston, Baltimore and Cincinnati.[17] The US EPA concluded that when soil is a significant source of lead in the child's environment, and in certain conditions, the abatement of that soil will result in a reduction in exposure and blood lead level (of around 1.3 μg/dL). For another opinion on the efficacy of soil remediation and blood lead, see Yeoh et al.[18] and mentioned in 'Health effects of lead exposure', below.

In recent years, the focus has again become dust, although this was well recognized as a critical source of exposure in the 1980s.[19–21] Several new studies have shown that the blood lead of children is strongly associated with interior dust lead loading and will be reflected in hand lead levels.[22] Both exterior soil and paint lead contribute to interior dust lead levels. Besides dust-loading in homes, Lanphear and Roghmann[23] and Lanphear et al.[24,25] found that the blood lead levels of children were related to race/ethnicity, soil lead levels, ingestion of soil or dirt, lead content and condition of painted surfaces, and water lead levels.

The hand-to-mouth activities of young children, coupled with the ease with which they absorb and retain lead, make children more vulnerable to lead exposure than adults. Nevertheless, in an occupational setting, employees may also be exposed through hand-to-mouth activities such as smoking or not washing their hands prior to eating or drinking. They may also contaminate their residences and family by 'taking home' the lead on their clothes and/or motor vehicles.[26]

Biomarkers of exposure

A comprehensive discussion of the biomarkers of lead exposure (dose) may be found in a publication by the National Research Council,[27] a critical review by Barbosa et al.[28] and publications by the Agency for Toxic Substances and Disease Registry (ATSDR)[2] and Hu et al.[29]

Various biomarkers are listed in Table 26.1, and some discussion of the half-lives (or residence times) of lead in these media is given in the following section. The current accepted biomarker is blood lead, and a so-called 'level of concern' is 10 μg/dL (0.48 μm/L). It is recognized that blood lead may only reflect recent exposure (e.g. less than 30 days), although Chen et al.[30] suggest that current blood lead provides as much if not more useful information than historical blood lead. In spite of the concerns about blood lead reflecting recent (acute) exposure, stable isotope studies show that 40–70 per cent of the lead in blood is derived from endogenous sources such as the skeleton,[31–33] and for environmentally exposed subjects, an equilibrium between skeletal lead and blood lead is reached in a matter of months.[32] In occupational settings, cumulative blood lead levels are the accepted measure,[34] along with bone lead measurement by K alpha X-ray fluorescence where possible.

An integrated longer-term biomarker is bone or tooth lead, but X-ray fluorescence bone measurements are currently not widely available, there may be inconsistencies in low bone lead values for environmentally exposed subjects, and there may be problems with children (or even adults) because of the need to minimize movement during the measurement.

Advances in detector design have partially rectified some of these problems.[35] The X-ray fluorescence system is still essentially at a research stage, with two groups in the USA (the Harvard group, formerly led by Howard Hu, whose main focus has been on subjects in the Normative Aging Study, and in Mexico City, the group of Andrew Todd and Brian Schwartz, whose main focus has been on occupationally exposed subjects, especially in Taiwan), two groups in Canada (led by David Fleming, and David Chettle and Fiona McNeill), which undertake studies in mining and smelting communities and environmentally exposed subjects, and one laboratory in the UK.[36,37]

Tooth lead measurements have declined in popularity in recent years as there is some uncertainty in the interpretation of the results.[38]

Table 26.1   Common biomarkers of lead exposure

Medium	Methods of analysis	Parameter	Advantages	Disadvantages
Blood lead	GFAAS/ICP-MS/TIMS	μg/dL	Accepted biomarker Easily collected (venous blood recommended) 10 μg/dL is considered to be the 'level of concern'	Indicator of short-term exposure ($<$100 days)
Urine	GFAAS/ICP-MS/TIMS	μg/L	Non-invasive About 10% of blood lead value Indicator of very short-term exposure although used in chelation provocation testing	No value guidelines Potential for contamination, especially young children
Plasma/serum	GFAAS/ICP-MS/TIMS	μg/L	Potentially more interesting toxicologically $<$0.3% of blood lead value	No guidelines Easily contaminated during analysis Problems of haemolysis
Bone	K alpha XRF	μg/g bone mineral	Non-invasive Indicator of long-term exposure Can measure trabecular and cortical bone to provide data on different exposures	No guidelines Limited access to XRF units Problems at low bone lead levels, with length of time of measurement (around 30 minutes) and with potential movement of patient
Teeth	GFAAS/ICP-MS/TIMS	μg/g	Non-invasive Indicator of long-term exposure Can measure enamel and dentine to provide data on different exposures, especially in deciduous teeth	No guidelines Different tooth types can have different lead concentrations
Nails	GFAAS/ICP-MS/TIMS	μg/g	Potentially longer period of exposure (months)	No guidelines Easily contaminated from exogenous sources
Hair	GFAAS/ICP-MS/TIMS	μg/g	Potentially longer period of exposure (months)	No guidelines Easily contaminated from exogenous sources
Sweat	GFAAS/ICP-MS/TIMS	μg/g	Potential indicator of short-term exposure	No guidelines Limited data Easily contaminated in collection
Breast milk	GFAAS/ICP-MS/TIMS	μg/L	Potential indicator of body burden and short-term exposure	No guidelines Limited data Easily contaminated in collection and analysis

GFAAS, graphite furnace atomic absorption spectroscopy; ICP-MS, inductively coupled plasma mass spectrometry; TIMS, thermal ionization mass spectrometry; XRF, X-ray fluorescence.

Absorption, distribution, metabolism and excretion

ABSORPTION

The absorption of lead is influenced by the route of exposure, chemical speciation, the physicochemical characteristics of the lead and exposure medium, and the age and physiological states of the exposed individual (e.g. fasting or nutritional status for elements such as calcium and iron). Inorganic lead can be absorbed by the inhalation of fine particles and by ingestion. Once absorbed, lead is distributed via blood to various organs (Figure 26.4).

Inhalation exposure

Estimates of inhalation exposure are available only for adult males. The rate of deposition of airborne lead in the

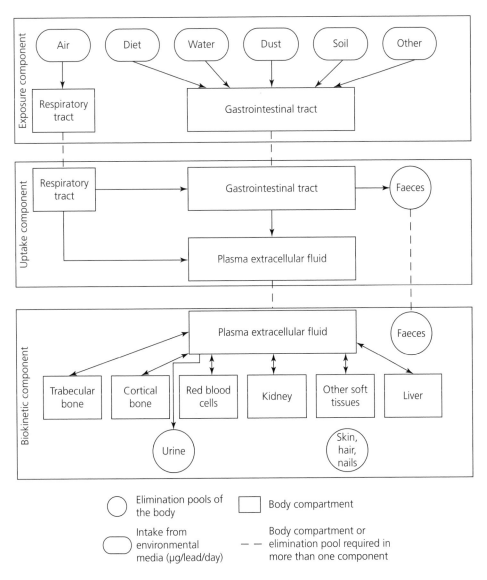

Figure 26.4 Structure of the integrated exposure uptake biokinetics model for lead in children. (Amended from US Environmental Protection Agency[1], with permission.)

lungs is approximately 30–50 per cent, with rate of deposition dependent on the size of the particles and the ventilation rate of the individual but independent of the absolute lead burden. The biological half-life for the retention of lead in the lungs is about 15 hours.[39] Once deposited in the lower respiratory tract, particulate lead is almost completely absorbed, and different chemical forms of lead are similarly absorbed.[1] Smaller particles (less than 1 μm in diameter) have been shown to have greater deposition and absorption rates than larger particles.[40]

Oral exposure

Gastrointestinal absorption of lead occurs primarily in the duodenum. The extent and rate of gastrointestinal absorption are influenced by physiological states such as age, fasting, nutritional elements including calcium, iron, copper, phosphorus and zinc, fat and calorie intake and the physicochemical characteristics of the medium ingested, such as particle size, mineralogy and solubility of the lead species.[41] The relationship between lead intake and blood lead concentration is curvilinear, i.e. the increment in

blood lead concentration per unit of lead intake decreases with increasing blood lead concentration.

Most data on absorption are available for adults, with very limited studies on children, and apart from metabolic studies undertaken in the 1970s when daily intakes and blood lead levels were orders of magnitude higher than in current times, more recent studies have been based on indirect evidence of absorption/retention. The experimental adult studies generally had small numbers of subjects and mainly employed radioactive tracers with other evidence, often indirect, coming from stable lead isotope methods and epidemiological studies (see Table 81 in reference [3]). There was a wide variation in absorption between individuals in most studies. In addition, estimates of absorption of ingested lead compounds are critically dependent on the timing of food intake.[42] In adults, the absorption of ingested lead is less than 10 per cent if a meal is consumed but can increase dramatically if in a fasting state.[42,43] In children, approximately 50 per cent of the ingested lead is absorbed, and retention is up to about 30 per cent.[44]

Nutritional factors affecting absorption

Mineral content is one factor contributing to the lower absorption of lead when lead is ingested with a meal. For example, the presence and amount of calcium and phosphorus in a meal depresses the absorption of ingested lead.[41,45,46] In children, an inverse relationship has been observed between dietary calcium intake and blood lead concentration,[44, 47] although Lanphear et al.[48] found that dietary iron but not calcium intake was inversely associated with blood lead level. A higher dietary intake of iron is associated with lower blood lead levels among children, and iron deficiency may result in a higher absorption of lead in both adults and children.[49–52] A positive association has been observed between blood lead in children and total and saturated fat and calorific intake,[53,54] although no relationship between fat and protein versus bone and blood lead was found in middle-aged to elderly men in the Normative Aging Study.[55] The relationships between ascorbic acid and blood lead are controversial.

Dermal exposure

Limited information on dermal exposure in humans is available, and it is generally regarded of little consequence; a more detailed discussion of dermal absorption is given in *Inorganic and Organic Lead Compounds*.[3]

DISTRIBUTION

Absorbed lead is distributed to various tissue compartments. Several models of lead pharmacokinetics are briefly outlined under 'Pharmacokinetic models', below.

Blood

Once absorbed, lead appears to be distributed in essentially the same manner regardless of the route of absorption.[56] In general, the distribution of lead appears to be similar in children and adults, although a larger fraction of the lead body burden of adults resides in bone.[57]

Blood lead concentrations change with age, commonly reaching a maximum in children at 2–3 years of age and then decreasing until later in life, when increases in the elderly may be due to bone resorption and the release of lead. As discussed below, recent neurodevelopmental studies suggest that not all damage from lead is done at 2–3 years of age and that current blood lead levels provide as much if not more useful information than historical blood lead levels.[30] The overwhelming data for blood lead are based on single measurements such as in cross-sectional studies (e.g. NHANES) and may not reflect the real body burden of lead.

Lead in blood is primarily located in the red blood cells (approximately 99 per cent) rather than the plasma.[1] The principal lead-binding protein is delta-aminolevulinic acid dehydratase (ALAD).[58] The human *ALAD* gene has two alleles: ALAD-1 and ALAD-2.[59] Whether or not this polymorphism in blood or bone may cause differential sensitivity to lead exposure is controversial.[60–65]

The half-life of lead in human blood has been mainly determined experimentally in adult males using radioactive or stable isotope tracers, although the results are based on small numbers of subjects (usually fewer than 10). There are very limited data for children. Large differences have been noted between individuals. The mean half-lives for environmentally exposed adult males range from 18 to 30 days (see Table 83 in *Inorganic and Organic Lead Compounds*[3]), and for female adults of child-bearing age a mean half-life of 59 days, standard deviation 6 days, almost double that of the males, has been reported.[66] Infants born to migrant mothers had apparent half-lives considerably longer than those of the female adults.[22,66] Apparent half-lives of lead in blood estimated for lead workers are commonly much longer than those environmentally exposed and reflect a complex elimination of lead from the blood and a remobilization of lead from bone compartments.[67–76]

Several authors have proposed that measurement of lead in serum or plasma may better reflect the fraction of circulatory lead that is more available for exchange with target organs such as the central nervous system and kidneys, and with the developing fetus.[77–83] The low concentrations of lead in plasma, relative to red blood cells, have made it extremely difficult to measure plasma lead concentrations accurately in humans, particularly at lower blood lead concentrations (i.e. less than $20\,\mu g/dL$). The percentage of serum lead/whole-blood lead is less than 0.3 per cent, and the relation is probably linear for blood lead levels below $10\,\mu g/dL$.

Soft tissues

In 32 deceased smelter workers with a known history of lead exposure, the major soft tissue organs of lead accumulation were, in decreasing order, the liver, kidney, lungs and brain.[84] The half-life of lead in these organs is similar to that in blood.[85]

Bone

In human adults, more than 90 per cent of the total body burden of lead is found in the skeleton, whereas bone lead accounts for around 70 per cent of the body burden in children.[57] Approximately 15 per cent of circulating lead per day is incorporated into bone,[86] where it substitutes for calcium in hydroxyapatite. Lead is not distributed uniformly in bone.[37,61,87,88] Lead accumulation is thought to occur predominantly in trabecular bone during childhood and in both cortical and trabecular bone in adulthood. Estimates of the half-life of lead in trabecular bone are partly dependent on the tissue analysed and the 'purity' of the trabecular component (patella, calcaneus or phalanx); current estimates range from about 2 to 8 years, although earlier estimates ranged from 12 to 19 years.[89,90] Earlier estimates for the half-life of lead in cortical bone ranged from 13 to 27 years.[86,89,90] The rate of removal of lead from bone throughout adulthood is controversial.[73,91–93]

Maternal patella bone lead levels have been shown to be superior to tibia bone lead levels in predicting lower infant birth weight[94] and lower growth velocity from birth to 1 month of age.[95] Bone lead levels correlate more strongly with serum/plasma lead than with whole-blood lead levels[78,83,96] and urine where it has been used as a proxy for serum.[97] Analyses of bone and teeth can provide an integrated biomarker of previous lead exposure and can be used in a variety of investigations. For example, using K alpha X-ray fluorescence analyses of bone, investigators have found strong associations between bone lead and hypertension/renal dysfunction, cognitive functioning[98–104] and delinquency.[105,106]

METABOLISM

Inorganic lead ion in the body is not known to be metabolized or biotransformed.[107]

EXCRETION

The excretion of lead is not dependent on the exposure pathway.[40] The major routes of excretion of absorbed lead are urinary and biliary clearance. Excretion of lead via the faeces is generally greater than excretion via the urinary route. For example, of the 85 per cent of ingested lead that was excreted, more than 90 per cent was found in the faeces of adult volunteers who ingested 0.3–3.0 mg lead as lead acetate in drinking water per day for 16–208 weeks.[56] At around 26 hours after ingestion by three subjects of a single dose of lead-204 tracer, Smith et al.[108] measured from 71 per cent to 97 per cent of the excreted tracer in the faeces. As mentioned previously, the retention of lead appears to be higher in children compared with adults.

MOBILIZATION OF LEAD

With greater than 90 per cent of the lead stored in the bones of adults, potential mobilization of lead from the skeleton could occur at times of physiological stress associated with enhanced bone remodelling, such as pregnancy and lactation,[31,109–112] menopause,[113] extended bed rest,[114] hyperparathyroidism,[115] and weightlessness.[116] This large pool of lead in adults can serve to maintain blood lead levels long after exposure has ended.[3,22,66–76]

Pregnancy and lactation

During pregnancy and lactation, there is increased bone resorption to meet the calcium requirements of the developing fetus, and earlier studies using only lead concentrations generally showed an increase in blood lead levels during the third trimester (see the references in reference [117]). Studies employing high-precision stable lead isotopes have confirmed that extra lead is released from the maternal skeleton during pregnancy and lactation in cynomolgus monkeys[79,110] and humans.[66,111,117–119]

Transplacental transfer/breast milk

The transplacental transfer of lead in humans has been demonstrated in a number of studies based mainly on umbilical cord–maternal relationships. The cord–maternal blood lead concentration ratio at delivery ranges from about 0.6 to 1.0 (see Table 7 and the reference list in reference [120]). The maternal-to-fetal transfer of lead appears to be related partly to the mobilization of lead from the maternal skeleton, as shown in the stable lead isotope studies in cynomolgus monkeys.[79,110] Likewise, strong evidence for placental transfer is shown by the correlation of 0.99 in lead isotopic ratios for maternal and cord blood and urinary isotopic ratios in newborn infants.[31,117]

Breast milk can also be a pathway of maternal excretion of lead. However, given the very low lead concentrations (e.g. 0.73 μg/kg, standard deviation 0.70 μg/kg; blood lead less than 5 μg/dL) and analytical difficulties arising from high fat contents in breast milk, their collection and analysis require careful attention.[121] Breast-fed infants are only at risk if the mother is exposed to high concentrations of contaminants from either endogenous sources such as the skeleton or exogenous sources. Arora et al.[122] found that a higher maternal dietary intake of polyunsaturated fatty acids may limit the transfer of lead from bone to breast milk.

Menopause

Increases in blood lead levels for postmenopausal women have been attributed to the release of lead from the skeleton associated with increased bone remodelling during menopause.[113,123–126] More recent investigations employing bone X-ray fluorescence measurements with supplemental blood lead values have supported an endogenous contribution of lead to blood.[75,101,127–129]

PHARMACOKINETIC MODELS

Several pharmacokinetic models for lead have been proposed to explain and predict physiological processes, including intercompartmental lead exchange rates, the retention of lead in various pools, and the relative rates of distribution among the tissue groups. One of the earliest models was a three-compartment model based on stable lead isotope tracer experiments and balance data on five healthy men.[85] Another is a physiologically based pharmacokinetic model developed initially for rats by O'Flaherty (see reference [130] for further references). Two other models in current use are compartmental pharmacokinetic models, including the integrated exposure uptake biokinetic model (Figure 26.4) for lead in children[131] and the Leggett model,[91] which simulate the same general processes as in the physiologically based pharmacokinetic model, although transfer rate constants and kinetic coefficients may not have precise physiological correlates. Comprehensive discussions of these models are given in *Air Quality Criteria for Lead*.[1]

HEALTH EFFECTS OF LEAD EXPOSURE

A brief summary of health effects is given below. A more detailed account is available in the US EPA[1] and the US ATSDR[2] documents.

General effects

The immediate health effects of high-level exposure to lead resulting in blood lead values of 70–100 μg/dL or above are clinical emergencies and may cause encephalopathy or severely affect neurological function. Symptoms include stomach pain, vomiting, convulsions (fitting), loss of consciousness and possibly death. Such cases of lead poisoning are now extremely rare.

Chronic occupational lead exposure was found to be associated with peripheral sensory nerve impairment, visuomotor and memory impairment, prolonged visual-evoked potentials and brainstem auditory-evoked potentials, and postural sway abnormalities. A possible threshold at blood lead levels 14 μg/dL or above was observed for these neurotoxic effects.[132–137]

Longer-term health effects

Long-term exposure to lead at levels less than those required to cause acute symptoms can result in effects on the peripheral nervous system, general fatigue, headaches, anaemia, small increases in blood pressure and reduced renal function. Associations between lead dose and reduced renal function were observed in most studies of the general population.[1,104,138–144] The public health significance of such effects is not clear, however, in view of the more serious signs of kidney dysfunction found in occupationally exposed workers only at much higher blood lead levels (over 30–40 μg/dL). There are many papers on the relationship between blood pressure and lead in blood and bone, the most recent being that of Weaver et al.;[145] these authors found that blood lead was more relevant to elevations in blood pressure than was patellar lead.

In adults, exposure to chronic low levels of environmental lead and its association with effects on the nervous system were examined in several populations originally followed to study conditions associated with ageing, especially cardiovascular/mortality: the Veterans Affairs Normative Aging Study population;[146–148] subjects in the Study of Osteoporotic Fractures;[123] participants in the Kungsholmen Project on ageing and dementia,[149] subjects in the second and third NHANES surveys (NHANES and NHANES III);[150,151] and organo-lead manufacturing workers.[152] More recent studies, especially those using data from NHANES III and the Normative Aging Study, have indicated increased cardiovascular/mortality rates at blood lead levels below 10 μg/dL.[153–156] However, the evidence for an association of lead with cardiovascular morbidity and mortality is limited but supportive.[1]

The World Health Organization's International Agency for Research on Cancer recently concluded that there is limited evidence in humans for the carcinogenicity of inorganic lead compounds, and inadequate evidence in humans for the carcinogenicity of organic lead compounds (such as those used in leaded petrol). The US ATSDR considers the evidence to be inconclusive.[2,3]

Recent studies have drawn attention to a possible increased risk of dental caries associated with lead,[157] although others[158] have found no association between lead, dental caries and neurobehavioural development.

Health effects on reproduction

High lead exposure may cause pregnant women to miscarry.[159] As lead is transferred to the unborn infant during pregnancy and a small amount may also arise from breast milk, women are especially advised to minimize their exposure to lead both before and during pregnancy and lactation. There is evidence that lead adversely affects sperm motility, size, number and quality in occupationally exposed males. The US EPA[1] and ATSDR[2] documents have excellent sections on reproductive outcomes.

Health effects in children

Children are more sensitive to the health effects of lead compared with adults as they absorb and retain more lead in their body than adults. Longitudinal studies undertaken over the last 30 years have shown that lead may impact adversely on the neurodevelopment of children at exposure levels well below those required to induce the acute signs and symptoms described above.[1,2] These effects have been assessed using ability scales, Intelligence Quotients (IQ) and standardized reports of emotional and behavioural problems.

There is, however, uncertainty over the extent to which low-level lead exposure is actually causing the neurodevelopmental deficits.[160] This uncertainty arises partly because there are other factors besides lead that can impact on a child's abilities and behaviour, such as genetics, major life-events (e.g. parental separation and divorce), early childhood experiences and learning, and the quality of parenting in the home environment. Thus, the relationship between lead exposure and children's abilities and behaviour becomes less certain when these factors are all taken into account. The variability in IQ scores of children that can be explained by lead exposure is of the order of 2–4 per cent.[161] In a study of 780 children with blood concentrations ranging between 20 and 44 μg/dL,[30] the proportion of variability attributable to lead was quite modest. There are no published estimates of what proportion of variability in emotional and behavioural problem scores can be explained by lead exposure.

The current opinion among researchers is that no threshold for the effects of lead on IQ has been identified,[1,2] although the nature of the dose–response relationship between lead exposure and the intellectual abilities and behaviour of children is contentious. Longitudinal studies undertaken in the 1980s and 90s indicated that an increase in lead exposure from 10 to 30 μg/dL was associated with an average decrease of 1–3 IQ points at a population level. However, two US studies, one from a highly disadvantaged community in Rochester New York,[162] and the other from a highly educated community in Boston,[163] have reported larger decreases in IQ as blood lead levels increase from 3 to 10 μg/dL.

Other studies supporting the negative effects of lead on neurodevelopmental parameters at blood lead levels of 10 μg/dL or less include the New England Children's Amalgam Trial[164] and studies from Saudi Arabia[165] and Mexico.[166,167] In spite of the increasing information indicative of negative effects of lead on neurodevelopmental parameters at blood lead levels of 10 μg/dL or less, the Centers for Disease Control and Prevention have retained a value of 10 μg/dL.[160] Although the above studies are relevant at a population level, they cannot be used to predict the responses of an individual child to a given lead exposure.

The neurodevelopmental deficits generally appear to persist into adolescence and young adulthood.[168–172] Attempts to reverse or limit lead-associated neurodevelopmental decrements with pharmacological or nutritional intervention strategies have thus far been ineffective.[173]

In another view of the effects of lead on neurodevelopment, Gulson[174] drew attention to the similar effects in children arising from pesticides, to the fact that there was an extensive use of pesticides, especially in the USA, at the same time as the prospective lead studies, and to the fact that the question of pesticide use was never addressed or documented in these studies, so pesticides might therefore perhaps account for some of the neurodevelopmental deficits. This posit was firmly rebutted by Lanphear et al.,[175] although these authors never addressed the pesticide question that was raised.

Nevertheless, it is important to consider the extensive supporting experimental animal evidence not compromised by the possibility of confounding in examining lead effects on health.[176,177]

MEDICAL MANAGEMENT OF LEAD EXPOSURE

There is insufficient space in this chapter to provide details of the management of lead exposure.

Industrial exposures are usually associated with the lead industry and are hence covered by regulations on blood lead levels and continuity of exposure. For example, in Australia, workers in the lead industry come under the auspices of the National Occupational Health and Safety Commission.[178] The frequency of monitoring is contingent on the results of the blood tests, which for medical removal in Australia are: 50 μg/dL for males and females not of reproductive capacity, 50 μg/dL for males of reproductive capacity, 20 μg/dL for females of reproductive capacity;

and 15 μg/dL for females who are pregnant or breast-feeding. There does, however, appear to be a dichotomy here between the factor of five differential in occupational exposure blood lead levels for the first category and those for the general population of 10 μg/dL. Lower limits have been suggested by Kosnett et al.:[179]

we recommend that individuals be removed from occupational lead exposure if a single blood lead concentration exceeds 30 μg/dL or if two successive blood lead concentrations measured over a 4-week interval are ≥20 μg/dL. Removal of individuals from lead exposure should be considered to avoid long-term risk to health if exposure control measures over an extended period do not decrease blood lead concentrations to <10 μg/dL or if selected medical conditions exist that would increase the risk of continued exposure. Recommended medical surveillance for all lead-exposed workers should include quarterly blood lead measurements for individuals with blood lead concentrations between 10 and 19 μg/dL, and semiannual blood lead measurements when sustained blood lead concentrations are <10 μg/dL. It is advisable for pregnant women to avoid occupational or a vocational lead exposure that would result in blood lead concentrations >5 μg/dL. Chelation may have an adjunctive role in the medical management of highly exposed adults with symptomatic lead intoxication but is not recommended for asymptomatic individuals with low blood lead concentrations.

With regard to chelation, a large study of the effects of chelation therapy using dimercaptosuccinic acid (DMSA or succimer) in US children aged 12 to 33 months with an average blood lead level of around 26 μg/dL did not yield sustainable changes in blood lead concentration or improve cognitive abilities, possibly because these compounds only remove a limited amount of lead (less than 10 per cent) from the skeleton, which may then release stored lead back into the bloodstream.[173]

As far as environmental exposures are concerned, epidemiological studies are reporting effects at blood lead levels for which there is no effective means of medical or secondary environmental intervention to avoid developmental morbidity. This thus emphasizes the importance of taking primary protective measures to substantially reduce and ultimately prevent the exposure of young infants and children to blood lead concentration at 7 years compared with one at 2 years of age.[1]

This is reinforced by the Cochrane Review by Yeoh et al.,[18] who state in their 'Implications for practice':

Based on review of the current evidence, there is no evidence that educational and dust control interventions are effective in reducing blood lead levels in children. Therefore, it is difficult to support the use of the interventions examined in this review as a general population health measure, given their cost and the lack of data showing positive reductions in blood lead levels. There is currently insufficient evidence that soil abatement or combination interventions reduce blood lead levels.

There are several excellent documents providing details for the management of lead exposure, especially around the home and for the clinician. Some of these are as follows:

- 'Managing Elevated Blood Lead Levels Among Young Children: Recommendations from the Advisory Committee on Childhood Lead Poisoning Prevention':[180] Chapters 2 ('Assessment and remediation of residential lead exposure'), 3 ('Medical assessment and interventions'), 4 ('Nutritional assessment and interventions'), 5 ('Developmental assessment and interventions') and 6 ('Educational interventions for caregivers').
- 'The Environmental Case Management of Lead-exposed Persons Guidelines for Public Health Units', Revised edition.[181]
- 'Interpreting and managing blood lead levels of less than 10 µg/dL in children and reducing childhood exposure to lead: recommendations of the Centers for Disease Control and Prevention Advisory Committee on Childhood Lead Poisoning Prevention'.[161] This paper includes a section on recommendations for clinicians.
- How can families reduce the risk of exposure to lead? Public Health Statement page 11.2.[2]
- 'Recommendations for medical management of adult lead exposure'.[179]
- Additional information can be obtained from the Global Lead Advice and Support Service via http://www.lead.org.au/cu.html.

In addition, there is possible advice for during pregnancy and lactation. An increased intake of calcium has been suggested as a preventative measure against the mobilization of extra lead during pregnancy and lactation (see the reference list in reference [118]). Using the lead isotope method, calcium supplementation at the recommended level of approximately 1 g of calcium per day lowered the extra amount of skeletal lead released during pregnancy, and this extra release was delayed to the second and third trimesters compared with a cohort having a very low calcium intake (a mean of approximately 300 mg per day). No benefit of calcium supplementation was found during lactation.[118]

In contrast, pregnancy and lactation studies using blood and bone lead measures and bone resorption markers in Mexico City have shown a significant benefit of calcium supplementation (1200 and 900 mg per day in two cohorts) during pregnancy as well as during lactation.[174,182–184]

Earlier studies employing bone mineral density and biochemical markers showed that there was a minimal impact on preventing bone resorption during lactation

from additional calcium.[185] Arora et al. measured lead in blood, breast milk and bone (patella and tibia) at 1 month postpartum in 310 women from Mexico City.[122] They found that a higher maternal dietary intake of polyunsaturated fatty acids might limit the transfer of lead from bone to breast milk.

REFERENCES

● = Key primary paper

◆ = Major review article

◆1. US Environmental Protection Agency. *Air Quality Criteria for Lead*. EPA/600/R-5/144aF. Washington, DC: EPA, 2006.

◆2. Agency for Toxic Substances and Disease Registry. *Toxicological Profile for Lead*. Washington, DC: US Department of Health and Human Services, Public Health Service, 2007.

◆3. International Agency for Research on Cancer. *Inorganic and Organic Lead Compounds*, Vol. 87. Lyon: IARC, 2006.

4. Zheng L, Wu K, Li Y et al. Blood lead and cadmium levels and relevant factors among children from an e-waste recycling town in China. *Environ Res* 2008; **108**: 15–20.

5. Cooper K, Noller B, Connell D et al. Public health risks from heavy metals and metalloids present in traditional Chinese medicines. *J Toxicol Environ Health A* 2007; **70**: 1694–9.

6. Weidenhamer JD, Clement ML. Evidence of recycling of lead battery waste into highly leaded jewelry. *Chemosphere* 2007; **69**: 1670–2.

7. Zabel TF. Diffuse sources of pollution by heavy metals. *J Inst Water Environ Manage* 1993; **7**: 513–20.

8. Laidlaw MAS, Filippelli GM. Resuspension of urban soils as a persistent source of lead poisoning in children: a review and new directions. *Appl Geochem* 2008; **23**: 2021–39.

9. Moschandreas DJ, Karuchit S, Berry MR et al. Exposure apportionment: ranking food items by their contribution to dietary exposure. *J Expo Anal Environ Epidemiol* 2002; **12**: 233–43.

10. Gulson BL, Mizon KJ, Korsch MJ, Taylor AJ. Changes in the lead isotopic composition of blood, diet and air in Australia over a decade: globalization and implications for future isotopic studies. *Environ Res* 2006; **100**: 130–8.

11. Miranda ML, Kim D, Hull AP, Paul CJ, Galeano MA. Changes in blood lead levels associated with use of chloramines in water treatment systems. *Environ Health Perspect* 2007; **115**: 221–5.

12. Singh AK, Singh M. Lead decline in the Indian environment resulting from the petrol-lead phase-out programme. *Sci Total Environ* 2006; **368**(2–3): 686–94.

13. Hwang YH, Ko Y, Chiang CD et al. Transition of cord blood lead level, 1985–2002, in the Taipei area and its determinants after the cease of leaded gasoline use. *Environ Res* 2004; **96**: 274–82.

14. Pino P, Walter T, Oyarzun MJ, Burden MJ, Lozoff B. Rapid drop in infant blood lead levels during the transition to unleaded gasoline use in Santiago, Chile. *Arch Environ Health* 2004; **59**: 182–7.

15. Yan C, Wu S, Shen X *et al.* The trends of changes in children's blood lead levels since the introduction of lead free gasoline in Shanghai. *Zhonghua Liu Xing Bing Xue Za Zhi* 2002; **23**: 172–4.

16. Stromberg U, Lundh T, Skerfving S. Yearly measurements of blood lead in Swedish children since 1978: the declining trend continues in the petrol-lead-free period 1995–2007. *Environ Res* 2008; **107**: 332–5.

17. US Environmental Protection Agency. *Urban Soil Lead Abatement Demonstration Project.* EPA600P93001. Washington, DC: EPA, Office of Research and Development, 1996.

♦18. Yeoh B, Woolfenden S, Wheeler D, Alperstein G, Lanphear B. Household interventions for prevention of domestic lead exposure. *Cochrane Database Syst Rev* 2008; (2): 1–41.

19. Roels HA, Buchet J, Lauwerys R *et al.* Exposure to lead by the oral and the pulmonary routes of children living in the vicinity of a primary lead smelter. *Environ Res* 1980; **22**: 81–94.

20. Charney E, Sayre J, Coulter M. Increased lead absorption in inner city children: where does the lead come from? *Pediatrics* 1980; **65**: 226–31.

21. Duggan MJ, Inskip MJ. Childhood exposure to lead in surface dust and soil: a community health problem. *Public Health Rev* 1985; **13**(1–2): 1–54.

●22. Manton WI, Angle CR, Stanek KL, Reese YR, Kuehnemann TJ. Acquisition and retention of lead by young children. *Environ Res* 2000; **82**: 60–80.

23. Lanphear BP, Roghmann KJ. Pathways of lead exposure in urban children. *Environ Res* 1997; **74**: 67–73.

●24. Lanphear BP, Burgoon DA, Rust SW, Eberly S, Galke W. Environmental exposures to lead and urban children's blood lead levels. *Environ Res* 1998; **76**: 120–30.

25. Lanphear BP, Hornung R, Ho M. Screening housing to prevent lead toxicity in children. *Public Health Rep* 2005; **120**: 305–10.

26. Chiaradia M, Gulson B, MacDonald K. Contamination of houses by workers occupationally exposed in a lead-zinc-copper mine and impact on blood lead concentrations in the families. *Occup Environ Med* 1997; **54**: 117–24.

♦27. National Research Council. *Measuring Lead Exposure in Infants, Children, and Other Sensitive Populations.* Washington, DC: National Academy Press, 1993.

28. Barbosa F, Tanus-Santos J E, Gerlach RF, Parsons PJ. A critical review of biomarkers used for monitoring human exposure to lead: advantages, limitations, and future needs. *Environ Health Perspect* 2005; **113**: 1669–74.

29. Hu H, Shih R, Rothenberg S, Schwartz BS. The epidemiology of lead toxicity in adults: measuring dose and consideration of other methodologic issues. *Environ Health Perspect* 2007; **115**: 455–62.

●30. Chen A, Dietrich KN, Ware JH, Radcliffe J, Rogan WJ. IQ and blood lead from 2 to 7 years of age: are the effects in older children the residual of high blood lead concentrations in 2-year-olds? *Environ Health Perspect* 2005; **113**: 597–601.

●31. Manton WI. Total contribution of airborne lead to blood lead. *Br J Ind Med* 1985; **42**: 168–72.

●32. Gulson BL, Mahaffey KR, Mizon KJ, Korsch MJ, Cameron MA, Vimpani G. Contribution of tissue lead to blood lead in adult female subjects based on stable lead isotope methods. *J Lab Clin Med* 1995; **125**: 703–12.

33. Smith DR, Osterloh JD, Flegal AR. Use of endogenous, stable lead isotopes to determine release of lead from the skeleton. *Environ Health Perspect* 1996; **104**: 60–6.

34. Chia SE, Chia HP, Ong CN, Jeyaratnam J. Cumulative blood lead levels and nerve conduction parameters. *Occup Med (Lond)* 1996a; **46**: 59–64.

35. Fleming DE, Mills CE. A 4 × 500 mm cloverleaf detector system for in vivo bone lead measurement. *Med Phys* 2007; **34**: 945–51.

●36. Somervaille LJ, Chettle DR, Scott MC *et al.* In vivo tibia lead measurements as an index of cumulative exposure in occupationally exposed subjects. *Br J Ind Med* 1988; **45**: 174–81.

37. Somervaille LJ, Nilsson U, Chettle DR *et al.* In vivo measurements of bone lead – a comparison of two X-ray fluorescence techniques used at three different bone sites. *Phys Med Biol* 1989; **34**: 1833–45.

38. Gulson BL, Mizon KJ, Davis JD, Palmer JM, Vimpani G. Identification of sources of lead in children in a primary zinc–lead smelter environment. *Environ Health Perspect* 2004; **112**: 52–60.

●39. Chamberlain AC, Heard MJ, Little P, Newton D, Wells AC, Wiffen RD. *Investigations into Lead from Motor Vehicles.* AERE-R9198. Harwell: United Kingdom Atomic Energy Authority, 1978.

♦40. Agency for Toxic Substances and Disease Registry. *Public Health Statement for Lead.* Washington, DC: US Department of Health and Human Services, Public Health Service, 1997.

♦41. Mushak P. Gastro-intestinal absorption of lead in children and adults: overview of biological and biophysico-chemical aspects. *Chem Spec Bioavail* 1991; **3**: 87–104.

●42. James HM, Hilburn ME, Blair JA. Effects of meals and meal times on uptake of lead from the gastrointestinal tract in humans. *Hum Toxicol* 1985; **4**: 401–7.

43. Rabinowitz MB, Kopple JD, Wetherill GW. Effect of food intake and fasting on gastrointestinal lead absorption in humans. *Am J Clin Nutr* 1980; **33**: 1784–8.

●44. Ziegler EE, Edwards BB, Jensen RL, Mahaffey KR, Fomon SJ. Absorption and retention of lead by infants. *Pediatr Res* 1978; **12**: 29–34.

●45. Heard MJ, Chamberlain AC, Sherlock JC. Uptake of lead by humans and effect of minerals and food. *Sci Total Environ* 1983; **30**: 245–53.

46. Blake KC, Mann M. Effect of calcium and phosphorus on the gastrointestinal absorption of 203Pb in man. *Environ Res* 1983; **30**: 188–94.

●47. Mahaffey KR, Gartside PS, Glueck CJ. Blood lead levels and dietary calcium intake in 1- to 11-year-old children: the Second National Health and Nutrition Examination Survey, 1976 to 1980. *Pediatrics* 1986; **78**: 257–62.

48. Lanphear BP, Hornung R, Ho M *et al.* Environmental lead exposure during early childhood. *J Pediatr* 2002; **140**: 40–7.

49. Watson WS, Morrison J, Bethel MI *et al.* Food iron and lead absorption in humans. *Am J Clin Nutr* 1986; **44**: 248–56.

●50. Mahaffey KR, Annest JL. Association of erythrocyte protoporphyrin with blood lead level and iron status in the second National Health and Nutrition Examination Survey, 1976–1980. *Environ Res* 1986; **41**: 327–38.

51. Hammad TA, Sexton M, Langenberg P. Relationship between blood lead and dietary iron intake in preschool children. A cross-sectional study. *Ann Epidemiol* 1996; **6**: 30–3.

52. Wright RO, Tsaih SW, Schwartz J, Wright RJ, Hu H. Association between iron deficiency and blood lead level in a longitudinal analysis of children followed in an urban primary care clinic. *J Pediatr* 2003; **142**: 9–14.

53. Lucas SR, Sexton M, Langenberg P. Relationship between blood lead and nutritional factors in preschool children: a cross-sectional study. *Pediatrics* 1996; **97**: 74–8.

54. Gallicchio L, Scherer RW, Sexton M. Influence of nutrient intake on blood lead levels of young children at risk for lead poisoning. *Environ Health Perspect* 2002; **110**: A767–72.

55. Cheng Y, Willett WC, Schwartz J, Sparrow D, Weiss S, Hu H. Relation of nutrition to bone lead and blood lead levels in middle-aged to elderly men. The Normative Aging Study. *Am J Epidemiol* 1998; **147**: 1162–74.

●56. Kehoe RA. Studies of lead administration and elimination in adult volunteers under natural and experimentally induced conditions over extended periods of time. *Food Chem Toxicol* 1987; **25**: 421–93.

●57. Barry PS, Mossman DB. Lead concentrations in human tissues. *Br J Ind Med* 1970; **27**: 339–51.

●58. Bergdahl IA, Grubb A, Schütz A *et al.* Lead binding to delta-aminolevulinic acid dehydratase (ALAD) in human erythrocytes. *Pharmacol Toxicol* 1997; **81**: 153–8.

●59. Battistuzzi G, Petrucci R, Silvagni L, Urbani FR, Caiola S. Delta-aminolevulinate dehydratase: a new genetic polymorphism in man. *Ann Hum Genet* 1981; **45**: 223–9.

60. Ziemsen B, Angerer J, Lehnert G, Benkmann HG, Goedde HW. Polymorphism of delta-aminolevulinic acid dehydratase in lead-exposed workers. *Int Arch Occup Environ Health* 1986; **58**: 245–7.

●61. Wittmers LE, Aufderheide AC, Wallgren J, Rapp G, Alich A. Lead in bone. IV: Distribution of lead in the human skeleton. *Arch Environ Health* 1988; **43**: 381–91.

62. Schwartz BS, Lee BK, Stewart W *et al.* Delta-aminolevulinic acid dehydratase genotype modifies four

hour urinary lead excretion after oral administration of dimercaptosuccinic acid. *Occup Environ Med* 1997; **54**: 241–6.

63. Smith CM, Hu H, Wang X, Kelsey KT. ALA-D genotype is not associated with HT or HB levels among workers exposed to low levels of lead. *Med Lav* 1995; **86**: 229–35.

64. Fleming DE, Chettle DR, Wetmur JG *et al.* Effect of the delta-aminolevulinate dehydratase polymorphism on the accumulation of lead in bone and blood in lead smelter workers. *Environ Res* 1998; **77**: 49–61.

65. Hu H, Wu MT, Cheng Y, Sparrow D, Weiss S, Kelsey K. The delta-aminolevulinic acid dehydratase (ALAD) polymorphism and bone and blood lead levels in community-exposed men: the Normative Aging Study. *Environ Health Perspect* 2001; **109**: 827–32.

♦66. Gulson BL, Mizon KJ, Korsch MJ, Palmer JM, Donnelly JB. Mobilization of lead from human bone tissue during pregnancy and lactation – a summary of long-term research. *Sci Total Environ* 2003; **303**(1–2): 79–104.

●67. O'Flaherty EJ, Hammond PB, Lerner SI. Dependence of apparent blood lead half-life on the length of previous lead exposure in humans. *Fundam Appl Toxicol* 1982; **2**: 49–54.

68. Hryhorczuk DO, Rabinowitz MB, Hessl SM *et al.* Elimination kinetics of blood lead in workers with chronic lead intoxication. *Am J Ind Med* 1985; **8**: 33–42.

●69. Schütz A, Skerfving S, Ranstam J, Christoffersson JO. Kinetics of lead in blood after the end of occupational exposure. *Scand J Work Environ Health* 1987; **13**: 221–31.

70. Christoffersson JO, Ahlgren L, Schütz A, Skerfving S, Mattsson S. Decrease of skeletal lead levels in man after end of occupational exposure. *Arch Environ Health* 1986; **41**: 312–18.

71. Nilsson U, Attewell R, Christoffersson JO *et al.* Kinetics of lead in bone and blood after end of occupational exposure. *Pharmacol Toxicol* 1991; **68**: 477–84.

●72. Erkkila J, Armstrong R, Riihimaki V *et al.* In vivo measurements of lead in bone at four anatomical sites: long term occupational and consequent endogenous exposure. *Br J Ind Med* 1992; **49**: 631–44.

●73. Fleming DE, Boulay D, Richard NS *et al.* Accumulated body burden and endogenous release of lead in employees of a lead smelter. *Environ Health Perspect* 1997; **105**: 224–33.

74. Fleming DE, Chettle DR, Webber CE, O'Flaherty EJ. The O'Flaherty model of lead kinetics: an evaluation using data from a lead smelter population. *Toxicol Appl Pharmacol* 1999; **161**: 100–9.

75. Popovic M, McNeill FE, Chettle DR, Webber CE, Lee CV, Kaye WE. Impact of occupational exposure on lead levels in women. *Environ Health Perspect* 2005; **113**: 478–84.

76. Morrow L, Needleman HL, McFarland C, Metheny K, Tobin M. Past occupational exposure to lead: association between current blood lead and bone lead. *Arch Environ Occup Health* 2007; **62**: 183–6.

77. Manton WI, Cook JD. High accuracy (stable isotope dilution) measurements of lead in serum and cerebrospinal fluid. *Br J Ind Med* 1984; **41**: 313–19.

78. Hernandez-Avila M, Smith D, Meneses F, Sanin LH, Hu H. The influence of bone and blood lead on plasma lead levels in environmentally exposed adults. *Environ Health Perspect* 1998; **106**: 473–7.

●79. O'Flaherty EJ, Inskip MJ, Franklin CA, Durbin PW, Manton WI, Baccanale CL. Evaluation and modification of a physiologically based model of lead kinetics using data from a sequential isotope study in cynomolgus monkeys. *Toxicol Appl Pharmacol* 1998; **149**: 1–16.

80. Smith DR, Ilustre RP, Osterloh JD. Methodological considerations for the accurate determination of lead in human plasma and serum. *Am J Ind Med* 1998; **33**: 430–8.

81. Hu H, Rabinowitz M, Smith D. Bone lead as a biological marker in epidemiologic studies of chronic toxicity: conceptual paradigms. *Environ Health Perspect* 1998; **106**: 1–8.

82. Bergdahl IA, Vahter M, Counter SA *et al.* Lead in plasma and whole blood from lead-exposed children. *Environ Res* 1999; **80**: 25–33.

83. Lamadrid-Figueroa H, Tellez-Rojo MM, Hernandez-Cadena L *et al.* Biological markers of fetal lead exposure at each stage of pregnancy. *J Toxicol Environ Health A* 2006; **69**: 1781–96.

84. Gerhardsson L, Englyst V, Lundstrom NG, Nordberg G, Sandberg S, Steinvall F. Lead in tissues of deceased lead smelter workers. *J Trace Elem Med Biol* 1995; **9**: 136–43.

●85. Rabinowitz M, Wetherill GW, Kopple JD. Kinetic analysis of lead metabolism in healthy humans. *J Clin Invest* 1976; **58**: 260–70.

86. Rabinowitz MB. Toxicokinetics of bone lead. *Environ Health Perspect* 1991; **91**: 33–7.

87. Todd AC, Parsons PJ, Tang S, Moshier EL. Individual variability in human tibia lead concentration. *Environ Health Perspect* 2001; **109**: 1139–43.

88. Hoppin JA, Aro A, Hu H, Ryan PB. Measurement variability associated with KXRF bone lead measurement in young adults. *Environ Health Perspect* 2000; **108**: 239–42.

89. Gerhardsson L, Attewell R, Chettle DR *et al.* In vivo measurements of lead in bone in long-term exposed lead smelter workers. *Arch Environ Health* 1993; **48**: 147–56.

90. Bergdahl IA, Stromberg U, Gerhardsson L, Schütz A, Chettle DR, Skerfving S. Lead concentrations in tibial and calcaneal bone in relation to the history of occupational lead exposure. *Scand J Work Environ Health* 1998; **24**: 38–45.

●91. Leggett RW. An age-specific kinetic model of lead metabolism in humans. *Environ Health Perspect* 1993; **101**: 598–616.

●92. O'Flaherty EJ. Physiologically based models for bone-seeking elements. IV: Kinetics of lead disposition in humans. *Toxicol Appl Pharmacol* 1993; **118**: 16–29.

93. Brito JA, McNeill FE, Stronach I *et al.* Longitudinal changes in bone lead concentration: implications for modelling of human bone lead metabolism. *J Environ Monit* 2001; **3**: 343–51.

94. Gonzalez-Cossio T, Peterson KE, Sanin LH *et al.* Decrease in birth weight in relation to maternal bone-lead burden. *Pediatrics* 1997; **100**: 856–62.

95. Sanin LH, Gonzalez-Cossio T, Romieu I *et al.* Effect of maternal lead burden on infant weight and weight gain at one month of age among breastfed infants. *Pediatrics* 2001; **107**: 1016–23.

96. Cake KM, Bowins RJ, Vaillancourt C *et al.* Partition of circulating lead between serum and red cells is different for internal and external sources of lead. *Am J Ind Med* 1996; **29**: 440–5.

97. Tsaih SW, Korrick S, Schwartz J *et al.* Influence of bone resorption on the mobilization of lead from bone among middle-aged and elderly men: the Normative Aging Study. *Environ Health Perspect* 2001; **109**: 995–9.

98. Cheng Y, Schwartz J, Sparrow D, Aro A, Weiss ST, Hu H. Bone lead and blood lead levels in relation to baseline blood pressure and the prospective development of hypertension: the Normative Aging Study. *Am J Epidemiol* 2001; **153**: 164–71.

99. Bergdahl IA, Vahter M, Counter SA *et al.* Lead in plasma and whole blood from lead-exposed children. *Environ Res* 1999; **80**: 25–33.

100. Rothenberg SJ, Manalo M, Jiang J *et al.* Blood lead level and blood pressure during pregnancy in South Central Los Angeles. *Arch Environ Health* 1999; **54**: 382–9.

101. Korrick SA, Schwartz J, Tsaih SW *et al.* Correlates of bone and blood lead levels among middle-aged and elderly women. *Am J Epidemiol* 2002; **156**: 335–43.

102. Gerr F, Letz R, Stokes L, Chettle D, McNeill F, Kaye W. Association between bone lead concentration and blood pressure among young adults. *Am J Ind Med* 2002; **42**: 98–106.

103. Peters JL, Kubzansky L, McNeely E *et al.* Stress as a potential modifier of the impact of lead levels on blood pressure: the normative aging study. *Environ Health Perspect* 2007; **115**: 1154–9.

104. Muntner P, Menke A, Batuman V, Rabito FA, He J, Todd AC. Association of tibia lead and blood lead with end-stage renal disease: a pilot study of African-Americans. *Environ Res* 2007; **104**: 396–401.

105. Hoppin JA, Ryan PB, Hu H, Aro AC. Bone lead levels and delinquent behavior. *JAMA* 1996; **275**: 1727, discussion 1728.

●106. Needleman HL, McFarland C, Ness RB, Fienberg SE, Tobin MJ. Bone lead levels in adjudicated delinquents. A case control study. *Neurotoxicol Teratol* 2002; **24**: 711–17.

◆107. US Environmental Protection Agency. *Air Quality Criteria for Lead.* EPA600883028F. Research Triangle Park, NC: US Environmental Protection Agency, Office of Research and Development, Office of Health and Environmental Assessment, Environmental Criteria and Assessment Office, 1986.

108. Smith DR, Markowitz ME, Crick J, Rosen JF, Flegal AR. The effects of succimer on the absorption of lead in adults determined by using the stable isotope 204Pb. *Environ Res* 1994; **67**: 39–53.

♦109. Silbergeld EK. Lead in bone: implications for toxicology during pregnancy and lactation. *Environ Health Perspect* 1991; **91**: 63–70.

●110. Franklin CA, Inskip MJ, Baccanale CL *et al*. Use of sequentially administered stable lead isotopes to investigate changes in blood lead during pregnancy in a nonhuman primate (*Macaca fascicularis*). *Fundam Appl Toxicol* 1997; **39**: 109–19.

111. Gulson BL, Jameson CW, Mahaffey KR, Mizon KJ, Korsch MJ, Vimpani G. Pregnancy increases mobilization of lead from maternal skeleton. *J Lab Clin Med* 1997; **130**: 51–62.

112. Hertz-Picciotto I, Schramm M, Watt-Morse M, Chantala K, Anderson J, Osterloh J. Patterns and determinants of blood lead during pregnancy. *Am J Epidemiol* 2000; **152**: 829–37.

●113. Silbergeld EK, Schwartz J, Mahaffey K. Lead and osteoporosis: mobilization of lead from bone in postmenopausal women. *Environ Res* 1988; **47**: 79–94.

114. Markowitz ME, Weinberger HL. Immobilization-related lead toxicity in previously lead-poisoned children. *Pediatrics* 1990; **86**: 455–7.

115. Kessler M, Durand PY, Huu TC *et al*. Mobilization of lead from bone in end-stage renal failure patients with secondary hyperparathyroidism. *Nephrol Dial Transplant* 1999; **14**: 2731–3.

116. Kondrashov VS. Cosmonauts and lead: resorption and increased blood lead levels during long term space flight. *J Med Toxicol* 2006; **2**: 172–3.

●117. Gulson BL, Mahaffey KR, Jameson CW *et al*. Mobilization of lead from the skeleton during the postnatal period is larger than during pregnancy. *J Lab Clin Med* 1998b; **131**: 324–9.

118. Gulson BL, Mizon KJ, Palmer JM, Korsch MJ, Taylor AJ, Mahaffey KR. Blood lead changes during pregnancy and postpartum with calcium supplementation. *Environ Health Perspect* 2004; **112**: 1499–507.

119. Manton WI, Angle CR, Stanek KL, Kuntzelman D, Reese YR, Kuehnemann TJ. Release of lead from bone in pregnancy and lactation. *Environ Res* 2003; **92**: 139–51.

120. al-Saleh I, Khalil MA, Taylor A. Lead, erythrocyte protoporphyrin, and hematological parameters in normal maternal and umbilical cord blood from subjects of the Riyadh region, Saudi Arabia. *Arch Environ Health* 1995; **50**: 66–73.

121. Gulson BL, Jameson CW, Mahaffey KR *et al*. Relationships of lead in breast milk to lead in blood, urine, and diet of the infant and mother. *Environ Health Perspect* 1998a; **106**: 667–74.

122. Arora M, Ettinger AS, Peterson KE *et al*. Maternal dietary intake of polyunsaturated fatty acids modifies the relationship between lead levels in bone and breast milk. *J Nutr* 2008; **138**: 73–9.

●123. Muldoon SB, Cauley JA, Kuller LH *et al*. Effects of blood lead levels on cognitive function of older women. *Neuroepidemiology* 1996; **15**: 62–72.

●124. Symanski E, Hertz-Picciotto I. Blood lead levels in relation to menopause, smoking, and pregnancy history. *Am J Epidemiol* 1995; **141**: 1047–58.

125. Weyermann M, Brenner H. Factors affecting bone demineralization and blood lead levels of postmenopausal women – a population-based study from Germany. *Environ Res* 1998; **76**: 19–25.

126. Hernandez-Avila M, Villalpando CG, Palazuelos E, Hu H, Villalpando ME, Martinez DR. Determinants of blood lead levels across the menopausal transition. *Arch Environ Health* 2000; **55**: 355–60.

127. Webber CE, Chettle DR, Bowins RJ *et al*. Hormone replacement therapy may reduce the return of endogenous lead from bone to the circulation. *Environ Health Perspect* 1995; **103**: 1150–3.

128. Garrido Latorre F, Hernandez-Avila M, Tamayo Orozco J *et al*. Relationship of blood and bone lead to menopause and bone mineral density among middle-age women in Mexico City. *Environ Health Perspect* 2003; **111**: 631–6.

129. Potula V, Kaye W. The impact of menopause and lifestyle factors on blood and bone lead levels among female former smelter workers: the Bunker Hill Study. *Am J Ind Med* 2006; **49**: 143–52.

●130. O'Flaherty EJ. Physiologically based models for bone-seeking elements. V: Lead absorption and disposition in childhood. *Toxicol Appl Pharmacol* 1995; **131**: 297–308.

♦131. US Environmental Protection Agency. *Guidance Manual for the Integrated Exposure Uptake Biokinetic Model for Lead in Children*. EPA540R93081, PB93963510. Washington, DC: US Environmental Protection Agency, 1994.

●132. Chia SE, Chua LH, Ng TP, Foo SC, Jeyaratnam J. Postural stability of workers exposed to lead. *Occup Environ Med* 1994; **51**: 768–71.

133. Osterberg K, Borjesson J, Gerhardsson L, Schütz A, Skerfving S. A neurobehavioural study of long-term occupational inorganic lead exposure. *Sci Total Environ* 1997; **201**: 39–51.

134. Kovala T, Matikainen E, Mannelin T *et al*. Effects of low level exposure to lead on neurophysiological functions among lead battery workers. *Occup Environ Med* 1997; **54**: 487–93.

135. Yokoyama K, Araki S, Yamashita K *et al*. Subclinical cerebellar anterior lobe, vestibulocerebellar and spinocerebellar afferent effects in young female lead workers in China: computerized posturography with sway frequency analysis and brainstem auditory evoked potentials. *Ind Health* 2002; **40**: 245–53.

●136. Bleecker ML, Ford DP, Celio MA, Vaughan CG, Lindgren KN. Impact of cognitive reserve on the relationship of lead exposure and neurobehavioral performance. *Neurology* 2007; **69**: 470–6.

137. Chuang HY, Schwartz J, Tsai SY, Lee ML, Wang JD, Hu H. Vibration perception thresholds in workers with long

term exposure to lead. *Occup Environ Med* 2000; **57**: 588–94.

138. Staessen JA, Lauwerys RR, Buchet JP *et al*. Impairment of renal function with increasing blood lead concentrations in the general population. The Cadmibel Study Group. *N Engl J Med* 1992; **327**: 151–6.

139. Staessen JA, Bulpitt CJ, Fagard R *et al*. Hypertension caused by low-level lead exposure: myth or fact? *J Cardiovasc Risk* 1994; **1**: 87–97.

●140. Staessen JA, Roels H, Fagard R. Hypertension and lead exposure. *JAMA* 1996; **276**: 1037–8.

141. Payton M, Hu H, Sparrow D, Weiss ST. Low-level lead exposure and renal function in the Normative Aging Study. *Am J Epidemiol* 1994; **140**: 821–9.

142. Wu MT, Kelsey K, Schwartz J, Sparrow D, Weiss S, Hu H. A delta-aminolevulinic acid dehydratase (ALAD) polymorphism may modify the relationship of low-level lead exposure to uricemia and renal function: the normative aging study. *Environ Health Perspect* 2003; **111**: 335–41.

143. Tsaih SW, Korrick S, Schwartz J *et al*. Lead, diabetes, hypertension, and renal function: the normative aging study. *Environ Health Perspect* 2004; **112**: 1178–82.

●144. Hu H, Aro A, Payton M *et al*. The relationship of bone and blood lead to hypertension. The Normative Aging Study. *JAMA* 1996; **275**: 1171–6.

145. Weaver VM, Ellis LR, Lee BK *et al*. Associations between patella lead and blood pressure in lead workers. *Am J Ind Med* 2008; **51**: 336–43.

146. Payton M, Riggs KM, Spiro A, Weiss ST, Hu H. Relations of bone and blood lead to cognitive function: the VA Normative Aging Study. *Neurotoxicol Teratol* 1998; **20**: 19–27.

147. Rhodes D, Spiro A, Aro A, Hu H. Relationship of bone and blood lead levels to psychiatric symptoms: the Normative Aging Study. *J Occup Environ Med* 2003; **45**: 1144–51.

148. Weisskopf MG, Proctor SP, Wright RO *et al*. Cumulative lead exposure and cognitive performance among elderly men. *Epidemiology* 2007; **18**: 59–66.

149. Nordberg M, Winblad B, Fratiglioni L, Basun H. Lead concentrations in elderly urban people related to blood pressure and mental performance: results from a population-based study. *Am J Ind Med* 2000; **38**: 290–4.

●150. Lustberg M, Silbergeld E. Blood lead levels and mortality. *Arch Intern Med* 2002; **162**: 2443–9.

151. Krieg EF Jr, Chrislip DW, Crespo CJ, Brightwell WS, Ehrenberg RL, Otto DA. The relationship between blood lead levels and neurobehavioral test performance in NHANES III and related occupational studies. *Public Health Rep* 2005; **120**: 240–51.

152. Schwartz BS, Stewart WF, Bolla KI *et al*. Past adult lead exposure is associated with longitudinal decline in cognitive function. *Neurology* 2000; **55**: 1144–50.

●153. Menke A, Muntner P, Batuman V, Silbergeld EK, Guallar E. Blood lead below 0.48 micromol/L (10 microg/dL) and mortality among US adults. *Circulation* 2006; **114**: 1388–94.

154. Park SK, Schwartz J, Weisskopf M *et al*. Low-level lead exposure, metabolic syndrome, and heart rate variability: the VA Normative Aging Study. *Environ Health Perspect* 2006; **114**: 1718–24.

●155. Schober SE, Mirel LB, Graubard BI, Brody DJ, Flegal KM. Blood lead levels and death from all causes, cardiovascular disease, and cancer: results from the NHANES III mortality study. *Environ Health Perspect* 2006; **114**: 1538–41.

◆156. Navas-Acien A, Guallar E, Silbergeld EK, Rothenberg SJ. Lead exposure and cardiovascular disease – a systematic review. *Environ Health Perspect* 2007; **115**: 472–82.

157. Campbell JR, Moss ME, Raubertas RF. The association between caries and childhood lead exposure. *Environ Health Perspect* 2000; **108**: 1099–102.

158. Martin D, Glass TA, Bandeen-Roche K, Todd AC, Shi W, Schwartz BS. Association of blood lead and tibia lead with blood pressure and hypertension in a community sample of older adults. *Am J Epidemiol* 2006; **163**: 467–78.

159. Lamadrid-Figueroa H, Tellez-Rojo MM, Hernandez-Avila M *et al*. Association between the plasma/whole blood lead ratio and history of spontaneous abortion: a nested cross-sectional study. *BMC Pregnancy Childbirth* 2007; **7**: 22.

◆160. Centers for Disease Control and Prevention. *Preventing Lead Poisoning in Young Children*. Atlanta, Georgia: CDC, 2005.

●161. Binns HJ, Campbell C, Brown MJ and for the Advisory Committee on Childhood Lead poisoning prevention. Interpreting and managing blood lead levels of less than 10 μ dl in children and managing reducing childhood exposure to lead: recommendations of the Centers for Disease Control and Prevention Advisory Committee on Childhood Lead Poisoning Prevention. *Pediatrics 2007;* **120e:** *1285–98.*

●162. Canfield RL, Henderson CR Jr, Cory-Slechta DA, Cox C, Jusko TA, Lanphear BP. Intellectual impairment in children with blood lead concentrations below 10 microg per deciliter. *N Engl J Med* 2003; **348**: 1517–26.

●163. Bellinger DC, Stiles KM, Needleman HL. Low-level lead exposure, intelligence and academic achievement: a long term follow-up study. *Pediatrics* 1992; **90**: 855–61.

164. Surkan PJ, Zhang A, Trachtenberg F, Daniel DB, McKinlay S, Bellinger DC. Neuropsychological function in children with blood lead levels < 10μg/dL. *Neurotoxicology 2007;8: 1170–7.*

165. al-Saleh I, Nester M, DeVol E, Shinwari N, Munchari L, al-Shahria S. Relationships between blood lead concentrations, intelligence, and academic achievement of Saudi Arabian schoolgirls. *Int J Hyg Environ Health* 2001; **204**(2–3): 165–74.

166. Tellez-Rojo MM, Bellinger DC, Arroyo-Quiroz C *et al*. Longitudinal associations between blood lead concentrations lower than 10μg/dL and neurobehavioral development in environmentally exposed children in Mexico City. *Pediatrics* 2006; **118**: e323–30.

167. Kordas K, Canfield RL, Lopez P *et al*. Deficits in cognitive function and achievement in Mexican first-graders with low blood lead concentrations. *Environ Res* 2006; **100**: 371–86.

168. Surkan PJ, Schnaas L, Wright RJ *et al.* Maternal self-esteem, exposure to lead, and child neurodevelopment. *Neurotoxicology* 2008; **29**: 278–85.

●169. Needleman HL, Schell A, Bellinger D, Leviton A, Allred EN. The long-term effects of exposure to low doses of lead in childhood. An 11-year follow-up report. *N Engl J Med* 1990; **322**: 83–8.

♦170. Lanphear BP, Hornung R, Khoury J *et al.* Low-level environmental lead exposure and children's intellectual function: an international pooled analysis. *Environ Health Perspect* 2005b; **113**: 894–9.

171. Jusko TA, Henderson CR, Lanphear BP, Cory-Slechta DA, Parsons PJ, Canfield RL. Blood lead concentrations < *10μg/dL and child intelligence at 6 years of age.* *Environ Health Perspect* 2008; **116**: 243–8.

172. Wright JP, Dietrich KN, Ris MD *et al.* Association of prenatal and childhood blood lead concentrations with criminal arrests in early adulthood. *PLOS Medicine* 2008; **5**: 732–40.

●173. Rogan WJ, Dietrich KN, Ware JH *et al.* The effect of chelation therapy with succimer on neuropsychological development in children exposed to lead. *N Engl J Med* 2001; **344**: 1421–6.

174. Gulson BL. Can some of the detrimental neurodevelopmental effects attributed to lead be due to pesticides? *Sci Total Environ* 2008; **396**(2–3): 193–5.

175. Lanphear BP, Hornung RW, Khoury J, Dietrich KN, Cory-Slechta DA, Canfield RL. The conundrum of unmeasured confounding: Comment on: "Can some of the detrimental neurodevelopmental effects attributed to lead be due to pesticides? by Brian Gulson". *Sci Total Environ* 2008; **396**(2–3): 196–200.

176. Bellinger DC. Assessing environmental neurotoxicant exposures and child neurobehavior: confounded by confounding? *Epidemiology* 2004; **15**: 383–4.

♦177. Davis JM, Otto DA, Weil DE, Grant LD. The comparative developmental neurotoxicity of lead in humans and animals. *Neurotoxicol Teratol* 1990; **12**: 215–29.

178. National Occupational Health and Safety Commission. *Control of Inorganic Lead at Work. National Standard for the Control of Inorganic Lead at Work.* NOHSC:1012. Canberra: NOHSC, 1994.

179. Kosnett MJ, Wedeen RP, Rothenberg SJ *et al.* Recommendations for medical management of adult lead exposure. *Environ Health Perspect* 2007; **115**: 463–71.

180. Harvey B (ed.) Managing Elevated Blood Lead Levels Among Young Children: Recommendations from the Advisory Committee on Childhood Lead Poisoning Prevention. Available from: http://www.cdc.gov./nceh/lead/casemanagement (accessed July 2009).

181. New Zealand Ministry of Health. The Environmental Case Management of Lead-exposed Persons Guidelines for Public Health Units, Revised edition. Available at: www.moh.govt.nz

182. Hernandez-Avila M, Gonzalez-Cossio T, Hernandez-Avila JE *et al.* Dietary calcium supplements to lower blood lead levels in lactating women: a randomized placebo-controlled trial. *Epidemiology* 2003; **14**: 206–12.

183. Tellez-Rojo MM, Hernandez-Avila M, Gonzalez-Cossio T *et al.* Impact of breastfeeding on the mobilization of lead from bone. *Am J Epidemiol* 2002; **155**: 420–8.

184. Janakiraman V, Ettinger A, Mercado-Garcia A, Hu H, Hernandez-Avila M. Calcium supplements and bone resorption in pregnancy. *Am J Prev Med* 2003; **24**: 260–4.

185. Kalkwarf HJ. Hormonal and dietary regulation of changes in bone density during lactation and after weaning in women. *J Mammary Gland Biol Neoplasia* 1999; **4**: 319–29.

MERCURY

LISA HILL, JON G. AYRES

EXPOSURE

Exposure to environmental mercury is an important potential cause of morbidity in human populations, the chief sources of exposure being ingestion of contaminated fish, dental amalgams and vaccines.[1] The burning of coal and of mercury amalgams used in gold and silver mining releases mercury vapour into the environment. This mercury then returns to the earth's surface in rainwater entering waterways, where it is converted by microorganisms to highly toxic methyl mercury which can contaminate fish, becoming further concentrated with each successive step up the food chain. A study by the United States Geological Survey in 2009 revealed mercury in all fish sampled, with concentrations exceeding the US Environmental Protection Agency human health criterion of 0.3 µg per gram wet weight in over a quarter of fish.[2] The main route of environmental mercury exposure is ingestion, but inhalation and transdermal uptake also occur. Dental amalgams release mercury vapour, which is inhaled and absorbed into the bloodstream. Ethyl mercury, the active ingredient of thiomersal, is a preservative used in many vaccines.

POISONING OUTBREAKS

There have been many epidemics of environmental poisoning with mercury, notably the devastating effects of environmental mercury exposure on the population of Minamata Bay in Japan. In the 1950s, a factory manufacturing vinyl chloride released inorganic mercury into a river feeding into the bay, resulting in the accumulation of mercury in fish – so-called Minamata disease. A total of 121 people living in villages around Minamata Bay were poisoned, 46 (38 per cent) of whom died.[3,4] Similar occurrences have been seen in gold-mining areas in the Amazon.[5]

TOXICITY

The toxic effects of mercury are dependent on both the route and the form of exposure, with uptake to and distribution within the tissues depending on the properties of the various forms of the metal.[6] Organic methyl mercury is particularly toxic to the nervous system as it crosses the blood–brain barrier and has a high affinity for thiol groups, enabling it to inhibit the enzyme glutathione peroxidase. Inorganic mercury is more toxic to the kidney, where it accumulates.

CLINICAL PRESENTATION

Classically, mercury poisoning has been seen in occupational groups such as hatters and mercury miners.

Exposure to corrosive mercury compounds causes inflammation, pain and tissue necrosis. Ingestion of mercury salts can result in colitis presenting with abdominal pain and bloody diarrhoea, while inhalation of mercury can result in cough, dyspnoea and, in severe cases, pulmonary oedema. Symptoms of acute toxicity have been reported after the inhalation of mercury vapour at concentrations of 1 part per million.

Chronic mercury toxicity most commonly presents with neurological symptoms such as paraesthesiae, visual field disturbances and ataxia, which are associated with the destruction of neurones in the visual cortex and cerebellum. The developing nervous system is particularly vulnerable to toxic insult, and mercury toxicity has been suggested by some to be a cause of autistic spectrum disorders.[7] Inorganic mercury accumulates in the glomeruli, which can result in nephrotic syndrome and can in large doses cause acute tubular necrosis. Mercury absorption through the skin can result in chronic toxicity as well as causing local symptoms of burns and blistering. There is some evidence for an association between methyl mercury exposure and cardiovascular dizease.[1]

Mercury concentrations in blood of above 95 mmol/L and in urine of above 120 nmol/mmol creatinine for inorganic compounds and 15 nmol/nmol creatinine for organic compounds are typical in chronic mercury poisoning.[3]

All forms of mercury, irrespective of route of exposure, carry the potential to have important effects on human health, with exposures largely occurring through releases to the environment from industrial activity. Approaches to the control of such sources are consequently through legislation encompassed within environmental protection law.

REFERENCES

♦ = Major review article

♦1. Clarkson TW, Magos L, Myers GJ. The toxicology of mercury – current exposures and clinical manifestations. *New Engl J Med* 2003; **349**: 1731–7.
2. Scudder BC, Chasar LC, Wentz DA *et al. Mercury in Fish, Bed Sediment, and Water from Streams Across the United States, 1998-2005.* Reston, VA: US Geological Survey, 2009.
3. Baxter PJ *et al. Hunter's Diseases of Occupations*, 10th edn. London: Arnold, 2010.

4. Kurland LT, Faro SN, Siedler H. minamata disease. The outbreak of a neurologic disorder in Minamata, Japan, and its relationship to the ingestion of seafood contaminated by mercuric compounds. *World Neurol* 1960; **1**: 370–95.
5. Malm O. Gold mining as a source of mercury exposure in the Brazilian Amazon. *Environ Res* 1998; **77**: 73–8.
6. Environmental Protection Agency. Mercury. Available from: http://www.epa.gov/mercury/effects.htm (accessed November 19, 2009).
7. Geier MR, Geier DA. Thimerosal in childhood vaccines, neurodevelopment disorders, and heart disease in the United States. *J Am Physician Surg* 2003; **8**: 6–11.

27

Cadmium

PAUL CULLINAN

INTRODUCTION AND ENVIRONMENTAL SOURCES

In the natural environment, cadmium is distributed widely but in low concentrations, almost always in conjunction with other elements such as zinc, lead, copper and sulphur. Its principle ore, greenockite, is generally found in conjunction with zinc sulphide (sphalerite). The pure metal – first isolated in 1817 – is bivalent, soft and silver-white in colour with a relatively low melting point (321 °C). Important cadmium compounds include cadmium oxide, cadmium sulphide, cadmium chloride and cadmium sulphate, the last two of which are soluble in water. The major producers of cadmium are currently in China, Japan and South Korea.

Industrially, cadmium has a variety of uses. It is applied to steel and some non-ferrous metals to produce corrosion-resistant plating, and used in welding, soldering and bearings in low-melting point, low-resistance alloys. Cadmium sulphide (yellow) and cadmium selenium sulphide (red) are used as pigments in plastics, fabrics, ceramics and glass. Heat- and light-stabilizers in plastics may also contain cadmium compounds. Nickel–cadmium batteries, for portable electronic equipment, use metallic cadmium as a negative electrode plate. Cadmium sulphide and cadmium telluride are used, in small quantities, in the manufacture of specialized mirrors and lenses.

Cadmium sulphide, cadmium selenide and cadmium telluride are photovoltaic and used in the manufacture of some solar fuel cells; they also have semi-conducting properties that are employed in a variety of electronic products. Cadmium-containing alloys are sometimes used in radiation detection equipment. High-phosphate fertilizers contain variable concentrations of cadmium, and in the past it was used as a weed-killer.

The main anthropogenic sources of environmental cadmium are contamination from non-ferrous metal smelting – especially zinc smelting – coal and oil combustion, battery manufacture and disposal, heavy fertilizer use and iron/steel manufacture. Cadmium in air, released primarily from industrial processes, occurs principally in the form of particulate cadmium oxide. Particles released from combustion processes are typically of respirable size and small enough to remain airborne for several days and over long distances.[1] Those produced during metal smelting tend to be larger and to be deposited more rapidly; conversely, smelting at very high temperatures can produce a non-particulate cadmium vapour. Cadmium in soil or water is in a variety of forms, some soluble others not.

EXPOSURES AND TEMPORAL TRENDS

Increased levels of cadmium in water and soil generally derive directly from industrial processes (chiefly metal smelting), by leaching from contaminated landfill or by agricultural run-off. A small proportion of cadmium in air arises from natural processes such as weathering, volcanic eruption and forest fires, but most is produced by the burning of fossil fuels and by industrial activity.

For humans, the most important routes of exposure are oral and respiratory; dermal absorption may occur in the workplace but is believed to be minimal outside exceptional circumstances. In the non-industrial setting, almost all cadmium exposure is through the ingestion of contaminated water or, more importantly, plants – vegetables, pulses and grains – grown in contaminated soils. Animals feeding off such material may concentrate cadmium in their livers and kidneys, and the (human) consumption of these meats – and of shellfish – may contribute to the total exposure. Most foods contain less than 0.02 µg/g cadmium, but levels may be much higher in contaminated areas. Typically, the total intake of dietary cadmium is between 10 and 35 µg per day, or 0.2–0.7 µg/kg body weight. Intakes for children may, on a weight-for-weight basis, be higher.

In most circumstances, the proportion of daily cadmium intake that is derived from drinking water is less than that from food. The concentration of cadmium in most potable groundwater is below 1 µg/L, and in these circumstances the total intake from drinking water would be around 2 µg per day. Contaminated supplies may have concentrations of cadmium 50 times higher.[1]

Tobacco grown in cadmium-rich soils is an important source of cadmium for smokers, and active smoking may increase a typical daily exposure by between 10 per cent and 100 per cent.[2–4] There is some evidence that smoking counterfeit cigarettes results in a greater exposure to cadmium (and other heavy metals) even after correcting for differences in nicotine composition.[5]

Concentrations of cadmium in air are dependent largely on emissions from local industry. In non-industrialized, rural environments, levels are around 1 ng/m³; urban concentrations may be up to 40 times higher, while those in close proximity to industrial sources can be as high as 10 µg/m³. In most settings, without local industrial sources, and in non-smokers, the total daily cadmium intake from air is less than 1.0 µg, less than a tenth of that from dietary sources.

TRENDS IN CADMIUM EXPOSURE

The production and use of cadmium is dependent not only on the specific industrial needs for the metal, but also on the production of zinc, of which it is a major by-product. While cadmium consumption for batteries grew steadily from the 1980s, its use in other materials, such as pigments, stabilizers and alloys, declined. The replacement of some nickel–cadmium batteries by lithium–ion and nickel–metal hydride types has reduced demand, a process furthered by increasing environmental regulation on the disposal of cadmium-containing materials. Reductions, in many but not all countries, in the use of coal and fuel oil combustion in electricity-generating plants have led to a decline in atmospheric emissions of cadmium. Nonetheless, industrial processes for at least a century have led to a legacy of heavy cadmium contamination in many parts of the world. As described below, these have sometimes had devastating health consequences for exposed populations.

TOXICOKINETICS

Absorption

- Ingested cadmium: Only a small proportion of ingested cadmium is absorbed, the remainder being excreted in the faeces. Absorption is increased in persons with iron or calcium deficiencies, and in those with high-fat diets.
- Respired cadmium: It is estimated that about 25 per cent of inhaled cadmium is absorbed, primarily through the alveoli. The proportion absorbed from tobacco smoking is believed to be far higher, probably because of the very small size of the particles in cigarette smoke. As a result, the whole-body burden of cadmium is about seven times higher in smokers than in non-smokers.[6]

Distribution and excretion

Following absorption through any route, cadmium is transported mainly within red blood cells. After cell death or haemolysis, it is released into the plasma, and a proportion is bound to a number of metal-binding proteins including albumin and metallothionein. Thereafter, it is distributed widely throughout the body, chiefly to the kidneys and liver, but also in skeletal muscle.

Metallothionein binding occurs mainly in the liver and only to a limited extent in the alveoli and gastrointestinal tract. Cadmium that is bound to metallothionein is filtered in the renal glomerulus but reabsorbed in the proximal tubule and accumulates in the renal cortex. The protein is inducible, with concentrations increased not only by cadmium, but also by exposure to related metals (notably zinc) and by some physiological or pathological factors including exercise and inflammation. The toxicity of cadmium may relate to the local, free concentration of metal that remains unbound to protein.

Renal and hepatic concentrations of cadmium are extremely low at birth, but both rise with age, with adult concentrations in the kidney (40–50 µg/g wet weight) being about 20–40 times higher than in the liver. Very heavy exposures may reverse these proportions. The half-life of cadmium in the kidney is estimated to be between 10 and 30 years and that in the liver between 5 and 10 years.[7] Cadmium may cross the placenta and is excreted, in relatively low concentrations, in breast milk.

BIOMONITORING OF CADMIUM EXPOSURE

Neutron activation or X-ray fluorescence techniques that measure the accumulation of cadmium in the liver or kidney are available but are impracticable in most circumstances, especially where general population exposures are being studied. Indirect markers of exposure include measurements of cadmium in the urine, blood, hair and faeces. Although the last of these is a good indicator of recently ingested cadmium, the collection of the appropriate material is relatively complicated. Cadmium in hair reflects not only the blood concentration of the metal during the its growth phase, but also cadmium that has been deposited directly from air.[8]

The half-life of cadmium in blood is around 3 months. Although blood cadmium concentrations are influenced by both the body burden and recent exposure, levels in most circumstances reflect only the latter. Reflecting this, blood cadmium levels show only a weak correlation with age,[9] and in occupationally exposed populations, blood cadmium values are proportional to average intensities of current exposure.[10] In non-smoking adults without workplace exposures, blood cadmium concentrations are generally less than 0.8 μg/L.[11,12] Values may be twice as high or higher in smokers.[12,13]

In contrast, urinary cadmium levels increase with age, indicating that they are a more faithful reflection of the total body burden of the metal, and particularly of that portion held in the kidneys. Only at very high levels of prolonged exposure, when cadmium-binding sites are saturated and absorbed cadmium is rapidly excreted, do urinary values reflect recent exposure. In circumstances of renal tubular damage consequent on cadmium toxicity – but possibly not that from other causes – there may be a considerable increase in the urinary excretion of the metal. In persons without occupational exposure to cadmium, urinary levels are generally below 1.0 μg/L creatinine.[12]

ADVERSE HEALTH EFFECTS

Renal disease

Cadmium accumulates in the kidney, and this organ is the main site of cadmium toxicity whether exposure is by ingestion or through inhalation. Early signs of damage are manifest by evidence of proximal tubular dysfunction, with increased levels of urinary low molecular mass (less than 40 kDa) proteins such as beta$_2$-microglobulin and retinol-binding protein.[14] With higher – or longer – exposures, there may be an increased excretion of larger proteins, indicative of further tubular or glomerular damage.[15,16] Although urinary protein and other measurements are often used as surrogates for whole-body cadmium burden, it is worth appreciating that the thresholds of cadmium exposure at which different urinary biomarkers are detectable are very variable, reflecting both different assay sensitivities and differential damage to specific parts of the tubular nephron.

Numerous surveys of both occupationally and environmentally exposed populations have demonstrated direct relationships between urinary cadmium excretion and a wide variety of proteinurias.[17] These relationships are probably modified by age, sex and possibly genotype.

Although there is a well-established risk of proteinuria at urinary cadmium levels of 10 μg/g or more of creatinine, the risk at lower levels is more uncertain. For an individual, the risk associated with levels below 10 μg/g creatinine is probably low;[14] some population surveys, however, have detected an increased rate of proteinuria at urinary cadmium levels of around 2–4 μg/g creatinine.[18–21] It is suggested that such levels may be reached by a daily intake of dietary cadmium of about 1 g/kg body weight continuously for 50 years, or a weekly intake of around 7 μg/kg body weight.[22]

These issues are further complicated by the fact that the kidney handles metallothionein-bound cadmium in the same manner as it does low molecular mass proteins. Thus any (other) cause of renal tubular dysfunction may increase urinary levels of both cadmium and microproteins. Some more recent surveys have accounted for the potential for such confounding by relating proteinuria to both urinary and blood levels of cadmium.[23]

The clinical significance of reduced tubular resorption of low molecular mass proteins is uncertain, as is the question of whether mild degrees of cadmium-related proteinuria are reversible.[24] Persistent proteinuria at levels of over 1000 μg/g creatinine (beta$_2$-microglobulin or retinol-binding protein) may increase the individual risk of renal failure. Reductions in glomerular filtration rate have been related to both proteinuria and body cadmium burdens in some occupationally exposed populations.[25] It is less clear whether environmental cadmium exposures carry a similar risk, although a case-referent study in Sweden suggested that patients with end-stage renal failure were more likely than controls to live in the vicinity of cadmium-emitting industries.[26]

Progressive cadmium-related nephropathy may further be accompanied by an increased urinary excretion of non-proteins such as glucose, uric acid, phosphorus and calcium. Hypercalciuria and renal stones have been described in some populations of cadmium-exposed workers.[27,28]

Evidence that cadmium exposure may affect kidney vitamin D metabolism with subsequent disturbances in calcium balance and bone density[18,29,30] suggests that decreased bone density, particularly in elderly women, may be a significant adverse effect of kidney cadmium accumulation.

Bone disease

Prolonged exposure to cadmium can cause a disturbance in bone metabolism, combined osteomalacia–osteoporosis and, in severe case, painful and multiple fractures. The mechanisms that give rise to these effects are probably complex and probably include not only the results of nephrotoxicity, including reduced activation of vitamin D, but also direct actions of cadmium on bone mineralization.[31]

The most notorious manifestation of cadmium bone disease was the outbreak of itai-itai disease in the Jinzu river basin in Japan. The inhabitants – particularly malnourished women over the age of 40 – of an area down-river from zinc and other mining operations who had for many years consumed rice grown in paddy fields heavily contaminated with cadmium developed multiple fractures and tender limb-bone deformities.[32] Lower levels of environmental cadmium contamination may also be associated with an increased risk of fracture, height loss and reduced bone density.[33–35]

Respiratory disease

Cadmium oxide is odourless and insoluble in water, and its adverse respiratory effects have a latency of several hours. It is not uncommon, therefore, in settings of high airborne concentrations for exposed persons to inhale large quantities of fumes without immediate adverse effect. At sufficiently high doses, a delayed toxic pneumonitis may ensue, in some cases accompanied by pulmonary oedema and even death. Survivors of high-intensity exposures may be left with permanent respiratory damage.[36]

Exposures at lower intensities for longer durations are associated with the development of emphysema. An increased risk of death from non-malignant respiratory disease, related to cadmium exposure, has been observed in several occupationally exposed cohorts,[37,38] and more detailed studies of working populations have observed direct relationships between cumulative cadmium exposure and functional or radiological evidence of pulmonary emphysema.[39–41] It is unlikely that these associations are wholly confounded by other workplace exposures or by cigarette-smoking. A biological explanation may lie in the ability of cadmium to reduce circulating levels of alpha$_1$-antitrypsin[42] and procollagen production by lung fibroblasts.[43]

It is less clear whether non-occupational exposures to cadmium are related to the development of obstructive lung disease. In a representative sample of US adults, for example, urinary cadmium levels were negatively associated with pulmonary function,[44] a relationship that could be explained by cadmium being an important agent in tobacco-related lung disease. More probably, however, in populations without significant occupational exposure, urinary cadmium levels – far lower than they are in working populations – are a reflection of accumulated cigarette-smoking.

Cancer

Cohort studies of employees with occupational exposure to cadmium initially suggested an increase in the risk of lung cancer; in 1993 (updated in 1997), the evidence was considered sufficiently strong for the International Agency for Cancer Research (IARC) to label cadmium and cadmium compounds as group I human carcinogens.[45] None of the studies included in this evaluation, however, was able to control adequately for potentially confounding exposures to cigarette smoke or other occupationally encountered carcinogens such as arsenic. Moreover,

information on exposure–response relationships was very limited. Subsequent studies of other working populations have not provided strong support for the IARC position.[37,46,47] A systematic review of environmentally exposed populations suggests no increase in the risk of lung cancer in this group.[48]

The position is similar with respect to cancers at other sites. Early reports of increased risks of prostatic cancer[49] have not been supported by subsequent studies.[50] Similarly, although there are several reports of increased rates of renal cancer in occupationally exposed populations,[51] there is very little convincing evidence that they can be attributed independently to cadmium exposure. Interestingly, the failure to demonstrate human carcinogenesis by cadmium in these sites is in stark contrast to the evidence from animal 'models', in which genitourinary tract cancers can be established with relative ease.

Reports of cadmium exposure causing human cancer in the bladder,[52] testicle,[53] breast[54] or colon[55] remain speculative.

REFERENCES

♦ = Major review article

♦1. US Department for Health and Human Services, Public Health Service Agency for Toxic Substances and Disease Registry. *Draft Toxicological Profile for Cadmium*. Washington, DC: US Department for Health and Human Services, 2008.
2. Elinder CG. *Cadmium: Uses, Occurrence and Intake. Cadmium and Health: A Toxicological and Epidemiological Appraisal*. Vol. I: *Exposure, Dose, and Metabolism. Effects and Response*. Boca Raton, FL: CRC Press, 1985: pp. 23–64.
3. Lewis GP, Coughlin LL, Jusko WJ, Hartz S. Contribution of cigarette smoking to cadmium accumulation in man. *Lancet* 1972; **1**: 291–2.
4. Massadeh AM, Alali FQ, Jaradat QM. Determination of cadmium and lead in different cigarette brands in Jordan. *Environ Monit Assess* 2005; 104(1–3): 163–70.
5. Pappas RS, Polzin GM, Watson CH, Ashley DL. Cadmium, lead, and thallium in smoke particulate from counterfeit cigarettes compared to authentic US brands. *Food Chem Toxicol* 2007; **45**: 202–9.
6. Franklin DM, Guthrie CJ, Chettle DR *et al*. In vivo neutron activation analysis of organ cadmium burdens. Referent levels in liver and kidney and the impact of smoking. In: Shrauzer G (ed.) *Biological Trace Elements Research* (pp. 401–6). Clifton, NJ: Humana Press, 1990.
7. Ellis KJ, Cohn SH, Smith TJ. Cadmium inhalation exposure estimates: their significance with respect to kidney and liver cadmium burden. *J Toxicol Environ Health* 1985; **15**: 173–87.
8. Nishiyama K, Nordberg GF. Adsorption and elution of cadmium on hair. *Arch Environ Health* 1972; **25**: 92–6.
9. Sartor FA, Rondia DJ, Claeys FD *et al*. Impact of environmental cadmium pollution on cadmium exposure and body burden. *Arch Environ Health* 1992; **47**: 347–53.

10. Lauwerys R, Roels H, Regniers M, Buchet JP, Bernard A, Goret A. Significance of cadmium concentration in blood and in urine in workers exposed to cadmium. *Environ Res* 1979; **20**: 375–91.

11. Minoia C, Sabbioni E, Apostoli P *et al.* Trace element reference values in tissues from inhabitants of the European community. I. A study of 46 elements in urine, blood and serum of Italian subjects. *Sci Total Environ* 1990; **95**: 89–105.

12. White MA, Sabbioni E. Trace element reference values in tissues from inhabitants of the European Union. X. A study of 13 elements in blood and urine of a United Kingdom population. *Sci Total Environ* 1998; **216**: 253–70.

13. Lauwerys RR, Bernard AM, Roels HA, Buchet JP. Cadmium: exposure markers as predictors of nephrotoxic effects. *Clin Chem* 1994; **40**(7 Pt 2): 1391–4.

♦14. Bernard A. Renal dysfunction induced by cadmium: biomarkers of critical effects. *Biometals* 2004; **17**: 519–23.

15. Mason HJ, Davison AG, Wright AL *et al.* Relations between liver cadmium, cumulative exposure, and renal function in cadmium alloy workers. *Br J Ind Med* 1988; **45**: 793–802.

16. Roels HA, Lauwerys RR, Buchet JP, Bernard AM, Vos A, Oversteyns M. Health significance of cadmium induced renal dysfunction: a five year follow up. *Br J Ind Med* 1989; **46**: 755–64.

♦17. Jarup L, Berglund M, Elinder CG, Nordberg G, Vahter M. Health effects of cadmium exposure – a review of the literature and a risk estimate. *Scand J Work Environ Health* 1998; **24**(Suppl. 1): 1–51.

18. Buchet JP, Lauwerys R, Roels H *et al.* Renal effects of cadmium body burden of the general population. *Lancet* 1990; **336**: 699–702.

19. Hayano M, Nogawa K, Kido T, Kobayashi E, Honda R, Turitani I. Dose-response relationship between urinary cadmium concentration and beta2-microglobulinuria using logistic regression analysis. *Arch Environ Health* 1996; **51**: 162–7.

20. Ishizaki M, Kido T, Honda R *et al.* Dose-response relationship between urinary cadmium and beta 2-microglobulin in a Japanese environmentally cadmium exposed population. *Toxicology* 1989; **58**: 121–31.

21. Jarup L, Hellstrom L, Alfven T *et al.* Low level exposure to cadmium and early kidney damage: the OSCAR study. *Occup Environ Med* 2000; **57**: 668–72.

22. World Health Organization. Cadmium. *Environmental Health Criteria*, Vol. 134. Geneva: WHO, 1992.

23. Jin T, Nordberg M, Frech W *et al.* Cadmium biomonitoring and renal dysfunction among a population environmentally exposed to cadmium from smelting in China (ChinaCad). *Biometals* 2002; **15**: 397–410.

♦24. Hotz P, Buchet JP, Bernard A, Lison D, Lauwerys R. Renal effects of low-level environmental cadmium exposure: 5-year follow-up of a subcohort from the Cadmibel study. *Lancet* 1999; **354**: 1508–13.

25. Jarup L, Persson B, Elinder CG. Decreased glomerular filtration rate in solderers exposed to cadmium. *Occup Environ Med* 1995; **52**: 818–22.

26. Hellstrom L, Elinder CG, Dahlberg B *et al.* Cadmium exposure and end-stage renal disease. *Am J Kidney Dis* 2001; **38**: 1001–8.

27. Elinder CG, Edling C, Lindberg E, Kagedal B, Vesterberg O. Assessment of renal function in workers previously exposed to cadmium. *Br J Ind Med* 1985; **42**: 754–60.

28. Jarup L, Elinder CG. Incidence of renal stones among cadmium exposed battery workers. *Br J Ind Med* 1993; **50**: 598–602.

29. Kido T, Nogawa K, Yamada Y *et al.* Osteopenia in inhabitants with renal dysfunction induced by exposure to environmental cadmium. *Int Arch Occup Environ Health* 1989; **61**: 271–6.

30. Nogawa K, Tsuritani I, Kido T, Honda R, Ishizaki M, Yamada Y. Serum vitamin D metabolites in cadmium-exposed persons with renal damage. *Int Arch Occup Environ Health* 1990; **62**: 189–93.

31. Kazantzis G. Cadmium, osteoporosis and calcium metabolism. *Biometals* 2004; **17**: 493–8.

32. Shigematsu I. The epidemiological approach to cadmium pollution in Japan. *Ann Acad Med Singapore* 1984; **13**: 231–6.

33. Nordberg G, Jin T, Bernard A *et al.* Low bone density and renal dysfunction following environmental cadmium exposure in China. *Ambio* 2002; **31**: 478–81.

34. Wang H, Zhu G, Shi Y, Weng S, Jin T, Kong Q, *et al.* Influence of environmental cadmium exposure on forearm bone density. *J Bone Miner Res* 2003; 18: 553–60.

35. Staessen JA, Roels HA, Emelianov D *et al.* Environmental exposure to cadmium, forearm bone density, and risk of fractures: prospective population study. Public Health and Environmental Exposure to Cadmium (PheeCad) Study Group. *Lancet* 1999; **353**: 1140–4.

36. Townshend RH. Acute cadmium pneumonitis: a 17-year follow-up. *Br J Ind Med* 1982; **39**: 411–12.

37. Sorahan T, Lister A, Gilthorpe MS, Harrington JM. Mortality of copper cadmium alloy workers with special reference to lung cancer and non-malignant diseases of the respiratory system, 1946–92. *Occup Environ Med* 1995; **52**: 804–12.

38. Armstrong BG, Kazantzis G. The mortality of cadmium workers. *Lancet* 1983; **1**: 1425–7.

39. Cortona G, Apostoli P, Toffoletto F *et al.* Occupational exposure to cadmium and lung function. In: Nordberg GF, Herber RFM, Alessio L (eds) *Cadmium in the Human Environment: Toxicity and Carcinogenicity* (pp. 205–10). Lyon: International Agency for Research on Cancer, 1992.

♦40. Davison AG, Fayers PM, Taylor AJ *et al.* Cadmium fume inhalation and emphysema. *Lancet* 1988; **1**: 663–7.

41. Smith TJ, Petty TL, Reading JC, Lakshminarayan S. Pulmonary effects of chronic exposure to airborne cadmium. *Am Rev Respir Dis* 1976; **114**: 161–9.

42. Chowdhury P, Louria DB. Influence of cadmium and other trace metals on human alpha1-antitrypsin: an in vitro study. *Science* 1976; **191**: 480–1.

43. Chambers RC, Laurent GJ, Westergren-Thorsson G. Cadmium inhibits proteoglycan and procollagen production

by cultured human lung fibroblasts. *Am J Respir Cell Mol Biol* 1998; **19**: 498–506.

44. Mannino DM, Holguin F, Greves HM, Savage-Brown A, Stock AL, Jones RL. Urinary cadmium levels predict lower lung function in current and former smokers: data from the Third National Health and Nutrition Examination Survey. *Thorax* 2004; **59**: 194–8.

45. International Agency for Research on Cancer. *Beryllium, Cadmium, Mercury, and Exposures in the Glass Manufacturing Industry.* IARC Monographs on the Evaluation of the Carcinogenic Risk of Chemicals to Humans. Vol. 58. Lyon: IARC, 1993.

46. Jarup L, Bellander T, Hogstedt C, Spang G. Mortality and cancer incidence in Swedish battery workers exposed to cadmium and nickel. *Occup Environ Med* 1998; **55**: 755–9.

47. Sorahan T, Esmen NA. Lung cancer mortality in UK nickel-cadmium battery workers, 1947–2000. *Occup Environ Med* 2004; **61**: 108–16.

48. Verougstraete V, Lison D, Hotz P. Cadmium, lung and prostate cancer: a systematic review of recent epidemiological data. *J Toxicol Environ Health B Crit Rev* 2003; **6**: 227–55.

49. Potts CL. Cadmium proteinuria – the health of battery workers exposed to cadmium oxide dust. *Ann Occup Hyg* 1965; **8**: 55–61.

50. Sahmoun AE, Case LD, Jackson SA, Schwartz GG. Cadmium and prostate cancer: a critical epidemiologic analysis. *Cancer Invest* 2005; **23**: 256–63.

51. Il'yasova D, Schwartz GG. Cadmium and renal cancer. *Toxicol Appl Pharmacol* 2005; **207**: 179–86.

52. Siemiatycki J, Dewar R, Nadon L, Gerin M. Occupational risk factors for bladder cancer: results from a case-control study in Montreal, Quebec, Canada. *Am J Epidemiol* 1994; **140**: 1061–80.

53. Rhomberg W, Schmoll HJ, Schneider B. High frequency of metalworkers among patients with seminomatous tumors of the testis: a case-control study. *Am J Ind Med* 1995; **28**: 79–87.

54. Antila E, Mussalo-Rauhamaa H, Kantola M, Atroshi F, Westermarck T. Association of cadmium with human breast cancer. *Sci Total Environ* 1996; **186**: 251–6.

55. Kjellstrom T, Friberg L, Rahnster B. Mortality and cancer morbidity among cadmium-exposed workers. *Environ Health Perspect* 1979; **28**: 199–204.

ALUMINIUM

FINLAY D. DICK

Aluminium, the most common metal in the earth's crust, is highly reactive and rarely found in its pure state in nature. The metal is widely used in engineering, construction and cookware, and aluminium sulphate is used as a water flocculant. The main exposure in man is by ingestion. Aluminium is poorly absorbed from the gut, and a high silica level in water may further reduce its bioavailability.

POSSIBLE HEALTH EFFECTS OF ENVIRONMENTAL ALUMINIUM EXPOSURE

Dialysis dementia, characterized by altered behaviour, seizures and speech problems, was described in 1970 and subsequently linked to high aluminium levels in dialysis water.[1] Whether aluminium is associated with other dementias is more controversial. One study[2] suggested that brain aluminium was increased in Alzheimer's disease, but a later study found no such difference.[3]

Studies have examined the risk of cognitive impairment, dementia or Alzheimer's disease with aluminium in water,[4–8] foodstuffs,[9,10] or antacids,[10,11] with conflicting results that have generated considerable debate.[12,13] One study[4] found an increased risk of probable Alzheimer's disease (based on computed tomography scan results) among the residents of areas with mean aluminium in water concentrations of 110 µg/L compared with those from areas with mean aluminium in water concentrations of 10 µg/L (relative risk [RR] 1.5, 95 per cent confidence interval [CI] 1.1–2.2). A Canadian study found an increased risk of pathologically confirmed Alzheimer's disease with aluminium in water concentrations of over 100 µg/L (odds ratio 2.6, 95 per cent CI 1.2–5.7).[6]

A pilot study of dietary aluminium found an association with Alzheimer's disease.[9] However, a small English study found no association between Alzheimer's disease and aluminium in water, food or medicines.[10] A later UK study also found no association between aluminium in water and Alzheimer's disease.[8] The PAQUID study[7] found an association between aluminium in water (over 100 µg/L) and incident Alzheimer's disease (RR 2.14, 95 per cent CI 1.21–3.80) but no dose–response relationship. It also found a protective effect for high silica in water (over 11.24 mg/L) on incident dementia (RR 0.74, 95 per cent CI 0.58–0.96). This inconsistent evidence does not support an association between aluminium ingestion and Alzheimer's disease.

THE CAMELFORD INCIDENT

On July 6th, 1988, a relief driver working for the water company emptied 20 tonnes of aluminium sulphate into the wrong tank at an unmanned water treatment plant, contaminating the drinking water of around 20000 people around the village of Camelford, Cornwall, UK. A retrospective study[14] found an association between aluminium exposure and a range of health effects, including joint pains. A follow-up of exposed expectant mothers found no excess of congenital abnormalities among their newborn.[14] There were no significant differences in schoolchildren's test performances before and after the event compared with unexposed children, suggesting no effect on cognitive decline.[14] In contrast, one study,[15] heavily criticized by others, found evidence of impaired cognitive function in a self-selected group of people who believed their memory had been affected.

There were no significant differences in mortality between those exposed to aluminium, at concentrations several hundred times above the European Community limit of 200 µg/L for 3 days, and those not exposed.[16] Eight years after the event, a woman exposed in the Camelford incident died of a rare form of dementia, aged 58 years,[17] the post mortem revealing increased brain aluminium, but whether this was causal or coincident is unclear.

The indirect effects of knowledge of an environmental exposure are difficult to separate from the direct consequences of that exposure: it is unlikely that aluminium sulphate directly affected Camelford residents' health, although some were undoubtedly exposed to high levels of aluminium over several days. Whether environmental exposure to aluminium is a cause of ill health thus remains unclear.

References

1. Alfrey AC, LeGendre GR, Kaehny WD. The dialysis encephalopathy syndrome. Possible aluminum intoxication. *N Engl J Med* 1976; **294**: 184–8.
2. Crapper DR, Krishnan SS, Quittkat S. Aluminum, neurofibrillary degeneration and Alzheimer's disease. *Brain* 1976; **99**: 67–80.
3. McDermott JR, Smith AI, Iqbal K, Wisniewski HM. Brain aluminium in aging and Alzheimer disease. *Neurology* 1979; **29**: 809–14.
4. Martyn CN, Barker DJP, Osmond C *et al.* Geographical relation between Alzheimer's disease and aluminium in drinking water. *Lancet* 1989; **i**: 59–62.
5. Neri LC, Hewitt D. Aluminium, Alzheimer's disease, and drinking water. *Lancet* 1991; **338**: 390.
6. McLachlan DRC, Bergeron C, Smith JE *et al.* Risk for neuropathologically confirmed Alzheimer's

disease and residual aluminum in municipal drinking water employing weighted residential histories. *Neurology* 1996; **46**: 401–5.

7. Rondeau V, Commenges D, Jacqmin-Gadda H, Dartigues J-F. Relation between aluminium concentrations in drinking water and Alzheimer's disease: an 8-year follow-up study. *Am J Epidemiol* 2000; **152**: 59–66.

8. Martyn CN, Coggon DN, Lacey RF *et al.* Aluminium concentrations in drinking water and risk of Alzheimer's disease. *Epidemiology* 1997; **8**: 281–6.

9. Rogers MAM, Simon DG. A preliminary study of dietary aluminium intake and risk of Alzheimer's disease. *Age Ageing* 1999; **28**: 205–9.

10. Forster DP, Newens AJ, Kay DWK, Edwardson JA. Risk factors in clinically diagnosed presenile dementia of the Alzheimer type: a case-control study in northern England. *J Epidemiol Comm Health* 1995; **49**: 253–8.

11. Graves AB, White E, Koepsell TD *et al.* The association between aluminium-containing products and Alzheimer's disease. *J Clin Epidemiol* 1990; **43**: 35–44.

12. Forbes WF, Hill GB. Is exposure to aluminium a risk factor for the development of Alzheimer disease? – yes. *Arch Neurol* 1998; **55**: 740–1.

13. Munoz DG. Is exposure to aluminium a risk factor for the development of Alzheimer disease? – no. *Arch Neurol* 1998; **55**: 737–9.

14. David AS, Wessely SC. The legend of Camelford: medical consequences of a water pollution accident. *J Psychosom Res* 1995; **39**: 1–9.

15. Altmann P, Cunningham J, Dhanesha U *et al.* Disturbances of cerebral function in people exposed to drinking water contaminated with aluminium sulphate: retrospective study of the Camelford water incident. *BMJ* 1999; **319**: 807–11.

16. Owen PJ, Miles DPB, Draper GJ, Vincent TJ. Retrospective study of mortality after a water pollution incident at Lowermoor in north Cornwall. *BMJ* 2002; **324**: 1189.

17. Exley C, Esiri MM. Severe cerebral congophilic angiopathy coincident with increased brain aluminium in a resident of Camelford, Cornwall, UK. *J Neurol Neurosurg Psychiatry* 2006; **77**: 877–9.

MANGANESE

MICHAEL ASCHNER

Manganese is required for normal growth, development and cellular homeostasis. There are a range of manganese-dependent enzyme families (e.g. oxidoreductases, transferases and hydrolases) and manganese metalloenzymes (e.g. arginase, glutamine synthetase and manganese superoxide dismutase). Manganese is required for normal immune function, the regulation of blood sugars and cellular energy, reproduction, digestion and bone growth, in defence mechanisms against free radicals and, in concert with vitamin K, to support blood clotting. An adequate intake of manganese for men and women is 2.3 and 1.8mg per day, respectively. Tissue levels are stably maintained through a tight regulation of its absorption and excretion.

EXPOSURES

An increased manganese body-burden is associated with maneb-adulterated food,[1] the administration of the manganese superoxide-dismutase mimetic, EUK-8,[2] the intravenous use of the euphoric stimulant methcathinone[3] and potassium permanganate.[4] Occupational exposures occur in mining, steel manufacturing and welding.[5,6] Environmental exposure to combustion products of the anti-knock agent methylcyclopentadienyl manganese

tricarbonyl has also been documented,[7] and high well-water manganese concentrations are known to occur.[8,9]

MANGANESE TRANSPORT

The transport of divalent manganese into the brain is regulated by the non-specific divalent metal transporter (DMT1), a symporter energized by the proton-motive force generated by the vacuolar ATPase.[10] Trivalent manganese is transported as a conjugate of transferrin. Voltage-gated and store-operated calcium channels, the glutamate ionotropic receptor and the solute carrier 39 family member ZIP8, as well as organic (citrate) carriers, have also been implicated in manganese transport into the brain.[10]

TOXICITY AND CLINICAL PICTURES

Manganese toxicity in humans is a well-recognized occupational hazard, and the inhalation of particulate manganese compounds (e.g. during welding) can lead to lung inflammation, causing cough, bronchitis, pneumonitis and impaired pulmonary function.[8] These effects may reflect an indirect response to inhaled particulate matter or may be associated with direct pulmonary toxicity induced by manganese.[9]

Impotence and loss of libido have also been reported in male workers with high manganese exposure,[10] but the main effects are on the central nervous system. Brain manganese overload is associated with not only environmental exposures, but also parenteral nutrition,[11] as well as with congenital diseases such as hepatic cirrhosis, congenital biliary atresia, primary biliary cirrhosis, congenital intrahepatic portosystemic shunt, Rendu–Osler–Weber syndrome and patent ductus venosus.[11] Manganese accumulates in the basal ganglia and a syndrome referred to as manganism, characterized by progressive Parkinsonism,[12] a dystonic gait disorder ('cock gait'), dystonia, psychosis and emotional lability, is well recognized although rare. At the tissue level, excessive manganese levels lead to cell loss and gliosis in the globus pallidus and to a lesser degree in the striatum.[13] However, it remains controversial whether manganese spares the substantia nigra pars compacta and results in Lewy body formation.

INVESTIGATION

Magnetic resonance imaging has been extensively used to localize manganese. Because manganese contains several unpaired electrons, it is highly effective as a paramagnetic relaxation agent that shortens both the T1 and T2 relaxation times of water molecules. In general, increased blood manganese levels occur in acutely exposed individuals. However, in chronic exposures, blood manganese levels are tightly controlled and are often indistinguishable from those in occupationally unexposed individuals. Hair samples have been used for manganese analyses, but it is arguable whether these reflect exposure.

TREATMENT AND PROGNOSIS

It is doubtful whether L-dopa offers therapeutic benefit in patients with manganism. Environmental exposure should result in the removal of subjects from the source. Chelation therapy has been used, but is controversial.[14]

References

●1. Ferraz HB, Bertolucci PH, Pereira JS, Lima JG, Andrade LA. Chronic exposure to the fungicide maneb may produce symptoms and signs of CNS manganese intoxication. *Neurology* 1988; **38**: 550–3.

●2. McDonald MC, d'Emmanuele di Villa Bianca R, Wayman NS *et al.* A superoxide dismutase mimetic with catalase activity (EUK-8) reduces the organ injury in endotoxic shock. *Eur J Pharmacol* 2003; **466**: 181–9.

●3. Stepens A, Logina I, Liguts V *et al.* A Parkinsonian syndrome in methcathinone users and the role of manganese. *N Engl J Med* 2008; **358**: 1009–17.

●4. Xu XR, Li HB, Wang WH, Gu JD. Decolorization of dyes and textile wastewater by potassium permanganate. *Chemosphere* 2005; **59**: 893–8.

♦5. Pal PK, Samii A, Calne DB. Manganese neurotoxicity: a review of clinical features, imaging and pathology. *Neurotoxicology* 1999; **20**: 227–38.

●6. Myers JE, teWaterNaude J, Fourie M *et al.* Nervous system effects of occupational manganese exposure on South African manganese mineworkers. *Neurotoxicology* 2003; **24**: 649–56.

●7. Sierra P, Loranger S, Kennedy G, Zayed J. Occupational and environmental exposure of automobile mechanics and nonautomotive workers to airborne manganese arising from the combustion of methylcyclopentadienyl manganese tricarbonyl (MMT). *Am Ind Hyg Assoc J* 1995; **56**: 713–16.

●8. Wasserman GA, Liu X, Parvez F *et al.* Water manganese exposure and children's intellectual function in Araihazar, Bangladesh. *Environ Health Perspect* 2006; **114**: 124–9.

●9. Roels H, Lauwerys R, Buchet JP *et al.* Epidemiological survey among workers exposed to manganese: effects on lung, central nervous system, and some biological indices. *Am J Ind Med* 1987; **11**: 307–27.

♦10. Agency for Toxic Substances and Disease Registry. Toxicological Profile for Manganese, U.S. Department of Health and Human Services Public Health Service. Available at: http://www.atsdr.cdc.gov/toxprofiles/tp151.html (accessed July 20, 2009).

♦11. Au C, Benedetto A, Aschner M. Manganese transport in eukaryotes: The role of DMT1. *Neurotoxicology* 2008; **29**: 569–76.

♦12. Perl DP, Olanow CW. The neuropathology of manganese-induced Parkinsonism. *J Neuropathol Exp Neurol* 2007; **66**: 675–82.

●13. Uchino A, Noguchi T, Nomiyama K *et al.* Manganese accumulation in the brain: MR imaging. *Neuroradiology* 2007; **49**: 715–20.

●14. Herrero Hernandez E, Discalzi G, Valentini C *et al.* Follow-up of patients affected by manganese-induced Parkinsonism after treatment with CaNa2EDTA. *Neurotoxicology* 2006; **27**: 333–9.

28

Arsenic

PAUL CULLINAN, GEOFF H. PIGOTT

INTRODUCTION AND ENVIRONMENTAL SOURCES

Arsenic is a 'metalloid' with properties intermediate between those of the metals and the non-metals. It shares several chemicophysical similarities with phosphorus – its predecessor in the periodic table – and indeed some aspects of its toxicity are a reflection of its ability to replace phosphorus in critical biochemical processes.

There are more than 150 arsenic-bearing minerals, the single most important of which is arsenopyrite ('mispickel'), the source of 'white arsenic'. The element is found in conjunction with metal ores, notably those of copper, silver, gold, lead and nickel, and with coal. The average concentration of arsenic in the earth's crust is low (around 5 mg/kg), but its distribution is very uneven, and in some parts of the world, such as Bangladesh, there are much higher naturally occurring concentrations. China is the major commercial producer of arsenic, a by-product of its gold mining operations; other important sources are in South America and North Africa.

There is a wide variety of inorganic and organic arsenic compounds, in which the element can exist in four oxidation states:

- as the free element 'arsenic', which is very rare in the natural environment;
- as an unstable gas with a valency of −3 ('arsine');
- as 'arsenite', a +3 valency state commonly abbreviated to As(III);
- as 'arsenate', a +5 valency state abbreviated to As(V).

These last two, especially the latter, are the most common forms of environmental arsenic. In surface water, an oxidizing environment, As(V) species predominate; by contrast, As(III) species are more important in the reducing environments of much groundwater. The speciation and oxidation state of arsenic in soil is variable and dependent in part on soil pH. Arsenic released from industrial sources is generally arsenic trioxide (white arsenic) in both particulate and vapour forms; less common forms are arsenic trisulphide and arsenic trichloride. Most cases of human toxicity from arsenic are associated with exposure to inorganic compounds.

The most important recent commercial use of arsenic has been in timber preservation; the mixture of copper–chrome–arsenate (CCA) imparts a green colour to treated wood and is an effective protection against fungi, insects and the weather. Concerns over the leaching of arsenic from preserved timber into adjacent soil or groundwater, and its release into the atmosphere during combustion, have led many countries to ban the use of CCA.

Other contemporary uses of arsenic are in the manufacture of gallium arsenide (a semi-conductor) and, in organic forms, in animal feeds and in some herbicide/pesticide mixtures (e.g. monosodium methyl arsenate) used in agriculture and horticulture. Other commercial uses of arsenic – for example as a pigment – are largely redundant. Many widely used medicinal products have traditionally contained arsenic, and others still do, both in conventional, Western practice (chiefly the treatment of some haematological malignancies) and in alternative approaches.[1]

EXPOSURES AND TEMPORAL TRENDS

Arsenic is released to soil and groundwater from the natural erosion of rocks, by the action of volcanoes or through a variety of anthropogenic sources. These last include the mining and smelting of non-ferrous metals (notably copper and gold), the burning of coal, the use of pesticides and the dumping of industrial, agricultural and building waste. Small quantities of arsenic may be found in vegetable beds (and the vegetables grown in them) constructed from CCA-treated timber.[2,3]

Non-occupational (oral) exposures result from drinking contaminated groundwater or eating food grown in contaminated soils; although some fish contain high levels of arsenic, it is usually in relatively low-toxicity organic forms (e.g. arsenobetaine, arsenocholine and dimethylarsinic acid). Levels of arsenic in water vary considerably from a 'background' concentration of less than $10\,\mu g/L$ to levels above $1\,mg/L$ in localities where there is geological or anthropogenic contamination. Soil concentrations are similarly determined and variable, with 'natural' levels between 1 and $40\,mg/kg$ but much higher levels close to sources of contamination.

The most important workplace exposures to (inorganic) arsenic are through inhalation and occur vicariously during the smelting of non-ferrous ores, especially copper and lead, or the burning of some types of coal in power plants. Respiratory (and dermal) exposure may also occur during the production, use and disposal of arsenical timber preservatives or pesticides.

As a result of such activities, atmospheric concentrations of arsenic in industrial areas may reach $100\,mg/m^3$; in remote areas they are more generally between 1 and $3\,ng/m^3$. Pesticides used in tobacco farming have in the past been responsible for high levels of arsenic in cigarette smoke; the practice is now largely prohibited.

For those without occupational contact, oral (and possibly dermal) exposures to arsenic are more important than those by inhalation.[4] Average dietary intakes of total arsenic are around $50\,\mu g$ per day,[5] perhaps 200 times higher than those from ambient air.

TRENDS IN ARSENIC EXPOSURES

Reductions in the use of arsenic and improvements in the control of industrial emissions and waste-handling have, in many countries, greatly reduced ongoing environmental contamination with arsenic compounds. However, this is not universally the case, and there is continuing and increasing cause for concern in many rapidly industrializing countries. Levels of arsenic in cigarettes have been greatly reduced by the prohibition of arsenical pesticides in tobacco production.

TOXICOKINETICS

Absorption and distribution

INGESTED ARSENIC

The absorption of arsenic after ingestion is probably by passive diffusion. Water-soluble forms are better absorbed than those which are insoluble; the latter include arsenic sulphides in soil. The bodily distribution of arsenic imbibed in drinking water may be age-dependent.[6]

RESPIRED ARSENIC

The absorption of arsenic after particle deposition on the respiratory mucosa is dependent on its solubility and on particle size. After the inhalation of soluble compounds such as arsenous oxide, most of the deposited arsenic is absorbed into the bloodstream from the digestive tract following respiratory clearance. Less soluble particles, including those of arsenic trisulphide, calcium arsenate, lead arsenate and gallium arsenide, tend to be retained to a greater extent in the lungs.[7,8]

Studies of workers with occupational exposure to inorganic arsenic trioxide[9] suggest that around half of an inhaled arsenic dose is absorbed. There are no human data on the body distribution of arsenic after inhaled exposures, but it is likely to be widespread; there are no data to indicate that the fate of inhaled arsenic in children is different from that in adults.

DERMAL

Dermal absorption seems to be less efficient than that following either oral or respiratory exposure.

Metabolism, distribution and excretion

The metabolism of arsenic – however it is introduced – consists chiefly of two processes: reduction/oxidation reactions that interconvert arsenate and arsenite; and methylation.[10] Methylation takes place mainly in the liver, converting arsenic to monomethylarsonic acid and dimethylarsinic acid, both of which have a lower affinity for tissue and thus a lower toxicity than arsenic. Arsenic and its metabolites appear to distribute to all organs in the body with no evidence of preferential distribution in human tissues. More than 75 per cent of absorbed arsenic is excreted in the urine;[11] smaller proportions are excreted via the faeces, hair and nails.

Toxicity

Although, despite intensive study, the mechanisms of the toxicity of arsenic are not entirely clear, they almost certainly are closely associated with vital metabolic processes. A useful review is provided by Hughes.[12]

Trivalent arsenic reacts with free thiols such as glutathione and cysteine; binding to critical thiol groups may lead to an inhibition of essential biochemical reactions and alterations in cellular redox status. Pentavalent arsenic is less reactive with tissue constituents but can substitute phosphate ions in various cellular enzyme-catalysed reactions, inhibiting or blocking energy metabolism and specifically oxidative phosphorylation. The genotoxic and carcinogenic effects of arsenic are probably multiple, reflecting its capacities to inhibit DNA repair, induce oncogene amplification and interfere with DNA synthesis.

BIOMONITORING OF ARSENIC EXPOSURE

Concentrations of arsenic in blood reflect only very recent exposures; although 'normal' blood levels are typically below 1 μg/L, those which follow acute poisoning may be as high as 1 mg/L or more. Urinary measurements, reflecting exposures over the previous 1–2 days, are far more commonly used and correlate with both industrial[13,14] and 'environmental'[15] sources of exposure. Not all species and metabolites of arsenic are harmful (e.g. arsenobetaine in fish), and the measurement of total urinary arsenic may overestimate the burden of toxic exposure. Speciation is possible but seldom used in routine screening. Spot urine measurements appear to be equivalent to 24 hour collections and are far easier to arrange.[15]

Since arsenic accumulates in hair and nails, its measurement in these tissues can provide a useful indicator of exposures over the previous 6–12 months, although the levels of exposure required to cause increased concentrations are uncertain. These methods have been used in studies of populations with occupational,[16] environmental[17] and dietary exposures.[18]

Measurement of total arsenic in biological and environmental samples is usually by atomic absorption photospectrometry or other spectrometric techniques; the speciation of separate inorganic or organic arsenic compounds is also possible, for example by high-performance liquid chromatography.

Where populations are geographically stable and there has been little variation in levels of arsenic contamination, a reasonably valid estimate of exposure to arsenic from drinking water can be achieved through time-weighted measurements of current arsenic concentrations (from all water sources). More refined estimates include assessments of past concentrations and measures of consumption, and may incorporate biomeasurements as above.[19]

ADVERSE HEALTH EFFECTS

Acute effects

High oral doses of arsenic are notoriously poisonous but are, despite popular belief, more often the result of an accidental ingestion of pesticides or insecticides than from murderous intent. Doses of 100 mg or more induce nausea, vomiting, colicky abdominal pain, excessive salivation and watery, bloody diarrhoea and death within 1–4 days. Other, less consistent, features include haematological abnormalities, renal failure, pulmonary oedema, psychosis, skin rash and cardiomyopathy. Survivors of acute poisoning may develop peripheral neuropathy (with a Guillain–Barré syndrome) and encephalopathy.

Acute exposures to toxic levels of airborne arsenic occur mainly in occupational settings, although research from China suggests that burning contaminated coal in domestic settings has also resulted in acute and chronic effects on health.[20] Exposure to As(III) dust causes irritation of the conjunctivae and upper respiratory tract and occasionally perforation of the nasal septum, occurring within days or weeks. Death from acute inhalation appears to be rare even with exposures up to 100 mg/m^3.[21]

Chronic effects

A large number and variety of adverse human health effects have been attributed to chronic arsenic exposure. In many cases, these relate to long-term oral exposures in parts of the world – such as Bangladesh, China, Mongolia and Taiwan – where there is heavy geological contamination of drinking water. Extensive exposures in China, involving both inhalational and dietary routes, have been associated with the domestic use of contaminated coal.[20] There are fewer studies of the human toxicity of inhaled arsenic, and almost all of them are of populations exposed in the workplace.

Ingested arsenic

SKIN

Non-malignant skin disorders are an easily recognized, apparently common feature of chronic poisoning by inorganic arsenic and are frequently used as a sensitive index of high community exposures. Typical are changes in pigmentation, hyperkeratosis (frequently on the palms or soles) and Bowen's disease. There is a large epidemiological literature describing such effects, much of it reporting clear dose–response relationships, and helpfully reviewed by Yoshida et al.[19] Community surveys – which need to take careful account of confounding exposures and biases in ascertainment – indicate that the minimum level of chronic arsenic contamination in water required to induce such skin disease is around 100 μg/L.[22]

In a similar manner, the chronic oral ingestion of arsenic can give rise to malignant skin disease, typically multiple squamous cell carcinomas arising, it seems, in areas of previous hyperkeratosis. Less commonly, basal cell carcinomas may develop. A large, ecological survey of Taiwanese villagers described a clear relationship between the prevalence of skin cancer and levels of arsenic in drinking water.[23]

INTERNAL MALIGNANCIES

Long-term, oral exposures to high concentrations of inorganic arsenic appear also to increase the risk of bladder cancers; this effect has been reported in both those whose exposure is through contaminated drinking water[24] and those with medicinal exposures to potassium arsenite, 'Fowler's solution'.[25] In the former group, it seems that only those with several decades of exposure are at an increased risk.[26]

Risks may also be increased for renal, hepatic, pulmonary and prostate cancers, but the evidence for these is weaker than that for skin and bladder malignancies.

CARDIOVASCULAR EFFECTS

The most striking circulatory association with chronic arsenic ingestion is 'blackfoot disease', a peripheral vascular condition of the feet and hands peculiar to areas of south-western Taiwan with elevated levels of inorganic arsenic in drinking water. The prevalence of blackfoot disease is associated with levels of cumulative exposure to arsenic; its incidence fell after the introduction of uncontaminated tap water to endemic villages.[27] The risk may be further increased in those with a reduced capacity to methylate arsenic, determined in part by age and sex as well as by ethnic group.[28]

Other adverse cardiovascular outcomes include prolongation of the Q–T interval on electrocardiography, an effect seen not only in patients with promyelocytic leukaemia who have been treated with high doses of arsenic trioxide,[29] but also in communities exposed over long periods to inorganic arsenic in drinking water.[30] Coronary artery disease, hypertension and stroke have also been related to chronic arsenic ingestion and are usefully reviewed by Navas-Acien et al.[31]

NEUROLOGICAL EFFECTS

The most characteristic neuropathic effect of chronic arsenic ingestion is a peripheral neuropathy affecting both motor and sensory nerves.[32] However, there is increasing concern that similar exposures may have an adverse effect on intellectual development in childhood. A small number

of studies – in Taiwan, Bangladesh, China and India – have succeeded in correlating intellectual performance with estimates of chronic arsenic ingestion in communities with geologically contaminated drinking water.[33–36] It remains unclear how far these associations are explained by residual confounding effects.

OTHER EFFECTS

Other adverse effects of chronic exposure include mild anaemia, hepatitis and portal fibrosis, and an increased risk of spontaneous abortion and other adverse reproductive outcomes. Studies of pregnancies in the Bengal region suggest that these effects are apparent at arsenic concentrations in drinking water of over 0.05 mg/L.[37–39]

Inhaled arsenic

The evidence relating to the adverse effects of long-term exposures to airborne arsenic is relatively limited, and much of it may be confounded by other relevant exposures, notably cigarette-smoking and other workplace toxins. Increased risks of peripheral neuropathy[40] and vasospasticity[41,42] have been described in copper smelter workers with an exposure to arsenic at levels above 50 mg/m^3. Dermatitis,[43] similar to that seen in communities with chronic oral exposures, and hypertension[44] have also been reported in occupational populations.

There is rather more evidence in relation to the risks of lung cancer from inhaled arsenic. Increased risks have been reported in cohorts of Swedish and US smelter workers with a wide range of cumulative exposures to arsenic[45–47] and in a case–control study of Chilean miners and smelters.[48] In each case, there was no adjustment for other potentially relevant occupational dust exposures and only limited adjustment for smoking; indeed, there may be important interactions between smoking and arsenic inhalation in the development of lung cancer.[49] Nonetheless, most agencies would accept that inhaled arsenic is a pulmonary carcinogen.

Studies of communities with airborne exposure from nearby industry are rare; two suggest an increase in risk of lung cancer[50] and stillbirths[51] in populations living close to a copper-smelting facility and a pesticide factory respectively.

REFERENCES

♦ = Major review article

1. Lynch E, Braithwaite R. A review of the clinical and toxicological aspects of 'traditional' (herbal) medicines adulterated with heavy metals. Expert Opin Drug Saf 2005; **4**: 769–78.

2. Katz SA, Salem H. Chemistry and toxicology of building timbers pressure-treated with chromated copper arsenate: a review. *J Appl Toxicol* 2005; **25**: 1–7.

3. Rahman FA, Allan DL, Rosen CJ, Sadowsky MJ. Arsenic availability from chromated copper arsenate (CCA)-treated wood. *J Environ Qual* 2004; **33**: 173–80.

4. Meacher DM, Menzel DB, Dillencourt MD *et al.* Estimation of multimedia inorganic arsenic intake in the U.S. population. *Human Ecol Risk Assess* 2002; **8**: 1697–721.

5. MacIntosh DL, Williams PL, Hunter DJ *et al.* Evaluation of a food frequency questionnaire-food composition approach for estimating dietary intake of inorganic arsenic and methylmercury. *Cancer Epidemiol Biomarkers Prev* 1997; **6**: 1043–50.

6. Meza MM, Yu L, Rodriguez YY *et al.* Developmentally restricted genetic determinants of human arsenic metabolism: association between urinary methylated arsenic and CYT19 polymorphisms in children. *Environ Health Perspect* 2005; **113**: 775–81.

7. Pershagen G, Lind B, Bjorklund NE. Lung retention and toxicity of some inorganic arsenic compounds. *Environ Res* 1982; **29**: 425–34.

8. Webb DR, Sipes IG, Carter DE. In vitro solubility and in vivo toxicity of gallium arsenide. *Toxicol Appl Pharmacol* 1984; **76**: 96–104.

9. Pinto SS, Varner MO, Nelson KW, Labbe AL, White LD. Arsenic trioxide absorption and excretion in industry. *J Occup Med* 1976; **18**: 677–80.

10. Vahter M. Mechanisms of arsenic biotransformation. *Toxicology* 2002; **181–182**: 211–17.

11. Marcus WL, Rispin AS. Threshold carcinogenicity using arsenic as an example. In: Cothern CR, Mehlmann MA, Marcus WL (eds) *Risk Assessment and Risk Management of Industrial and Environmental Chemicals.* pp. 133–58. Princeton, NJ: Princeton Science & Technology, 1988.

♦12. Hughes MF. Arsenic toxicity and potential mechanisms of action. *Toxicol Lett* 2002; **133**: 1–16.

13. Milham S, Strong T. Human arsenic exposure in relation to a copper smelter. *Environ Res* 1974; **7**: 176–82.

14. Polissar L, Lowry-Coble K, Kalman DA *et al.* Pathways of human exposure to arsenic in a community surrounding a copper smelter. *Environ Res* 1990; **53**: 29–47.

♦15. Calderon RL, Hudgens E, Le XC, Schreinemachers D, Thomas DJ. Excretion of arsenic in urine as a function of exposure to arsenic in drinking water. *Environ Health Perspect* 1999; **107**: 663–7.

16. Agahian B, Lee JS, Nelson JH, Johns RE. Arsenic levels in fingernails as a biological indicator of exposure to arsenic. *Am Ind Hyg Assoc J* 1990; **51**: 646–51.

17. Bencko V, Symon K. Health aspects of burning coal with a high arsenic content. I: Arsenic in hair, urine, and blood in children residing in a polluted area. *Environ Res* 1977; **13**: 378–85.

18. Kurttio P, Komulainen H, Hakala E, Kahelin H, Pekkanen J. Urinary excretion of arsenic species after exposure to arsenic present in drinking water. *Arch Environ Contam Toxicol* 1998; **34**: 297–305.

♦19. Yoshida T, Yamauchi H, Fan SG. Chronic health effects in people exposed to arsenic via the drinking water: dose-response relationships in review. *Toxicol Appl Pharmacol* 2004; **198**: 243–52.

20. Dong A, Dasheng L, Liang Y, Jing Z. Unventilated indoor coal-fired stoves in Guizhou province, China: Reduction of arsenic exposure through behaviour changes resulting from mitigation and health education in populations with arsenicosis. *Environ Health Perspect* 2007; **115**: 659–62.

♦21. Agency for Toxic Substances and Disease Registry. Toxicological Profile: Arsenic. Available from: http://www.atsdr.cdc.gov/toxprofiles/tp2.html (accessed July 28, 2009).

22. Haque R, Mazumder DN, Samanta S *et al.* Arsenic in drinking water and skin lesions: Dose-response data from West Bengal, India. *Epidemiology* 2003; **14**: 174–82.

23. Tseng WP, Chu HM, How SW, Fong JM, Lin CS, Yeh S. Prevalence of skin cancer in an endemic area of chronic arsenicism in Taiwan. *J Natl Cancer Inst* 1968; **40**: 453–63.

24. Bates MN, Rey OA, Biggs ML *et al.* Case-control study of bladder cancer and exposure to arsenic in Argentina. *Am J Epidemiol* 2004; **159**: 381–9.

25. Cuzick J, Sasieni P, Evans S. Ingested arsenic, keratoses, and bladder cancer. *Am J Epidemiol* 1992; **136**: 417–21.

26. Chiou HY, Chiou ST, Hsu YH *et al.* Incidence of transitional cell carcinoma and arsenic in drinking water: A follow-up study of 8,102 residents in an arseniasis-endemic area in northeastern Taiwan. *Am J Epidemiol* 2001; **153**: 411–18.

♦27. Tseng CH. An overview on peripheral vascular disease in blackfoot disease-hyperendemic villages in Taiwan. *Angiology* 2002; **53**: 529–37.

28. Tseng CH, Huang YK, Huang YL *et al.* Arsenic exposure, urinary arsenic speciation, and peripheral vascular disease in blackfoot disease-hyperendemic villages in Taiwan. *Toxicol Appl Pharmacol* 2005; **206**: 299–308.

29. Westervelt P, Brown RA, Adkins DR *et al.* Sudden death among patients with acute promyelocytic leukemia treated with arsenic trioxide. *Blood* 2001; **98**: 266–71.

30. Mumford JL, Wu K, Xia Y *et al.* Chronic arsenic exposure and cardiac repolarization abnormalities with QT interval prolongation in a population-based study. *Environ Health Perspect* 2007; **115**: 690–4.

♦31. Navas-Acien A, Sharrett AR, Silbergeld EK *et al.* Arsenic exposure and cardiovascular disease: A systematic review of the epidemiologic evidence. *Am J Epidemiol* 2005; **162**: 1037–49.

32. Chakraborti D, Hussam A, Alauddin M. Arsenic: Environmental health aspects with special reference to groundwater in South Asia. *J Environ Sci Health* 2003; **38**: xi–xv.

33. Tsai SY, Chou HY, The HW, Chen CM, Chen CJ. The effects of chronic arsenic exposure from drinking water on the

neurobehavioral development in adolescence. *Neurotoxicology* 2003; **24**(4–5): 747–53.

34. von Ehrenstein OS, Poddar S, Yuan Y *et al.* Children's intellectual function in relation to arsenic exposure. *Epidemiology* 2007; **18**: 44–51.

35. Wang SX, Wang ZH, Cheng XT *et al.* Arsenic and fluoride exposure in drinking water: Children's IQ and growth in Shanyin county, Shanxi province, China. *Environ Health Perspect* 2007; **115**: 643–7.

36. Wasserman GA, Liu X, Parvez F *et al.* Water arsenic exposure and children's intellectual function in Araihazar, Bangladesh. *Environ Health Perspect* 2004; **112**: 1329–33.

37. Ahmad SA, Sayed MH, Barua S *et al.* Arsenic in drinking water and pregnancy outcomes. Environ *Health Perspect* 2001; **109**: 629–31.

38. Milton AH, Smith W, Rahman B *et al.* Chronic arsenic exposure and adverse pregnancy outcomes in Bangladesh. *Epidemiology* 2005; **16**: 82–6.

39. von Ehrenstein OS, Guha Mazumder DN, Hira-Smith M *et al.* Pregnancy outcomes, infant mortality, and arsenic in drinking water in West Bengal, India. *Am J Epidemiol* 2006; **163**: 662–9.

40. Lagerkvist BJ, Zetterlund B. Assessment of exposure to arsenic among smelter workers: A five-year follow-up. *Am J Ind Med* 1994; **25**: 477–88.

41. Lagerkvist B, Linderholm H, Nordberg GF. Vasospastic tendency and Raynaud's phenomenon in smelter workers exposed to arsenic. *Environ Res* 1986; **39**: 465–74.

42. Lagerkvist BE, Linderholm H, Nordberg GF. Arsenic and Raynaud's phenomenon. Vasospastic tendency and excretion of arsenic in smelter workers before and after the summer vacation. *Int Arch Occup Environ Health* 1988; **60**: 361–4.

43. Mohamed KB. Occupational contact dermatitis from arsenic in a tin-smelting factory. *Contact Derm* 1998; **38**: 224–5.

44. Jensen GE, Hansen ML. Occupational arsenic exposure and glycosylated haemoglobin. *Analyst* 1998; **123**: 77–80.

45. Enterline PE, Day R, Marsh GM. Cancers related to exposure to arsenic at a copper smelter. *Occup Environ Med* 1995; **52**: 28–32.

46. Jarup L, Pershagen G, Wall S. Cumulative arsenic exposure and lung cancer in smelter workers: A dose-response study. *Am J Ind Med* 1989; **15**: 31–41.

47. Lee-Feldstein A. Cumulative exposure to arsenic and its relationship to respiratory cancer among copper smelter employees. *J Occup Med* 1986; **28**: 296–302.

48. Ferreccio C, Gonzalez C, Solari J, Noder C. [Bronchopulmonary cancer in workers exposed to arsenic: a case control study.] *Rev Med Chil* 1996; **124**: 119–23.

49. Hertz-Picciotto I, Smith AH. Observations on the dose-response curve for arsenic exposure and lung cancer. *Scand J Work Environ Health* 1993; **19**: 217–26.

50. Pershagen G. Lung cancer mortality among men living near an arsenic-emitting smelter. *Am J Epidemiol* 1985; **122**: 684–94.

51. Ihrig MM, Shalat SL, Baynes C. A hospital-based case-control study of stillbirths and environmental exposure to arsenic using an atmospheric dispersion model linked to a geographical information system. *Epidemiology* 1998; **9**: 290–4.

29

Fluorine

PETER J. BAXTER

Fluorine is the most reactive non-metal and almost never occurs in its elemental state. Combined with elements in the form of fluoride, fluorine is ubiquitous and occurs in plants and animals in trace amounts. If excess fluoride in the environment is ingested or inhaled, it can cause dental mottling starting in childhood and, at higher levels, abnormal bone growth at any stage of life, which, with prolonged exposure, may become deforming and crippling. Fluorine enters the hydrosphere by the leaching of soils and minerals into groundwater, and can enter vegetation through plant roots or by the absorption of gaseous or particulate fluorides in the air and in rain falling on leaves.[1] It arises in the atmosphere through volcanic activity, by the entrainment of soil and water particles by wind action, and from industrial emissions.

Industrial processes such as aluminium manufacture, the kiln-firing of brick and ceramic materials, and glass-making are some of the many industrial activities that can release fluoride into the environment in particulate or gaseous form. Hydrogen fluoride is the greatest single fluoride air pollutant and requires stringent emission controls to protect local populations and the environment.

In Western societies, the main sources of fluoride intake are food and water, and fluoride-containing dental products. Excess fluoride intake from drinking water or other sources is principally associated around the world with two conditions: dental fluorosis and skeletal fluorosis. Dental fluorosis is commonly found wherever water supplies contain naturally elevated amounts of fluoride. In the USA, some 200000 people have concentrations exceeding 4 mg/L in their water sources, a level at which severe dental fluorosis occurs in on average 10 per cent of children in US communities.[2] Skeletal fluorosis is, however, rare in the USA and most developed countries, but it is a major public health problem in India, China and northern, eastern and southern Africa, most commonly because of fluoride in geological strata that contaminate groundwater and surface waters used for drinking.

The practice of adding fluoride to drinking water in order to improve dental health has been endorsed by many national and international bodies, including the World Health Organization (WHO), but it has not attained universal acceptance on either ethical or scientific safety grounds.[3] Supplementation of drinking water with fluoride has been practised in some countries since 1945. In England and Wales, several local authorities introduced schemes for fluoridating water supplies between 1964 and 1975, covering about 9 per cent of the total population.

A large epidemiological literature exists on the health effects of water fluoridation. Two influential reviews of the evidence were made by the National Health Service Centre for Review and Dissemination at the University of York[4] and the Medical Research Council.[5] These confirmed the beneficial effect of water fluoridation on dental caries, at the expense of a small increase in the prevalence of mild fluorosis (mottled teeth). An association with water fluoride and disorders such as cancer, bone fracture and Down's syndrome was not found, but both reports emphasized the poor quality of much of the evidence that underlies the fluoridation debate.

GENERAL SOURCES OF FLUORIDE

Where water supplies are deliberately fluoridated as a public health measure to protect against dental caries, drinking water probably remains the most important source of fluoride intake. Up until the 1960s, it represented the bulk of fluoride exposure for both adults and children, but since then the availability of fluoride from other sources, such as toothpastes and dentifrices, leaves fluoride in drinking water as just one component of an individual's total fluoride intake in developed countries.[6] In the early 1990s, public health approaches were introduced to limit the exposure to systemic fluoride from toothpaste and supplements.

The parts of the world with endemic fluorosis are marked by having extensive geographical belts associated with fluoride-bearing geological formations: sediments of marine origin in mountainous areas; volcanic rocks; and granitic and gneissic rocks. Some of the highest concentrations of fluoride ever recorded have been found in lakes and groundwater of the Great Rift Valley system, stretching from northern Syria through Sudan, Ethiopia, Uganda, Kenya and Tanzania, to Mozambique, where there are well-documented areas with high rates of severe dental and skeletal fluorosis.[7] This is mainly due to the contact of water bodies with hyperalkaline volcanic rocks enriched in fluoride, as well as from high-fluoride geothermal solutions; fine-grained ashes are also particularly reactive.[7]

The worst affected region is in the East African Rift Valley, where some lakes, bore holes and wells may have fluoride levels high enough to cause acute toxic symptoms if the water is consumed (>30 mg/L).[8] In this region, water scarcity is a problem, and the warming climate can lead to drought, while burgeoning populations, migrations and conflicts can add further pressure on the limited available sources of safe drinking water.

In China, the indoor burning of fluoride-rich coal (with exposure to hydrogen fluoride) for heating and cooking also contributes to the high overall fluoride intake.[1] The preparation of foodstuffs in water containing increased fluoride and/or the consumption of specific foodstuffs naturally rich in fluoride (such as tea) are also significant dietary sources.

Certain industries using raw materials containing even small amounts of fluoride have the potential to pollute the air and soils of surrounding areas; notably, these industries include coal-fired power stations, coke production, brick, phosphate fertilizer and glass manufacture, and primary aluminium production. Point sources of fluoride emissions (industrial processes and volcanoes) can multiply soil fluoride concentrations 2–20 times for distances up to 10–20 km downwind.[9] Soluble fluoride species deposited on the ground by dry or wet deposition can remain in the surface soil indefinitely.

Contaminated soils pose a particular hazard to children, because of both hand-to-mouth behaviour and the intentional ingestion of soil (pica), as well as indoor dust contamination.[10] Grazing animals may also be at risk of developing chronic fluorosis in polluted areas. The widespread farming practice in many parts of the world of applying fluoride-rich phosphate fertilizers derived from natural phosphate rock deposits is another

well-recognized cause of fluorosis in grazing animals.[9] The disease manifestations are not unlike those observed in humans.

The main natural sources of hydrogen fluoride are degassing and erupting volcanoes. A catastrophic volcanic eruption that lasted 8 months at the Laki fissure in southern Iceland in 1783–84 produced immense gas and ash emissions with a high fluoride content, which poisoned grazing sheep, horses and cattle, and stunted vegetation. The mainly subsistence farmers had little food to fall back on after the loss of their animals and crops, and around 20 per cent of the total population of Iceland (about 50 000) died in the ensuing famine.[11] Reports of sickness and deaths in livestock due to acute and chronic fluoride intoxication have been associated with Iceland's Hekla volcano ever since the first human encounter with one of its eruptions in 1104.[12]

Forage contaminated with fluoride-enriched ash after an eruption of Lonquimay volcano, Chile, in 1988 acutely poisoned cattle,[13] but outside Iceland outbreaks of fluoride poisoning in livestock after volcanic eruptions are uncommon, and reports of animal deaths are more likely to be due to starvation or lack of water in fields covered with deep blankets of ash.

ENVIRONMENTAL EXPOSURE TO FLUORIDE

Exposure to fluoride can vary widely, and various types of study have attempted to estimate the mean daily intake of fluoride in Western societies. Most have found intakes of 0.01–0.13 mg/kg body weight, with mean intake values between 0.03 and 0.04 mg/kg body weight in non-fluoridated areas and 0.04 and 0.06 mg/kg body weight in fluoridated areas.[4] Individual intakes in children can, however, greatly exceed the mean value, owing to ingestion of dentifrice,[5,6] with some subgroups in the population having levels of dietary intake of fluoride considerably higher than the mean estimates. Beverages can be a significant source of fluoride intake in children. Further information in relation to recommended dietary intakes in children and adults is available.[1,14]

Fluoride is generally well absorbed in the gastrointestinal tract, from where it is rapidly distributed to all organs and tissues: a substantial amount is accumulated in bone, the rest being excreted in the urine. Bone deposition of fluoride occurs to the extent of 50 per cent in growing children but only 10 per cent in adults.[15] The bioavailability of ingested fluoride is important, however, and remains poorly understood:[5] calcium, magnesium and aluminium can form insoluble complexes with fluoride that can substantially reduce its absorption.[1]

Even with a low intake of fluoride from water, a certain level of dental fluorosis of the permanent teeth will be found arising from exposure during dental enamel formation and tooth development from birth to 6–8 years of age. Milder forms of mottling of the teeth are not noticeable, but more severe forms might be objectionable on aesthetic or cosmetic grounds.[16] Historically, a low prevalence of the milder forms of fluorosis has been accepted as a 'reasonable and minor consequence' balanced against the substantial protection from dental caries afforded by the use of fluoridated drinking water, dietary fluoride supplements and oral care products.

Establishing a discernible threshold for the development of dental fluorosis is problematic when the available studies do not record all sources of exposure to fluoride. In a meta-analysis performed in a systematic review of water fluoridation by the NHS Centre for Review and Dissemination,[17] an estimated 12.5 per cent (95 per cent confidence interval 7.0–21.5 per cent) of exposed people had fluorosis of aesthetic concern at a fluoride level in drinking water of 1 part per million (ppm), with an overall prevalence of detectable dental fluorosis of 18 per cent. This finding was made in comparison with a theoretical low fluoride concentration of 0.4 ppm, even though many areas in Britain may have fluoride levels lower than 0.4 ppm. The quality of the studies on which this estimate was based was, however, acknowledged to be low.

Skeletal fluorosis is usually restricted to tropical and subtropical regions, and an intake of 10–20 mg per day (equivalent to 5–10 ppm in the drinking water, for a person who ingests 2 L per day) for at least 10 years is often stated to be necessary for its development.[1] There is wide individual variation, and the problem of determining water fluoride levels and other sources of exposure to fluoride over years of intake makes it difficult for studies to demonstrate an exposure–response relationship or allow reliable estimates to be made of the global burden of this disease.

Skeletal fluorosis was first diagnosed in the Danish cryolite industry in 1932, where workers were exposed to elevated levels of hydrogen fluoride in the working atmosphere.[12] Cryolite (Na_3AlF_6) is used in the manufacture of aluminium. Today, populations living near uncontrolled industrial sources of hydrogen fluoride may be exposed to elevated levels of fluoride in the air, and vegetables and fruits may contain higher levels of fluoride, particularly from fluoride-containing dust settling on the plants. In a coal-burning area in China, endemic dental fluorosis was attributed to air pollution causing environmental contamination, including the contamination of broad-leaf vegetables and stored water.[1,18]

Although fluorides are emitted to the atmosphere in both gaseous and particulate forms, studies typically only report total fluoride content. In heavily polluted areas, typical daily inhalation intakes are in the range 10–40 µg per day (0.5–2 µg per m^3) and in some cases are as high as 60 µg per day (3 µg/m^3).[15]

According to one laboratory animal study, the absorption of hydrogen fluoride from the upper respiratory tract approaches 100 per cent.[19] Mean urinary fluoride levels are linearly related to the hydrogen fluoride concentration in the air in occupational settings.[20] No data are available regarding the distribution of fluoride in the body following exposure to hydrogen fluoride only.[10] The major route of fluoride excretion is via the kidneys and urine, and urine-testing for fluoride is a useful measure of recent exposure.

The available data on chronic toxicity from hydrogen fluoride inhalation are mainly limited to studies of workers exposed to levels exceeding 2–2.5 mg/m^3, or a daily exposure to a worker of 20–25 mg. The Health and Safety Commission[21] has set an 8 hour time-weighted average work exposure limit of 1.5 mg/m^3.

HUMAN HEALTH CONSEQUENCES OF EXCESS FLUORIDE INTAKE

The term 'fluoride' is frequently used to cover all combined forms of the element, with an assumption that the different forms of fluorine and its compounds have the same uptakes, distribution and retention, as well as health consequences, which is questionable. It is, for example, still uncertain whether there are differences in bioavailability between artificially and naturally fluoridated water.[5] Other factors to consider include age, health, exposure to other toxic substances (e.g. cigarette smoke), diet and poor nutrition.

Dental fluorosis

Enamel fluorosis (mottled teeth) is a hypomineralization of enamel, characterized by greater surface and subsurface porosity than normal enamel. It manifests in the permanent dentition as small white areas in the enamel or in more severe forms as staining and pitting. Enamel deposition is completed with the laying down of an insoluble form of calcium phosphate, $Ca_{10}(PO_4)_6(OH)_2$, similar to the rock apatite. In fluorosis, some of the fluoride present in drinking water is incorporated into the apatite crystal lattice of the tooth enamel during the formative stages: if F^- replaces OH^- as a major presence, it forms fluoroapatite. The condition does not arise once the permanent teeth have been established and therefore cannot develop in adults even when their intake of fluoride is raised through dietary sources or industrial exposures

In endemic areas, early changes include the gradual loss of translucency of the teeth, becoming more severe in association with an increase in the chalky-white opaqueness of the enamel in some and eventually all the teeth. The surfaces become subject to attrition and wear, and brown staining. Severe fluorosis is marked by the general form of the tooth being affected by hypoplasia, with discrete or confluent pitting and widespread brown stains (Figure 29.1).

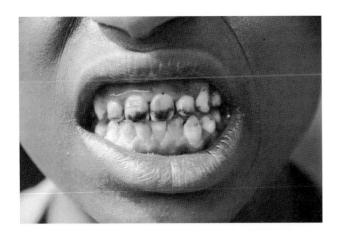

Figure 29.1 Severe dental fluorosis in a teenage boy living in an endemic area in the Southern Ethiopian Highlands (Great Rift Valley; see text).

Although the main consequences are due to disfigurement, the teeth also become more susceptible to caries in the advanced stages of the condition.

Skeletal fluorosis

Skeletal fluorosis is a condition that typically develops after many years of living in an endemic area and is not confined to those exposed in early life; unlike dental enamel, dietary fluoride is avidly incorporated into bone at all stages of life. The condition is marked by the onset of the pathological changes of osteosclerosis (bone thickening), resulting in marked limb and spinal deformities that become disabling or very painful in the advanced stages. The spinal changes can lead to neurological complications in the lower limbs.

In contrast, severe skeletal changes, such as bow legs, knock knees and sabre shins, have been reported to arise in childhood and the early teens in endemic areas in association with malnutrition.[22-24] Clinically, the deformities may be indistinguishable from those of rickets (vitamin D deficiency is the main cause of rickets, and calcium deficiency contributes in communities where little milk is consumed[25]) and remains poorly understood; radiological findings may reveal a spectrum of bone changes, including osteoporosis.

The early symptomless stage of the condition can be detected by finding dense bone changes on radiological examination.[26] Diagnosis is made on the basis of radiological bone changes in an endemic area, and can be confirmed by measurement of bone fluoride content, which constitutes a good reflection of long-term exposure. Histological examination of bone biopsies reveals line formation defects and periosteocytic lacunae. X-ray diffraction confirms the presence of fluoroapatite in the denser bone material.[27] The radiological findings in advanced cases typically include diffuse thickening or osteosclerosis, most marked in the pelvis, spine, ribs and lower limbs, with bone exostoses, and calcification of the tendons and ligaments, which may lead to an inflexible spine (kyphosis) in the most severely affected patients.[26] As well as osteosclerosis, two patterns of osteopenia are also seen: an osteoporotic type with overall decreased bone density, and an osteomalacic type that combines osteoporotic features with bone deformity. Nutritional status and calcium intake may be important determinants of the bone abnormalities in a particular patient.[26]

Fluoride is a potent stimulus to bone formation, resulting in a net increase in bone mass in skeletal fluorosis. For this reason, high doses have been used for the treatment of osteoporosis (in a recommended dose of 50 mg sodium fluoride daily, i.e. 22.6 mg of fluoride ion, for at least 2 years, together with calcium and vitamin D).[27]

Other adverse health outcomes

Studies of individuals undergoing fluoride treatment for osteoporosis, epidemiological studies of communities with naturally high levels of fluoride in drinking water and community-based studies of populations with fluoridated water supplies have examined the possible relationship between exposure to fluoride and alterations in bone mineral density and/or the risk of bone fractures, especially of the hip. A Medical Research Council (2002) report concluded that a small increase (or decrease) in risk cannot be ruled out.[5] Other potential effects that have been suggested by some include cancer, reproductive and developmental defects, and effects on the immune system, kidney and gastrointestinal tract, but no links with water fluoridation have been established.[5] Nonetheless, the Medical Research Council report recommended an updated analysis of UK data on fluoridation and cancer rates.[5]

CONTROL OF EXPOSURE TO FLUORIDE

The WHO guideline value for drinking water of 1.5 mg/L was set in 1984 and was last reviewed in 1996, when it was not changed.[1] This value is higher than that recommended for the fluoridation of water supplies (about 1 mg/L in temperate climes). For tropical countries, where the average daily water intake may exceed 2 L per day, a lower guideline value has been frequently suggested.[28]

In communities with endemic fluorosis, the first option is to find alternative water supplies, but where this is not possible defluoridation should be considered. Although many filter media and water-treatment methods are available for removing excessive fluoride from water, none has been widely adopted, and many initiatives have failed in the past for a variety of reasons.[8] Where alternative sources of drinking supplies are not available, a health risk assessment will be needed, and as a minimum the fluoride levels should be monitored and the population examined for signs of excessive fluoride exposure (moderate-to-severe dental fluorosis and clinically significant skeletal fluorosis), while taking account of the nutritional status of the population.[8] Water fluoride levels above 30 mg/L are acutely toxic (>1 mg/kg body weight)[8] and are unlikely to be tolerated for long periods, the first symptoms being nausea, diarrhoea and a bad taste in the mouth.

The UK government's Expert Panel on Air Quality Standards found, in setting a guideline value based on the acute irritant effects of hydrogen fluoride on the respiratory system, that, even at this low level (0.16 mg/m^3), the amount of fluoride inhaled by the lungs as a result of living near an emitting point source of hydrogen fluoride could be sufficient to double the average intake of fluoride in adults and also add significantly to the intake in children.[29] The panel concluded that, at an air concentration below 0.016 mg/m^3 over a long-term averaging period, the daily intake from this source would be about 10 per cent of the recommended total daily intake in children aged 1–3 years and would represent a non-significant risk in a child of developing dental fluorosis of aesthetic concern.[30,31] This level corresponds to a daily intake in an adult of about 0.3 mg per day, which would be a negligible addition as far as the systemic effects on skeletal bone are concerned.

According to WHO guidelines,[15] ambient air levels of hydrogen fluoride should be less than 1 μg/m^3 to prevent harmful effects on livestock and plants.

REFERENCES

♦ = Major review article

♦1. World Health Organization/International Programme on Chemical Safety. *Fluorides*. Environmental Health Criteria No.227. Geneva: WHO, 2002.

♦2. National Academy of Sciences. *Fluoride in Drinking Water: A Scientific Review of EPA's Standards*. Washington, DC: National Academies Press, 2006.

3. Cheng KK, Chalmers I, Sheldon TA. Adding fluoride to water supplies. *BMJ* 2007; **395**: 699–702.

♦4. NHS Centre for Review and Dissemination. *A Systematic Review of Public Water Fluoridation*. CRD Report No.18. York: University of York, 2000.

♦5. Medical Research Council. *Water Fluoridation and Health*. London: MRC, 2002.

6. Warren JJ, Levy SM. Systemic fluoride - sources, amounts, and effects of ingestion. *Dent Clin North Am* 1999; **43**: 695–711.

7. Edmunds M, Smedley P. Fluoride in natural waters. In: Selinius O, Alloway BJ, Ceneteno JA *et al.* (eds) *Essentials of Medical Geology* (pp. 301–29). Amsterdam: Elsevier, 2005.

♦8. Fawell J, Bailey K, Chilton J, Dahi E, Fewtrell L, Magara Y; World Health Organization. *Fluoride in Drinking Water*. London: IWA Publishing, 2006.

9. Cronin SJ, Manoharan V, Hedley MJ, Loganathan P. Fluoride: A review of its fate, bioavailability, and risks of fluorosis in grazed-pasture systems in New Zealand. *N Z J Agric Res* 2000; **43**: 295–321.

♦10. Agency for Toxic Substances and Disease Registry. *Toxicological Profile for Fluorides, Hydrogen Fluoride and Fluorines*. Atlanta: ATSDR, 2001.

11. Thordason T, Self S. Atmospheric and environmental effects of the 1783–1784 Laki eruption: A review and reassessment. *J Geophys Res* 2003; **108**(D1): 4011.

12. Roholm KAJ. *Fluorine Intoxication*. London: HK Lewis, 1937.

13. Araya O, Wittwer A, Villa A, Ducom C. Bovine fluorosis following volcanic activity in the southern Andes. *Vet Rec* 1990; **12**: 641–2.

14. European Food Safety Authority. Opinion of the Scientific Panel on Dietetic Products, Nutrition and Allergies on a request from the Commission related to the tolerable upper intake level of fluoride. *EFSA J* 2005; **192**: 1–65.

15. World Health Organization. *Air Quality Guidelines for Europe*, 2nd edn. Copenhagen: WHO, 2000.

16. Centers for Disease Control. Surveillance for dental caries, dental sealants, tooth retention, edentulism, and enamel fluorosis – United States, 1988–1994 and 1992–2002. *MMWR* 2005; **54**(SS-3): 1–43.

♦17. McDonagh MS, Whiting PF, Wilson PM *et al.* Systematic review of water fluoridation. *BMJ* 2000; **321**: 855–9.

18. Yixin C, Meiqi L, Zhaolong HE *et al.* Air pollution-type fluorosis in the region of Pingxiang, Jiangxi, Peoples' Republic of China. *Arch Environ Health* 1993; **48**: 246–9.

19. Morris, JB, Smith FA. Regional deposition and absorption of inhaled hydrogen fluoride in the rat. *Toxicol Appl Pharmacol* 1982; **62**: 81–9.

20. Lund K, Ekstrand J, Boe J, Sorstrand P, Kongerud J. Exposure to hydrogen fluoride: an experimental study in humans of concentrations of fluoride in plasma, symptoms, and lung function. *Occup Environ Med* 1997; **54**: 32–7.

21. Health and Safety Commission. List of Approved Workplace Exposure Limits (as Consolidated with Amendments October 2007). EH40/2005. Available from: http://www.hse.gov.uk/coshh/table1.pdf (accessed November 20, 2009).

22. Christie DP. The spectrum of radiographic bone changes in children with fluorosis. *Radiology* 1980; **136**: 85–90.

23. Krishnamachari KAVR, Krishnaswamy K. Genu valgum and osteoporosis in an area of endemic fluorosis. *Lancet* 1973; **2**: 877–9.

24. Teotia M, Teotia SPS, Kunwar KB. Endemic skeletal fluorosis. *Arch Dis Child* 1971; **46**: 686–91.

25. Wharton B, Bishop N. Rickets. *Lancet* 2003; **362**: 1389–99.

26. Wang Y, Yin Y, Gilula LA, Wilson AJ. Endemic fluorosis of the skeleton: Radiographic features in 127 patients. *Am J Radiol* 1994; **162**: 93–8.

27. Bouvin G, Meunier PJ. Fluoride and bone: Toxicological and therapeutic aspects. In: Lewis B, Alberti KGMM, Denman AM (eds) *The Metabolic and Molecular Basis of Acquired Diseases* (pp. 1803–23). London: Ballière Tindall, 1990.

28. Brouwer ID, Backer Dirks O, De Bruin A, Hautvast JGAJ. Unsuitability of World Health Organization guidelines for fluoride concentrations in drinking water in Senegal. *Lancet* 1988; **1**: 223–5.

29. Expert Panel on Air Quality Standards. *Halogens and Hydrogen Halides.* London: Defra, 2006.

30. Expert Panel on Air Quality Standards. *Addendum to Guidelines for Halogens and Hydrogen Halides.* London: Defra, 2009.

31. World Health Organization. *Trace Elements in Human Nutrition and Health.* Geneva: WHO, 1996.

30

Toxicity of ingested radionuclides

JOHN HARRISON

Marie Curie discovered polonium and radium in 1898[1,2] and died of aplastic anaemia or leukaemia in 1934. At the time, the toxic effects of ionizing radiation were poorly understood. A century later, a lot more is known of the carcinogenic properties of radiation and its ability to cause gross tissue damage and death at high doses.[3–5] A striking recent example of radionuclide toxicity was the death in 2006 of Alexander Litvinenko, thought to have been due to the ingestion of polonium-210.[6]

Our knowledge of the properties of radionuclides and the radiations that they emit allows us to make predictions about their potential to cause cancer and death. Exposures can occur from external sources of photon radiation (gamma and X-rays) and following the intake of radionuclides into the body. The toxicity of radionuclides that decay by the emission of short-range alpha and beta particles is largely dependent on their intake into the body and their direct irradiation of the organs and tissues in which they deposit.[4,7,8]

Their potential to cause particular types of cancer depends on their physical properties and on the chemical properties that determine their distribution and retention in organs and tissues. Thus, the potential to cause leukaemia will depend on the irradiation of haematopoietic tissue in red bone marrow, and evidence suggests that regional irradiation within bone marrow may be important.[8,9] The dose to the haematopoietic tissue will also be an important determinant of the potential of a radionuclide to kill.[10] Polonium-210 and radium-226 both decay by the emission of alpha particles, which have a range in body tissues of a few tens of micrometres, traversing only a few cell widths. The skeleton is an important site of deposition of both radionuclides, but differences in their distribution within the skeleton lead to differences in bone marrow irradiation that can be related to differences in toxicity.

Radiation doses from the intake of radionuclides are estimated using biokinetic and dosimetric models.[8] Biokinetic models are mathematical representations of the movement of elements and their radioisotopes within the body and their uptake and retention in organs and tissues. They are used to calculate the number of radioactive disintegrations occurring in individual organs and tissues. Dosimetric models represent the geometrical relationships of body structures and are used to calculate energy deposition, and hence dose, in so-called 'target regions' (organs and tissues) per disintegration occurring in 'source regions'. The internationally recognized source of such models is the International Commission on Radiological Protection (ICRP). ICRP models consider intakes of radionuclides by ingestion and inhalation, taking account of doses to the alimentary and respiratory tracts as well as to other organs and tissues following absorption to blood.[11,12]

This chapter provides a brief explanation of the use of biokinetic and dosimetric models to calculate organ and tissue doses. Specific examples of the health effects of radionuclide intake are then examined, considering cases of known or possible radionuclide ingestion. Alpha-emitting isotopes of radium were used in the early decades of the twentieth century as luminizers on instrument dials, leading to a clear excess of bone sarcomas in the mainly female workforce who ingested radium as they tipped their brushes.[13,14] Beta-emitting isotopes of strontium were among the radionuclides discharged to the Techa River in massive quantities during the early years of operation of the Russian Mayak plutonium plant. An excess of leukaemia has been reported in Techa River residents.[15] Evidence from these and other studies, together with an examination of differences in the behaviour of radionuclides in the body, are used to compare their toxicity, concentrating on the effects of bone marrow irradiation, from the certainty of death at high levels of ingested activity to a low estimated risk of leukaemia induction at normal environmental levels of exposure.

BIOKINETIC AND DOSIMETRIC MODELS

The ICRP has published biokinetic models that consider intakes of radionuclides by ingestion and inhalation, by adults and children.[11,12] Models have also been developed for the transfer of radionuclides to the fetus following maternal intake[16] and also the transfer of radionuclides in breast milk.[17] Models of the alimentary tract (Figure 30.1) and respiratory tract are used to define the movement of radionuclides within these systems, resulting in absorption to the blood and/or loss from the body.[18,19]

The behaviour of radionuclides absorbed to the blood is described by element-specific systemic models[20] that

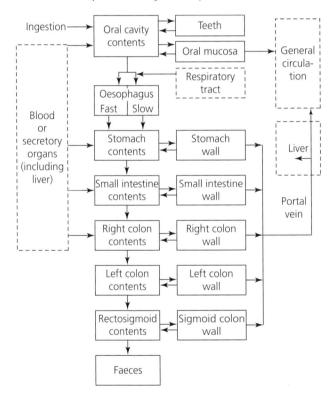

Figure 30.1 The biokinetic model of the human alimentary tract produced by the International Commission on Radiological Protection.[19] The model depicts the transit of ingested radionuclides through regions of the alimentary tract, retention in the various regions and absorption to blood. In most cases, calculations will be performed using standard values for transit times through the tract and values for absorption to blood, assumed to take place exclusively in the small intestine unless other information is available. (Reproduced from International Commission on Radiological Protection,[19] with permission.)

range in complexity from very simple models that assume uniform whole-body distribution (e.g. caesium) to multicompartment recycling models that take account of movement within and between body organs and tissues (e.g. strontium, radium and plutonium). The most complex models are those developed for the bone-seeking alkaline earth elements (Figure 30.2) and actinide elements.

The reliability of biokinetic models ultimately depends on the quality of the data on which they are based, including the availability of human data, as well as on the realism of the model developed from these data. Whereas ICRP models have been developed primarily to calculate equivalent and effective doses for use within the ICRP framework of radiological protection,[3,4] they are also used for other purposes, including the estimation of absorbed organ and tissue doses in epidemiological studies[21,22] and medical applications. In such cases, it is important that the applicability of models to the specific circumstances of exposure is carefully considered. Thus, for example, to calculate doses from the ingestion of strontium-90 in water from the Techa River (see below), a modification of the ICRP biokinetic model was developed using data relating specifically to the local population in the South Urals.[22]

Dose calculations involve the use of nuclear decay data[23] and anthropomorphic phantoms that describe the geometric relationship between different tissues and organs.[24-27] Doses from 'crossfire' radiation between source and target organs and tissues are important for penetrating photon radiation. For 'non-penetrating' alpha and beta particle radiations, energy will be largely deposited in the tissue in which the radionuclide is deposited, but in a number of important cases it is necessary to take account of the distribution of the radionuclide relative to target cells within the tissues. Such cases include the calculation of doses to target regions in the gut and skeleton.[4,7,19,28]

Biokinetic models for individual elements and their radioisotopes are used to calculate the total number of radioactive decays (transformations) occurring within specific tissues, organs or body regions (source regions) during a given period of time (usually to age 70 years). Dosimetric models are used to calculate the deposition of energy in all important organs/tissues (targets) for transformations occurring in each source region, taking account of the energies and yields of all emissions. The *absorbed* dose in grays (1 Gy = 1 J/kg) can then be calculated, knowing the number of decays occurring in source regions and energy deposition in the target regions.

For the purposes of radiation protection, including comparison with dose limits, the ICRP[3,4] calculates equivalent and effective dose in sieverts (Sv). The *equivalent* dose is intended to allow for differences between radiation types in their effectiveness per Gy in causing cancer and is obtained by multiplying absorbed dose in Gy by radiation weighting factors (e.g. 1 for gamma rays and beta particles, and 20 for alpha particles).

The *effective* dose provides a single quantity that allows for differences between organs and tissues in their

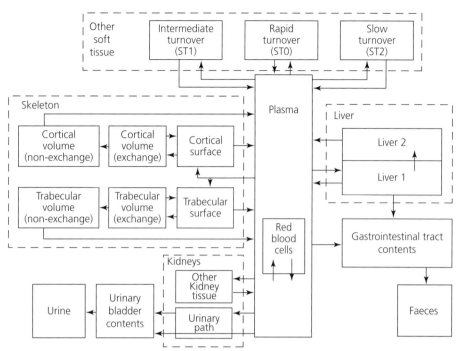

Figure 30.2 The systemic model of the International Commission on Radiological Protection for the behaviour of alkaline earth (including strontium and radium) and similar elements absorbed to the blood.[20] The model depicts uptake and retention in the skeleton and excretion in the urine and faeces. Skeletal uptake and retention distinguishes between cortical and trabecular bone, and between bone surfaces and volume. Note that the liver is included with other soft tissues in the cases of strontium and radium. Liver 1 and 2 represent shorter- and longer-term components of retention. ST, soft tissues. (Adapted from International Commission on Radiological Protection,[20] with permission.)

contributions to the total radiation detriment from cancer and hereditary effects following uniform external irradiation of the body. Thus, the effective dose is obtained by summing the values of equivalent doses to the various organs and tissues after multiplying them by tissue weighting factors. The cancer risk estimates on which the tissue weighting factors are based are derived principally from follow-up studies of the survivors of the atomic bombings at Hiroshima and Nagasaki[3,4], exposed mainly to gamma rays.

The ICRP scheme is an elegant solution to the problem of addition of doses from external sources and from radionuclide intakes that may result in very different patterns of dose delivery, both between organs and over time. However, the ICRP protection quantities were not intended for calculations of doses and risks to individuals and defined population groups. For such applications, absorbed dose (Gy) should be used, together with the best available information on the relative biological effectiveness of different radiations for the health effect under consideration, as well as age- and sex-specific risk factors.[4,7,8]

MARIE CURIE – THE DISCOVERY OF POLONIUM AND RADIUM

The discovery of polonium and radium was reported in 1898.[1,2] Marie Curie was awarded the Nobel Prize for Physics in 1903 and for Chemistry in 1911. She is reported to have died of either aplastic anaemia or leukaemia in 1934. At the time of the pioneering work of the Curies, there was no understanding of the toxic effects of radiation exposure. More than a century later, we know a great deal, and it is possible to comment on the contribution that radiation from external and internal sources may have

made to the death of Marie Curie. However, we are still far from having all the answers.

We know that the radionuclides discovered by the Curies in the uranium ore pitchblende were [210]Po and [226]Ra, both alpha particle emitters, decaying with half-lives of 138 days and 1600 years, respectively. Both are quite well absorbed from the intestinal tract following ingestion (around 10–20 per cent), and similar fractions would be absorbed to the blood from the respiratory tract following inhalation. Figure 30.2 shows the ICRP systemic model applied to radium and other alkaline earth elements absorbed to the blood. Figure 30.3 shows a systemic model for polonium developed by Leggett and Eckerman[29] which is more physiologically realistic than the current ICRP[20] model and is likely to be adopted by the ICRP for future dose calculations.

The skeleton is an important site of deposition of both polonium and radium. However, there are important differences in their distribution within the skeleton and hence the pattern of dose delivered to haematopoietic tissue in bone marrow. Radium is deposited exclusively on bone surfaces and, with time, deposits in bone mineral become more uniform. In contrast, animal data show that polonium deposits throughout bone marrow as well as on bone surfaces. Thus, alpha particles from [226]Ra irradiate only peripheral marrow within a few tens of micrometres of bone surfaces, whereas alpha particles from [210]Po are emitted throughout the red bone marrow.

The targets for radiation-induced leukaemias are likely to be haematopoietic stem cells or early lineage-committed precursor cells. There is same evidence for two locations or niches for haematopoietic stem cells in red bone marrow.[30] It has been established that osteoblasts function as a key component of the stromal microenvironment for the long-term maintenance of quiescent haematopoietic stem cells.[31–33]

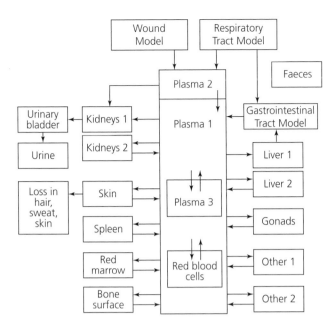

Figure 30.3 Leggett and Eckerman's[21] systemic model for polonium. The diagram also shows the entry of polonium into blood from wounds and from the alimentary and respiratory tracts. The systemic model depicts uptake and retention in a number of organs and tissues, including red bone marrow and liver, and excretion from the body via the kidneys, the alimentary tract and the skin. Numbers represent different components of retention in organs or blood plasma. (Adapted from Leggett and Eckerman,[21] with permission.)

A second niche, identified as being involved in the short-term maintenance of haematopoietic stem cells, involves endothelial cells in vascular sinusoids within the red bone marrow.[34,35] The available evidence suggests that cell division in the osteoblastic niche may release cells that relocate to the vascular niche, which regulates proliferation, differentiation and mobilization. This implies that stem cells in the osteoblastic niche have a higher self-renewal capacity than those in the central marrow vascular niche, although uncertainty remains over the relationship between niche location.[36]

It appears that [226]Ra on bone surfaces will preferentially irradiate the adjacent peripheral marrow, which contains the most primitive haematopoietic stem cells. Polonium-210, and external sources of radiation, will result in a more uniform distribution of dose throughout the bone marrow, potentially irradiating all cell types, including haematopoietic stem cells in the osteoblastic and vascular niches. Before commenting further on the possible health effects resulting from these different patterns of irradiation of haematopoietic tissue, we should examine epidemiological evidence from studies including those of the radium dial painters and Techa River residents who ingested beta particle-emitting isotopes of strontium.

THE RADIUM DIAL PAINTERS

An increased incidence of bone tumours has been observed in people exposed to long-lived alpha-emitting isotopes of radium, particularly in painters of luminous dials, but also in radium chemists and in people treated with radium salts in the belief that their effect was therapeutic.[13]

In the USA, almost 5000 workers, mainly female, were employed in the luminizing industry, mainly between 1915 and 1954. By the end of 1983, 62 cases of bone sarcoma and 32 cases of head sinus carcinoma had occurred in a total of 2352 people who had been measured to obtain an estimate of their body content and hence dose.[13] In addition, [224]Ra (an alpha emitter, half-life 3.62 days, decaying to radon-220) was used in Germany as a treatment for arthritis, ankylosing spondylitis and bone tuberculosis in the 1940s and 50s. Reports of cancer in patients exposed to high levels of [224]Ra (a mean cumulative bone surface dose of around 30 Gy) have included 899 individuals exposed as adults or children.[37–40] A total of 56 malignant bone tumours have occurred (0.3 being expected), with more recent observations of a lower number of other malignancies but no clear excess of leukaemia. Thus, it appears that alpha-emitting isotopes of radium are effective in causing bone cancer but not leukaemia.

However, the picture is complicated by observations after lower levels of [224]Ra administration to adult patients with ankylosing spondylitis (a typical mean cumulative bone surface dose of about 5 Gy). The most recent report included 1462 patients[41] and reported five cases of malignant disease of the bone and bone marrow but a notable increase in leukaemias (16 being observed but seven expected).

TECHA RIVER RESIDENTS

In the late 1940s and 50s, many thousands of people living in rural villages on the Techa River, now in Russia, received protracted external and internal radiation exposures as a result of discharges of radionuclides from the Mayak plutonium production complex, particularly during the early years of its operation.[15,42] The dominant source of the dose to red bone marrow, and hence the major determinant of the risk of leukaemia, was the intake by ingestion of beta particle-emitting isotopes of strontium, principally [90]Sr.[42] Strontium-90 and its immediate decay product, yttrium-90, emit beta particles with mean energies of about 0.2 and 1 MeV, respectively, and ranges in soft tissue of up to 2 and 10 mm, respectively.

Krestinina et al.[15] reported a preliminary analysis of cancer mortality in a cohort of almost 30 000 people born before 1950 who lived near the river some time between 1950 and 1960. Further work is required to provide improved estimates of the doses received by cohort members. However, based on 1842 solid cancer deaths and 61 deaths from leukaemia, it was estimated that 2.5 per cent of solid cancers and 63 per cent of leukaemia deaths were attributable to radiation.[15] Because the dose to red bone marrow was dominated by ^{90}Sr, this study provides direct evidence of the induction of leukaemia by beta particles from ^{90}Sr and [90]Y.

The workers at the Russian Mayak nuclear complex were exposed to very high levels of external and internal radiation, including plutonium exposure. Levels were particularly high during the early years of plant operation in the late 1940s to mid-1950s. Although dose reconstruction for both external and internal exposure is difficult and further work is required to improve dose estimates, clear excesses of plutonium-239-attributable lung, liver and bone cancers have been reported.[43–48] In a detailed assessment of the risk of cancer mortality from external radiation exposure in Mayak workers, Shilnikova et al.[49] demonstrated a significant dose–response effect for leukaemia induction, but with no indication of an effect of plutonium exposure. Positive dose–response relationships were also obtained for lung, liver and bone cancer, but these were sensitive to assumptions regarding plutonium exposure. Thus, it appears that skeletal deposits of ^{239}Pu, and the resulting alpha particle irradiation, result in bone cancer but are ineffective in causing leukaemia.

Overall, the available epidemiological evidence indicates that peripheral alpha irradiation of marrow from ^{239}Pu and radium isotopes is effective in causing bone cancer but has limited potential to cause leukaemia. However, there is clear evidence of leukaemia induction following a more uniform irradiation of marrow by external radiation or beta particles from ^{90}Sr/^{90}Y in bone.

POLONIUM AS A POISON

Radiation at sufficiently high doses is lethal due to massive cell-killing in the organs and tissues of the body. Organs and tissues vary substantially in their sensitivity to damage by radiation. Particularly sensitive is the haematopoietic tissue of the bone marrow, followed by the epithelial lining of the alimentary tract. Information on the acute effects of radiation relates mainly to exposure to external radiation.[50–55]

Considering the acute effects of ingested Po, animal data for a number of mammalian species are consistent with death occurring within 20 days of an uptake to the

blood of about 1–4 MBq/kg or more.[56,57] These data show haematological changes characteristic of bone marrow failure. They also show gross damage to other organs, including the kidneys and liver, and to the gut mucosa after oral administration.[58] An uptake to blood of 1–4 MBq/kg corresponds to an absorption of about 0.1–0.3 GBq in a 70 kg man and an intake by ingestion of 1–3 GBq, assuming 10 per cent absorption. Table 30.1 shows an estimate of doses to the organs and tissues as Gy per GBq ingested, calculated using the Leggett and Eckerman[21] model and assuming 10 per cent absorption to blood.

A knowledge of the nature of the acute effects of radiation indicates that most have a dose threshold below which no effect will be detectable without conducting a clinical test. Dose–response relationships are expressed in terms of LD_{50} values (the lethal dose for 50 per cent of individuals) with LD_0–LD_{100} ranges. The LD_{50} for bone marrow irradiation following the ingestion of 2 GBq of ^{210}Po and the absorption to blood of 200 MBq was estimated as about 2.5 Gy with minimal medical care and 3.5–4 Gy with good supportive medical care.[10] These estimates took account of the relative biological effectiveness (RBE) of alpha particles compared with gamma or X-rays[59,60] and of the possible effect of dose protraction.[53,61,62] The data in Table 30.1 show that, following the ingestion of 2 GBq, the LD_{50} of 3.5–4 Gy with supportive medical treatment would be reached after about 10 days, and the LD_{100} value of about 5 Gy within 2 weeks. Although these dose estimates and LD values should be recognized as uncertain, their comparison indicates that bone marrow failure is a likely short-term consequence of an intake by ingestion of 2 GBq ^{210}Po.

Damage to tissues other than the bone marrow is likely to contribute to early death. In particular, estimated dose rates for the kidneys and liver of about 4 and 2 Gy per day, respectively, over the first few days after intake compare with estimated LD_{50} values of 6 and 8 Gy, respectively.[10] The available evidence suggests that the ingestion of around one-tenth of this amount (i.e. 200 MBq) might

Table 30.1 Cumulative doses to the organs/tissues of a reference adult male after ingesting polonium-210, assuming 10 per cent absorption to the blood, calculated using the Leggett and Eckerman systemic model (see Figure 30.3)

Time after intake (days)	Cumulative absorbed dose (Gy/GBq ingested)						
	Red bone marrow	Gut	Liver	Kidneys	Spleen	Skin	Testes
1	0.2	0.04	1.1	1.9	0.7	0.1	0.2
2	0.4	0.09	2.5	4.1	1.5	0.3	0.4
3	0.6	0.1	3.8	6.2	2.2	0.5	0.7
4	0.8	0.2	5.1	8.2	3.0	0.6	0.9
5	1.0	0.2	6.3	10	3.7	0.8	1.2
10	2.0	0.5	12	18	7.1	1.8	2.6
15	2.8	0.6	16	25	10	2.9	4.2
20	3.6	0.8	20	30	13	4.0	5.9
25	4.2	0.9	23	35	15	5.2	7.7
30	4.8	1.0	25	39	16	6.4	9.4

prove fatal over a period of months, primarily due to kidney failure.[10]

DISCUSSION AND CONCLUSION

This chapter has provided a brief description of the use of biokinetic and dosimetric models to calculate radiation doses to the organs and tissues of the body, concentrating on specific examples of radionuclide ingestion and associated health effects. At normal environmental levels of exposure, the health effect of concern is cancer, with the risk of specific cancer types being dependent on the distribution and retention of individual radionuclides and on the characteristics of the radiation that they emit. However, we also know that sufficiently high activities can cause gross tissue damage, organ failure and death.

Doses to the gut from ingested radionuclides are generally less important than doses to other organs and tissues following absorption to the blood because movement through the gut is relatively rapid and target cells are situated at some depth within the epithelial lining.[19,28] Thus, for example, the ingestion of alpha-emitting isotopes of radium results in their deposition in the skeleton, and the dominant health effect is bone cancer.

Taking the example of the ability of radionuclides to cause leukaemia, the available epidemiological evidence indicates that beta irradiation of bone marrow from ^{90}Sr in bone mineral is more effective than peripheral alpha irradiation of marrow from bone deposits of radium and plutonium isotopes. These observations might be taken to indicate that the primary targets for the induction of leukaemia are stem cells in the vascular niche and associated lineage-committed precursor cells, located away from bone surfaces, rather than primitive haematopoietic stem cells in the osteoblastic niche adjacent to the bone surfaces. However, the observation that lower activities of ^{224}Ra preferentially induce leukaemia rather than bone cancer suggests the possibility that haematopoietic stem cells near to bone surfaces are particularly sensitive to cell killing. Support for this conclusion comes from experimental and epidemiological evidence of a low RBE for alpha-induced leukaemia,[9] attributable to cell killing by alpha particles. It seems likely on current evidence that cell killing and regional irradiation are important factors determining the risk of leukaemia from skeletal deposits of alpha-emitting radionuclides.

The skeleton is an important site of deposition of ^{210}Po but unlike the bone-seeking alpha-emitting isotopes of radium and plutonium, it deposits throughout bone marrow as well as on bone surfaces. This distribution is a key factor in determining the toxicity of ^{210}Po at high administered levels of activity, enabling the complete destruction of haematopoietic tissue with lethal consequences. It is also likely that ^{210}Po at lower doses is a more effective leukaemogen than are the bone-seeking alpha emitters, including ^{226}Ra. Thus, we now know a good deal about the behaviour and toxicity of the radionuclides

discovered by Marie Curie, and although ^{210}Po cannot, of course, be identified definitively as the cause of her death, it is a highly plausible contributor.

We all ingest ^{210}Po in our diets, and it may be instructive to end this chapter by examining the risk that this entails. The average annual intake in the UK is about 40 Bq;[63] the dose to red bone marrow from this intake is about 5 μGy. Since each cell that is hit by an alpha particle receives a dose of around 0.5 Gy,[64] an annual dose of 5 μGy means that an average of 1 in 100 000 cells in the bone marrow are hit during the year. Assuming a low alpha particle RBE for leukaemia induction and using a lifetime risk factor for leukaemia of 1×10^{-2}/Gy,[9] the risk from 5 μGy is 1 in 1 million after 20 years' intake. Similarly small risks can be calculated for other cancer types.

However, such risk estimates depend on the assumption of a linear non-threshold dose–response relationship. Although this is a reasonable assumption for radiation protection purposes, it is unlikely to apply uniformly to all cancer types, and arguments are advanced for supra-linear low-dose responses and for thresholds and/or hormetic effects.[64–67] The ICRP[4] concludes that the true validity of the linear non-threshold model may prove to be beyond definitive resolution for the foreseeable future. Whereas we are able to predict the health effects of radionuclide exposures at higher doses with some confidence, more accurate assessments of risks at the lowest doses will require improvements in our understanding of the mechanisms of radiation carcinogenesis.

REFERENCES

● = Key primary paper

◆ = Major review article

●1. Curie P, Curie P Mme. Sur une nouvelle substance dans le pithblende [On a new substance in pitchblende]. *C R Acad Sci Gen* 1898; **127**: 175–6.

●2. Curie P, Curie P Mme, Bemont G. Sur une nouvelle substance fortement radioactive dans le pithblende [On a new strongly radioactive substance in pitchblende]. *C R Acad Sci Gen* 1898; **127**: 1215–17.

3. International Commission on Radiological Protection. 1990 Recommendations of the International Commission on Radiological Protection. ICRP Publication 60. *Annals of the ICRP* 1991; **21**(1–3).

4. International Commission on Radiological Protection. The 2007 Recommendations of the International Commission on Radiological Protection. ICRP Publication 103. *Annals of the ICRP* 2007; **37**(2–4).

◆5. United Nations Scientific Committee on the Effects of Atomic Radiation. Sources and Effects of Ionizing Radiation. *2000 Report to the General Assembly, with Scientific Annexes*. New York: United Nations, 2000.

6. Commons Hansard. Alexander Litvinenko (Case Update): The Secretary of State for Foreign and Commonwealth

Affairs (David Milliband). Columns 21–2, July 16, 2007. London: House of Commons.

7. Harrison JD, Streffer C. The ICRP protection quantities, equivalent and effective dose: their basis and application. *Radiat Prot Dosim* 2007; **127**: 12–18.

♦8. Harrison JD, Day P. Radiation doses and risks from internal emitters. *J Radiol Prot* 2008; **28**: 137–59.

●9. Harrison JD, Muirhead CR. Quantitative comparisons of cancer induction in humans by internally deposited radionuclides and external radiation. *Int J Radiat Biol* 2003; **79**: 1–13.

●10. Harrison JD, Leggett RW, Lloyd DC, Phipps AW, Scott BR. Polonium-210 as a poison. *J Radiol Prot* 2007; **27**: 17–40.

11. International Commission on Radiological Protection. Dose Coefficients for Intake of Radionuclides by Workers. ICRP Publication 68. *Annals of the ICRP* 1994; **24**(4).

12. International Commission on Radiological Protection. Age-dependent Doses to Members of the Public from Intake of Radionuclides Part 5: Compilation of Ingestion and Inhalation Dose Coefficients. ICRP Publication 72. *Annals of the ICRP* 1996; **26**(1).

13. Rundo J, Keane AT, Lucas HF, Schlenker RA, Stebbings JH, Stehney AF. Current (1984) status of the study of ^{226}Ra and ^{228}Ra in humans at the Center for Human Biology. In: Proc. Symp. The Radiobiology of Radium and Thorotrast (Eds. W. Gössner, G.B. Gerber, U. Hagan, A. Luz). *Strahlentherapie* 1986; **80**(Suppl.): 14–21.

●14. Fry SA. Studies of US radium dial workers: an epidemiological classic. *Radiat Res* 1998; **150**: S21–29.

●15. Krestinina LY, Preston DL, Ostroumova EV *et al.* Protracted radiation exposure and cancer mortality in the Techa River Cohort. *Radiat Res* 2005; **164**: 602–11.

16. International Commission on Radiological Protection. Doses to the Embryo and Fetus from Intakes of Radionuclides by the Mother. ICRP Publication 88. *Annals of the ICRP* 2001; **31** (1–3). Corrected version issued May 2002.

17. International Commission on Radiological Protection. Doses to Infants from Ingestion of Radionuclides in Mothers' Milk. ICRP Publication 95. *Annals of the ICRP* 2004; **34**(3–4).

18. International Commission on Radiological Protection Human Respiratory Tract Model for Radiological Protection. ICRP Publication 66. *Annals of the ICRP* 1994; **24**(1–3).

19. International Commission on Radiological Protection. Human Alimentary Tract Model for Radiological Protection. ICRP Publication 100. *Annals of the ICRP* 2006; **36**(1/2).

20. International Commission on Radiological Protection. Age-dependent Doses to Members of the Public from Intake of Radionuclides. Part 2: Ingestion Dose Coefficients. ICRP Publication 67. *Annals of the ICRP* 1993; **23**(3/4).

●21. Leggett RW, Eckerman KF, Khokhryakov VF, Suslova KG, Krahenbuhl MP, Miller SC. Mayak worker study: an improved biokinetic model for reconstructing doses from internally deposited plutonium. *Radiat Res* 2005; **164**: 111–22.

22. Shagina NB, Tolstykh EI, Fell TP, Harrison JD, Phipps AW, Degteva MO. *In utero* and postnatal haemopoietic tissue doses resulting from maternal ingestion of strontium isotopes from the Techa River. *Radiat Prot Dosim* 2007; **127**: 497–501.

23. Endo A, Yamaguchi Y, Eckerman KF. Development and assessment of a new radioactive decay database use for dosimetry calculation. *Radiat Prot Dosim* 2003; **105**: 565–9.

24. Cristy M, Eckerman KF. Specific *Absorbed Fractions of Energy at Various Ages from Internal Photon Sources*. ORNL/TM-8381/V1–7. Oak Ridge, TN: Oak Ridge National Laboratory, 1987.

25. Fill UA, Zankl M, Petoussi-Henss N, Siebert M, Regulla D. Adult female voxel models of different stature and photon conversion coefficients for radiation protection. *Health Phys* 2004; **86**: 253–72.

26. Zankl M, Petoussi-Henss N, Fill U, Regulla D. The application of voxel phantoms to the internal dosimetry of radionuclides. *Radiat Prot Dosim* 2003; **105**: 539–48.

27. Zankl M, Eckerman K, Bolch WE. Voxel-based models representing the male and female ICRP reference adult – the skeleton. *Radiat Prot Dosim* 2007; **127**: 174–86.

28. Harrison JD, Fell TP, Phipps AW, Smith TJ. The new ICRP model of the human alimentary tract: target cell assumptions and colon doses from ingested alpha- and beta- emitting radionuclides. In: *Proceedings of the 9th International Conference on Health Effects of Incorporated Radionuclides: Emphasis on Radium, Thorium, Uranium and their Daughter Products. HEIR 2004.* Neuherberg, Germany: GSF, 2005: 293–300.

●29. Leggett RW, Eckerman KF. A systemic biokinetic model for polonium. *Science Total Environ* 2001; **275**: 109–25.

♦30. Yin T, Li L. The stem cell niches in bone. *J Clin Invest* 2006; **116**: 1195–201.

31. Moore KA. Recent advances in defining the haematopoietic stem cell niche. *Curr Opin Hematol* 2004; **11**: 107–11.

32. Taichman RS. Blood and bone: two tissues whose fates are intertwined to create the haemopoietic stem-cell niche. *Blood* 2005; **105**: 2631–9.

33. Passegue E, Wagers AJ, Giuriato S, Anderson WC, Weisman IL. Global analysis of proliferation and cell cycle gene expression in the regulation of hematopoietic stem and progenitor cell fates. *J Exp Med* 2005; **202**: 1599–611.

34. Kiel MJ, Yilmaz OH, Iwashita T, Terhorst C, Morrison SJ. SLAM family receptors distinguish hematopoietic stem and progenitor cells and reveal endothelial niches for stem cells. *Cell* 2005; **121**: 1109–21.

35. Kopp HG, Avecilla ST, Hooper AT, Rafii S. The bone marrow vascular niche: home of HSC differentiation and mobilization. *Physiology (Bethesda)* 2005; **20**: 349–56.

36. Kiel MJ, Morrison SJ. Uncertainty in the niches that maintain haematopoeitic stem cells. *Nat Rev Immunol* 2008; **8**: 290–301.

37. Spiess H. The Ra-224 study: past, presence and future. In: van Kaick G, Karaoglou A, Kellerer AM (eds) *Health Effects of Internally Deposited Radionuclides: Emphasis on Radium and Thorium*. Singapore: World Scientific, 1995: 157–63.

38. Nekolla EA, Kellerer AM, Kuse-Isingschulte M, Eder E, Spiess H. Malignancies in patients treated with high doses of radium-224. *Radiat Res* 1999; **152**: S3–7.

●39. Nekolla EA, Kreisheimer M, Kellerer AM, Kuse-Isingschults M, Gössner W, Spiess H. Induction of malignant bone tumours in radium-224 patients: risk estimates based on the improved dosimetry. *Radiat Res* 2000; **153**: 93–103.

40. Nekolla EA, Walsh L, Schottenhammer G, Spiess H. Malignancies in patients treated with high doses of radium-224. In: *Proceedings of the 9th International Conference on Health Effects of Incorporated Radionuclides: Emphasis on Radium, Thorium, Uranium and their daughter products. HEIR 2004.* Neuherberg, Germany: GSF, 2005: 67–74.

41. Wick RR, Nekolla EA. Long term investigation of the late effects in ankylosing spondylitis patients treated with radium-224. In: *Proceedings of the 9th International Conference on Health Effects of Incorporated Radionuclides: Emphasis on Radium, Thorium, Uranium and their daughter products. HEIR 2004.* Neuherberg, Germany: GSF, 2005: 75–81.

42. Degteva MO, Shagina NB, Tolstykh EI *et al.* An approach to reduction of uncertainties in internal dose reconstructed for the Techa River population. *Radiat Prot Dosim* 2007; **127**: 480–5.

43. Koshurnikova NA, Shilnikova NS, Okatenko PV *et al.* The risk of cancer among nuclear workers at the "Mayak" Production Association: preliminary results of an epidemiological study. In: Boice JD (ed.) *Implications of New Data on Radiation Cancer Risk.* NCRP Proceedings No. 18. Bethesda, MD: NCRP, 1997: 113–22.

44. Koshurnikova NA, Bolotnikova MG, Illyin LA *et al.* Lung cancer risk due to exposure to incorporated plutonium. *Radiat Res* 1998; **149**: 366–71.

45. Koshurnikova NA, Shilnikova NS, Okatenko PV *et al.* Characteristics of the cohort of workers at the Mayak nuclear complex. *Radiat Res* 1999; **152**: 352–63.

46. Gilbert ES, Koshurnikova NA, Sokolnikov ME *et al.* Liver cancers in Mayak workers. *Radiat Res* 2000; **154**: 246–52.

●47. Gilbert ES, Koshurnikova NA, Sokolnikov ME *et al.* Lung cancer in Mayak workers. *Radiat Res* 2004; **162**: 505–16.

48. World Health Organization International Agency for Research on Cancer. *Ionizing Radiation.* Part 2: *Some Internally Deposited Radionuclides.* IARC Monographs on the Evaluation of Carcinogenic Risks to Humans, Vol. 78. Lyon: IARC Press, 2001.

●49. Shilnikova NS, Preston DL, Ron E *et al.* Cancer mortality risk among workers at the Mayak nuclear complex. *Radiat Res* 2003; **159**: 797–8.

50. United Nations Scientific Committee on the Effects of Atomic Radiation. Sources, Effects and Risks of Ionizing Radiation. *United Nations Scientific Committee on the Effects of Atomic Radiation. 1988 Report to the General Assembly with Annexes.* Annex: *Early Effects in Man of High Doses of Radiation.* New York: United Nations, 1988: 545–647.

51. Stather JW, Muirhead CR, Edwards AA, Harrison JD, Lloyd DC, Wood NR. *Health Effects Models Developed from the 1988 UNSCEAR Report.* NRPB-R226. Available from Health Protection Agency, Chilton, Didcot, Oxfordshire, 1988.

52. Scott BR, Hahn FF. Early occurring and continuing effects. In: Evans JS, Moeller JW, Cooper DW (eds) *Health Effects Models for Nuclear Power Plant Accident Consequence Analysis.* NUREG/CR-4214 (SAND85-7185). Washington, DC: Nuclear Registry Commission, 1985.

53. Scott BR, Hahn FF. Early occurring and continuing effects. In: Evans JS, Moeller JW, Cooper DW (eds) *Health Effects Models for Nuclear Power Plant Accident Consequence Analysis.* NUREG/CR-4214 (SAND85-7185), Rev. 1, Part II. Washington, DC: Nuclear Registry Commission, 1989.

54. Scott BR. Early occurring and continuing effects. In: *Modification of Models Resulting from Addition of Effects of Exposure to Alpha-Emitting Nuclides.* NUREG/CR-4214. Rev. 1, Part II. Addendum 2 (LMF-136). Washington, DC: Nuclear Registry Commission, 1993.

◆55. Edwards AA, Lloyd DC. *Risk from Deterministic Effects of Ionising Radiation.* Doc. NRPB 1996; **7**(3). Available from Health Protection Agency, Chilton, Didcot, Oxfordshire, UK.

56. Della Rosa RJ, Stannard JN. Acute toxicity as a function of route of administration. *Radiat Res Suppl* 1964; **5**: 205–15.

57. Cohen N, Fellman AL, Hickman DP, Ralston LG, Ayres LS. *Primate Polonium Metabolic Models and their use in Estimation of Systemic Radiation Doses from Bioassay Data.* Miamisburg, OH: Mound Laboratory, 1989.

58. Stannard JN, Casarett GW. Concluding comments on biological effects of alpha particle emitters in soft tissues as exemplified by experiments with polonium-210. *Radiat Res Suppl* 1964; **5**: 398–434.

59. Scott BR. Early occurring and continuing effects. In: *Modification of Models Resulting from Addition of Effects of Exposure to Alpha-Emitting Nuclides.* NUREG/CR-4214, Rev. 1, Part II. Addendum 2 (LMF-136). Washington, DC: Nuclear Registry Commission, 1993.

60. Scott BR. Health risks from high-level radiation exposures from radiological weapons. *Radiat Prot Manag* 2004; **21**: 9–25.

61. Scott BR, Dillehay LE. A model for hematopoietic death in man from irradiation of bone marrow during radioimmunotherapy. *Br J Radiol* 1990; **63**: 862–70.

62. Haskin FE, Goossens LHJ, Harper FT, Kraan BCP. *Probabilistic Accident Consequence Uncertainty Analysis. Early Health Effects Uncertainty Analysis.* Vol. 2: *Appendices.* NUREG/CR-6545, EUR 16775. Washington DC: Joint Report of US Nuclear Regulatory Commission and Commission of the European Communities, 1997.

63. Hughes JS. *Ionising Radiation Exposure of the UK Population: 1999 Review.* NRPB-R311. London: Stationery Office, 1999.

◆64. Committee Examining Radiation Risks of Internal Emitters. Report of the Committee Examining Radiation Risks of Internal Emitters. Available from: http://www.cerrie.org/pdfs/cerrie_report_e-book.pdf (accessed July 30, 2009).

65. Feinendegen LE, Paretzke H, Neumann RD. Two principal considerations are needed after low doses of ionizing radiation. *Radiat Res* 2008; **169**: 247–8.

66. Tubiana M, Aurengo A. La relation dose-effet et l'estimation des effets cancérogè;nes des faibles doses de rayonnement ionisants [The dose–response relationship and estimation of the carcinogenic effects of weak doses of ionising radiation]. Available from: http://www.academie-sciences.fr/publications/rapports/pdf/dose_effet_07_04_05.pdf (accessed July 30, 2009).

67. Tubiana M, Aurengo A, Averbeck D, Masse R. Low-dose risk assessment: the debate continues. *Radiat Res* 2008; **169**: 246–7.

SECTION D

Diseases related to the ingestion of infectious agents

31

The sources and environmental origins
of gastrointestinal pathogens

GORDON NICHOLS, KÅRE MØLBAK

HISTORY AND BURDEN

Throughout history, mankind has been subject to a large variety of infections and intoxications associated with the consumption of contaminated food or water, or with the transmission of infection from direct or indirect contact with animals or other infected humans. Epidemics of typhoid and pandemics of cholera have been significant causes of morbidity and mortality throughout the world over the last two centuries, and in poor areas of the world still are. Diarrhoeal diseases remain a leading cause of infant and childhood mortality in developing countries, and parasitic worm burdens can cause important delays in both the physical and mental development of children.

Although a modern understanding of the epidemiology of many of the pathogens is well developed and public health measures to prevent them are part of the infrastructure and legislation of developed countries, some infections can still be remarkably common. In developing countries, diarrhoeal diseases from a variety of pathogens are often common in childhood, and as a consequence a high proportion of the adult population has usually been exposed to infection with many of the common pathogens. This means complete or partial immunity to some pathogens, which makes asymptomatic or mildly symptomatic infection in adults common.

Travel from developed to developing countries with inadequate food and water hygiene and sanitation carries with it increased risks of diarrhoeal diseases and other gastrointestinal infections. Some pathogens (e.g. enterotoxigenic *Escherichia coli* and *Vibrio cholerae*) remain largely restricted to developing countries, but imported produce from such countries may occasionally be contaminated and thus pose a more global threat to consumers. Outbreaks of diarrhoeal diseases including *Shigella* infections and cholera have been particularly associated with famine, flooding and other disasters, displaced populations, refugee camps and war.

Many of the gastrointestinal infections that cause diarrhoea in humans are thought to have evolved from infections in animals. Moreover, many are acquired from animals and are therefore called zoonotic. The epidemiology of the various pathogens differs, based on the sources, transmission routes, abilities to grow outside the host, survival in the environment and behaviour of people.

GASTROINTESTINAL PATHOGENS

The range of pathogens related to food, water and environmental transmission through the oral route is diverse (Tables 31.1 and 31.2). This includes (with examples in brackets):

- organisms causing diarrhoeal diseases (*Shigella sonnei*);
- organisms infecting the gastrointestinal tract without causing diarrhoea (*Helicobacter pylori*);

- organisms infecting people through the consumption of food and causing diarrhoea (*Salmonella enterica*);
- organisms infecting people through the consumption of food and not causing diarrhoea (*Listeria monocytogenes* and *Toxoplasma gondii*);
- organisms infecting people through the consumption of water (*Cryptosporidium hominis*);
- organisms producing a toxin in food that causes diarrhoea when consumed (*Clostridium perfringens* and *Staphylococcus aureus*);
- organisms producing a toxin in food that does not cause diarrhoea (*Alexandrium* spp. – paralytic shellfish poisoning);
- organisms producing a toxin in food that does not cause immediate illness but may cause long-term disease (*Aspergillus flavus*);
- gastrointestinal parasites that do not complete their life-cycles within man but do cause disease (*Anisakis* spp.);
- gastrointestinal parasites that complete their life-cycles within man but are not transmitted through food or drinking water (*Schistosoma mansoni*);
- food-borne parasites that complete their life-cycles within man but do not cause gastrointestinal disease (*Trichinella spiralis*);
- waterborne parasites that complete their life-cycles within man but do not cause gastrointestinal disease (*Dracunculus medinensis*);
- syndromic diseases that have no confirmed association with a pathogen but may be infectious in origin (ulcerative colitis, Crohn's disease and Brainerd diarrhoea);
- gastrointestinal diseases caused by organisms that are not readily cultivable (*Tropheryma whipplei*, causing Whipple's disease);
- gastrointestinal illness resulting from the diet and normal bowel flora (diverticulosis);
- gastrointestinal illness resulting from disruption of the normal bowel flora (*Clostridium difficile*);
- gastrointestinal infections that can cause cancer and other chronic diseases (*Helicobacter pylori*);
- food poisoning caused by poisonous foods or the inadequate handling of foods with natural poisons (poisonous mushrooms, red kidney beans, red whelks, cassava, etc.);
- gastrointestinal infections primarily associated with immunocompromised patients (*Mycobacterium avium*).

***Salmonella* spp.** are one of the most common causes of bacterial infectious diarrhoea. *Salmonella enterica* is classified into more than 2500 serotypes, a few of which are restricted to man (*Salmonella* Typhi and Paratyphi). However, most serotypes are zoonotic and are common causes of food-borne infections. In industrialized countries, serotypes *enteritidis* and *typhimurium* are most common.

Infection usually follows 12–48 hours after eating contaminated foods, and infection can last for 10 days with carriage for up to a month (some carriage lasting for months). The higher incidence in the summer is thought to reflect an ability to grow in ready-to-eat foods at warmer temperatures, and also reflects a higher burden of (most often) asymptomatic *Salmonella* infections in food animals during summer time. Most of the cases present as acute gastroenteritis, but less commonly there can be septicaemia, meningitis or abscess formation in organs.

Infection derives from animal and vegetable sources and less commonly through person-to-person transmission. *Salmonella* Enteritidis in particular has been associated with zoonotic spread in layer chickens that has passed to other animals and led to a large epidemic in the late 1980s and 1990s, associated with a zoonotic infection in chickens and contamination of their eggs. The reduction in disease in the UK has followed the vaccination of chickens, whereas other countries have adopted control strategies based on *Salmonella*-free parent and 'grandparent' animals and a number of biosecurity measures applied at farms and slaughterhouses. *Salmonella* Typhimurium is found in a variety of agricultural animals, but infection is commonly linked to pork and broiler chickens. *Salmonella* can survive in dried products (coconut and peanuts), in some seeds (bean sprouts) and in fruit, vegetables and dairy products.

***Campylobacter* spp.** first came to be regarded as intestinal pathogens in the 1970s when methods for their isolation from faeces became available, and they are now the most common bacterial cause of diarrhoea in many industrialized countries. Illness (diarrhoea that can be bloody, abdominal pain, fever and lethargy) usually occurs 2–5 days after eating contaminated food, and infection can last for 10 days. Uncommon complications include bacteraemia, reactive arthritis and peripheral paralysis (Guillain–Barré syndrome).

Campylobacter infection has a marked seasonality, although the cause of this remains unclear. It has been suggested that increased environmental transmission of *Campylobacter* in warm periods (e.g. by insects) to houses can in part explain this seasonality. Compared with *Salmonella*, there are relatively few outbreaks; contaminated raw meats, particularly chicken, remain the most important sources. The pathogenic *Campylobacter* spp. (*C. jejuni*, *C. coli*, *C. lari* and *C. hyointestinalis*) and related *Arcobacter* spp. are widely distributed in the environment, as are a variety of species that do not cause diarrhoea in humans.

***Shigella* spp.** cause dysentery or diarrhoea and are frequently associated with poor standards of hygiene. There are four species (*S. dysenteriae*, *S. boydii*, *S. flexneri* and *S. sonnei*). *Shigella sonnei* outbreaks can be common in child-care institutions and schools, and this and the other species are common in war, refugee camps and developing countries where hygiene is poor. *Shigella* invades the intestinal mucosa and can cause ulceration. There is no natural animal reservoir and the source of human

Table 31.1 Agents (viral, eubacterial, cyanobacterial, diatom, dinoflagellate, protozoan and fungal) involved with gastrointestinal or food-borne diseases

Pathogen	Disease/syndrome/symptoms	Diarrhoea toxins preformed in food/water	Diarrhoea toxins generated in situ	Usually invades beyond mucosa	Usual incubation period	Death in cases (risk factor)	Disease duration	Transmission via faeces	Similar disease in animals	Sources
Adenovirus (st 40, 41)	Diarrhoea	No	No	No		Rare	8–12 days	Yes	Yes	H
Alexandrium spp.	PSP	Yes	No	No	10 Mins–3 hours	1–12%	3–4 days	No	Yes	S
Alternaria spp.	ATA	Yes	No	No	24 hours	3%	Prolonged	No	Yes	P
Arcobacter spp.	Diarrhoea	No	No	No		Rare		Yes		A
Aspergillus spp.	BEN	Yes	No	No		Yes (cancer)	Acute + chronic	No		P
Astrovirus	Diarrhoea	No	No	No				Yes		H
Campylobacter Fetus	Diarrhoea/septicaemia	No	No	Yes				Yes	Yes	A, H
Campylobacter upsaliensis	Diarrhoea	No	No	No				Yes	Yes	A, H
Bacillus anthracis	Anthrax	No	No	Yes	15–72 hours	25–60%		No	Yes	A
Bacillus cereus group*	Diarrhoea	Yes	No	No	2–3 hours		12–24 hours	No	Yes	E
Balantidium coli	Dysentery	No	No	No	2–14 days	up to 30%	Variable	Yes	Yes	A
Blastocystis hominis	Diarrhoea	No	No	No		No	Prolonged	Yes		E, H
Brucella spp.	Brucellosis	No	No	Yes				No	Yes	A
Campylobacter coli	Diarrhoea	No	No	No	1–3 days	Rare	10 days	Yes	No	A, H
Campylobacter jejuni	Diarrhoea	No	No	No	1–3 days	Rare	10 days	Yes	No	A, H
Cladosporium spp.	ATA	Yes	No	No	24 hours	3%	Prolonged	No	Yes	P
Claviceps purpurea	Ergotism	Yes	No	No		10–60%		No	Yes	P
Clostridium botulinum	Paralysis	Yes	No	No	18–36 hours	Common	Months	No	Yes	E, A, F
Clostridium difficile	Diarrhoea	No	No	No		Common		Yes	Yes	H, E
Clostridium perfringens toxin A	Diarrhoea	Yes	Yes	No	12–18 hours		12–48 hours	No	Yes	H, A
Clostridium perfringens toxin C	Pigbel	Yes	Yes	Yes	12–18 hours	Yes (Malnutrition)	Acute	No	Yes	A
Cryptosporidium hominis	Diarrhoea	No	No	No	5–7 days	(HIV)	2–10 days	Yes	Yes	H
Cryptosporidium meleagridis	Diarrhoea	No	No	No	5–7 days	(HIV)	2–10 days	Yes	Yes	H, B

(Continued)

Table 31.1 (Continued)

Pathogen	Disease/syndrome/symptoms	Diarrhoea toxins preformed in food/water	Diarrhoea toxins generated in situ	Usually invades beyond mucosa	Usual incubation period	Death in cases (risk factor)	Disease duration	Transmission via faeces	Similar disease in animals	Sources
Cryptosporidium parvum	Diarrhoea	No	No	No	5–7 days	(HIV)	2–10 days	Yes	Yes	H, A
Cylindrospermopsis raciborskii	CN	Yes	No	No	NK			No	Yes	W
Cyclospora cayetanensis	Diarrhoea	No	No	Yes	2–14 days	(HIV)	5–30 days	No	Yes	H
Dientamoeba fragilis	Diarrhoea	No	No	No	No	No	NK	Yes	No	H, A
Dinophysis spp.	DSP	Yes	No	No	0.5–a few hours	No	3 days	No		S
Encephalitozoon hellem	Microsporidiosis	No	No	Yes	Days to weeks	(HIV)		Yes		A
Encephalitozoon intestinalis	Microsporidiosis	No	No	No		(HIV)		Yes		A, H
Entamoeba histolytica	Dysentery	No	No	Yes	Days to weeks	Rare		Yes		H
Enterocytozoon bieneusi	Microsporidiosis	No	No	No				Yes		H, A
E. coli AEEC	Diarrhoea	No	No	No		Rare		Yes	No	A, H
E. coli AIEC	Link to Crohn's disease	No	No	No	NK	No	NK	Yes	No	NK
E. coli DAEC	Diarrhoea	No	No	No		Rare		Yes	No	A, H
E. coli EIEC	Diarrhoea	No	No	No	12–72 hours	Rare		Yes	No	H
E. coli EPEC	Diarrhoea	No	No	No		Rare (infant)		Yes	No	H
E. coli ETEC	Diarrhoea	No	Yes	No	<24 hours	Rare		Yes	Yes	H
E. coli VTEC	Diarrhoea	No	Yes	No	3–4 days	10%	14 days	Yes	No	A, H
Enterovirus echovirus	Encephalitis	No	No	Yes				Yes		H
Enterovirus poliovirus	Paralytic polio	No	No	Yes	1–2 weeks		Prolonged	Yes		H
Enterovirus coxsackievirus A	Hand, foot + mouth disease	No	No	No				Yes		H
Enterovirus coxsackievirus B	Encephalitis	No	No	Yes	2–35 days	Occasional	2 weeks	Yes		H
Gambierdiscus spp.	CFP	Yes	No	No	0.25–24 hours	<12%	2–14 days	No		F
Giardia lamblia	Diarrhoea	No	No	No	1–2 weeks	Rare	Days to months	Yes	No	H, A

Organism	Disease				Incubation		Duration			
Gonyaulax tamarensis	CFP	Yes	No	No	0.25–24 hours		2–3 days	No		F
Gymnodinium spp.	PSP	Yes	No	No	0.5–3 hours	1–12%	3–4 days	No		S
Helicobacter heilmannii	Gastritis	No	No	No	Years	(Cancer)	Years	No	Yes	H
Helicobacter pylori	Gastritis	No	No	No	NK	(Cancer)	Years	No		H
Hepatitis A virus	Hepatitis	No	No	Yes	15–45 days		3 weeks	Yes		H
Hepatitis E virus	Hepatitis	No	No	Yes	15–60 days	(Pregnancy)	1–4 weeks	Yes	Yes	H, A
Isospora spp.	Diarrhoea	No	No	Yes	NK			NK		H, A
Karenia spp.	NSP	Yes	No	No	1–3 hours	Rare	2–3 days	No		S
Listeria monocytogenes	Fever	No	No	Yes	1–90 days	Yes (elderly, pregnant)	Acute	No	Yes	E
Microcystis aeruginosa	CN	Yes	No	No	Variable	(Dialysis)	Variable	No	Yes	W
Mycobacterium avium	Mycobacterial	No	No	Yes	NK	(HIV)	Chronic	NK		E, W
Mycobacterium bovis	Mycobacterial	No	No	Yes	NK		Chronic	No		A
Norovirus	Vomiting	No	No	No	12–24 hours	Rare	1–2 days	Yes	No	H
Oscillatoria spp.	CN	Yes	No	No				No	Yes	W
Ostreopsis spp.	CFP, PTP	Yes	No	No	0.25–24 hours	<12%	2–14 days	No		F
Plesiomonas shigelloides	Diarrhoea	No	No	No	NK	Rare		Yes		E
Procentrum spp.	CFP, DSP	Yes	No	No	0.25–24 hours	<12%	3 days	No		F, S
Protoperidinium crassipes	AZP	Yes	No	No				No		S
Protoceratium reticulatum	NSP	Yes	No	No	1–3 hours	Rare	2–3 days	No		S
Pseudo-nitzschia spp.	ASP	Yes	No	No	<24 hours	Yes	Days to weeks	No		S
Pyrodinium spp.	PSP	Yes	No	No	3 hours	<12%	3–4 days	No		S
Rotavirus	Diarrhoea	No	No	No	48 hours	Yes (poor)	3–8 days	Yes	Yes	H
Salmonella enterica Paratyphi	Paratyphoid	No	No	Yes				Yes	Rare	H
Salmonella enterica serotypes†	Diarrhoea	No	No	Some	12–48 hours	1%	10 days	Yes	Yes	A, H
Salmonella enterica Typhi	Typhoid	No	No	Yes	10–14 days	Yes	3 weeks	Yes	No	H
Sapovirus	Diarrhoea	No	No	No	2–5 days	Rare		Yes		H

(Continued)

Table 31.1 (Continued)

| Pathogen | Disease/syndrome/symptoms | Diarrhoea toxins | | Usually invades beyond mucosa | Usual incubation period | Death in cases (risk factor) | Disease duration | Transmission via faeces | Similar disease in animals | Sources |
		preformed in food/water	generated in situ							
Sarcocystis spp.	Sarcocystosis	No	No	Yes	NK	NK	Protracted	No	Yes	A
Shigella spp.†	Dysentery	No	No	No	12–96 hours	Rare (poor)		Yes	No	H
Staphylococcus aureus	Vomiting	Yes	No	No	2–6 hours	Rare	8–12 hours	No	No	H
Toxoplasma gondii	Toxoplasmosis	No	No	Yes		Yes		No	Yes	A, B
Tropheryma whipplei	Whipple's disease	No	No	Yes	Months to years	Yes	Years	NK	No	E
Vibrio cholerae	Cholera	No	Yes	No	12–72 hours	Yes	Acute	Yes	No	E, H, S
Vibrio parahaemolyticus	Diarrhoea	No	Yes	No	12–24 hours	Rare		No		S
Vibrio vulnificus	Necrosis	No	Yes	Yes	12–72 hours	30% (liver)		No		S
Yersinia enterocolitica	Diarrhoea	No	No	Yes	1–10 days	Rare		Yes	Yes	A
Yersinia pseudotuberculosis	Lymphadenitis	No	No	Yes		Rare (liver)	1–3 weeks	Yes	Yes	A

A, animal; AEEC, attaching and effacing *Escherichia coli*; AIEC, adherent–invasive *Escherichia coli*; ATA, alimentary toxic aleukia; ASP, amnesic shellfish poisoning; AZP, azaspiracid poisoning (nausea, vomiting, severe diarrhoea and stomach cramps); B, birds; CFP, ciguatera fish poisoning (mixed symptoms including gastrointestinal, neurological, cardiovascular and general symptoms); CN, cyanobacterial poisoning; DAEC, diffusely adherent *Escherichia coli*; DSP, diarrhoeic shellfish poisoning; E, environment; EIEC, enteroinvasive *Escherichia coli*; EPEC, enteropathogenic *Escherichia coli*; ETEC, enterotoxigenic *Escherichia coli*; F, fish; H, human; NK, not known; NSP, neurotoxic shellfish poisoning; P, plants; PSP, paralytic shellfish poisoning (symptoms include a tickling sensation of the lips, mouth and tongue, numbness of the extremities, gastrointestinal problems, difficulty breathing and a sense of dissociation followed by complete paralysis); PTP, palytoxin poisoning; S, shellfish; VTEC, verocytotoxigenic *Escherichia coli*; W, water.

*The *Bacillus cereus* group includes *B. cereus*, *B. subtilis*, *B. licheniformis*, *B. amyloliquefaciens* and *B. pumilis*, all of which can cause gastroenteritis.

†There are two species (*S. enterica* and *S. bongori*) and over 2500 *Salmonella* serotypes. There are six subspecies of *S. enterica*, with almost all human cases belonging to *S. enterica* subsp. *enterica* (*S. enterica* subsp. *enterica* serotype Enteritidis phage type 4 usually being abbreviated to S. Enteritidis PT4).

‡There are four *Shigella* spp.: *S. sonnei* (1 serotype), *S. flexneri* (6 serotypes), *S. boydii* (18 serotypes) and *S. dysenteriae* (12 serotypes).

Table 31.2 Human helminth infections (intestinal and other)

Parasitic helminths	Occurrence	Distribution	Clinical presentation	Infection sources
Ancylostoma braziliense	Rare	South America	Hookworm	Soil
Ancylostoma caninum	Rare	Australia	Hookworm	Soil
Ancylostoma ceylanicum	Rare	Asia, Far East	Hookworm	Soil
Ancylostoma duodenale	Common	Africa	Hookworm	Soil
Angiostrongylus cartonensis	Rare	SE Asia, Pacific	Eosinophilic meningitis	Crabs or snails
Angiostrongylus costaricensis	Uncommon	South America	Intestinal granulanas	Slug, rat
Anisakis spp.	Uncommon	Worldwide	Stomach pain	Sea fish
Ascaris lumbricoides	Common	Worldwide	Intestinal obstruction	Human faeces
Baylisascaris procyonis	Uncommon	North America	Visceral larva migrans	Raccoon faeces
Bertiella spp.	Rare	Africa, Asia, Middle East	Tapeworm	Monkeys
Bunostomum	Rare	Worldwide	Hookworm	Sheep and goats
Capillaria philippinensis	Rare	Far East	Chronic diarrhoea	Fish and shellfish
Diphyllobothrium latum	Uncommon	Worldwide	Diarrhoea, epigastric pain, nausea, vomiting	Sea fish
Dracunculus medinensis	Uncommon	Africa	Guinea worm	Cyclops in water
Echinococcus granulosus	Uncommon	Worldwide	Hydatid cyst	Dogs and water
Echinococcus multilocularis	Uncommon	Europe, North America	Hydatid cyst	Dogs and water
Echinococcus oligarthrus	Rare	South America	Hydatid cyst	Wild cats
Echinococcus vogeli	Uncommon	South America	Hydatid cyst	Bush dogs
Echinostoma spp.	Rare	Asia and Far East	Intestinal flukes	Snails
Enterobius vermicularis	Common	Worldwide	Itchy anus. Pinworm	Children
Fasciola gigantica	Rare	Asia, Africa, Hawaii	Liver fluke	Aquatic plants
Fasciola hepatica	Uncommon	Middle East, Africa, Asia	Liver fluke	Aquatic plants
Fasciolopsis buski	Uncommon	Far East, India	Liver fluke	Aquatic plants
Gnathostoma spp.	Uncommon	South-East Asia	Migrating erythema and pruritus	Fish and frogs
Gongylonema pulchrum	Rare	Europe, US, Asia, N Africa	Oral discomfort	Cattle and insects
Haplorchis spp.	Rare	North Thailand	Intestinal fluke	Dogs, cats, pigs
Heterophyes heterophyes	Rare	Japan, N Africa	Diarrhoea and abdominal pain. Fluke	Freshwater fish
Hymenolepis nana	Uncommon	Worldwide	Dwarf tapeworm	Insects
Inermicapsifer madagascariensis	Rare	Africa	Mild abdominal symptoms	Rodents
Lagochilascaris minor	Rare	South America	Chronic abscesses	Rodents
Mammomonogamus laryngeus	Rare	Brazil and West Indies	Respiratory syngamosis	
Moniliformis moniliformis	Rare	Worldwide	Acanthocephalan	Rodents
Nanophyetus salmincola	Rare	North-West USA	Gastrointestinal discomfort	Salmon, trout
Necator americanus	Common	North America	Hookworm	Soil
Oesophagostomum bifurcum	Common	West Africa	Abdominal pain, obstruction, mass	Monkeys
Opisthorchis spp.	Uncommon	Asia	Liver fluke	Fish
Paragonimus spp.	Uncommon	Asia, Africa, America	Lung fluke	Fish, wild boar
Pelodera strongyloides	Rare	US, Central Europe	Cutaneous larva migrans	Soil
Pseudoterranova spp.	Uncommon	Worldwide	Stomach pain	Raw marine fish
Schistosoma haematobium	Common	Africa, Middle East, India	Schistosomiasis	Water contact, snails
Schistosoma intercalatum	Uncommon	Africa	Schistosomiasis	Water contact, snails
Schistosoma japonicum	Common	China, Japan	Katayama fever, liver disease	Water contact, snails
Schistosoma malayensis	Rare	South East Asia	Schistosomiasis	Water contact, snails
Schistosoma mansoni	Common	S America, Africa, Caribbean	Intestinal schistosomiasis	Water contact, snails
Schistosoma mekongi	Uncommon	South East Asia	Schistosomiasis	Water contact, snails
Schistosoma spindale	Uncommon	India, SE Asia	Cercarial dermatitis	Water contact, snails
Spirometra spp.	Rare	SE Asia, E Africa	Sparganosis	Cyclops in water, frogs
Strongyloides fülleborni	Uncommon	Africa and Asia	Intestinal and larva migrans	Soil
Strongyloides fuelliborni	Rare	Central Africa	Intestinal, larva migrans	Soil

(Continued)

Table 31.2   (*Continued*)

Parasitic helminths	Occurrence	Distribution	Clinical presentation	Infection sources
Strongyloides kellyi	Rare	Papua New Guinea	Intestinal, larva migrans	Soil
Strongyloides stercoralis	Uncommon	Africa, Asia, S America	Intestinal and larva migrans	Soil
Taenia brauni	Rare	Africa	Cysts in muscle, eye, CNS	Dog
Taenia multiceps	Rare	Worldwide	Cysts in muscle, eye, CNS	Dog
Taenia saginata	Uncommon	Worldwide	Tapeworm	Cattle
Taenia solium	Uncommon	Worldwide	Tapeworm, cysticercosis	Pigs
Ternidens deminutus	Uncommon	East Africa	Hookworm	Soil
Toxocara canis	Common	Worldwide	Visceral larva migrans, eye/brain	Dogs
Toxocara cati	Common	Worldwide	Visceral larva migrans, eye/brain	Cats
Trichinella pseudospiralis	Uncommon		Trichinosis	Pig and game
Trichinella spiralis	Uncommon	Worldwide	Trichinosis	Pig and horse
Trichobilharzia regenti	Uncommon	Europe, USA	Cercarial dermatitis	Water contact
Trichostrongylus spp.	Rare	Worldwide	Abdominal pain, nausea	Herbivores
Trichuris trichiura	Common	Worldwide	Diarrhoea, anaenia	Human faeces
Uncinaria spp.	Rare	Spain, South America	Larva migrans	Wildlife

CNS, central nervous system.

infections is other people, commonly children, or contaminated food products or water. *Shigella dysenteriae* produces Shiga toxin, which can cause haemolytic–uraemic syndrome (HUS) and systemic effects.[1]

Escherichia coli are bacteria that contain both non-pathogenic and pathogenic strains that are an important cause of diarrhoeal disease and have been termed enterovirulent or diarrhoeagenic *E. coli*. Several classes have been defined based on the possession of distinct virulence factors. From the perspective of industrialized countries, the most important is verocytotoxin-producing *E. coli*, and diarrhoea can progress to HUS and thrombotic thrombocytopenic purpura, with a high mortality rate. The majority of infections are caused by serogroup O157, but other serogroups, including O26, O103, O111 and O145, have been involved. Infection can derive from contaminated food (in particular beef or beef products), drinking or recreational water or through person-to-person transmission. Agricultural animals (ruminants) can be infected, and cross-contamination between raw meat and ready-to-eat foods can be a cause.

Other enterovirulent *E. coli* are the enteropathogenic *E. coli*, which belong to a small number of defined serotypes and cause sporadic cases and outbreaks of diarrhoea in children, usually under the age of 2 years, as well as occasional sporadic cases and outbreaks affecting adults. Enterotoxigenic *E. coli* are a major cause of diarrhoea among children in developing countries and in addition cause travellers' diarrhoea. Enteroinvasive *E. coli* resemble *Shigella* infections in their presentation, invading the epithelia and causing bloody diarrhoea. They are usually travel related. Enteroaggregative *E. coli* cause sporadic cases and outbreaks affecting all ages; many clinical and epidemiological aspects are less understood than for the other types of enterovirulent *E. coli* mentioned

above. The diffusely adherent *E. coli* do not appear to be an important cause of diarrhoea.

Yersinia enterocolitica causes diarrhoea, abdominal pain and fever, and the mesenteric lymphadenitis it produces can sometimes resemble appendicitis. Infection can persist for up to 2 weeks and it occasionally causes systemic infections (meningitis, bacteraemia and endocarditis) in patients suffering from pre-existing diseases (immunosuppression, iron-overload, cirrhosis, severe anaemia, diabetes mellitus or malnutrition). Sequelae include Reiter's syndrome, particularly reactive arthritis and erythema nodosum. There are strains of *Y. enterocolitica* that are not implicated in human diarrhoeal disease, and in Europe the pathogenic serotypes are O:3, O:9, and O:5,27, with O:8 in North America. Human infection is most commonly associated with pigs but other animals (rodents, cattle, horses, rabbits, sheep and dogs) can act as natural reservoirs.

Yersinia pseudotuberculosis can cause symptoms that are similar to those of *Y. enterocolitica* infections, with diarrhoea, abdominal pain and fever, mesenteric lymphadenitis and reactive arthritis. Infection can be acquired from wild or domesticated animals and also from raw vegetables and untreated water. Both species can grow at refrigeration temperatures.

Cholera is caused by *V. cholerae* and is covered in Chapter 33.

Vibrio parahaemolyticus infections produce a watery diarrhoea and usually derive from contaminated shellfish. *Vibrio vulnificus* infection can be from eating shellfish grown in subtropical areas or from wound infections derived from seawater. Infection usually occurs in older men with impaired liver function, causes diarrhoea and necrotic wound infections and, although uncommon, has a high mortality.[2] The factor that reduces risk in women is thought to be oestrogen.

Listeria monocytogenes causes septicaemia and meningitis, particularly in people who are more susceptible to infection (pregnant women, unborn or newly delivered infants, those who are immunosuppressed and the elderly). The organism can grow in foods with an extended shelf-life at refrigeration temperature, relatively high water activity and near-neutral pH. The foods associated with transmission are usually ready-to-eat products that are able to support the multiplication of *Listeria monocytogenes*. Infection in pregnancy is rare before 20 weeks' gestation, and symptoms – if they occur – include chills, fever, back pain, sore throat and headache. The outcome for the mother is benign, but abortion, stillbirth and early-onset neonatal disease are common; death in utero is more common early in gestation. Most other cases are in elderly and/or immunosuppressed patients receiving steroid or cytotoxic therapy, or people being treated for malignancies.

Listeria monocytogenes is common in the environment, and most disease is transmitted by the consumption of contaminated foods. There is microbiological and epidemiological evidence for associations with fish, shellfish, cooked meats, vegetables and dairy products, both in sporadic disease and in outbreaks. Preventing contamination and complying with shelf-life recommendations through the food production chain are important in reducing disease.

TOXINS PRODUCED IN FOODS

Clostridium perfringens type A food poisoning causes diarrhoea, abdominal pain and nausea (but rarely vomiting) that usually begins 12–18 hours after eating contaminated foods. It usually results from growth of the organism in cooked foods that have been contaminated after cooking and left at ambient temperature. A more severe and life-threatening form of food poisoning caused by *Clostridium perfringens* type C called enteritis necroticans (pigbel) is an occasional problem in New Guinea and in parts of Africa, Asia and the South Pacific, where it affects children with severe protein malnutrition.[3,4] The disease is characterized by haemorrhagic, inflammatory or ischaemic necrosis of the jejunum. Vaccination can prove effective in reducing the condition.[5] In the elderly, there can also be outbreaks of *Clostridium perfringens* infection that result from the growth of toxin-producing strains in the intestine rather than the consumption of contaminated food.[6,7] Infection can also follow antibiotic treatment.[8]

Clostridium botulinum strains produce seven different heat-labile neurotoxins (A to G) that cause paralysis. Types A, B, E and occasionally F cause human disease.[9,10] Botulism is usually caused by the inadequate cooking of home-preserved meat, fish, vegetables and mushrooms, where the spores can germinate and grow through extended storage. The growth conditions for these pathogens are well understood, and regulation of the preservation conditions has proved effective in preventing outbreaks. Acute bilateral cranial neuropathy with symmetrical descending muscle weakness and paralysis occurs 18–36 hours after food consumption. Death results from paralysis of the respiratory muscles and diaphragm. Infant botulism (intestinal botulism) results from growth of *Clostridium botulinum* within the developing bowel flora of babies (less than 6 months old).[11,12] The organism can derive from contaminated honey or corn syrup.

Bacillus cereus has two distinct clinical presentations with emetic and diarrhoeal syndromes that are associated with different toxins. The foods normally implicated include rice, meat or vegetable dishes and sauces. The emetic syndrome, caused by the heat-stable toxin cereulide, begins 1–6 hours after food is consumed and includes nausea, vomiting, stomach cramps and diarrhoea that rarely last more than 12 hours. The diarrhoeal syndrome, however, begins 8–16 hours after eating and can last for a day. Disease is prevented through the refrigerated storage of cooked foods.

Staphylococcus aureus produces 19 heat-stable enterotoxins (A to E, G to R, U and V) that cause nausea, vomiting, abdominal pain and diarrhoea 2–6 hours after eating contaminated food. Recovery is usually within 24 hours. Outbreaks have been associated with cooked pies, preserved meats, poultry, fish, shellfish, dairy products and desserts.

OTHER BACTERIAL INFECTIONS

Clostridium difficile is the main cause of pseudomembranous colitis and antibiotic-associated diarrhoea. *Clostridium difficile* can be a normal part of the gut flora, and disease is caused by cytotoxin-producing strains that are resistant to a variety of antimicrobial drugs. Symptomatic infection therefore usually follows antibiotic treatment. *Clostridium difficile* is an important cause of nosocomial infection, and preventing outbreaks of diarrhoea in hospitals requires control of the environmental contamination and an antibiotic policy.

Clostridium difficile is covered in detail in Chapters 43, p. 463.

Helicobacter pylori infects the stomach lining and is associated with gastritis, gastric and duodenal ulcers and gastric cancer.[13,14] The reservoir of *Helicobacter pylori* is the digestive tracts of humans and some primates. Transmission is thought to be predominantly from person to person (probably oral–oral), although there is some evidence for faeco-oral transmission through drinking water in developing countries. *Helicobacter pylori* is shed in the faeces after turnover of the gastric mucosa and has been detected by PCR in sewage in Peru. Drinking water pollution is therefore a possible route of transmission.[15] *Helicobacter heilmannii* (syn. *Gastrospirillum hominis*) is larger and more tightly helical than *Helicobacter pylori* and is associated with a small percentage of patients with gastritis. *Helicobacter bilis* is regarded as an enteric *Helicobacter* and has been implicated in liver disease, particularly biliary tract cancer.[16]

Mycobacterium avium complex organisms include *Mycobacterium avium*, *Mycobacterium intracellulare* and *Mycobacterium scrofulaceum*, the three species being difficult to differentiate within the laboratory. They can cause intestinal infection, septicaemia and wasting in patients with untreated acquired immune deficiency syndrome (AIDS), up to 50 per cent of whom may develop *Mycobacterium avium* complex bacteraemia. Where the isolates have been speciated, they have been found to be predominantly *Mycobacterium avium*. Isolates recovered from water are a source of human infection.

Tropheryma whipplei is a non-culturable Gram-positive bacterium that causes rare systemic infections, infects the gastrointestinal tract and causes a polyarthritis.[17,18] The disease is usually diagnosed by the demonstration of periodic acid–Schiff (PAS) positive macrophages in histology, and a PCR technique is available for confirmation of the diagnosis. Carriage can be relatively common.[19]

Brachyspira spp. are anaerobic spirochaetes that infect the colon of man, pigs and birds and have been thought to cause chronic diarrhoea in man.[20,21] Human infection is more common in developing countries and among men who have sex with men. *Brachyspira aalborgi* has been associated with human intestinal spirochaetosis, and *Brachyspira pilosicoli* (syn. *Serpulina pilosicoli*) has been associated with human intestinal spirochaetosis and disease in pigs.

Arcobacter butzleri is a *Campylobacter*-like bacterium that is associated with watery diarrhoea. *Arcobacter skirrowii* can cause persistent diarrhoea. *Arcobacter cryaerophilus* is a third species found in human infections. *Arcobacter* spp. can be isolated from animals, birds, food, water and the environment.

FRESHWATER AND MARINE BLOOMS

The impact of toxic algae, diatoms and dinoflagellates is covered in Chapter 34.

PARASITIC INFECTIONS TRANSMITTED BY FOOD AND WATER

A number of protozoan parasites are associated with diarrhoea in humans; these include *Cryptosporidium* spp., *Isospora belli*, *Sarcocystis* spp., *Giardia intestinalis*, *Entamoeba histolytica*, *Cyclospora cayetanensis*, *Blastocystis hominis* and the microsporidia *Enterocytozoon bieneusi* and *Septata intestinalis* (microsporidia being classified as of fungal origin but possessing properties that resemble those of protozoa).[22] In addition, *Toxoplasma gondii* infects through the gastrointestinal tract but does not usually cause diarrhoea.

Cryptosporidium spp. can cause diarrhoea in humans. *Cryptosporidium hominis*, *Cryptosporidium parvum* and *Cryptosporidium meleagridis* are the most commonly encountered.[23,24] Infection begins 5–7 days after exposure, and the disease usually resolves within 1–2 weeks. In patients with untreated human immunodeficiency virus (HIV) infection and in cancer patients on chemotherapy, a chronic watery diarrhoea can occur that is life-threatening.[25] In addition, children in developing countries may suffer from severe disease due to this parasite, for which there is not yet an established treatment.[26] The resistance of *Cryptosporidium* oocysts to chlorine and many other disinfectants is the reason that outbreaks of cryptosporidiosis associated with mains drinking water have occurred throughout the world.[27] *Cryptosporidium parvum* is common in young calves and lambs, and their faeces can, along with human faeces and sewage, be important sources of infection. *Cryptosporidium hominis* is predominantly acquired from other humans as agricultural animals are rarely affected. Infections can derive from swimming pools, educational farms and child care.

Cyclospora cayetanensis is a tropical infection that causes diarrhoea, infection being restricted to man and other primates. The oocysts excreted in the faeces need to mature in the environment for 10 days before they become infectious. Outbreaks have been associated with the importing of fresh fruit and vegetables from developing countries.[28,29] Soil may be important in transmission.[30]

Isospora belli can cause diarrhoeal illness in humans but is not common in the UK and is regarded as a tropical infection.[31] Infection is through the ingestion of the oocysts in contaminated food or water. The main symptoms are watery diarrhoea, abdominal pain, malabsorption and fever. In immunocompetent individuals, symptoms are usually mild and self-limiting, although in some patients symptoms may be recurrent or even chronic.[32,33] Infection can be more severe in people with a compromised immune system (Hodgkin's disease, non-Hodgkin's lymphoma and acute lymphoblastic leukaemia) and occurs in patients with HIV/AIDS, particularly in Africa, South America and South-East Asia. In these cases, infection may be more severe, may be more likely to be recurrent or chronic and may involve extraintestinal sites such as the liver, spleen and gall bladder. Infection is probably transmitted through the contamination of food or water by the faeces of an infected patient. The infection can be controlled with trimethoprim–sulphamethoxazole, although symptoms may recur when treatment is stopped, particularly in AIDS patients.

Sarcocystis spp. can cause both diarrhoea and intramuscular cysts, depending upon whether meat or sporocysts are eaten.[22,34] The parasite requires two hosts to complete its life-cycle. Human diarrhoeal infection through the consumption of uncooked infected meat is uncommon in developed countries, but both *Sarcocystis hominis* and *Sarcocystis suihominis* can cause human illness. An acute non-diarrhoeal illness contracted through the accidental consumption of oocysts is characterized by fever, myalgias, bronchospasm, transient pruritic rashes, lymphadenopathy, subcutaneous nodules, eosinophilia and a raised erythrocyte sedimentation rate and muscle creatine kinase level.

Toxoplasma gondii occurs in a wide range of warm-blooded animals. The only definitive host in which the full sexual cycle has been observed is members of the cat family (Felidae). Disseminated infection is a particular problem in pregnancy and in immunocompromised patients. Oocysts from cat faeces can be directly infectious to humans and can contaminate drinking water, causing waterborne outbreaks; alternatively, people can be infected from the tissue cysts by the consumption of undercooked or raw meat.

Giardia are flagellated protozoan parasites that attach to the small intestinal wall and cause malabsorption. Infections have been commonly acquired from recreational water activity and from drinking water that is not properly treated. *Giardia* are common in agricultural and domestic animals and these have been thought to be one of the sources of human infection. However, much human disease seems to be associated with types that do not occur in these animals so human sources may be more important.

Entamoeba histolytica causes amoebic dysentery. The scientific literature requires interpretation because the originally described 'species' contains two species, one of which is a significant pathogen (*Entamoeba histolytica*) and the other a non-pathogen (*Entamoeba dispar*); they are morphologically similar on routine microscopy.[35,36] Amoebic dysentery is a tropical disease that causes bloody diarrhoea and abscess formation in the liver and other organs. Infection is predominantly from other infected people living in conditions of poor hygiene.

Blastocystis hominis is a very common parasite with a debated pathogenicity. It can be isolated from roughly 25 per cent of patients suspected of intestinal parasitosis. At least 10 subtypes have been isolated from humans and animals, and recent data demonstrate that the pathogenicity of the parasite is subtype dependent. Symptoms may include persistent or intermittent diarrhoea or more subtle gastrointestinal complaints.

Microsporidia are a particular problem in patients with untreated HIV who have low CD4 counts; two main intestinal species are involved (*Encephalitozoon intestinalis* and *Enterocytozoon bieneusi*). *Enterocytozoon bieneusi* infection is usually confined to the intestines and is not associated with disseminated infection. It has been detected in pigs, cats, dogs and a rhesus monkey. Although its transmission is not well understood, it is likely that *Enterocytozoon bieneusi* is transmitted via the usual faeco-oral pathways, including via food and water.

A large number of helminthic species are transmitted in the environment; some have a global distribution, whereas others are restricted to specific geographical regions (see Table 31.2 for an overview). The burden of illness of worm infections remains highest in developing countries and is associated with nutritional deficiencies, failure to thrive and delayed mental development.

ENTERIC VIRUSES

Gastrointestinal viruses are covered in Chapter 35.

POTENTIAL PATHOGENS

There are a range of enteric organisms that are recognized as non-pathogens, including the enteric protozoa *Entamoeba coli*, *Endolimax nana*, *Iodamoeba butschlii* and *Retortamonas*. In addition, a variety of potential or opportunistic pathogens have yet to have their status as diarrhoea-producing agents better understood. These include *Aeromonas* spp., *Edwardsiella tarda*, enterotoxigenic *Bacteroides fragilis*,[37,38] *Plesiomonas shigelloides*, *Laribacter hongkongensis*,[39–41] *Dientamoeba fragilis* and *Brachyspira* spp. The production of virulent and non-pathogenic strains of a range of pathogens has made this more difficult. This has been true for *Yersinia* spp., *Campylobacter* spp., *E. coli* subtypes, *Clostridium difficile* and a few *Salmonella* serotypes.

The process of demonstrating a clear association between a potential enteric pathogen and a gastrointestinal disease has been on the basis of Koch's postulates and the Bradford Hill guidelines. However, some pathogens (e.g. *Aeromonas hydrophila*) can have a large body of evidence associated with their relation to diarrhoeal disease while still providing relatively poor evidence that the disease is caused by the pathogen.

LONG-TERM SEQUELAE

Bacterial intestinal infections can lead to autoimmune reactions, including the condition called Reiter's syndrome, characterized by arthritis, urethritis and conjunctivitis. Arthritis is particularly common in *Yersinia enterocolitica* infections. A high percentage of patients with Reiter's syndrome are HLA-B27 positive. In addition, HLA-B27 disease (ankylosing spondylitis) is thought to result from autoantibodies to *Klebsiella* in the bowel flora that cross-react with spinal collagen types I, III and IV.

Autoimmunity can follow *Helicobacter pylori* gastritis, producing autoantibodies to parietal cells and intrinsic factor; this leads to atrophic body gastritis and pernicious anemia. Cobalamin (vitamin B$_{12}$) deficiency can also result from infection with the tapeworm *Diphyllobothrium latum*, which competes for cobalamin. Cobalamin deficiency can also result from small intestinal bacterial overgrowth syndrome, in which a mixture of faecal flora organisms overgrow the small bowel and prevent the absorption of cobalamin.

Guillain–Barré[42,43] and Miller Fisher[44,45] syndromes are acute inflammatory demyelinating polyneuropathies causing paralysis through demyelination of the nerve axons. It is postulated that the disease results from molecular mimicry between epitopes on bacteria, particularly *Campylobacter*, and nerve cell gangliosides.

Chronic diarrhoeal side-effects of acute diarrhoea linked to travel overseas have been termed tropical sprue.[46,47] The disease can be similar in presentation to *Giardia* infection or coeliac disease and is characterized by diarrhoea, weight loss, anorexia, macrocytic anaemia and partial villous atrophy. A cause is not usually identified, but treatment with folic acid and tetracycline can be effective. Chronic diarrhoea occurring as an outbreak has been termed Brainerd diarrhoea. Although no aetiological agent has been associated with it, outbreak epidemiology has implicated food and water sources.[48–50]

It is postulated that infections at an early age may predispose to coeliac disease, also as a result of the development of autoantibodies. Toxic megacolon can be a problem following *Trypanosoma cruzi* in Chagas disease. There can be enteric infection or symptoms in a variety of diseases that are usually non-diarrhoeal, including tuberculosis, anthrax, syphilis and Legionnaires' disease.

DIAGNOSIS, SURVEILLANCE, EPIDEMIOLOGY, OUTBREAKS, RESPONSE AND PREVENTION

The full understanding of gastrointestinal infectious diseases, as with other infectious diseases, comes from good diagnosis and systematic local and national reporting that allows the early detection and investigation of outbreaks and the analysis of time trends. All types of infection are subject to incomplete ascertainment, with well-investigated infections (e.g. *Salmonella*) and very severe diseases (e.g. botulism) generally having better ascertainment. Specific studies of pathogen-specific underascertainment can be useful in the investigation of the burden of infectious intestinal diseases. Age, sex, social, economic, climatic and seasonal factors can differ between pathogens and can help contribute to an understanding of sources and transmission routes.

BARRIERS TO INFECTION AND IMMUNE RESPONSE

All humans are exposed to gastrointestinal infections from time to time, and the likelihood that this exposure will result in infection (which can be symptomatic or subclinical) depends on a number of factors. Important factors are:

- the pathogen itself;
- the host;
- the conditions under which exposure takes place;
- the number of infectious agents (i.e. the dose at exposure).

The 'cocktail' of virulence factors and the expression and regulation of these varies between different pathogens, and are even described together. For example, verocytotoxigenic *E. coli* contains a number of virulence factors, the types and composition of which are important in predicting whether a specific strain is able to give rise to HUS. The serotype (e.g. O157:H7) is merely a marker for these virulence factors, useful for surveillance, but may not by itself be important.

In addition to virulence factors, other factors are important, for example the ability to survive environmental stress such as low water activity and sensitivity to variations in pH and temperature. Some *Salmonella* serotypes have been able to adapt to extreme environments and may thus be associated with outbreaks caused by unusual vehicles. *Salmonella* Agona, for example, has caused outbreaks with desiccated products such as cereals and milk powder as vehicles.

Host factors are important in several ways. The acidity of the stomach is a natural barrier for most gastrointestinal infections, and ingested pathogens must pass the acid barrier of the stomach. An important factor that increases the risk of infection is reduced gastric acidity due to, for example, achlorhydria, antacid use or gastric surgery. Neonates and infants may be at high risk of infection because of their relative achlorhydria and the buffering capacity of breast milk or formula feed. Therapy with antimicrobial drugs has been shown to be a risk factor for *Salmonella* infections. The recent administration of antimicrobials may provide a relative advantage for the Gram-negative flora, a so-called competitive effect. In addition, if the *Salmonella* is resistant to the drug, it has a selective advantage compared with other bacteria in the gut. In addition to extremes of age, chronic illness, including immunosuppressive disease, malignant disease and diabetes, may also decrease the number of bacteria needed to cause infection.

Natural and specific immunity will develop to most pathogens after a number of exposures. This immunity may not be sterile, as seen following many systemic infections, but rather a time-limited reduction in the disease-to-infection ratio; that is, after repeated exposures, the risk of becoming ill decreases.

The conditions under which exposure takes places are also of importance. If *Salmonella* or *E. coli* organisms are suspended in a lipophilic vehicle, the kill from the acid barrier is reduced, and consequently more bacteria may pass on into the intestine. Hence, the infectious dose is reduced when the bacteria are protected in vehicles such as ice-cream, several other types of dessert, some sauces and chocolate.

Furthermore, the average dose of infection varies greatly between pathogens. Whereas the old medical literature often suggests a minimum dose of infection, risk-modellers now often apply a single-hit model, in which one exposure can in principle cause infection. This property depends on the pathogen as well as the factors mentioned above.

It is important to realize that control and prevention are most easily achieved for pathogens that cause infection at high doses (e.g. enterotoxigenic *E. coli* and *V. cholerae*) than those with a medium or low dose (e.g. *Shigella*), particularly if there is also a widespread environmental or animal reservoir (e.g. *Campylobacter* and verocytotoxinogenic *E. coli*). This notion is important for understanding why some infections have been eliminated by the sanitary revolution of the industrialized countries, whereas at the same time and in the same countries, there are great challenges for the food safety systems or in the control of nosocomial infections.

REFERENCES

♦ = Major review article

1. Mark TC. Enterohaemorrhagic *Escherichia coli* and *Shigella dysenteriae* type 1-induced haemolytic uraemic syndrome. *Pediatr Nephrol* 2008; **23**: 1425–31.
2. Oliver JD. Wound infections caused by *Vibrio vulnificus* and other marine bacteria. *Epidemiol Infect* 2005; **133**: 383–91.
3. Murrell TG, Walker PD. The pigbel story of Papua New Guinea. *Trans R Soc Trop Med Hyg* 1991; **85**: 119–22.
4. Murrell TG. Pigbel in Papua New Guinea: An ancient disease rediscovered. *Int J Epidemiol* 1983; **12**: 211–14.
5. Lawrence GW, Lehmann D, Anian G et al. Impact of active immunisation against enteritis necroticans in Papua New Guinea. *Lancet* 1990; **336**: 1165–7.
6. Wada A, Masuda Y, Fukayama M et al. Nosocomial diarrhoea in the elderly due to enterotoxigenic *Clostridium perfringens. Microbiol Immunol* 1996; **40**: 767–71.
7. Brett MM, Rodhouse JC, Donovan TJ, Tebbutt GM, Hutchinson DN. Detection of *Clostridium perfringens* and its enterotoxin in cases of sporadic diarrhoea. *J Clin Pathol* 1992; **45**: 609–11.
8. Modi N, Wilcox MH. Evidence for antibiotic induced *Clostridium perfringens* diarrhoea. *J Clin Pathol* 2001; **54**: 748–51.
9. Brook I. Botulism: The challenge of diagnosis and treatment. *Rev Neurol Dis* 2006; **3**: 182–9.
10. McLauchlin J, Grant KA, Little CL. Food-borne botulism in the United Kingdom. *J Public Health (Oxf)* 2006; **28**: 337–42.
♦11. Domingo RM, Haller JS, Gruenthal M. Infant botulism: Two recent cases and literature review. *J Child Neurol* 2008; **23**: 1336–46.
12. Brook I. Infant botulism. *J Perinatol* 2007; **27**: 175–80.
13. Brenner H, Rothenbacher D, Arndt V. Epidemiology of stomach cancer. *Methods Mol Biol* 2009; **472**: 467–77.
14. Hatakeyama M. *Helicobacter pylori* and gastric carcinogenesis. *J Gastroenterol* 2009; **44**: 239–48.
15. Dube C, Tanih NF, Ndip RN. *Helicobacter pylori* in water sources: A global environmental health concern. *Rev Environ Health* 2009; **24**: 1–14.

16. Murata H, Tsuji S, Tsujii M et al. *Helicobacter bilis* infection in biliary tract cancer. *Aliment Pharmacol Ther* 2004; **20**(Suppl. 1): 90–4.
17. Freeman HJ. *Tropheryma whipplei* infection. *World J Gastroenterol* 2009; **15**: 2078–80.
18. Jackuliak P, Koller T, Baqi L et al. Whipple's disease-generalized stage. *Dig Dis Sci* 2008; **53**: 3250–8.
19. Fenollar F, Trani M, Davoust B et al. Prevalence of asymptomatic *Tropheryma whipplei* carriage among humans and nonhuman primates. *J Infect Dis* 2008; **197**: 880–7.
20. Margawani KR, Robertson ID, Hampson DJ. Isolation of the anaerobic intestinal spirochaete *Brachyspira pilosicoli* from long-term residents and Indonesian visitors to Perth, Western Australia. *J Med Microbiol* 2009; **58**(Pt 2): 248–52.
21. Calderaro A, Bommezzadri S, Gorrini C et al. Infective colitis associated with human intestinal spirochetosis. *J Gastroenterol Hepatol* 2007; **22**: 1772–9.
♦22. Nichols GL. Food-borne protozoa. *Br Med Bull* 2000; **56**: 209–35.
23. Pedraza-Diaz S, Amar CF, McLauchlin J et al. *Cryptosporidium meleagridis* from humans: Molecular analysis and description of affected patients. *J Infect* 2001; **42**: 243–50.
24. McLauchlin J, Amar C, Pedraza-Diaz S, Nichols GL. Molecular epidemiological analysis of *Cryptosporidium* spp. in the United Kingdom: Results of genotyping *Cryptosporidium* spp. in 1,705 fecal samples from humans and 105 fecal samples from livestock animals. *J Clin Microbiol* 2000; **38**: 3984–90.
♦25. Hunter PR, Nichols G. Epidemiology and clinical features of *Cryptosporidium* infection in immunocompromised patients. *Clin Microbiol Rev* 2002; **15**: 145–54.
26. Mølbak K, Andersen M, Aaby P et al. *Cryptosporidium* infection in infancy as a cause of malnutrition: A community study from Guinea-Bissau, west Africa. *Am J Clin Nutr* 1997; **65**: 149–52.
27. Semenza JC, Nichols G. Cryptosporidiosis surveillance and water-borne outbreaks in Europe. *Euro Surveill* 2007; **12**: E13–14.
28. Cann KJ, Chalmers RM, Nichols G, O'Brien SJ. *Cyclospora* infections in England and Wales: 1993 to 1998. *Commun Dis Public Health* 2000; **3**: 46–9.
29. Chalmers RM, Nichols G, Rooney R. Foodborne outbreaks of cyclosporiasis have arisen in North America. Is the United Kingdom at risk? *Commun Dis Public Health* 2000; **3**: 50–5.
30. Chacin-Bonilla L. Transmission of *Cyclospora cayetanensis* infection: A review focusing on soil-borne cyclosporiasis. *Trans R Soc Trop Med Hyg* 2008; **102**: 215–16.
31. Lindsay DS, Dubey JP, Blagburn BL. Biology of *Isospora* spp. from humans, nonhuman primates, and domestic animals. *Clin Microbiol Rev* 1997; **10**: 19–34.
32. Jongwutiwes S, Putaporntip C, Charoenkorn M, Iwasaki T, Endo T. Morphologic and molecular characterization of *Isospora belli* oocysts from patients in Thailand. *Am J Trop Med Hyg* 2007; **77**: 107–12.

33. Mirdha BR, Kabra SK, Samantray JC. Isosporiasis in children. *Indian Pediatr* 2002; **39**: 941–4.

34. Fayer R. *Sarcocystis* spp. in human infections. *Clin Microbiol Rev* 2004; **17**: 894–902.

35. Ximénez C, Morán P, Rojas L, Valadez A, Gómez A. Reassessment of the epidemiology of amebiasis: State of the art. *Infect Genet Evol* 2009; **9**: 1023–32.

36. Diamond LS, Clark CG. A redescription of *Entamoeba histolytica* Schaudinn, 1903 (Emended Walker, 1911) separating it from *Entamoeba dispar* Brumpt, 1925. *J Eukaryot Microbiol* 1993; **40**: 340–4.

37. Marcos LA, DuPont HL. Advances in defining etiology and new therapeutic approaches in acute diarrhea. *J Infect* 2007; **55**: 385–93.

38. Myers LL, Shoop DS, Stackhouse LL *et al.* Isolation of enterotoxigenic *Bacteroides fragilis* from humans with diarrhea. *J Clin Microbiol* 1987; **25**: 2330–3.

♦39. Schlenker C, Surawicz CM. Emerging infections of the gastrointestinal tract. *Best Pract Res Clin Gastroenterol* 2009; **23**: 89–99.

40. Woo PC, Lau SK, Teng JL, Yuen KY. Current status and future directions for *Laribacter hongkongensis*, a novel bacterium associated with gastroenteritis and traveller's diarrhoea. *Curr Opin Infect Dis* 2005; **18**: 413–19.

41. Woo PC, Kuhnert P, Burnens AP *et al. Laribacter hongkongensis*: A potential cause of infectious diarrhea. *Diagn Microbiol Infect Dis* 2003; **47**: 551–6.

42. Vucic S, Kiernan MC, Cornblath DR. Guillain–Barré syndrome: An update. *J Clin Neurosci* 2009; **16**: 733–41.

43 Winer JB. Guillain–Barré syndrome. *Mol Pathol* 2001; **54**: 381–5.

44. Overell JR, Willison HJ. Recent developments in Miller Fisher syndrome and related disorders. *Curr Opin Neurol* 2005; **18**: 562–6.

45. Li H, Yuan J. Miller Fisher syndrome: Toward a more comprehensive understanding. *Chin Med J (Engl)* 2001; **114**: 235–9.

46. Khokhar N, Gill ML. Tropical sprue: Revisited. *J Pak Med Assoc* 2004; **54**: 133–4.

47. Westergaard H. Tropical sprue. *Curr Treat Options Gastroenterol* 2004; **7**: 7–11.

48. Kimura AC, Mead P, Walsh B *et al.* A large outbreak of Brainerd diarrhea associated with a restaurant in the Red River Valley, Texas. *Clin Infect Dis* 2006; **43**: 55–61.

49. Bryant DA, Mintz ED, Puhr ND, Griffin PM, Petras RE. Colonic epithelial lymphocytosis associated with an epidemic of chronic diarrhea. *Am J Surg Pathol* 1996; **20**: 1102–9.

50. Osterholm MT, MacDonald KL, White KE *et al.* An outbreak of a newly recognized chronic diarrhea syndrome associated with raw milk consumption. *JAMA* 1986; **256**: 484–90.

32

The causes of waterborne disease

PAUL R. HUNTER

Waterborne diseases are estimated to be one of the most important environmental causes of disease and early death globally. In 2001, diarrhoeal disease was responsible for about 1.8 million deaths in all age groups, or about 3.7 per cent of all deaths worldwide.[1] In terms of years of life lost, diarrhoeal diseases came a close sixth behind lower respiratory tract infections, ischaemic heart disease, perinatal conditions, human immunodeficiency disease (HIV) and cardiovascular disease. The vast majority of these deaths (about 90 per cent) occur in children under the age of 5 years in developing countries. Diarrhoeal disease was the second most common cause of death in children under 5 years old in 2001, second only to respiratory disease and rather more than malaria or road traffic accidents.

Some 88 per cent of cases of diarrhoeal disease are estimated to be due to unsafe drinking water, sanitation and hygiene. In low- and middle-income countries in 2001, unsafe water, sanitation and hygiene practices were estimated to be the fifth major contributing factor to disease burden as measure by disability-adjusted life-years, behind malnutrition, high blood pressure, unsafe sex and smoking.[1] In children under 5 years of age, unsafe water, sanitation and hygiene is second only to malnutrition as a contributor to disease burden.

However, in this author's opinion, the global burden of disease study underestimates the contribution that unsafe water has on disease burden. Calculations are based almost entirely on acute diarrhoeal disease and deaths from diarrhoea. As Guerrant et al. have pointed out, the adverse impacts on health can go well beyond the acute episode of diarrhoea.[2] Diarrhoea in the first 2 years of life is associated with impaired fitness, growth shortfalls, cognitive impairment and reduced school performance months and years later. This association remains even after possible confounding variables such as maternal education, socio-economic factors and breast-feeding are controlled for.

The probably synergistic interaction between poverty, protein–energy malnutrition, diarrhoeal disease and unsafe water, sanitation and hygiene, and failure to thrive is not adequately understood. Other infectious diseases that do not cause diarrhoea but may be associated with unsafe water such as hepatitis A and hepatitis E, toxoplasmosis, *Helicobacter pylori* and mycobacterial infections are not included. Neither are non-infectious diseases such as arsenic and fluoride poisoning in many low-income communities reliant on boreholes for their drinking water. Also, the possible impacts on the musculoskeletal system of having to carry heavy containers of water from an early age are not present in any estimates of disease burden.

Taking all these issues together, in low- and middle-income countries, unsafe water, sanitation and hygiene are one of the top two major causes of disease and loss of life opportunities that are entirely preventable with current scientific knowledge and technology. Yet, despite much recent effort, we are barely able to manage to keep pace with population growth, and the millennium development goal target of reducing by half the number of people without access to safe water and sanitation by 2015 is not going to be met by a long way.[3]

The burden of disease therefore falls mostly on low- and middle-income countries. However, waterborne disease is still a recurrent problem in high-income countries such as the USA and the countries of Western Europe. Here, the focus tends to be not on endemic disease but on the occurrence of outbreaks due to failures in water treatment and distribution.[4–6]

This chapter will focus on the classic waterborne diseases, i.e. those diseases which are acquired by drinking water that has been contaminated by the faeces of animals or other humans. The main waterborne pathogens will be briefly listed. The chapter will then address recent data and causes of outbreaks, as well as the epidemiological evidence estimating the incidence of waterborne disease in high-income countries. Finally, a range of current topical issues will be discussed, including problems with small rural water supplies, evidence on the effectiveness of interventions to reduce waterborne disease, and finally the potential impact of climate change.

WATERBORNE PATHOGENS

Waterborne pathogens include examples of viruses, bacteria and protozoa (Table 32.1).[7] Most cause self-limiting diarrhoeal illness that lasts a few days to a few weeks at most. Some of the infections, especially cryptosporidiosis and giardiasis, have been known to cause illness lasting several weeks before recovery.

In immunocompromised patients, such as people living with HIV/acquired immune deficiency disease (AIDS), the disease can be particularly severe. This is the case for cryptosporidiosis in patients with HIV/AIDS.[8] In this group, the infection carries a substantial mortality when CD4 T-cell counts are low. The illness may be very severe with high fluid loss, dehydration and rapid death, or it more commonly becomes chronic, leading to weight loss with the patient literally wasting away over a period of months. Prior to the widespread use of antiretroviral therapy, cryptosporidiosis in a patient with AIDS was almost universally fatal.

Many waterborne diseases are emerging infectious diseases and were largely unknown to medical science until relatively recently. *Cryptosporidium, Cyclospora,*

Table 32.1   Examples of pathogens implicated in waterborne disease

Organism	Disease	Clinical features
Protozoa		
Giardia duodenalis	Giardiasis	Diarrhoea and abdominal pain, weight loss and failure to thrive
Cryptosporidium parvum	Cryptosporidiosis	Diarrhoea, often prolonged
Cyclospora cayetanensis	Cyclosporiasis	Diarrhoea and abdominal pain, weight loss and failure to thrive
Entamoeba histolytica	Amoebiasis	Diarrhoea, may be severe dysentery
Toxoplasma gondii	Toxoplasmosis	Glandular fever, fetal damage in pregnant women
Bacteria		
Vibrio cholerae	Cholera	Watery diarrhoea, may be severe
Salmonella spp.	Salmonellosis	Diarrhoea, colicky abdominal pain and fever
Salmonella typhi	Typhoid	Fever, malaise and abdominal pain with high mortality
Shigella spp.	Shigellosis (bacillary dysentery)	Diarrhoea, frequently with blood loss
Campylobacter spp.	Campylobacteriosis	Diarrhoea, frequently with blood loss
Enterotoxigenic *Escherichia coli*		Watery diarrhoea
Enterohaemorrhagic *Escherichia coli*		Bloody diarrhoea and haemolytic–uraemic syndrome in children
Yersinia spp.	Yersiniosis	Fever, diarrhoea and abdominal pain
Francisella tularensis	Tularaemia	Typhoid-like or mucocutaneous with suppurative skin lesions
Helicobacter pylori		Gastritis that can progress to gastric cancer
Mycobacteria spp. but **not** *M. tuberculosis*	Varies	Varies, includes respiratory disease, wound infections and skin disease
Viruses		
Hepatitis A, hepatitis E	Viral hepatitis	Hepatitis
Various, especially Norovirus	Viral gastroenteritis	Vomiting and diarrhoea
Enteroviruses	Various, including poliomyelitis	Various

Adapted from Hunter (2003)[39].

Campylobacter, noroviruses, hepatitis E virus and enterohaemorrhagic *Escherichia coli* were all unknown in the early 1970s. Many of these agents were unknown because they could not be identified by routine microbiological methods, but enterohaemorrhagic *E. coli* is almost certainly a new species that evolved about 30 years ago.

OUTBREAKS OF WATERBORNE DISEASE

In the high-income countries of the Western world, the main driver of research and policy change relating to water safety has been the detection and reporting of outbreaks of waterborne disease. The most important outbreaks in the UK in this regard have been the outbreaks of cryptosporidiosis in Oxfordshire and the south west of England, the Milwaukee outbreak of cryptosporidiosis in the USA and the Walkerton outbreak of enterohaemorrhagic *E. coli* in Canada.[9–12] All these outbreaks had significant political and policy impacts in their countries. The Walkerton outbreak in particular had substantial political repercussions. One of the main factors behind the outbreak was deemed to be a reduction in the funding of regulatory oversight in Canada. The outbreak resulted in resignation of the State Premier.

Although such outbreaks have been known for many years, it was only in recent years that reports of outbreaks began to be systematically collected by national disease surveillance centres. Probably the first national surveillance scheme was in the USA from the early 1970s, with one in England and Wales from the early 1990s. It is notable that there has in both countries been a fairly noticeable decline in detected outbreaks some 10 years after the start of national surveillance. It is tempting to speculate that this decline has been in part driven by the realization that failures in water treatment that pose a risk to human health are more likely to be identified than in the past. The number of outbreaks reported differs quite dramatically from one country to another, even in Western Europe.[6] However, the main driver of this variation is more likely to be differences in infectious disease diagnostic and surveillance approaches between countries than real differences in the actual number of outbreaks after correction for population size.

One of the very important values of detecting and investigating outbreaks is that the process can highlight the failings in water system management that led to the outbreak. Risebro *et al.* have used an adaptation of fault tree analysis to study reports of waterborne outbreaks in Europe in an attempt to determine the main failings.[6] One of the main advantages of this approach compared with some others is that the fault tree method allows multiple factors to be identified and their relative importance assessed.

Risebro *et al.* categorized factors into those affecting the source water, those affecting treatment, those affecting distribution and those affecting the ability of the water utilities to detect a problem. Examples of problems with the source included allowing livestock into close proximity to the extraction point, heavy rainfall and the poor design and situation of water extraction points. Problems in treatment included lack of adequate filtration or failures in disinfection. The authors found that for a source problem to lead to an outbreak, there usually also had to be a problem with the water treatment. So a poorly located extraction point located close to cattle would not cause an outbreak of cryptosporidiosis unless there was also a problem with the filtration system of the water treatment works. In the outbreaks that Risebro *et al.* reviewed, about two-thirds were due to a combination of source and treatment problems. The remaining one-third were primarily due to distribution problems and included such issues as low pressure and damaged distribution pipes or cross-connections with contaminated water.

The issues associated with the fourth category (the ability to detect a problem) were never the primary problem but often exacerbated the outbreak by delaying the realization that the water system was no longer safe. Examples of this include water staff not reporting poor results rapidly enough and people actually being ignorant of the health risks associated with their level of treatment.

The links between rainfall events and outbreaks, as mentioned above, had been identified and reported on by other workers. In particular, a review of 548 waterborne outbreaks in the USA from 1948 to 1994 found that 51 per cent of these outbreaks had been preceded by a heavy rainfall event.[13] This observation was mirrored in a review of 89 outbreaks in England and Wales that found a significant excess rainfall in the 7 days prior to the outbreak compared with the same time period in the previous 5 years, as well as a significant excess of low rainfall in the 3 weeks prior to the outbreak week.[14]

It is noteworthy that the recent decline in the number of waterborne outbreaks in the UK and USA has been predominantly in outbreaks due to contaminated water leaving the water treatment works. This reflects an increased awareness in the water industry of the risks due to cryptosporidiosis where contaminated source waters are not subject to adequate filtration. Problems due to contamination in distribution networks are more difficult to control, especially given the old and decaying distribution networks in many cities around the world. It is likely that, over the coming decades, distribution problems will become the dominant source of outbreaks of waterborne disease.

THE INCIDENCE OF ENDEMIC WATERBORNE DISEASE

By contrast with the situation in low- and middle-income countries, knowledge about the likely prevalence of waterborne disease in high-income countries is uncertain.

This may be in part because there was until relatively recently a widespread belief that existing water treatment was safe. This belief was badly dented by the major outbreaks discussed above. However, it remains uncertain what the exact level of sporadic endemic disease actually is.

Some of this endemic disease is in fact likely to be due to undetected outbreaks. Hunter *et al.* retrospectively reviewed reports of cryptosporidiosis in areas that had recently experienced two large waterborne outbreaks.[15] In contrast to other areas, there had been multiple times where case numbers had increased but an outbreak had not been declared. This suggested that many outbreaks of waterborne disease go undetected.

There have also been several randomized controlled trials in which volunteers have been provided with point-of-use devices to remove pathogens at the kitchen tap. The first of these was in Canada, where the subjects in one study arm had domestic reverse osmosis filters fitted on their kitchen tap and were then asked to report all episodes of gastroenteritis.[16] Based on the difference in reporting rates between the volunteers with and without a filter, the authors estimated that about 50 per cent of diarrhoeal disease was due to exposure to tap water. Since then, there have been two other similar studies, one in Australia and the other in the USA, that used a double-blind approach in that the control group were fitted with sham filters.[17,18] In neither of these studies did illness rates differ between the intervention and control groups.

Another approach has been to do time series analyses on diarrhoeal illness rates and measures of drinking water quality, especially turbidity. The first such study reported an association between drinking water turbidity and emergency visits and admissions to the Children's Hospital of Philadelphia for gastrointestinal illness.[19] However, this study was criticized by several other authors on grounds such as the measurement uncertainty in turbidity meters.[20]

In a second early study from France, the authors demonstrated an association between turbidity and over-the-counter sales of antidiarrhoeal medicine.[21] The water system studied took water from a karstic aquifer that had substantial turbidity spikes after heavy rainfall. The authors estimated that about 10 per cent of cases of gastroenteritis in the community were associated with these peaks of turbidity. Finally, in a systematic review of the issue, Mann *et al.* concluded from a review of eight papers that an 'association between turbidity and [gastrointestinal] illness exists in some settings or over a certain range of turbidity'.[22]

More recently, attention has turned towards potential problems in drinking water distribution systems. In a case–control study from Sweden, the authors identified an association between the risk of *Campylobacter* infection and distance from the water treatment works.[23] It is not clear whether this association was due to bacterial regrowth in the distribution network or to increased opportunities for contamination in the network.

Recent work from the USA has highlighted the potential risk associated with pressure loss in distribution.[24] Water in distribution is invariably under some pressure so that if leaks occur, water will flow out rather than contaminants flow in. However, two recent studies have demonstrated an association between low pressure at the kitchen tap and a subsequent risk of gastroenteritis. In the first study, the authors compared reporting of low pressure by people with self-reported gastroenteritis.[25] They estimated that up to 15 per cent of all cases of diarrhoea were associated with reports of low water pressure. However, as the authors pointed out, the primary study had not been designed to test this hypothesis.

This issue was further investigated in a prospective cohort study that followed up communities 1 week after they had suffered a loss of water supply, either because of a pipe break or because of maintenance.[26] The authors compared these communities with other communities that did not have such a recent history. They found that gastrointestinal illness rates in the study households were 1.6 times higher than in the control households, and that the risk was highest in households with an above-average water consumption. The evidence certainly points to the suggestion that a loss of water supply poses a risk of gastroenteritis, probably because pathogens can gain access to the supply.

By contrast to the studies from high-income countries, there have been many more studies from low-income countries. However, it is still not possible to be certain of the real incidence of waterborne disease in the setting of developing countries, in part because it is difficult to define control groups with no risk. In addition, other transmission pathways, such as inadequate sanitation or poor hygiene, are commonly found in settings with inadequate drinking water. Even the use of randomized controlled trials of water quality interventions as reported above do not give a true picture. These are discussed further below.

TOPICAL ISSUES IN WATERBORNE DISEASE

Health issues with small rural water supplies

Although most people who live in the developed world take their drinking water from large municipal supplies, up to 10 per cent of people are reliant on small or very small supplies, most of which supply drinking water to fewer than 50 people and often to just a single household. These very small supplies are most often taken from shallow groundwater or spring water. They are much more likely to be prone to faecal contamination than are larger water supplies. For example, although in the UK less than 0.1 per cent of water samples from mains drinking water are positive for *E. coli*, almost 20 per cent of samples from small rural waster supplies are positive.[27] These supplies are also highly likely to be contaminated by human pathogens including *Campylobacter*, *Giardia*, *Cryptosporidium* and enteroviruses.[28]

There are a number of temporal and geographical factors that affect the likelihood of small rural water supplies being contaminated. Very small supplies are more likely to take water from contaminated sources (surface or spring waters) and then not be adequately treated or indeed treated at all.[27] Rainfall in the previous few days is an important driver of contamination, as is the presence of livestock close to the source. Supplies are most likely to have high indicator organism counts in the early autumn and least likely in the first months of the year.

Despite the difficulties of detecting outbreaks in very small populations, people reliant on these waters are also more likely to be involved in outbreaks of waterborne disease.[29] However, as with mains water supplies, there remains uncertainty over what the burden of endemic disease is. Two of the first studies to attempt to identify the burden of endemic waterborne disease in high-income countries were in France. The first was a prospective follow-up study on illness rates in 48 villages that had untreated ground water as their drinking water.[30] The authors found a relationship between faecal streptococcal counts and acute gastrointestinal disease.

In a second study, the same group reported a study of 24 villages.[31] In 13 villages, the source water met microbiological criteria and was distributed without treatment. In the other 11 villages, water was chlorinated as the source water yielded indicator bacteria. Even after chlorination, the diarrhoea was about 1.4 times more common in the villages that drank contaminated source waters even though water at the tap was negative for indicator bacteria. A study in Canada of very small supplies did not find a significant association between indicator bacteria and risk of diarrhoea, although the study was underpowered and the mid-point risk assessment was actually similar to the findings of the French studies.

Interventions aimed at reducing waterborne disease in developing countries

In his pioneering review of the evidence up until that point, Esrey *et al.* put forward two arguments:[32] first, that water quantity was more important than water quality to reduce waterborne disease in developing country settings; and second, that the full impact of improving water quality/quantity on disease reduction could not be achieved unless sanitation was simultaneously improved. These two beliefs are still widespread and have almost become dogma. However, recent systematic reviews have cast doubt on these views.[33,34] The Clasen review was particularly thorough and was unable to find a difference in the impact of interventions that focused on improving water quality and those that focused on improving water availability. Furthermore, this review did not find an effect of simultaneous sanitation interventions.

Of particular interest in the Clasen review was the comparison of in-home point-of-use water treatment

systems and community interventions. The main in-home interventions are chlorination, solar disinfection and various filtration devices. An initial assessment of the evidence in the systematic review would suggest that in-home interventions are more effective than community-level interventions. However, as Clasen pointed out, most of the studies of in-home interventions had very short follow-up periods compared with community interventions, which had much longer follow-up.

A much greater problem though is whether the current evidence does indeed support the view that in-home water treatment reduces diarrhoeal disease burden. One of the major problems with trials of in-home water treatment is that very few studies have blinded volunteers to whether or not they have received the intervention. Consequently, it is plausible that inadequate concealment of allocation will have biased the findings of most studies. In a recent study, it was reported that inadequate allocation concealment would lead to an erroneous odds ratio of 0.69 (95 per cent confidence interval [CI] 0.59–0.82) increased effect compared with adequate concealment for subjective health outcomes.[35] This bias impact is very similar to the effects of in-home water treatment described in the meta-analyses of water interventions. In a subsequent meta-analysis of in-home water treatment in poor populations, the authors investigated the impact of blinding on heterogeneity.[36] Unblinded studies found an overall effect on diarrhoeal disease reduction (risk ratio 0.51, 95 per cent CI 0.38–0.69). However, in blinded studies, there was no effect on diarrhoeal disease reduction, with relative risk being greater than 1.

There is also a further concern, and this is about whether or not people continue to use in-home devices over the months and years after the study. Several studies have now investigated the longer-term use and impact of these systems, and the evidence that they are still being used by the great majority of the targeted population over subsequent years is frequently not good.[37,38] To this author, the balance of evidence does not currently support the hypothesis that in-home water treatment has an important role in controlling waterborne diarrhoeal disease. There is, however, a clear need for more research, although this research must be better designed than much of the published research to date. The literature already has too many poorly designed randomized trials that were not blinded and were assessed by totally inadequate follow-up periods.

The health benefits of point-of-use devices in high-income countries are even more uncertain, although there has been very little reliable research on this.

Climate change and waterborne disease

Climate change could impact on the quantity or quality of drinking water in several ways.[39] Heavy rainfall events may become more frequent and seasonal, there may be longer periods of drought between rainfall events leading to seasonal aridification, and finally water temperatures may increase.

As already mentioned, rainfall is a significant driver of poor water quality in small supplies, and extreme rainfall events have been identified as an important driver of outbreaks of waterborne disease. This is most obvious when the rainfall has led to flooding, but it is not restricted to flooding. The seasonal aridification that may also accompany climate change can also adversely affect source water quality as levels in rivers and lakes fall. The most obvious example of this is the appearance of cyanobacterial blooms.[40] Although it is difficult to generalize, extreme heat and reduced flow can also negatively impact on other aspects of source water quality.[41]

In its recent paper on climate change and water, the Intergovernmental Panel on Climate Change concluded that current water management practices may not be robust enough to cope with the impact of climate change on the reliability of water supplies.[42] It is likely that the main impacts of climate change will fall on those water supplies that have an inadequate infrastructure. In other words, the main brunt of the effect in high-income countries will largely be restricted to small and very small supplies.

CONCLUSION

Globally, waterborne disease remains a major cause of ill health and premature mortality. Although most of this disease burden falls on children in low-income countries, drinking water still poses a risk to the health of certain people living in high-income countries. One of the most obvious risks is associated with the large number of very small water supplies, especially in rural settings. Another major area of concern is the old and decaying distribution networks that are present in many of the developed world's major cities. It is likely that, for people on mains drinking water, the risks associated with distribution problems will in the future outweigh the risks from source or treatment problems. The impact of climate change on waterborne disease risks is unclear, although these risks will fall mostly on low-income countries and on very small supplies in the developed world.

REFERENCES

● = Key primary paper
◆ = Major review article

1. Lopez AD, Mathers CD, Ezzati M, Jamison DT, Murray CJL. Global and regional burden of disease and risk factors, 2001: Systematic analysis of population health data. *Lancet* 2006; **367**: 1747–57.

2. Guerrant RL, Kosek M, Lima AAM, Lorntz B, Guyatt HL. Updating the DALYs for diarrhoeal disease. *Trends Parasitol* 2002; **18**: 191–3.

3. United Nations. *The Millennium Development Goals Report 2007*. New York: United Nations, 2007.

4. Schuster CJ, Ellis AG, Robertson WJ *et al*. Infectious disease outbreaks related to drinking water in Canada, 1974–2001. *Can J Publ Hlth* 2005; **96**: 254–8.

5. Craun GF, Craun MF, Calderon RL, Beach MJ. Waterborne outbreaks reported in the United States. *J Water Hlth* 2006; **4**(Suppl. 2): 19–30.

6. Risebro HL, Doria MF, Andersson Y *et al*. Fault tree analysis of the causes of waterborne outbreaks. *J Water Hlth* 2007; **5**(Suppl. 1): 1–18.

7. Hunter PR. *Waterborne Disease: Epidemiology and Ecology*. Chichester: Wiley, 1997.

◆8. Hunter PR, Nichols G. The epidemiology and clinical features of cryptosporidium infection in immune-compromised patients. *Clin Microbiol Rev* 2002; **15**: 145–54.

9. Richardson AJ, Frankenberg RA, Buck AC, Selkon JB, Colbourne JS. An outbreak of waterborne cryptosporidiosis in Swindon and Oxfordshire. *Epidemiol Infect* 1991; **107**: 485–95.

10. Harrison SL, Nelder R, Hayek L, MacKenzie IF, Casemore DP, Dance D. Managing a large outbreak of cryptosporidiosis: How to investigate and when to decide to lift a 'boil water' notice. *Commun Dis Publ Hlth* 2002; **5**: 230–9.

●11. MacKenzie WR, Hoxie NJ, Proctor ME *et al*. A massive outbreak in Milwaukee of *Cryptosporidium* infection transmitted through the public water supply. *N Engl J Med* 1994; **331**: 161–7.

12. Hrudey SE, Payment P, Huck PM, Gillham RW, Hrudey EJ. A fatal waterborne disease epidemic in Walkerton, Ontario: Comparison with other waterborne outbreaks in the developed world. *Water Sci Technol* 2003; **47**: 7–14.

●13. Curriero FC, Patz JA, Rose JB, Lele S. The association between extreme precipitation and waterborne disease outbreaks in the United States, 1948–1994. *Am J Publ Hlth* 2001; **91**: 1194–9.

14. Nichols G, Lane C, Asgari N, Verlander NQ, Charlett A. Rainfall and outbreaks of drinking water related disease and in England and Wales. *J Water Health* 2009; **7**: 1–8.

15. Hunter PR, Syed Q, Naumova EN. Possible undetected outbreaks of cryptosporidiosis in areas of the North West of England supplied by an unfiltered surface water source. *Commun Dis Publ Hlth* 2001; **4**: 136–8.

●16. Payment P, Richardson L, Siemiatycki J, Dewar R, Edwardes M, Franco E. A randomized trial to evaluate the risk of gastrointestinal disease due to consumption of drinking water meeting current microbiological standards. *Am J Publ Hlth* 1991; **81**: 703–8.

17. Hellard ME, Sinclair MI, Forbes AB, Fairley CK. A randomized, blinded, controlled trial investigating the gastrointestinal health effects of drinking water quality. *Env Health Perspect* 2001; **109**: 773–8.

18. Colford JM, Wade TJ, Sandhu SK *et al*. A randomized, controlled trial of in-home drinking water intervention to reduce gastrointestinal illness. *Am J Epidemiol* 2005; **161**: 472–82.

19. Schwartz J, Levin R, Hodge K. Drinking water turbidity and pediatric hospital use for gastrointestinal illness in Philadelphia. *Epidemiol* 1997; **8**: 615–20.

20. Sinclair MI, Fairley CK: Drinking water and endemic gastrointestinal illness. *J Epidemiol Comm Hlth* 2000, **54**: 728.

21. Beaudeau P, Payment P, Bourderont D *et al.* A time series study of anti-diarrhoeal drug sales and tap-water quality. *Int J Env Health Res* 1999; **9**: 293–312.

22. Mann AG, Tam CC, Higgins CD, Rodrigues LC. The association between drinking water turbidity and gastrointestinal illness: A systematic review. *BMC Publ Hlth* 2007; **7**: 256.

23. Nygard K, Andersson Y, Rottingen JA *et al.* Association between environmental risk factors and *Campylobacter* infections in Sweden. *Epidemiol Infect* 2004; **132**: 317–25.

24. Le Chevallier MW, Gullick RW, Karim MR, Friedman M, Funk JE. The potential for health risks from intrusion of contaminants into the distribution system from pressure transients. *J Water Health* 2003; **1**: 3–14.

25. Hunter PR, Chalmers RM, Hughes S, Syed Q. Self reported diarrhea in a control group: A strong association with reporting of low pressure events in tap water. *Clin Infect Dis* 2005; **40**: e32–4.

26. Nygard K, Wahl E, Krogh T *et al.* Breaks and maintenance work in the water distribution systems and gastrointestinal illness: A cohort study. *Int J Epidemiol* 2007; **36**: 873–80.

27. Richardson HY, Nichols G, Lane C, Lake IR, Hunter PR. Microbiological surveillance of private water supplies in England – the impact of environmental and climate factors on water quality. *Water Res* 2009; **43**: 2159–68.

28. Kay D, Watkins J, Francis CA *et al.* The microbiological quality of seven large commercial water supplies in the United Kingdom. *J Water Health* 2007; **5**: 523–8.

29. Said B, Wright F, Nichols GL, Reacher M, Rutter M. Outbreaks of infectious disease associated with private drinking water supplies in England and Wales 1970–2000. *Epidemiol Infect* 2003; **130**: 469–79.

●30. Ferley JP, Zmirou D, Collin JF, Charrel M. Etude longitudinale des risques liés à la consommation d'eaux non conformes aux normes bactériologiques [Longitudinal study on the risks associated with the consumption of water not conforming to bacteriological standards]. *Rev Epidemiol Sante Publique* 1986; **34**: 89–99.

●31. Zmirou D, Rey S, Courtois X *et al.* Residual microbiological risk after simple chlorine treatment of drinking ground water in small community systems. *Eur J Public Hlth* 1995; **5**: 75–81.

◆32. Esrey SA, Potash JB, Roberts L, Shiff C. Effects of improved water supply and sanitation on ascariasis, diarrhoea, dracunculiasis, hookworm infection, schistosomiasis, and trachoma. *Bull World Hlth Org* 1991; **69**: 609–21.

◆33. Clasen T, Schmidt WP, Rabie T, Roberts I, Cairncross S. Interventions to improve water quality for preventing diarrhoea: Systematic review and meta-analysis. *Br Med J* 2007; **334**: 782–5.

34. Fewtrell L, Kaufmann RB, Kay D, Enanoria W, Haller L, Colford JM. Water, sanitation, and hygiene interventions to reduce diarrhoea in less developed countries: A systematic review and meta-analysis. *Lancet Infect Dis* 2005; **5**: 42–52.

35. Wood L, Egger M, Gluud LL *et al.* Empirical evidence of bias in treatment effect estimates in controlled trials with different interventions and outcomes: Meta-epidemiological study. *Br Med J* 2008; **336**: 601–5.

36. Schmidt WP, Cairncross S. Household water treatment in poor populations: Is there enough evidence for scaling up now? *Environ Sci Technol* 2009; **43**: 986–92.

37. Clasen TF, Brown J, Collin SM. Preventing diarrhoea with household ceramic water filters: Assessment of a pilot project in Bolivia. *Int J Environ Hlth Res* 2006; **16**: 231–9.

38. Luby SP, Mendoza C, Keswick BH, Chiller TM, Hoekstra RM. Difficulties in bringing point-of-use water treatment to scale in rural Guatemala. *Am J Trop Med Hyg* 2008; **78**: 382–7.

39. Hunter PR. Climate change and waterborne and vector-borne disease. *J Appl Microbiol* 2003; **94**: 37S–46S.

40. Hunter PR. Cyanobacterial toxins and human health. *J Appl Bacteriol* 1998; **84**(Suppl): 35S–40S.

41. Senhorst HA, Zwolsman JJ. Climate change and effects on water quality: A first impression. *Water Sci Technol* 2005: **51**: 53–9.

42. Bates B, Kundzewicz ZW, Wu S, Palutikof J (eds). *Climate Change and Water. Technical Paper of the Intergovernmental Panel on Climate Change.* Geneva: IPCC Secretariat, 2008.

33

Cholera

KELLEY LEE, ADAM KAMRADT-SCOTT

Despite significant advances in modern medicine over the past century, cholera is still today one of the most feared infectious diseases in public health. It is an acute diarrhoeal infection caused by the ingestion of food or water contaminated with the bacterium *Vibrio cholerae* (over 100 serotypes of *V. cholerae* exist but only two – O1 and O139 – cause cholera). When ingested, the organism produces an enterotoxin composed of A and B protein subunits that binds to the surface of intestinal enterocytes. The A subunit enters the cell and alters the G protein, resulting in cyclic AMP production. This leads to the secretion of water and electrolytes into the lumen of the small intestine, resulting in rapid dehydration and voluminous diarrhoea and vomiting.

Compared with other infectious diseases, cholera has a very short incubation period, usually between 2 hours and 5 days. In its most severe form, the disease can rapidly lead to death due to acute dehydration and kidney failure, and without effective medical treatment, cholera is fatal in approximately 50 per cent of cases. Affected individuals are highly contagious, yet almost 75 per cent of people infected with cholera fail to develop symptoms. Whether or not individuals are symptomatic, the organism can remain in their faeces for 7–14 days post infection. This allows the pathogen to be shed back into the environment, resulting in the contamination of food and water, and thus continuing the chain of transmission.

Since *V. cholerae* was first identified by Robert Koch in 1883, medical knowledge of the disease and how to treat it has expanded considerably. The development of oral rehydration therapy during the 1960s and 70s, arguably the most important public health intervention of the twentieth century, led to remarkable reductions in mortality from acute diarrhoeal disease. Where individuals are appropriately treated with fluid and electrolyte replacement, mortality can be reduced to less than 1 per cent.[1] The entire DNA sequence of *V. cholerae* has also been mapped,[2] yielding an understanding of how the O139 strain changed to become lethal, and how effective various treatments (including the use of antibiotic and oral cholera vaccine) have prove to be.

At the same time, cholera presents ongoing challenges in the twenty-first century as a consequence of an increasingly globalized world. Global change is influencing the broader determinants of health, which are central to the way in which the disease has persisted and adapted over time. Since 1961, the world has been experiencing its seventh cholera pandemic. Caused by a different biotype of *V. cholerae* O1, known as El Tor, the current pandemic has behaved quite differently from previous pandemics and shows no sign of abating. In the early 1990s, the first non-O1 serotype of cholera to cause epidemic disease, *V. cholerae* O139 Bengal, began spreading in what may become an eighth pandemic.

This chapter explores how environmental factors have facilitated the spread of cholera over the past two centuries. Following a brief history of the disease and its pandemic spread from the nineteenth century, we will discuss how contemporary processes of globalization are influencing the spread of the disease in the developing world.

A BRIEF HISTORY OF CHOLERA PANDEMICS

Until 1817, cholera was a disease that was largely limited to South Asia. Epidemics of cholera-like illnesses were recorded on the Indian subcontinent as early as the sixteenth century, with occasional outbreaks among

China's coastal populations (via trading ships) and the Middle East (via pilgrims travelling to Mecca). Earlier accounts by Hippocrates and in Sanskrit writings indicate, however, that human interaction with the disease extends back much further. From the nineteenth century, the geographical reach of the disease changed dramatically as a result of the intensification of human interaction through trade, imperialism, military conflict and migration.

The first cholera pandemic (1817–23), mostly affecting the Far and Middle East, has been attributed to South Asia's integration into the British Empire. This process led to the construction of poorly draining irrigation canals for raising cash crops (e.g. tea and opium), the impoverishment of local populations by land reforms and increased taxation, and mass migration due to economic hardship.[3]

From 1826, cholera spread beyond the region as a consequence of military expansionism, trade and migration. Early European imperialism focused on the search for riches in the Orient. From the early nineteenth century, European commercial pursuits prompted huge movements of traders, military personnel, camp followers and immigrants between Europe and Asia. Along with the use of military means, such as 'gunboat diplomacy', to forcibly open and maintain new markets, conflict grew among European countries competing for economic and political power. During the Crimean War (1853–56), for example, military personnel lived in appalling conditions, becoming effective carriers of diseases such as syphilis, tuberculosis, typhus, typhoid fever and cholera.[4]

Similarly, social conditions created by rapid European industrialization facilitated the spread of cholera. Large-scale urbanization, particularly in Europe, was accompanied by poor sanitation, housing and nutrition, and a lack of healthcare. Until Koch identified the bacillus responsible for the disease in 1883, this close association between cholera and social deprivation led to the disease being attributed to immorality and a lack of 'proper habits'.[2] Political movements were also inspired by the disease, focusing on social inequalities and improving basic living conditions. The historic removal of the Broad Street pump handle by John Snow in 1832, demonstrating cholera as a waterborne disease spread by the faeco-oral route, remains perhaps the most enduring example of the relationship between social environment and disease.[5]

Finally, prevailing modes of transportation influenced the spread of cholera worldwide. For centuries, cholera was limited to population movements on foot or by draught animals and sailing ships. With the advent of steam power during the nineteenth century, infectious diseases such as cholera could spread more rapidly across greater distances. Other technological developments, such as the opening of the Panama Canal, further hastened the spread of cholera into South America.

Overall, the geographical pattern of the six cholera pandemics from 1817 to 1923 closely mirrors changes in social and natural environments.[6] The intercontinental spread and consolidation of economic and political links during this period generated economic development and growth, benefiting many. At the same time, resultant environmental changes created conditions within which cholera could spread.

CHOLERA IN A GLOBALIZING WORLD

The history of cholera shows that although contaminated food and water is the primary means by which the disease is spread, the social and natural environment directly influences the capacity to prevent and control outbreaks. Cholera outbreaks no longer occur in the industrialized world for three reasons:

1. It is now known that, compared with other enteric pathogens, a large number of *V. cholerae* must be swallowed before illness occurs.
2. Improvements in housing, water (especially chlorinated) and sanitation prevent exposure to faeces.
3. Despite individual infection with cholera, there is little opportunity for onward transmission either to other people or to the coastal environment and its shellfish.

For the developing world, however, cholera remains a potential threat. In 1961, the seventh pandemic began in Indonesia involving a different biotype known as *V. cholerae* O1 El Tor (named after the El Tor quarantine camp on the Sinai peninsula where it was first isolated in pilgrims to Mecca in 1905). El Tor cholera then spread worldwide, replacing the more virulent and lethal classical biotype, and behaving distinctly from the first six pandemics in several respects.

First, the pandemic has been more geographically widespread, including regions where the disease has never been present or has not been present for some time. Although India and Bangladesh have remained seasonally affected by the disease (related to survival of the organism in coastal waters, the rise in sea temperature and the consequent increase in phytoplankton densities), the range of countries affected has far exceeded that of previous pandemics, with an increasing number showing disease that has become endemic. Second, the spatial pattern of outbreaks has not been linear. Major outbreaks have occurred, for example in South America (1991–94), South Africa (2000–01), Angola (2005), Iraq (2007–08) and Zimbabwe (2008–09). Third, the seventh pandemic has been the longest in duration to date, eclipsing the longest previous – sixth – pandemic (24 years).

Although the less virulent nature of El Tor cholera has contributed to its spread and persistence worldwide (as less serious illness allows a greater mobility of human hosts and an enhanced ability to infect others over a longer period of time), environmental factors have been fundamentally important. In relation to the natural environment, there is some evidence that global climate change may be a significant factor in the epidemiology of cholera. In relation to the South American outbreak of the early 1990s, warmer temperatures caused by El Niño may have led to higher than average phytoplankton blooms upon which zooplankton feed. A proliferation of zooplankton may, in turn, have resulted in an increased number of vibrios. The result may have been an infectious load of *V. cholerae* that can infect people who drink fresh water inhabited with zooplankton or contaminated seafood. As Belkin and Colwell write, 'The disease cholera can no longer be considered a simple equation of bacteria and human host, but represents a complex network that includes global weather patterns, aquatic reservoirs, phages, zooplankton, collective behaviour of surface-attached cells, an adaptable genome, and the deep sea inter alia.'[7]

Human impacts on the natural environment remain central to understanding why and where cholera outbreaks occur. In the Celebes Islands of Indonesia, an overpopulation of urban peripheries, military operations and other human disturbances of the environment, along with certain cultural practices (e.g. the use of night soil), are believed to have led to the initial cholera outbreak of the early 1960s. From South-East Asia, El Tor cholera spread further afield wherever human populations overstressed their social and natural environments. There are also suggestions that worldwide transmission is due to the large scale transport of water via ships' ballast.

This close relationship between cholera and the environment remains most evident in countries where political and economic instability have undermined basic living standards along with public health capacities. This may be due to conflict (e.g. Angola and Iraq), economic transition (e.g. the former Soviet Union) or the introduction of policies that undermine access (e.g. South Africa). In South Africa, for example, the worst cholera epidemic in the country's recorded history began in 2000 resulting in some 106 151 cases and approximately 232 deaths primarily in KwaZulu-Natal province. The outbreak was also subsequently linked to others in neighbouring countries, notably Mozambique, Swaziland and Zambia, accounting for 73 per cent of Africa's entire cholera cases that year.[8]

Demonstrating how political decisions can negatively impact on environmental management practices, the cause of South Africa's cholera epidemic has been widely attributed to the privatization of the country's water industry.[9] Following the collapse of the Apartheid regime in 1994, the newly elected South African government sought the assistance of the World Bank and other international financial institutions such as the International Monetary Fund in the rebuilding of the country.[10,11] One of the key recommendations of the World Bank was to encourage private investment,[12] which informed the government's adoption of the Growth, Employment & Redistribution (GEAR) policy in 1996.[13] In accordance with GEAR, barriers to certain public services such as water and sanitation were removed to encourage private

investment and thereby the 'self-sustainability' of these services.[14]

In 1997, the KwaZulu-Natal provincial authorities initiated a programme to install a purified 'pay-as-you-use' water service based on the full-cost recovery principles of GEAR. In addition, while the new service was reportedly an improvement on the existing (free) system of nine communal taps and a series of boreholes (that were later removed), the new system was installed without sufficient community consultation. On top of that, the new system increased the costs associated with obtaining fresh water, adding to community dissatisfaction. Resistance to the new system then grew even further as the company installing the new service experienced a number of difficulties, and when the new water service broke down entirely for a 3 week period in August 2000, leaving whole communities without access to clean water, residents had little option but to source water from a local river – later identified to be the source of the outbreak.

Another example is the 2008–09 outbreak in Zimbabwe, where cholera has been an annual occurrence for more than a decade.[15] Although the frequency of these outbreaks has been an ongoing concern, the number of people affected each year has, by and large, been relatively small. The epidemic of cholera that commenced in August 2008, however, was substantively different, spreading throughout the entire country to infect more than 98 424 people (4276 deaths).[16]

In the decade leading up to the epidemic, Zimbabwe was a country with significant political turmoil and economic instability.[17] This instability, in turn, decimated the country's infrastructure, including its sewage systems and water supplies. Coupled with a lack of refuse collection, due to power cuts and fuel shortages,[18] an environment has been created in which infectious disease can flourish. Added to this, the country's health system has also progressively deteriorated due to severe financial constraints, declining infrastructure and, with inflation reaching 231 million per cent, an inability to procure essential medicines, supplies and equipment.[19] Correspondingly, as the epidemic spread, the health system was inadequately prepared to respond. The outbreak has not only been the worst epidemic in Zimbabwe's history, but has also been the single most devastating cholera epidemic in Africa to date.

The ease with which cholera can spread across national boundaries is one of the key reasons why effective global health governance is crucial in containing infectious diseases. The World Health Organization (WHO) is central to this work, coordinating international outbreak responses to prevent diseases such as cholera from spreading. Historically, lower-income countries that lack an adequate infrastructure are particularly at risk and, on average, experience a higher proportion of cholera outbreaks than middle- and high-income countries. The actions (or inaction) of one country in containing an outbreak of cholera can, however, have widespread implications for others. In recognition of this fact, cholera remains a disease subject to the revised International Health Regulations (2005). Under the terms of this treaty, national authorities are required to assess every outbreak of cholera for its potential to spread beyond their borders and notify the WHO accordingly.[20] Although underreporting is acknowledged to be an ongoing problem owing to concerns over trade and travel sanctions, it has in recent years regrettably been African countries that have continued to report the highest number of cholera cases worldwide.[21] In 2005, for instance, 31 (78 per cent) of the 40 countries that notified the WHO of indigenous cholera cases were located within Sub-Saharan Africa. Some 14 of those West African countries accounted for 58 per cent of the world's cholera cases.[22]

CONCLUSION

Although improved medical knowledge, a basic infrastructure and the availability of effective treatments have somewhat tempered fears of cholera in the industrialized world, the disease remains a harbinger of deterioration in social and natural environments. During the twentieth century, cholera was removed as a serious threat in developed countries as a result of access to clean water and sanitation. Where such conditions remain absent, where the social and natural environments become overstressed by human activities, or where access to life-saving treatments such as oral rehydration therapy is inadequate,[23] cholera remains a much-feared risk.

ACKNOWLEDGEMENTS

This research has been made possible through funding from the European Research Council under the European Community's Seventh Framework Programme – Ideas Grant 230489. All the views expressed remain those of the authors.

REFERENCES

◆ = Major review article
● = Key primary paper

◆1. Nalibow Ruxin J. Magic bullet: The history of oral rehydration therapy. *Med Hist* 1994; **38**: 363–97.
2. Schoolnik GK, Yildiz FH. The complete genome sequence of *Vibrio cholerae*: A tale of two chromosomes and of two lifestyles. *Genome Biol* 2000; **1**: REVIEWS1016.
●3. Watts S. Cholera and civilization: Great Britain and India, 1817 to 1920. In: Watts S (ed.) *Epidemics and History, Disease, Power and Imperialism* (pp. 167–212). New Haven: Yale University Press, 1997.
4. Bray RS. *Armies of Pestilence. The Effects of Pandemics in History.* Cambridge: Lutterworth Press, 1996.
5. Lee K. The global dimensions of cholera. *Glob Change Hum Health* 2001; **2**: 2–15.
●6. Speck RS. Cholera. In: Kiple F (ed.) *The Cambridge World History of Human Diseases.* Cambridge: Cambridge University Press, 1993: 642–8.
◆7. Belkin S, Colwell R. *Global Microbial Ecology of* Vibrio cholerae. New York: Springer, 2006.
8. World Health Organization. Cholera, 2001. *Wkly Epidemiol Rec* 2002; **77**: 257–68.
9. Pauw J. The politics of underdevelopment: Metered to death – how a water experiment caused riots and a cholera epidemic. *Int J Health Serv* 2003; **33**: 819–30.
10. World Bank. *South Africa Country Assistance Strategy: Building a Knowledge Partnership.* South Africa: World Bank, 1999.
11. Padayachee V. Debt, development and democracy: The IMF in post-Apartheid South Africa. *Rev Afr Polit Econ* 1994; **21**: 585–97.
12. World Bank. *South Africa Economic Performance and Policies: Discussion Paper.* South Africa: World Bank, 1994.
13. McKinley DT. The struggle against water privatization in South Africa. In: Balanya B, Brennan B, Hoedeman O, Kishimoto S, Terhorst P (eds) *Reclaiming Public Water: Achievements, Struggles and Visions from Around the World.* Amsterdam: Transnational Institute and Corporate Europe Observatory, 2005: 181–9.
14. Deedat H, Cottle E. Cost recovery and prepaid water meters and the cholera outbreak in KwaZulu-Natal. In: McDonald DA, Pape J (eds) *Cost Recovery and the Crisis of Service Delivery in South Africa.* London: HSRC Publishers, 2002: 81–97.
15. World Health Organization. Cholera Country Profile: Zimbabwe (6 March 2009). *Global Task Force on Cholera Control.* Geneva: WHO, 2009.
16. World Health Organization. Cholera in Zimbabwe – update 4. *Disease Outbreak News* 9 June 2009. Available from: http://www.who.int/csr/don/2009_06_09/en (accessed January 4, 2010).
17. Human Rights Watch. Zimbabwe: Fast track land reform in Zimbabwe. *Hum Rights Watch* 2002; **14**: 8–10.
18. Chambers K. Zimbabwe's battle against cholera. *Lancet* 2009; **373**: 993.
19. Mason PR. Zimbabwe experiences the worst epidemic of cholera in Africa. *J Infect Dev Ctries* 2009; **3**: 148.
20. World Health Organization. *International Health Regulations, Annex 2,* 2nd edn. Geneva: WHO, 2005.
21. Bhattacharya S, Black R, Bourgeois L *et al.* The cholera crisis in Africa. *Science* 2009; **324**: 885.
22. World Health Organization. Cholera 2005. *Wkly Epidemiol Rec* 2006; **31**: 297.
●23. Guerrant RL, Carneiro-Filho A, Dillingham RA. Cholera, diarrhea, and oral rehydration therapy: Triumph and indictment. *Clin Infect Dis* 2003; **37**: 398–405.

34

Human health risks from toxic cyanobacteria, dinoflagellates and diatoms

GORDON NICHOLS

There are a diverse range of freshwater and seawater microorganisms that produce potent toxins capable of causing both acute and chronic disease in mammals, including man. With many of these toxic algae, dinoflagellates and diatoms, exposure is commonly to a mixture of species, each of which can produce a variety of toxins. As a consequence, the combination of symptoms can be different between incidents.

These microbes have evolved potent toxins to survive and reproduce within their aquatic niches, but many dinoflagellate species, when present in sufficient numbers, can cause substantial fish loss. There are a number of species that have not been associated with human disease but have either been shown to produce potent toxins in the laboratory or been implicated in disease in animals, that are potentially able to cause human disease. There are also blooms of some known toxic species that do not produce toxin. Some of the toxins are very much more toxic by the intravenous or intraperitoneal route in experimental mice than when given orally.

CYANOBACTERIA (BLUE-GREEN ALGAE)

Cyanobacteria commonly grow as blooms or mats within freshwater bodies, being more commonly found in eutrophic inland waters (eutrophic waters having a high concentration of nutrients).

Human health risks can arise if heavily contaminated water is consumed untreated, if people bathe or participate in water contact sports in waters with a scum or heavy bloom, and particularly if contaminated water is used in renal dialysis. There have been some notable outbreaks of

disease associated with cyanobacterial toxins with a high mortality rate in dialysis patients. There are also associations between exposure to cyanobacterial toxins through drinking contaminated water and long-term health risks including cancer.

Microcystis aeruginosa is one of the most common cyanobacterium species found in eutrophic waters. Blooms and scums of this species are typically highly toxic due to the production of a family of microcystin toxins. These are hepatotoxic tumour promoters. *Microcystis* can cause hepatic failure in man and a wide range of other animals, as well as diarrhoea. Associations have been found between drinking water contaminated with *M. aeruginosa* in New South Wales, Australia, and raised liver enzymes in the population, as well as between drinking microcystin-contaminated water and primary liver cancer in China.

Cylindrospermopsis raciborskii includes strains that produce the potent hepato- and genotoxin cylindrospermopsin. Palm Island Mystery Disease in Queensland, Australia caused 140 children to be hospitalized with a variety of symptoms including malaise, anorexia, vomiting, headache, painful liver enlargement and constipation followed by bloody diarrhoea and kidney damage. Water from a dam contaminated with *C. raciborskii* was thought to have been responsible.

Anabaena spp. have caused liver damage and deaths in waterfowl, sheep, cattle and other agricultural animals. The genus *Anabaena* includes species that can produce saxitoxins, microcystins, anatoxin a and anatoxin-a(s). As with other cyanobacterial genera, the production of individual classes of these toxins is not uniform, and variations occur. *Vibrio cholerae* has been found to survive for long periods inside the sheath material of *A. variabilis*.

Oscillatoria **spp.** are freshwater cyanobacteria that produce anatoxin-a, which can cause neurotoxicity leading to respiratory failure. The consumption of water contaminated with the toxin has been associated with acute respiratory failure and death in dogs and waterbirds. In surface water, *Oscillatoria* spp. are often present in mixtures with other cyanobacteria.

Nodularia spumigena has caused fatalities of cattle, sheep, dogs and waterfowl via oral exposure. This illness is thought to be due to nodularin, another potent hepatotoxin, which has carcinogenic and tumour-promoting actions.

Phormidium favosum produces anatoxin-a and has been associated with neurotoxicosis in dogs. Toxin-producing strains have been found in water from reservoirs in Australia and several lakes in Scotland where dog deaths attributed to anatoxin-a have occurred.

Other freshwater species include *Aphanizomenon* spp., *Planktothrix* spp., *Raphidiopsis mediterranea*, *Anabaenopsis milleri*, *Anacystis nidulans*, *Cylindrospermum* spp. and *Umezakia natans*, a cyanobacterium from Japanese waters. *Nostoc* spp. are cyanobacteria that can grow as symbionts within plant roots. The amino acid beta-methylamino L-alanine produced by *Nostoc* spp. has been implicated in the neurological disease amyotrophic lateral sclerosis and Parkinsonism–dementia complex found in Guam. Several *Nostoc* species grow in symbiotic associations with fungi, to form lichens, and with representatives of each of the major phylogenetic groups of plants.

Marine cyanobacteria are less common. *Trichodesmium erythraeum* is a marine cyanobacterium that is reported to produce a neurotoxin and hepatotoxin related to, if not identical with, microcystin. It has also been suggested that these organisms may contribute to some ciguatera toxin accumulation in fish. Debromoaplysiatoxin has been isolated from *Lyngbya gracilis* and has dermonecrotic activity; it may be the dermatitis-producing substance in *L. majuscula*, the causative agent of outbreaks of 'swimmers' itch' in Hawaiian waters.

DINOFLAGELLATES AND DIATOMS

Dinoflagellates and diatoms are protozoan organisms that can produce a range of potent toxins. They occur predominantly in saltwater and can, under the right conditions, produce blooms in seawater ('red tides'), potentially causing toxic effects in fish and other sea life. The toxins can accumulate within shellfish and in fish, where they are concentrated up the food chain, resulting in some carnivorous fish that are toxic to man and cause ciguatera poisoning, clupeotoxism and palytoxin poisoning. There are a number of types of shellfish poisoning that result from the accumulation of the toxins of dinoflagellates or diatoms within shellfish, including paralytic shellfish poisoning (PSP), diarrhoeic shellfish poisoning (DSP), amnesic shellfish poisoning (ASP), neurotoxic shellfish poisoning (NSP), and azaspiracid shellfish poisoning

(AZP) (see also chapter 23). Not all blooms form red tides, not all red tides are toxic, and not all dinoflagellate-related disease is linked to blooms. However, some blooms can occasionally cause symptoms in bathers.

A number of different organisms in this group are toxic or potentially toxic.

Dinophysis **spp.** are dinoflagellates that form red tides and cause DSP through the accumulation of the toxins, particularly okadaic acid and its derivatives, in bivalve molluscs.

Prorocentrum **spp.**, notably *P. borbonicum*, produce compounds (probably neurotoxic) that can be fatal in mice, and while other species are of questionable toxicity, *P. minimum* extracts are toxic to mice and molluscs, while *P. arabianum* produces two cytotoxic compounds, one of which is fatal to fish.

Alexandrium **spp.** are dinoflagellates that form blooms in seawater and cause PSP and can cause mass fish kills. *Gymnodinium catenatum* is responsible for red tides as well as high mortality in fish, and also produces PSP toxin and causes human disease. The dinoflagellate *Pyrodinium* spp. can cause red tides, and *Pyrodinium bahamense* var. *compressa* has also been implicated in PSP. Bivalve molluscs, crabs and snails that feed on coral reef seaweed can concentrate NSP toxin.

Karenia **spp.** are toxin-producing dinoflagellates that produce red tides and can cause NSP associated with the consumption of shellfish. They can also cause high mortality in fish, invertebrates, marine animals and plants, as well as respiratory distress and eye and skin irritation in humans. Most species produce brevetoxin in culture.

Nitzschia **spp. and** *Pseudo-nitzschia* **spp.** are diatoms that cause ASP through the production of the neurotoxin domoic acid. Symptoms include dizziness, nausea, vomiting, cramps, diarrhoea, headache, seizures, disorientation, short-term memory loss, respiratory difficulty and coma. Blooms of *Pseudo-nitzschia australis* have been implicated in the deaths of fish and sea lions. *Nitzschia navis-varingica* are diatoms that produce domoic acid, and outbreaks of ASP in humans have been attributed to the consumption of contaminated mussels. *Amphora coffeaeformis* is another diatom that produces domoic acid, but its role in human disease is unclear.

Protoperidinium crassipes is a dinoflagellate that produces azaspiracid, which gives DSP-like symptoms in humans but a mixture of DSP-and neurotoxin-like effects in mice. This toxin is the cause of AZP.

Pfiesteria piscicida is a dinoflagellate that resides in estuarine waters and is responsible for mass fish kills. It has been associated with skin and neurological problems in humans exposed to the toxins under the name of 'possible estuary-associated syndrome'. *Pfiesteria shumwayae* can cause mass fish kills in estuarine waters, but no human illness has yet been associated with this organism.

Hematodinium **spp.** are dinoflagellates that cause bitter crab disease and pink crab disease in crabs, making them

Table 34.1 The toxins of cyanobacteria, diatoms and dinoflagellates

Toxin group	Primary target in mammals	Group (toxin-producing genus)
1,5-norlyngbyapeptin A	Unknown	Cyanobacteria (*Lyngbya*)
Anatoxin-a	Neurotoxic	Cyanobacteria (*Anabaena, Aphanizomenon, Phormidium, Planktothrix, Oscillatoria*)
Anatoxin-a (s)	Neurotoxic	Cyanobacteria (*Anabaena*)
Antillatoxins A and B	Neurotoxic	Cyanobacteria (*Lyngbya*)
Aplysiatoxins	Skin	Cyanobacteria (*Lyngbya, Planktothrix, Oscillatoria, Schizothriix*)
Azaspiracid	Gastrointestinal, organ damage (AZP)	Dinoflagellates (*Protoperidinium*)
Beta-methylaminoalanine	Neurotoxic	Cyanobacteria (All)
Brevetoxin	Neurotoxic, partial paralysis, respiratory distress, eye irritation, skin irritation (NSP)	Dinoflagellates (*Karenia*)
Ciguatoxin	Gastrointestinal, neurological, muscle pain, paraesthesia	Dinoflagellates (*Amphidinium, Coolia, Gonyaulax, Ostreopsis, Prorocentrum, Gambierdiscus*)
Cylindrospermopsins	Liver	Cyanobacteria (*Aphanizomenon, Cylindrospermopsis, Phormidium, Umezakia*)
Decarbamoylsaxitoxin	Neurotoxic	Dinoflagellates (*Gymnodinium*)
Dinophysistoxins 1 and 2	Gastrointestinal (DSP)	Dinoflagellates (*Dinophysis, Prorocentrum*)
Gonyautoxin	Neurotoxic	Dinoflagellates (*Gonyaulax*)
Goniodomin A	Liver	Dinoflagellates (*Alexandrium*)
Homoanatoxin-a	Neurotoxic	Cyanobacteria (*Anabaena, Phormidium, Oscillatoria*)
Kalkitoxin	Neurotoxic	Cyanobacteria (*Lyngbya*)
Lipopolysaccharides	Potentially irritant affecting any exposed tissue	Cyanobacteria (All)
Lyngbyabellin D	Cytotoxin	Cyanobacteria (*Lyngbya*)
Lyngbyatoxin-a	Skin, gastrointestinal	Cyanobacteria (*Lyngbya*)
Maitotoxin	Haemolysin, cytotoxin, neurotoxin	Dinoflagellates (*Amphidinium, Coolia, Gonyaulax, Ostreopsis, Prorocentrum, Gambierdiscus*)
Malyngamide T	Toxic to fish (unknown toxicity to mammals)	Cyanobacteria (*Lyngbya*)
Mascarenotoxins A and B	Gastrointestinal, neurotoxic	Dinoflagellates (*Ostreopsis*)
Microcystins	Liver	Cyanobacteria (*Anabaena, Anabaenopsis, Hapalosiphon, Microcystis, Nostoc, Phormidium, Planktothrix, Oscillatoria*)
Neosaxitoxin	Neurotoxic	Dinoflagellates (*Alexandrium*)
Nodularin	Liver	Cyanobacteria (*Nodularia*)
Okadaic acid	Gastrointestinal (DSP)	Dinoflagellates (*Prorocentrum*)
Ostreocin D	Neurotoxin	Dinoflagellates (*Ostreopsis*)
Palau'amide	Cytotoxic	Cyanobacteria (*Lyngbya*)
Palytoxin	Haemolysin, cytotoxin, neurotoxin (clupeotoxism)	Dinoflagellates (*Ostreopsis*)
Pectenotoxin-2	Liver	Dinoflagellates (*Dinophysis*)
Prorocentrolide	Fast-acting toxin lethal to mice	Dinoflagellates (*Prorocentrum*)
Saxitoxins*	Neurotoxic (PSP)	Cyanobacteria (*Anabaena, Aphanizomenon, Cylindrospermopsis, Phormidium, Planktothrix, Lyngbya*) Dinoflagellates (*Alexandrium, Gymnodynium*)
Spirolide	Neurotoxic	Dinoflagellates (*Alexandrium*)
Yessotoxin	Neurotoxin	Dinoflagellates (*Protoceratium, Lingulodinium, Gonyaulax*)

See text for abbreviations.
*Saxitoxins are also found in puffer fish.

unpalatable. There is little evidence for a health risk associated with the consumption of infected crabs. A variety of other species are potentially toxic, but their role in human disease remains unclear. Examples are *Heterocapsa circularisquama*, which forms red tides and can cause mass fish kills, and *Protoceratium reticulatum*, which produces yessotoxin that may accumulate in bivalves and is toxic to mice.

Ciguatera food poisoning

Dinoflagellate species including *Ostreopsis* spp., *Gonyaulax* and *Gambierdiscus* cause ciguatera poisoning in people who have eaten fish and shellfish contaminated by the toxins they produce. Ciguatera food poisoning produces gastrointestinal, neurological and cardiovascular symptoms, including diarrhoea, vomiting, abdominal pain, reversal of temperature sensation, muscular aches, dizziness, anxiety, sweating, and a numbness and tingling of the mouth and digits. The contamination occurs due to the accumulation of toxins as they pass up the food chain, and large predatory fish growing in tropical waters can contain dangerous amounts of toxin. Ciguatera poisoning is a particular problem in carnivorous finfish (e.g. barracuda and grouper) in tropical and subtropical waters.

Gambierdiscus spp. produce ciguatoxin or maitotoxin, which acts by activating voltage-dependent sodium and calcium channels, respectively, by indirect membrane depolarization.

Ostreopsis lenticularis is the presumed vector of ciguatera poisoning in the Caribbean. *Ostreopsis siamensis* is a benthic dinoflagellate that produces ostreocin D, a palytoxin analogue. It has been implicated in clupeotoxism, a fatal form of human intoxication due to the ingestion of clupeoid fish (sardines, anchovies and herring). *Ostreopsis mascarenensis* may be responsible for palytoxin poisoning, which in humans results in cramps, nausea, diarrhoea, etc., after eating of crabs and certain fish. *Ostreopsis ovata* is also a toxin producer and has been associated with the toxic effects of bathing in a bloom of this organism (nausea, breathing difficulties, high fever, stomach cramps, irritation of the eyes, vomiting and diarrhoea) in Italy.

CONCLUSION

The wide range of potent toxins found in these aquatic microbes might put many people off bathing in natural waters and eating fish and shellfish. However, the risks from cyanobacteria, dinoflagellates and diatoms are confined to particular situations. They do not usually appear as major public health issues in developed countries, although outbreaks do occur. The increase in foreign travel and the global sourcing of food means that exposure may increase. Shellfish toxins are controlled by monitoring

shellfish beds that have exhibited problems in the past, and well-managed drinking water treatment can remove cyanobacteria and their toxins. The consumption of fish such as barracuda that can be subject to ciguatera toxin accumulation is controlled by import restrictions and is primarily a problem with tropical waters. However, this remains an emerging area, and the burden of acute and chronic disease in developing countries remains unclear.

REFERENCES

♦ = Major review article

1. Burgess V, Shaw G. Pectenotoxins – an issue for public health: a review of their comparative toxicology and metabolism. *Environ Int* 2001; **27**: 275–83.
2. Camargo JA, Alonso A. Ecological and toxicological effects of inorganic nitrogen pollution in aquatic ecosystems: a global assessment. *Environ Int* 2006; **32**: 831–49.
3. Dittmann E, Wiegand C. Cyanobacterial toxins – occurrence, biosynthesis and impact on human affairs. *Mol Nutr Food Res* 2006; **50**: 7–17.
♦4. Funari E, Testai E. Human health risk assessment related to cyanotoxins exposure. *Crit Rev Toxicol* 2008; **38**: 97–125.
5. Haider S, Naithani V, Viswanathan PN, Kakkar P. Cyanobacterial toxins: a growing environmental concern. *Chemosphere* 2003; **52**: 1–21.
6. Mos L. Domoic acid: a fascinating marine toxin. *Environ Toxicol Pharmacol* 2001; **9**: 79–85.
7. Papapetropoulos S. Is there a role for naturally occurring cyanobacterial toxins in neurodegeneration? The beta-N-methylamino-L-alanine (BMAA) paradigm. *Neurochem Int* 2007; **50**(7–8): 998–1003.
8. Pearson LA, Neilan BA. The molecular genetics of cyanobacterial toxicity as a basis for monitoring water quality and public health risk. *Curr Opin Biotechnol* 2008; **19**: 281–8.
9. Schmidt W, Bornmann K, Imhof L, Mankiewicz J, Izydorczyk K. Assessing drinking water treatment systems for safety against cyanotoxin breakthrough using maximum tolerable values. *Environ Toxicol* 2008; **23**: 337–45.
10. Stewart I, Seawright AA, Shaw GR. Cyanobacterial poisoning in livestock, wild mammals and birds – an overview. *Adv Exp Med Biol* 2008; **619**: 613–37.
11. Swinker M, Tester P, Koltai AD, Schmechel D. Human health effects of exposure to *Pfiesteria piscicida*: a review. *Microbes Infect* 2002; **4**: 751–62.
♦12. Wang DZ. Neurotoxins from marine dinoflagellates: a brief review. *Mar Drugs* 2008; **6**: 349–71.
13. Watkins SM, Reich A, Fleming LE, Hammond R. Neurotoxic shellfish poisoning. *Mar Drugs* 2008; **6**: 431–55.
♦14. Zurawell RW, Chen H, Burke JM, Prepas EE. Hepatotoxic cyanobacteria: a review of the biological importance of microcystins in freshwater environments. *J Toxicol Environ Health B Crit Rev* 2005; **8**: 1–37.

35

Enteric viruses

JIM GRAY, MIREN ITURRIZA-GÓMARA

Enteric virus infections are responsible for a considerable burden of disease worldwide, and the associated mortality is particularly significant in young children. The incidence of rotavirus gastroenteritis is similar in both industrialized and developing countries, suggesting that improvements in water supply, hygiene and sanitation have little impact on the incidence of rotavirus infection. Although every child throughout the world will have experienced at least one rotavirus infection by the age of 5, the mortality associated with infection is concentrated in developing countries, with over 600 000 children dying per year as a result of dehydration associated with rotavirus infection.[1]

In an epidemic in Taiwan associated with enterovirus 71 in 1998, physicians reported 129 106 cases of hand, foot and mouth disease, or herpangina, 405 patients having severe disease characterized by encephalitis, aseptic meningitis, acute flaccid paralysis or myocarditis. Ninety-one per cent of the 71 patients who died were 5 years of age or younger.[2]

The burden of disease associated with norovirus infection is high in children, and outbreaks of gastroenteritis among adults are common. Outbreaks in semi-closed communities such as hospitals, nursing homes and care homes are associated with ward closures, staff illness, reductions in planned admissions and a restriction on patient movement. This places a considerable burden on health resources, and it is estimated to cost the National Health Service in England in excess of £100 million per year.[3]

Epidemics of hepatitis in tropical and subtropical counties and associated with hepatitis E virus infection are predominantly waterborne. The size of the outbreaks can be considerable, with tens of thousands affected. The death rate is 0.5–3.0 per cent in young adults and 15–20 per cent in pregnant women.[4]

Enteric viruses are commonly transmitted among infants and young children, and immunity from disease is associated with multiple infections. Asymptomatic infection in children is common, and young adults are often infected by their own children and may present with symptoms.

Viruses infecting the gut, such as rotaviruses, noroviruses, sapoviruses, astroviruses, enteric adenoviruses and kobuviruses, are often associated with sporadic cases and outbreaks of gastroenteritis. Enteroviruses, including polioviruses, coxsackieviruses, echoviruses, parechoviruses and enterovirus 71, are associated with systemic infections with symptoms ranging from asymptomatic infection, mild respiratory illness and rash illness to aseptic meningitis, poliomyelitis and neonatal multiorgan failure (Table 35.1). Hepatitis A and E viruses are spread via the faeco-oral route and may result in outbreaks of acute hepatitis if transmission is associated with environmental contamination (Table 35.1). Other viruses such as toroviruses, coronaviruses, parvoviruses, bocavirus and picobirnaviruses, have been found in the human gut, but their role in enteric disease has yet to be confirmed.

Enteric viruses can be transmitted directly through contact with human excreta or the ingestion of contaminated drinking water or vegetables, shellfish or other foods exposed to contaminated water or soil. Food may be contaminated in the growing area before harvest, by field workers during harvest or by infected food handlers during food preparation.[5]

The accidental ingestion of contaminated water during swimming or recreational activities and contact with surfaces contaminated with vomitus or human excreta are also associated with the transmission of enteric viruses. In swimming pools, the infection risk is related to the quality

Table 35.1 Enteric viruses transmitted through the ingestion of contaminated food or water or through contact with contaminated surfaces or infected people

Virus	Family	Genome	Symptoms	Incubation period	Duration of illness†	Detection				Characterization
						Clinical sample	Food	Water	Environment	
Rotavirus	*Reoviridae*	Segmented dsRNA	Gastroenteritis Encephalopathy	2 days	3–8 days	EM or EIA RT-PCR	RT-PCR	RT-PCR	RT-PCR	RT-PCR Sequencing
Norovirus	*Caliciviridae*	ssRNA pos sense	Gastroenteritis	24–48 hours	12–60 hours	RT-PCR	RT-PCR	RT-PCR	RT-PCR	Sequencing
Sapovirus	*Caliciviridae*	ssRNA pos sense	Gastroenteritis	24–36 hours	1–4 days	RT-PCR	RT-PCR	RT-PCR	RT-PCR	Sequencing
Astrovirus	*Astroviridae*	ssRNA pos sense	Gastroenteritis	24–36 hours	1–4 days	RT-PCR	RT-PCR	RT-PCR	RT-PCR	Sequencing
Enteric adenovirus	*Adenoviridae*	dsDNA	Gastroenteritis	3–10 days	>7 days	EIA or PCR	PCR	PCR	PCR	Sequencing
Kobuvirus	*Picornaviridae*	ssRNA pos sense	Travellers' diarrhoea	24–48 hours	2–4 days	RT-PCR	RT-PCR	RT-PCR	RT-PCR	Sequencing
Coxsackie A viruses	*Picornaviridae*	ssRNA pos sense	Meningitis, HFM	3–10 days	2–10 days	RT-PCR	RT-PCR	RT-PCR	RT-PCR	Sequencing
Coxsackie B viruses	*Picornaviridae*	ssRNA pos sense	Meningitis, myocarditis	3–10 days	2–10 days	Cell culture or RT-PCR	Cell culture or RT-PCR	Cell culture or RT-PCR	Cell culture or RT-PCR	Neutralization or Sequencing
Echoviruses	*Picornaviridae*	ssRNA pos sense	Meningitis	3–10 days	2–10 days	Cell culture or RT-PCR	Cell culture or RT-PCR	Cell culture or RT-PCR	Cell culture or RT-PCR	Neutralization or Sequencing
Polioviruses	*Picornaviridae*	ssRNA pos sense	Poliomyelitis, meningitis	3–10 days	2–10 days*	Cell culture or RT-PCR	Cell culture or RT-PCR	Cell culture or RT-PCR	RT-PCR	Neutralization or Sequencing
Enterovirus 71	*Picornaviridae*	ssRNA pos sense	Meningitis, HFM, AFP	3–10 days	7–10 days	RT-PCR	RT-PCR	RT-PCR	RT-PCR	Sequencing
Hepatitis A	*Picornaviridae*	ssRNA pos sense	Hepatitis	10–50 days	36–391 days	RT-PCR or Serology	RT-PCR	RT-PCR	RT-PCR	Sequencing
Hepatitis E	*Caliciviridae*	ssRNA pos sense	Hepatitis	10–60 days	20 days	RT-PCR or Serology	RT-PCR	RT-PCR	RT-PCR	Sequencing

AFP, acute flaccid paralysis; ds, double-stranded; EIA, enzyme immunoassay; EM, electron microscopy; HFM, hand, foot and mouth disease; pos sense, positive sense; RT-PCR, reverse transcription-polymerase chain reaction; ss, single-stranded.

†Virus may still be excreted for some days after the illness has resolved

*Poliomyelitis symptoms lasting more than 6 months are significantly associated with permanent neuronal damage.

of the water source, the pool design including drainage and filters, the operation and maintenance and type of water treatment and most importantly disinfection. Risk is also influenced by the age, health and hygiene of the bathers, their number and the duration of use each day. The quality of recreational waters such as river and seawater is influenced by run-off from animal waste, annual rainfall, storm surges, upstream sewage treatment and the presence of sea outfalls.[6]

Patterns of gastrointestinal disease include endemic diarrhoea, which occurs in children and is predominantly associated with rotaviruses, adenoviruses, noroviruses, sapoviruses and astroviruses. However, epidemic viral gastroenteritis affects both children and adults and is primarily associated with noroviruses worldwide, and often with an identifiable source of contamination such as water, food or the environment. Disease transmission may be associated with the ability of the virus to survive for prolonged periods of time in the environment, the low infectious dose required, a lack of long-term protective immunity and, in the case of rotavirus, the ability to infect across the species barrier.

VIRUS DETECTION AND CHARACTERIZATION

Viruses in clinical samples can be detected through their growth in susceptible mammalian cell cultures, by the detection of virus-specific antigens or through detection of the virus genome. Virus particles in water, food or the environment are present in much lower concentrations, and samples need to be subjected to pre-treatment in order to purify and concentrate the virus before detection methods can be applied. Some viruses replicate poorly or not at all in mammalian cell cultures and so are more usually detected by molecular methods. It is important to note that, unlike cell culture, molecular methods do not determine the viability of the virus particles.

The polymerase chain reaction (PCR) and reverse transcription (RT)-PCR are highly sensitive and specific methods used to detect DNA and RNA virus genomes, respectively, and have sensitivities ranging between 10 and 10 000 genome copies. It should be noted that, with infectious doses of around 10–100 virus particles for norovirus and rotavirus, RT-PCR may be negative in the presence of a significant number of contaminating virus particles.

The detection of viruses in food and water samples is hampered by the need to remove toxins and bacteria that may interfere with cell culture systems, as well as inhibitors of PCR that may produce false-negative results in molecular assays. There is also a need to concentrate large sample volumes in order to maximize the recovery of virus particles. Purification is often associated with immobilizing the virus particles on charged or antibody-coated surfaces, allowing the removal, by washing, of particulate matter, bacteria and toxins, followed by elution of the virus particles and concentration by precipitation

Table 35.2 Methods used for food preparation prior to virus isolation and/or genome detection

Food	Methods used	Reference
Vegetables	Elution with glycine buffer and microfiltration	30
Tomato sauce	Acidic adsorption, elution and concentration	31
Strawberries	Acidic adsorption, elution and concentration	32
Oysters	Acidic adsorption, elution, polyethylene glycol precipitation, threonine–chloroform extraction	33
Oysters	Glycine buffer pH 9.0, polyethylene glycol precipitation, sonication at pH 9.0, adjust to pH 7.4	34
Oysters	Dissect out hepatopancreas, proteinase K treatment, centrifugation	35

and/or centrifugation. Preparation methods for foodstuffs are shown in Table 35.2, and detailed descriptions of methods used for the detection of viruses in water are described in reviews by Wyn-Jones and Sellwood[7] and Fong and Lipp.[8]

FOOD

Food-borne viral pathogens are present in low numbers and may be non-randomly dispersed in food matrices contaminated by a food handler. However, faecal contamination may allow viruses to be incorporated within the food during processing. Outbreaks of gastroenteritis associated with food contaminated with faeces/sewage are often associated with multiple viral pathogens, multiple genotypes of the same virus or a mixture of viral and bacterial pathogens.[9–11] Contamination usually arises during cultivation and is primarily of ready-to-eat foods such as salad vegetables, berries or bivalve molluscs. Food-borne outbreaks reported in the USA in 2006 by the Centers for Disease Control in which the vehicle was identified and with confirmed norovirus aetiologies ($n = 198$) were predominantly associated with the consumption of salad vegetables (36.4 per cent), sandwiches (13.6 per cent), seafood (8.6 per cent) and fruit (7.1 per cent).[12]

WATER

A range of viruses can be isolated from or detected in water. The contamination of swimming pools, swimming holes and bathing beaches by enteroviruses has been associated with outbreaks of viral meningitis.[13–15] Norovirus outbreaks have been associated with recreational waters and activities such as canoeing, with the attendant submersion and swallowing of water being particular risk factors.[16,17] Interestingly, frequent users of recreational waters report fewer episodes of gastroenteritis than novices, which is likely to be associated with the regular boosting of virus-specific immunity.

Survival rates of virus in water are variable and are dependent on temperature, the turbidity of the water and the penetration of ultraviolet light. Poliovirus and hepatitis A virus have been shown to survive for 30 days in seawater with little inactivation at 5 °C but with pronounced decay at 25 °C.[18] Suspended solids hinder the diffusion of virus-inactivating ultraviolet rays, and the presence of cations protects enteroviruses from thermal inactivation. Enteric viruses are inactivated in alkaline solution and in sunlight at wavelengths of below 370 nm.[19]

ENVIRONMENT

Viruses are frequently isolated from environmental surfaces, and their persistence has been associated with prolonging outbreaks. In hospitals, environmental contamination is associated with hand contact, and viruses are found often on light switches, door handles, toilet flush handles, wash hand basin taps, computer keyboards and telephones.[20] Bed curtains, soft furnishings and carpets have also been implicated in harbouring infectious virus.[21]

It should be noted that the asymptomatic excretion of enteric viruses is not uncommon,[22] and a lack of good hygiene practices such as hand-washing will exacerbate environmental contamination. An observational study of carers and child hygiene revealed that child carers washed their hands with soap after changing a dirty nappy on 42 per cent of occasions and that 1 in 5 toilet users did not wash their hands with soap afterwards.[23] The impact of poor hygiene during child care was reflected in the results of the Infectious Intestinal Disease study, which showed a significant incidence of symptomatic and asymptomatic infection with rotavirus (19.5 per cent) and norovirus (25.6 per cent) in young adults 20–29 years of age.[22]

In studies of viral survival, it has been shown that poliovirus, echovirus and coxsackievirus can remain viable for more than 12 days on painted surfaces, glass and cotton. Rotavirus RNA has been found on the surface of a variety of laundry equipment as well as damp textiles and folded laundry.[24] Data on the survival of noroviruses in food, water or the environment are not available as no culture system exists. However, repeated outbreaks in the same location detected as new populations in hotels, on cruise ships, and in military training camps, succumb to gastroenteritis would suggest that this virus is stable in its biological matrix in the environment.[25]

PREVENTION

Enteric viruses are widespread in the population, particularly in young children, and the prevention of transmission of enteric viruses in food, water or the environment is dependent on several factors. Transmission via food could be reduced if high-risk agricultural practices such as the use of sewage sludge or untreated waste water were abandoned and food handlers maintained a good level of hand hygiene. Hepatitis E virus seropositivity was 34.8 per cent in Turkish workers who used untreated waste water in agriculture compared with 4.4 per cent in a non-exposed control group,[26] although this has not been confirmed in studies in other countries.[27] Transmission via water could be interrupted if raw sewage were prevented from entering water courses or the sea. This would also prevent transmission via bivalve molluscs contaminated through sewage passing over shellfish feeding beds. Effective vaccines are available for poliovirus and rotavirus but are live-attenuated oral vaccines, whose delivery in developing countries is problematic.

The inter-relationships between risks associated with norovirus outbreaks in hospitals and the measures adopted to reduce these risks are described in Figure 35.1. The mutability of enteric viruses, the low infectious dose required and the nature of symptoms such as projectile vomiting all contribute to their efficient transmission. Reduced staffing associated with staff illness, high bed occupancy rates, unrestricted visiting and admissions are

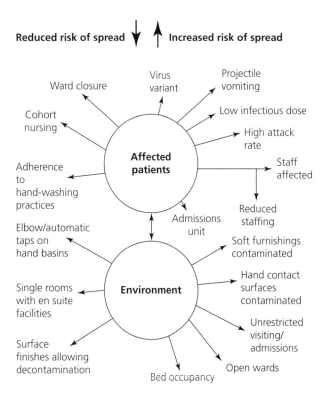

Figure 35.1 Factors associated with increased and reduced risk of spread of enteric viruses in hospitals or semi-closed communities.

likely to prolong an outbreak. Ward closure, cohort nursing and adherence to hand-washing policies will result in fewer staff affected and will reduce the duration of the outbreak.[28,29] Environmental measures such as the provision of elbow or automatic taps on wash basins, single rooms with en suite toilet facilities and surface finishes that allow rapid decontamination may all help to interrupt virus transmission.

REFERENCES

● = Key primary paper

◆ = Major review article

1. Parashar UD, Hummelman EG, Bresee JS, Miller MA, Glass RI. Global illness and deaths caused by rotavirus disease in children. *Emerg Infect Dis* 2003; **9**: 565–72.

2. Ho M, Chen E-R, Hsu K-H *et al.* An epidemic of enterovirus 71 infection in Taiwan. *N Engl J Med* 1999; **341**: 929–35.

3. Lopman BA, Reacher MH, Vipond IB *et al.* Epidemiology and cost of nosocomial gastroenteritis, Avon, England, 2002–2003. *Emerg Infect Dis* 2004; **10**: 1827–34.

◆ 4. Mushahwar IK. Hepatitis E virus: molecular virology, clinical features, diagnosis, transmission, epidemiology and prevention. *J Med Virol* 2008; **80**: 646–58.

5. Iturriza-Gomara M, Gallimore CI, Gray J. Gastroenteric viruses. In: Simjee S (ed.) *Foodborne Diseases* (pp. 215–32). New Jersey: Humana Press, 2007.

6. Schernewski G, Julich WD. Risk assessment of virus infections in the Oder estuary (southern Baltic) on the basis of spatial transport and virus decay simulations. *Int J Hyg Environ Health* 2001; **203**: 317–25.

◆ 7. Wyn-Jones AP, Sellwood J. Enteric viruses in the aquatic environment. *J Appl Microbiol* 2001; **91**: 945–62.

◆ 8. Fong TT, Lipp EK. Enteric viruses of humans and animals in aquatic environments: health risks, detection, and potential water quality assessment tools. *Microbiol Mol Biol Rev* 2005; **69**: 357–71.

● 9. Gallimore CI, Pipkin C, Shrimpton H *et al.* Detection of multiple enteric viruses within a foodborne outbreak of gastroenteritis: an indication of the source of contamination. *Epidemiol Infect* 2005; **134**: 41–7.

10. Gallimore CI, Cheesbrough JS, Lamden K, Bingham C, Gray JJ. Multiple norovirus genotypes characterised from an oyster-associated outbreak of gastroenteritis. *Int J Food Microbiol* 2005; **103**: 323–30.

11. Gallimore CI, Gajraj R, Nye K *et al.* Dual *Salmonella* and norovirus gastroenteritis in linked food outlets caused by contaminated lettuce. Unpublished data. 2003.

12. Centers for Disease Control and Prevention. Outbreak Surveillance Data. Available from: http://www.cdc.gov/foodborneoutbreaks/outbreak_data.htm

13. Aseptic meningitis outbreak associated with echovirus 9 among recreational vehicle campers – Connecticut, 2003. *Morb Mortal Wkly Rep* 2004; **53**: 710–13.

14. Faustini A, Fano V, Muscillo M *et al.* An outbreak of aseptic meningitis due to echovirus 30 associated with attending school and swimming in pools. *Int J Infect Dis* 2006; **10**: 291–7.

15. Hauri AM, Schimmelpfennig M, Walter-Domes M *et al.* An outbreak of viral meningitis associated with a public swimming pond. *Epidemiol Infect* 2005; **133**: 291–8.

●16. Gray JJ, Green J, Cunliffe C *et al.* Mixed genogroup SRSV infections among a party of canoeists exposed to contaminated recreational water. *J Med Virol* 1997; **52**: 425–9.

17. Kappus KD, Marks JS, Holman RC *et al.* An outbreak of Norwalk gastroenteritis associated with swimming in a pool and secondary person-to-person transmission. *Am J Epidemiol* 1982; **116**: 834–9.

◆ 18. Rzezutka A, Cook N. Survival of human enteric viruses in the environment and food. *FEMS Microbiol Rev* 2004; **28**: 441–53.

19. Fujioka RS, Yoneyama BS. Sunlight inactivation of human enteric viruses and fecal bacteria. *Water Sci Technol* 2002; **46**(11–12): 291–5.

● 20. Gallimore CI, Taylor C, Gennery AR *et al.* Environmental monitoring for gastroenteric viruses in a primary immunodeficiency unit. *J Clin Microbiol* 2006; **44**: 395–9.

21. Boone SA, Gerba CP. Significance of fomites in the spread of respiratory and enteric viral disease. *Appl Environ Microbiol* 2007; **73**: 1687–96.

●22. Amar CF, East CL, Gray J, Iturriza-Gomara M, Maclure EA, McLauchlin J. Detection by PCR of eight groups of enteric pathogens in 4,627 faecal samples: re-examination of the English case-control Infectious Intestinal Disease Study (1993–1996). *Eur J Clin Microbiol Infect Dis* 2007; **26**: 311–23.

●23. Curtis V, Biran A, Deverell K, Hughes C, Bellamy K, Drasar B. Hygiene in the home: relating bugs and behaviour. *Soc Sci Med* 2003; **57**: 657–72.

24. Fijan S, Steyer A, Poljsak-Prijatelj M, Cencic A, Sostar-Turk S, Koren S. Rotaviral RNA found on various surfaces in a hospital laundry. *J Virol Methods* 2008; **148**(1–2):66–73.

25. Cheesbrough JS, Green J, Gallimore CI, Wright PA, Brown DW. Widespread environmental contamination with Norwalk-like viruses (NLV) detected in a prolonged hotel outbreak of gastroenteritis. *Epidemiol Infect* 2000; **125**: 93–8.

26. Ceylan A, Ertem M, Ilcin E, Ozekinci T. A special risk group for hepatitis E infection: Turkish agricultural workers who use untreated waste water for irrigation. *Epidemiol Infect* 2003; **131**: 753–6.

27. Jeggli S, Steiner D, Joller H, Tschopp A, Steffen R, Hotz P. Hepatitis E, *Helicobacter pylori*, and gastrointestinal symptoms in workers exposed to waste water. *Occup Environ Med* 2004; **61**: 622–7.

●28. Chadwick PR, Beards G, Brown D *et al.* Management of hospital outbreaks of gastro-enteritis due to small round structured viruses. *J Hosp Infect* 2000; **45**: 1–10.

● 29. Lopman BA, Andrews N, Sarangi J, Vipond IB, Brown DW, Reacher MH. Institutional risk factors for outbreaks of nosocomial gastroenteritis: survival analysis of a cohort of hospital units in South-west England, 2002–2003. *J Hosp Infect* 2005; **60**: 135–43.

30. Le Guyader FS, Schultz AC, Haugarreau L *et al.* Round-robin comparison of methods for the detection of human enteric viruses in lettuce. *J Food Prot* 2004; **67**: 2315–19.

31. Love DC, Casteel MJ, Meschke JS, Sobsey MD. Methods for recovery of hepatitis A virus (HAV) and other viruses from processed foods and detection of HAV by nested RT-PCR and TaqMan RT-PCR. *Int J Food Microbiol* 2008; **126**(1–2): 221–6.

32. Andino R, Rieckhof GE, Achacoso PL, Baltimore D. Poliovirus RNA synthesis utilizes an RNP complex formed around the 5′-end of viral RNA. *Embo J* 1993; **12**: 3587–98.

33. Mullendore JL, Sobsey MD, Carol Shieh Y. Improved method for the recovery of hepatitis A virus from oysters. *J Virol Methods* 2001; **94**(1–2): 25–35.

34. Lees DN, Henshilwood K, Dore WJ. Development of a method for detection of enteroviruses in shellfish by PCR with poliovirus as a model. *Appl Environ Microbiol* 1994; **60**: 2999–3005.

35. Jothikumar N, Lowther JA, Henshilwood K, Lees DN, Hill VR, Vinje J. Rapid and sensitive detection of noroviruses by using TaqMan-based one-step reverse transcription-PCR assays and application to naturally contaminated shellfish samples. *Appl Environ Microbiol* 2005; **71**: 1870–5.

36

The oral acquisition of nematode, cestode and trematode parasites

SIMON BROOKER, JEROEN H.J. ENSINK

Nematode, cestode and trematode parasites are helminth (worm) infections and are among the most ubiquitous and widely distributed of all pathogens in humans (Table 36.1, page 395).[1] Infection typically occurs by exposure to infective stages either present in the external environment or ingested in contaminated food. For many of the major intestinal nematode species, transmission is direct from mature eggs or larval stages to the mouth via fingers contaminated from infected soil. Transmission in some settings can additionally occur through the practice of geophagia – the eating of soil. Cestode infections are acquired via the ingestion of raw or undercooked meat contaminated with adult stages, while a number of trematode species can be contracted from eating raw fish or vegetables or by drinking contaminated water. Since the transmission of these groups of parasites depends on faecal contamination of the environment, these parasites tend to be most prevalent and cause the largest disease burden in areas of poverty and inadequate sanitation and hygiene in the humid tropics of the developing world.

The ubiquity of these parasites has stimulated numerous large-scale control programmes, with a number of countries achieving successful and sustained control. For example, Japan's national programme reduced the nationwide overall prevalence of intestinal nematodes from over 75 per cent in 1949 to less than 1 per cent in the 1990s.[2] Recent progress in helminth control has also been made in a number of Latin American and Asian countries.[3,4] A principal tool used in successful control programmes has been population-based anthelmintic drug treatment, but environmental control measures aimed at reducing transmission, including improved water and sanitation, enhanced hygiene behaviour and adequate food inspection, have also been important, and represent the ultimate control measure.

This chapter focuses on the major intestinal nematodes (the soil-transmitted helminths [STHs] or geohelminths), the tissue nematodes *Dracunculus medinensis* and *Trichinella spiralis* spp. and the major cestode (tapeworm) and trematode (fluke) infections. The aim of the chapter is to highlight the public health importance of orally acquired helminth infections in developing countries, to examine the role of environmental factors in the epidemiology of infection and to examine the potential of environmental control measures in reducing transmission. For each group of parasites, an examination is made of life-cycles, exposure-related risk factors, patterns of human infection and disease, and individual-level, population-level and environmental control measures that can reduce transmission rates.

INTESTINAL NEMATODES

Nematodes are non-segmented roundworms belonging to the phylum Nematoda, the most common of which are four STHs: the roundworm *Ascaris lumbricoides*, the whipworm *Trichuris trichiura* and the hookworms *Necator americanus* and *Ancylostoma duodenale*. STHs are most prevalent in warm and humid areas of the tropics and subtropics.[5] In temperate climates, the most prevalent intestinal nematode is the pinworm *Enterobius vermicularis*. This also occurs in developing countries, although its true prevalence is unknown, largely because the diagnosis of infection requires a technique that is rarely employed in population surveys.

Life-cycle and transmission

The life-cycle of intestinal nematodes follows a general pattern, with adult worms inhabiting either the small intestine (*Ascaris lumbricoides* and *Ancylostoma duodenale*) or the colon (*Trichuris trichiura* and *Enterobius vermicularis*), where they mate and produce eggs. These are passed in human faeces and deposited in the external environment. Infection with *Ascaris lumbricoides* and *Trichuris trichiura* occurs exclusively through the ingestion of embryonated eggs. Oral acquisition is considered to be a secondary mode of transmission for the hookworm *Ancylostoma duodenale*, which predominantly infects humans by infective larvae penetrating unprotected skin; the hookworm *Necator americanus* is only acquired through skin penetration. The transmission of *Enterobius vermicularis* occurs through female worms migrating down to the anus, from which they emerge to deposit eggs on the perianal skin and on the perineum. Scratching of the anal area transfers faecal material and eggs to under the fingernails, from where they are ingested.

Risk factors

A number of specific behavioural, household and environmental factors have been identified that affect the risk of acquiring STH infection. For example, studies demonstrate that the risk is greater among individuals living in a household without sanitary latrine facilities.[6,7] For school-aged children, the risk is further enhanced by attending schools with inadequate sanitary facilities.[8] Occupation-related exposure is also important: STH infection has been shown to be more common in households that use waste water and human excreta in agriculture and aquaculture.[7,9,10] The risk of *Enterobius vermicularis* is generally similar across population groups.

Infection and disease

Patterns of infection with age are similar among the major intestinal nematode species, exhibiting a rise in childhood to a relatively stable plateau in adulthood. Maximum prevalence is typically attained before 5 years of age for *Ascaris lumbricoides*, *Trichuris trichiura* and *Enterobius vermicularis*, and in young adults for hookworm infection.

However, the prevalence provides little indication of the underlying morbidity associated with infection. This is because the severity of morbidity is strongly related to the number of intestinal nematodes harboured by an individual (the intensity of infection): the intestinal blood loss caused by hookworm infection,[11] the growth stunting due to *Ascaris lumbricoides*,[4,12] and the dysentery and colitis due to *Trichuris trichiura*[13] are all related to worm burden. The intensity of infection is also a key determinant of the overall rate of nematode transmission within a community.[14] For *Ascaris lumbricoides* and *Trichuris trichiura*, maximum worm burdens occur among 5–10-year-olds, and for hookworms they occur during early adulthood.[15]

An important epidemiological feature of nematodes is that infections have an aggregated distribution in human communities such that most worms are harboured by a minority of individuals in a community and the majority harbour no or few worms.[16] There is also evidence of clustering of infection within households and families.[17] Similarly, infection with *Enterobius vermicularis* clusters in families and in institutions, such as schools and asylums.

Chronic infections with *Ascaris lumbricoides* and *Trichuris trichiura* can contribute to malnutrition and dramatically affect physical and cognitive development in children.[12,18] Hookworm is an important cause of intestinal blood loss, which can contribute to anaemia, especially among children and pregnant women.[11,19] Infection with *Enterobius vermicularis* is generally symptomless, although it can cause insomnia, restlessness and, in rare cases, non-specific childhood colitis.[20]

Control

Current efforts to control STHs focus mainly on chemotherapy, using benzimidazole anthlemintics – most commonly albendazole and mebendazole – which treat infections effectively.[21] The primary goal of current chemotherapy programmes is to reduce the morbidity associated with infection. As such, attention needs to be paid to the age-specificity of the infection.

The World Health Organization (WHO) identifies three key groups who are more vulnerable than others to the harmful effects of chronic infections, namely school-age children, preschool children and pregnant women. Operational research shows that school-based chemotherapy programmes are extremely cost-effective in controlling the disease burden of STH even in environments where transmission is high.[22,23] Treatment programmes for preschool children and pregnant women have been developed as part of child health days and maternal health programmes. *Enterobius vermicularis* is effectively treated with albendazole, mebendazole or pyrantel pamoate (pyrantel embonate), often given in a family context.

A drawback of chemotherapy is that individuals in endemic areas often reacquire infection, necessitating regular re-treatment. In the long term, therefore, only universal sanitation and clean water offer the potential for sustainable control and the eradication of infection. Such measures are, however, only likely to be achieved in developing countries over an extended period. The provision of improved sanitation and clean water does not necessarily mean that these facilities will be used or properly maintained and cleaned. For example, past studies show that latrines constructed without proper involvement of the local community or the household quickly fall into disuse and can even become focal points for the transmission of infection.[24] In addition, an individual or household ownership of sanitary facilities will not necessarily prevent the household from contracting STHs if latrine or sewerage collection coverage is low in the surrounding community.[7,8,25]

Such practical challenges mean that the impact of introducing sanitation on infection levels may only be evident after decades,[26] and even then it may not be completely effective. For example, in one study, hookworm prevalence declined by only 4 per cent after the introduction of latrines.[27] In El Salvador, the use of solar-powered, urine-diverting desiccating latrines was effective in reducing the transmission of enteric protozoa, but was not fully effective in removing the more environmentally persistent ova of *Ascaris lumbricoides* and *Trichuris trichiura*.[28] It has been suggested that water and sanitation interventions need to reach a certain coverage threshold before there is a significant reduction in the transmission of intestinal nematodes.[29] It is also clear that health education to promote appropriate hygiene behaviour and ensure that sanitary facilities are properly used is an essential component of any control strategy aimed at reducing the transmission of nematode infection.[30,31]

In areas of water scarcity or with poor soil fertility, the use of urban sewage, night-soil or sewage sludge in agriculture is common practice and often encouraged as a cheap form of waste water disposal and treatment; as indicated, however, this practice is associated with an increased risk of infection. In order to protect farmers and consumers from possible adverse health impacts, the WHO has developed a guideline for the safe use of waste water in agriculture and aquaculture, recommending that water with more than one helminth egg per litre is not used for the irrigation of crops that are consumed uncooked.[32] The investment in waste water treatment systems and sewage systems required to reduce the risk of infection is, however, beyond the means of many developing countries.

Nematodes causing visceral larva migrans

Certain nematode species are incapable of growing to maturity in humans, but their larvae wander in the body, resulting in a variety of clinical manifestations. Cutaneous larva migrans is caused by nematodes that enter the body through skin penetration, such as *Strongyloides* and zoonotic hookworms (*Ancylostoma braziliense*, *Ancylostoma caninum* and *Uncinaria stenocephala*); it is characterized by serpiginous burrows appearing most frequently on the feet, buttocks and abdomen. Visceral larva migrans (VLM),

on the other hand, results from the ingestion of eggs, leading to larvale wandering through the viscera (internal organs), sometimes with serious results.

The most important cause of VLM is toxocariasis caused by the dog ascarid *Toxocara canis* or the cat ascarid *Toxocara cati*.[33] Infection is orally acquired, typically by children playing in soil or playgrounds contaminated with *Toxocara* eggs passed by infected animals. VLM occurs mainly in young children and presents as fever, enlargement of the liver and asthma. *Toxocara* can also cause ocular larval migrans, occasionally resulting in visual impairment. Control focuses upon the treatment of infection in animals and health education on reducing human exposure to contaminated soil.

TISSUE NEMATODES

Of the major nematodes that residue in human tissues, only *Dracunculus medinensis* (dracunculiasis or Guinea worm) and *Trichinella spiralis* spp. are acquired orally. Previously endemic in 20 countries in the developing world in the 1980s, the global incidence of dracunculiasis has, thanks to a global eradication programme, fallen from an estimated 3.5 million cases in 1986 to fewer than 10 000 in 2007.[34] As of 2009, only five countries continue to have indigenous cases of dracunculiasis: Ghana, Mali, Niger, Nigeria and Sudan. Infection with *Trichinella spiralis* spp. is cosmopolitan, with various subspecies occupying distinct geographical foci.[35]

Life-cycle and transmission

Humans become infected with *Dracunculus medinensis* by swallowing copepods (water fleas) containing larvae, usually in drinking water. Upon reaching the small intestine, stomach acid kills the copepods and the released larvae penetrate the stomach wall and migrate through the connective tissues, maturing to adults along the way. Egg-laden (gravid) females migrate through the subcutaneous tissue of the lower extremities, where they cause painful blisters that burst and expose the anterior end of the worm. Infected individuals try to relieve the burning sensation caused at the site of blister by cooling it in a local water source. This results in the release of first-stage larvae into the water that are ingested by copepods, thereby completing the life-cycle. Humans are the only reservoir.

Human infection with *Trichinella* occurs by eating undercooked meat containing larvae: *Trichinella spiralis spiralis* from pork, *Trichinella spiralis nativa* from bear and walrus meat, and *Trichinella spiralis nelsoni* from bush pig or wart-hog. Humans are not the normal host so there is no outward transmission; transmission occurs from one carnivore to another when the cysts are digested in the stomach and eventually find their way to striated muscle tissue.

Infection and disease

Age- and sex-specific patterns of dracunculiasis show a strong variation according to locality, which is determined primarily by water contact patterns. Infection can result in intensely painful blisters, which can be accompanied by fever, nausea and vomiting. Up to half of all cases suffer from secondary infections and become incapacitated, with resultant economic and social consequences in terms of days lost from work and school absenteeism. The economic impact of the disease is further reinforced by the seasonality of infection, with female worms typically appearing during the peak seasons of agricultural activity.[36] Trichinella is most common among adults and can cause nausea, vomiting and diarrhoea, followed by oedema. Larvae in the muscle may result in transient cardiac and pulmonary manifestations.[37]

Risk factors

The key risk factor for dracunculiasis is the choice of source of drinking water, along with related behavioural factors such as fetching water, travelling and farming.[38,39] Trichinella infection in humans is related to cultural dietary habits, the eating of raw or undercooked meat being the most important risk factor.

Control

The main environmental measures for the prevention and control of dracunculiasis include:

- filtering drinking water to remove copepods using simple cloth and polyester filters;
- treating contaminated drinking water with larvicides that kill copepods;
- providing alternative, safe drinking water;
- educating individuals with blisters and ulcers not to enter water sources.

Since its initiation in 1980, the global Dracunculiasis Eradication Program has implemented village-based surveillance, health education and the distribution of cloth filters, as well as providing larvicides and soliciting operational support for digging wells. The programme has seen a precipitous decline in the global incidence of dracunculiasis, along with reduction in school absenteeism and economic losses due to infection.[34] The dracunculiasis eradication programme is one of today's global health success stories.

The main method of preventing Trichinella is the thorough cooking of all meat, regular meat inspection and the storage of meat in deep freezes.

CESTODES

Cestodes (tapeworms) are flat, segmented worms belonging to the phylum Platyhelminthes, which inhabit the intestinal tract. Taenia saginata (beef tapeworm) is the most prevalent cestode infection, occurring predominantly in pastoral communities in Africa and in both farming communities and cities in Latin America (see Table 36.1). Infection rarely results in morbidity. In contrast, Taenia solium (pork tapeworm) infection, although less common, can result in severe neurological consequences. Human fascioliasis, caused by Echinococcus granulosus and Echinococcus multilocularis, is an important health problem in the Andean countries, Iran, Egypt and parts of Europe.

The fish tapeworm Diphyllobothrium latum was previously common throughout lakes in Scandinavia and North America but has mainly been controlled through improved sanitation. Today, however, it is becoming increasingly common in Brazil, Russia and Japan.[40] In light of the limited distribution of Diphyllobothrium latum infection in developing countries and the fact that infection rarely causes pathology, this parasite is not considered further here.

Life-cycle and transmission

Infection with Taenia in humans occurs by the ingestion of raw or undercooked beef (Taenia saginata) or pork (Taenia solium) that contains encapsulated juvenile stages, called cysticerci. These cysticerci enter the small intestine, where they develop into adults. Gravid segments (proglottids) of worms are passed in the faeces, and a cow (Taenia saginata) or pig (Taenia solium) then ingests the proglottids. Eggs embedded within the proglottids hatch in the small intestine, and the resultant larvae migrate through the vasculature and eventually infect striated skeletal muscle tissue. Here, the larvae develop into cysticerci, which are ingested by humans via the consumption of raw or undercooked meat. Humans are occasionally infected with Taenia solium by ingesting embryonated eggs. Eggs can also contaminate water, which, if used to irrigate agriculture, can be ingested with the contaminated food.

Echinococcus parasites live as adults in the small intestine of dogs and other carnivores. Infective eggs are released in faeces that are subsequently ingested by sheep and other domestic animals as well as humans.

Infection and disease

Infection is common among all age groups although, because of their dietary habits, adults are often at greater risk of infection. Most cases of Taenia saginata or Taenia solium infection are asymptomatic; transient abdominal pain, nausea and vomiting can occasionally occur.

Table 36.1   The major orally acquired nematode, cestode and trematode infections of humans[1,34,50,51,56]

Species	Common name	Estimated population infected in 2007	Major endemic regions
Intestinal nematodes*			
Ascaris lumbricoides	Roundworm infection	884–1221 million	Sub-Saharan Africa, South and Central America, Asia
Trichuris trichiura	Whipworm infection	634–795 million	
Necator americanus and *Ancylostoma duodenale*	Hookworm infection	616–740 million	
Enterobius vermicularis	Pinworm infection	NA	Worldwide
Larva migrans[†]			
Toxocara canis and *Toxocara cati*	Arrowhead worm	NA	Worldwide
Tissue nematodes[‡]			
Dracunculus medinensis	Guinea worm	<10 000 cases	Ghana, Nigeria, Sudan
Trichinella spiralis spp.	Trichina worm	11 million	North America, China, Mexico, Argentina, Chile, Baltic States
Cestodes[§]			
Taenia saginata	Beef tapeworm	45 million	Sub-Saharan Africa, South and Central America
Taenia solium	Pork tapeworm	5 million	South and Central America, Indian subcontinent, South-East Asia, west and southern Africa
Diphyllobothrium latum	Fish tapeworm	NA	Scandinavia, North America, Russia, Japan, Chile, Brazil
Echinococcus granulosus	Cystic echinococcosis or hydatid disease	NA	Mediterranean countries, Africa, Asia, South America
Echinococcus multilocularis	Alveolar echinococcosis	NA	The Arctic, central and southern Europe, Central Asia, China, Canada
Trematodes[#]			
Opisthorchis viverrini	Liver fluke	63 million at risk	China, Korea, South-East Asia, Russia
Opisthorchis felineus	Liver fluke	12.5 million at risk	Russia, Kazakhstan, Ukraine, South-East Asia, Russia
Clonorchis sinensis	Chinese liver fluke	7 million cases, with 600 million at risk	China, Russia, Taiwan, Vietnam
Paragonimus westermani	Oriental lung fluke	21 million cases, with 293 million at risk	China, South Korea, South-East Asia, parts of Africa and South America
Fasciola hepatica and *Fasciola gigantica*	Intestinal flukes	3 million cases, 90 million at risk	Europe, Bolivia and Peru, Iran, Egypt
Fasciolopsis buski	Busk's fluke infection	NA	China, South-East Asia, Bangladesh, India

NA, relevant data not available, no estimate provided.

*Other orally acquired human intestinal nematodes of minor medical importance include *Capillaria hepatica* (syn. *Calodium hepaticum*), *Capillaria philippinensis*, *Lagochilascaris minor*, *Mammomonogamus laryngeus*, *Marshallagia marshalli*, *Oesophagostomum bifurcum*, *Parastrongylus cantonensis*, *Ternidens deminutus* and *Trichostrongylus* spp.

[†]Other orally acquired nematodes that cause visceral larva migrans in humans include *Angiostrongylus* spp., *Anisakis* spp., *Baylisascaris procyonis* and *Gnathostoma* spp.

[‡]Other orally acquired tissue nematodes include *Aonchotheca philippinensis*, *Capillaria hepatica* (syn. *Calodium hepaticum*) and *Trichinella pseudospiralis*.

[§]Rarer orally acquired cestodes include *Bertiella* spp., *Dipylidium caninum*, *Echinococcus oligarthrus*, *Echinococcus vogeli*, *Hymenolepis diminuta*, *Hymenolepis* (*Rodentolepis*) *nana*, *Inermicapsifer madagascariensis*, *Mathevotaenia symmetrica*, *Spirometra* spp., *Taenia brauni* and *Taenia multiceps* (syn. *Taenia serialis*, *Multiceps multiceps*).

[#]Other, rarer trematodes infecting humans include *Alaria* spp., *Brachylaima cribbi*, *Echinostoma* spp., *Fischoederius elongates*, *Haplorchis* spp., *Heterophyes heterophyes*, *Gastrodiscoides hominis*, *Gymnophalloides seoi*, *Metagonimus yokogawai*, *Nanophyetus salmincola*, *Nanophyetus schikhobalowi*, *Neodiplostomum seolense* and *Watsonius watsoni*.

There can, however, be more serious consequences of *Taenia solium* infection, associated with the ingestion of eggs shed in the faeces of humans or pigs. Larval cysts can form in human tissues, and when these occur in the brain or central nervous system, they may result in neurocysticercosis.[41,42] This disease is one of the main causes of adult-onset epileptic seizures in the developing world and is also increasingly seen in more developed countries because of immigration from endemic areas. The maximum severity of neurocysticercosis generally occurs 3–5 years after exposure.

Infection with the intermediate cystic stage of *Echinococcus* spp. can cause disease and incapacity in animals and humans, and, in the most serious cases, the death of the host.[43]

Risk factors

Owning to their life-cycle, *Taenia saginata* and *Taenia solium* are most prevalent among communities that have an inadequate disposal of faeces, undertake cattle or pig husbandry, and eat raw or undercooked meat.[44,45] Infection with *Echinococcus* spp. is most prevalent in areas of sheep and cattle husbandry.

Control

Taeniasis due to infection with *Taenia saginata* or *Taenia solium* is effectively treated using the anthelmintic praziquantel. By contrast, the treatment of neurocysticercosis is more difficult, with varying success achieved with anthelmintics (praziquantel or albendazole) and corticosteroids.[46] The significant global disease burden of cysticercosis prompted the WHO in 2003 to recommend the identification and treatment of individuals harbouring adult tapeworms in combination with population-based treatment with praziquantel.

The long-term, successful control of taeniasis and cysticercosis is more likely when anthelmintic chemotherapy programmes are integrated with a wider programme of environmental control. Specific environmental control strategies for cestodes include the appropriate disposal of human faeces, improved animal husbandry and meat inspection, and the thorough cooking of all meat or its thorough freezing prior to cooking. Cysticerci are destroyed by storage at −15°C for 10 days, −20°C for 5 days, −25°C for 3 days, and immediately by quick freezing at −37°C. Veterinary sanitary measures, including appropriate legislation and regular and strict meat inspection, have helped to control infection in many developed countries, but inspection is often inadequate in many developing countries.

Environmental control measures for *Echinococcus* spp. include the avoidance of eggs passed by dogs as well as the sanitary disposal of infected organs of sheep and other animals, thereby preventing dogs eating these organs.[47]

TREMATODES

Trematodes (flukes) are found in the bile ducts, lungs and blood of humans. The trematodes that are the most prevalent and cause of greatest burden are the schistosomes (*Schistosoma haematobium*, *S. intercalatum*, *S. mansoni*, *S. mekongi* and *S. japonicum*, and very rarely *S. guineensis* and *S. malayensis*; for a recent review see Gryseels *et al.*[48]). Infection occurs when humans enter fresh water containing the infective stages (cercariae), which can penetrate the skin. Because of their cutaneous mode of transmission, schistosomes are not considered further here.

The trematodes that are acquired orally include a number of fish-borne (*Opisthorchis* and *Clonorchis*), crustacean-borne (*Paragonimus*) and plant-borne (fasciolid) species.[49] Owing to poor hygiene behaviours and inadequate sanitation in many developing countries, people infected with these trematodes typically pass parasite eggs in their faeces into water bodies, infecting intermediate host snail species, which then release infective stages called cercariae. These stages either infect cyprinoid fish or attach themselves to the surfaces of vegetables. As with most helminth species, light infections are of no clinical consequence, but heavy, long-standing infection can result in diarrhoea, abdominal pain, dyspepsia and nausea, as well as a number of hepatobiliary diseases.[50]

Liver fluke infection caused by *Opisthorchis viverrini*, *Opisthorchis felineus* and *Clonorchis sinensis* is an important public health problem in East Asia and Eastern Europe, where it is common to eat raw fish. The risk of infection is greatest among communities living near freshwater and engaged in aquaculture.[51] The lung fluke *Paragonimus westermani* occurs throughout Asia, infecting a wide range of reservoir hosts, with freshwater crabs and crayfish being the most common food-borne source of infection.[52] Hygienic waste disposal and the thorough cooking of food prevents infection; in practice, however, traditional dietary preferences hinder effective control.

The main plant-borne trematode species known to infect humans are *Fasciola hepatica*, *Fasciola gigantica* and *Fasciolopsis buski*.[53] The number of reports of human infections and the endemic range has been increasing in recent years due, in part, to the expansion of aquaculture.[51] *Fasciola hepatica* predominantly infects sheep and cattle, but humans can occasionally become infected by eating infected salad vegetables. Prevalence rates are highest in Europe, central Asia and the Andean areas of Bolivia and Peru. *Fasciola gigantica* is a common trematode of cattle and camels, occurring mainly in Africa and Asia. *Fasciolopsis buski* is most prevalent in Asia and is typically contracted by eating contaminated water vegetables. Control measures against these fasciolid species include preventing domestic livestock from polluting commercial vegetable beds and the peeling and washing of vegetables.

THE FUTURE

An improved understanding of the public health significance of nematode and cestode infections, coupled with the cost-effectiveness of intervention strategies, has led to a renewed interest in implementing control programmes. For intestinal nematodes, the focus of control is on carefully targeting chemotherapy to those individuals in most need and most likely to benefit from treatment. Numerous national governments and international organizations are currently including anthelmintic treatment in their public health programmes, with demonstrable health benefits. In addition, dracunculiasis has been virtually eradicated due to global control efforts.

Despite these achievements, there remains an essential role for environmental control measures, including the adequate disposal of human faeces, the provision of safe drinking water and improved veterinary sanitation. In many developing countries, however, coverage rates from these measures are often unacceptably low. For example, in 2008 – the International Year of Sanitation[54] – an estimated 1.1 billion people globally did not have access to clean water supplies, and there were 2.4 billion people with no access to adequate sanitation. In addition, it is estimated that over 80 per cent of all globally produced sewage is disposed of untreated or partially treated into rivers, irrigation canals and lakes, and approximately 20 million hectares worldwide are irrigated with untreated or insufficiently treated waste water.[55] The reasons for such numbers are self-evident: low socioeconomic status, a lack of government resources, poor hygiene behaviour and inadequate sanitation in public places such as schools. It is apparent that a high level of effort and investment is still required to ensure that environmental health measures are an integral component of helminth control efforts.

REFERENCES

♦ = Major review article

1. Muller R. *Worms and Human Disease*. Wallingford, UK: CABI, 2002.
2. Kobayashi A, Hara T, Kajima J. Historical aspects for the control of soil-transmitted helminthiases. *Parasitol Int* 2006; **55**(Suppl.): S289–91.
3. de Silva NR, Brooker S, Hotez PJ, Montresor A, Engels D, Savioli L. Soil-transmitted helminth infections: Updating the global picture. *Trends Parasitol* 2003; **19**: 547–51.
4. Montresor A, Cong DT, Sinuon M *et al.* Large-scale preventive chemotherapy for the control of helminth infection in Western pacific countries: Six years later. *PLoS Negl Trop Dis* 2008; **2**: e278.
5. Brooker S, Bundy DAP. Soil-transmitted helminths (geohelminths). In: Cook GC, Zumla AL (eds) *Manson's Tropical Diseases* (pp. 1515–48). London: Elsevier, 2008.
6. Chongsuvivatwong V, Pas-Ong S, McNeil D, Geater A, Duerawee M. Predictors for the risk of hookworm infection: Experience from endemic villages in southern Thailand. *Trans R Soc Trop Med Hyg* 1996; **90**: 630–3.
7. Do TT, Molbak K, Phung DC, Dalsgaard A. Helminth infections among people using wastewater and human excreta in peri-urban agriculture and aquaculture in Hanoi, Vietnam. *Trop Med Int Health* 2007; **12**(Suppl. 2): 82–90.
8. Ekpo UF, Odoemene SN, Mafiana CF, Sam-Wobo SO. Helminthiasis and hygiene conditions of schools in Ikenne, Ogun State, Nigeria. *PLoS Negl Trop Dis* 2008; **2**: e146.
9. Humphries DL, Stephenson LS, Pearce EJ, The PH, Dan HT, Khanh LT. The use of human faeces for fertilizer is associated with increased intensity of hookworm infection in Vietnamese women. *Trans R Soc Trop Med Hyg* 1997; **91**: 518–20.
10. Ensink JH, Blumenthal UJ, Brooker S. Wastewater quality and the risk of intestinal nematode infection in sewage farming families in Hyderabad, India. *Am J Trop Med Hyg* 2008; **79**: 561–7.
11. Stoltzfus RJ, Albonico M, Chwaya HM *et al.* Hemoquant determination of hookworm-related blood loss and its role in iron deficiency in African children. *Am J Trop Med Hyg* 1996; **55**: 399–404.
12. O'Lorcain P, Holland CV. The public health importance of *Ascaris lumbricoides*. *Parasitology* 2000; **121**(Suppl.): S51–71.
13. Cooper ES, Bundy DA, Henry FJ. Chronic dysentery, stunting, and whipworm infestation. *Lancet* 1986; **2**: 280–1.
14. Anderson RM, May RM. Helminth infections of humans: mathematical models, population dynamics and control. *Adv Parasitol* 1985; **24**: 1–101.
♦15. Bundy DA. Population ecology of intestinal helminth infections in human communities. *Philos Trans R Soc Lond B Biol Sci* 1988; **321**: 405–20.
16. Anderson RM. The population dynamics and epidemiology of intestinal nematode infections. *Trans R Soc Trop Med Hyg* 1986; **80**: 686–96.
17. Forrester JE, Scott ME, Bundy DA, Golden MH. Clustering of *Ascaris lumbricoides* and *Trichuris trichiura* infections within households. *Trans R Soc Trop Med Hyg* 1988; **82**: 282–8.
18. Jukes MCH, Drake LJ, Bundy DAP. *Health, Nutrition and Education for all: Levelling the Playing Field*. Wallingford: CABI, 2008.
19. Brooker S, Hotez PJ, Bundy DAP. Hookworm-related anaemia among pregnant women: A systematic review. *PLoS Negl Trop Dis* 2008; **2**: e291.
20. Jardine M, Kokai GK, Dalzell AM. *Enterobius vermicularis* and colitis in Children. *J Pediatr Gastroenterol Nutr* 2006; **43**: 610–12.
♦21. Keiser J, Utzinger J. Efficacy of current drugs against soil-transmitted helminth infections: Systematic review and meta-analysis. *JAMA* 2008; **299**: 1937–48.
22. Bundy DAP, Shaeffer S, Jukes M *et al.* School-based health and nutrition programs. In: Jamison DEA (ed.) *Disease*

Control Priorities in Developing Countries (pp. 1091–108). New York: World Bank/Oxford University Press, 2006.

23. Hotez PJ, Bundy DAP, Beegle K *et al.* Helminth infections: Soil-transmitted helminth infections and schistosomiasis. In: Jamison DEA (ed.) *Disease Control Priorities in Developing Countries* (pp. 467–97). New York: World Bank/Oxford University Press, 2006.

24. Schad GA, Nawalinski TA, Kochar V. Human ecology and the distribution and abundance of hookworm populations. In: Croll NA, Cross JH (eds) *Human Ecology and Infectious Disease* (pp. 187–223). New York: Academic Press, 1983.

25. Moraes LR, Cairncross S. Environmental interventions and the pattern of geohelminth infections in Salvador, Brazil. *Parasitology* 2004; **129**: 223–32.

26. Esrey SA, Potash JB, Roberts L, Shiff C. Effects of improved water supply and sanitation on ascariasis, diarrhoea, dracunculiasis, hookworm infection, schistosomiasis, and trachoma. *Bull World Health Organ* 1991; **69**: 609–21.

27. Huttly SR. The impact of inadequate sanitary conditions on health in developing countries. *World Health Stat Q* 1990; **43**: 118–26.

28. Corrales LF, Izurieta R, Moe CL. Association between intestinal parasitic infections and type of sanitation system in rural El Salvador. *Trop Med Int Health* 2006; **11**: 1821–31.

29. Asaolu SO, Ofoezie IE, Odumuyiwa PA, Sowemimo OA, Ogunniyi TA. Effect of water supply and sanitation on the prevalence and intensity of *Ascaris lumbricoides* among pre-school-age children in Ajebandele and Ifewara, Osun State, Nigeria. *Trans R Soc Trop Med Hyg* 2002; **96**: 600–4.

30. Asaolu SO, Ofoezie IE. The role of health education and sanitation in the control of helminth infections. *Acta Tropica* 2003; **86**: 283–94.

31. Albright JW, Hidayati NR, Basaric-Keys J. Behavioral and hygienic characteristics of primary schoolchildren which can be modified to reduce the prevalence of geohelminth infections: A study in central Java, Indonesia. *Southeast Asian J Trop Med Public Health* 2005; **36**: 629–40.

32. World Health Organization. *Guidelines for the Safe Use of Wastewater in Agriculture.* Geneva: WHO, 2006.

33. Despommier D. Toxocariasis: Clinical aspects, epidemiology, medical ecology, and molecular aspects. *Clin Microbiol Rev* 2003; **16**: 265–72.

34. Tayeh A, Cairncross S. Dracunculiasis eradication by 2009: Will endemic countries meet the target? [Editorial] *Trop Med Int Health* 2007; **12**: 1403–8.

35. Pozio E, Darwin Murrell K. Systematics and epidemiology of trichinella. *Adv Parasitol* 2006; **63**: 367–439.

36. Smith GS, Blum D, Huttly SR, Okeke N, Kirkwood BR, Feachem RG. Disability from dracunculiasis: Effect on mobility. *Ann Trop Med Parasitol* 1989; **83**: 151–8.

37. Capo V, Despommier DD. Clinical aspects of infection with *Trichinella* spp. *Clin Microbiol Rev* 1996; **9**: 47–54.

38. Tayeh A, Cairncross S, Maude GH. Water sources and other determinants of dracunculiasis in the northern region of Ghana. *J Helminthol* 1993; **67**: 213–25.

39. Etard JF, Kodio B, Traore S, Audibert M. Water contacts in dracunculiasis-infected patients in Mali: Transmission risk activities. *Bull Soc Pathol Exot* 2002; **95**: 295–8.

40. Dick TA, Nelson PA, Choudhury A. Diphyllobothriasis: Update on human cases, foci, patterns and sources of human infections and future considerations. *Southeast Asian J Trop Med Public Health* 2001; **32**(Suppl. 2): 59–76.

◆41. Garcia HH, Gonzalez AE, Evans CA, Gilman RH. *Taenia solium* cysticercosis. *Lancet* 2003; **362**: 547–56.

42. Willingham AL III, Engels D. Control of *Taenia solium* cysticercosis/taeniosis. *Adv Parasitol* 2006; **61**: 509–66.

43. Jenkins DJ, Romig T, Thompson RC. Emergence/re-emergence of *Echinococcus* spp. – a global update. *Int J Parasitol* 2005; **35**: 1205–19.

44. Wandra T, Depary AA, Sutisna P *et al.* Taeniasis and cysticercosis in Bali and North Sumatra, Indonesia. *Parasitol Int* 2006; **55**(Suppl.): S155–60.

45. Prasad KN, Prasad A, Gupta RK, Pandey CM, Singh U. Prevalence and associated risk factors of *Taenia solium* taeniasis in a rural pig farming community of north India. *Trans R Soc Trop Med Hyg* 2007; **101**: 1241–7.

46. Del Brutto OH, Roos KL, Coffey CS, Garcia HH. Meta-analysis: Cysticidal drugs for neurocysticercosis: albendazole and praziquantel. *Ann Intern Med* 2006; **145**: 43–51.

◆47. Craig PS, McManus DP, Lightowlers MW *et al.* Prevention and control of cystic echinococcosis. *Lancet Infect Dis* 2007; **7**: 385–94.

48. Gryseels B, Polman K, Clerinx J, Kestens L. Human schistosomiasis. *Lancet* 2006; **368**: 1106–18.

49. Marcos LA, Terashima A, Gotuzzo E. Update on hepatobiliary flukes: Fascioliasis, opisthorchiasis and clonorchiasis. *Curr Opin Infect Dis* 2008; **21**: 523–30.

50. Toledo R, Esteban JG, Fried B. Immunology and pathology of intestinal trematodes in their definitive hosts. *Adv Parasitol* 2006; **63**: 285–365.

51. Keiser J, Utzinger J. Emerging foodborne trematodiasis. *Emerg Infect Dis* 2005; **11**: 1507–14.

52. Liu Q, Wei F, Liu W, Yang S, Zhang X. Paragonimiasis: An important food-borne zoonosis in China. *Trends Parasitol* 2008; **24**: 318–23.

◆53. Mas-Coma S, Bargues MD, Valero MA. Fascioliasis and other plant-borne trematode zoonoses. *Int J Parasitol* 2005; **35**: 1255–78.

54. UN-Water. Tackling a global crisis: International Year of Sanitation 2008. Available from: http://esa.un.org/iys/docs/IYS_flagship_web_small.pdf (accessed January 5, 2010).

55. Scott CA, Faruqui NI, Raschid-Sally L. Wastewater use in irrigated agriculture: Management challenges in developing countries. In: Scott CA, Faruqui NI, Raschid-Sally L (eds) *Wastewater Use in Irrigated Agriculture: Confronting the Livelihood and Environmental Realities* (pp. 1–10). Wallingford: CABI, 2004.

◆56. Bethony J, Brooker S, Albonico M *et al.* Soil-transmitted helminth infections: Ascariasis, trichiuriasis, and hookworm. *Lancet* 2006; **367**: 1521–32.

MYCOBACTERIUM AVIUM SUBSPECIES *PARATUBERCULOSIS*, JOHNE'S DISEASE AND CROHN'S DISEASE

ROGER W. PICKUP, GLENN RHODES, JOHN HERMON-TAYLOR

MYCOBACTERIUM AVIUM SUBSPECIES *PARATUBERCULOSIS*

Mycobacterium avium subspecies *paratuberculosis* (MAP) is a member of the *M. avium* complex.[1] The total GC-rich genome sequence comprises 4.83 mega base pairs encoding a predicted 4350 open reading frames. A little over 96 per cent of its DNA is virtually identical in sequence and genetic organization to that of the generally non-pathogenic *M. avium*. The remainder of the genome, comprising fewer than 200 open reading frames, is either unique to MAP or homologous to genes associated with pathogenicity in other organisms.[2]

MAP has diversified into multiple bovine (type II) and ovine (type I) strains, with evidence of the emergence of humanized strains.[3] Some strains, particularly from sheep and humans, may be almost impossible to isolate and maintain in culture. Others, particularly bovine strains, may require prolonged incubation.[4]

JOHNE'S DISEASE IN ANIMALS

Unlike other *M. avium* complexes, MAP has the specific ability to cause Johne's disease in many animal species, including primates.[5] Johne's disease is a systemic infection whose principal clinicopathological manifestation is chronic inflammation of the intestine.[5] The disease in animals ranges from pluribacillary to paucimicrobial-like leprosy in humans.[5]

Johne's disease was first reported in 1895 in Europe and in 1908 in North America. Currently, there is an extensive prevalence of ovine/bovine subclinical MAP infection worldwide.[3] Infected animals secrete MAP in their milk and faeces. MAP has been detected in retail pasteurized milk supplies (in the UK, Czech Republic and USA) and in the environment.[3]

CROHN'S DISEASE IN HUMANS

Crohn's disease in humans is a systemic disorder whose principal clinicopathological manifestation is chronic inflammation of the intestine. It is a 'new' disease that first emerged in Europe and North America between 1940 and 1950, with generally increasing incidence and prevalence since then.[3,6] Crohn's disease has also emerged and is increasing in former low-incidence areas. In Europe, the incidence of the disease in adults is increasing by about 25 per cent per decade, while the rise in the incidence of Crohn's disease in children in recent years has averaged fivefold per decade.[3]

MAP INFECTION IN CROHN'S DISEASE

MAP infection in humans is paucimicrobial and extremely difficult to detect. When optimized methods are used, most people with Crohn's disease are found to be infected with MAP.[3,7] MAP is an established multi-host pathogen with the proven ability to cause chronic inflammation of the intestine in many species including primates. Although the causes of Crohn's disease remain subject to disagreements within the scientific literature, the specific association with Crohn's disease makes MAP a strong candidate for disease causation.[7]

References

● = Key primary paper

◆ = Major review article

◆1. Harris ND, Barletta RG. *Mycobacterium avium* subspecies *paratuberculosis* in veterinary medicine. *Clin Microbiol Rev* 2001; **14**: 489–512.

●2. Li LL, Bannantine JP, Zhang Q *et al.* The complete genome sequence of *Mycobacterium avium* subspecies *paratuberculosis*. *Proc Natl Acad Sci USA* 2005; **102**: 12344–9.

◆3. Hermon-Taylor J, El-Zaatari FAK. The *Mycobacterium avium* subspecies *paratuberculosis* problem and its relation to the causation of Crohn's disease. In: Bartram J, Cotruvo J, Dufour A, Rees G, Pedley S (eds) *Pathogenic Mycobacteria in Water: A Guide to Public Health Consequences, Monitoring and Management* (pp. 74–94). London: IWA Publishing, 2004.

●4. Pickup RW, Rhodes G, Arnott S *et al. Mycobacterium avium* subsp *paratuberculosis* in the catchment area and water of the river Taff in South Wales, United Kingdom, and its potential relationship to clustering of Crohn's disease cases in the city of Cardiff. *Appl Environ Microbiol* 2005; **71**: 2130–9.

◆5. Chacon O, Bermudez LE, Barletta RG. Johne's disease, inflammatory bowel disease, and *Mycobacterium paratuberculosis*. *Ann Rev Microbiol* 2004; **58**: 329–63.

●6. Gearry RB, Richardson A, Frampton CM *et al.* Environmental factors associated with Crohn's disease: a population-based case-control study. *Gastroenterology* 2006; **130**: A621–A.

●7. Feller M, Huwiler K, Stephan R *et al. Mycobacterium avium* subspecies *paratuberculosis* and Crohn's disease: a systematic review and meta-analysis. *Lancet Infect Dis* 2007; **7**: 607–13.

SECTION E

Vector and skin-borne diseases

37

Environmental factors that affect vector-borne pathogen transmission

SARAH E. RANDOLPH

BASIC PRINCIPLES

Many pathogenic organisms of different types, from viruses to macroparasites, have evolved to exploit the significant transmission potential offered by vectors. By definition, a vector is an animal that picks up a pathogen from one host (usually a vertebrate) and passes it directly on to another host, without the pathogen having any free-living stage in the environment outside the bodies of either the vector or the host. The vector itself is therefore a host, and the pathogen must be adapted to survive in its two very different types of host alternately. For this direct transmission, the vector typically feeds on the fluid tissues of vertebrates; most vectors are indeed blood-feeding (i.e. parasitic) arthropods, either insects or ticks, but bats may also transmit pathogens, although, curiously, leeches appear to have limited, if any, capacity to do so.

Some vectors act merely as 'flying pins', carrying pathogens mechanically from host to host on mouthparts contaminated with infected blood. This occurs most effectively with vectors such as large tabanid flies; these commonly have painful bites and so, being disturbed before completing their meal, transfer quickly to another host, typically within herds of ungulates. In the majority of vectors, more specialized for completing their meal at one sitting, pathogens undergo a complex biological development cycle: after arriving (and surviving) in the gut, they must exit through the gut wall and transfer to the salivary glands to be ready for reinjection when the vector feeds again. This passage is accompanied by metamorphosis to distinct sequential stages, and multiplication, often involving sexual

reproduction among more complex parasites. This cycle takes time, characterized as the extrinsic incubation period (i.e. extrinsic to the vertebrate host).

Thus the transmission potential of vector-borne pathogens (VBP) depends on a number of biological processes directly involving each member of the pathogen–vector–host triangle and interactions between them (Figure 37.1).[1] Each process operates at a variable rate under different conditions, most obviously increasing (or decreasing) at higher temperatures. Thus, a wide variety of patterns arise from a small handful of the same processes,

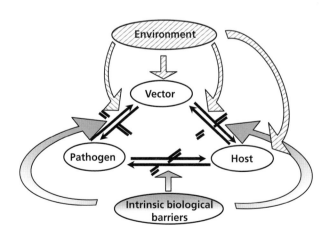

Figure 37.1 The triangle of host–vector–pathogen interactions, showing the points of action of the intrinsic biological barriers to transmission and the extrinsic environmental factors. (Reproduced from Randolph,[1] with permission.)

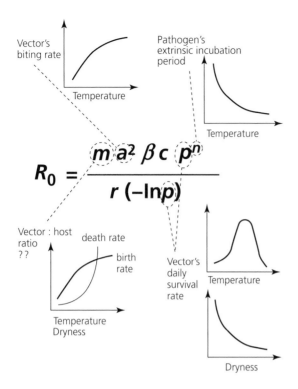

$$R_0 = \frac{m\,a^2\,\beta\,c\,p^n}{r\,(-\ln p)}$$

Figure 37.2   The quantitative biological basis for the impact of climatic factors on the transmission potential of insect-borne pathogens.

The basic reproduction number, R_0, is the central concept in quantitative analytical epidemiology. It expresses the mean number of new cases of infection that arise from the introduction of one index case into a totally susceptible population, i.e. before any immunity has developed. It is thus a measure of the intrinsic transmission potential. Most of the parameters refer to characteristics of the vectors, and most vary with environmental conditions of temperature and rainfall [2].

- n, the extrinsic incubation period, the delay between the insect taking an infected blood meal and being able to transmit infectious pathogens to new hosts, decreases with temperature.

- p, the vector's daily survival probability, increases with temperature until it gets too hot, when survival decreases again; it also decreases with increasing dryness. This determines the insect's lifespan $(1/(-\ln p))$, and also the proportion of the vector population that lives long enough to survive the extrinsic incubation period (p_n).

- a, the vector's daily biting rate, increases with temperature and dryness as insects use up their energy and fluid faster. The term is squared because an insect must bite twice, once to acquire and again to transmit pathogens. Biting rates vary very little (up to about 2-fold) under natural conditions, as insects minimize the danger of contact with defensive hosts, so even squaring this term has relatively little effect on the value of R_0.

- m, the ratio of vectors to hosts, is the single most variable term, varying by up to several orders of magnitude between places, years and seasons. Vector density is very hard to predict because it is the outcome of birth and death rates, both of which are highly sensitive to both temperature and dryness.

- β, c, and r refer to the transmission coefficients from vertebrate to vector and *vice versa*, and the rate of loss of infection by the vertebrate hosts, respectively. They are not known to vary with climate.

Temperature and moisture co-vary so that any increases due to rising temperatures may be (more than) offset by decreases due to greater dryness.

depending on environmental factors that vary in space and time. For insect-borne pathogens, the essential parameters are captured in a simple equation for the basic reproduction number, R_0 (Figure 37.2).[2] The equivalent model for tick-borne pathogens must take account of the very different biology of ticks:[3,4] hard ticks (Ixodidae) take one very large, prolonged meal per life stage, as a larva, nymph and adult at long intervals, while soft ticks (Argasidae) take smaller meals and feed several times as nymphs.

The rates of three critical vector processes – birth, death and feeding – vary with temperature and moisture conditions, but not linearly and not unidirectionally. Thus, for example, an arthropod's birth rate commonly increases with temperature, while its death rate (the reciprocal of survival rate) decreases but then increases again as temperatures rise. At the same time, the death rate increases with dryness, which itself commonly co-varies with temperature (e.g. cool and moist, or hot and dry). In addition, these effects operate differentially on the immature (larval and/or pupal) and adult stages. The outcome in terms of adult vector abundance is unpredictable without a fully parameterized population model, which has been achieved only for tsetse flies as a basis for modelling the transmission dynamics of African trypanosomes[5] and an African tick, *Rhipicephalus appendiculatus*, the vector of *Theileria parva*, which causes East Coast fever in cattle.[6] This gap in our predictive toolbox is unfortunate given the extreme variability of vector density (Figure 37.1).

The rate of pathogen development within the vector also increases with rising ambient temperature. An insect's lifespan is typically short, often not much longer on average than the pathogen's extrinsic incubation period, so that only a small proportion of insects survive long enough to become infectious (i.e. with mature salivary gland infections). Any environmentally driven change in the balance between these two time spans will affect the transmission potential non-linearly.

RISK AND EXPOSURE TO RISK

Any complex system must first be dissected into its component parts before being built up again into a clear description and predictive model. With all infectious diseases, there are two sides to the coin: risk of infection (the presence and abundance of the infectious agents) and exposure to that risk (contact between infectious agents and susceptible hosts). For pathogens whose primary host is humans, a susceptible human who becomes infected soon becomes infectious, so both sides of the coin may be governed by similar factors, those of the R_0 equation. This is true of human malaria.

Many VBPs, however, are zoonotic; they are maintained in cycles between vectors and wildlife host populations, into which humans may intrude accidentally when bitten

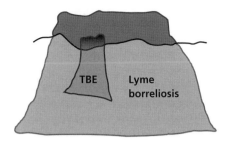

Figure 37.3 The zoonotic iceberg. Wildlife cycles are largely hidden beneath the surface, with exposure varying in time and space. The incidence in humans depends on the bulk (natural transmission potential) and the relative exposure (human contact rates) of the iceberg. Lyme borreliosis, for example, is more prevalent than tick-borne encephalitis (TBE) because it has a greater bulk but the same relative exposure via the same tick vectors. (Reproduced from Randolph and Šumilo,[7] with permission.)

by an infected vector. Humans are dead-end hosts, unable to transmit the pathogen back to vectors. In this case, the risk of infection is governed by the biological factors of the R_0 equation, whereas exposure to that risk is governed by human sociodemographic factors, behaviour, etc. This distinction can be portrayed by the simple analogy of the zoonotic iceberg (Figure 37.2):[7] the risk is equivalent to the submerged bulk of the iceberg, whose size varies with the transmission potential within the enzootic cycles, while exposure to risk is equivalent to the relative size of the visible tip of the iceberg. The size of these two parts may vary independently.

The incidence of infection in humans is thus determined by a nexus of interacting factors, operating with differential force in space and time, which inevitably generates epidemiological heterogeneity. This nexus includes a range of abiotic and biotic environmental factors, together with human behaviour determined by socioeconomic conditions. One or other set of factors, purely biological enzootic or human behavioural, may play the more significant role, but there is an explicit causal linkage from one to the other because environmental conditions may both affect and be affected by human activities.

RELEVANT ASPECTS OF THE ENVIRONMENT

Climate

Temperature is commonly presented as annual means (even on a global scale), to which virtually no creature on earth is exposed or adapted. Instead, organisms respond to a number of specific thermal conditions, any one of which may be limiting, for example the daily minimum, daily maximum, the sum of day–degrees above a threshold value, etc. Furthermore, VBP systems are exquisitely sensitive to seasonal patterns, so that conditions in a

seasonal or weekly period may be critical. In the tropics, the hot dry season may be critical to mosquito survival, whereas in temperate zones, cold winter conditions may impose a demographic bottleneck. For each specific system, the most significant determinant of epidemiological patterns, and therefore past and possible future changes in those patterns, depends on the biological basis of the transmission potential and the timing of maximum human exposure to risk.

Various methods can identify these salient climatic factors, many based on the fact that such factors are correlated with the distribution and/or incidence of infection. Specific statistical methods[8,9] can identify the best correlates of the spatial or temporal variation in incidence. The environmental data (e.g. climatic and land cover) for these exercises may be derived from ground measurements, but these suffer from inadequate numbers of observation stations on continental or even national scales. The alternative is to use surrogate measures remotely sensed from satellites. The latest versions can give either extremely high spatial resolution, down to less than 1 m, but at relatively long time intervals (a few times per year) with each expensive image covering a limited area, or lower spatial resolution, down to less than 1 km, at 10 day or monthly intervals, freely available over the entire globe.[10,11] The latter are most useful for capturing seasonal climate; summary statistics characterizing the seasonal features in each place (each geo-referenced pixel within a geographical information system) over selected years can be extracted using temporal Fourier analysis.[11,12] Satellite data, however, lack long-term continuity, as successive generations of satellites and sensors replace each other.

The moisture conditions to which arthropod vectors are so sensitive are equally specific but are rarely measured directly other than at small scales. Water loss through the cuticle causes decreased activity and risk of death that vary with saturation deficit, a non-linear combination of temperature and relative humidity that determines the drying power of the atmosphere. Relative humidity varies even more than temperature in different parts of the vector's microhabitat, which makes standardized records from a Stevenson's screen (1.33 m above mown grass) useful only for relative degrees of moisture stress. Rainfall may be a more reliable ground-based index of variation over wider areas and longer periods. Within any one type of habitat, the Normalized Difference Vegetation Index (NDVI), a remotely sensed measure of photosynthetic activity in plants, is usefully correlated with saturation deficit and also with insect mortality rates,[13] and can be used to estimate the months suitable for malaria transmission.[14] Although vapour pressure deficit can now be derived from remotely sensed data, it is a somewhat crude index of dubious reliability. The test of all these approximate measures of such an important climatic factor is whether a credible signal emerges more strongly than the background noise.

Land cover and land use

Because both vectors and vertebrate hosts usually occupy specific habitat types according to microclimate and food requirements, land cover has long been recognized as a significant correlate for the presence of a wide variety of VBPs. Land cover maps may be derived from satellite images, again commonly based on the NDVI, whose value and seasonality vary with different plant types. An early example of broad-scale epidemiological use was to establish the strong association of anopheline mosquitoes, and therefore malaria, with rice fields and other places with the standing water required by the mosquito larvae.[15]

Anthropogenic changes can have marked unintended consequences on the risk of VBPs. The abundance of mosquito vectors of both malaria and West Nile virus in the Camargue, an extensive wetland in south-west France, can be related to the historical fluctuations in rice production and chemical pest control in that area, as a consequence of the Marshall Plan (price guarantee) after World War II, the European Common Agricultural Policy in 1963, invasion by the striped rice borer in 1971, the French support plan in 1981, limited subsidies in 1994 under the General Agreement on Tariffs and Trade, and finally the introduction of pest-resistant rice varieties in 2000.[16] As the authors wrote, 'this story highlights the inter-twined importance of historical, political, environmental, technical and social factors in explaining agricultural changes ... contributed to variation in the abundance of [mosquito] populations, with possible consequences for vector-borne diseases.' On the other side of the world, biting rates by *Anopheles darlingi* were higher in areas with more deforestation in the Amazon rainforest due less to the greater presence of humans there than to the mosquito's preference for this more open habitat for breeding sites.[17]

Likewise, because the European tick *Ixodes ricinus* requires the high mid-summer humidity and host density (see below) provided by woodlands, the presence of tick-borne pathogens can be predicted by mapping different types of tree cover.[18] Other tick-borne disease systems are associated with other habitat characteristics. The dry-adapted African bont tick *Amblyomma variegatum*, principal vector of the cattle disease heartwater caused by the rickettsia *Cowdria ruminantium*, was introduced to the Caribbean, where it spread into dry, rough grazing land that had expanded due to land and grazing mismanagement.[19,20]

Land use as distinct from land cover is also important in determining human exposure to risk. In Estonia, Latvia and Slovenia, woodlands that cover about 40–60 per cent of each country have increased in area only gradually since 1970, but their use changed abruptly from the early 1990s. The local incidence of tick-borne encephalitis (TBE) in Latvia is related to different patterns of exploitation, management and access in state-owned and private forests.[21]

Biotic aspects – host availability

Biotic elements are as much a part of the environment as abiotic factors. For any vector that feeds predominantly on wild animals, the presence and density of appropriate species can drive epidemiological events. The decline and final demise of malaria in England (and other northern European and American regions) in the mid-twentieth century has been attributed partially to winter fodder crops allowing larger livestock herds that diverted *Anopheles atroparvus* (the most competent vector) from feeding on humans.[22]

Conversely, the introduction of and increase in deer populations following reforestation in north-east USA during the twentieth century is the most likely explanation for the rise in Lyme disease there,[23,24] because deer, although not competent to transmit the causative *Borrelia burgdorferi* s.l., are essential hosts for adult *Ixodes scapularis* ticks. Recent increases in deer and other large hosts for *Ixodes ricinus* throughout Europe may have helped to drive the apparent increase in both Lyme disease and TBE. At the same time, however, the more hosts there are, the sooner ticks can find one, thereby leaving the questing tick population and reducing their threat to humans.

IMPACTS OF WEATHER ON HUMAN EXPOSURE

In addition to the all-important impact of abiotic factors on all the partners in the enzootic cycle (vectors, wildlife hosts and pathogens), human responses to the weather on short time scales may cause abrupt changes in exposure to risk of infection. Passive exposure to insect bites increases simply by people wearing fewer clothes and opening more windows in hot weather. The spike in TBE incidence in 2006 in Switzerland, Germany, Slovenia and the Czech Republic has been related to the exceptionally warm, dry summer and autumn of that year, interrupted by a cool wet August.[25,26] In addition to a general increase in outdoor recreational activities, conditions were perfect for the growth and harvest of mushrooms from (tick-infested) woodlands, which is a major cultural leisure pursuit in central and eastern Europe[25] and a major risk factor in this disease system.[27] In other countries (Lithuania and Poland), with similar weather but no unusual TBE spike in 2006, the local economic significance of mushrooms as a new cash crop since the advent of the free market may constrain people to harvest mushrooms vigorously whatever the weather.[26]

CONCLUSION

It is clear that a wide range of environmental factors have both direct and indirect impacts on the complex interactions that determine the dynamics of VBP transmission. It is important to distinguish between the effects of weather on short-term fluctuations in incidence, the effects of climate on more or less stable patterns of the distribution and prevalence of infection, and finally the impact of recent and future human-induced climate (and biotic) changes on long-term shifts in distribution and prevalence. Because climate change is the back-drop to all events over recent decades, crude correlations in time with epidemiological changes are inevitable. When tested for causality, however, factors other than climate change, for example variation in vector control, drug effectiveness, wildlife host populations, socioeconomic conditions and human activities, have almost always provided better explanations for recent epidemiological events that include decreases as well as increases in infection rates.

REFERENCES

● = Key primary paper
◆ = Major review article

1. Randolph SE. Dynamics of tick-borne disease systems: minor role of recent climate change. In: de la Roque S (ed.) *Climate Change: The Impacts on the Epidemiology and Control of Animal Diseases*. Paris: Office International des Epizooties, 2008: 367–81.
◆2. Rogers DJ, Randolph SE. Climate change and vector-borne diseases. *Adv Parasitol* 2006; **62**: 345–81.
3. Randolph SE. Ticks are not insects: consequences of contrasting vector biology for transmission potential. *Parasitol Today* 1998; **14**: 186–92.
4. Hartemink NA, Randolph SE, Davis SA, Heesterbeek JAP. The basic reproduction number for complex disease systems: defining R_0 for tick-borne infections. *Am Nat* 2008; **171**: 743–54.
5. Rogers DJ. Satellites, space, time and the African trypanosomiases. *Adv Parasitol* 2000; **47**: 130–73.
6. Randolph SE, Rogers DJ. A generic population model for the African tick *Rhipicephalus appendiculatus*. *Parasitology* 1997; **115**: 265–79.
7. Randolph SE, Šumilo D, Tick-borne encephalitis in Europe: dynamics of changing risk. In: Takken W, Knols BGJ (eds) *Emerging Pests and Vector-borne Disease in Europe*. Wageningen: Wageningen Academic Publishers, 2007: 187–206.
◆8. Hay SI, Graham AJ, Rogers DJ (eds). *Global Mapping of Infectious Diseases: Methods, Examples and Emerging Applications*. London: Academic Press, 2006.
9. Elith J, Graham CH, Anderson RP *et al.* Novel methods improve prediction of species' distributions from occurrence data. *Ecography* 2006; **29**: 129–51.
10. Atkinson PM, Graham AJ. Issues of scale and uncertainty in the global remote sensing of disease. *Adv Parasitol* 2006; **62**: 80–118.
11. Hay SI, Tatem AJ, Graham AJ *et al.* Global environmental data for mapping infectious disease distribution. *Adv Parasitol* 2006; **62**: 37–77.
12. Rogers DJ, Hay SI, Packer MJ. Predicting the distribution of tsetse flies in West Africa using temporal Fourier processed meteorological satellite data. *Ann Trop Med Parasitol* 1996; **90**: 225–41.
●13. Rogers DJ, Randolph SE. Mortality rates and population density of tsetse flies correlated with satellite imagery. *Nature* 1991; **351**: 739–41.
14. Hay SI, Omumba JA, Craig MH, Snow RW. Earth observation, geographic information systems and *Plasmodium falciparum* malaria in sub-saharan Africa. *Adv Parasitol* 2000; **47**: 174–215.
15. Wood BL, Washino R, Beck LR *et al.* Distinguishing high and low anopheline-producing rice fields using remote sensing and GIS technologies. *Prev Vet Med* 1991; **11**: 277–88.
●16. Poncon N, Balenghien T, Toty C *et al.* Effects of local anthropogenic changes on potential malaria vector *Anopheles hyrcanus* and West Nile virus vector *Culex modestus*, Camargue, France. *Emerg Infect Dis* 2007; **13**: 1810–15.
17. Vittor AY, Gilman RH, Tielsch J *et al.* The effect of deforestation on the human-biting rate of *Anopheles darlingi*, the primary vector of falciparum malaria in the Peruvian Amazon. *Am J Trop Med Hyg* 2006; **74**: 3–11.
18. Daniel M, Kolar J, Zeman P *et al.* Predictive map of *Ixodes ricinus* high-incidence habitats and a tick-borne encephalitis risk assessment using satellite data. *Exp Appl Acarol* 1998; **22**: 417–33.
19. Hugh-Jones M, O'Neil P. The epidemiological uses of remote sensing and satellites. In: *4th International Symposium on Veterinary Epidemiology and Economics*. Singapore, 18–22 November, 1985.
20. Hugh-Jones M, Barre N, Nelson G *et al.* Landsat-TM identification of *Amblyomma variegatun* (Acari: Ixodidae) habitats in Guadeloupe. *Rem Sens Environ* 1992; **40**: 43–55.
21. Vanwambeke SO, Šumilo D, Bormane A, Lambin EF, Randolph SE. Landscape predictors of tick-borne encepalitis in Latvia: land cover, land use and land ownership. *Vector Borne Zoonotic Dis* DOI: 10.1089/vbz.2009.0116.
22. Reiter P. From Shakespeare to Defoe: malaria in England in the little ice age. *Emerg Infect Dis* 2000; **6**: 1–11.
23. Spielman A, Wilson ML, Levine JF, Piesman J. Ecology of *Ixodes dammini*-borne human babesiosis and Lyme disease. *Ann Rev Entomol* 1985; **30**: 439–60.
24. Fish D, Daniels TJ, Frank DH, Falco RC. Ecology of Lyme disease in the suburban residential landscape of southern New York State. In: Munderloh UG, Kurtti TJ (eds) *Tick-borne Pathogens at the Host–Vector Interface: An Agenda for Research*. Saint Paul, MN: University of Minnesota, 1992: 274–81.

25. Daniel M, Kriz B, Danielova V, Benes C. Sudden increase in tick-borne encephalitis cases in the Czech Republic, 2006. *Int J Med Microbiol* 2008; **298**(S1): 81–7.

26. Randolph SE, Asokliene L, Avsic-Zupanc T *et al.* Variable spikes in TBE incidence in 2006 independent of variable tick abundance in relation to weather. *Parasit Vectors* 2008; **1**: 44.

27. Šumilo D, Asokliene L, Avsic-Zupanc T *et al.* Behavioural responses to perceived risk of tick-borne encephalitis: vaccination and avoidance in the Baltics and Slovenia. *Vaccine* 2008; **26**: 2580–8.

38

Flavivirus epidemiology, evolution, dispersal and survival: the influence of anthropology

ERNEST A. GOULD, STEPHEN HIGGS

INTRODUCTION

Viruses that infect and are transmitted by arthropods to vertebrate hosts are known as arboviruses (arthropod-borne viruses). With very few exceptions, humans are incidental hosts of arboviruses, i.e. these viruses are naturally sustained and transmitted between vertebrates and arthropod vectors without the need for human infections. There are more than 500 recognized arboviruses, and because arthropods are so sensitive to environmental changes of temperature and humidity, they are excellent indicators for the prediction of emerging arbovirus disease.

The genus *Flavivirus* is growing rapidly but currently represents a group of about 70 closely related flaviviruses several of which cause fever, encephalitis and/or haemorrhagic disease in humans and other animal species. They are enveloped RNA viruses with a diameter of approximately 50 nm. They have a positive-sense genome of about 10.5 kb. The open-reading frame encodes three structural proteins (envelope, capsid and membrane) and seven non-structural proteins (NS1, NS2a, NS2b, NS3, NS4a, NS4b and NS5).[1–4] The 5′ and 3′ terminal flanking regions of the viral genome encode untranslated regions (UTRs) that function as promoters and enhancers of virus replication. These UTRs fold to form secondary structures that provide a structural scaffold for the assembly of the viral and cellular proteins that represent the virus replication complex. Detailed comparative manual alignments of flavivirus UTR sequences and computer-simulated predictions of RNA secondary structure have revealed a range of repeat sequences referred to as direct repeats that represent surviving elements of ancestral RNA. These repeated sequences can be used to define relationships between widely disparate flaviviruses, providing new insights into flavivirus survival and evolution.[5–10]

TYPES OF FLAVIVIRUS

The first flaviviruses were isolated in the early 1930s,[11] and as more were discovered and characterized, it became clear that the natural transmission cycles of some mosquito-borne flaviviruses (MBFVs) were primarily associated with *Aedes* spp. mosquitoes, whereas others were typically associated with *Culex* spp.[12] Subsequent studies of flavivirus antigenic relationships using neutralization tests demonstrated their subdivision into tick-borne, mosquito-borne and no-known vector viruses.[13,14] These findings were confirmed and further elaborated using phylogenetic analyses, initially based on partial sequences representing the highly conserved non-structural (NS5) polymerase and the variable envelope (E) gene.[15,16]

The phylogenies defined two specific clades of MBFV, i.e. viruses primarily associated with *Culex* spp. mosquitoes and viruses primarily associated with *Aedes* spp. mosquitoes, correlating closely with the antigenic and ecological interpretations (Figure 38.1). These subdivisions are not absolute; for example, some *Culex* spp.-associated viruses can also infect and be transmitted by *Aedes* spp. mosquitoes, and vice versa. However, the vector with which each virus is primarily associated conforms to the reported antigenic and phylogenetic patterns. Thus, the

412   Flavivirus epidemiology, evolution, dispersal and survival: the influence of anthropology

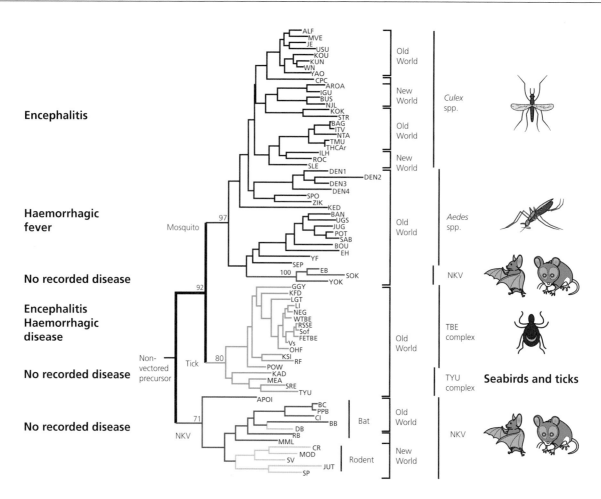

Figure 38.1 Phylogenetic tree showing the association between the groups of related viruses with their invertebrate vectors, vertebrate hosts and geographical distribution. ALF, Alfuy; MVE, Murray Valley encephalitis; JE, Japanese encephalitis; USU, Usutu; KOU, Koutango; KUN, Kunjin; WN, West Nile; YAO, Yaounde; CPC, Cacipacore; ARO, Aroa; IGU, Iguape; BUS, Bussuquara; NJL, Naranjal; KOK, Kokobera; STR, Stratford; BAG, Bagaza; IT, Israel Turkey meningoencephalomyelitis virus; NTA, Ntaya; TMU, Tembusu; THCAr, strain of Tembusu; ILH, Ilheus; ROC, Rocio; SLE, St Louis encephalitis; DEN, dengue; SPO, Spondweni; ZIK, Zika forest; KED, Kedougou; BAN, Banzi; UGS, Uganda S; JUG, Jugra; POT, Potiskum; SAB, Saboya; BOU, Bouboui; EH, Edge Hill; YF, Yellow fever; SEP, Sepik; EB, Entebbe bat; SOK, Sokoluk; YOK, Yokose; GGY, Gadgets Gully; KFD, Kyasanur Forest disease; LGT, Langat; LI, Louping ill; NEG, Negishi; WTBE, Western European TBE; RSSE, Russian spring and summer encephalitis; Sof, Sofjin; FETBE, far eastern TBE; Vs, Vasilchenko; OHF, Omsk haemorrhagic fever; KSI, Karshi; RF, Royal Farm; POW, Powassan; KAD, Kadam; MEA, Meaban; SRE, Saumarez Reef; TYU, Tyuleniy; APOI, Apoi; BC, Batu Cave; PPB, Phnom Penh bat; CI, Carey Island; BB, Bukalasa bat; DB, Dakar bat; RB, Rio Bravo; MML, Montana myotis leukoencephalitis; CR, Cowbone Ridge; MOD, Modoc; SV, Sal Vieja; JUT, Jutiapa; SP, San Perlita; NKV, viruses with no known vector; TBE, tick-borne encephalitis. (Adapted from Gould and Solomon,[1] with permission.)

findings based on molecular epidemiological studies are compatible with virological and ecological data.

In this chapter, we focus on selected medically important viruses that can be divided into two categories: tick-borne flaviviruses (TBFVs), which include tick-borne encephalitis virus (TBEV), Omsk haemorrhagic fever virus (OHFV) and Kyasanur Forest disease virus (KFDV); and the MBFV that subdivide into those associated primarily with *Aedes* spp. mosquitoes, i.e. yellow fever virus (YFV) and dengue virus (DENV), or with *Culex* spp. mosquitoes, i.e. Japanese encephalitis virus (JEV), St Louis encephalitis virus (SLEV) and Murray Valley encephalitis virus.[16]

FLAVIVIRUSES TRANSMITTED BY TICKS

The mammalian TBFVs were originally known as the 'tick-borne encephalitis antigenic complex' because they all share close antigenic relationships. The prototype TBEV, designated Russian spring and summer encephalitis virus (RSSEV), was isolated in far-east Asia in 1937.[17] In a recent survey covering the past 30 years, there has been a reported overall increase in incidence of tick-borne encephalitis in Europe and Russia from a total of approximately 3000 to about 9000 cases per year.[18] Related but less virulent strains of TBEV are found in western and west-central Europe, causing between 2000 and 3000 cases of encephalitis annually.

Louping ill virus (LIV) is the UK form of TBEV. LIV was first described in 1930[19] and, in common with closely related strains in Spain, Turkey and Greece, is primarily associated with encephalomyelitis in sheep, rather than humans. This is primarily explained by the low frequency of human exposure to infected ticks, rather than inherent virus properties.

Human infections with TBFV are frequently asymptomatic but can produce a wide range of clinical manifestations, including subclinical infections, biphasic fever, chronic disease and encephalitis, which may result in paresis or fatal infection. OHFV, KFDV and Alkhurma virus (ALKV) are characteristically associated with fatal haemorrhagic fever. In general, however, the haemorrhagic fever viruses do not cause major epidemics, probably because human exposure to infected ticks rarely, if ever, occurs on an epidemic scale. Nevertheless, serological surveys suggest between 70 per cent and 95 per cent of TBEV human infections are subclinical,[20–22] indicating frequent exposure to infected ticks.

An unusual feature of tick-borne encephalitis is seen when whole families contract biphasic fever during local epidemic outbreaks.[23] This form of disease is associated with the consumption of goat's milk or cheese. Although it was first recognized immediately following World War II, this type of infection is still recorded in many parts of Eurasia. Apparently, the milk of the infected goats remains infectious for weeks.

Arthropod vectors of the TBEV group include hard ticks in the genera *Ixodes*, *Haemaphysalis* and *Dermacentor*, with a life-cycle that may last from a few months to several years depending on the prevailing climatic conditions.[24] They feed only three times during their life-cycle: once as larvae, once as nymphs and once as adults, prior to laying the eggs that produce the next generation (Figure 38.2). If they become infected as larvae, they may remain infected throughout their life-cycle. Thus, the virus spends most of its time replicating in the invertebrate rather than the vertebrate host.

This protracted life-cycle has a major impact on the evolution, dispersal and survival of the TBFV. Vertebrates become infected when they are fed upon by TBFV-infected ticks and may develop a viraemia that provides an infectious blood meal for uninfected feeding ticks. Thus, the cycle of virus transmission between ticks and vertebrates is maintained through viraemic infection of the vertebrate host. Importantly, for reasons discussed below, viral replication may result in viraemia while the transmitting ticks are still feeding. In contrast, with MBFV, replication occurs long after the transmitting mosquito has left the host. However, although viraemic transmission and associated disease undoubtedly occur in susceptible humans and some animal species,[1,25] this is not the primary mechanism by which TBFVs survive long-term in the wild. Most TBEV group viruses are associated with ticks and wild animals such as rodents and deer in forest environments.[1,26] Disease is rarely associated with these animals, although serological evidence confirms exposure to TBEV group viruses. Thus the viruses continue to cycle even in the absence of symptomatic and viraemic infections.

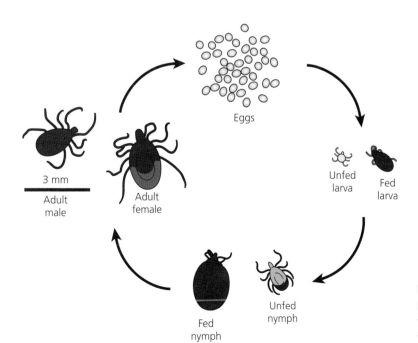

Figure 38.2 Life cycle of *Ixodes ricinus* ticks, represented by the individual stages through which the tick passes from the egg to the engorged adult female. The complete cycle may last up to 5 years.

The discovery of non-viraemic transmission of LIV[27] and of TBEV[28] between co-feeding nymphs and larvae provides a rational explanation for how these viruses may survive in nature. Since non-viraemic transmission can take place between ticks co-feeding on susceptible or insusceptible animals and even on immune animals, this mode of transmission can be sustained by a wide variety of vertebrates including those which some virologists regard as dead-end hosts. Non-viraemic transmission therefore ensures a wide variety of potential hosts to maintain the virus.[1,29]

Moreover, the virus does not need to replicate significantly in the exposed vertebrate for co-feeding transmission to occur. This has implications for the genetic variation of the virus, which is known to vary according to the host in which the virus replicates.[22] Therefore, the rates of evolution and of dispersal of TBFV group viruses are primarily determined by the protracted generation time of the tick and its limited movement across the forest undergrowth.[3] Indeed, molecular epidemiological comparisons of evolution rates estimated that the mosquito-transmitted flaviviruses evolve at approximately 2.5 times the rate of the TBFVs. This is largely explained by the fact that mosquitoes have much shorter generation times and replicate virus to high titres within a few days.[30]

Evidence based on phylogenetic analysis and population dynamics supports the concept that the TBFVs have gradually evolved across the Old World forests of the northern hemisphere over an estimated period of about 2000 years.[30–32] This correlation of increasing genetic distance with time and geographical dispersal is known as clinal evolution and is illustrated in Figure 38.3.

Omsk haemorrhagic fever virus

OHFV is closely related to the far-east Asian strains of TBEV, and although it is primarily associated with haemorrhagic fever in humans, sporadic cases of encephalitis may also be seen with this virus. OHFV occupies a different ecological niche from forest-associated TBEV. Epidemic foci characteristically occur in the Omsk and Novosibirsk regions of West Siberia, associated with the forest-steppe. There are also recent reports of emerging Omsk haemorrhage fever-like clinical manifestations in the Ukraine, Smolensk, North Kazakhstan and Orenburg, although this information requires confirmation.

Historically, sporadic human haemorrhagic fever outbreaks were associated with epizootics in muskrats (*Ondatra zibethica*) that were reintroduced into the Omsk region in 1928 from Canada to replace the locally extinct species. Prior to the introduction of muskrats, which are highly susceptible to the disease, Omsk haemorrhage fever was probably very rare in humans. Muskrats were hunted by the local farmers, who became infected with OHFV

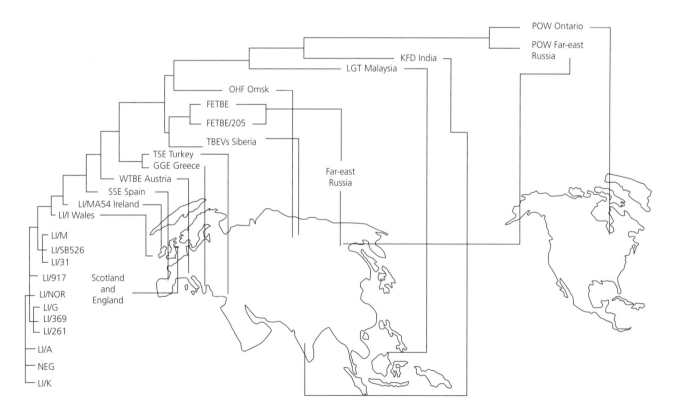

Figure 38.3 Illustration of the clinal evolution of viruses in the tick-borne encephalitis virus complex. LI, louping ill; NEG, Negishi; SSE, Spanish sheep encephalitis; WTBE, Western European tick-borne encephalitis; GGE, Greek goat encephalitis; TSE, Turkish sheep encephalitis; TBEV, tick-borne encephalitis virus; FETBE, far Eastern tick-borne encephalitis; OHF, Omsk haemorrhagic fever; LGT, Langat; KFD, Kyasanur Forest disease; POW, Powassan. (Adapted from Zanotto *et al.*,[31] with permission.)

when they skinned the animals. It is presumed that the farmers transmitted the virus to their close relatives possibly by direct contact. However, the indigenous small mammalian species (rats, voles, mice, hamsters, polecats and birds) are much less susceptible to infection by OHFV,[33] and it is likely that the virus circulates naturally among some of all of these indigenous species.

The onset of human infection is marked by fever, headache, myalgia and cough, which progress to bradycardia, dehydration, hypotension and gastrointestinal symptoms. The most marked pathological signs of the disease are focal visceral haemorrhages in the mucosa of the nose, gums, uterus and lungs. Clinical symptoms also include diffuse encephalitis, which disappears during the recovery period. Convalescence is usually uneventful without residual effects; fatal cases are also registered, but rarely (0.5–3 per cent).[33]

Kyasanur Forest disease virus

Although the transmission cycle of KFDV has not been studied as exhaustively as that of TBEV, their genetic similarity makes it reasonable to assume that there are many common features between these viruses. Kyasanur Forest disease was first recognized in January 1957 as a febrile illness at the Primary Health Centre at Ulvi in the Shimoga district of Karnataka State in India.[34] Preceding the human epidemic, a large number of sick and dead monkeys had been noticed in the nearby forest area. The virus was isolated from dead monkeys, sick patients and from *Haemaphysalis* spp. ticks. This emergent virus was shown to be genetically closely related to the other TBFVs[35] and, based on the subsequent discovery of the clinical evolution and dispersal of the TBFVs, described above, as well as the discovery of ALKV (see below), it seems likely that the introduction of KFDV into this region of India was partly the result of commercial animal transportation and partly a natural process of dispersal and adaptation to ground-dwelling wildlife species.[26] The outbreaks of haemorrhagic disease that were first recognized in monkeys from 1957 in India probably arose as the result of environmental perturbation through land reclamation, urbanization and deforestation. Under these different conditions, scavenging arboreal monkeys descended to the forest floor and encountered KFDV-infected ticks.[26,35,36] Humans entering these tick-infested areas were similarly exposed to the virus.

Cases of haemorrhagic disease due to KFDV are now observed annually in or near the forest regions of Karnataka State. Moreover, serological evidence of the presence of KFDVs has also been found in Gujarat State[36] on the western coast of India directly facing the Arabian Peninsula. It is therefore logical to assume that KFDV or a closely related virus is also present in other states, such as Maharashtra State, which separates the states of Karnataka and Gujarat. Indeed, the fact that KFDV has not been reported does not mean that it is not present in that state. Its detection reflects the rate of exposure to infected ticks, which may differ in different states.

Alkhurma virus

A virus closely related to KFDV, designated 'Alkhurma virus', was discovered in 1992 in the Arabian Peninsula. This virus causes haemorrhagic disease indistinguishable from that caused by KFDV in humans. It was first identified in butchers and associated workers who handled sheep and camels imported into Saudi Arabia to feed the millions of people who make the annual pilgrimage to Mecca.[37] Although infectious ALKV was never isolated from ticks removed from these animals, a molecular analysis of ticks collected from camels and camel resting places in three different locations in western Saudi Arabia revealed ALKV.

Whether or not ALKV was introduced into the Arabian Peninsula by ticks associated with these imported animals is unknown. However, animal trading which is common between Gujarat State and the Arabian Peninsula could explain the genetic closeness of ALKV and KFDV. These viruses are also closely related to other viruses found in Africa and Asia.[3,15,38] Thus, the annual large-scale introduction of livestock into the Arabian Peninsula from surrounding African and Asian regions could explain how ALKV and KFDV have evolved and dispersed from ancestral African or Asian viruses.

FLAVIVIRUSES TRANSMITTED BY MOSQUITOES

Yellow fever virus

The Latin word *flavus* means 'yellow', and thus the term *Flavivirus* reflects the type species of the genus, i.e. 'yellow fever virus', so named because the skin of infected individuals may appear yellow (from jaundice) due to infection of the liver.

On the basis of phylogenetic analysis (see Figure 38.1) and vector–host relationships, the mosquito-transmitted flaviviruses were divided into two major groups: flaviviruses primarily associated with *Aedes* spp. mosquitoes, and those primarily associated with *Culex* spp. mosquitoes.[16] However, with the frequent publication of new flavivirus sequences, further subdivisions will be required in future. Nevertheless, these general groupings and their ecological and geographical correlations provide a fascinating and highly informative interpretation of the evolutionary history of flaviviruses. In many cases, the phylogenies can explain the epidemiological characteristics of the flaviviruses.[26,30,39]

The most frequently reported estimates for yellow fever infections are 200 000 cases per year, of which up to

30 000 may result in death, but in view of the poor accessibility to many of the cases that occur in remote regions of Africa, such data are presumed to be an underestimate.[40] However, recent World Health Organization (WHO) records show a lower frequency of cases.[41] It seems unlikely that this reflects human immunity resulting from the administration of live attenuated YF 17D vaccine, since despite the demonstrated success of the vaccine, relatively few people in areas endemic for yellow fever are routinely immunized against the virus. Human serological studies show that many infections result in asymptomatic or very mild disease, which is unlikely to be reported. This background immunity could lessen the impact of virus spread and thus its epidemicity. In severe cases, infection is followed by an incubation period of 3–6 days.

Two phases of clinical symptoms are recognized. The 'acute' phase is normally characterized by fever, muscle pain (with prominent backache), headache, shivers, loss of appetite, nausea and/or vomiting. The high fever is often paradoxically associated with a slow pulse. After 3–4 days, the condition of most of these patients improves, and their symptoms disappear. However, about 15 per cent enter a 'toxic phase' within 24 hours. Fever reappears, and the patient may rapidly develop jaundice and abdominal pain accompanied by vomiting. Bleeding can occur from the mouth, nose, eyes and/or stomach, and blood appears in the vomit and faeces. Kidney function deteriorates; this can range from abnormal protein levels in the urine (albuminuria) to complete kidney failure with no urine production (anuria). Up to 60 per cent of these patients may die within 10–14 days. The remainder recover without significant organ damage.[40]

The tropical jungles of central/west Africa, South America and some Caribbean islands provide natural habitats for YFV. In the African jungles, the 'sylvatic' life-cycle of YFV involves transmission of the virus between *Aedes africanus* mosquitoes and monkeys. The female mosquitoes feed at dusk and dawn, and at this time the monkeys rest and sleep in the canopy (tree tops) of the forests. Since, in general, relatively few humans visit the African jungles, human infections are only rarely recorded as being 'jungle fever'.

However, an 'intermediate' life-cycle involves the neighbouring savannah regions, particularly where human agricultural activity occurs, and monkeys often forage for food. *Aedes simpsoni* is highly competent to reproduce and transmit YFV and is commonly found in these savannah regions; it will feed on either humans or monkeys, thus bridging the gap between the sylvan and rural/urban environments. Human epidemics are frequently seen in the rural villages. Infected humans occasionally then carry the virus to accessible urban areas, i.e. small towns or even cities, where *Aedes aegypti* is the predominant anthropophilic (human-biting) mosquito species. The introduction of YFV into the urban environment results in epidemics of varying intensity depending on the prevailing climatic conditions and the resultant mosquito densities. These cases are known as 'urban fever'.[42]

Generally speaking, in Africa, disease is rarely seen in the monkeys in the jungles, implying that this natural monkey–mosquito virus cycle has existed for many years. Moreover, serological studies have shown that, in sylvatic endemic areas, many monkeys develop immunity to YFV during their early years of life. It is therefore possible that the primary transmission mechanism for YFV is that it cycles among mosquitoes and immunologically naive monkeys. An alternative would be for the virus to circulate among the immune monkeys and mosquitoes, but this would require a mechanism such as non-viraemic transmission to occur, because immune monkeys would presumably not develop viraemic infections. A third possibility is that the virus survives long-term by circulating among other forest animals and mosquitoes. Although YFV has been isolated from other species in jungles, none of these alternative possibilities has been adequately investigated.

A similar situation exists in Latin America, but there are important differences. First, YFV-infected monkeys in Latin America often develop fatal haemorrhagic disease. The most plausible explanation for this is that these monkeys are neither resistant nor immune to the virus, possibly because the virus was introduced into Latin America relatively recently when compared with YFV in Africa. Second, in Latin American jungles, and in regions equivalent to those of the savannah in Africa, YFV is associated most frequently with *Haemagogus* spp. mosquitoes. In Latin America, yellow fever is most frequently associated with humans entering the forests and neighbouring areas, seeking food, farming or cutting down trees in the forests, which exposes them to the *Haemagogus* spp. that normally inhabit the forest canopy. Alternatively, monkeys sick and dying from YFV infection do occasionally introduce the virus into mosquito species associated with the small communities in the savannah regions. Human cases of urban fever are seen much less frequently than in Africa, and urban epidemics are rarely recorded these days in Latin America.

Max Theiler was awarded the Nobel Prize for his work on the development of a yellow fever vaccine. He first reported evidence that the African and Latin American strains of YFV were very closely related.[43,44] Indeed, he used the same virus to develop a vaccine against both African and Latin American YFV. However, they are genetically distinct and have clearly been geographically separated for a significant amount of time. Historical records provide the most plausible explanation for why YFV has this relatively restricted geographical distribution, i.e. Africa and Latin America. In addition to the ecological characteristics of YFV in Africa, phylogenetic evidence supports historical records implying that YFV emerged in Africa during the past few millenia.[26,44]

Nevertheless, during the past 400–500 years, many cases of yellow fever infection were recorded in the tropical and subtropical regions of Latin America. Until the beginning of the twentieth century, these New World cases of yellow fever almost always coincided with the arrival of ships carrying slaves from Africa to the New World. The records show that many slaves died with yellow fever as they were moved from central Africa to the western coast prior to transportation across the Atlantic Ocean. Others died on the ships during transportation or even after arriving in the New World.[26,45,46] Indeed, even though yellow fever is not endemic in North America, quite frequent epidemics occurred in the Mississippi region and even New York and Boston during the most intensive periods of slave trading with Africa.[46] It is believed that repeated introductions of *Aedes aegypti* and YFV-infected humans from the slave ships refuelled the outbreaks of yellow fever among local residents.[47]

As the accompanying *Aedes aegypti*, introduced from Africa, became established in Latin America, YFV became endemic among humans in urban and semi-urban regions, although it has in general remained most closely associated with forest and savannah regions within tropical South America. There are also records of local outbreaks of yellow fever in northern Europe when ships carrying sick passengers returned from the Caribbean.[45] Presumably these localized and usually very short-term outbreaks in the cooler northern European regions could not be sustained by the indigenous mosquitoes, which were insufficiently competent and/or abundant to maintain replication and transmission of the virus between humans.

Dengue virus

With 50–100 million estimated dengue infections occurring annually,[48] dengue fever presents a different epidemiological picture from yellow fever even though both viruses cause haemorrhagic disease and are transmitted between humans by the same mosquito species, i.e. *Aedes aegypti*. First, the four DENV serotypes (DENV-1, DENV-2, DENV-3 and DENV-4) are distributed much more widely than YFV, causing disease in all tropical regions of the world, and they are particularly prominent in Asia and south east Asia.[49]

Second, although sylvatic cycles are recognized for DENV in Africa and Asia, in contrast with YFV, given the vectors and susceptible humans, dengue epidemics may be sustained for long periods and over wide geographical regions of the tropics without the requirement of virus replenishment from forest/savannah reservoirs. Indeed, different DENV serotypes may overlap geographically and contribute independently to outbreaks of disease among dense human populations, a characteristic known as hyperendemicity.[50] In other words, DENV is transmitted highly efficiently between humans by *Aedes aegypti*. In contrast, whereas *Aedes aegypti* is almost entirely responsible for the human transmission of YFV during epidemics, the efficiency of transmission appears to be lower than for DENV, possibly due to a combination of lower vector competence, shorter viraemic periods and lower viraemias in humans.

Third, DENV shows much higher levels of genetic variability than YFV, so, in addition to the existence of four genetically distinct serotypes, there are several genotypes within the serotypes, and significant strain variation within the genotypes is also recognized.[51] This genetic variability may provide DENV with the capacity to circumvent the protective barrier of human immunity.

Fourth, in addition to *Aedes aegypti*, DENV can also be transmitted by *Aedes albopictus*,[52,53] the so-called 'Tiger mosquito', so named because of its striped appearance. In contrast, YFV is not normally associated with transmission by *Aedes albopictus*. The significance of this mosquito species in the epidemiology of DENV is currently not fully understood, but because of its semi-rural nature, it may contribute to the provision of a long-term survival strategy for DENV during interepidemic periods. Moreover, the alphavirus Chikungunya virus has recently greatly increased its geographical dispersal as the result of adaptation to *Aedes albopictus* by a single mutation in the envelope glycoprotein.[54,55] A similar type of adaptation by any or all of the four DENV serotypes could have major implications for their epidemiology and dispersal.

Finally, serological evidence shows that, in young children, most human dengue fever results in a nonspecific febrile illness. In older children and adults, the disease presents as a classic fever–arthralgia–rash syndrome, with skin eruptions, an abrupt onset of fever and muscle and joint pains, usually with retro-orbital pain, photophobia and lymphadenopathy. In severe cases of dengue fever, the patient may experience severe joint pains, originally described by a Spanish physician in Puerto Rico in 1771 as 'quebrantahuesos', i.e. 'breakbone'. The word 'dengue' is attributed to the Queen of Spain who, in 1801, used the word to describe the acute febrile illness with bone and joint pains, haemorrhage and jaundice. Petechiae, bleeding from the gums, nose or gastrointestinal tract, leukopenia and mild thrombocytopenia are often observed.

Most patients recover rapidly, but depression is common after infection. However, depending on the previous history of DENV in a particular geographical area, up to 1–2 per cent of infections may result in more severe forms of the disease, defined as dengue haemorrhagic fever or dengue shock syndrome, resulting in fatal infections with a frequency of up to 1 per cent[48] if high-quality medical intervention is not readily available.

Dengue haemorrhagic fever presents as increased vascular permeability with plasma leakage into the tissues, accompanied by thrombocytopenia and bleeding manifestations. Dengue shock syndrome takes place if the leakage or bleeding, or both, are sufficient to induce shock. In children, a reduced difference between systolic and diastolic pressures is common (shown by a narrowing of the pulse pressure). The syndrome is treated by prompt restoration of plasma volume. WHO guidelines[56] recommend the replacement of plasma losses with crystalloid solutions, followed by colloids for patients with recurrent or refractory shock.

Over the past 30 years, co-circulation of the four antigenically related but distinct serotypes has become widespread. This has coincided with a marked increase in the global number of reported cases of dengue fever and an almost six-fold increase in the number of countries reporting dengue haemorrhagic fever. Rapid and unplanned urbanization, increased human movement and ineffective mosquito control strategies are among the many factors that have contributed to this increased number of cases.[57]

There is still considerable debate concerning the factors that lead to the development of dengue haemorrhagic fever in humans. It has been suggested that dengue haemorrhagic fever arises when strains having increased virulence cause a human epidemic,[58] and there are also reports implying that some humans may be genetically predisposed to the development of dengue haemorrhagic fever/dengue shock syndrome.[59,60] This is to some extent supported by the evidence that black-skinned humans of African descent appear to be less susceptible to the development of dengue haemorrhagic fever/dengue shock syndrome than caucasians.[61]

Regardless of these various observations and interpretations, there is good evidence to show that, some years after primary infection with one DENV serotype, residual low-level non-neutralizing antibodies reacting with a second infecting DENV serotype can enhance virus infectivity by targeting the virus–antibody complex to Fc-receptors on the antigen-presenting macrophages. This results in the activation of pre-existing cross-reactive DENV-specific T-lymphocytes from the primary flavivirus infection.[62,63] This self-amplifying cascade can then lead to the release of cytokines and chemical mediators that may cause plasma leakage.[64]

There are currently no vaccines or antiviral agents with which to control the epidemiology of DENV. However, several different strategies are currently being employed to develop live attenuated vaccines. The major difficulties anticipated are, first, the need to demonstrate that the vaccine can simultaneously immunize humans against all four DENV serotypes, and second, the problem of logistics, i.e. how to deliver the vaccine to those in most need of protection.

Japanese encephalitis virus

Japanese encephalitis is both endemic and epidemic in the subtropical and tropical regions of Asia. This virus is estimated to cause at least 50 000 cases of encephalitis each year, with a fatality rate of about 25 per cent.[65] As shown in Figure 38.1, viruses included in the JEV antigenic complex are primarily associated with *Culex* spp., mosquitoes that feed on birds, humans, pigs, horses, rodents, reptiles and even amphibians. The most important JEV vectors are *Culex tritaeniorhynchus, Culex annulus,*

Culex fuscocephala, Culex gelidus and mosquitoes in the *Culex vishnui* complex. *Culex* spp. breed in rice paddy fields and in new irrigation projects that support agricultural development, both of which increase the number of mosquitoes and the risk of disease outbreaks.[66]

In horses in endemic regions of Asia, most JEV infections are asymptomatic but may progress to encephalitis, although the mortality rate is relatively low. Horses appear to be dead-end hosts for the virus, whereas pigs, which may suffer reproductive failure (stillbirth, mummification, embryonic death and infertility), can act as amplifying hosts for the virus. A seasonal cycle of transmission exists in the temperate regions of Asia: mosquitoes appear in late spring, horses and swine become infected during the summer, and human cases peak during August and September. Although JEV is primarily maintained in the environment by transmission between birds and mosquitoes, the birds apparently do not show signs of infection.

Analysis of the phylogenetic trees based on nucleotide and amino acid sequence data implies that the JEV complex viruses have their evolutionary origins in Africa, since the ancestral lineage of this clade is descended from more divergent lineages that contain mostly African flaviviruses. However, the strains of JEV that currently cause human epidemics in the Old World through India, Sri Lanka, Pakistan, Bangladesh, southern China, Malaysia, Vietnam, Indonesia, Thailand, Northern Marianna Islands, Papua New Guinea and occasionally Japan, probably emerged from an ancestral African virus lineage that was introduced by birds into south-east Asia. In this geographical region, all year round high temperatures and humidity provide ideal environmental conditions for high densities of competent vectors to feed on highly susceptible vertebrates.

Although the extensive geographical distribution of JEV throughout large regions of southern Asia primarily reflects dispersal by migratory birds, the commercial transportation of animals and other goods such as scrap car tyres or plants are also recognized as efficient methods of dispersing mosquitoes.[47] An important consequence of these dispersal mechanisms is that virtually identical and also substantially different strains of JEV can be isolated either at the same site or at sites thousands of miles apart,[39,67,68] thus complicating the interpretation of data relating to the evolution, dispersal, epidemiology and pathogenesis of JEV.

Disease following infection with JEV is more common in children than in adults because children usually do not have immunity to the virus. The disease has an incubation period varying from about 5 to 15 days. Early symptoms may include headache, cough, coryza, nausea, vomiting, diarrhoea and rigors. Alternatively, patients may present with aseptic meningitis or acute flaccid paralysis and have no encephalopathic features. Japanese encephalitis typically includes a syndrome similar to Parkinson's disease, with facial expressions that are mask-like with wide unblinking eyes,[1] tremor and cogwheel rigidity. Other abnormal movements, such as upper motor neurone and cerebellar signs, and cranial nerve palsies, may also be seen. Seizures are common, especially in children. About 30 per cent of patients who develop severe disease have frank persistent motor deficits or more subtle sequelae such as learning difficulties and behavioural problems.[1]

Theoretically, the most effective method for the control of diseases such as Japanese encephalitis would be to eradicate the mosquito vectors. This is, however, an almost impossible task except perhaps in localized urban areas with well-developed infrastructures. Vaccines are currently the most effective alternative to vector eradication in horses, pigs and humans. This strategy has proved reasonably successful in countries such as Japan, Korea and Taiwan, and even in a country as large as China, the widespread use of inactivate and live attenuated vaccines has significantly reduced the incidence of Japanese encephalitis in children. In many other Asian countries, such as India, Malaysia, Sri Lanka, Indonesia and Burma, vaccine usage has been less effectively coordinated. However, recent attempts to develop a structured programme of human immunization in India, partly funded by The Bill & Melinda Gates Foundation, using 13 million doses of vaccine supplied by China at a substantially reduced price, offer hope for the future.[1]

St Louis encephalitis virus

St Louis encephalitis virus is a member of the JEV complex,[2,11] and although it is antigenically and genetically closely related to JEV,[14–16,69] it is found exclusively in the New World, i.e. the Americas, and is thus geographically isolated from JEV, which is currently found only in the Old World, i.e. Asia and Australasia. Human cases of St Louis encephalitis in the USA were first recorded in 1933, and the virus was named after an epidemic that occurred in St Louis, Missouri.[70–72] There have been at least 41 recorded outbreaks in North America since that time.

The natural virus–vector transmission cycle involves a wide range of bird species and mosquitoes in the genus *Culex*. On the basis of serological evidence, humans and other mammals are often infected but rarely develop clinical disease.[71] In general, they are considered to be dead end hosts for SLEV. An average of 128 cases of St Louis encephalitis are recorded annually in North America. In temperate areas, St Louis encephalitis cases occur primarily in the late summer or early fall. However, in the southern USA, where the climate is warm throughout the year, infections occur all year round.[72] Fatality rates increase with age, with humans below 49 years old exhibiting mortality rates of 5 per cent, but those above 70 years of age showing a rate of 23 per cent.[71] Interestingly, it has recently been suggested that the presence of West Nile virus in the USA may be reducing the incidence of infections caused by SLEV.[73]

Infections due to SLEV that may result in encephalitis often go unrecognized because of the lack of awareness of its circulation.[74] For example, in the summer of 1989, in Kern County, southern California, a sudden increase in hospital admissions presenting with encephalitis coincided with high seroconversion rates in sentinel chickens. This led to follow-up tests on blood samples of patients discharged after central nervous system disease, approximately 30 per cent of whom had elevated immunoglobulin M titres against SLEV, indicating recent SLEV infection.[71,75] In the absence of immunity, clinical disease is most severe and frequent among the elderly, although in endemic areas where acquired immunity rates are highest in older residents, clinical illness has been shown to peak in children rather than the elderly.[76]

Clinical disease may present as one of three distinct syndromes:

- headache with fever, headache associated with nausea or vomiting, and no central nervous system illness;
- aseptic meningitis with a high fever and stiff neck;
- encephalitis (including meningoencephalitis and encephalomyelitis) with a high fever, altered consciousness and/or neurological dysfuntion.

The onset may be sudden (less than 4 days) and acute, rapidly leading to encephalitis or insidious progression through all three syndromes. Symptoms may resolve spontaneously during any stage of the illness with full recovery. Acute illness may be followed by 'convalescent fatigue syndrome' in fewer than 50 per cent of patients, with complaints of general weakness, depression and an inability to concentrate. Other sequelae include disturbances in gait and memory loss.[74,77–79]

A combination of phylogenetic studies and historical evidence provides the basis for a rational explanation for how SLEV circulates among birds and mosquitoes in the New World but is genetically closely related to other JEV complex viruses that are found solely in the Old World.[1,15,16,80] It appears most likely that one or more of the ancestral lineages to the JEV complex viruses was dispersed to the Americas via transportation from Africa, where ancestral lineages that include YFV are known to circulate. Evidence for this assumption is now compelling. First, the main vectors of SLEV are *Culex* spp. mosquitoes, and all the evidence suggests that this mosquito species was introduced into the Americas from the Old World.[81] Second, the most likely method of dispersal of these mosquitoes to the New World was via ships.[47] Third, there is also genetic evidence that humans introduced lice from the Old World to the New World at least 1000 years ago, i.e. before the voyage of Columbus to the New World,[82] reinforcing the evidence of the movement of humans and associated species across the Atlantic Ocean to the Americas. Thus, SLEV and many other related flaviviruses were almost certainly introduced to the Americas, from Africa, in this manner.

Additional evidence for this argument is based on sequence data and a phylogenetic analysis (Figure 38.4) of a wide range of strains of SLEV.[39] All viruses at the root of the tree were isolated from South America, whereas most of the more recent lineages were derived from Central and North America, suggesting that SLEV was introduced from Africa into South America and subsequently dispersed northwards, carried by infected migratory birds. This interpretation has now been independently supported by an additional recent publication.[83]

In common with all other flaviviruses, there are no recognized effective antiviral drugs with which to treat human infections caused by SLEV, and no vaccines have been developed, presumably because the relatively low incidence of clinical disease in North America does not justify the cost of developing a vaccine. Control measures are therefore confined to avoidance of being bitten by *Culex* spp. mosquitoes, both by avoiding exposure during peak mosquito feeding times and by the use of appropriate insect repellents.

Murray Valley encephalitis virus

Murray Valley encephalitis virus is both antigenically[14,67] and genetically[3,15,39] very closely related to JEV and is most likely a descendant lineage of the virus that emerged as JEV in Asia.[26,39] Murray Valley encephalitis virus is endemic to northern Australia and Papua New Guinea. It circulates among water birds (Ciconiiformes) including herons and cormorants, and *Culex* spp. mosquitoes, particularly *Culex annulirostris*. Other mosquito vectors include *Culex australicus* and some *Ochlerotatus* spp. Cases of Murray Valley encephalitis have been reported from all mainland states of Australia and also Papua New Guinea,[84] presumably reflecting its dispersal via migratory birds. However, in its endemic form, MVEV is generally restricted to the north-western region of Australia, with virus activity being recorded from the tropical Kimberley region in most years. It is most active, with an increased risk of human infection, during

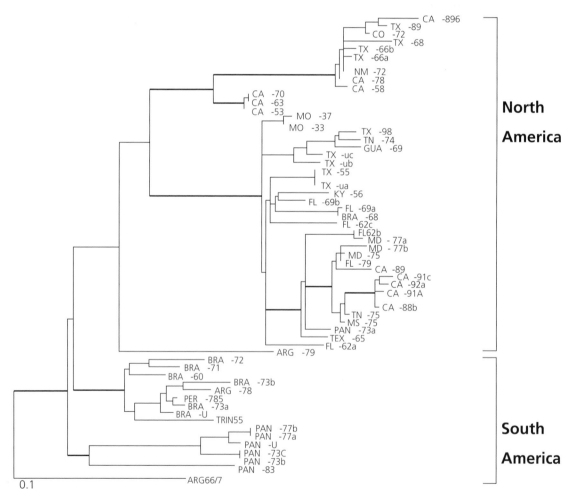

Figure 38.4 Maximum likelihood phylogenetic tree based on the complete envelope gene sequence of representative strains of St Louis encephalitis virus. The topology of the tree shown is based on a tree rooted with a virus closely related to the basal cluster. Emboldened branches correspond to bootstrap values *of over* 75 per cent. The tree was developed in PAUP*. Variable parameters were estimated using MODEL TEST. Parameters were estimated from the data, the optimal model being TrN + I + Γ. All codon positions were included. (Adapted from Gould *et al.*,[39] with permission.)

particularly wet years in which extensive flooding is involved.

Most infections are usually asymptomatic, but rare cases of clinical illness may have devastating consequences.[85] The clinical picture of Murray Valley encephalitis in humans resembles Japanese encephalitis. Treatment is confined to supportive therapy. There are no vaccines for MVEV, but it is reasonable to assume that immunity to JEV would confer at least a level of cross-immunity to MVEV. Control measures involve the avoidance of *Culex* spp. and the use of repellents.

CONCLUSION

In summary, these arboviruses have evolved long-term survival strategies that primarily depend upon their arthropod vectors. In the case of the TBFVs, non-viraemic transmission provides an increased range of potential vertebrate hosts that can facilitate virus survival without necessarily involving clinical illness in the relatively passive vertebrate species. Evolution and dispersal appears to be a gradual process, interrupted only by anthropological disturbance. The viraemic transmission of TBFV is, however, often associated with disease among non-native, immunologically and genetically naive introduced vertebrates where the TBFV naturally circulate harmlessly in the indigenous vertebrates.

In contrast, MBFVs exhibit a 'discontinuous' evolutionary pattern with little geographical structure and frequent lineage extinction. This may reflect the fact that the vector lifespan in this case is significantly shorter, typically measured in days. Evolutionary dynamics will also be affected by other differences between these two vector groups, including the number and volume of blood meals during the vector lifespan, the number of different hosts, vector mobility and the likelihood of vertical transmission.[30]

With the application of reverse transcriptase polymerase chain reaction technology, new arboviruses are now being discovered with increasing frequency. This will undoubtedly lead to new discoveries in the context of flavivirus evolution and dispersal, but the overriding message is that anthropological impacts will continue to influence flavivirus epidemiology.

REFERENCES

● = Key primary paper
♦ = Major review article

♦1. Gould EA, Solomon TS. Pathogenic flaviviruses. *Lancet* 2008; **371**: 500–9.
2. Heinz FX, Collett MS, Purcell RH et al. In: MHV van Regenmortel CF, DHL Bishop, EB Carstens, MK Estes et al. (eds) *Virus Taxonomy, VIIth Report of the International Committee on Taxonomy of Viruses.* San Diego: Academic Press, 2000; 859–78.
♦3. Gould EA, de Lamballerie X, Zanotto PMA, Holmes EC. Evolution, epidemiology and dispersal of flaviviruses revealed by molecular phylogenies. *Adv Virus Res* 2001; **57**: 71–103.
♦4. Lindenbach BD, Rice CM. *Flaviviridae*: The viruses and their replication. In: Knippe DM, Howley PM (eds) *Fields Virology*, Vol. 1. London: Lippincott Williams & Wilkins, 2001; 991–1042.
●5. Gritsun TS, Gould EA. The 3' untranslated region of tick-borne flaviviruses originated by the duplication of long repeat sequences within the open reading frame. *Virology* 2006; **354**: 217–23.
6. Gritsun TS, Gould EA. Direct repeats in the 3' untranslated regions of mosquito-borne flaviviruses: Possible implications for virus transmission. *J Gen Virol* 2006; **87**: 3297–305.
7. Gritsun TS, Gould EA. The 3' untranslated regions of Kamiti River virus and cell fusing agent virus originated by self-duplication. *J Gen Virol* 2006; **87**: 2615–19.
8. Gritsun TS, Gould EA. Direct repeats in the flavivirus 3' untranslated region: A strategy for survival in the environment? *Virology* 2007; **358**: 258–65.
♦9. Gritsun TS, Gould EA. Origin and evolution of 3'UTR of flaviviruses: Long direct repeats as a basis for the formation of secondary structures and their significance for virus transmission. *Adv Virus Res* 2007; **69**: 203–48.
10. Gritsun TS, Gould EA. Origin and evolution of flavivirus 5'UTRs and panhandles: Trans-terminal duplications? *Virology* 2007; **366**: 8–15.
♦11. Calisher CH, Gould EA. Taxonomy of the virus family *Flaviviridae. Adv Virus Res* 2003; **59**: 1–17.
♦12. Theiler M, Downs WG. *The Arthropod-borne Viruses of Vertebrates: An Account of the Rockefeller Foundation Virus Program (1951–1970).* London: Yale University Press, 1973.
♦13. Porterfield JS. Antigenic characteristics and classification of Togaviridae. In: Schlesinger RW (ed.) *The Togaviruses.* New York: Academic Press, 1980: 13–46.
14. Calisher CH, Karabatsos N, Dalrymple JM et al. Antigenic relationships between flaviviruses as determined by cross-neutralization tests with polyclonal antisera. *J Gen Virol* 1989; **70**: 37–43.
●15. Kuno G, Chang GJ, Tsuchiya KR et al. Phylogeny of the genus Flavivirus. *J Virol* 1998; **72**: 73–83.
●16. Gaunt MW, Sall AA, de Lamballerie X et al. Phylogenetic relationships of flaviviruses correlate with their epidemiology, disease association and biogeography. *J Gen Virol* 2001; **82**: 1867–76.
17. Silber LA. The spring (spring summer) tick-borne endemic encephalitis. *Arch Sci Biol* 1939; **56**: 37.
18. Suss J. Tick-borne encephalitis in Europe and beyond – the epidemiological situation as of 2007. *Eurosurveillance* 2008; **13**: ii, 18916.
19. Pool WA, Brownlee A, Wilson RD. The etiology of louping ill. *J Comp Pathol Ther* 1930; **43**: 253–90.

20. Pogodina VV, Frolova MP, Erman BA. Chronic tick-borne encephalitis. In: Zasukhina GD, Nepomnyashikh LM, (eds) *Chronic Tick-borne Encephalitis*. Moscow: Nauka, 1986.

21. Gritsun TS, Lashkevich VA, Gould EA. Tick-borne encephalitis. *Antiviral Res* 2003; **57**: 129–46.

22. Růžek D, Gritsun TS, Forrester NL *et al*. Mutations in the NS2B and NS3 genes affect mouse neuroinvasiveness of a Western European field strain of tick-borne encephalitis virus. *Virology* 2008; **374**: 249–55.

23. Shapoval AN. The outbreaks of tick-borne encephalitis in Karelia and their significance for studies of disease. In: *Tick-borne Encephalitis*. Leningrad: Pasteur Institute of Epidemiology and Microbiology, 1989: 49–56.

24. Loomis EC. Life histories of ticks under laboratory conditions (Acarina: Ixodidae and Argasidae). *J Parasitol* 1961; **47**: 91–9.

◆25. Reid HW. Epidemiology of louping ill. In: Mayo MA, Harrap KA (eds) *Vectors in Virus Biology*. London: Academic Press, 1984; 161–78.

◆26. Gould EA, de Lamballerie X, Zanotto PM, Holmes EC. Origins, evolution, and vector/host coadaptations within the genus Flavivirus. *Adv Virus Res* 2003; **59**: 277–314.

●27. Jones LD, Gaunt M, Hails RS *et al*. Transmission of louping ill virus between infected and uninfected ticks co-feeding on mountain hares. *Med Vet Entomol* 1997; **11**: 172–6.

28. Labuda M, Kozuch O, Zuffova E *et al*. Tick-borne encephalitis virus transmission between ticks cofeeding on specific immune natural rodent hosts. *Virology* 1997; **235**: 138–43.

●29. Higgs S, Schneider BS, Vanlandingham DL *et al*. Nonviremic transmission of West Nile virus. *Proc Natl Acad Sci USA* 2005; **102**: 8871–4.

◆30. Zanotto PM, Gould EA, Gao GF *et al*. Population dynamics of flaviviruses revealed by molecular phylogenies. *Proc Natl Acad Sci USA* 1996; **93**: 548–53.

●31. Zanotto PM, Gao GF, Gritsun T *et al*. An arbovirus cline across the northern hemisphere. *Virology* 1995; **210**: 152–9.

32. Marin MS, Zanotto PM, Gritsun TS, Gould EA. Phylogeny of TYU, SRE, and CFA virus: Different evolutionary rates in the genus Flavivirus. *Virology* 1995; **206**: 1133–9.

◆33. Kharitonova NN, Leonov YA. *Omsk Hemorrhagic Fever. Ecology of the Agent and Epizootiology*. New Delhi: Amerind Publishing, 1985.

34. Work TH, Trapido H. Kyasanur Forest disease, a new virus disease in India. *Indian J Med Sci* 1957; **11**: 341–5.

35. Venugopal K, Gritsun T, Lashkevich VA, Gould EA. Analysis of the structural protein gene sequence shows Kyasanur Forest disease virus as a distinct member in the tick-borne encephalitis virus serocomplex. *J Gen Virol* 1994; **75**: 227–32.

36. Boshell J. Kyasanur Forest disease: Ecologic considerations. *Am J Trop Med Hyg* 1969; **18**: 67–80.

37. Zaki AM. Isolation of a flavivirus related to the tick-borne encephalitis complex from human cases in Saudi Arabia. *Trans R Soc Trop Med Hyg* 1997; **91**: 179–81.

38. Grard G, Moureau G, Charrel RN *et al*. Genetic characterization of tick-borne flaviviruses: New insights into evolution, pathogenetic determinants and taxonomy. *Virology* 2006; 361: 80–92.

39. Gould EA, Moss SR, Turner SL. Evolution and dispersal of encephalitic flaviviruses. *Arch Virol* 2004; Suppl.(18): 65–84.

40. World Health Organization. *Yellow Fever*. Fact Sheet No. 100. Geneva: WHO, 2001.

41. World Health Organization. The yellow fever situation in Africa and South America in 2004. *Wkly Epidemiol Rec* 2005; **80**: 249–56.

◆42. Strode GK. *Yellow Fever*. New York: McGraw-Hill, 1951.

43. Theiler M, Sellards AW. Immunological relationship of yellow fever as it occurs in West Africa and South America. *Ann Trop Med* 1928; **22**: 449–60.

44. Bryant JE, Holmes EC, Barrett ADT. Out of Africa: A molecular perspective on the introduction of yellow fever virus into the Americas. *PLoS Pathog* 2007; **3**: e75.

45. Smith CE, Gibson ME. Yellow fever in South Wales. *Med Hist* 1986; **30**: 322–40.

◆46. Bloom KJ. *The Mississippi Valley's Great Yellow Fever Epidemic of 1878*. Baton Rouge, Louisiana: Louisiana State University Press, 1993.

◆47. Lounibos LP. Invasions by insect vectors of human disease. *Ann Rev Entomol* 2002; **47**: 233–66.

◆48. Gubler DJ. Dengue/dengue haemorrhagic fever: History and current status. *Novartis Found Symp* 2006; **277**: 3–16; discussion 16–22, 71–3, 251–3.

49. Tomashek KM. Dengue fever (DF) and dengue hemorrhagic fever (DHF). Available from: http://wwwnc.cdc.gov/travel/yellowbook/2010/chapter-5/dengue-fever-dengue-hemorrhagic-fever.aspx (accessed January 23, 2010).

50. Halstead SB, Streit TG, Lafontant JG *et al*. Haiti: Absence of dengue hemorrhagic fever despite hyperendemic dengue virus transmission. *Am J Trop Med Hyg* 2001; **65**: 180–3.

51. Twiddy SS, Farrar JJ, Vinh Chau N *et al*. Phylogenetic relationships and differential selection pressures among genotypes of dengue 2 virus. *Virology* 2002; **298**: 63–72.

52. Ibanez-Bernal S, Briseno B, Mutebi JP *et al*. First record in America of *Aedes albopictus* naturally infected with dengue virus during the 1995 outbreak at Reynosa, Mexico. *Med Vet Entomol* 1997; **11**: 305–9.

53. Shroyer DA. *Aedes albopictus* and arboviruses: A concise review of the literature. *J Am Mosq Control Assoc* 1987; **2**: 424–8.

●54. Tsetsarkin KA, Vanlandingham DL, McGee CE, Higgs S. A single mutation in Chikungunya virus affects vector specificity and epidemic potential. *PLoS Pathog* 2007; **3**: e201.

●55. de Lamballerie X, Leroy E, Charrel RN *et al*. Chikungunya virus adapts to tiger mosquito via evolutionary convergence: A sign of things to come? *Virol J* 2008; **5**: 33.

56. World Health Organization. *Dengue Haemorrhagic Fever. Diagnosis, Treatment, Control*. Geneva: WHO, 1997.

◆57. Mackenzie JS, Gubler DJ, Petersen LR. Emerging flaviviruses: The spread and resurgence of Japanese encephalitis, West Nile and dengue viruses. *Nature Med* 2004; **10**: S98–109.

58. Vaughn DW, Green S, Kalayanarooj S *et al.* Dengue viremia titer, antibody response pattern, and virus serotype correlate with disease severity. *J Infect Dis* 2000; **181**: 2–9.

59. Fernández-Mestre MT, Gendzekhadze K, Rivas-Vetencourt P, Layrisse Z. TNF-α-308A allele, a possible severity risk factor of hemorrhagic manifestation in dengue fever patients. *Tissue Antigens* 2004; **64**: 469–72.

60. Stephens HA, Klaythong R, Sirikong M *et al.* HLA-A and -B allele associations with secondary dengue virus infections correlate with disease severity and infecting viral serotype in ethnic Thais. *Tissue Antigens* 2002; **60**: 309–18.

61. Bravo JR, Guzman MG, Kouri GP. Why dengue haemorrhagic fever in Cuba? 1: Individual risk factors for dengue haemorrhagic fever/dengue shock syndrome (DHF/DSS). *Trans R Soc Trop Med Hyg* 1987; **81**: 816–20.

62. Kurane I, Meager A, Ennis FA. Dengue virus-specific human T cell clones. Serotype crossreactive proliferation, interferon gamma production, and cytotoxic activity. *J Exp Med* 1989; **170**: 763–75.

63. Green S, Vaughn DW, Kalayanarooj S *et al.* Early immune activation in acute dengue illness is related to development of plasma leakage and disease severity. *J Infect Dis* 1999; **179**: 755–62.

64. Kurane I, Innis BL, Nimmannitya S *et al.* Activation of T lymphocytes in dengue virus infections. High levels of soluble interleukin 2 receptor, soluble CD4, soluble CD8, interleukin 2, and interferon-gamma in sera of children with dengue. *J Clin Invest* 1991; **88**: 1473–80.

◆65. Mackenzie JS, Johansen CA, Ritchie SA *et al.* Japanese encephalitis as an emerging virus: The emergence and spread of Japanese encephalitis virus in Australasia. *Curr Top Microbiol Immunol* 2002; **267**: 49–73.

66. Peiris JS, Amerasinghe FP, Amerasinghe PH *et al.* Japanese encephalitis in Sri Lanka – the study of an epidemic: Vector incrimination, porcine infection and human disease. *Trans R Soc Trop Med Hyg* 1992; **86**: 307–13.

67. Solomon T, Ni H, Beasley DW *et al.* Origin and evolution of Japanese encephalitis virus in southeast Asia. *J Virol* 2003; **77**: 3091–8.

68. Uchil PD, Satchidanandam V. Phylogenetic analysis of Japanese encephalitis virus: Envelope gene based analysis reveals a fifth genotype, geographic clustering and multiple introductions of the virus into the Indian subcontinent. *Am J Trop Med Hyg* 2001; **65**: 242–51.

69. Porterfield JS. Arboviruses – structure and classification (author's transl.). *Med Trop (Mars)* 1980; **40**: 493–8.

70. Howitt BF. Viruses of equine and St. Louis encephalitis in relationship to human infections in California 1937–1938. *Am J Public Health*; **29**: 1083–97.

◆71. Reisen WK. Epidemiology of St Louis encephalitis virus. *Adv Virus Res* 2003; **61**: 139–83.

72. Day JF. Predicting St. Louis encephalitis virus epidemics: Lessons from recent, and not so recent, outbreaks. *Annu Rev Entomol* 2001; **46**: 111–38.

73. Reisen WK, Lothrop HD, Wheeler SS *et al.* Persistent West Nile virus transmission and the apparent displacement of St. Louis encephalitis virus in southeastern California, 2003–2006. *J Med Entomol* 2008; **45**: 494–508.

◆74. Tsai TF. St Louis encephalitis. In: Monath TP (ed.) *The Arboviruses, Epidemiology and Ecology.* Boca Raton, FL: CRC Press, 1989: 431–58.

75. Tueller JE. An outbreak of illness due to St Louis encephalitis virus in the southern San Joaquin Valley, California, 1989. *Proc Californian Mosq Vector Control Assoc* 1990; **58**: 12.

76. Reeves WC, Hammon W. Epidemiology of the arthropod-borne viral encephalitides in Kern County, California, 1943–1952. *Univ Calif Berkeley Public Health* 1962; **4**: 1–257.

◆77. Brinker KR, Monath TP. The acute disease. In: Monath TP (ed.) *St Louis Encephalitis.* Washington, DC: American Public Health Association, 1980; 503–34.

78. Bredeck JF, Broun GO, Hemplemann TC *et al.* Follow-up studies of the 1933 St Louis epidemic of encephalitis. *J Am Med Assoc* 1938; **111**: 15–18.

79. Palmer RJ, Finlay KH. Sequelae of encephalitis: Report of a study of a clinical follow-up study in California. *Calif Med* 1956; **84**: 98–100.

◆80. Gould EA, Zanotto PM, Holmes EC. The genetic evolution of flaviviruses. In: Saluzzo JF, Dodet B (eds) *Factors in the Emergence of Arbovirus Disease.* Amsterdam: Elsevier, 1997; 51–63.

81. Fonseca DM, Keyghobadi N, Malcolm CA *et al.* Emerging vectors in the *Culex pipiens* complex. *Science* 2004; **303**: 1535–8.

82. Raoult D, Reed DL, Dittmar K *et al.* Molecular identification of lice from pre-Columbian mummies. *J Infect Dis* 2008; **197**: 535–43.

83. Baillie GJ, Kolokotronis S-O, Waltari E *et al.* Phylogenetic and evolutionary analyses of St. Louis encephalitis virus genomes. *Mol Phylogenet Evol* 2008; **47**: 717–28.

◆84. MacKenzie JS, Lindsay MD, Coelen RJ *et al.* Arboviruses causing human disease in the Australasian zoogeographic region. *Arch Virol* 1994; **136**: 447–67.

85. Broom AK, Lindsay MD, Plant AJ *et al.* Epizootic activity of Murray Valley encephalitis virus in an aboriginal community in the southeast Kimberley region of Western Australia: Results of cross-sectional and longitudinal serologic studies. *Am J Trop Med Hyg* 2002; **67**: 319–23.

39

Trypanosomes, leishmania and lymphatic filariasis

EDWIN MICHAEL

It is becoming accepted wisdom that variations in climate-associated exogenous factors may represent primary or first-order determinants governing the global spatial distribution of vector-borne diseases in human populations.[1,2] An important outcome from this perspective is that global climate change could, by affecting the transmission dynamics of vector-borne diseases, result in an expansion of these tropical diseases into areas currently unsuited to disease transmission,[3] making reliable environmental risk assessments for climate-driven disease spread an increasingly significant topic of study in current public health research.[4]

This interest has led to numerous empirical studies on spatial and temporal associations between climate/environmental variables, vector abundance and disease incidence in the field,[5,6] and many quantitative studies of the effects of climate variables on the biological processes that govern vector and pathogen population dynamics in the laboratory.[7,8] More recently, it has also led to the development of climate-related, process-based mathematical models of disease transmission for predicting the effects of climate variability and change on vector and pathogen transmission, as well as for quantifying disease risk levels from climate and environmental variations.[9,10]

These studies have reinforced the expectation that climate may play a fundamental role in influencing habitat suitability and hence the transmission of vector-borne diseases in communities where the diseases are endemic, particularly through the effects of factors such as temperature and rainfall on vector and pathogen development and survival rates. There has also, in parallel, been a growing appreciation that the link between climate and vector-borne disease transmission may not be direct, but that human activities in particular can moderate the ultimate risk of disease from climate variability and change.[2,11,12] This has resulted in recent calls for a need to take a broader integrated socioecological approach that combines the ecology and sociology of pathogen transmission to evaluate human health risk from vector-borne diseases as a result of global climate change.[2]

A feature in the assessments carried out so far of the impact that climate and/or the environment may have on vector-borne disease transmission and epidemiology is that the focus has been mostly on malaria, and to a lesser extent on dengue fever. The consequence of this is that little is currently known about how climate/environmental variability may affect the transmission ecology of the other major vector-borne diseases.[6] This gap in knowledge is particularly true for those vector-borne diseases, such as trypanosomiasis, leishmaniasis and lymphatic filariasis, that belong to the so-called neglected tropical diseases. This lacuna exists for these diseases despite the increasing recognition of their potentially large health and developmental impacts on countries where they are endemic, and the growing calls to achieve their global control.[13]

This chapter will review the published studies that have looked at the links between climate/environmental variables and the transmission ecology of the major 'neglected' vector-borne parasitic infections to assess the impact that these factors could play on their epidemiology and transmission. For each disease, an attempt has been made to assess the impact that climatic and environmental factors may have on the observed incidence of the disease in the community, and the impact that climate variables may have on the transmission parameters and vital processes of the relevant vector and parasite population. The results are discussed in terms of the current evidence on the likely effect that climate/environmental variability and change may have in influencing pathogen transmission, and the nature of further studies required to assess the impact of climate on the future extent and burden of these diseases.

TRYPANOSOMIASIS

The disease

Trypanosomiasis is a protozoan disease caused by several species of *Trypanosoma*. Infection with *Trypanosoma brucei* causes two forms of sleeping sickness in humans: acute infection of the East African type, caused by *Trypanosoma brucei rhodesiense*, and a more chronic infection caused by *Trypanosoma brucei gambiense* (West African type). Chagas disease, caused by *Trypanosoma cruzi* infection and occurring only in Central or South America, on the other hand, progresses over many years into the disease state.

African trypanosomiasis is transmitted by the tsetse fly, *Glossina* spp., which is found across Africa in regions south of the Sahara and north of the Kalahari Desert (14° north and 29° south of the equator). Infection occurs through insect bites. The number of individuals thought to be infected with African trypanosomiasis is estimated at 0.3–0.5 million.[14] Early symptoms are red sores where the tsetse fly has bitten, and the development of fever, swollen lymph glands, aching muscles and joints, headaches and irritability within a few weeks. In advanced stages, the disease attacks the central nervous system, leading to personality changes, slurred speech, seizures and difficulty with walking and talking. These problems can develop over many years in the *gambiense* form and some months in the *rhodesiense* form; if not treated, the person will die.

Chagas disease is spread through the faeces of the blood-sucking triatomine bugs that live in cracks in house walls, in thatched roofs or in palm trees. There are two phases of Chagas disease: the acute and the chronic phase. Both phases can be symptom-free or life-threatening. The acute phase lasts for the first few weeks or months of infection. It usually occurs unnoticed because it is symptom-free or exhibits only mild symptoms and signs, such as fever, fatigue, body aches, headache, rash, loss of appetite, diarrhoea and vomiting. The most recognized marker of acute Chagas disease is called Romaña's sign, which includes swelling of the eyelids on the side of the face near the bite wound or where the bug faeces have been deposited or accidentally rubbed into the eye. Although the symptoms resolve, the infection persists if untreated.

During the chronic phase, the infection may remain silent for decades or even for life. However, some people can develop cardiac complications, which can include an enlarged heart (cardiomyopathy), heart failure, altered heart rate or rhythm, and cardiac arrest (sudden death). Intestinal complications, which can include an enlarged oesophagus (mega-oesophagus) or colon (megacolon), can occur and can lead to difficulties with eating or with passing stool.

Climate and disease distribution

The main focus of previous studies on climate and trypanosomiasis has been to demonstrate the potential of using remotely sensed satellite data in uncovering vector–environment relationships relevant to mapping the co-distribution and spread of vectors and the disease.[15] Thus, Kitron *et al.* analysed tsetse fly catches from sets of traps set in the Lambwe Valley of Western Kenya during 1988–90 and found that high-resolution Landsat Thematic Mapper imagery data were able to explain most of the variance in fly catch density.[16] In particular, wavelength band 7 of the Landsat Thematic Mapper imagery, which is associated with soil water content, was found to be consistently highly correlated, reflecting the importance of soil moisture in tsetse fly survival.

In contrast, Rogers and Randolph explored the utility of Global Area Coverage (GAC) normalized difference vegetation index (NDVI) data derived from the National Oceanic and Atmospheric Administration's (NOAA) Advanced Very High Resolution Radiometer (AVHRR) as a proxy for studying tsetse fly ecology and distribution in West Africa, since they considered the NDVI to integrate a variety of environmental factors of importance to tsetse survival.[17,18] They found an inverse relationship between the monthly NDVI and the fly mortality rate in the Yankari game reserve in Nigeria, and significant non-linear relationships between tsetse fly abundance and NDVI in the northern part of Cote d'Ivoire.

Rogers and Randolph focused on a 700 km transect running north–south through Cote d'Ivoire and Burkina Faso. This area is of particular epidemiological interest since sleeping sickness is found only in the central region of the transect, despite the local vector (*Glossina palpalis*) occurring throughout the area. The analysis showed that this focalized transmission was a result of differences in overall fly size. During the wet season, the NDVIs across the transect were all high, and fly size was uniformly large. In the dry season, however, fly size was strongly correlated with NDVI, with flies in the drier north being significantly smaller than those in the wetter south. Since fly mortality increases with decreasing fly size in tsetse, these data were interpreted as indicating a geographical gradient in the degree of human–fly contact and thus West African trypanosome transmission potential.

In the south, low mortality rates resulted in high densities of flies, but the flies were not nutritionally stressed (even seasonally) so did not often resort to biting humans, who are not favoured hosts. Conversely, in the north, fly populations suffered too high a mortality to pose a serious health risk. Only in the central areas was there an intermediate density of sufficiently stressed flies, resulting in a regional and seasonal focus of disease transmission. This study showed that, although at relatively small spatial scales both tsetse distribution and abundance, and disease incidence and prevalence, could be related to the low-resolution NDVI, interpretation of the data required a knowledge of local conditions and fly biology from ground studies.

Rogers and Williams extended the above analysis by applying NOAA–AVHRR GAC–NDVI data and synoptic meteorological temperature data to the problem of predicting the larger scale distribution of *Glossina morsitans* in Zimbabwe, Kenya and Tanzania.[19] Temperature data (a critical climatic variable in determining the survival of tsetse fly) were included in the analysis by interpolating data from meteorological stations to grid squares covering the whole of Zimbabwe. When these data were combined with NDVI variables in a linear discriminant analysis, the historical distribution of *Glossina morsitans* in Zimbabwe was predicted with an accuracy of over 80 per cent, thereby indicating the utility of remote sensed data in predicting fly distributions at broader spatial scales.

However, the statistical difficulties of selecting apparently important climatic and remotely sensed variables for determining the observed distribution pattern were highlighted by Rogers and Randolph.[20] These authors reassessed the distributions of *Glossina morsitans* in Zimbabwe, Kenya and Tanzania via predictions from a discriminant analysis of several components of the NDVI (monthly mean, minimum, maximum and range), elevation and synoptic temperature data. Although they were able to predict the distribution to an overall accuracy of 82 per cent, the key variables contributing most to the prediction varied between the countries. This could suggest that, at the very least, the environment–vector abundance relationship varies on a regional scale, thereby precluding the building of general global predictive models. Alternatively, the results may indicate difficulties with the analysis of complex multivariate data. Recent work investigating the application of temporal Fourier analysis[19] and multivariate techniques based on likelihood principles[21] to climate and remotely sensed vegetation data for predicting fly distributions has attempted to address this issue.

The above and other similar studies have allowed the identification of tsetse habitats supporting *Trypanosoma brucei* transmission on the African continent.[20,22,23] They have also demonstrated how when such multivariate models are combined with data on elevation and human densities along with estimates of agricultural activity and cattle numbers, it is possible to establish decision models that are useful for prioritizing areas for tsetse control.[24,25] Similarly, work in north-eastern Brazil has shown that using just annual mean minimum temperature and annual mean rainfall as the major climate variables can help to distinguish distinctly different populations of the *Triatoma brasiliensis* vector responsible for transmitting *Trypanosoma cruzi*.[26]

A more recent study from West Africa, however, combined long-term data on sleeping sickness incidence and changes in annual rainfall and human movements. This highlighted the complex interactions occurring between biophysical factors and human activity that could govern changes in the spatial distribution of a vector-borne disease.[27] The key finding from this study was that human African trypansomiasis no longer seems to occur in regions where the annual rainfall was less than 1200 mm per year, which was not the case at the beginning of the twentieth century. The authors suggest that a decrease in annual rainfall associated or coupled with increasing human densities or activities in these areas has had an impact on land use and hence tsetse fly distribution.

Climatic factors and transmission processes

Understanding the effects of climatic factors on disease transmission processes is critical for reliably predicting how changes in these exogenous variables can dynamically alter the intensity and spatial extent of pathogen transmission.[10] For vector-borne diseases, the first step in developing this understanding is through evaluating the direct effects of key climatic factors on the vital biological processes connected with pathogen transmission, which include vector development, feeding frequency and survival, and the rate of pathogen development within the vector host.

For trypanosomiasis, the majority of experimental work investigating such effects appears to have been carried out for *Trypanosoma cruzi* and its vectors (summarized in Carcavallo[28]). As for other vector-borne diseases, this work has shown that temperature and humidity may significantly affect *Trypanosoma cruzi* transmission, by effects on vector embryonic development, generation time, survival rate and feeding frequency, and the development rate of the protozoan in the digestive tube of the *Triatoma infestans* vector (Table 39.1).

The overall evidence suggests that higher temperatures would tend to extend the geographical distribution of the vectors while lower humidity may act to shorten the vector life-cycle, although several authors have highlighted the importance of microclimate in *Trypanosoma cruzi* transmission. In particular, Pifano showed how the temperature inside the palm tree *Scheelea humboldtiana* can be a constant 22–23 °C, while on the external leaves it can vary from 16 to 30 °C, with a corresponding 40–95 per cent variation in humidity.[29] Triatomine bugs (especially *Rhodnius*) can counter macroscale seasonal climatic variations in both temperature and humidity by choosing optimal conditions through moving around the tree. Similar microhabitat variations in relative humidity inside and outside dwelling structures may also be exploited by *Triatoma infestans* to counteract seasonal changes.

Table 39.1 The impact of climate factors on transmission processes in Chagas disease

Study	Process	Impact
Nevia (1913)[65]	Vector embryogenesis	Experimental warming accelerates the embryonic period of *Triatoma infestans*
Hack (1955)[66]	Vector life-cycle/generation time	High temperatures result in two generations per year for *Triatoma infestans*, whereas it results in only one per year in temperate areas
Carcavallo and Martinez (1972)[67]		Life-cycles are shorter in three species of *Triatoma* reared at permanent high temperature (27–28 °C) compared with specimens reared outdoors at variable temperatures
Zeledon *et al.* (1970)[68]		*Triatoma dimidiate* eggs hatched at 29 days at 22–24 °C and at 23 days when reared at 26 °C
Silva and Silva (1986a, b, c, 1988)[69–72]		Completion of life cycles of *Triatoma matogrossensis* took 248 and 190 days when reared at 25 and 30 °C, whereas for the same temperatures it was 145 and 114 days for *Rhodnius nasutus*, 230 and 186 days for *Triatoma vitticeps*, 181 and 152 days for *Panstrongylus megistus*, and 181 and 134 days for *Triatoma infestans*
Blaksley and Carcavallo (1968)[73]	Vector resistance to cold	Only a few specimens from nine species of *Triatoma* died after 4 hours at −2 °C, with no mortality in the case of *Triatoma platensis* even at −4 °C, although mortality was high (83%) even at −2 °C in the case of *Triatoma rubrovaria*
Catala (1991)[74]	Vector feeding frequency	The proportion of *Triatoma infestans* bugs feeding on chickens was low, at only 0.014, in July (winter), whereas it was significantly higher, at 0.470, in December (spring/summer)
Asin and Catala (1995)[75]	Pathogen development rate	High temperatures accelerate the development of *Trypanosoma cruzi* in the digestive tube of *Triatoma infestans*: when reared at 28 °C, trypomastigotes were seen in the faeces 32 days after an infective meal, whereas in specimens reared at 30 °C, trypomastigotes appeared on the 24th day

LEISHMANIASIS

The disease

Leishmaniasis is a disease complex caused by 17 different species of protozoan parasites belonging to the genus *Leishmania*. The parasites are transmitted between mammalian hosts by phlebotomine sandflies. An estimated 12 million humans are infected, with an incidence of 0.5 million cases for the visceral form of the disease and 1.5–2.0 million cases for the cutaneous form of the disease.[30]

Leishmaniasis has a worldwide distribution with important foci of infection in Central and South America, southern Europe, North and East Africa, the Middle East and the Indian subcontinent. The main foci of visceral leishmaniasis are currently in Sudan and India, and those of cutaneous leishmaniasis (CL) are in Afghanistan, Syria and Brazil. In addition to these two major clinical forms of the disease, there are other cutaneous manifestations, including mucocutaneous leishmaniasis, diffuse CL, recidivans leishmaniasis and post-kala-azar dermal leishmaniasis.[30,31]

Cutaneous forms of the disease normally produce skin ulcers on the exposed parts of the body, such as the face, arms and legs. A large number of such lesions can be produced, causing serious disability and invariably leaving the patient permanently scarred. Visceral leishmaniasis, also known as kala-azar, is characterized by irregular bouts of fever, substantial weight loss, swelling of the spleen and liver and anaemia (occasionally serious). If left untreated, patients die after weeks to months of illness.[31]

Climate and disease distribution

The geographical distribution of leishmania transmission foci has long suggested climatic effects on disease transmission – disease foci are usually located below a latitude of 45° north and below 400–600 m above sea level.[32] It has also long been known that ecosystem disturbances, particularly changes in forest proximity and deforestation, urbanization and new agricultural practices, can positively affect the transmission of both CL and visceral leishmaniasis.[33–36] Given that leishmaniasis is the only tropical vector-borne disease that has been endemic to southern Europe for decades, there is also concern that it could re-emerge on that continent, particularly in the more lethal zoonotic visceral form, as a result of climate change.[34]

Preliminary modelling studies have confirmed that the distribution of sandfly vectors and disease transmission in Italy are significantly influenced by temperature.[35–37] Few studies have, however, explicitly quantified such linkages between environment and disease incidence. It is therefore difficult to estimate by how much changes in environmental or climatic factors can affect disease transmission. However, Wasseberg et al. undertook field experiments to show that the gradual and continuous increase in the incidence of CL in southern Israel over the past 20 years or so may be related to anthropogenic disturbances, particularly agricultural development, that enhance both water availability to vectors and quality of food to the rodent hosts of Leishmania major.[35]

More recently, Chaves and Pascaul analysed monthly data on the incidence of CL in Costa Rica from 1991 to 2001.[38] They demonstrated that CL in Costa Rica has cycles of approximately 3 years that are associated with those of mean temperature fluctuations and El Niño Southern Oscillation (ENSO) indices (sea surface temperature 4 and multivariate ENSO index). Indeed, linear models using temperature and multivariate ENSO index have been shown to be able to predict the incidence of CL up to 12 months ahead, with an accuracy of between 72 and 77 per cent. The complexity of the link between environmental and climatic factors and disease transmission was, however, underscored by Chaves et al., who showed that social factors, particularly social exclusion and marginality, may modulate the effect of forest proximity and the temporal effects of ENSO on disease patterns at small spatial scales.[39]

Petersen and Shaw also investigated the impact that climate change may have on Leishmania transmission using ecological niche modelling techniques to uncover the ecological basis for the distributional differences between three species of Lutzomyia vectors for CL in Southern Brazil.[40] Their results showed that while Lutzomyia whitmani tended to be most tropical in distribution (high precipitation, high temperature, wet climates and high vapour pressure), Lutzomyia migonei tended towards the opposite extreme, whereas Lutzomyia intermedia sensu lato lay in the middle of these climate ranges. When these results were used in conjunction with two climate scenarios (HHGSDX50, the Hadley Centre general circulation model HadCM2 assuming a 0.5 per cent per year increase in carbon dioxide, and HHGGAX50, the HadCM2 model assuming a 15 per cent per year increase in carbon dioxide), the authors found that all three species could experience some degree of improvement as a result of changes in diurnal temperature range in their habitats in south-eastern Brazil.

Climatic factors and transmission processes

Very few studies have investigated the direct effects of climate or environmental variables on transmission processes in leishmaniasis. However, two important findings are:

- that the optimal temperature for the development of both sandflies and Leishmania parasites is approximately 25 °C;[41,42]
- that the biting activity of sandflies, at least in Europe, is strongly seasonal, being restricted to the summer months in most areas.[32]

LYMPHATIC FILARIASIS

The disease

Lymphatic filariasis is a major cause of acute and chronic morbidity for humans in the tropical and subtropical areas of Asia, Africa, the Western Pacific and some parts of the Americas. Over 1.2 billion people live in areas where they are at risk of infection with filarial parasites.

In the estimated 120 million individuals with lymphatic filariasis currently living in 83 endemic countries, 91 per cent of cases are caused by the filarial worm Wuchereria bancrofti, while Brugia malayi and Brugia timori infections account for the other 9 per cent.[43] Brugia timori is only known to be endemic in Timor and the Flores islands of the Indonesian archipelago. These lymphatic-dwelling parasites cause damage to the lymphatic system that leads to lymphoedema, genital pathology (especially hydroceles) and elephantiasis in some 41 million men, women and children. A further 76 million have hidden infection, most often with microfilariae in their blood and hidden internal damage to their lymphatic and renal systems.[44]

The filarial parasites have biphasic life-cycles involving the definitive mammalian host and various species of mosquito vector including Anopheles, Aedes, Culex, Mansonia and Ochlerotatus species. Wuchereria bancrofti seems to be exclusively a human parasite, whereas Brugia spp. are zoonotic in limited situations. Parasite transmission occurs through the bite of an infective mosquito containing third-stage infective (L3) larvae that have developed through two intermediate stages (L1 and L2) from microfilariae ingested with the blood meal taken by female mosquitoes of a susceptible vector species during a previous blood feed on an infected human.

Climate and disease distribution

Surprisingly, quite a lot is known about climate and filariasis transmission or spatial distribution.[45] An early publication by Acton and Rao highlighted the fact that mosquito infection rates in the wild fluctuated throughout the year as a result of seasonal variations in humidity.[46] These authors showed that a relative humidity of 60 per cent and over and a temperature between 26.6 and 32.2 °C were most conducive to parasite transmission. Indeed, based on this information, they divided filarious areas in India into low, moderate and hyperendemic with varying degrees of infection and disease, and also of types of disease processes.

Rao and Sukhatme established a statistically significant correlation between season and the incidence of acute filarial cases in Calcutta.[47] They showed that disease incidence increased significantly during the monsoon period, i.e. at a time when climatic conditions were hot and humid. This finding is supported by more recent studies of seasonal links between rainfall and acute disease in East Africa.[48]

Several authors have also remarked upon the relationship between altitude and filariasis endemicity. Raghavan, for example, noted that infection and disease due to *Wuchereria bancrofti* and *Brugia malayi* may occur in places up to an altitude of 600 m in India,[49] whereas *Wuchereria bancrofti* in Nepal and Africa has been shown to occur up to a height of 1300 m.[50,51]

More recent work has sought to quantify the relationship between climate/environmental variables and the community prevalence of filariasis using spatial analysis and geographical information systems (GIS)/remote sensing technology. Thomson *et al.* used remotely sensed data on diurnal temperature differences (dT) in conjunction with spatial data on case prevalences from 297 villages within the Southern Nile Delta and showed that this environmental variable might underlie the observed spatial distribution of lymphatic filariasis at least within their study region.[52] Diurnal temperature differences indicate surface and subsurface moisture contained in soil and plant canopy, and hence may act as a surrogate for the abundance of the mosquito vector *Culex quinquefasciatus*.

Satellite image data from NOAA-AVHRR were analysed to determine dTs for the southern Nile Delta, while the case prevalence and location data for each of the 297 villages were inputted into a GIS. Point dT values for each village were obtained by averaging the values for 3 × 3 pixel areas (10 km²) centred on the corresponding longitude and latitude of each village. The digitized filariasis prevalence data were superimposed on the dT map and assigned to each of four prevalence categories of 0.5, 5, 15 and 25 per cent, respectively. The association between village dT value and prevalence category was investigated using stepwise polychotomous logistic regression, which indicated a significant relationship between the two variables.

Similarly, in the same region, Sowilem *et al.* used remotely sensed data and GIS functions to show that the most important environmental elements that differentiated between filarious and non-filarious villages in Egypt were water-related variables and different types of vegetation.[53]

Finally, Lindsay and Thomas used community prevalence data in conjunction with climate layers and a logistic regression model to predict the prevalence of lymphatic filariasis across sub-Saharan African.[54] Their model predicted with 76 per cent accuracy whether or not sites had microfilaraemiac patients across Africa, with the accuracy improving to 84.1 per cent in the case of Egypt. The most significant variables associated with infection in the case of Africa were precipitation/potential evapotranspiration, minimum annual temperature and maximum annual temperature, whereas for the Egyptian sites the corresponding variables were precipitation/potential evapotranspiration and minimum and maximum temperatures.

Climatic factors and transmission processes

A great deal is also known about how climate can influence the density, longevity and biting activities of filariasis vectors, as well as the parasite's extrinsic incubation period in these vectors. Thus, Rao and Iyengar corroborated findings from seasonal adult catches of *Culex fatigans* from various parts of Culcatta with experimental studies indicating that the monsoon temperature range of 26.6–35.0 °C and a relative humidity of 84 per cent were optimum for filariasis transmission in terms of their combined effects on mosquito longevity and the extrinsic incubation period.[55] In Travancore, Iyengar also found that, although mosquito density was low during the monsoon, infection levels were high as a result of a shortened extrinsic incubation period.[56]

Ray showed that that the low mosquito density during the monsoon period could be explained by a flushing of breeding sites as well as a dilution of organic matter in these sites (important for *Culex fatigans* development), but that the favourable humidity levels might increase the longevity and infection rates in the remaining vectors.[57] Shlenova also demonstrated that the gonotrophic cycle in filarial vectors can be affected by climatic factors.[58] Thus, in anophelines, blood digestion was accentuated up to 30.0 °C but retarded at 35.0 °C. Above 15 °C, it was increased by high humidity. Bates noted that the percentage of *Anopheles* sp. laying eggs varied with temperature.[59] An important early finding was additionally that, in the case of *Culex fatigans*, mosquito biting activity was increased at temperatures nearing that of the host's body.[60]

A more recent experimental study by Lardeux and Cheffort has provided important information about the developmental rates for *Wuchereria bancrofti* larvae maturing in the vector *Aedes polynesiensis*.[61] These authors analysed stage–frequency data consisting of counts of larval stages in mosquitoes reared at 20, 22.5, 25, 27.5, 30 and 32 °C, and showed that lower temperature thresholds required for stage-specific development were approximately 12.5 °C for microfilariae in the thorax, around 17 °C for stage L1, 15.5 °C for L2 and 16.5 °C for L3, while the corresponding upper thresholds were 29.3 °C for microfilariae, 29.1 °C for L1, 32.2 °C for L2 and 31.5 °C for L3, respectively. These relationships were non-linear in form, but a linear degree–day model was shown to hold for temperatures below 27–28 °C.

CONCLUSION

The population dynamics of infections are highly complex, and there are many factors that make it difficult to reliably predict the outcome of climate change on disease incidence. This review has, on the one hand, supported the general expectation that exogeneous factors related to climate and the environment will play important roles in the transmission dynamics and hence spatial distribution of vector-borne diseases, including the neglected diseases studied here. On the other hand, it has also highlighted the fragmented nature of the available studies. In particular, a systematic framework for combining insights into how climate variables relate to the vital rates of vectors (larval development and survival rates, biting rate and adult survivorship) and the vital rates of the pathogen (development rate in the vector), with habitat suitability results determined using correlative climate mapping studies, are still lacking not only for the present diseases, but also for infectious diseases in general.

A comprehensive framework that links the two approaches would facilitate a more reliable prediction of how climate and environmental factors may govern the distribution and spread of these diseases. This could be through providing information on the realized versus fundamental niches for disease transmission,[62] and on interaction effects arising from prevailing human socioeconomic systems.[11] The studies on leishmaniasis reviewed here[38,39] show how such social factors may moderate climatic factors in disease transmission and highlight the need to develop socioecological approaches that reliably predict the effect of climate change on these diseases.

Nonetheless, this review shows that there has been a relatively large amount of work carried out on the potential relationship between climate/environment and the transmission of trypanosomiasis, leishmaniasis and lymphatic filariasis. These studies have highlighted how key environmental factors such as temperature, rainfall, humidity and altitude (as well as spatial scale of study), as in the case generally for vector-borne diseases, can not only govern the observed distributions of these diseases, but also affect important vital rates of vectors and implicated pathogens. For example, it is already possible to predict that *Leishmania* is likely to be able to invade currently cooler European regions more readily than other organisms involved in vector-borne diseases as a result of global warming if social conditions (inadequate health systems and adaptive capacity) are favourable. This is because of the lower range of optimal temperatures required for vector and pathogen development for this vector–pathogen system.[34,37]

It is also suggested that the data on the impact of pathogen development rates available for lymphatic filariasis can be combined with those from studies of the impact of climate variables, such as temperature and humidity, on vector vital rates carried out, in particular, on *Anopheles* mosquitoes in the context of malarial infections; this will allow the development of more fundamental process-based models for describing the effects of climate variability and change on the transmission and spatial distribution of this parasitic disease.

The control of infectious diseases remains important in improving the public health of people in endemic areas. The data summarized in this review point to a very real risk that climate change can potentially extend the ranges of these diseases, and may thus further complicate and hamper their proposed control. Assessing how real this growing climate-related risk will be will ultimately depend on our ability to successfully develop and apply investigative frameworks that combine theories of ecological niche with integrated assessment approaches that merge the disciplines of pathogen transmission dynamics and ecological and sociological forces.[11,63,64] The initiation of such work has now become urgent if current initiatives to achieve control of these diseases are to be successfully accomplished.

REFERENCES

● = Key primary paper

◆ = Major review article

1. Patz JA, Graczyk TK, Geller N, Vittor AY. Effects of environmental change on emerging parasitic diseases. *Int J Parasitol* 2000; **30**: 1395–405.
◆2. Sutherst RW. Global change and human vulnerability to vector-borne diseases. *Clin Microbiol Rev* 2004; **17**: 136–73.

3. Epstein PR. Is global warming harmful to health? *Sci Am* 2000; **283**: 50–7.

4. Institute of Medicine. *Vector-borne Diseases: Understanding the Environmental, Human Health, and Ecological Connections.* Washington DC: National Academies Press, 2008.

5. Kovats RS, Campbell-Lendrum DH, Reid C, Martens P. *Climate and Vector-borne Disease: An Assessment of The Role of Climate in Changing Disease Patterns.* Maastricht: ICIS/LSHTM/UNEP, 2000.

♦6. McMichael AJ, Campbell-Lendrum DH, Kovats S *et al.* (eds). *Global and Regional Burden of Diseases Attributable to Selected Major Risk Factors*, Vol. 2. Geneva: World Health Organization, 2004.

●7. Martens WJM. Health impacts of climate change and ozone depletion: An ecoepidemiologic modelling approach. *Environ Health Perspect* 1998; **106**: 241–51.

8. Mossad E, Forattini OP. Modelling the temperature sensitivity of some physiological parameters of epidemiologic significance. *Ecosystem Health* 1998; **4**: 119–29.

●9. Depinay J-M, Mbogo CM, Killeen G *et al.* A simulation model of African *Anopheles* ecology and population dynamics for the analysis of malaria transmission. *Malar J* 2003; **3**: 29.

●10. Martens WJ, Jetten JH, Rotmans J, Niessen LW. Climate change and vector-borne diseases: A global modelling perspective. *Glob Environ Change* 1995; **5**: 195–209.

♦11. Eisenberg JN, Desai MA, Levy K *et al.* Environmental determinants of infectious disease: A framework for tracking causal links and guiding public health research. *Environ Health Perspect* 2007; **115**: 1216–23.

12. Patz JA, Epstein PR, Burke TA, Balbus JM. Global climate change and emerging infectious diseases. *JAMA* 1996; **275**: 217–23.

13. Hotez PJ, Bottazzi ME, Franco-Paredes C, Ault SK, Periago MR. The neglected tropical diseases of Latin America and the Caribbean: A review of disease burden and distribution and a roadmap for control and elimination. *PLoS Negl Trop Dis* 2008; **2**: e300.

14. Krishna S, Stich A. Trypanosomiasis: African and American. *Medicine* 2005; **33**: 50–3.

15. Hay SI, Packer MJ, Rogers DJ. The impact of remote sensing on the study and control of invertebrate intermediate hosts and vectors of disease. *Int J Remote Sens* 1997; **18**: 2899–930.

16. Kitron U, Otien LH, Hungerford LL *et al.* Spatial analysis of the distribution of tsetse flies in the Lambwe Valley, Kenya, using Landsat TM satellite imagery and GIS. *J Ecol* 1996; **65**: 371–80.

●17. Rogers DJ, Randolph SE. Mortality rates and population density of tsetse flies correlated with satellite imagery. *Nature* 1991; **351**: 739–41.

18. Rogers DJ, Randolph SE. Satellite imagery, tsetse flies, and sleeping sickness in Africa. *Sistema Terra* 1994; **3**: 40–3.

19. Rogers DJ, Williams BG. Monitoring trypanosomiasis in space and time. *Parasitology* 1993; **106**: 77–92.

20. Rogers DJ, Randolph SE. Distribution of tsetse and ticks in Africa, past, present and future. *Parasitol Today* 1993; **9**: 266–71.

21. Robinson TP, Rogers DJ, Williams B. Mapping tsetse habitat suitability in the common fly belt of southern Africa using multivariate analysis of climate and remotely sensed vegetation data. *Med Vet Entomol* 1977; **11**: 235–45.

22. Hendrickx G, Napala A, Dao B *et al.* A systematic approach to area-wide tsetse distribution and abundance maps. *Bull Entomol Res* 1999; **89**: 231–44.

♦23. Rogers DJ. Satellites, space, time and the African trypanosomiasis. *Adv Parasitol* 2000; **47**: 129–71.

●24. Hendrickx G, de La Rocque S, Reid R, Wint W. Spatial trypanosomiasis management: From data-layers to decision making. *Trends Parasitol* 2001; **17**: 35–41.

●25. Robinson TP. Geographic information systems and the selection of priority areas for control of tsetse-transmitted trypanosomiasis in Africa. *Parasitol Today* 1998; **14**: 457–61.

26. Costa J, Peterson AT, Beard CB. Ecologic niche modeling and differentiation of populations of *Triatoma brasiliensis neiva*, 1911, the most important Chagas' disease vector in northeastern Brazil (Hemiptera, Reduviidae, Triatominae). *Am J Trop Med Hyg* 2002; **67**: 516–20.

●27. Courtin F, Jamonneau V, Duvallet G *et al.* Sleeping sickness in West Africa (1906–2006): Changes in spatial repartition and lessons from the past. *Trop Med Int Health* 2008; **13**: 334–44.

28. Carcavallo RU. Climatic factors related to Chagas disease transmission. *Mem Inst Oswaldo Cruz* 1999; **94**(Suppl. 1): 367–69.

29. Pifano CFR. *Algunos Aspectos en la Ecologia y Epidemiologia de las Enfermedades Endemicas con Focos Naturales en el Area Tropical, Especialmente en Venezuela.* [*Some Aspects of the Ecology and Epidemiology of Endemic Illnesses with Natural Centres in a Tropical Area, Especially in Veneuela.*] Caracas: Office Public Bibliotheque en Archieves Ministrie Sanitation Asistance Social, 1969.

30. Croft SL, Sundar S, Fairlamb AH. Drug resistance in leishmaniasis. *Clin Microbiol Rev* 2006; **19**: 111–26.

31. Davidson RN. Leishmaniasis. *Medicine* 2005; **33**: 43–6.

32. Campbell-Lendrum DH, Wilkinson P, Kuhn K *et al.* Monitoring the health impacts of global climate change. In: Martens P, McMichael AJ (eds) *Environmental Change, Climate and Health Issues and Research Methods.* Cambridge: Cambridge University Press, 2002: 253–89.

33. Desjeux P. The increase in risk factors for leishmaniasis worldwide. *Trans R Soc Trop Med Hyg* 2001; **95**: 239–43.

34. Dujardin JC, Campino L, Canavate C *et al.* Spread of vector-borne diseases and neglect of leishmaniasis, Europe. *Emerg Infect Dis* 2008; **14**: 1013–18.

35. Wasserberg G, Abramsky Z, Kotler BP, Ostfeld RS, Yarom I, Warburg A. Anthropogenic disturbances enhance occurrence of cutaneous leishmaniasis in Israeli deserts: Patterns and mechanisms. *Ecol Appl* 2003; **13**: 868–81.

36. Wijeyaratne PM, Arsenault LK, Murphy CJ. Endemic disease and development: The leishmaniases. *Acta Trop* 1994; **56**: 349–64.

37. Kuhn KG. Global warming and leishmaniasis in Italy. *Bull Trop Med Int Health* 1999; **7**: 1–2.

●38. Chaves LF, Pascual M. Climate cycles and forecasts of cutaneous leishmaniasis, a nonstationary vector-borne disease. *PLoS Med* 2006; **3**: e295.

●39. Chaves LF, Cohen JM, Pascual M, Wilson ML. Social exclusion modifies climate and deforestation impacts on a vector-borne disease. *PLoS Negl Trop Dis* 2008; **2**: e176.

40. Peterson AT, Shaw J. *Lutzomyia* vectors for cutaneous leishmaniasis in Southern Brazil: Ecological niche models, predicted geographic distributions, and climate change effects. *Int J Parasitol* 2003; **33**: 919–31.

41. Killick-Kendrick R, Killick-Kendrick M. The laboratory colonization of *Phlebotomus ariasi* (Diptera: Psychodidae). *Ann Parasitol Hum Comp* 1987; **62**: 354–6.

42. Rioux JA, Aboulker JP, Lanotte G, Killick-Kendrick R, Martini-Dumas A. [Ecology of leishmaniasis in the south of France. 21: Influence of temperature on the development of *Leishmania infantum* Nicolle, 1908 in *Phlebotomus ariasi* Tonnoir, 1921. Experimental study]. *Ann Parasitol Hum Comp* 1985; **60**: 221–9.

43. Michael E, Bundy DA, Grenfell BT. Re-assessing the global prevalence and distribution of lymphatic filariasis. *Parasitology* 1996; **112**(Pt 4): 409–28.

44. World Health Organization. Lymphatic filariasis: Progress of disability prevention activities. *Wkly Epidemiol Rec* 2004; **47**: 417–24.

45. Raghavan NGS. Climate and filaria. *Bull Natl Soc India Malar Other Mosq Borne Dis* 1958; **6**: 137–45.

46. Acton HW, Rao SS. Factors which determine the differences in the types of lesions produced by *Filaria bancrofti* in India. *Indian Med Gaz* 1930; **65**: 620–9.

47. Roa SS, Sukhatme PV (1941). Cited in Peterson AT, Shaw J. *Lutzomyia* vectors for cutaneous leishmaniasis in Southern Brazil: Ecological niche models, predicted geographic distributions, and climate change effects. *Int J Parasitol* 2003; **33**: 919–31.

48. Gasarasi DB, Premji ZG, Mujinja PG, Mpembeni R. Acute adenolymphangitis due to bancroftian filariasis in Rufiji district, south east Tanzania. *Acta Trop* 2000; **75**: 19–28.

49. Raghavan NGS. Clinical manifestations and associated epidemiological factors of filariasis. *J Commun Dis* 1969; **1**: 75–102.

50. Bowie JH. Filariasis. *Edinb Med J* 1950; **57**: 561–71.

51. Jordan P. Bancroftian filariasis in Tanganyika: Observations on elephantiasis, microfilarial density, genital filariasis and microfilaraemia rates. *Ann Trop Med Parasitol* 1960; **54**: 132–40.

52. Thompson DF, Malone JB, Harb M *et al.* Bancroftian filariasis distribution and diurnal temperature differences in the southern Nile delta. *Emerg Infect Dis* 1996; **2**: 234–35.

53. Sowilem MM, Bahgat IM, el-Kady GA, el-Sawaf BM. Spectral and landscape characterization of filarious and non-filarious villages in Egypt. *J Egypt Soc Parasitol* 2006; **36**: 373–88.

54. Lindsay SW, Thomas CJ. Mapping and estimating the population at risk from lymphatic filariasis in Africa. *Trans R Soc Trop Med Hyg* 2000; **94**: 37–45.

55. Rao SS, Iyengar MOT (1929). Cited in Peterson AT, Shaw J. *Lutzomyia* vectors for cutaneous leishmaniasis in Southern Brazil: Ecological niche models, predicted geographic distributions, and climate change effects. *Int J Parasitol* 2003; **33**: 919–31.

56. Iyengar MOT. *Studies on Epidemiology of Filariasis in Travancore.* Calcutta: Thacker Spink, 1938.

57. Ray AP (1957). Cited in Peterson AT, Shaw J. *Lutzomyia* vectors for cutaneous leishmaniasis in Southern Brazil: Ecological niche models, predicted geographic distributions, and climate change effects. *Int J Parasitol* 2003; **33**: 919–31.

58. Shlenova MF (1938). Cited in Peterson AT, Shaw J. *Lutzomyia* vectors for cutaneous leishmaniasis in Southern Brazil: Ecological niche models, predicted geographic distributions, and climate change effects. *Int J Parasitol* 2003; **33**: 919–31.

59. Bates M (1941). Cited in Peterson AT, Shaw J. *Lutzomyia* vectors for cutaneous leishmaniasis in Southern Brazil: Ecological niche models, predicted geographic distributions, and climate change effects. *Int J Parasitol* 2003; **33**: 919–31.

60. van Thiel PH (1939). Cited in Peterson AT, Shaw J. *Lutzomyia* vectors for cutaneous leishmaniasis in Southern Brazil: Ecological niche models, predicted geographic distributions, and climate change effects. *Int J Parasitol* 2003; **33**: 919–31.

61. Lardeux F, Cheffort J. Temperature thresholds and statistical modelling of larval *Wuchereria bancrofti* (Filariidea: Onchocercidae) developmental rates. *Parasitology* 1997; **114**: 123–34.

●62. Soberon J. Grinnellian and Eltonian niches and geographic distributions of species. *Ecol Lett* 2007; **10**: 1115–23.

●63. Chan NY, Ebi KL, Smith F, Wilson TF, Smith AE. An integrated assessment framework for climate change and infectious diseases. *Environ Health Perspect* 1999; **107**: 329–37.

64. Ebi KL, Patz JA. Epidemiological and impacts assessment methods. In: Martens P, McMichael AJ (eds) *Environment Change, Climate and Health Issues and Research Methods.* Cambridge: Cambridge University Press, 2002: 120–43.

65. Neiva A. Informacoes sobre a biologia da vinchuca [Information on the biology of the vinchuca], *Triatoma infestans* Klug. *Mem Inst Oswaldo Cruz* 1913; **5**: 24–31.

66. Hack W. Estudios sobre biologia del *Triatoma infestans* [Studies on the biology of *Triatoma infestans*] (Klug, 1834) (Hemiptra, Reduviidae). *Ann Inst Med Reg* 1955; **4**: 125–47.

67. Carcavallo RU, Martinez A. Life cycles of some species of *Triatoma* (Hemiptera, Reduviidae). *Can Entomol* 1972; **104**: 699–704.

68. Zeledon R, Guardia VM, Zuniga A, Swartzwelder JC. Biology and ethology of *Triatoma dimidiata* (Latreille, 1811). I: Life cycle, amount of blood ingested, resistance to starvation, and size of adults. *J Med Entomol* 1970; **7**: 313–19.

69. Silva IG, Silva HHG. Influencia da temperatura na biologia de Triatomineos. [Influence of temperature on the biology of the triatomines.] V: *Rhodnius riasutus* Stal, 1859 (Hemiptera, Reduviidae). *Mem Inst Oswaldo Cruz* 1986; **81**(Suppl): 163.

70. Silva IG, Silva HHG. Influencia da temperatura na biologia de Triatomineos. [Influence of temperature on the biology of the triatomines.] IV: *Triatoma infestans* (Klug, 1834) (Hemiptera, Reduviidae). *Ann Soc Entomol Bras* 1986; **17**: 443–55.

71. Silva IG, Silva HHG. Influencia da temperatura na biologia de Triatomineos. [Influence of temperature on the biology

72. Silva IG, Silva HHG. Influencia da temperatura na biologia de Triatomineos. [Influence of temperature on the biology of the triatomines.] III: *Panstrongylus megistus* (Burmeister, 1835) (Hemiptera, Reduviidae). *Rev Bras Entomol* 1988; **37**: 489–96.

73. Blaksley JC, Carcavallo RU. *La Enfermedad de Chagas-Mazza en la Argentina.* [*Chagas–Mazza Disease in Argentina.*] Buenos Aires: Ministerio Salud, 1968.

74. Catala S. The biting rate of *Triatoma infestans* in Argentina. *Med Vet Entomol* 1991; **5**: 325–33.

75. Asin S, Catala S. Development of *Trypanosoma cruzi* in *Triatoma infestans*: Influence of temperature and blood consumption. *J Parasit* 1995; **81**: 1–7.

of the triatomines.] X: *Triatoma vitticeps* Stal 1859 (Hemiptera, Reduviidae). *Rev Goiana Med* 1986; **34**: 39–45.

40

Disease transmission by non-biting flies

GORDON L. NICHOLS

INTRODUCTION

Non-biting flies have been implicated in the transmission of a wide variety of pathogens over the last century[1–5] and are still regarded as important vectors for the direct transmission of pathogens from one infected patient to another, as well as for the transmission from faeces to food, the eye or the mouth.[6] However, epidemiological evidence supporting disease transmission in this way is poor for a number of reasons (Table 40.1).

In developing countries transmission of organisms requiring a high infective dose, such as *Vibrio cholerae* and *Salmonella*, has been reported, implying heavy contamination through the fly-borne route. Within developed countries, transmission is likely to be from animal faeces or raw meats to ready-to-eat food and is more likely to be the result of individual transmission by a single fly, with few examples of outbreaks. In such situations, the transmission of organisms that are common in animal faeces and can cause human infections with a low infecting dose, such as *Campylobacter*, might be expected.

However, analytical studies in this area can be difficult to undertake, and intervention studies can be population-based and intrusive. Overall, there is no convincing body of information indicating the burden of disease related to non-biting flies. Unlike the evidence for the transmission of infectious diseases by biting flies and other arthropods, for which the bite is the principal transmission route, with non-biting flies the pathogens can also be transmitted by a variety of other routes of infection.

The evidence linking flies to human disease is diverse and patchy, with much of the evidence dating from past years when the epidemiological data were limited and the microbiological evidence lacked modern molecular biological back-up (Table 40.2). The best evidence comes from outbreaks and from studies that have looked at the impact of interventions to reduce fly populations. There is a particular limitation resulting from the rarity of outbreaks caused by flies because outbreaks can provide good evidence of transmission. However, the rarity of outbreaks also reflects the sporadic nature of this transmission route. There have been a large number of publications demonstrating the presence of particular pathogens on or in different fly species. Although these provide circumstantial evidence implicating them in transmission, the epidemiological evidence needs to be improved before their role will be widely accepted.

WARFARE

The importance of fly-borne transmission first came to light in the latter part of the nineteenth century in military situations.[2] Armies used large numbers of horses and, when camped, the faeces of these animals provided a fertile breeding ground for a range of fly species. The flies landed on animal and human faeces and were thus able to fly directly on to food just before consumption. As a consequence, outbreaks of dysentery were attributed to transmission by flies. Control through manure management was effective

Table 40.1   Transmission by non-biting flies – evidence and limitations

Source of evidence	Evidence for transmission	Limitations
Historical publications	Much useful work on flies and diarrhoeal diseases was conducted in the first half of the twentieth century	The pre-Medline evidence is microbiologically suspect Many hypothesized associations have been superseded by improved knowledge about the epidemiology
Individual transmission	Experimental studies indicate that infected flies can infect animals	Because transmission could be through an infective dose carried by an individual fly, the source can be difficult to identify
Outbreaks	Outbreaks linked to non-biting flies are uncommon. Outbreak investigation has highlighted pathogens that are probably transmitted by flies that would not otherwise have been thought to be fly-borne	Most fly-borne disease is likely to be sporadic The investigation of outbreaks can involve other transmission routes People involved in the investigation of outbreaks have not usually been able to test flies for the pathogen There is often a suspicion that other routes of infection (e.g. water and food) may not have been investigated with sufficient rigour
Microbiological surveys	Many studies have shown the natural carriage of a wide variety of pathogenic microorganisms by many fly species	Natural contamination of flies is likely to reflect recent access to contaminated faeces. Such contamination may therefore vary dramatically over short distances
Body of research	There is a large body of work on the microbiological contamination of flies	There is remarkably little good work on the epidemiology of non-biting fly-borne diseases
Experimental microbiology	Under experimental conditions, it is possible to contaminate newly hatched flies and monitor how contamination changes over time	Some studies have demonstrated the growth of pathogens in flies Other studies have shown their gradual elimination from surface and gut
Fly pools	The microbiological examination of fly pools can give percentages positive for particular pathogens. Collections of flies (fly pools) provide a useful way of monitoring pathogens in natural fly populations	This can imply that the number of flies that are positive is low and therefore that the risk is low As with food and water, when investigating an outbreak contamination of the source of infection may no longer be present, even though the flies remain
Seasonal and geographical differences	The local and seasonal differences in fly populations and human disease can be triggers for suspecting an association	The microbiological analysis of flies can vary by location and season, and snapshot studies may give a false overall picture
Delicate pathogens	There is strong evidence for *Chlamydia trachomatis* transmission by flies. Associations with *Treponema pertenue* and *Neisseria gonorrhoeae* also suggest that delicate pathogens can be transmitted under the right conditions	Focus on enteric pathogens can create the impression that it is predominantly robust organisms that are transmitted by flies
Epidemiological methods	A few studies have shown clear associations between disease and flies	Many of the epidemiological studies have been methodologically flawed, for instance because of confounding or lack of control populations
Intervention in transmission	Evidence for fly reduction causing disease reduction in developing countries	Fly reduction programmes are difficult to sustain over time There have been few deliberate intervention studies in developed countries

(*Continued*)

Table 40.1 *(Continued)*

Source of evidence	Evidence for transmission	Limitations
Kitchen transmission	There is a strong environmental health rationale for controlling flies in kitchens	The evidence of the burden of disease associated with fly-borne transmission within kitchens is limited
Food-borne route	The contamination of ready-to-eat foods is understandable, feasible and is part of environmental health training	Traditional case–control studies that look at 'risk foods' will be unlikely to identify food contaminated by flies
Infective dose	Many of the pathogens thought to be fly-borne are those requiring only a low infective dose to cause infection	There is limited evidence on the numbers of organisms that can be transmitted by a single fly in real-life situations
Source–pathway–receptor	Evidence of source–pathway–receptor: animal faeces–fly–food, human faeces–fly–food, eye–fly–eye, wound–fly–wound	Sources can be diverse
Seasonal changes in disease may reflect changes in source contamination as well as fly prevalence
Textbooks	Simple advice is given in environmental health textbooks	There is little evidence or advice in most microbiology textbooks
Industry investment	Flies are common in animal production and may be involved in the transmission of infections in animals, which might be regarded as a market for industry	No industry supporting research
Research expertise	There is little evidence of major research groups working on this area	Such work should involve entymologists, epidemiologists and microbiologists. The design of good epidemiological studies is a limiting factor

and is still preferable to insecticide use in fly management because of the development of insecticide resistance.

HISTORICAL EVIDENCE LINKING FLIES WITH HUMAN DISEASE

Work published by Niven in 1910 showed a relationship between the number of flies caught in Manchester in the summer months between 1904 and 1909 and deaths from childhood summer diarrhoea (Figure 40.1). A relationship was shown between ground temperature and fly numbers in this study.[7]

In another study, a relationship was reported between the annual summer deaths from diarrhoea per 100 000 population and the number of horse-drawn vehicles licensed per year (Figure 40.2).[5] The decline in diarrhoeal deaths in England and Wales between 1906 and 1929 was thus attributed to a reduction in the number of flies that breed in the horse manure as a result of there being fewer horses.

There is a group of fly species that can regularly be found growing near human activity, and these flies are termed synanthropic (living near, and benefiting from, an association with humans and their habitats). The synanthropic fly species linked to human infections are broadly grouped into houseflies, blowflies and flesh flies.

Synanthropic flies are particularly associated with poverty, dislocation and disaster, where large numbers of flies have access to faeces and people are outside for most of the time.

NON-ENTERIC BACTERIAL INFECTIONS

Flies can transmit a variety of non-enteric pathogens to humans. These include *Haemophilus aegyptius*[33] and *Chlamydia trachomatis*.[8,12,34,35] Some seasonality in the occurrence of flies has been linked to cases of trachoma.[8,11,12,36]

Trachoma

Eye-seeking flies are important trachoma vectors.[37–39] One study examined the prevalence of, magnitude of and factors influencing the transmission and severity of trachoma in Saudi Arabia.[40] A stratified multistage random cluster design selected primary sampling units of 50–60 houses in both metropolitan and non-metropolitan communities. Evidence of trachoma (active and inactive) was found among 22.2 per cent of the Saudi population in 1984, with 6.2 per cent having evidence of active trachoma, 17.4 per cent having conjunctival scarring, and 1.5 per cent having entropion or trichiasis. In 1994, this had reduced to 10.7 per cent with evidence of trachoma (active and inactive), 2.6 per cent with active trachoma, 8.1 per cent with conjunctival scarring, and 0.2 per cent with entropion and trichiasis. The prevalence of trachoma in households was directly related to the presence of children, the presence of flies and the appearance rating of the household itself.

Trachoma (*Chlamydia trachomatis*) has been identified as a major cause of morbidity in Australian Aboriginal

Table 40.2   Epidemiological evidence of associations between flies and disease

Organism/disease	Location	Date	Epidemiological evidence	Reference
Comparison of seasonal variations in flies and trachoma	West Kimberley, Australia	1996	Correlations between seasonal incidence of trachoma and fly numbers	8
Outbreak of *Neisseria gonorrhoeae* conjunctivitis	Northern Territories, Western Australia, South Australia	1997	Outbreak of gonococcal conjunctivitis (447 cases) with large fly populations at the start	52
Nursery school outbreak of *Escherichia coli* O157: H7 enterohaemorrhagic colitis	Japan	1999	Organism isolated from patients and flies	9
Childhood diarrhoea	Pakistan	1995–1996	Community randomized intervention study – two cohorts	10
Trachoma and diarrhoea	The Gambia	1997–1998	Community randomized intervention study – two cohorts	11, 12
Shigella, Escherichia coli, norovirus (NLV) and diarrhoea	Israel	1988–1989	Prospective cross-over intervention study	13, 14
A large outbreak of *Neisseria gonorrhoeae* severe pustular conjunctivitis	Ethiopia (9000 cases) over 8 months	1987–1988	Intense crowding, lack of water and flies were thought to be important in transmission. Lack of face-washing was identified as a household risk factor in a case–control study	15
Annual outbreak of *Corynebacterium pyogenes* granulomatous leg ulcers	Thailand	1987	It was hypothesized that infection followed skin injury and was transmitted by Oriental-eye flies	16
Diarrhoeal disease	Thailand	1981	Correlation between fly numbers and disease	17
Gastrointestinal diseases	Thailand	1976	Correlation between fly density and disease	18
Diarrhoeal disease	India	1975	Correlation between fly density and diarrhoeal episodes	19
Shigella dysenteriae type 1	St Martin island	1973	The average attack rate was high. A common source outbreak was unlikely, and flies may have been involved in transmission	20
Dysentery	Georgia	1969	Comparison of fly rates with cases of dysentery	21
Diarrhoeal disease	Venezuela	1969	Fly numbers did not correlate well with diarrhoeal diseases	22
Shigella	Phoenix, Arizona	1955	Descriptive evidence	23
Diarrhoeal disease	Guatemala	1956–1959	Increase in diarrhoea at the end of the rains, and flies are very common at this period	24
Shigella	Sacaton and Guadelupe, Arizona	1954–1955	Comparison of *Shigella* types isolated from people and flies	108
Salmonella and *Shigella*	Georgia, USA	1949–1951	Community randomized intervention study – two cohorts	25
Salmonella and *Shigella*	Texas, USA	1947–1948	Community randomized intervention study – two cohorts	26
Shigella outbreak	Not known	1944	Cases increased and decreased in line with fly numbers. *Shigella* was isolated from flies	27
Deaths	China	1929	Death rates and fly densities rose and fell in parallel	109

(Continued)

Table 40.2 (*Continued*)

Organism/disease	Location	Date	Epidemiological evidence	Reference
Bacillary dysentery	Salonica	1916–1918	Circumstantial descriptive information	28
Dysentery	Mesopotamia	1917	Correlations between seasonal incidence of dysentery and fly numbers	29
Summer diarrhoea deaths	England and Wales	1906–1927	Relationship between deaths from diarrhoea and horse-drawn vehicles	5
Epidemic diarrhoea and dysentery	Poona, India	1912–1915	Relationship shown between the early part of the annual diarrhoea epidemic and fly numbers. The absence of a relationship in the late summer suggested water was important	110
Summer diarrhoea deaths	England and Wales	1902–1909	Descriptive evidence linking deaths from diarrhoea, climate and flies	30
Conjunctivitis, summer diarrhoea, typhoid, yaws and cholera			Descriptive review	31
Summer diarrhoea deaths	England and Wales	1904–1909	Descriptive weekly evidence linking deaths from diarrhoea, climate and flies	32

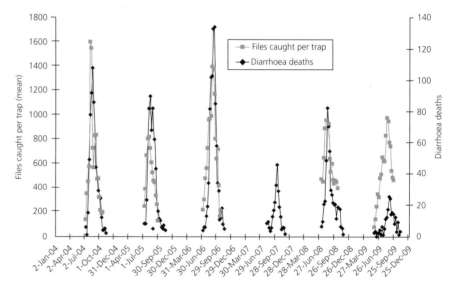

Figure 40.1   Deaths from diarrhoea in Manchester 1904–09.

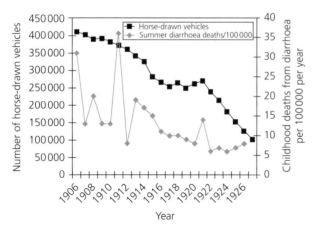

Figure 40.2   Relationship between summer deaths from diarrhoea in England and Wales and the number of horse-drawn vehicles licensed per year.

communities, particularly among younger age groups.[8] The World Health Organization has launched a programme (GET 2020) for the elimination of trachoma, the leading cause of preventable blindness.[41] GET 2020 has adopted the SAFE strategy, a set of control measures including Surgery, Antibiotics, Facial cleanliness and Environmental improvements such as fly control and access to clean water.[42,43]

One study compared the prevalence of trachoma between three Aboriginal communities, with differences in adult bush fly (*Musca vetustissima*) populations between the wet and dry seasons.[8] Preschool and school-aged children were screened for trachoma using the World Health Organization method for clinical assessment. Flies were trapped fortnightly using a wind-orientated fly trap. There was a significantly higher rate of trachoma during the wet season (46–69 per cent) compared with the dry season (14–59 per cent). Populations of bush fly significantly increased during the wet season (ranging from 6 to 146 flies per hectare per month).

The fly *Musca sorbens* transmits *Chlamydia trachomatis* in rural Gambia, causing trachoma. *Musca sorbens* usually breeds in isolated human faeces on the soil surface, but not in covered pit latrines.[44] Experimental studies indicate that *Musca sorbens* can develop within human, calf, cow, dog and goat faeces, but not in horse faeces, composting kitchen scraps or a soil control. After adjusting for mass of medium, the greatest number of flies emerged from human faeces (1426 flies/kg). Median time for emergence was 9 (interquartile range 8–9.75) days post oviposition. Of all flies emerging from faeces, 81 per cent were *Musca sorbens*. Male and female flies emerging from human faeces were larger than those from other media. Female flies caught from children's eyes were of a similar size to those from human faeces but larger than those from other faeces. Improvements in basic sanitation, with the removal of human and animal faeces from the environment, is likely to reduce fly density, eye contact and hence trachoma transmission.

Several species of fly were caught in traps placed in villages in The Gambia, but only two species, *Musca sorbens* and *Musca domestica*, were caught from the eyes of children.[12] All fly species were more numerous in the wet season than the dry season. Children's eyes are the main reservoir of *Chlamydia trachomatis*, flies exhibit frequent fly–eye contacts (three every 15 minutes), and children with ocular or nasal discharge had twice as many fly–eye contacts compared with children with no discharge. *Chlamydia* DNA was demonstrated by polymerase chain reaction in two of 395 flies caught from the eyes of children with a current active trachoma infection.

A study examined two pairs of villages, one pair in the 1997 wet season, and one pair in the 1998 dry season.[11] Deltamethrin was sprayed for 3 months to control flies in one village, while the other was used as a control. Fly populations were monitored with traps. Fly control reduced muscid flies numbers by around 75 per cent in the intervention villages compared with controls. Trachoma prevalence was similar at the start, but after 3 months of fly control there were 75 per cent fewer new cases of trachoma in the intervention villages, with a 22 per cent reduction in childhood diarrhoea in the wet season and 26 per cent less diarrhoea in the dry season compared with controls.

A community-based 'Flies and Eyes' project used a cluster-randomized intervention trial in a rural area of The Gambia.[36] Twenty-one clusters, of 300–550 people, were recruited in groups of three. The study was designed to prove whether flies are mechanical vectors of trachoma, to quantify the relative importance of flies as vectors of trachoma, and to test the effectiveness of insecticide spraying and the provision of latrines in trachoma control.

A national trachoma disease prevalence survey was conducted in Mali in 1996 and 1997 and examined its prevalence and potential risk factors.[45] A representative sample of 30 clusters in Mali's regions were taken from the general population. All children under 10 years of age were examined. A total of 15 187 children under 10 years of age were examined. Aridity/environmental dryness was a risk factor influencing the geographical distribution of trachoma, and small villages had a higher prevalence than larger ones. The presence of a dirty face was strongly associated with trachoma (odds ratio 3.67), as was the presence of flies on the child's face (odds ratio 3.62). Trachoma prevalence increased with the distance to a water source and decreased with a higher frequency of both face-washing and bathing. Studies in Tanzania have also shown associations between flies on the face and disease,[46] and identified face-washing as protective.[37,47]

Yaws

Yaws is a form of non-sexually acquired syphilis (*Treponema pallidum* subsp. *pertenue*) that causes deforming lesions in skin, cartilage and bone. The organism is related to the similar treponemal infections bejel (*T. pallidum* subsp. *endemicum*), syphilis (*T. pallidum* subsp. *pallidum*) and pinta (*T. carateum*). Yaws was the subject of an effective worldwide eradication campaign in the 1950s, because of its sensitivity to penicillin, but this has since faltered.[48,49] Although it can be transmitted from person to person, it can also be mechanically transmitted by eye flies (*Hippelates pallipes*) feeding at wounds, and in the West Indies this was thought to be the main transmission route.[50] The spirochaetes remain motile in the fly pharynx and oesophageal diverticula for several hours, but are apparently immobilized in the midgut and do not develop in the fly. They have been shown to pass through house flies. The absence of any reference to fly-borne transmission in recent decades does not appear to reflect any counterevidence showing that this is not an important transmission route. It is perhaps more a reflection of the limited utility of this evidence for eradication as a single treatment with penicillin will treat the disease effectively.

Neisseria gonorrhoeae

A large outbreak of severe pustular conjunctivitis (9000 cases) caused by *Neisseria gonorrhoeae* occurred over 8 months in 1987–88 in one district in Ethiopia.[15] The outbreak affected all age groups and sexes, and particularly affected children under 5 years of age with few neonatal cases. Although the epidemic curve suggested person-to-person transmission, there was no concurrent genital gonorrheal outbreak, and genital transmission could not explain the community-wide outbreak. Two peaks in transmission coincided with recent rain. In the setting of intense crowding and a relative lack of water, flies were thought to be important in transmission. Lack of face-washing was identified as a household risk factor in a case–control study.

The risk of fly-borne gonococcal conjunctivitis in Australia has been recognized,[51] and an outbreak of non-sexually transmitted gonococcal conjunctivitis among Aboriginal children in Central Australia in 1997 implicated high numbers of flies at the time of the outbreak.[52] There was also an increase in conjunctivitis caused by *Haemophilus* spp. at the start of the outbreak.

The evidence of large outbreaks of gonococcal infection associated with possible transmission by face fly species is not conclusive but provides further tantalizing evidence for the direct transmission of delicate organisms from person to person by flies. It suggests the possibility that meningococcal meningitis caused by *Neisseria meningitidis* might also be transmitted by this mechanism in a developing country setting, and that this hypothesis might be worth examining in the meningitis belt in Africa, where the cause of epidemics remains elusive. Evidence suggests that epidemics of meningococcal disease are seasonal and may be linked to climate.[53] However, there is no published evidence supporting an association between meningococcal disease and flies.

ENTERIC BACTERIAL PATHOGENS

There is circumstantial, microbiological and analytical evidence of human enteric pathogens being transmitted by flies.[5,54–56] This includes enterotoxigenic *Escherichia coli*,[17,57–59] *Escherichia coli* O157,[60] *Vibrio cholerae* non-O1,[17,71] *Vibrio cholerae* O1,[61,62] *Vibrio cholerae* O139,[63] *Vibrio fluvialis*,[17] *Campylobacter* spp.,[64,66,68,70] *Helicobacter pylori*,[66–68] *Shigella* spp.,[13,17,58,59] *Salmonella* spp.,[58,59,69–71] *Salmonella typhi*,[1,72,73] *Staphylococcus aureus*,[69] hepatitis A[21] and hepatitis E viruses.[74]

Campylobacter spp.

Flies are commonly contaminated with *Campylobacter* spp.[54,56,59,64,65,75] and could contribute to disease transmission through direct transmission from faeces to mouth, from faeces to food or through cross-contamination from raw foods to ready-to-eat food. It has been argued that the levels of contamination in flies are insufficient to commonly cause human disease.[65] Their abundance does change with the time of year, being less common in the winter and more common in the late spring to late autumn period.

Chicken is the most commonly identified risk factor for human *Campylobacter* infection. The *Campylobacter* contamination of chicken flocks has been a problem that is thought to be attributable to the introduction of infection on boots or by rodents, and improved animal biosecurity has been emphasized.[76] Animal biosecurity can be defined as preventing the ingress of human or animal pathogens into agricultural animal populations through containment

measures. There is evidence that flies can gain access to chicken houses through ventilation ducts, and improved fly screening has been shown to reduce flock contamination.[77–79] Although *Campylobacter* carriage can be short-lived, there is a rationale for believing that flies are able to breach animal biosecurity around *Campylobacter*-negative flocks.[80] Logistic regression modelling was used to demonstrate that a lower prevalence of *Campylobacter* in Icelandic flocks occurred following periods that had temperatures not conducive to fly growth.[81,82]

The marked seasonal distribution of human *Campylobacter* infection has been hypothesized to be attributable to direct transmission of the organism from animal and bird faeces to ready-to-eat foods,[83,84] thereby bypassing all of the farm-to-fork protection offered by traditional hazard analysis critical control point approaches to food safety. *Campylobacter* infections in England and Wales occur as a late spring to summer epidemic (with a large increase from May to the peak in June) every year. These appear to result from an unidentified driver that is the cause of the geographically sporadic cases that have the temporal appearance of an outbreak.[83]

There are few outbreaks of *Campylobacter* gastroenteritis,[85,86] and most cases are thought to be sporadic. A hypothesis suggests that this pattern reflects a multiple-vehicle epidemic caused by direct or indirect contamination of people by packets (quanta) of infected material carried by flies that have been in contact with faeces.[83] The local pattern of human illness appears as if chosen at random, while having a defined geographical and temporal distribution that is a function of the growth kinetics of one or more fly species and access to contaminated faeces. There are differing seasonal distributions of human *Campylobacter* infections in many countries around the world,[87–89,111] and it is predicted that these can be largely explained by changes in fly populations.[83]

Flies can carry *Campylobacter* and have the potential to infect both humans and animals.[54,59,90] A variety of synanthropic fly species could be involved, including house flies (e.g. *Musca* spp. and *Fannia* spp.), blowflies (e.g. *Calliphora* spp., *Lucilia* spp., *Pollenia* spp., *Cynomya* spp. and *Phormia* spp.) and other dung-related flies (e.g. *Sarcophaga* spp. and *Drosophila* spp.).[91] These flies exhibit different behaviour, ecology, physiology and temporal and geographical distributions, which can influence whether they occur in kitchens, on human or animal faeces and on food. *Musca domestica* are commonly found in houses and food-processing establishments and are likely to be involved. However, larger flies (e.g. *Calliphora* spp.) may be able to transmit larger doses of *Campylobacter*.

The increase in fly populations in England and Wales in May and June is hypothesized to result from rainy weather and an increase in temperature that shortens the fly life-cycle and causes a big increase in fly numbers over a short time period. The decline in fly numbers in late summer to autumn is less dramatic and defined than the spring increase, possibly because fly mortality is not as acutely temperature dependent as larval development, and travel-related *Campylobacter* infection is more common in the late summer. It remains possible that another driver may be found that explains the seasonality of *Campylobacter* infections. The dramatic change in *Campylobacter* contamination of chickens through the seasons might be the best alternative explanation. However, the fly hypothesis remains conjectural in the absence of good scientifically conducted studies.

Shigella spp.

Houseflies feed in human excrement and can act as mechanical vectors, transmitting *Shigella* and possibly enterotoxigenic *Escherichia coli*. *Shigella* spp. have been isolated from flies.[13,17,58,59] Because shigellosis is a strictly human disease and the organism is rarely found in wild or domestic animals, transmission is predominantly from person to person through poor hygiene, particularly among schoolchildren. Seasons during which both flies and cases of dysentery are prevalent often coincide.[29] Intervention studies in the USA in the 1940s provided evidence of the role of houseflies in the transmission of shigellae. The inoculum required to transmit shigellosis is low ($10–10^2$ organisms). Since houseflies co-habit with humans, they can readily contaminate food and eating utensils.

A prospective cross-over intervention study at two military field bases several kilometers apart was conducted in 1988.[13] Intensive fly control measures including baiting and trapping were introduced on one base, while the other served as a control. There was 11 weeks of intervention at one site and then at the other. The study was repeated the following year. Fly counts were 64 per cent lower on the bases exposed to fly control measures ($P=0.024$). There was a corresponding drop in clinic visits by 42 per cent ($P=0.146$) for diarrhoeal diseases and by 85 per cent for shigellosis ($P=0.015$); there were also falls in the rate of *Shigella* seroconversion, by 76 per cent ($P=0.024$), and in antibodies to enterotoxigenic *Escherichia coli* by 57 per cent ($P=0.006$).

Shigella were isolated from 4.8 per cent of pools of 10 flies in a town in Myanmar.[58] All enteric bacterial pathogens were more frequently isolated from flies collected at refuse dumps and animal pens than those collected from kitchens. More pathogens were isolated in the hot, wet season than at other times. A study of fly populations in a village in north-eastern Thailand in 1981 found that fly number (predominantly *Musca domestica*) increased in kitchens and animal pens in the hot dry spring, and this was also when the incidence of diarrhoea was highest in the village. Enterotoxigenic *Escherichia coli*, *Shigella* spp., non-O1 *Vibrio cholerae* and *Vibrio fluvalis* were isolated from fly pools in yards (69 per cent), animal pens (38 per cent), bathrooms (35 per cent) and kitchens (8 per cent).[17]

In the summer and early autumn of 1974, flies were trapped in districts of Beirut.[92] *Musca domestica*, *Muscina stabulans*, *Calliphora vicina*, *Phormia regina*, *Phaenicia sericata*, Sarcophagidae and *Fannia canicularis* were identified. The rural areas had higher densities of *Musca domestica*, while higher densities of Calliphoridae were found in the Slaughter House, Quarantine and Burj-Hammoud districts. Out of 72 batches of Muscidae and 84 Calliphoridae, 10 had *Shigella* spp. and 19 *Salmonella* spp.

An epidemic of *Shigella dysenteriae* type 1 broke out in St Martin Island in the Bay of Bengal between May and July 1973.[20] The average attack rate was high (32.9 per cent), and the outbreak could not be controlled by treatment with antibiotics. The age-specific attack rate was highest in the age group 1–4 years (52.2 per cent) and in smaller families, suggesting that person-to-person spread was not the principal route of transmission. There was little evidence for contaminated water being the source of infection. There was a significant death rate (2.1 per cent), particularly in children less than a year old. A common-source outbreak was unlikely, and flies may have played an active role in transmission.

Arcanobacterium (Corynebacterium) pyogenes

An annual outbreak of endemic leg ulcers in Thailand suggested that skin injury followed by infection with *Arcanobacterium pyogenes* caused the development of granulomatous leg ulcers, and infection was hypothesized to be transmitted by Oriental-eye flies.[16] *Arcanobacterium pyogenes* can also cause mastitis in cattle, and flies may be involved in transmission.

PROTOZOA

A study of risk factors for *Toxoplasma gondii* in Panama city found a significantly increased relative risk in children living in an environment with many flies.[93] *Giardia* may be transmitted by flies,[94,95] as may *Entamoeba histolytica*,[96] and it has been suggested that *Cryptosporidium* may be transmitted by this route.[95,97–99]

HELMINTHS

Eye worm infections by members of the nematode *Thelazia* genus can occur in a variety of animal species and can result from transmission by non-biting face flies; human infections can also occur.[100,101] In animal populations, *Musca autumnalis* has been implicated in transmission, but other species have been involved, There have been a small number of human cases in Europe, where dogs appear to be the principal reservoir, but infection is more common in the Far East.

A large variety of gastrointestinal helminth ova have been recovered from captured flies, and it is presumed that transmission by this route may be common in developing country settings. The ova of several intestinal nematodes, including *Ascaris lumbricoides*, *Strongyloides stercoralis*, *Ancylostoma caninum* and *Toxocara canis*, have been recovered from the outside surface of flies and from their intestine and crop.[102–104] The ova are thought to survive better in the crop than on the outer fly surface.[103]

A study of helminth contamination of flies captured in the Zoological Garden of Rio de Janeiro between 1996 and 1998 trapped 41 080 flies. *Chrysomya megacephala* and *Musca domestica* had human and animal helminth eggs on their body surface and in their intestinal contents, including *Ascaris*, *Toxascaris*, *Toxocara*, *Trichuris*, *Capillaria*, Oxyuridae, Trichostrongylidae and *Acanthocephala*. Helminth larvae were also recovered from the body surface of flies. A study of flies in an urban slum in the Philippines examined 1016 flies for the presence of helminth ova attached to their external surfaces, with *Ascaris* and *Trichuris trichiura* ova being most common.[104]

Another study at four sites in Malaysia found ova of *Ascaris lumbricoides*, *Trichuris trichiura* and hookworm on the adult external body surface and in the gut lumen of the dominant fly species *Chrysomya megacephala* as well as *Chrysomya rufifacies* and *Sarcophaga* spp.[105]

A study examined the viability of hookworm and *Ascaris lumbricoides* ova when fed to *Musca vicina* and *Musca domestica* in infected faeces.[106] There was no difference in the developmental periods of ova recovered from the house flies up to 2 hours post ingestion and those in the faeces. Flies fed hookworm larvae carried these for up to 8 hours after ingestion.

FLIES AND FARMING

Because many fly species breed in the faeces of agricultural animals and such animals are commonly surrounded by flies, it is unrealistic to expect animals reared outdoors to be free from flies. For poultry and agricultural animals grown indoors, the reduction in fly numbers may usefully contribute to reductions in the carriage of some infectious diseases through improving animal biosecurity.

OTHER AREAS

The decomposition of faecal waste and the associated pathogens carried therein relies on processing by insect larvae that use the faeces as a growth medium. This is an area that has had limited research investment. Flies can also cause nuisance if they are present in large numbers, such as around landfill sites or where a large amount of vegetation is decomposing.

A variety of different fly species can infect humans and cause myiasis. They can be separated into **obligatory** (e.g. *Chrysomya bezziana*, *Dermatobia hominis* and *Cordylobia*

anthropophaga), which require a host for the larvae to grow in, **facultative** (e.g. *Lucilia cuprina*, *Calliphora* spp. and *Sarcophaga* spp.), whose larvae develop in decaying vegetation but can grow in open wounds, and **accidental** (*Musca domestica* and *Fannia* spp.), whose larvae develop in decaying vegetation but can grow in food or within the oral or genital environment.[155] Infections can be cutaneous, nasopharyngeal, urogenital, ocular or intestinal, and can be difficult to diagnose. Myiasis can cause economic disease in sheep (strike) where the larvae of *Lucilia* spp. grow in wool contaminated with faeces (facultative) and then create wounds that lead to toxaemia, weakness and death. Flies can also be used in forensic work to estimate the time of death, and larvae can be used in cleaning necrotic wounds.

INVESTIGATION OF FLIES AND INFECTIOUS DISEASES

In investigating any associations between flies and disease, some consideration needs to be given to the biology and ecology of the different fly species implicated. Where do the flies land, and how does this change with climate, season, time of day and location? What is the likelihood of flies landing on faeces, food and faces, what parts of the fly (exterior, crop or intestine) are contaminated, and for how long does the pathogen survive there? Can the pathogen be present in numbers that are high enough to cause transmission to people? Are the epidemiological methods for investigating the problem likely to be able to prove or disprove the transmission by flies? Can the pieces of evidence for disease being due to non-biting flies be accommodated within the Bradford Hill guidelines on causality?

There is a lot of evidence that flies are commonly contaminated with human pathogens and can carry these for short periods in a wide variety of settings. There is evidence that a number of pathogens have been experimentally transmitted to animals by flies. There is also good evidence that this can occasionally cause outbreaks, but these are difficult to investigate. However, the majority of transmission is probably occurring as sporadic disease, and the epidemiological studies have provided good evidence for associations with disease in comparatively few cases.[107] The reason for this could reflect an absence of infectious disease transmission by non-biting flies or a problem in conducting epidemiological studies in this area. If there are genuine associations, they may not translate into useful interventions, but without good epidemiological and microbiological investigation, the true nature of disease transmission may not be identified and interventions in other areas may have limited effects.

There is a strong case for developing new analytical approaches that utilize modern molecular epidemiology in the investigation of transmission through non-biting flies.

Flies could play an important role in a number of animal diseases such as foot-and-mouth disease and bovine tuberculosis through airborne transmission, although these are not areas that have been studied. Fly-borne transmission within catering establishments remains important, and control by environmental health departments remains relevant. Although the impact of fly-borne transmission in both developed and developing countries remains unclear, there is a burden and it may be larger than is currently understood.

REFERENCES

● = Key primary paper

◆ = Major review article

1. Graham-Smith GS. *Flies and Disease – Non-bloodsucking Flies.* Cambridge: Cambridge University Press, 1913.
2. Shipley AE. *Flies. The Minor Horrors of War.* London: Smith, Elder, 1915: 57–86.
3. Busvine J. Houseflies and blowflies. In: Busvine J (ed.) *Insects and Hygiene.* London: Methuen, 1951: 1–17.
4. Riley WA, Johannsen OA. House flies and their allies. In: Riley WA, Johannsen OA (eds) *Medical Entomology.* New York: McGraw-Hill, 1938: 321–463.
5. Graham-Smith GS. The relation of the decline in the number of horse-drawn vehicles, and consequently of the urban breeding grounds of flies, to the fall in the summer diarrhoea death rate. *J Hyg (Lond)* 1929; **29**: 132–8.
6. Scott JG, Liu N, Kristensen M, Clark AG. A case for sequencing the genome of *Musca domestica* (Diptera: Muscidae). *J Med Entomol* 2009; **46**: 175–82.
7. Niven J. Summer diarrhoea and enteric fever. *Proc R Soc Med* 1910; **III** (Epidem. Sect.): 131–216.
8. da Cruz L, Dadour IR, McAllister IL, Jackson A, Isaacs T. Seasonal variation in trachoma and bush flies in north-western Australian Aboriginal communities. *Clin Experiment Ophthalmol* 2002; **30**: 80–3.
9. Kobayashi M, Sasaki T, Saito N *et al.* Houseflies: Not simple mechanical vectors of enterohemorrhagic *Escherichia coli* O157: H7. *Am J Trop Med Hyg* 1999; **61**: 625–9.
10. Chavasse DC, Shier RP, Murphy OA, Huttly SR, Cousens SN, Akhtar T. Impact of fly control on childhood diarrhoea in Pakistan: Community-randomised trial. *Lancet* 1999; **353**: 22–5.
11. Emerson PM, Lindsay SW, Walraven GE *et al.* Effect of fly control on trachoma and diarrhoea. *Lancet* 1999; **353**: 1401–3.
12. Emerson PM, Bailey RL, Mahdi OS, Walraven GE, Lindsay SW. Transmission ecology of the fly *Musca sorbens*, a putative vector of trachoma. *Trans R Soc Trop Med Hyg* 2000; **94**: 28–32.
13. Cohen D, Green M, Block C *et al.* Reduction of transmission of shigellosis by control of houseflies (*Musca domestica*). *Lancet* 1991; **337**: 993–7.

14. Cohen D, Monroe SS, Haim M *et al.* Norwalk virus gastroenteritis among Israeli soldiers: Lack of evidence for flyborne transmission. *Infection* 2002; **30**: 3–6.
15. Mikru FS, Molla T, Ersumo M *et al.* Community-wide outbreak of *Neisseria gonorrhoeae* conjunctivitis in Konso district, North Omo administrative region. *Ethiop Med J* 1991; **29**: 27–35.
16. Kotrajaras R, Tagami H. *Corynebacterium pyogenes.* Its pathogenic mechanism in epidemic leg ulcers in Thailand. *Int J Dermatol* 1987; **26**: 45–50.
17. Echeverria P, Harrison BA, Tirapat C, McFarland A. Flies as a source of enteric pathogens in a rural village in Thailand. *Appl Environ Microbiol* 1983; **46**: 32–6.
18. Sucharit S, Tumrasvin W, Vutikes S. A survey of houseflies in Bangkok and neighboring provinces. *Southeast Asian J Trop Med Public Health* 1976; **1**: 85–90.
19. Anjaneyulu G, Banerji SC, Indrayan A. A study of fly density and meteorological factors in occurrence of diarrhoea in a rural area. *Indian J Public Health* 1975; **19**: 115–21.
20. Khan M, Rahaman MM, Aziz KM, Islam S. Epidemiologic investigation of an outbreak of *Shiga bacillus* dysentery in an island population. *Southeast Asian J Trop Med Public Health* 1975; **6**: 251–6.
21. Spotarenko SS, Tikhomirov ED, Kikodze SL. [Evaluation of the role of flies in the epidemiology of dysentery and infectious hepatitis.] *Zh Mikrobiol Epidemiol Immunobiol* 1969; **46**: 43–8.
22. Wolff HL, van Zijl WJ, Roy M. Houseflies, the availability of water, and diarrhoeal diseases. *Bull World Health Organ* 1969; **41**: 952–9.
23. Coleman PJ, Maier P. Investigation of diarrhoea in a migrant labor camp. *Public Health Rep* 1955; 1242.
24. Bruch HA, Ascoli W, Scrimshaw NS *et al.* Studies of diarrhoeal diseases in Central America. V: Environmental factors in the origin and transmission of acute diarrheal disease in four Guatamalan villages. *Am J Trop Med Hyg* 1963; **12**: 567–679.
25. Lindsay DR, Stewart WH, Watt J. Effect of fly control on diarrhoeal disease in an area of moderate morbidity. *Public Health Rep* 1953; **68**: 361–7.
26. Watt J, Lindsay DR. Diarrhoeal disease control studies. 1: Effect of fly control in a high morbidity area. *Public Health Rep* 1948; **63**: 1319–34.
27. Kuhns DM, Anderson TG. A fly-borne bacilliary dysentery epidemic in a large military organisation. *Am J Public Health* 1944; **34**: 750–5.
28. Boyd JSK. Dysentery: Some personal experiences and observations. *Trans R Soc Trop Med Hyg* 1957; **51**: 471–7.
◆29. Levine OS, Levine MM. Houseflies (*Musca domestica*) as mechanical vectors of shigellosis. *Rev Infect Dis* 1991; **13**: 688–96.
30. Nash JTC. House flies as carriers of disease. *J Hyg (Lond)* 1909; **9**: 10–169.
31. Hewitt CG. *House Flies and how they Spread Disease.* Cambridge: Cambridge University Press, 1912.
32. Tondella ML, Paganelli CH, Bortolotto IM *et al.* [Isolation of *Haemophilus aegyptius* associated with Brazilian purpuric

fever, of Chloropidae (Diptera) of the genera Hippelates and Liohippelates.] *Rev Inst Med Trop Sao Paulo* 1994; **36**: 105–9.

33 da Cruz L, Dadour IR, McAllister IL, Jackson A, Isaacs T. Seasonal variation in trachoma and bush flies in north-western Australian Aboriginal communities. *Clin Experiment Ophthalmol* 2002; **30**: 80–3.

34. Datta P, Frost E, Peeling R *et al.* Ophthalmia neonatorum in a trachoma endemic area. *Sex Transm Dis* 1994; **21**: 1–4.

35. West SK, Congdon N, Katala S, Mele L. Facial cleanliness and risk of trachoma in families. *Arch Ophthalmol* 1991; **109**: 855–7.

36. Emerson PM, Lindsay SW, Walraven GE, Dibba SM, Lowe KO, Bailey RL. The Flies and Eyes project: Design and methods of a cluster-randomised intervention study to confirm the importance of flies as trachoma vectors in The Gambia and to test a sustainable method of fly control using pit latrines. *Ophthalmic Epidemiol* 2002; **9**: 105–17.

37. Forsey T, Darougar S. Transmission of chlamydiae by the housefly. *Br J Ophthalmol* 1981; **65**: 147–50.

38. Salim AR, Sheikh HA. Trachoma in the Sudan. An epidemiological study. *Br J Ophthalmol* 1975; **59**: 600–4.

39. Gupta CK, Gupta UC. Flies and mothers as modes of transmission of trachoma and associated bacterial conjunctivitis. *J All India Ophthalmol Soc* 1970; **18**: 17–22.

40. Tabbara KF, al Omar OM. Trachoma in Saudi Arabia. *Ophthalmic Epidemiol* 1997; **4**: 127–40.

41. Bailey R, Lietman T. The SAFE strategy for the elimination of trachoma by 2020: Will it work? *Bull World Health Organ* 2001; **79**: 233–6.

42. Emerson PM, Cairncross S, Bailey RL, Mabey DC. Review of the evidence base for the 'F' and 'E' components of the SAFE strategy for trachoma control. *Trop Med Int Health* 2000; **5**: 515–27.

43. Pruss A, Mariotti SP. Preventing trachoma through environmental sanitation: a review of the evidence base. *Bull World Health Organ* 2000; **78**: 258–66.

44. Emerson PM, Bailey RL, Walraven GE, Lindsay SW. Human and other faeces as breeding media of the trachoma vector *Musca sorbens. Med Vet Entomol* 2001; **15**: 314–20.

45. Schemann JF, Sacko D, Malvy D *et al.* Risk factors for trachoma in Mali. *Int J Epidemiol* 2002; **31**: 194–201.

46. Brechner RJ, West S, Lynch M. Trachoma and flies. Individual vs environmental risk factors. *Arch Ophthalmol* 1992; **110**: 687–9.

47. West S, Munoz B, Lynch M *et al.* Impact of face-washing on trachoma in Kongwa, Tanzania. *Lancet* 1995; **345**: 155–8.

48. Rinaldi A. Yaws: A second (and maybe last?) chance for eradication. *PLoS Negl Trop Dis* 2008; **2**: e275.

49. Asiedu K, Amouzou B, Dhariwal A *et al.* Yaws eradication: Past efforts and future perspectives. *Bull World Health Organ* 2008; **86**: 499–499A.

50. Langley PA. Pathogen transmission in relation to feeding and digestion by haematophagous arthropods. *Acta Trop* 1975; **32**: 116–24.

51. Weinstein P. The Australian bushfly (*Musca vetustissima* Walker) as a vector of *Neisseria gonorrhoeae* conjunctivitis. *Med J Aust* 1991; **155**: 717.

52. Matters R, Wong I, Mak D. An outbreak of non-sexually transmitted gonococcal conjunctivitis in Central Australia and the Kimberley region. *Commun Dis Intell* 1998; **22**: 52–6.

53. Thomson MC, Molesworth AM, Djingarey MH, Yameogo KR, Belanger F, Cuevas LE. Potential of environmental models to predict meningitis epidemics in Africa. *Trop Med Int Health* 2006; **11**: 781–8.

●54. Rosef O, Kapperud G. House flies (*Musca domestica*) as possible vectors of *Campylobacter fetus* subsp. *jejuni. Appl Environ Microbiol* 1983; **45**: 381–3.

55. Simango C, Rukure G. Potential sources of *Campylobacter* species in the homes of farmworkers in Zimbabwe. *J Trop Med Hyg* 1991; **94**: 388–92.

56. Rosef O, Kapperud G, Lauwers S, Gondrosen B. Serotyping of *Campylobacter jejuni, Campylobacter coli,* and *Campylobacter laridis* from domestic and wild animals. *Appl Environ Microbiol* 1985; **49**: 1507–10.

57. Giugliano LG, Bernardi MG, Vasconcelos JC, Costa CA, Giugliano R. Longitudinal study of diarrhoeal disease in a peri-urban community in Manaus (Amazon-Brazil). *Ann Trop Med Parasitol* 1986; **80**: 443–50.

58. Khin NO, Sebastian AA, Aye T. Carriage of enteric bacterial pathogens by house flies in Yangon, Myanmar. *J Diarrhoeal Dis Res* 1989; **7(3–4)**: 81–4.

59. Khalil K, Lindblom GB, Mazhar K, Kaijser B. Flies and water as reservoirs for bacterial enteropathogens in urban and rural areas in and around Lahore, Pakistan. *Epidemiol Infect* 1994; **113**: 435–44.

60. Zhang J, Xia S, Shen G *et al.* [A study on acute renal failure after an outbreak of diarrhea in Suixian county, Henan province.] *Zhonghua Liu Xing Bing Xue Za Zhi* 2002; **23**: 105–7.

61. Fotedar R. Vector potential of houseflies (*Musca domestica*) in the transmission of *Vibrio cholerae* in India. *Acta Trop* 2001; **78**: 31–4.

62. Broza M, Gancz H, Halpern M, Kashi Y. Adult non-biting midges: Possible windborne carriers of *Vibrio cholerae* non-O1 non-O139. *Environ Microbiol* 2005; **7**: 576–85.

63. Sengupta PG, Sircar BK, Mandal SK *et al.* Epidemiology of *Vibrio cholerae* O139 with special reference to intrafamilial transmission in Calcutta. *J Infect* 1995; **31**: 45–7.

64. Ruble R. Flies and *Campylobacter. Am J Public Health* 1986; **76**: 1457.

65. Wright EP. The isolation of *Campylobacter jejuni* from flies. *J Hyg (Lond)* 1983; **91**: 223–6.

66. Brown LM. *Helicobacter pylori*: Epidemiology and routes of transmission. *Epidemiol Rev* 2000; **22**: 283–97.

67. Osato MS, Ayub K, Le HH, Reddy R, Graham DY. Houseflies are an unlikely reservoir or vector for *Helicobacter pylori. J Clin Microbiol* 1998; **36**: 2786–8.

68. Grubel P, Cave DR. [Flies – reservoirs and vectors of *Helicobacter pylori.*] *Fortschr Med* 1997; **115**: 35–6.

69. Akinboade OA, Hassan JO, Adejinmi A. Public health importance of market meat exposed to refuse flies and

air-borne microorganisms. *Int J Zoonoses* 1984; **11**: 111–14.

70. Olsen AR, Hammack TS. Isolation of *Salmonella* spp. from the housefly, *Musca domestica* L., and the dump fly, *Hydrotaea aenescens* (Wiedemann) (Diptera: Muscidae), at caged-layer houses. *J Food Prot* 2000; **63**: 958–60.

71. Totescu E, Popescu-Pretor I, Schirer E. [Reconsideration of the role of synanthropic flies in the diffusion of *Salmonella* germs in present conditions of salmonellosis.] *Microbiol Parazitol Epidemiol (Bucur)* 1973; **18**: 345–50.

72. Altynbekov MA. [Dynamics of typhoid–paratyphoid infection morbidity in Chimkent Province.] *Zh Mikrobiol Epidemiol Immunobiol* 1982; (6): 35–8.

73. Sakdisiwasdi O, Achananuparp S, Limsuwan A, Nanna P, Barnyen L. *Salmonella* and *Shigella* carrier rates and environmental sanitation in a rural district, Central Thailand. *Southeast Asian J Trop Med Public Health* 1982; **13**: 380–4.

74. Tomar BS. Hepatitis E in India. *Zhonghua Min Guo Xiao Er Ke Yi Xue Hui Za Zhi* 1998; **39**: 150–6.

75. Forster M, Sievert K, Messler S, Klimpel S, Pfeffer K. Comprehensive study on the occurrence and distribution of pathogenic microorganisms carried by synanthropic flies caught at different rural locations in Germany. *J Med Entomol* 2009; **46**: 1164–6.

76. Stern NJ, Hiett KL, Alfredsson GA *et al. Campylobacter* spp. in Icelandic poultry operations and human disease. *Epidemiol Infect* 2003; **130**: 23–32.

77. Hald B, Skovgard H, Pedersen K, Bunkenborg H. Influxed insects as vectors for *Campylobacter jejuni* and *Campylobacter coli* in Danish broiler houses. *Poult Sci* 2008; **87**: 1428–34.

78. Hald B, Sommer HM, Skovgard H. Use of fly screens to reduce *Campylobacter* spp. introduction in broiler houses. *Emerg Infect Dis* 2007; **13**: 1951–3.

79. Hald B, Skovgard H, Bang DD *et al*. Flies and *Campylobacter* infection of broiler flocks. *Emerg Infect Dis* 2004; **10**: 1490–2.

80. Wales AD, Carrique-Mas JJ, Rankin M, Bell B, Thind BB, Davies RH. Review of the carriage of zoonotic bacteria by arthropods, with special reference to *Salmonella* in mites, flies and litter beetles. *Zoonoses Public Health* 2009. DOI 10.1111/j.1863-2378.2008.01222.

81. Guerin MT, Martin SW, Reiersen J *et al*. Temperature-related risk factors associated with the colonization of broiler-chicken flocks with *Campylobacter* spp. in Iceland, 2001–2004. *Prev Vet Med* 2008; **86**(1–2): 14–29.

82. Guerin MT, Martin W, Reiersen J *et al*. House-level risk factors associated with the colonization of broiler flocks with *Campylobacter* spp. in Iceland, 2. *BMC Vet Res* 2007; **3**: 30.

83. Nichols GL. Fly transmission of *Campylobacter*. *Emerg Infect Dis* 2005; **11**: 361–4.

84. Ekdahl K, Normann B, Andersson Y. Could flies explain the elusive epidemiology of campylobacteriosis? *BMC Infect Dis* 2005; **5**: 11.

85. Frost JA, Gillespie IA, O'Brien SJ. Public health implications of campylobacter outbreaks in England and Wales, 1995–9: Epidemiological and microbiological investigations. *Epidemiol Infect* 2002; **128**: 111–18.

86. Furtado C, Adak GK, Stuart JM, Wall PG, Evans HS, Casemore DP. Outbreaks of waterborne infectious intestinal disease in England and Wales, 1992–5. *Epidemiol Infect* 1998; **121**: 109–19.

87. Kapperud G, Aasen S. Descriptive epidemiology of infections due to thermotolerant *Campylobacter* spp. in Norway, 1979–1988. *APMIS* 1992; **100**: 883–90.

88. Nylen G, Dunstan F, Palmer SR *et al*. The seasonal distribution of campylobacter infection in nine European countries and New Zealand. *Epidemiol Infect* 2002; **128**: 383–90.

89. Sopwith W, Ashton M, Frost JA *et al*. Enhanced surveillance of campylobacter infection in the north west of England 1997–1999. *J Infect* 2003; **46**: 35–45.

90. Shane SM, Montrose MS, Harrington KS. Transmission of *Campylobacter jejuni* by the housefly (*Musca domestica*). *Avian Dis* 1985; **29**: 384–91.

91. Kettle DS. *Medical and Veterinary Entomology*, 2nd edn. Wallingford, Oxon: CABI, 2000.

92. Bidawid SP, Edeson JF, Ibrahim J, Matossian RM. The role of non-biting flies in the transmission of enteric pathogens (*Salmonella* species and *Shigella* species) in Beirut, Lebanon. *Ann Trop Med Parasitol* 1978; **72**: 117–21.

93. Frenkel JK, Hassanein KM, Hassanein RS, Brown E, Thulliez P, Quintero-Nunez R. Transmission of *Toxoplasma gondii* in Panama City, Panama: A five-year prospective cohort study of children, cats, rodents, birds, and soil. *Am J Trop Med Hyg* 1995; **53**: 458–68.

94. Kasprzak W, Majewska A. [Transmission of *Giardia* cysts. I: Role of flies and cockroaches.] *Wiad Parazytol* 1981; **27**(4-5): 555–63.

95. Graczyk TK, Grimes BH, Knight R, Da Silva AJ, Pieniazek NJ, Veal DA. Detection of *Cryptosporidium parvum* and *Giardia lamblia* carried by synanthropic flies by combined fluorescent in situ hybridization and a monoclonal antibody. *Am J Trop Med Hyg* 2003; **68**: 228–32.

96. Obiamiwe BA. The pattern of parasitic infection in human gut at the Specialist Hospital, Benin City, Nigeria. *Ann Trop Med Parasitol* 1977; **71**: 35–43.

97. Clavel A, Doiz O, Morales S *et al*. House fly (*Musca domestica*) as a transport vector of *Cryptosporidium parvum*. *Folia Parasitol* (*Praha*) 2002; **49**: 163–4.

98. Graczyk TK, Fayer R, Knight R *et al*. Mechanical transport and transmission of *Cryptosporidium parvum* oocysts by wild filth flies. *Am J Trop Med Hyg* 2000; **63**(3–4): 178–83.

99. Graczyk TK, Fayer R, Cranfield MR *et al*. Filth flies are transport hosts of *Cryptosporidium parvum*. *Emerg Infect Dis* 1999; **5**: 726–7.

100. Otranto D, Dutto M. Human thelaziasis, Europe. *Emerg Infect Dis* 2008; **14**: 647–9.

101. Otranto D, Traversa D. Thelazia eyeworm: An original endo- and ecto-parasitic nematode. *Trends Parasitol* 2005; **21**: 1–4.

102. Umeche N, Mandah LE. *Musca domestica* as a carrier of intestinal helminths in Calabar, Nigeria. *East Afr Med J* 1989; **66**: 349–52.

103. Oyerinde JP. The role of the house fly (*Musca domestica*) in the dissemination of hookworm. *Ann Trop Med Parasitol* 1976; **70**: 455–62.

104. Monzon RB, Sanchez AR, Tadiaman BM *et al.* A comparison of the role of *Musca domestica* (Linnaeus) and *Chrysomya megacephala* (Fabricius) as mechanical vectors of helminthic parasites in a typical slum area of Metropolitan Manila. *Southeast Asian J Trop Med Public Health* 1991; **22**: 222–8.

105. Sulaiman S, Sohadi AR, Yunus H, Iberahim R. The role of some cyclorrhaphan flies as carriers of human helminths in Malaysia. *Med Vet Entomol* 1988; **2**: 1–6.

106. Dipeolu OO. Laboratory investigations into the role of *Musca vicina* and *Musca domestica* in the transmission of parasitic helminth eggs and larvae. Int *J Zoonoses* 1982; **9**: 57–61.

107. Esrey S. Interventions for the control of diarrhoeal diseases among young children: fly control. 1991. World Health Organization Disease Control Programme. WHO/CDD/91.37.

108. Richards CS, Jackson WB, DeCapito TM, Maier PP. Studies on rates of recovery of *Shigella* from domestic flies and from humans in south-western United States. *Am J Trop Med Hyg* 1916; **10**: 44–8.

109. Yao HY, Yuan IC, Hiue D. The relation of flies, beverages and well-water to gastro-intestinal diseases in Peiping. *Natl Med J China* 1929; **15**: 410–18.

110. Morison J, Keyworth WD. Flies and their relation to epidemic diarrhoea and dysentery in Poona. *Indian J Med Res* 1916; **3**: 619–27.

111. Kovats RS, Edwards SJ, Charron D, Cowden J, D'Souza RM, Ebi KL, *et al.* Climate variability and Campylobacter infection: an international study. *Int J Biometeorol* 2005; **49**(4): 207–14.

41

Tick-borne disease – changing patterns and effective interventions

CAIRNS SMITH, MUTUKU A. MWANTHI

INTRODUCTION

Tick-borne diseases are an important cause of morbidity and occasionally mortality, with infection usually passing zoonotically from animal hosts to humans. The nature and extent of tick-borne disease can change in distribution as a result of changes in habitat, vectors and reservoirs, as well as through host population movement and alterations in agricultural, industrial and leisure activities. The diseases are also sensitive to climate and may therefore either decrease or increase under the effects of climate change. These dynamically changing patterns of disease, along with increased international travel, mean that medical practitioners need to be aware of the potential diagnosis of tick-borne disease as there can be serious clinical consequences of misdiagnosis or delayed detection.

EPIDEMIOLOGY

Tick-borne disease is global, and the patterns of infections are complex and evolving. Clinical presentation varies by host and by agent, and includes both acute and chronic presentations. Trends are difficult to interpret and may result from an increased awareness on the part of doctors and communities, misdiagnoses and improved diagnostic methods, as well as real changes in epidemiological patterns. Rapid travel makes a good travel history an essential component of clinical practice, as is an awareness of the potential diagnosis. The risk of disease is higher in certain occupational groups such as forestry workers,[1] migrants from endemic to non-endemic areas, dog-owners, rural residents and those who work on or are exposed to farms.[2]

The tick-borne diseases that are prevalent in Europe include Lyme disease, Mediterranean spotted fever, tularaemia, tick-borne relapsing fever and tick-borne encephalitis. In America, Lyme disease is the most common tick-borne disease, but there are also rickettsial diseases such as Rocky Mountain spotted fevers, babesiosis and human granulocytic anaplasmosis. In Africa, there are spotted fevers as well tick-borne relapsing fevers and African tick-borne fever. The epidemiology in Asia is less well documented but includes both rickettsial disease and tularaemia.

AGENTS

A very wide range of agents is implicated in tick-borne diseases, including viruses, bacteria, protozoa and toxins. Tick-borne viral agents are responsible for encephalitis, Colorado tick fever and Crimean–Congo haemorrhagic fever.[3] Bacterial agents[4] responsible for tick-borne diseases include *Borrelia* spp., *Francisella tularensis*, *Rickettsia* spp.[5] and Anaplasmacae. *Babesia* spp. are protozoa, and tick paralysis is thought to be caused by a toxin found in tick saliva.

PREVENTION AND CONTROL

The main measures for prevention and control relate to addressing the animal reservoirs and the ticks, preventing tick bites, the prompt removal of ticks and increased awareness leading to early detection and treatment.

Landscape management and interventions such as deer fencing and the re-routing of walking paths are important measures to reduce transmission. In certain circumstances, pesticides can be used to control ticks, or repellents, although their effectiveness may be short term,[6] and protective clothing can be employed in endemic areas to prevent bites. Daily checks for ticks and their prompt removal in prevalent areas is also recommended, and community-wide education programmes have been shown to be effective.[7] Improved livestock management and the control of animal movement are also used to control disease. In a number of countries, surveillance and control measures have significantly reduced mortality from tick-borne disease,[8] whereas elsewhere measures such as reducing deer populations have had no effect on incidence of Lyme disease.[9]

A vaccine is a further method for preventing some tick-borne diseases. A vaccine had been developed for Lyme disease, but the manufacturer discontinued production in 2002. Vaccines for preventing tick-borne encephalitis[10] have been shown to be strongly antigenic and rapidly induce high antibody titres.[11] A recent Austrian study showed 99 per cent efficacy of such a vaccine,[12] but this study was based on a retrospective review of cases. Further research based on evidence from randomized controlled trials is recommended by the most recent Cochrane Systematic Review to properly establish clinical protection.[10]

DIAGNOSIS AND TREATMENT

There are a large number of tick-borne diseases (Table 41.1), and this section will focus on the more common and important diseases. Information on exposures and a history of tick bites are critical for the detection and diagnosis of tick-borne disease. Guidance on the diagnosis and treatment of tick-borne diseases[4,13] is produced and regularly updated by the European Society of Clinical Microbiology and Infectious Diseases and the Infectious Diseases Society of America. Readers are recommended to visit their websites for details of specific treatments, as these are continually revised to include new evidence and recommendations can become outdated.

Lyme disease

Lyme borreliosis caused by *Borrelia burgdorferi* s.l. is the most common tick-borne disease in Europe and in North America. The tick usually needs to feed for over 24 hours for transmission to occur. The incubation from infection to the appearance of skin lesions is usually 7–14 days. The early signs are the target skin lesions of erythema migrans, fever and malaise. Musculoskeletal and neurological symptoms may in some cases develop during the phase of disseminated infection.[14] Early diagnosis is usually clinical, although both serological and molecular diagnostic methods are available.[15]

Antibiotics are the treatment of choice, but the recommended regimen depends on the stage of the disease and the clinical manifestations.[13] The long-term rather than short-term outcomes of treatment are important,[16] and there can be residual long-term sequelae that resemble chronic fatigue syndrome.[17]

Relapsing fever

Tick-borne relapsing fever is caused by *Borrelia duttonii* and occurs in Europe, Asia,[18] Africa[19] and North America.[20] The onset of symptoms occurs 4–14 days following transmission and consists of fever, headache, malaise and muscle and joint pain lasting around 3 days; this is then followed by recurrent episodes. The primary host varies between settings and includes wild rodents such as mice, rats, chipmunks and squirrels but may also include domestic animals.[21] Relapsing fever often occurs in travellers and is underdiagnosed.

The spirochaete infection responds to a number of antibiotics, and there is no evidence of antibiotic resistance. A randomized controlled trial showed that post-exposure treatment with doxycycline was highly effective after exposure to ticks in high-risk environments.[22]

Rickettsial diseases

Tick-borne rickettsioses occur worldwide and are responsible for spotted fevers. In the last 25 years, multiple distinct spotted fever group rickettsioses have been recognized, with distinct regional patterns.[5]

Rocky Mountain spotted fever was first described over 100 years ago and is still a potentially life-threatening condition.[23] The clinical manifestations present about 7 days after transmission and can be non-specific, making diagnosis difficult at a time when treatment may be most effective. The illness presents with a sudden onset of fever with headache, malaise and a rash. The rash appears as small erythematous macules at the wrists and ankles before spreading to the soles and palms and then more centrally in the body. Early antibiotic treatment is highly recommended even before laboratory confirmation as the disease can progress rapidly.

New molecular methods have identified several new spotted fever group rickettsioses in South Africa responsible for African tick bite fever, a generally mild, self-limiting condition presenting with non-specific flu-like symptoms.[24]

Table 41.1 Tick-borne disease, organisms, ticks, reservoirs and distribution

Diseases	Organisms	Tick	Animal reservoirs	Geographical distribution
Lyme disease[13–17]	*Borrelia burgdorferi* and other species	Hard deer ticks *Ixodes scapularis* and *pacificus*	Deer and other mammals	North America, Europe and Asia
Relapsing fever[18–22]	*Borrelia* including around 15 species	Soft ticks *Ornithodoros*	Wild rodents	Africa, North and South America, Asia and Europe
Rickettsial disease – spotted fevers[6,23–25]	*Rickettsia rickettsii* (Rocky Mountain) and *conorii* (Mediterranean) spotted fever and others	Various ticks, including *Ixodidae*, *Dermacentor*, *Rhipicephalus* and *Amblyomma*	Various wild and domestic mammals, including rodents and dogs	Global
Babesiosis[26,27]	*Babesia microti* (USA) and *divergens* (Europe)	Hard ticks – *Ixodes scapularis*, *Ixodes ricinus* and others	Various mammals including rodents (USA) and cattle (Europe)	North America and Europe; also Africa and Asia
Tularaemia[28,29]	*Francisella tularensis*	Four genera: *Amblyomma*, *Dermacentor*, *Haemaphysalis* and *Ixodes*	Mammals such as hares, mink and prairie dogs	Northern hemisphere
Tick-borne encephalitis[30,31]	*Flavivirus*	*Ixodes ricinus* and *persulcatus*	Mammals and birds	Western Europe to Japan
Crimean–Congo haemorrhagic fever[32,33]	*Nairovirus*	*Hyalomma*	Small mammals and domestic animals	Africa, Asia and East Europe

African tick bite fever is associated with rural areas and contact with cattle and wild game.

In contrast, Mediterranean spotted fever is associated with urban areas and is a more serious condition with a mortality rate of around 2 per cent.[25] It presents with sudden fever, flu-like symptoms and a black eschar at the site of the tick bite. Antibiotic treatment is recommended and effective.

Babesiosis

Babesiosis is a haemolytic disease caused by protozoa of the genus *Babesia*. It occurs worldwide and is being increasingly reported because of increased awareness. Several new *Babesia* parasites have recently been recognized, and the disease is being diagnosed in areas where it was not previously known.[26] The clinical manifestations can be non-specific, but anaemia and thrombocytopenia are common, and the parasite can been seen in red blood cells on thin blood smears. Babesiosis may be misdiagnosed as malaria, but antimalarial drugs are not effective and combined therapy regimes are recommended.[27]

Tularaemia

Tularaemia is a zoonotic disease caused by *Francisella tularensis* and it is also known as rabbit or deer fly fever.

It occurs throughout Europe, North America and Asia, and there are three subspecies of *Francisella tularensis* that differ in pathogenicity. Transmission is associated with rabbits, sheep, beavers and muskrats and is often linked to watercourses. The clinical form of the disease is dependent on the route of acquisition.[28] Fever, ulceration at the site of the bite and lymph node enlargement are common features. Serological confirmation is seen as the gold standard, but molecular methods are available. Early recognition and appropriate antibiotic therapy are essential. Tularaemia can occur in outbreaks.[29]

Viral disease

Tick-borne encephalitis caused by a flavivirus is one of the most dangerous human infections to occur in Europe and Asia (see Chapter 38). Cases present with meningoencephalitis, and many patients have long-lasting neurological sequelae.[30] There is no specific treatment, and prevention includes the prevention of tick bites. Effective vaccines are available.[11] New vaccine schedules to provide rapid antibody responses are being investigated as possible post-exposure interventions.[31]

Crimean–Congo haemorrhagic fever is another tick-borne viral disease that is often fatal and has been reported from around 30 countries in Africa and Asia. Humans are infected through ticks as well as by direct contact with blood or tissues from infected livestock.[32] The disease presents as rapidly progressive haemorrhage with myalgia and fever. Early supportive therapy and actions to prevent nosocomial infection, such as barrier precautions, are recommended as there is a serious risk to healthcare workers. A recent study to assess the effectiveness of oral ribavirin treatment has not shown any improvement in survival rate.[33]

CONCLUSION

Tick-borne diseases occur worldwide and are responsible for considerable morbidity and mortality. There is a range of diseases including viral, bacterial and protozoan, and presentations are highly variable and often non-specific. The global patterns of tick-borne diseases are continually changing owing to changes in the complex biological cycles that maintain infection in tick populations (which may include climate change but has not yet been shown to do so), in addition to changes in human activities responsible for exposure to infected ticks. In many areas, there is an increase in tick-borne disease, and new tick-borne pathogens are being identified. Awareness is critical for prevention, early diagnosis and appropriate treatment. Important risk factors include travel, exposure to high-risk environments and certain occupations.

ACKNOWLEDGEMENT

We wish to acknowledge the contribution of Carrie Stewart who conducted the systematic literature search an tick-borne disease for this chapter and, along with the authors, critically appraised the evidence.

REFERENCES

♦ = Major review article

1. Cisak E, Chmielewska-Badora J, Zwoliński J, Wójcik-Fatla A, Polak J, Dutkiewicz J. Risk of tick-borne bacterial diseases among workers of Roztocze National Park (South-eastern Poland). Ann Agric Environ Med 2005; 12: 127–32.
2. Jones TF, Garman RL, LaFleur B, Stephan SJ, Schaffner W. Risk factors for tick exposure and suboptimal adherence to preventive recommendations. Am J Prev Med 2002; 23: 47–50.
♦3. Charrel RN, Attoui H, Butenko AM et al. Tick-borne virus diseases of human interest in Europe. Clin Microbiol Infect 2004; 1: 1040–55.
♦4. Brouqui P, Bacellar F, Baranton G et al. Guidelines for the diagnosis of tick-borne bacterial diseases in Europe. Clin Microbiol Infect 2004; 10: 1108–32.
♦5. Parola P, Paddock CD, Raoult D. Tick-borne rickettsioses around the world: Emerging diseases, challenging old concepts. Clin Microbiol Rev 2005; 18: 719–56.

6. Jensenius M, Pretorius AM, Clarke F, Myrvang B. Repellent efficacy of four commercial DEET lotions against Amblyomma hebraeum (Acari: Ixodidae), the principal vector of Rickettsia africae in southern Africa. Trans R Soc Trop Med Hyg 2005; 99: 708–11.
7. Gould LH, Nelson RS, Griffith KS et al. Knowledge, attitudes, and behaviors regarding Lyme disease prevention among Connecticut residents, 1999–2004. Vector Borne Zoonotic Dis 2008; 8: 769–77.
8. Chinikar S, Goya MM, Shirzadi MR et al. Surveillance and laboratory detection system of Crimean-Congo haemorrhagic fever in Iran. Transbound Emerg Dis 2008; 55: 200–4.
9. Jordan RA, Schulze TL, Jahn MB. Effects of reduced deer density on the abundance of Ixodes scapularis (Acari: Ixodidae) and Lyme disease incidence in a Northern New Jersey endemic area. J Med Entomol 2007; 44: 752–7.
♦10. Demicheli V, Debalini MG, Rivetti A. Vaccines for preventing tick-borne encephalitis. Cochrane Database Syst Rev 2009; (1): CD000977.
11. Schöndorf I, Beran J, Cizkova D, Lesna V, Banzhoff A, Zent O. Tick-borne encephalitis (TBE) vaccination schedule. Vaccine 2007; 25: 1470–5.
12. Heinz FX, Holzmann H, Essl A, Kundi M. Field effectiveness of vaccination against tick-borne encephalitis. Vaccine 2007; 25: 7559–67.
♦13. Wormser GP, Dattwyler RJ, Shapiro ED et al. The clinical assessment, treatment, and prevention of Lyme disease, human granulocytic anaplasmosis, and babesiosis: Clinical practice guidelines by the Infectious Diseases Society of America. Clin Infect Dis 2006; 43: 1089–134.
14. Bratton RL, Whiteside JW, Hovan MJ, Engle RL, Edwards FD. Diagnosis and treatment of Lyme disease. Mayo Clin Proc 2008; 83: 566–71.
15. Ekerfelt C, Ernerudh J, Forsberg P et al. Lyme borreliosis in Sweden – diagnostic performance of five commercial Borrelia serology kits using sera from well-defined patient groups. Acta Pathol Microbiol Immunol Scand 2004; 112: 74–8.
16. Oksi J, Nikoskelainen J, Hiekkanen H et al. Duration of antibiotic treatment in disseminated Lyme borreliosis: A double-blind, randomized, placebo-controlled, multicenter clinical study. Eur J Clin Microbiol Infect Dis 2007; 26: 571–81.
17. Treib J, Grauer MT, Haass A, Langenbach J, Holzer G, Woessner R. Chronic fatigue syndrome in patients with Lyme borreliosis. Eur Neurol 2000; 43: 107–9.
18. Rebaudet S, Parola P. Epidemiology of relapsing fever borreliosis in Europe. FEMS Immunol Med Microbiol 2006; 48: 11–15.
19. Vial L, Diatta G, Tall A et al. Incidence of tick-borne relapsing fever in west Africa: Longitudinal study. Lancet 2006; 368: 37–43.
20. Dworkin MS, Shoemaker PC, Fritz CL, Dowell ME, Anderson DE. The epidemiology of tick-borne relapsing fever in the United States. Am J Trop Med Hyg 2002; 66: 753–8.

21. McCall PJ, Hume JC, Motshegwa K, Pignatelli P, Talbert A, Kisinza W. Does tick-borne relapsing fever have an animal reservoir in East Africa? *Vector Borne Zoonotic Dis* 2007; **7**: 659–67.

22. Hasin T, Davidovitch N, Cohen R *et al*. Postexposure treatment with doxycycline for the prevention of tick-borne relapsing fever. *N Engl J Med* 2006; **355**: 148–55.

◆23 Dantas-Torres F. Rocky Mountain spotted fever. *Lancet Infect Dis* 2007; **7**: 724–32.

24. Pretorius A, Jensenius M, Birtles RJ. Update on spotted fever group rickettsiae in South Africa. *Vector Borne Zoonotic Dis* 2004; **4**: 249–60.

25. Brouqui P, Parola P, Fournier PE, Raoult D. Spotted fever rickettsioses in southern and eastern Europe. *FEMS Immunol Med Microbiol* 2007; **49**: 2–12.

26. Hunfeld KP, Hildebrandt A, Gray JS. Babesiosis: Recent insights into an ancient disease. *Int J Parasitol* 2008; **38**: 1219–37.

27. Krause P. Babesiosis diagnosis and treatment. *Vector Borne Zoonotic Dis* 2003; **3**: 45–51.

◆28. World Health Organization. WHO Guidelines on Tularaemia. http://whqlibdoc.who.int/publications/2007/9789241547376_eng.pdf (accessed December 30, 2009).

29. Leblebicioglu H, Esen S, Turan D *et al*. Outbreak of tularemia: A case–control study and environmental investigation in Turkey. *Int J Infect Dis* 2008; **12**: 265–69.

◆30. Lindquist L, Vapalahti O. Tick-borne encephalitis. *Lancet* 2008; **371**: 1861–71.

31. Bröker M, Kollaritsch H. After a tick bite in a tick-borne encephalitis virus endemic area: Current positions about post-exposure treatment. *Vaccine* 2008; **26**: 863–68.

◆32. Ergönül Ö. Crimean-Congo haemorrhagic fever. *Lancet Infect Dis* 2006; **6**: 203–14.

33. Elaldi N, Bodur H, Ascioglu S *et al*. Efficacy of oral ribavirin treatment in Crimean-Congo haemorrhagic fever: A quasi-experimental study from Turkey. *J Infect* 2009; **58**: 238–44.

WEBSITES

- European Society of Clinical Microbiology and Infectious Diseases: http://www.escmid.org/escmid_library/medical_guidelines/
- Infectious Diseases Society of America: http://www.idsociety.org/Content.aspx?id=9088

42

Haemorrhagic fevers: the natural reservoirs of Ebola, Marburg and Lassa viruses

LORENZO PEZZOLI, NATASHA S. CROWCROFT

INTRODUCTION

Ebola, Marburg and Lassa viruses cause severe haemorrhagic fevers in humans. They are highly infectious and occur in explosive outbreaks with high mortality. The viruses are endemic in tropical Africa, where they have the potential to cause large epidemics because of person-to-person spread, and are the archetypal zoonotic emerging infectious diseases.[1–3] *Marburgvirus* and *Ebolavirus* generally occur in outbreaks affecting tens of individuals with high case fatality. Lassa fever has lower case fatality but infects thousands of individuals each year. They are of high public health importance in countries where they are endemic, and pose a threat internationally due to high-speed worldwide travel and their potential as bio-terrorism weapons.[4,5] The natural reservoir of these diseases has been probably identified for Lassa fever, but, despite intense research, many uncertainties remain with regards to the reservoirs of Ebola and Marburg viruses, although recent studies indicate bats as plausible candidates.[6,7]

EBOLA AND MARBURG VIRUSES

Ebola and Marburg viruses are single-stranded, negative-sense RNA viruses of the family **Filoviridae**. They cause the most severe forms of haemorrhagic fever with probably the highest mortality rate of any infectious disease, and have been known since 1967, when an outbreak of *Marburgvirus* was linked to primates imported into Germany.[8]

One species of *Marburgvirus* is described, while *Ebolavirus* seems to exist in distinct species: *Zaire, Sudan,* *Ivory-Coast, Bundibugyo* and *Reston.*[9] The first four are known to be pathogenic in all primates, whereas the latter is thought to affect only Asian monkeys (*Macaca fascicularis*), but not African monkeys or humans.[10] *Zaire ebolavirus* is the most virulent in humans, with a case fatality rate of 80–90 per cent.[11,12] *Bundibugyo ebolavirus* was described for the first time in Uganda in late 2007, when it caused an outbreak characterized by an atypical and less haemorrhagic clinical presentation.[9,13–15] *Reston ebolavirus* was discovered in 1989 in monkeys exported from the Philippines; since then it has never caused disease in humans, but it has recently been isolated from pigs, causing concern that its passage through swine may allow the virus to diverge and shift its potential to pathogenicity.[16]

Outbreaks of Ebola and Marburg viruses have occurred largely across Africa.[17–20] Most of the primary cases have lived in or near rainforest, with a seroprevalence of *Ebolavirus* antibodies in people living in rural villages of 9.3 per cent, compared with 2.2 per cent for urban residents,[21] suggesting that the source of these viruses lies in the natural environment. Patients with primary infection tend to have visited or worked in forests,[22–25] caves[26,27] or mines.[17,28] During human outbreaks, concurrent epidemics have been described in animal populations (e.g. gorillas, chimpanzees and duikers), and patients have reported contact with animal species known to be susceptible to infection.[29–31] In particular, several outbreaks were linked to hunters who had contact with wildlife[22,32–34] or to individuals who had handled[28,32,35] or consumed dead animals.[28,32,33,36] These findings suggest that the infection has been acquired either through contact with an infected animal reservoir or with another species that is, like humans, a dead-end host.

More is known about how Ebola and Marburg viruses are spread after they are introduced into human populations. A high risk of infection is associated with direct or household contact with an infected individual or with their body after death, such as through washing the body in preparing for a funeral, and with nosocomial transmission.[11,37,38] Poorly resourced medical facilities, where infection control measures are difficult to establish, play a major role in amplifying transmission.[4]

Ecology

The geographical distribution of filoviruses gives clues about possible animal reservoirs. They spread across the African tropics, but viral types from particular locations appear to cluster together phylogenetically. Ebola viruses seem usually to be restricted to the humid rainforests of Central and Western Africa, whereas the related Marburg viruses are usually more common in the drier areas of Central and East Africa.[39] *Marburgvirus* seems to have a greater potential, compared with *Ebolavirus*, to occur in areas where filovirus disease has not previously been described.[39] Furthermore, *Zaire ebolavirus* and *Ivory-Coast ebolavirus* may occupy a geographical area different from that of *Sudan ebolavirus*.[40] Interestingly, this corresponds to the closer phylogenetic relationship between *Zaire ebolavirus* and *Ivory-Coast ebolavirus*, which group together on a separate branch from *Sudan ebolavirus* and *Reston ebolavirus*.[41] This correspondence suggests a similar ecological distribution, providing clues on the origin of *Reston ebolavirus*, which is the only one thought to have an Asian origin.[39]

Human outbreaks of filoviruses tend to occur in the tropical rainy season,[42,43] whereas animal epizootics are more common in the dry season.[44] This could be explained by increased contacts between animal species during periods of food scarcity typical of the dry season.[7,40] Food scarcity may also increase the likelihood that a reservoir sustains viraemia.[45] There is some evidence that seasonality is virus specific, and a pattern favouring wet months seems more pronounced in *Sudan ebolavirus*, whereas outbreaks of *Zaire ebolavirus* and *Ivory-Coast ebolavirus* are often associated with periods of declining rainfall.[40]

If the origin is zoonotic, the geographical variations of filovirus occurrence suggest a correlation with specific animal taxa that would inhabit the areas where outbreaks of filoviruses have occurred, but all belonging to a related group of animals distributed more broadly across Africa and South-East Asia.[39]

Two possible scenarios are currently envisaged, one in which the virus exists within a specific reservoir species for long periods of time, emerging episodically in areas with the appropriate conditions, and another that suggests that the virus spreads between adjacent susceptible host populations in a wave-like fashion.[40]

In considering the epidemiology of filoviral haemorrhagic fevers, some assumptions can be made on the nature of the reservoir. It is probably a mammal that has co-evolved with the viruses to develop a sustainable host–parasite relationship, and is most likely divided into local groups associated with a specific viral type.[3] It is also likely to support persistent and asymptomatic infection to allow maintenance of the viruses in the environment.[3]

Many animal species, including primates, bats, birds, reptiles, molluscs, arthropods, and even plants, have been experimentally infected with Marburg and Ebola,[44] and signs of infection (specific antibodies or viral RNA) have been found in non-human primates,[8,10,12,40,46–48] bats,[6,7,44,45] duikers,[12] rodents,[49,50] dogs,[51] pigs[16] and one shrew.[50]

ARTHROPODS

An arthropod vector has been considered for filoviruses because other viral haemorrhagic fevers, notably dengue and yellow fever, are transmitted by this route.[43] Anecdotal evidence indicated that haemorrhagic fever followed an insect bite in the index case in the 1975 Marburg fever outbreak in Johannesburg.[20] Ebola virus survival has been experimentally demonstrated in *Aedes aegypti* mosquitoes,[52] but extensive in vivo studies have failed to isolate filoviruses in arthropods.[53,54] Despite some exceptions,[55] most filovirus human epidemics can be traced to origination from a single primary case. If arthropod vectors were to carry filoviruses, multiple primary cases would be more common.

RODENTS

Early experimental inoculation of hamsters[49] and the detection of Ebola RNA in mice (*Mus setulosus* and *Praomys* spp.) from the Central African Republic[50] led to rodents becoming a suspect reservoir, but these findings have not been confirmed by alternative methodologies (i.e. serology, antigen detection or virus isolation) or by other studies.[40] Given the specific epidemiological patterns of filoviral disease occurrence, it is unlikely that species commensal to humans, such as rodents, would be the reservoir because, in this case as well, multiple primary cases would be observed.[3]

PRIMATES

Ebola and Marburg fevers in non-human primates are well documented,[10,12,40,46–48] including the first description in Germany[8] and a role as possible reservoirs.[56]

A study on the presence of *Ebolavirus*-specific antibodies in non-human primates in Cameroon, Gabon and the Republic of the Congo found seropositivity for *Zaire ebolavirus* in chimpanzees (*Pan troglodytes*), drills (*Mandrillus leucophaeus*), gorillas (*Gorilla gorilla*), one baboon (*Papio anubis*), one mandrill (*Mandrillus sphinx*) and one De Brazza's monkey (*Cercopithecus neglectus*).[21] Only wild-born primates presented detectable antibody levels, indicating that, like humans, primates can survive natural infection.[21] Nevertheless, outbreaks of Ebola in recent years have carried such high mortality that they may threaten conservation of many of the already endangered African great ape species.[12,47,57]

The observation that the natural habitats of drills and baboons are located in areas of Cameroon, where no human cases of Ebola have been described,[21] and that some positive samples have been found in non-human primates before outbreaks occurred in the human population[40] could indicate that future outbreaks may occur anywhere in the central African region. These viruses may have been present for a long time in the forests of central Africa, breaking out only when particular environmental conditions are met, infecting great apes with a pattern similar to that of human infections, including spread in social groups;[21,58] in fact, non-human primate epidemics also seem to begin with single primary cases.[39] It is also possible that cross-reactive non-pathogenic filoviruses may be present.[21]

Evidence shows that non-human primates succumb to infection following a disease likely to be fatal, suggesting that these animals are not the primary reservoir.[40] The habitat of the natural reservoir probably coincides with that of certain non-human primates; perhaps they feed on the same vegetation at the same time, with infection occurring through direct contact.[21]

A phylogenetic analysis of *Reston ebolavirus* in non-human primates has discovered that recent lineages emerged only in the 1970s, and also indicates recombination between lineages.[59] These observations do not support there being a long-term stable local reservoir, but may indicate another process such as movement of a reservoir that may be accompanying other ecological change. Outbreaks have tended to spread east, which is consistent with the hypothesis of a moving reservoir range.[58,59] Vaccine candidates with the potential to interrupt the transmission of Ebola and Marburg to both non-human and human primates are under development,[60,61] but viral recombination may present a challenge to vaccine development.[59]

BATS

Bats have been a suspected source of filovirus infection for many years as they harbour a wide range of other viral infections, including rabies. In 1975, Marburg haemorrhagic fever developed in two tourists who had slept in rooms with insectivorous bats in Zimbabwe.[62] In addition, observations during the 1976 Ebola outbreaks in the Democratic Republic of the Congo and Sudan implicated bats as the source of infection,[63] and the monkeys associated with the first outbreak of Marburg fever were kept in a holding facility on a island in Lake Victoria characterized by the presence of a large number of fruit bats.[62]

Leroy *et al.* found evidence of asymptomatic Ebola infection in three species of fruit bats (*Hypsignathus monstrosus*, *Epomops franqueti* and *Myonycteris torquata*),[7]

and signs of filovirus infection have been documented in bats several times.[6,7,44] During the *Ebolavirus* outbreak in Luebo (Democratic Republic of the Congo) in 2007, the investigators were able to show that the putative first human victim bought freshly killed bats from hunters to eat.[64] There is also anecdotal evidence that *Reston ebolavirus* may have been spread to pigs in the Philippines by bat droppings falling into the pigs' feed.[65] Phylogenetic analysis of these viruses indicates, however, that the strains are of recent origin, which may argue against bats being a long-standing stable reservoir species.[66] Alternatively, there may be something in the dynamics or the life-cycle of bats that has placed a bottleneck on the evolution of the virus.[66]

Following the occurrence of Marburg fever in the mining village of Durba, Democratic Republic of the Congo, the fauna of the mine associated with the outbreak[55] was examined.[6] Marburg viral RNA was found in two species of insectivorous bat (*Rhinolophus eloquens* and *Miniopterus inflatus*) and one of fruit bat (*Rousettus aegyptiacus*); the seroprevalence of *Marburgvirus* antibody was higher in the fruit bats (20.5 per cent) than in the insectivorous bats (9.7 per cent).[6] Marburg fever has also been associated with a mine in the Kamwenge district in western Uganda, in or around which approximately five million bats have been reported living.[67]

A report published in 2007 has found Marburg viral RNA and specific antibodies in fruit bats (*Rousettus aegyptiacus*) from an area of Gabon where *Marburgvirus* had never been detected, suggesting that filoviruses may not be necessarily confined to areas where outbreaks occurred, but may have a wider distribution.[68]

The prevalence of antibodies to *Zaire ebolavirus* in bats decreased from approximately 5 per cent to 1 per cent in regions previously affected by outbreaks. This suggests that epidemic periods may coincide with periods of higher rates of infection in bats, necessary for the passage of the virus from bats to other species (e.g. human and non-human primates), and that levels fall after the outbreak as new bats are born who have not been infected.[44] These viruses may in fact be present throughout the forested countries of central Africa and could wax and wane depending on unidentified forces affecting the immunological status of the reservoirs,[69] maybe die-offs in the bat population due to disease, or reduced reproduction in affected animals.[44]

In the Durba outbreak, many genetically distinct variants of *Marburgvirus* were detected in bats and humans.[6] In contrast to *Ebolavirus*, analysis of the divergence of the viral nucleotide sequences of *Marburgvirus* indicated a long relationship between the virus and the bats. At the same time, there was diversity that indicated either the circulation and evolution of strains confined to subpopulations of the same bat species, or that bats are not the reservoir.[6,17,55] These discrepancies may mean that, while many virus types are present in bats, a combination of factors may trigger the passage of an eventual outbreak strain from bats to humans.[6]

Bats could infect humans directly or indirectly by infecting intermediate animals.[7] Terrestrial mammals may feed on fallen fruits possibly contaminated by bats or may be in contact with bat excreta, suggesting a chain of events leading to viral transmission from bats to incidental hosts.[31] Bats have not been found to have antibodies and be viraemic, so the natural history may be more complex.[66] Non-human primates and bat populations compete for food during the dry season when fruit is scarce, creating opportunities for closer and more frequent contact between the species.[44] The dry season is also the birthing period for bats, and changes in immune function due to pregnancy as well as food scarcity may lead to a resurgence of viral replication or a higher likelihood that a bat will become ill and die rather than remaining asymptomatic, which could lead to transmission.[44] Adult bats presented a higher seroprevalence of *Ebolavirus* antibodies, suggesting that horizontal rather than vertical transmission is more likely, but sample sizes were too small for significant statistical analysis.[44]

The fact that two fruit bat species (*Epomophorus* and *Talarida*) developed viraemia for almost 4 weeks after intravenous inoculation with *Ebolavirus* without displaying clinical signs[44] is consistent with the notion that the natural reservoir would have to support persistent and largely asymptomatic filovirus infection.[3]

Whether insectivorous bats, fruit bats or both are the likely source of infection and whether particular species are involved with the secondary transmission of infection to other species is unclear. An evolutionary distinction may exist between cave-roosting bats as hosts of *Marburgvirus* and forest bats as hosts of *Ebolavirus*.[6] Moreover, the ultimate source of infection could prove to be external, such as bat parasites (e.g. *Streblidae* or *Nycteribiidae* flies)[43] or insects in the bats' diet.[6]

Up to now, live *Ebolavirus* or *Marburgvirus* has not been cultured from wild bats, a biological indication that transmission is possible. The presence of virus nucleic material has required highly sensitive polymerase chain reaction detection methods. Virus titres may be too low in asymptomatic carriers to be detected, and specific physiological or environmental stimuli may be necessary to produce apparent infection.[6,7] Antibody and viral RNA detection may be incidental, and more evidence on the natural progression of filoviral infection in bats is needed to prove that they are the primary reservoir.[68]

In July 2008, a tourist died of Marburg fever after being exposed to bats while visiting a cave in Uganda, increasing the suspicion that these animals might actually be the reservoir.[70] This evidence may still be circumstantial, and more epidemiological studies are needed.

LASSA VIRUS

Lassa virus is often considered alongside Ebola and Marburg viruses, but is in reality quite different in many ways. Lassa virus is an RNA virus from the *Arenaviridae* family. Haemorrhagic fevers caused by arenaviruses usually occur in Africa and the Americas.[71] Lassa fever is endemic in western Africa, where it is estimated to affect 300 000 people annually, mainly in Sierra Leone, Guinea, Liberia and Nigeria.[72–74] Viral strain variation has been observed across this region.[75] Although the disease has been known since the 1950s, Lassa virus was first described as its agent in 1969, when two nurses died from it in Lassa, Nigeria.[76,77]

Arenaviruses are usually transmitted through contact with the excreta of murids.[73] The natural host of Lassa fever was identified as the natal multimammate mouse (*Mastomys natalensis*),[78] found in many regions of Africa.[79] Person-to-person transmission has occurred through household, sexual and nosocomial contact, but is a much less important mode.

A study conducted among wild murid species sampled in Guinea from 2002 to 2005 identified traces of Lassa virus RNA only in *Mastomys natalensis*.[80] Following rodent-trapping, *Mastomys natalensis* was not found in the coastal regions of Guinea, where the lowest seroprevalence of human Lassa virus (0–6 per cent) has been reported, and only *Mastomys erythroleucus* was captured. In contrast, in the forest regions, where the highest seroprevalence of up to 55 per cent has been found in some villages, only *Mastomys natalensis* was trapped. Both species were captured in the savannah regions, where the seroprevalence was 2–42 per cent, but *Mastomys natalensis* was captured more frequently. Despite a massive trapping effort, *Mastomys huberti* was not detected in the regions of Guinea bordering Sierra Leone that had a high human seroprevalence of Lassa virus.[80] Although *Mastomys erythroleucus* and *Mastomys huberti* were also proposed as hosts in Sierra Leone,[78] and Lassa virus antigens were also detected in *Rattus* and *Mus* genera, raising the possibility that other rodents could be involved in transmission,[81] the conclusion of the study was that *Mastomys natalensis* is very likely the only reservoir of Lassa virus in Guinea.[80] This is supported by its low pathogenicity, indicating co-evolution of the host and pathogen.

The taxonomy of the genus *Mastomys* is considered unresolved, and species determination remains problematic, with eight distinct species currently recognized and coexisting in Lassa fever endemic areas.[82,83] *Mastomys natalensis* and *Mastomys huberti* have an identical number of chromosomes,[73,82] making species differentiation very difficult. It is therefore possible that the study that identified *Mastomys erythroleucus* and *Mastomys huberti* as hosts for Lassa fever[78] misclassified the species.

Studies conducted in Sierra Leone, where the seropositivity of Lassa virus ranged from 8 per cent to 52 per cent in the human population,[83] also found associations between *Mastomys natalensis* and Lassa fever. Keenlyside *et al.* found that 39 per cent of the *Mastomys* sampled in the houses of cases of Lassa fever were viraemic, compared with 3.7 per cent in the houses where no cases of Lassa fever were reported.[84] In addition, *Mastomys natalensis* constituted 50–60 per cent of the rodents captured in domestic settings but only 10–20 per cent of those captured in surrounding agriculture and bush areas, suggesting that houses are the most important location for transmission.[83] This is especially important in Lassa fever endemic countries, where the socioeconomic situation does not generally promote good hygiene of housing and the surroundings, and where refugee camps, settings prone to outbreak occurrence, are a common sight.[75,85]

Humans are probably infected via the excreta of the mice, but food-borne transmission has also been hypothesized.[77] Mice are a traditional food speciality in Lassa virus endemic areas, and a study demonstrated that Lassa antibodies after a febrile illness occurred in twice as many people who consumed mice compared with those who did not eat them.[86] Also, deafness, a common symptom of Lassa fever, occurred four times more frequently in patients reporting rodent consumption.[86]

Once primary cases have been infected, person-to-person transmission may follow via direct contact.[77] Nosocomial exposure, also a confirmed risk factor for secondary transmission, is of much less importance for Lassa fever compared with Ebola and Marburg fevers.[87]

If *Mastomys natalensis* is confirmed to be the only host for Lassa virus, we could be observing a phenomenon similar to that described for Bolivian haemorrhagic fever caused by Machupo virus, which has its natural reservoir only in specific genetic lineages of the mouse *Calomys callosus*.[80,88] When such a specific correlation exists between host and infectious agent, the term 'natural nidality' is used.[88] With the exception of Sabia virus, for which no natural reservoir is known, and Tacaribe virus, which was isolated from *Artibeus* bats, it is in fact believed that all arenaviruses follow the rule of natural nidality, because they all seem to be univocally associated with a specific lineage of *Muridae*.[89]

Table 42.1 Agents causing viral haemorrhagic fever, the animal species in which they were reported, and the location and year of human outbreaks

Family	Genus	Species	Host/Suspected reservoir (number of cases)	Locations and years of human outbreaks (number of cases)
Filoviridae	*Ebolavirus*	Zaire	Human (*Homo sapiens sapiens*)[91]; gorilla (*Gorilla gorilla gorilla*)[48]; chimpanzee (*Pan troglodytes*)[48]; drill (*Mandrillus leucophaeus*)[21]; baboon (*Papio anubis*)[21]; mandrill (*Mandrillus sphinx*)[21]; De Brazza's monkey (*Cercopithecus neglectus*)[21]; Duiker (*Cephalophus* spp.)[12]; dog (*Canis lupus familiaris*)[51]; rodents (*Mus setulosus, Praomys* sp1 *and Praomys* sp2)[92]; shrew (*Sylvisorex ollula*)[92] / **Fruit bats (*Hypsignathus monstrosus, Epomops franqueti, Myonycteris torquata*)**[7]	Zaire 1976[91]; Gabon 1994[93]; DRC 1995[94]; Gabon 1996[95]; Gabon 2001[96]; RC 2001[96]; RC 2003[34]; RC 2005[97]; DRC 2007[64]
		Ivory Coast	Human (*Homo sapiens sapiens*)[98]; chimpanzee (*Pan troglodytes*)[99]	Ivory Coast 1994[100]; Liberia 1995[98]
		Reston	Crab-eating macaque (*Macaca fascicularis*)[101]; pig (*Sus scrofa*)[16]	None to date
		Sudan	Human (*Homo sapiens sapiens*)[102]	Sudan 1976[102]; Sudan 1979[63]; Uganda 2000[103]; Sudan 2004[104]
		Bundibugyo	Human (*Homo sapiens sapiens*)[9]	Uganda 2007[9]
	Marburgvirus	Marburg	Human (*Homo sapiens sapiens*)[102]; vervet monkey (*Cercopithecus aethiops*)[105] / **Insectivorous bats (*Rhinolophus eloquens, Miniopterus inflatus*)**[54]; fruit bat (*Rousettus aegyptiacus*)[26]	Germany 1967 (ex-Uganda)[105]; Zimbabwe 1975[106]; South Africa 1975[107]; Kenya 1980[108]; Kenya 1987[27]; DRC 1999[109]; Angola 2005[110]; Uganda 2007[67]
Arenaviridae	*Arenavirus*	Lassa	Human (*Homo sapiens sapiens*)[76] / **Multimammate mouse (*Mastomys natalensis*)**[78]	Nigeria 1969[76]; Sierra Leone 1970[111]; Liberia 1972[112]; Sierra Leone 1973[113]; Guinea, Sierra Leone and Liberia 1980[114]; currently highly endemic in West Africa[115]

DRC, Democratic Republic of the Congo; RC, Republic of the Congo.

CONCLUSION

Many uncertainties remain with regard to the natural reservoirs of *Ebolavirus* and *Marburgvirus*, although the hypothesis of a bat reservoir is most likely to be true. The source of Lassa virus is one specific rodent reservoir, but other animals cannot be definitively excluded.

The epidemiology of these African viral haemorrhagic fevers is consistent. Filoviral fevers occur in sporadic outbreaks affecting a low number of cases and can be explained by contact with a species that is not commensal with humans, such as bats, whereas Lassa fever affects thousands of people every year in the endemic areas, showing a pattern typical of rodent-borne diseases with multiple primary cases. Individuals contracting Lassa fever probably live in close contact with the reservoir and share the same dwellings. This raises the larger context in which such infections emerge when the ecology is permissive. We must not ignore the role of poverty in increasing risk to human populations because of exposure, in the case of Lassa fever, to rodents, or, in the case of Ebola and Marburg viruses, to infected wildlife. In addition, the role of environmental change through non-sustainable farming and global warming must be taken into account.

The epidemiology and ecology of these diseases in human and animal populations requires further investigation and multidisciplinary collaboration if we are to understand them fully,[90] identify possibly epidemic-prone areas and prevent the occurrence of outbreaks. In central Africa, the chimpanzee population level is estimated to have fallen by 80 per cent,[12] so, in addition to its importance to human health, establishing the reservoirs of these viruses will benefit threatened African ape populations and protect the biodiversity on which we all depend. On the other hand, conducting more studies on the reservoir may adversely affect the captured species, and sampling endangered species raises ethical questions if reservoir population control is to be considered as a preventative measure for viral haemorrhagic fevers.

ACKNOWLEDGEMENTS

The authors wish to acknowledge Dr Dilys Morgan, Dr Amanda Walsh and Dr Dominik Zenner (Health Protection Agency, UK) for their expertise and support.

REFERENCES

1. Jones KE, Patel NG, Levy MA *et al.* Global trends in emerging infectious diseases. *Nature* 2008; **451**: 990–3.
2. Saijo M. [Clinical aspects of viral hemorrhagic fever.] *Nippon Rinsho* 2005; **63**: 2161–6.
3. Peterson AT, Carroll DS, Mills JN, Johnson KM. Potential mammalian filovirus reservoirs. *Emerg Infect Dis* 2004; **10**: 2073–81.
4. Crowcroft NS, Morgan D, Brown D. Viral haemorrhagic fevers in Europe – effective control requires a co-ordinated response. *Euro Surveill* 2002; **7**: 31–2.
5. Crowcroft NS, Meltzer M, Evans M *et al.* The public health response to a case of Lassa fever in London in 2000. *J Infect* 2004; **48**: 221–8.
6. Swanepoel R, Smit SM, Rollin PE *et al.* Studies of reservoir hosts for Marburg virus. *Emerg Infect Dis* 2007; **13**: 1847–51.
7. Leroy EM, Kumulungui B, Pourrut X *et al.* Fruit bats as reservoirs of Ebola virus. *Nature* 2005; **438**: 575–6.
8. Hennessen W. A hemorrhagic disease transmitted from monkeys to man. *Natl Cancer Inst Monogr* 1968; **29**: 161–71.
9. Towner JS, Sealy TK, Khristova ML *et al.* Newly discovered ebola virus associated with hemorrhagic fever outbreak in Uganda. *PLoS Pathog* 2008; **4**: e1000212.
10. Morikawa S, Saijo M, Kurane I. [Current knowledge on the lower virulence of Reston Ebola virus.] *Comp Immunol Microbiol Infect Dis* 2007; **30**(5–6): 391–8.
11. Formenty P, Libama F, Epelboin A *et al.* [Outbreak of Ebola hemorrhagic fever in the Republic of the Congo, 2003: A new strategy?]. *Med Trop (Mars)* 2003; **63**: 291–5.
12. Leroy EM, Rouquet P, Formenty P *et al.* Multiple Ebola virus transmission events and rapid decline of central African wildlife. *Science* 2004; **303**: 387–90.
13. Outbreak news. Ebola haemorrhagic fever, Uganda – end of the outbreak. *Wkly Epidemiol Rec* 2008; **83**: 89–90.
14. Alsop Z. Ebola outbreak in Uganda "atypical", say experts. *Lancet* 2007; **370**: 2085.
15. Mason C. The strains of Ebola. *CMAJ* 2008; **178**: 1266–7.
16. Barrette RW, Metwally SA, Rowland JM *et al.* Discovery of swine as a host for the Reston ebolavirus. *Science* 2009; **325**: 204–6.
17. Bausch DG, Nichol ST, Muyembe-Tamfum JJ *et al.* Marburg hemorrhagic fever associated with multiple genetic lineages of virus. *N Engl J Med* 2006; **355**: 909–19.
18. Colebunders R, Sleurs H, Pirard P *et al.* Organisation of health care during an outbreak of Marburg haemorrhagic fever in the Democratic Republic of Congo, 1999. *J Infect* 2004; **48**: 347–53.
19. Towner JS, Khristova ML, Sealy TK *et al.* Marburgvirus genomics and association with a large hemorrhagic fever outbreak in Angola. *J Virol* 2006; **80**: 6497–516.
20. Gear JS, Cassel GA, Gear AJ *et al.* Outbreak of Marburg virus disease in Johannesburg. *Br Med J* 1975; **4**: 489–93.
21. Leroy EM, Telfer P, Kumulungui B *et al.* A serological survey of Ebola virus infection in central African nonhuman primates. *J Infect Dis* 2004; **190**: 1895–9.
22. Ebola haemorrhagic fever. A summary of the outbreak in Gabon. *Wkly Epidemiol Rec* 1997; **72**(1–2):7–8.
23. Guimard Y, Bwaka MA, Colebunders R *et al.* Organization of patient care during the Ebola hemorrhagic fever epidemic in Kikwit, Democratic Republic of the Congo, 1995. *J Infect Dis* 1999; **179**(Suppl. 1): S268–73.
24. Bwaka MA, Bonnet MJ, Calain P *et al.* Ebola hemorrhagic fever in Kikwit, Democratic Republic of the Congo: Clinical observations in 103 patients. *J Infect Dis* 1999; **179**(Suppl. 1): S1–7.

25. Muyembe T, Kipasa M. Ebola haemorrhagic fever in Kikwit, Zaire. International Scientific and Technical Committee and WHO Collaborating Centre for Haemorrhagic Fevers. *Lancet* 1995; **345**: 1448.

26. Smith DH, Johnson BK, Isaacson M *et al.* Marburg-virus disease in Kenya. *Lancet* 1982; **1**: 816–20.

27. Johnson ED, Johnson BK, Silverstein D *et al.* Characterization of a new Marburg virus isolated from a 1987 fatal case in Kenya. *Arch Virol Suppl* 1996; **11**: 101–14.

28. Georges AJ, Leroy EM, Renaut AA *et al.* Ebola hemorrhagic fever outbreaks in Gabon, 1994–1997: Epidemiologic and health control issues. *J Infect Dis* 1999; **179**(Suppl. 1): S65–75.

29. Feldmann H, Jones S, Klenk HD, Schnittler HJ. Ebola virus: From discovery to vaccine. *Nat Rev Immunol* 2003; **3**: 677–85.

30. Nkoghe D, Formenty P, Leroy EM *et al.* [Multiple Ebola virus haemorrhagic fever outbreaks in Gabon, from October 2001 to April 2002.] *Bull Soc Pathol Exot* 2005; **98**: 24–9.

31. Gonzalez JP, Pourrut X, Leroy E. Ebolavirus and other filoviruses. *Curr Top Microbiol Immunol* 2007; **315**: 363–87.

32. Outbreak(s) of Ebola haemorrhagic fever, Congo and Gabon, October 2001–July 2002. *Wkly Epidemiol Rec* 2003; **78**: 223–8.

33. Outbreak of Ebola haemorrhagic fever in Yambio, south Sudan, April–June 2004. *Wkly Epidemiol Rec* 2005; **80**: 370–5.

34. Outbreak(s) of Ebola haemorrhagic fever in the Republic of the Congo, January–April 2003. *Wkly Epidemiol Rec* 2003; **78**: 285–9.

35. Le Guenno B, Formenty P, Boesch C. Ebola virus outbreaks in the Ivory Coast and Liberia, 1994–1995. *Curr Top Microbiol Immunol* 1999; **235**: 77–84.

36. Boumandouki P, Formenty P, Epelboin A *et al.* [Clinical management of patients and deceased during the Ebola outbreak from October to December 2003 in Republic of Congo.] *Bull Soc Pathol Exot* 2005; **98**: 218–23.

37. Kunii O, Kita E, Shibuya K. [Epidemics and related cultural factors for Ebola hemorrhagic fever in Gabon.] *Nippon Koshu Eisei Zasshi* 2001; **48**: 853–9.

38. Fisher-Hoch SP. Lessons from nosocomial viral haemorrhagic fever outbreaks. *Br Med Bull* 2005; **73–74**: 123–37.

39. Peterson AT, Bauer JT, Mills JN. Ecologic and geographic distribution of filovirus disease. *Emerg Infect Dis* 2004; **10**: 40–7.

40. Groseth A, Feldmann H, Strong JE. The ecology of Ebola virus. *Trends Microbiol* 2007; **15**: 408–16.

41. Georges-Courbot MC, Sanchez A, Lu CY *et al.* Isolation and phylogenetic characterization of Ebola viruses causing different outbreaks in Gabon. *Emerg Infect Dis* 1997; **3**: 59–62.

42. Pinzon JE, Wilson JM, Tucker CJ, Arthur R, Jahrling PB, Formenty P. Trigger events: Enviroclimatic coupling of Ebola hemorrhagic fever outbreaks. *Am J Trop Med Hyg* 2004; **71**: 664–74.

43. Monath TP. Ecology of Marburg and Ebola viruses: Speculations and directions for future research. *J Infect Dis* 1999; **179**(Suppl. 1): S127–38.

44. Pourrut X, Delicat A, Rollin PE, Ksiazek TG, Gonzalez JP, Leroy EM. Spatial and temporal patterns of Zaire ebolavirus antibody prevalence in the possible reservoir bat species. *J Infect Dis* 2007; **196**(Suppl. 2): S176–83.

45. Wong S, Lau S, Woo P, Yuen KY. Bats as a continuing source of emerging infections in humans. *Rev Med Virol* 2007; **17**: 67–91.

46. Schou S, Hansen AK. Marburg and Ebola virus infections in laboratory non-human primates: A literature review. *Comp Med* 2000; **50**: 108–23.

47. Walsh PD, Abernethy KA, Bermejo M *et al.* Catastrophic ape decline in western equatorial Africa. *Nature* 2003; **422**: 611–14.

48. Bermejo M, Rodriguez-Teijeiro JD, Illera G, Barroso A, Vila C, Walsh PD. Ebola outbreak killed 5000 gorillas. *Science* 2006; **314**: 1564.

49. Zlotnik I, Simpson DI. The pathology of experimental vervet monkey disease in hamsters. *Br J Exp Pathol* 1969; **50**: 393–9.

50. Morvan JM, Deubel V, Gounon P *et al.* Identification of Ebola virus sequences present as RNA or DNA in organs of terrestrial small mammals of the Central African Republic. *Microbes Infect* 1999; **1**: 1193–201.

51. Allela L, Boury O, Pouillot R *et al.* Ebola virus antibody prevalence in dogs and human risk. *Emerg Infect Dis* 2005; **11**: 385–90.

52. Kunz C, Hofmann H, Aspock H. [Propagation of "Marburg virus" (Vervet monkey disease agent) in *Aedes aegypti.*] *Zentralbl Bakteriol* 1968; **208**: 347–9.

53. Reiter P, Turell M, Coleman R *et al.* Field investigations of an outbreak of Ebola hemorrhagic fever, Kikwit, Democratic Republic of the Congo, 1995: Arthropod studies. *J Infect Dis* 1999; **179**(Suppl. 1): S148–54.

54. Swanepoel R, Leman PA, Burt FJ *et al.* Experimental inoculation of plants and animals with Ebola virus. *Emerg Infect Dis* 1996; **2**: 321–5.

55. Bausch DG, Borchert M, Grein T *et al.* Risk factors for Marburg hemorrhagic fever, Democratic Republic of the Congo. *Emerg Infect Dis* 2003; **9**: 1531–7.

56. Jahrling PB, Geisbert TW, Dalgard DW *et al.* Preliminary report: isolation of Ebola virus from monkeys imported to USA. *Lancet* 1990; **335**: 502–5.

57. Feldmann H, Wahl-Jensen V, Jones SM, Stroher U. Ebola virus ecology: A continuing mystery. *Trends Microbiol* 2004; **12**: 433–7.

58. Real LA, Biek R. Spatial dynamics and genetics of infectious diseases on heterogeneous landscapes. *J R Soc Interface* 2007; **4**: 935–48.

59. Wittmann TJ, Biek R, Hassanin A *et al.* Isolates of Zaire ebolavirus from wild apes reveal genetic lineage and recombinants. *Proc Natl Acad Sci USA* 2007; **104**: 17123–7.

60. Swenson DL, Warfield KL, Larsen T, Alves DA, Coberley SS, Bavari S. Monovalent virus-like particle vaccine protects guinea pigs and nonhuman primates against infection with multiple Marburg viruses. *Expert Rev Vaccines* 2008; **7**: 417–29.

61. Swenson DL, Wang D, Luo M et al. Vaccine to confer to nonhuman primates complete protection against multistrain Ebola and Marburg virus infections. Clin Vaccine Immunol 2008; 15: 460–7.

62. Conrad JL, Isaacson M, Smith EB et al. Epidemiologic investigation of Marburg virus disease, Southern Africa, 1975. Am J Trop Med Hyg 1978; 27: 1210–15.

63. Baron RC, McCormick JB, Zubeir OA. Ebola virus disease in southern Sudan: Hospital dissemination and intrafamilial spread. Bull World Health Organ 1983; 61: 997–1003.

64. Leroy EM, Epelboin A, Mondonge V et al. Human ebola outbreak resulting from direct exposure to fruit bats in Luebo, Democratic Republic of Congo, 2007. Vector Borne Zoonotic Dis 2009; 9: 723–8.

65. Cyranoski D. Ebola outbreak has experts rooting for answers. Nature 2009; 457: 364–5.

66. Biek R, Walsh PD, Leroy EM, Real LA. Recent common ancestry of Ebola Zaire virus found in a bat reservoir. PLoS Pathog 2006; 2: e90.

67. Nakazibwe C. Marburg fever outbreak leads scientists to suspected disease reservoir. Bull World Health Organ 2007; 85: 654–6.

68. Towner JS, Pourrut X, Albarino CG et al. Marburg virus infection detected in a common African bat. PLoS ONE 2007; 2: e764.

69. Dimitrov DT, Hallam TG, Rupprecht CE, McCracken GF. Adaptive modeling of viral diseases in bats with a focus on rabies. J Theor Biol 2008; 255: 69–80.

70. Enterlein S, Schmidt KM, Schumann M et al. The marburg virus 3′ noncoding region structurally and functionally differs from that of ebola virus. J Virol 2009; 83: 4508–19.

71. Enria DA, Pinheiro F. Rodent-borne emerging viral zoonosis. Hemorrhagic fevers and hantavirus infections in South America. Infect Dis Clin North Am 2000; 14: 167–84, x.

72. Ogbu O, Ajuluchukwu E, Uneke CJ. Lassa fever in West African sub-region: An overview. J Vector Borne Dis 2007; 44: 1–11.

73. Lecompte E, Brouat C, Duplantier JM, Galan M, Granjon L, Loiseau A. Molecular identification of four cryptic species of Mastomys. Biochem Syst Ecol 2005; 33: 681–9.

74. Gunther S, Lenz O. Lassa virus. Crit Rev Clin Lab Sci 2004; 41: 339–90.

75. Fair J, Jentes E, Inapogui A et al. Lassa virus-infected rodents in refugee camps in Guinea: A looming threat to public health in a politically unstable region. Vector Borne Zoonotic Dis 2007; 7: 167–71.

76. Muggia A. [The tragic story of the discovery of the Lassa fever virus.] Minerva Med 1970; 26(Suppl.): 16.

77. Richmond JK, Baglole DJ. Lassa fever: Epidemiology, clinical features, and social consequences. BMJ 2003; 327: 1271–5.

78. Monath TP, Newhouse VF, Kemp GE, Setzer HW, Cacciapuoti A. Lassa virus isolation from Mastomys natalensis rodents during an epidemic in Sierra Leone. Science 1974; 185: 263–5.

79. Granjon L, Lavrenchenko L, Corti M, Coetzee N, Rahman EA. Mastomys natalensis. In: International Union for the Conservation of Nature and Natural Resources, IUCN Red List of Threatened Species, Version 2009.2. Available from: http://www.iucnredlist.org/apps/redlist/details/12868/0 (accessed January 14, 2010).

80. Lecompte E, Fichet-Calvet E, Daffis S et al. Mastomys natalensis and Lassa fever, West Africa. Emerg Infect Dis 2006; 12: 1971–4.

81. Wulff H, Fabiyi A, Monath TP. Recent isolations of Lassa virus from Nigerian rodents. Bull World Health Organ 1975; 52(4–6): 609–13.

82. Granjon L, Duplantier J-M, Catalan J, Britton-Davidian J. Systematics of the genus Mastomys. Belg J Zool 1997; 127: 7–18.

83. McCormick JB, Webb PA, Krebs JW, Johnson KM, Smith ES. A prospective study of the epidemiology and ecology of Lassa fever. J Infect Dis 1987; 155: 437–44.

84. Keenlyside RA, McCormick JB, Webb PA, Smith E, Elliott L, Johnson KM. Case-control study of Mastomys natalensis and humans in Lassa virus–infected households in Sierra Leone. Am J Trop Med Hyg 1983; 32: 829–37.

85. Bonner PC, Schmidt WP, Belmain SR, Oshin B, Baglole D, Borchert M. Poor housing quality increases risk of rodent infestation and Lassa fever in refugee camps of Sierra Leone. Am J Trop Med Hyg 2007; 77: 169–75.

86. Ter Meulen J, Lukashevich I, Sidibe K et al. Hunting of peridomestic rodents and consumption of their meat as possible risk factors for rodent-to-human transmission of Lassa virus in the Republic of Guinea. Am J Trop Med Hyg 1996; 55: 661–6.

87. Helmick CG, Webb PA, Scribner CL, Krebs JW, McCormick JB. No evidence for increased risk of Lassa fever infection in hospital staff. Lancet 1986; 2: 1202–5.

88. Salazar-Bravo J, Dragoo JW, Bowen MD, Peters CJ, Ksiazek TG, Yates TL. Natural nidality in Bolivian hemorrhagic fever and the systematics of the reservoir species. Infect Genet Evol 2002; 1: 191–9.

89. Salazar-Bravo J, Ruedas LA, Yates TL. Mammalian reservoirs of arenaviruses. Curr Top Microbiol Immunol 2002; 262: 25–63.

90. Daszak P, Epstein JH, Kilpatrick AM, Aguirre AA, Karesh WB, Cunningham AA. Collaborative research approaches to the role of wildlife in zoonotic disease emergence. Curr Top Microbiol Immunol 2007; 315: 463–75.

91. Ebola haemorrhagic fever in Zaire, 1976. Bull World Health Organ 1978; 56: 271–93.

92. Morvan JM, Deubel V, Gounon P et al. Identification of Ebola virus sequences present as RNA or DNA in organs of terrestrial small mammals of the Central African Republic. Microbes Infect 1999; 1: 1193–201.

93. Georges AJ, Leroy EM, Renaut AA et al. Ebola hemorrhagic fever outbreaks in Gabon, 1994–1997: Epidemiologic and health control issues. J Infect Dis 1999; 179(Suppl. 1): S65–75.

94. Outbreak of Ebola viral hemorrhagic fever – Zaire, 1995. MMWR Morb Mortal Wkly Rep 1995; 44: 381–2.

95. Ebola haemorrhagic fever. A summary of the outbreak in Gabon. Wkly Epidemiol Rec 1997; 72(1–2):7–8.

96. Outbreak(s) of Ebola haemorrhagic fever, Congo and Gabon, October 2001–July 2002. *Wkly Epidemiol Rec* 2003; **78**: 223–8.

97. Outbreak news. Ebola virus haemorrhagic fever, Democratic Republic of the Congo – update. *Wkly Epidemiol Rec* 2007; **82**: 345–6.

98. Le GB, Formenty P, Boesch C. Ebola virus outbreaks in the Ivory Coast and Liberia, 1994–1995. *Curr Top Microbiol Immunol* 1999; **235**: 77–84.

99. Formenty P, Boesch C, Wyers M *et al.* Ebola virus outbreak among wild chimpanzees living in a rain forest of Cote d'Ivoire. *J Infect Dis* 1999; **179**(Suppl. 1): S120–6.

100. Formenty P, Hatz C, Le GB, Stoll A, Rogenmoser P, Widmer A. Human infection due to Ebola virus, subtype Cote d'Ivoire: Clinical and biologic presentation. *J Infect Dis* 1999; **179**(Suppl. 1): S48–53.

101. Geisbert TW, Jahrling PB. Use of immunoelectron microscopy to show Ebola virus during the 1989 United States epizootic. *J Clin Pathol* 1990; **43**: 813–16.

102. Ebola haemorrhagic fever in Sudan, 1976. Report of a WHO/International Study Team. *Bull World Health Organ* 1978; **56**: 247–70.

103. Sanchez A, Rollin PE. Complete genome sequence of an Ebola virus (Sudan species) responsible for a 2000 outbreak of human disease in Uganda. *Virus Res* 2005; **113**: 16–25.

104. Onyango CO, Opoka ML, Ksiazek TG *et al.* Laboratory diagnosis of Ebola hemorrhagic fever during an outbreak in Yambio, Sudan, 2004. *J Infect Dis* 2007; **196**(Suppl. 2): S193–8.

105. Bonin O. The *Cercopithecus* monkey disease in Marburg and Frankfurt (Main), 1967. *Acta Zool Pathol Antverp* 1969; **48**: 319–31.

106. Gear JH. The hemorrhagic fevers of Southern Africa with special reference to studies in the South African Institute for Medical Research. *Yale J Biol Med* 1982; **55**(3–4): 207–12.

107. Gear JS, Cassel GA, Gear AJ *et al.* Outbreake of Marburg virus disease in Johannesburg. *Br Med J* 1975; **4**: 489–93.

108. Bukreyev AA, Volchkov VE, Blinov VM, Dryga SA, Netesov SV. The complete nucleotide sequence of the Popp (1967) strain of Marburg virus: A comparison with the Musoke (1980) strain. *Arch Virol* 1995; **140**: 1589–600.

109. Colebunders R, Sleurs H, Pirard P *et al.* Organisation of health care during an outbreak of Marburg haemorrhagic fever in the Democratic Republic of Congo, 1999. *J Infect* 2004; **48**: 347–53.

110. Roddy P, Marchiol A, Jeffs B *et al.* Decreased peripheral health service utilisation during an outbreak of Marburg haemorrhagic fever, Uige, Angola, 2005. *Trans R Soc Trop Med Hyg* 2009; **103**: 200–2.

111. Fraser DW, Campbell CC, Monath TP, Goff PA, Gregg MB. Lassa fever in the Eastern Province of Sierra Leone, 1970–1972. I: Epidemiologic studies. *Am J Trop Med Hyg* 1974; **23**: 1131–9.

112. Monath TP, Mertens PE, Patton R *et al.* A hospital epidemic of Lassa fever in Zorzor, Liberia, March–April 1972. *Am J Trop Med Hyg* 1973; **22**: 773–9.

113. Keane E, Gilles HM. Lassa fever in Panguma Hospital, Sierra Leone, 1973–6. *Br Med J* 1977; **1**: 1399–402.

114. Knobloch J, McCormick JB, Webb PA, Dietrich M, Schumacher HH, Dennis E. Clinical observations in 42 patients with Lassa fever. *Tropenmed Parasitol* 1980; **31**: 389–98.

115. Fichet-Calvet E, Rogers DJ. Risk maps of Lassa fever in west Africa. *PLoS Negl Trop Dis* 2009; **3**: e388.

Nosocomial diseases – hospitals and institutions

Clostridium difficile

J. S. BRAZIER

In common with certain other bacterial genera, the genus *Clostridium* evolved a process to promote the long-term survival of member species. The process is called sporulation, which in simple terms can be described as the ability of a bacterial cell to wrap up its DNA in a protective coat in times of nutrient depletion or exposure to other adverse conditions. Apart from a few aerotolerant members of the genus, clostridia must be in an inert state to survive in the atmospheric environment, since oxygen is to them a poisonous gas from which they must be protected. Clostridial spores (Figure 43.1), unlike their vegetative cell counterparts, can withstand indefinite exposure to oxygen in addition to prolonged resistance to certain heat and disinfection processes that would kill non-sporing cells.

A bacterial spore is, however, inert, and in order for this survival strategy to be effective, the spore must undergo the process called germination, whereby a vegetative cell emerges from the spore into an environment in which it can replicate. For an anaerobic organism, this environment must be devoid of, or have very low concentrations of, oxygen, and for those clostridia which are of importance to human and animal health and form part of their normal flora, this anaerobic environment is commonly the lower intestinal tracts.

One could almost consider the clostridial species that inhabit the human or animal gut as having a life-cycle. They flourish in the warm nutritious anaerobic environment of the mammalian large bowel, undergoing massive multiplication to approximately 10^9 per gram of faecal material, before being voided into the cooler and aerobic atmosphere where only those bacilli that undergo sporulation will survive. From here, they must survive an indefinite period until they gain access to another anaerobic environment such as the human or mammalian gut, usually by means of ingestion. The spores then must first survive exposure to gastric acidity and are then stimulated to germinate by exposure to bile acids in the small bowel before completing their cycle in the lower intestinal tracts.

Since dirt, dust and soil containing dried human and animal waste products are not uncommon in the general environment, it is not surprising that clostridial spores are ubiquitous in nature. From a very early age, most children are told by their parents that those cuts and scratches obtained as part of childhood play must be cleaned of dirt for fear of infection. Although most parents are probably unaware of it, a major part of the threat of wound contamination by dirt, dust and foreign bodies comes from clostridial infections such as gas gangrene and tetanus. These diseases are caused by members of the

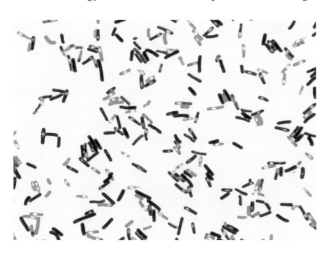

Figure 43.1 Gram stain of *Clostridium difficile* showing spores.

genus *Clostridium*, such as *C. perfringens* and *C. tetani*, which, in common with the other pathogenic species, produce exotoxins that are responsible for the symptoms of disease in man.

In evolutionary terms, however, clostridia and the exotoxins they produce evolved long before man existed, and their pathogenic effects to humans are usually a result of spores gaining access to tissues that are in some way compromised, thus allowing germination and toxin production. The clostridia are great opportunists, and the process of sporulation confers on the clostridia a survival, and ultimately an evolutionary, advantage that is key to their opportunism. Examples of opportunistic clostridial infections in humans are those in injecting drug users who inadvertently inject clostridial spore-contaminated heroin intramuscularly, soldiers who suffer contaminated high-velocity bullet and shrapnel wounds in theatres of war, and hospital patients receiving certain broad-spectrum antibiotics when exposed to *C. difficile* spores in the hospital ward.

Hence, it is the wider environment that is, by and large, the reservoir of clostridial spores. This chapter will focus on the role of the environment in the epidemiology of a very important member of the genus that causes much nosocomial morbidity and mortality, namely *C. difficile*.

CLOSTRIDIUM DIFFICILE AND ITS DISCOVERY

The organism was first described in 1935 by the American workers Hall and O'Toole,[1] who gave it the name *Bacillus difficilis*. They found it in the faeces and meconium of healthy newborns as part of the normal bacterial flora, and demonstrated that most strains produced exotoxins, postulating that it might be the cause of certain conditions such as febrile convulsions and the formation of occult blood in young infants. As the organism was an obligate anaerobic, Gram-positive, spore-bearing bacillus, it was subsequently classified as belonging to the genus *Clostridium*, and for the next few decades fell into obscurity, only making fleeting appearances in the literature. McBee[2] isolated *C. difficile* from the gut of a Weddel seal, and Smith and King,[3] looking specifically for reports of *C. difficile* in human infections, noted eight incidents of extraintestinal infection in which they concluded that it was not playing a pathogenic role. The second report of an animal origin was that of Stevenson,[4] who found *C. difficile* in the gut contents of a desert locust.

Three independent studies, all concluded in 1974, provided the platform from which *C. difficile* was shown to be an important cause of disease in man, ironically mainly at the opposite end of our lifespan than that envisaged by Hall and O'Toole. In the USA, Green[5] described a cytotoxin that was present in the stools of guinea-pigs that developed gut disease after receiving penicillin. Tedesco *et al.*,[6] also in the USA, found a significant association between patients

receiving clindamycin and the development of pseudomembranous colitis, coining the term 'clindamycin-associated colitis'. At this stage, neither group knew the aetiology of their observations.

Meanwhile in Leeds, UK, a PhD student completed his thesis on *C. difficile* and its toxicity[7] but was totally unaware at the time that the organism he was studying was responsible for the toxic effects noted by the workers in America. These independent publications were a catalyst to studies by Bartlett *et al.*[8] who described a clindamycin-induced colitis in hamsters. From hamster faeces, they isolated an unidentified *Clostridium* species that was eventually confirmed as *C. difficile*, and this was proven to cause the symptoms. Larson *et al.*[9] demonstrated that a cytotoxin could also be detected in the stools of humans in five out of six patients with histologically proven pseudomembranous colitis. There soon followed several studies that provided confirmation of the causal association of *C. difficile* with gut infection in man.[10,11]

Clostridium difficile is normally a harmless environmental organism, and, as is the case with a number of other bacterial species, it is man's intervention and the opportunistic nature of clostridia that have facilitated the conditions whereby they may cause significant human morbidity and mortality. In the case of *C. difficile* disease, it is the disturbance of the barrier to colonization by *C. difficile* afforded by the complex normal human gut flora, usually by antimicrobial agents, that facilitates infection by *C. difficile*. As ingestion of the spores of *C. difficile* is required for infection, an external source of the organism must exist. Autoinfection is one possibility, whereby the contaminated human hand transfers spores from the person's own faecal flora or skin to the oral cavity, but the environment is another obvious source.

CLOSTRIDIUM DIFFICILE IN ANIMALS AND THE GENERAL ENVIRONMENT

The first major study to screen specifically for *C. difficile* in the inanimate environment was that of Hafiz,[7] who isolated the organism from soil, sand and mud from a river bank, and from hay. He also found it in dung samples from a camel, a donkey, a cow and a horse. Others had also found the organism in soil in Poland,[12] although some only found it in sites related geographically or temporally to human sewage or patients with active *C. difficile* infection, while others completely failed to isolate it from soil samples.[13,14] This suggests either irregular environmental distribution or, more likely, that the results were affected by variable sampling methodology.

To date, the largest single study of the environment as a source of *C. difficile* has been that of Al Saif and Brazier,[15] who examined over two and a half thousand environmental samples in the Cardiff area of South Wales, UK. Their survey included samples of river and sea water, swimming pool water, raw vegetables, soil, and farm and pet animal faeces, in addition to general surfaces in homes, hospitals and veterinary clinics that were examined using a methodology designed to maximize spore recovery. Their results showed an overall positivity rate of 7.1 per cent with largely expected positive results for soil (21 per cent), pets (7 per cent) and hospitals (20 per cent). The most significant finding was that 87.5 per cent of river waters and 46.7 per cent of lake waters were positive for *C. difficile*, as well as 50 per cent of swimming pool samples. Logically, however, this should not have been too much of a surprise, since virtually all faecal material from patients suffering from *C. difficile* infection in hospital ends up in the sewage system, and from sewage treatment plants some spores will undoubtedly eventually enter the water cycle. Once in the water cycle, the levels of chlorine used to make water potable are much too low to affect the viability of clostridial spores.

The methodology used in examining water samples in the South Wales study may have been a key factor in its success, as a protocol of 5 days' incubation using a medium designed to enhance spore germination was used. This often resulted in isolation of *C. difficile* after 3–5 days' incubation from cultures that were culture negative at 48 hours. Such environmental data may explain how the population in the general community could be exposed to *C. difficile* from time to time and henceforth carry the organism into hospitals.

Until quite recently, there was little evidence that *C. difficile* disease in man could have zoonotic origins. Although numerous animal reservoirs have been recognized and a great variety of wild, farmed and domesticated species may carry the organism,[16–18] there has been no evidence that the strains found in animals were the same at those found in humans. Carriage in animals in the human food chain was also investigated by Al Saif and Brazier,[15] who sampled 524 faecal or gut contents from cattle, sheep, pigs, fish and poultry, with isolation rates ranging from zero to 1.6 per cent, concluding that neither meat nor fish was an important reservoir. However, the samples were not taken from intensively reared animals, so the results from factory-farmed stock could have been different.

Disease due to *C. difficile* infection in animals has been recognized, initially in hamsters treated with clindamycin.[8] Horses too, can suffer *C. difficile* infection, as in one study of hospitalized horses who developed diarrhoea after becoming colonized with toxigenic strains within a 2 day period.[19] Enteritis and enterotoxaemia due to *C. difficile* have also been reported in captive ostriches.[20] One report attributed chronic diarrhoea in dogs to *C. difficile*,[21] although Struble *et al.*[22] could find no direct association between toxin-positive isolates and dogs with diarrhoea in a veterinary teaching hospital, and Borriello *et al.*[16] found no association between carriage and diarrhoea in household pets. *Clostridium difficile* infection in mammals usually requires the same disturbance of gut flora by antibiotics as in man. Broiler chickens have been shown to

be a potential source of infection in Zimbabwe,[23] with 29 per cent of chicken faeces positive for *C. difficile*. In a separate study, Simango[24] had previously demonstrated toxigenic *C. difficile* in 37 per cent of soil samples and 6 per cent of water samples, and although a high percentage of these isolates were proven to be toxigenic, no typing studies were performed.

Molecular typing methods such as polymerase chain reaction (PCR) ribotyping[25,26] have been applied to isolates of *C. difficile* from farm animals such as piglets and calves. Rodriguez-Palacios *et al.*[27] in Canada examined 31 isolates of *C. difficile* from calves and found eight distinct ribotypes, seven of which have been found in humans. Two of these, PCR ribotypes 017 and 027, have been associated with outbreaks of disease in several countries. Another study from North America showed that PCR ribotype 078 accounted for 83 per cent of the strains found in neonatal pigs and 94 per cent of those in calves.[28] This same strain can also cause infections in humans, and in a surveillance study in England during 2007–08, PCR ribotype 078 accounted for 2.2 per cent of 677 hospital patient isolates. These studies raise the possibility that *C. difficile* may be in the human food chain, and indeed a recent investigation into ground (minced) beef in Canada demonstrated *C. difficile* in 20 per cent of samples.[29] An unpublished pilot study of retail minced meats on sale in South Wales, however, could not reproduce this finding (personal observation).

A body of evidence exists, therefore, to explain how the population in the community may from time to time be exposed to *C. difficile*, but in the absence of known risk factors such as antibiotic exposure, in general healthy people in the community rarely develop disease. Entry to hospital with underlying disease, and a subsequent exposure to certain antibiotics or other risk factors, could though enable a colonized patient to become symptomatic. More commonly, however, it is generally believed that they acquire the organism while in hospital from the ward environment.

CLOSTRIDIUM DIFFICILE IN THE HOSPITAL ENVIRONMENT

Levels of environmental contamination with spores of *C. difficile* are likely to be much higher in hospital wards that have had cases of active disease than anywhere else. Studies of newborn babies by Bolton *et al.*[30] and Sherertz and Sarubbi[31] showed that exposure in the nosocomial environment, rather than vertical transmission, was the most likely source of *C. difficile* acquisition. This was supported by the findings of Malamou–Ladas *et al.*,[32] who found *C. difficile* spores in 3 per cent of environmental samples in a neonatal unit. Fekety *et al.*[33] sampled the hospital environment in detail and isolated spores from floors, toilets, mops, bedding and furniture, although they did not find any spores on walls or in air samples or food.

In terms of establishing a relationship between exposure and disease, a correlation has been shown between the presence or absence of symptomatic patients and the levels of environmental contamination.[34] However, the methodology used for environmental sampling is important[35] as an incorporation of spore-germinating compounds such as sodium taurocholate in the selective medium gave a superior result compared with medium without them. Spore recovery from environmental sources is vital since vegetative cells of *C. difficile* only survive for 15 minutes in air.[35] Acquisition of *C. difficile* from the ward environment was shown to be a source of infection by Kaatz *et al.*[36] who found the same strains typed by bacteriophage–bacteriocin typing to be in the ward environment after cases of infection with the same strains had been identified in infected patients. They also demonstrated the efficacy of hypochlorite solutions in removing *C. difficile* spores from the environment.

More recently, the air in a hospital ward was implicated as possibly important in the dissemination of *C. difficile* spores. Using a portable air sampler, Roberts *et al.*[37] sampled the air in an elderly care ward over 2 days and found *C. difficile* in 23 samples, with mean counts of 53–426 colony-forming units per cubic metre of air. Twenty-two of these isolates belonged to the same strain, called PCR ribotype 001.

There is thus evidence that the spores of *C. difficile* are plentiful in our environment, both inside and outside hospitals. It is reasonable to surmise, therefore, that an individual may occasionally ingest a few spores, but, without the concomitant disturbance of his or her healthy gut flora afforded mainly by antibiotics, symptoms do not develop. Future research will probably show whether certain strains of *C. difficile* such as PCR ribotype 027 have superior environmental survival properties that may explain why they are so successful in causing disease.

RECOMMENDATIONS FOR THE MANAGEMENT OF *CLOSTRIDUM DIFFICILE* INFECTION IN HOSPITALS

There are three main principles for the prevention and control of *C. difficile* disease in hospitals:

1. good antimicrobial husbandry, which means reducing or replacing the often unnecessary use of broad-spectrum antibiotics, or courses of multiple antibiotics, with short courses of targeted narrow-spectrum agents wherever possible;
2. adherence to good infection control policies such as staff hand-washing and the isolation of infected patients in order to prevent the spread of infection within a ward or hospital;

3. the provision of a clean ward environment that will reduce the reservoir of *C. difficile* spores and therefore reduce the threat of infection.

For the most recent and comprehensive recommendations for the control and management of *C. difficile* disease compiled by a panel of experts in the field, the reader is referred to the Department of Health report *Clostridum difficile Infection: How to Deal with the Problem.*[38]

REFERENCES

● = Key primary paper
◆ = Major review article

1. Hall IC, O'Toole E. Intestinal flora in newborn infants with a description of a new pathogenic anaerobe, *Bacillus difficilis*. *Am J Dis Child* 1935; **49**: 390–402.
2. McBee RH. Intestinal flora of Antarctic birds and mammals. *J Bacteriol* 1960; **79**: 311–12.
3. Smith LDS, King EO. Occurrence of *Clostridium difficile* in infections of man. *J Bacteriol* 1962; **84**:65–7.
4. Stevenson JP. The normal bacterial flora of the alimentary canal of laboratory stocks of the desert locust *Schistocera gregaria (Forskal)*. *J Invertbr Pathol* 1966; **8**: 205–11.
5. Green RH. The association of viral activation with penicillin toxicity in guinea pigs and hamsters. *Yale J Biol Med* 1974; **3**: 166–81.
6. Tedesco FJ, Barton RW, Alpers DH. Clindamycin-associated colitis. *Ann Intern Med* 1974; **81**: 429–33.
7. Hafiz S. *Clostridium difficile* and its toxins. PhD thesis, Department of Microbiology, University of Leeds, 1974.
8. Bartlett JG, Onderdonk AB, Cisneros RL, Kasper DL. Clindamycin associated colitis due to a toxin-producing species of *Clostridium* in hamsters. *J Infect Dis* 1977; **136**: 701–5.
9. Larson HE, Parry JV, Price AB, Davies DR, Dolby J, Tyrell DA. Undescribed toxin in pseudomembranous colitis. *Br Med J* 1977; **1**: 1246–8.
●10. Bartlett JG, Chang TW, Gurwith M, Gorbach SL, Onderdonk AB. Antibiotic associated pseudomembranous colitis due to toxin producing clostridia. *N Engl J Med* 1978; **298**: 531–4.
11. George WL, Sutter VL, Goldstein EJC, Ludwig SL, Finegold SM. Etiology of antimicrobial agent associated colitis. *Lancet* 1978; **i**: 802–3.
12. Blawat F, Chylinski G. Pathogenic clostridia in soil and faeces of domestic animals in the Gdansk region. *Bull Inst Marine Med (Gdansk)* 1958; **9**: 117–26.
13. Kim KH, Fekety R, Batts DH, Brown D, Cudmore M, Silver J Jr. Isolation of *Clostridium difficile* from the environment of contacts of patients with antibiotic-associated colitis. *J Infect Dis* 1981; **143**: 42–50.
14. Riley TV. The epidemiology of *Clostridium difficile* associated diarrhoea. *Rev Med Microbiol* 1994; **5**: 117–26.

15. Al Saif N, Brazier JS. The distribution of *Clostridium difficile* in the environment of South Wales. *J Med Microbiol* 1996; **45**: 133–7.

16. Borriello SP, Honour P, Turner T, Barclay F. Household pets as a reservoir for *Clostridium difficile*. *J Clin Pathol* 1983; **36**: 84–7.

17. Riley TV, Adams JE, O'Neill GL, Bowman RA. Gastrointestinal carriage of *Clostridium difficile* in cats and dogs attending veterinary clinics. *Epidemiol Infect* 1991; **107**: 659–65.

18. Levett PN. *Clostridium difficile* in habitats other than the human gastro-intestinal tract. *J Infect* 1986; **12**: 253–63.

19. Madewell BR, Tang YJ, Jang S, Madigan JE, Hirsh DC, Gumerlock PH. Apparent outbreaks of *Clostridium difficile* associated diarrhoea in horses in a veterinary medical teaching hospital. *J Vet Diagn Invest* 1995; **7**: 343–6.

20. Frazier KS, Herron AJ, Hines ME, Gaskin JM, Altman NH. Diagnosis of enteritis and enterotoxemia due to *Clostridium difficile* in captive ostriches (*Struthio camelus*). *J Vet Diagn Invest* 1993; **5**: 623–5.

21. Berry AP, Levett PN. Chronic diarrhoea in dogs associated with *Clostridium difficile* infection. *Vet Rec* 1986; **118**: 102–3.

22. Struble AL, Tang YJ, Kass PH, Gumerlock PH, Madewell BR, Silva J Jr. Fecal shedding of *Clostridium difficile* in dogs: a period of prevalence survey in a veterinary medical teaching hospital. *J Vet Diagn Invest* 1994; **6**: 342–7.

23. Simango C, Mwakurudza S. *Clostridium difficile* in broiler chickens sold at market places in Zimbabwe and their antimicrobial susceptibility. *Int J Food Microbiol* 2008; **124**: 268–70.

24. Simango C. Prevalence of *Clostridium difficile* in the environment in a rural community in Zimbabwe. *Trans R Soc Trop Med Hyg* 2006; **100**: 1146–50.

25. O'Neill GL, Ogunsola FT, Brazier JS, Duerden BI. Modification of a PCR ribotyping method for application as a routine typing scheme for *Clostridium difficile*. *Anaerobe* 1996; **2**: 205–9.

•26. Stubbs SLJ, Brazier JS, O'Neill GL, Duereden BI. PCR targeted to the 16S–23S rRNA gene intergenic spacer region of *Clostridium difficile* and the construction of a library consisting of 116 different PCR ribotypes. *J Clin Microbiol* 1999; **37**: 461–3.

27. Rodriguez-Palacios A, Staempfli HR, Duffield T *et al.* *Clostridium difficile* PCR ribotypes in calves, Canada. *Emerg Infect Dis* 2006; **12**: 1730–6.

28. Keel K, Brazier JS, Post KW, Weese JS, Songer JG. Prevalence of PCR ribotypes among *Clostridium difficile* isolates from pigs, calves and other species. *J Clin Microbiol* 2007; **45**: 1963–4.

29. Rodriguez-Palacios A, Staempfli HR, Duffield T, Weese JS. *Clostridium difficile* in retail ground meat, Canada. *Emerg Infect Dis* 2007; **13**: 485–7.

30. Bolton RP, Tait SK, Dear PRF, Lowsosky MS. Asymptomatic neonatal colonisation by *Clostridium difficile*. *Arch Dis Child* 1984; **59**: 466–72.

31. Sherertz RJ, Sarubbi MD. The prevalence of *Clostridium difficile* and toxin in a nursery population: a comparison between patients with necrotizing enterocolitis and an asymptomatic group. *J Pediatr* 1982; **100**: 435–9.

32. Malamou-Ladas H, O'Farrell SO, Nash JQ, Tabaqchali S. Isolation of *Clostridium difficile* from the patients and the environment of hospital wards. *J Clin Pathol* 1983; **36**: 88–92.

33. Fekety R, Kim KH, Brown D, Batts DH, Cudmore M, Silva J Jr. Epidemiology of antibiotic associated colitis: isolation of *Clostridium difficile* from the hospital environment. *Am J Med* 1981; **70**: 906–8.

34. Kim KH, Fekety R, Batts DH *et al.* Isolation of *Clostridium difficile* from the environment and contacts of patients with antibiotic associated colitis. *J Infect Dis* 1981; **143**: 42–50.

35. Buggy BP, Wilson KH, Fekety R. Comparison of methods for recovery of *Clostridium difficile* from an environmental surface. *J Clin Microbiol* 1983; **18**: 348–52.

36. Kaatz GW, Gitlin SD, Schaberg DR *et al.* Acquisition of *Clostridium difficile* from the hospital environment. *Am J Epidemiol* 1988; **127**: 1289–94.

37. Roberts K, Smith CF, Snelling AM *et al.* Aerial dissemination of *Clostridium difficile* spores. *BMC Infect Dis* 2008; **8**: 7.

◆38. Department of Health. Clostridium difficile *Infection: How to Deal with the Problem.* The Hawkey Report. London: DH Publications, 2009.

44

The emergence of antibiotic resistance in the hospital environment

ALAN JOHNSON

The discovery of different classes of antibiotic from the late 1940s onwards and their introduction into clinical use was a major breakthrough in the fight against bacterial infections. Their initial success was so dramatic that, in the 1960s, the US Surgeon General William H. Stewart is reputed to have declared that 'it is time to close the book on infectious diseases'.[1] Four decades later, and with the benefit of hindsight, it is evident that such optimism was entirely misplaced. The reality is that infectious disease remains the second most common cause of death worldwide,[2] and in terms of bacterial infections, our failure to control these diseases is related in large part to the emergence of antibiotic resistance.

Antibiotic resistance can arise in individual strains of bacteria through the mutation of genes that encode target sites to which antibiotics bind, with the result that antibiotic-binding is reduced (e.g. mutations in the gene encoding RNA polymerase reducing the binding of rifampicin, and thus rendering strains resistant).[3] However, resistance is often encoded by transferable genetic elements including plasmids and transposons, which can move not only between different strains of the same bacterial species, but between different bacterial species and even genera.[3] These transferable genetic elements contain genes that encode a range of resistance mechanisms including enzymes that degrade antibiotics (e.g. beta-lactamases and chloramphenicol acetyltransferase), efflux proteins, and mechanisms for modifying antibiotic-binding sites (e.g. the *erm* and *tet* genes, which encode proteins that modify bacterial ribosomes, giving resistance to macrolides and tetracyclines, respectively).[3]

In terms of the epidemiology of antibiotic resistance, the extent of the problem in any particular patient population is thus a reflection of both the spread of resistant strains and the interstrain and interspecies spread of the genes encoding resistance. The relative importance of each will vary among different species of bacteria and in different settings.

ANTIBIOTIC RESISTANCE IN THE HOSPITAL ENVIRONMENT

It is now well recognized that antibiotic resistance is a significant problem in the hospital environment. Many patients in hospital are prone to infection either as a result of undergoing invasive procedures (e.g. surgery, renal dialysis, intravenous therapy or artificial ventilation), which provide a portal through which bacteria can enter the body, or as a result of receiving drugs that depress the immune system. In addition, a number of underlying illnesses (e.g. cancer and diabetes) can increase the vulnerability of patients to infection and impair the ability of their antimicrobial immune defences. Further to this, the close proximity of many hospitalized patients allows bacteria to spread between them, either through environmental contamination, via contaminated fomites or on the hands of healthcare workers, which may be colonized with pathogenic bacteria following physical contact with infected or colonized patients.

As patients in hospital are prone to developing infections, they frequently receive antibiotics either for the treatment of established infections or as prophylaxis to stop infections developing. It is this intense use of antibiotics in the hospital environment that is believed to provide the selective pressure for the emergence and spread of antibiotic-resistant bacteria. In essence, it is an extreme example of Darwinian evolution ('survival of the fittest') in that, in the face of widespread antibiotic use, antibiotic-susceptible bacteria will tend to be eliminated, while resistant strains will persist.

Surveillance

In order to define the extent of the problem posed by antibiotic-resistant pathogens in hospitals and to develop strategies for controlling and ideally reducing their occurrence, it is necessary to undertake surveillance. This requires the systematic and regular screening of patients for infection and/or colonization with antibiotic-resistant bacteria. Surveillance is also essential for the optimal management of patients with infections as knowledge of local rates of resistance is an important part of the decision-making process when deciding on which antibiotics should be used for empirical treatment.

Surveillance can be undertaken in the whole hospital or at the level of individual units such as intensive care units (ICUs). In addition, in some countries, the surveillance of antibiotic resistance in hospitals is coordinated at a national level. For example, in England, the Department of Health has made it mandatory for all hospitals to report cases of bacteraemia due to meticillin-resistant *Staphylococcus aureus* (MRSA).[4] It is crucially important to remember that surveillance is not an end in its own right, but should be regarded as providing 'information for action', and to this end the government has used the baseline data on MRSA rates in individual hospitals to set targets for reductions in the rates of MRSA bacteraemia.[5]

Surveillance is also invaluable for defining the detailed epidemiology of antibiotic resistance within the hospital environment. This knowledge can then be used to aid the rational development of strategies to control the problem and can indicate where resources need to be preferentially deployed. As an example, surveillance in many hospitals has shown that the problem of antibiotic resistance is not uniformly distributed but is frequently particularly acute in high-dependency units such as ICUs.[6] This almost certainly relates to the fact that ICUs have a higher proportion of patients who are highly vulnerable to infection, who as a result experience higher levels of antibiotic usage. This in turn exerts a stronger selection pressure for the emergence, spread and persistence of antibiotic-resistant bacteria than is seen in other areas of the hospital.

THE INTERFACE BETWEEN THE HOSPITAL ENVIRONMENT AND THE COMMUNITY

For a long time, the problem of infection with antibiotic-resistant bacteria was thought mainly to affect patients in hospital. Although patients may be transferred between hospitals (e.g. for specialist treatment or diagnostic tests), many patients enter hospital from the community and are discharged back into the community at the end of their treatment. If such patients are colonized with antibiotic-resistant bacteria, either at the time of admission or at discharge, there is clearly a possibility of the resistant bacteria being transported between the two settings. One antibiotic-resistant pathogen whose occurrence in both the hospital environment and the community is currently causing much interest is MRSA.

The occurrence of MRSA in the hospital environment and the community

A number of surveillance schemes have monitored trends in MRSA bacteraemia, as this has been widely used as a proxy marker for rates of healthcare-associated infection (HCAI). In many of these schemes, blood cultures positive for MRSA taken within 48 hours of admission are presumed to reflect community-associated infections (of sufficient severity that the patient was admitted to hospital), while positive blood cultures obtained 48 hours or more after admission are taken as indicative of hospital-acquired infection.[7,8] However, a study in two hospitals in the UK showed that about a quarter of the MRSA bacteraemias were seen in patients admitted from the community.[9] Crucially, this study highlighted that although these patients were living in their own homes prior to admission, they were predominantly elderly and often had a history of hospital contact (the median time since discharge being 46 days).

A similar picture was seen for hospitals in England as a whole from data obtained as part of the national mandatory surveillance scheme,[8] where 27 per cent of cases of MRSA bacteraemia were detected within 2 days of admission, with a further 6 per cent of cases (comprising regular attenders such as patients undergoing renal dialysis, Accident and Emergency patients, outpatients and day patients) not admitted at the time the blood specimen was taken. The authors of this report stressed that it was not possible to assess the percentage of community-acquired MRSA bacteraemias from these two groups of patients, as patients may have recently visited a healthcare facility prior to detection at the reporting Trust.

A further study confirmed that prior hospitalization is a major risk factor for bacteraemia due to MRSA (and other pathogens) at the time of hospital admission, although it was not clear from the study whether this could be explained by the acquisition of pathogens from the hospital environment, or by co-morbidities or other factors.[10] A molecular characterization of MRSA isolates from patients admitted from the community showed that the majority belonged to one or other of the two epidemic MRSA (EMRSA-15 and EMRSA-16) clones associated with HCAI in the UK.[11] The implication from these studies is that hospitalized patients may be colonized with MRSA at the time of discharge and are subsequently readmitted if an invasive MRSA infection develops, although further work is required to validate this likely clinical scenario.

As patients may be discharged from hospital while colonized with MRSA, it had long been assumed that MRSA might 'escape' from the hospital environment, probably initially to nursing and residential homes, and possibly thereafter become established in the general community. However, a number of reports of serious and sometimes fatal infections in the community, often involving children, from diverse regions of the world including various European countries, the USA and Australia, revealed that many of the patients affected had no demonstrable epidemiological links to a hospital or nursing home setting.[12,13] Moreover, characterization of the isolates showed that they differed from typical hospital-associated strains, and as a result such strains have been commonly designated community-acquired (later changed to community-associated) MRSA (CA-MRSA).

Interestingly, CA-MRSA from a number of different regions characteristically contained a gene encoding a putative virulence determinant, the Panton–Valentine leucocidin.[13] However, the epidemiological picture has become more complex in that, following the admission of patients infected with CA-MRSA to hospital, these strains have on occasion spread to become established in the hospital environment (thus becoming 'hospital-associated' strains), with the result that the epithet 'CA-MRSA' is a misnomer in this situation.[14]

STRATEGIES TO REDUCE ANTIBIOTIC RESISTANCE IN HOSPITALS

Antibiotic stewardship

As antibiotic usage is believed to be a major driver of antibiotic resistance, there is currently much interest in optimizing antibiotic prescribing. This entails a difficult balancing act of trying to reduce antibiotic use without compromising patient safety. The problem facing clinicians trying to reduce the hospital prescribing of antibiotics is that failure to initiate adequate antibiotic therapy when needed is associated with a higher level of adverse outcomes, including increased mortality and prolonged

length of patient stay, with the associated social and economic costs.[15,16]

One approach to addressing this issue is the concept of antibiotic stewardship, in which multidisciplinary teams (ideally including an infectious disease physician, a clinical microbiologist and a clinical pharmacist) strive to optimize the prescribing of antimicrobial therapy to hospitalized patients.[17] The objective of antibiotic stewardship is to ensure that antibiotic usage improves patients' outcomes and is cost-effective without promoting the spread of bacterial resistance. Antibiotic stewardship comprises multiple strategic components, including producing evidenced-based prescribing guidelines, improving staff education concerning antibiotic use, auditing antibiotic use and providing feedback to staff, and formulary restrictions for specific classes of antibiotics. Computerized decision support programs have also been used as part of antimicrobial stewardship and can be a powerful tool.[18,19]

An additional benefit of optimizing antibiotic usage in hospitals is that it will help to minimize the occurrence of gastrointestinal infections caused by *Clostridium difficile*. This bacterium is found in the human intestine, where it may cause disease due to the production of exotoxins that attack the gut mucosa. *Clostridium difficile* is usually kept in check by the competing microbial flora found in the intestine, a phenomenon known as 'colonization resistance'. However, in patients receiving broad-spectrum antibiotics that inhibit or kill bacteria in the large intestine, the resulting disruption to the microecology of the gut allows the small numbers of *C. difficile* present to increase in number, which may result in the signs and symptoms of infection. Gastrointestinal infection ranges from mild diarrhoea to severe inflammatory colitis to pseudomembranous colitis. Aspects of control thus include prudent antibiotic prescribing to minimize the unnecessary use of broad-spectrum antibiotics, although infection control measures such as the isolation of infected patients and high standards of hospital hygiene to prevent interpatient spread are also important.

Antibiotic cycling

As discussed above, the ICU is often the setting within the hospital environment where the problem of antibiotic resistance can be exceptionally acute. A particular strategy that has been advocated for aiding ICU physicians in their choice of therapy is the concept of antibiotic cycling. This involves the deliberate scheduled removal and substitution of an antibiotic with another, usually of a different class but with the same spectrum of antibacterial activity (e.g. a cephalosporin might be replaced by a quinolone). After a period of time, the second antibiotic is withdrawn from use to be replaced by another and so on. At some point, the original drug is reintroduced and the cycle recommences.

The rationale for cycling is that if resistance to a particular antibiotic emerges during the time it is used, cessation of its use will remove the selective pressure for persistence of the resistant bacterial strains. In addition, the introduction of the second antibiotic should, in principle, allow the successful treatment of patients with infections caused by bacteria resistant to the first drug. Although antibiotic cycling seems in principle to be a not unreasonable intervention for controlling antibiotic resistance in the ICU (and possibly other clinical settings), clinical experience has varied, and its effectiveness at achieving this objective remains the subject of much debate.[20,21] This probably reflects, at least in part, the fact that studies to date have not been standardized but have varied with regard to both the number and classes of antibiotic used and the duration of their use.

Infection control

A number of measures can be implemented with a view to minimizing the spread of antibiotic-resistant bacteria in the hospital environment (Box 44.1).[22,23] These are focused on preventing the transmission of microorganisms between patients and preventing their introduction during invasive procedures or other treatments, and as such are not specific for resistant bacteria but are aimed at all pathogens capable of causing HCAIs. Hospitals will usually have infection control teams whose function is to work with clinical and other staff in the hospital to ensure that

> **BOX 44.1: Measures for controlling the spread of antibiotic-resistant bacteria and other pathogens in the hospital environment**
>
> - Prevent the transfer of microorganisms between patients by washing or decontaminating the hands between contact with patients, especially before undertaking a procedure that may risk introducing infection to the patient (e.g. inserting an intravenous catheter or dressing a wound)
> - Have systems in place to ensure that the greatest possible care is taken to avoid introducing or transmitting infection during invasive procedures (e.g. the use of sterile supplies and decontamination of equipment)
> - Use protective clothing to protect healthcare workers from exposure to microorganisms from the patient, and minimize the risk that they will be transferred on clothing
> - By regular cleaning, ensure that microorganisms are not allowed to build up in the environment
> - Optimize the use of antibiotics to minimize the risk of antibiotic-resistant bacteria emerging

best practice is observed with a view to minimizing the spread of HCAIs. The responsibility for minimizing the spread of HCAIs does not, however, rest solely with the infection control team, but applies to all hospital staff. In England, this shared responsibility is now enshrined in law following enactment of The Health Act 2006: Code of Practice for the Prevention and Control of Healthcare Associated Infections.[24]

Although much effort is currently being expended in trying to reduce the burden of infection due to antibiotic-resistant pathogens, it may be naive to think that the problem will be eliminated. Being realistic, we may need to accept the fact that, to paraphrase the title of a recent report, antibiotic resistance in the hospital environment is 'inevitable but not unmanageable'.[25]

REFERENCES

1. The Office of the Public Health Historian. Frequently asked questions. US Public Health Service, Office of the Librarian. Available from: http://lhncbc.nlm.nih.gov/apdb/phsHistory/faqs.html (accessed November 11, 2009).
2. World Health Organization. World Health Report 2004. Deaths by Cause, Sex and Mortality Stratum in WHO Regions, Estimates for 2002. Available from: http://www.who.int/whr/2004/annex/topic/en/annex_2_en.pdf (accessed November 11, 2009).
3. Greenwood D, Finch R, Davey P, Wilcox M (eds). *Antimicrobial Chemotherapy*, 5th edn. Oxford: Oxford University Press, 2007.
4. Department of Health. CMO Update 30. Surveillance of Healthcare Associated Infections. Available from: http://www.dh.gov.uk/en/Publicationsandstatistics/Lettersandcirculars/CMOupdate/DH_4003623 (accessed November 11, 2009).
5. Department of Health. Bloodborne MRSA Infection Rates To Be Halved by 2008 – Reid. Available from: http://www.dh.gov.uk/en/Publicationsandstatistics/Pressreleases/DH_4093533 (accessed November 25, 2009).
6. Fridkin SK. Increasing prevalence of antimicrobial resistance in intensive care units. *Crit Care Med* 2001; **29**: N64–8.
7. Naimi TS, LeDell KH, Como-Sabetti K *et al*. Comparison of community- and health care-associated methicillin-resistant *Staphylococcus aureus* infection. *JAMA* 2003; **290**: 2976–84.
8. Health Protection Agency. Surveillance of Healthcare Associated Infections Report 2007. Available from: http://www.hpa.org.uk/web/HPAwebFile/HPAweb_C/1196942169446 (accessed November 11, 2009).
9. Wylie DH, Peto TE, Crook D. MRSA bacteraemia in patients on arrival in hospital: a cohort study in Oxfordshire 1997–2003. *BMJ* 2005; **331**:992.

10. Wylie DH, Walker AS, Peto TEA, Crook DW. Hospital exposure in a UK population, and its association with bacteraemia. *J Hosp Infect* 2007; **67**: 301–7.

11. Miller R, Esmail H, Peto T, Walker S, Crook D, Wylie D. Is MRSA admission bacteraemia community-acquired? A case control study. *J Infect* 2008; **56**: 163–70.

12. Alliance for the Prudent Use of Antibiotics. Focus: MRSA in the community (CMRSA). *APUA Newslett* 2003; **21**: 1–6. Available from: http://www.tufts.edu/med/apua/Newsletter/APUA_v21n2.pdf (accessed November 11, 2009).

13. Boucher HW, Corey GR. Epidemiology of methicillin-resistant *Staphylococcus aureus. Clin Infect Dis* 2008; **46**(Suppl. 5): 344–9.

14. Maree CL, Daum RS, Boyle-Vavra S, Matayoshi K, Miller LG. Community-associated methicillin-resistant *Staphylococcus aureus* isolates causing healthcare-associated infections. *Emerg Infect Dis* 2007; **13**: 236–42.

15. Kollef MH, Sherman G, Ward S, Fraser VJ. Inadequate antimicrobial treatment of infections: A risk factor for hospital mortality among critically ill patients. *Chest* 1999; **115**: 462–74.

16. Ibrahim EH, Sherman G, Ward S, Fraser VJ, Kollef MH. The influence of inadequate antimicrobial treatment of bloodstream infections on patient outcomes in the ICU setting. *Chest* 2000; **118**: 146–55.

17. Dellit, TH, Owens RC, McGowan JE Jr *et al.* Infectious Diseases Society of America; Society for Healthcare Epidemiology of America. Infectious Diseases Society of America and the Society for Healthcare Epidemiology of America guidelines for developing an institutional program to enhance antimicrobial stewardship. *Clin Infect Dis* 2007; **44**: 59–77.

18. Paul M, Andreassen S, Tacconelli E *et al.*, on behalf of the TREAT Study Group. Improving empirical antibiotic treatment using TREAT, a computerized decision support system: cluster randomized trial. *J Antimicrob Chemother* 2006; **58**: 1238–45.

19 Buising KL, Thursky KA, Robertson MB *et al.* Electronic antibiotic stewardship – reduced consumption of broad-spectrum antibiotics using a computerized antimicrobial approval system in a hospital setting. *J Antimicrob Chemother* 2008; **62**: 608–16.

20. Brown EM, Nathwani D. Antibiotic cycling or rotation: A systematic review of the evidence of efficacy. *J Antimicrob Chemother* 2005; **55**: 6–9.

21. Masterton RG. Antibiotic cycling: More than it might seem. *J Antimicrob Chemother* 2005; **55**: 1–5.

22. Centers for Disease Control and Prevention. Infection Control Guidelines. Available from: http://www.cdc.gov/ncidod/dhqp/guidelines.html (accessed November 11, 2009).

23. Health Protection Agency. Healthcare Associated Infections – What Are They and Why Do They Occur? Available from: http://www.hpa.org.uk/webw/HPAweb&HPAwebStandard/HPAweb_C/1195733802872?p=1191942126527 (accessed November 11, 2009).

24. Department of Health. The Health Act 2006: Code of Practice for the Prevention and Control of Healthcare Associated Infections. Available from: http://www.dh.gov.uk/en/Publicationsandstatistics/Publications/PublicationsPolicyAndGuidance/DH_081927 (accessed November 11, 2009).

25. Health Protection Agency. Antibiotic Resistance: Inevitable but not Unmanageable. Available from: http://www.hpa.org.uk/webw/HPAweb&HPAwebStandard/HPAweb_C/1202115622795?p=1158945066450 (accessed November 11, 2009).

Accidental and deliberate environmental contamination

45

CBRN contamination

ROBERT P. CHILCOTT

INTRODUCTION

The deliberate release of toxic materials to inflict injury or death is not a modern phenomenon. Indeed, it is likely that humans have utilized nature's readily available bounty of poisons for nefarious purposes since time immemorial. However, a major development occurred during World War I. Prior to this, poisons based on simple inorganic chemicals or derivatives of toxic fauna and flora were mainly limited to weapons of assassination. The industrial capabilities of the main combatants in World War I, however, led to a rapid escalation in the complexity and effectiveness of chemical weapons on an immense scale: suddenly, it was possible to simultaneously expose thousands of individuals in an open environment to toxic concentrations of harmful substances. This led to great public opprobrium, and subsequently, a number of international agreements to ban such means of warfare were implemented (with varying degrees of success). The most significant development in recent times has been the willingness of certain factions to engage in activities that deliberately seek to expose unprotected members of the public to chemical, biological, radiological or nuclear (CBRN) hazards. This presents a new and major challenge to medical personnel.

The purpose of this chapter is to provide a basic overview of chemical, biological and radiological materials and to summarize the physiological effects and available medical countermeasures for a small selection of chemicals. The emphasis herein on chemical hazards merely reflects the trend of recent terrorist attacks; clearly, it is necessary to adopt a generic readiness that encompasses the entire spectrum of CBRN threat.

OVERVIEW OF HAZARDOUS MATERIALS

In theory, there is a vast array of materials that could potentially be used to contaminate the environment with the aim of achieving adverse health effects. Paracelsus (Theophrastus Phillippus Aureolus Bombastus von Hohenheim, 1493–1541) was among the first to recognize that all substances are capable of eliciting a toxic response if the exposure exceeds a threshold dose: 'sola dosis facit venenum' (the dose makes the poison).[1] This chapter is necessarily limited to a small number of representative hazards (Table 45.1).

Many of the chemicals represented in Table 45.1 have either been used as chemical warfare agents or were developed specifically for such purposes. For example, tabun, sarin, soman, VX, sulphur mustard and lewisite have no application other than for chemical warfare. Other substances such as chlorine, phosgene, arsine, hydrogen cyanide and cyanogen chloride, although previously used as chemical warfare agents, are representative of a class of compounds frequently referred to as toxic industrial chemicals due to their extensive industrial use(s) and inherent toxicity. The health effects and medical treatment of casualties exposed to chemical agents are discussed in more detail later.

Biological agents may be empirically categorized according to the causative organism (bacteria and viruses), some of which may also release toxins after infecting the host (Table 45.1). When considering a deliberate release (terrorist) incident, it should be noted that toxins are most likely to be used in purified form. In addition to bacteria and viruses, toxins can be extracted from a wide range of

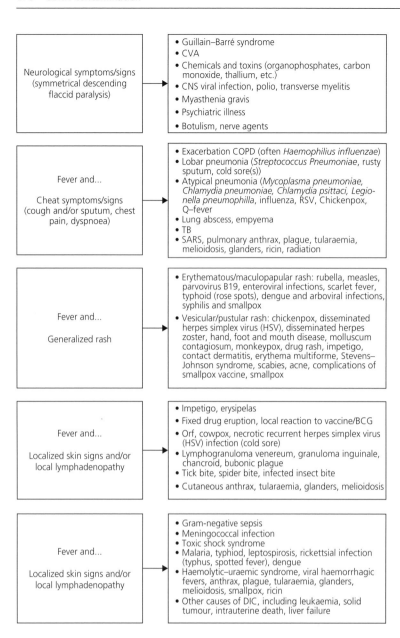

Figure 45.1 Biological agents – differential diagnosis for some important syndromic presentations. BCG, Bacille Calmette–Guerin; CNS, central nervous system; COPD, chronic obstructive pulmonary disease; CVA, cerebrovascular accident; DIC, disseminated intravascular coagulation; RSV, respiratory syncytial virus; SARS, severe acute respiratory syndrome; TB, tuberculosis. (Adapted from Health Protection Agency,[44] with permission.)

fauna and flora. For example, ricin and abrin are plant toxins, saxitoxin is derived from certain marine plankton (dinoflagellates) and batrachotoxins come from 'poison arrow' frogs. Interestingly, the word 'toxin' is derived from the Greek word *toxikon* (a poison) in which arrows were dipped prior to being fired from bows (*toxa*). Although extremely potent, many toxins have found a diverse range of clinical applications.[2]

The onset of signs and symptoms of exposure to biological agents may be preceded by a significant latent period (dependent on the particular pathogen) and can often be non-specific in presentation. However, clinical diagnosis may be assisted by the judicious use of appropriate clinical algorithms (see, for example, Figure 45.1). A more detailed account of the medical aspects of biological agents can be found elsewhere.[3,4]

Radioisotopes of relevance (see Table 45.1) may occur naturally in the environment or as a result of anthropogenic activities. In particular, there is concern over uncontrolled radioactive sources (arising from medical or nuclear industry sources) being used as starting material for 'dirty bombs', although a number of country-specific and international activities are in progress to limit or prevent the acquisition and distribution of such materials. Exposure to radioisotopes may cause non-specific and extensive damage to biomolecules such as DNA through various free radical-mediated reactions. The signs and symptoms of radiation exposure vary according to dose (Figure 45.2), and it is essential to seek early specialist advice if exposure is suspected. Further information on the health effects and medical management of radiation exposures is available elsewhere.[5]

Table 45.1 A representative selection of potentially hazardous materials

Category	Subcategory	Examples
Chemical	Nerve	Tabun (GA), sarin (GA), soman (GD), VX
	Vesicating (blistering)	Sulphur mustard (HD), nitrogen mustards (HN1, HN2, HN3), lewisite (L), phosgene oxime (CX)
	Lung (choking)	Chlorine, phosgene (CG), diphosgene (DP), sulphur dioxide
	Blood	Hydrogen cyanide (AC), cyanogen chloride (CK), arsine (SA)
	Riot control	CS gas (*o*-chlorobenzylidinemalonitrile), CN (chloroacetophenone), CR (dibenzoxazepine)
Biological	Bacterial	Anthrax, brucellosis, cholera, glanders, melioidosis, plague, salmonella, tularaemia, typhoid
	Viral	Ebola, influenza, Lassa fever, Marburg fever, Q-fever, Rift Valley fever, smallpox, Venezuelan equine encephalitis, yellow fever
	Toxins	Abrin, ricin, botulinum, saxitoxin, *Staphylococcus* enterotoxins
Radioisotopes		Americium-241, caesium-137, cobalt-60, iodine-131, plutonium (238 and 239), polonium-210, radium-226, strontium-90, technetium-99m, thorium-232, tritium (3H), uranium (233 and 238)

Letters in brackets refer to standard military designations.

<1 sievert	1–8 sievert	6–20 sievert	>20 sievert
Usually asymptomatic	**Haematopoetic syndrome**	**Gastrointestinal syndrome**	**CNS/CVS syndrome**
• Symptoms mild (or absent)	• Anorexia nausea, vomiting, fatigue: 1–4 hours post exposure (timing and severity dose related)	• Early nausea, vomiting, diarrhoea, anorexia, fatigue	• Almost immediate projectile vomiting, explosive bloody diarrhoea, headache, collapse, confusion, loss of consciousness, agitation, burning sensation on skin
• Episodic nausea, vomiting in first 48 hours in 1–10%		• Latent period: hours–1 week	
• Mildly depressed WBC at 2–4 weeks	• Latent period 2 days–4 weeks	• Severe GI symptoms (fever, abdominal pain, cramps, watery diarrhoea, haemorrhage. Electrolyte imbalance, dehydration) coupled with bone marrow suppression	• May be lucid interval (hours)
• No fetal effects if effective dose <100 millisievert	• Bone marrow depression: leukopenia – infection; low platelets – bleeding, bruising		• Neurobiological and cardiovascular symptoms predominate: convulsions, coma, hypotension, shock
	• Serial lymphocyte counts in first 48 hours predict severity	• LD_{100} is 10 sievert, death usually within 2 weeks	• Death within 2–3 days
	• 3–4 sievert: hair loss 2–3 weeks post exposure		
	• LD_{50} is 4.5 sievert in absence of treatment		

Figure 45.2 Signs and symptoms of radiation exposure according to dose. CNS, central nervous system; CVS, cardiovascular system; GI, gastrointestinal; LD_{50}, LD_{100} lethal dose for 50 and 100 per cent of the population, respectively; WBC, white blood cells. (Adapted from Health Protection Agency,[44] with permission.)

GENERIC EMERGENCY PROCEDURES

For the purpose of emergency preparedness, it is essential to have generic procedures available to counter the hazard posed by a chemical, biological or radiological incident. Fortunately, during the early stages of a confirmed deliberate release incident, the model response for all three categories of agent should be essentially the same: disrobe, decontaminate and corral up-wind (to prevent re-exposure) prior to transport to a holding area or medical facility.

Disrobing (Figure 45.3) at the earliest possible moment is a simple and effective countermeasure that can reasonably be expected to remove the majority of a contaminant from a casualty. However, great care should be exercised to avoid spreading contamination from clothing to the casualty. Ideally, clothes should be cut away, particularly items that are normally passed over the head (such as T-shirts, jumpers, vests, etc.).

Quantitatively, it is often stated that the act of disrobing can remove 80 per cent of contamination. It is not clear

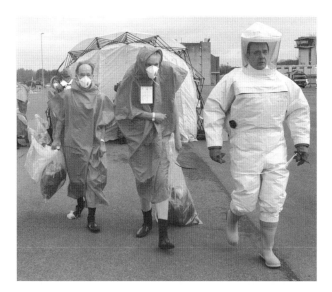

Figure 45.3 Disrobe procedure: casualties wearing a standard UK disrobe pack (a hooded poncho, oronasal particle mask, socks and shoes). Personal belongings are carried in a tagged, sealed bag. The casualties are being led to a decontamination unit by a medical officer in full personal protective ensemble. (© Health Protection Agency (2008),[44] reproduced with permission.)

whether this figure has been derived from experimental evidence or has simply attained authoritative status through multiple citations. However, using the simple 'rule of nines' for calculating body surface area and assuming negligible penetration of clothing by a toxic material, the figure of 80 per cent does not seem unrealistic, although the actual amount removed will be primarily dependent on the nature of the contaminant: liquid chemicals are likely to penetrate clothing to a greater extent than particles, so a correspondingly smaller proportion of the liquid contaminant is likely to be removed. Furthermore, the quantity of penetrating chemical removed is likely to be inversely proportional to the length of time between contamination and the onset of disrobing.

The aim of decontamination is to remove hazardous materials from the hair, nail and skin surfaces of affected individuals and serves three main purposes:

1. to prevent further systemic absorption and so limit the severity of intoxication;
2. to prevent the spread of hazardous material from a contaminated area ('hot zone') to a clean environment ('cold zone');
3. to protect emergency responders from the risk of secondary contamination.[6]

There is a common misconception that a delay following contamination will necessarily render the act of decontamination ineffective. This assumption arises from the military doctrine of implementing personal decontamination procedures within 2 minutes of exposure. It should be noted that the military objective of decontamination is to ensure that combatants continue to be fit to fight, so rapid action is required to prevent any overt signs of intoxication. From a public health perspective, a delay prior to the onset of decontamination is inevitable. Although this may potentially result in the onset of pathological sequelae, decontamination will remain to be of benefit to the patient, especially in the case of chemicals that form a reservoir within the superficial skin layer (stratum corneum) such as sulphur mustard and VX.[7–10]

There are clear benefits to removing this adsorbed material even after some considerable delay. First, extraction of the reservoir will prevent further systemic absorption. Second, the reservoir provides a source for off-gassing (the vaporization of adsorbed material from the skin to the environment, which can result in toxicologically significant concentrations being established within enclosed or unventilated environments) after exposure.[11,12] Finally, the reservoir represents a significant contact hazard to unprotected individuals, and this has been demonstrated in previous studies using human volunteers exposed to sulphur mustard.[13] In summary, the primary aim of decontaminating civilians is to save lives, not maintain an effective fighting force! Therefore, a distinction should be made when considering these two disparate objectives of decontamination.

The majority of mass casualty decontamination systems utilize water to which excipients such as detergents and bleach (hypochlorite) may be added. The incorporation of a detergent is important in order to facilitate the dissolution of hydrophobic chemicals (such as sulphur mustard) and thus improve effectiveness. Historically, bleach has been widely used, but its actual biocidal or chemical-neutralizing properties are questionable at the relatively low concentrations required to avoid dermal and ocular irritation.

In the UK, two main types of decontamination unit are available for deployment to CBRN incidents. The Fire and Rescue Service operate mass casualty decontamination tents that can quickly process large numbers of individuals (Figure 45.4) or a smaller number of non-ambulant casualties (Figure 45.5). In comparison, the Ambulance Service has smaller units that are designed for a lower throughput of non-ambulant patients and walking wounded, either at the scene of an incident or following deployment to casualty-receiving hospitals (Figure 45.6). In both types of system, casualties are showered with warm (37 °C) water containing up to 5 per cent detergent for 3–10 minutes, with the effluent being diverted to bunds for appropriate disposal to prevent environmental contamination. Although providing a generic capability across the CBRN spectrum, more specific decontamination procedures are available for some chemicals.[14]

There has been some debate about the relevance of disrobe and decontamination procedures following exposure to vapours and gases. It has consistently been assumed that such a practice is unnecessary: removal to a clean environment was deemed sufficient to remove traces

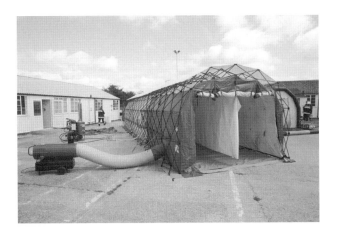

Figure 45.4 A UK mass casualty decontamination unit operated by the UK Fire and Rescue Service. Air and water heaters supply the re-robing area (foreground) and shower area (background), respectively. (© Health Protection Agency (2008),[44] reproduced with permission.)

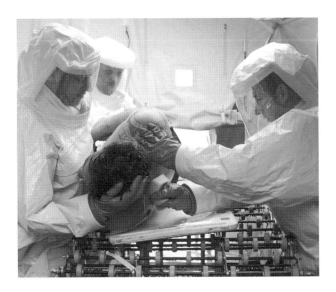

Figure 45.5 Ambulance Service staff conducting the decontamination of non-ambulant casualties within a mass casualty decontamination facility. (© Health Protection Agency (2008),[44] reproduced with permission.)

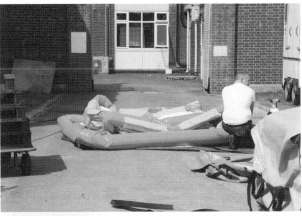

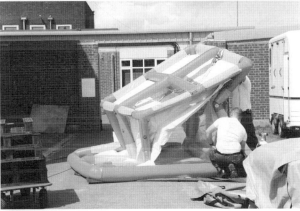

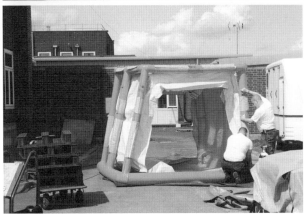

Figure 45.6 An example of a UK National Health Service rapid deployment decontamination unit. This series of photographs was taken over 1 minute. The unit is inflated using compressed air. Following erection, the unit is then connected to standard water hydrant water, which is passed through a water heater to the shower heads. Effluent is pumped to a collection bund (not shown). (© Health Protection Agency (2008),[44] reproduced with permission.)

of contaminant. However, the unexpectedly high incidence of secondary contamination of medical staff at hospitals receiving casualties from the Tokyo subway incident (from casualties exposed only to sarin vapour) has clearly challenged this dogma.[15,16] Thus, it may be prudent in cases of exposure to toxic vapours or gases to conduct a 'dry decontamination' procedure, that is, disrobing in the absence of decontamination to reduce secondary contamination.

There is an often overlooked problem to consider before conducting disrobe and decontamination procedures, especially in cooler climates – that of hypothermia. There

have been many instances during training exercises where role-playing casualties have required medical treatment for hypothermia following decontamination. It has not been uncommon for this to occur in otherwise fit and healthy adults. Therefore, the decision to conduct disrobe and decontamination should not be taken lightly, and guidance has recently been developed[17] that incorporates a decision-making algorithm for incident managers (Figure 45.7).

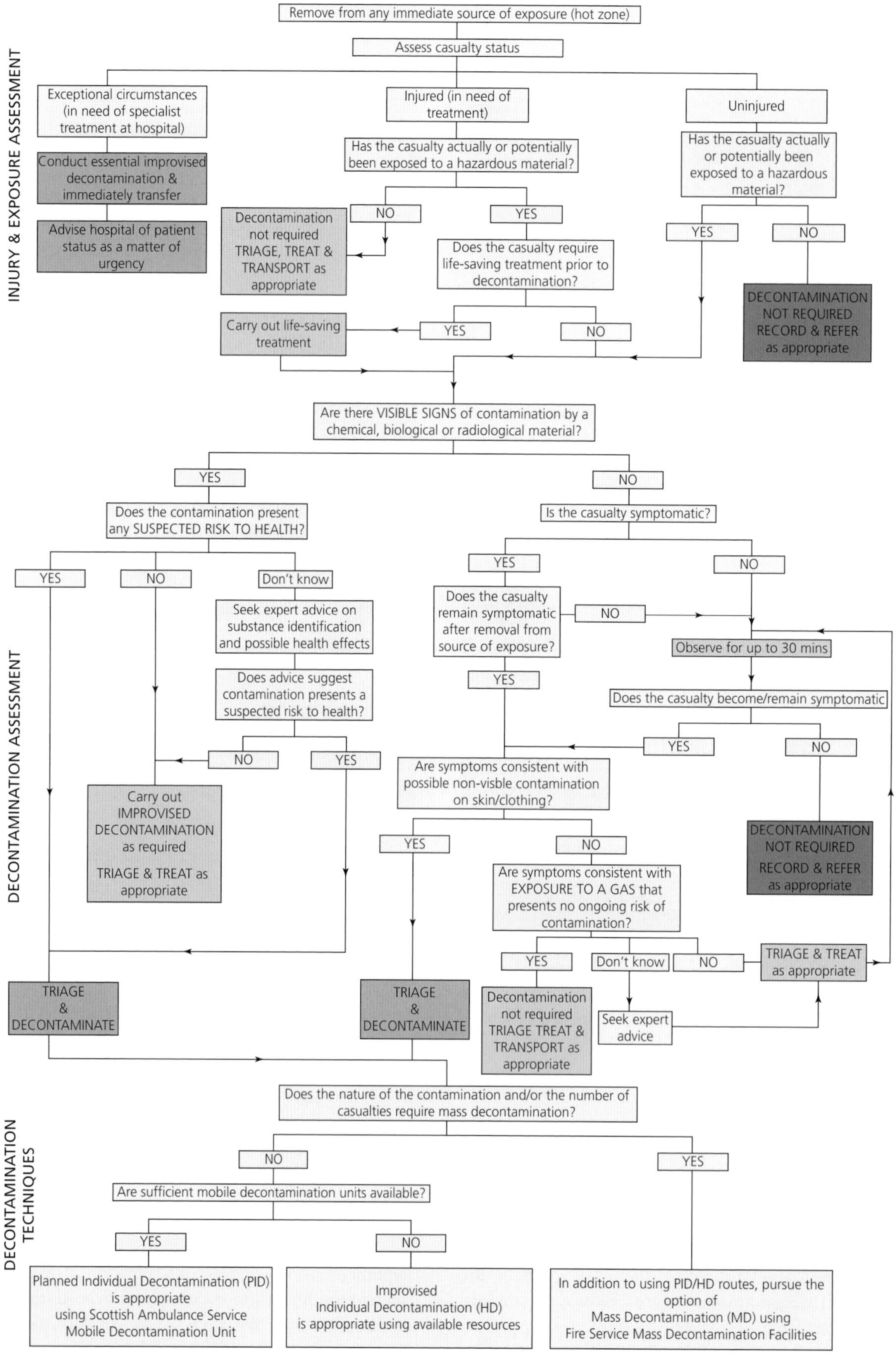

Figure 45.7 Scottish CBRN and Hazmat Decontamination Algorithm. (Reproduced from Health Protection Scotland,[17] with permission.)

It is worth giving brief consideration here to the 'worried well' and the corresponding phenomena of mass psychogenic pathology. Although not necessarily requiring decontamination, a dose of warm soapy water may be an effective antidote for such patients and certainly provides reassurance that 'something is being done'.

Following disrobing, decontamination and triage, casualties requiring further treatment should be transported under controlled conditions to an appropriate medical facility. Control of this process will facilitate immediate treatment without the need for further decontamination. However, it is likely that a number of potentially exposed individuals may self-present, so decontamination facilities should be available at hospitals.[18] Such on-site facilities may be integrated into the construction of a medical facility or, where this is impractical, rapid-deployment units should be available. In the UK, the latter are provided as inflatable structures with staff operating in full protective equipment (see Figure 45.6 above).

OVERVIEW OF THE TOXICOLOGY AND TREATMENT OF SOME CHEMICAL WARFARE AGENTS

This section will mainly concentrate on chemical warfare agents, specifically nerve, blister and lung-damaging agents; more comprehensive texts are available.[19,20] During the early stages of a deliberate release incident, the causative agent may not be identified. Indeed, the incident itself may not have become apparent. However, this is unlikely to preclude the administration of standard emergency therapies, such as oxygen for suspected exposure to lung-damaging and choking agents (subject to normal contraindications, for example suspected exposure to paraquat) or 'triple therapy' of oxime, an anticonvulsant and atropine for anticholinesterase exposure. Diagnostic algorithms (Figure 45.8) may be a useful aide-memoir during these early stages and the subsequent diagnosis, if indicative only of exposure to a certain class of chemical rather than to a specific material, may provide vital 'medical intelligence' for others coordinating or managing the incident response.

Nerve (anticholinesterase) agents

'Nerve agent' is the collective term for chemicals that cause a cholinergic crisis. This effect is primarily mediated through an inhibition of acetylcholinesterase (AChE), the enzyme responsible for the normal clearance of neurotransmitter (acetylcholine) from the neuromuscular junction and synaptic clefts of cholinergic systems.

Nerve agents were first synthesized in Germany prior to World War II, these being referred to as G-agents. During the 1950s, a second series of nerve agents was discovered by workers in the UK that were generally more toxic than G-agents. These became known as V-agents ('V' for venomous) and include VE, VM and VX, the latter of which was stockpiled by a number of countries.[21] Although they are mainly considered as chemical warfare agents, the genre of nerve agents can potentially include a number of organophosphate and carbamate-based insecticides that have notable human toxicity.[22,23] Nerve agents gained further notoriety in 1995 following the use of GB (sarin) by terrorists on the Tokyo subway system, which resulted in a number of deaths and several thousand cases of poisoning.[24] This was preceded by several months by an attack on three individuals by the same terrorist group using VX.[25]

Nerve agents are among the most toxic chemicals ever produced on an industrial scale, with estimates for human inhalation toxicity ranging from 10 to 400 mg per minute per m^3. Under normal environmental conditions, nerve agents can be encountered as solids, liquids or vapours. Liquid agents can readily penetrate skin and mucous membranes. Nerve agent vapour does not penetrate skin in substantial quantities but can be absorbed across the cornea to produce miosis. Absorption of vapour by the lung is generally more rapid in terms of onset of signs and symptoms than dermal absorption following liquid contamination.

The clinical features of nerve agent exposure reflect the cholinergic crisis arising from an accumulation of acetylcholine at the muscarininc and nicotininic receptors of the peripheral and central nervous systems (Table 45.2), the onset and severity of which are dependent on the route of entry and dose. For more volatile nerve agents (such as sarin, soman and tabun), exposure to vapour is the most likely scenario, so initial effects will be rapid (seconds to minutes) and initially limited to the eyes (miosis) and respiratory system (bronchospasm, bronchorrhoea and rhinorrhoea). In contrast, the effects of dermal exposure to liquid nerve agents (which include less volatile materials such as VX and carbamate/organophosphate pesticides) can be delayed by minutes to hours and may initially include localized signs such as sweating and fasciculations of the underlying muscles.

If the patient is untreated, systemic effects may develop. These include general muscle weakness, abdominal cramps, nausea, vomiting, involuntary micturition/defecation, anxiety, pallor, headache and confusion followed by convulsions and respiratory arrest (apnoea). It should be noted that paradoxical responses may (occasionally) occur that are inconsistent with cholinergic crisis, for example mydriasis, hypertension and tachycardia (Table 45.2).

Although it is standard clinical practice to measure plasma or erythrocyte AChE activity in patients presenting with signs and symptoms of nerve agent poisoning, AChE inhibition should be considered only as an indicator of intoxication and not as a prognostic aid or guide to therapy.[26–28]

A potentially fatal consequence of nerve agent exposure is respiratory failure: the maintenance of respiration

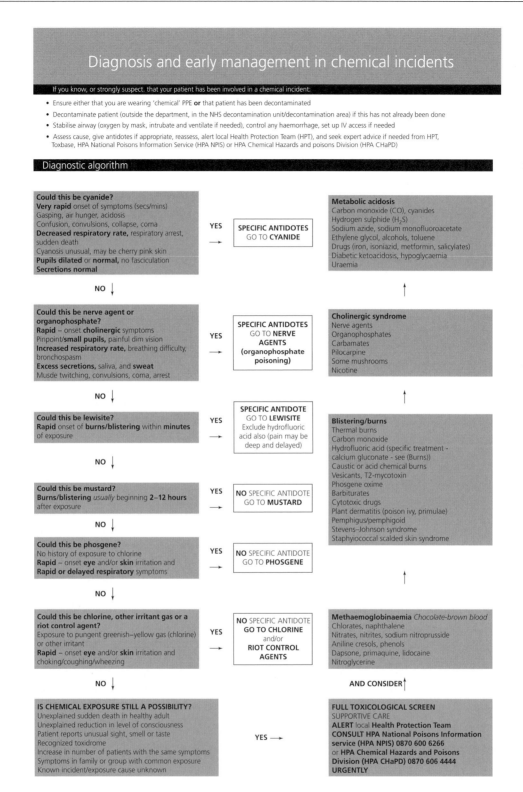

Diagnosis and early management in chemical incidents

If you know, or strongly suspect, that your patient has been involved in a chemical incident:

- Ensure either that you are wearing 'chemical' PPE **or** that patient has been decontaminated
- Decontaminate patient (outside the department, in the NHS decontamination unit/decontamination area) if this has not already been done
- Stabilise airway (oxygen by mask, intubate and ventilate if needed), control any haemorrhage, set up IV access if needed
- Assess cause, give antidotes if appropriate, reassess, alert local Health Protection Team (HPT), and seek expert advice if needed from HPT, Toxbase, HPA National Poisons Information Service (HPA NPIS) or HPA Chemical Hazards and poisons Division (HPA CHaPD)

Diagnostic algorithm

Could this be cyanide?
Very rapid onset of symptoms (secs/mins)
Gasping, air hunger, acidosis
Confusion, convulsions, collapse, coma
Decreased respiratory rate, respiratory arrest, sudden death
Cyanosis unusual, may be cherry pink skin
Pupils dilated or **normal,** no fasciculation
Secretions normal

YES → SPECIFIC ANTIDOTES GO TO **CYANIDE**

Metabolic acidosis
Carbon monoxide (CO), cyanides
Hydrogen sulphide (H_2S)
Sodium azide, sodium monofluoroacetate
Ethylene glycol, alcohols, toluene
Drugs (iron, isoniazid, metformin, salicylates)
Diabetic ketoacidosis, hypoglycaemia
Uraemia

NO ↓

Could this be nerve agent or organophosphate?
Rapid – onset **cholinergic** symptoms
Pinpoint/**small pupils,** painful dim vision
Increased respiratory rate, breathing difficulty, bronchospasm
Excess secretions, saliva, and **sweat**
Muscle twitching, convulsions, coma, arrest

YES → SPECIFIC ANTIDOTES GO TO **NERVE AGENTS (organophosphate poisoning)**

Cholinergic syndrome
Nerve agents
Organophosphates
Carbamates
Pilocarpine
Some mushrooms
Nicotine

NO ↓

Could this be lewisite?
Rapid onset of **burns/blistering** within **minutes** of exposure

YES → SPECIFIC ANTIDOTE GO TO **LEWISITE** Exclude hydrofluoric acid also (pain may be deep and delayed)

Blistering/burns
Thermal burns
Carbon monoxide
Hydrofluoric acid (specific treatment - calcium gluconate - see (Burns)
Caustic or acid chemical burns
Vesicants, T2-mycotoxin
Phosgene oxime
Barbiturates
Cytotoxic drugs
Plant dermatitis (poison ivy, primulae)
Pemphigus/pemphigoid
Stevens–Johnson syndrome
Staphylococcal scalded skin syndrome

NO ↓

Could this be mustard?
Burns/blistering *usually* beginning **2–12 hours** after exposure

YES → NO SPECIFIC ANTIDOTE GO TO **MUSTARD**

NO ↓

Could this be phosgene?
No history of exposure to chlorine
Rapid – onset **eye** and/or **skin** irritation and
Rapid or delayed respiratory symptoms

YES → NO SPECIFIC ANTIDOTE GO TO **PHOSGENE**

NO ↓

Could this be chlorine, other irritant gas or a riot control agent?
Exposure to pungent greenish–yellow gas (chlorine) or other irritant
Rapid – onset **eye** and/or **skin** irritation and choking/coughing/wheezing

YES → NO SPECIFIC ANTIDOTE **GO TO CHLORINE** and/or **RIOT CONTROL AGENTS**

Methaemoglobinaemia *Chocolate-brown blood*
Chlorates, naphthalene
Nitrates, nitrites, sodium nitroprusside
Aniline cresols, phenols
Dapsone, primaquine, lidocaine
Nitroglycerine

AND CONSIDER ↑

NO ↓

IS CHEMICAL EXPOSURE STILL A POSSIBILITY?
Unexplained sudden death in healthy adult
Unexplained reduction in level of consciousness
Patient reports unusual sight, smell or taste
Recognized toxidrome
Increase in number of patients with the same symptoms
Symptoms in family or group with common exposure
Known incident/exposure cause unknown

YES →

FULL TOXICOLOGICAL SCREEN
SUPPORTIVE CARE
ALERT local **Health Protection Team**
CONSULT HPA National Poisons Information service (HPA NPIS) 0870 600 6266
or **HPA Chemical Hazards and Poisons Division (HPA CHaPD) 0870 606 4444**
URGENTLY

Figure 45.8 Example of a diagnostic algorithm for putative chemical exposures. HPA, Health Protection Agency; IV, intravenous; NHS, National Health Service; PPE, personal protective equipment. (Reproduced from Health Protection Agency,[44] with permission.)

(concomitant with the administration of antidotes) may significantly improve the chances of recovery, so an effective ventilation strategy (using oxygen) is important.

The standard treatment for nerve agent poisoning is the immediate administration of a 'triple therapy' comprising a cholinolytic, an oxime reactivator and an anticonvulsant. (It should be noted that the term 'cholinolytic', although widely used to describe the effects of antidotes such as muscarinic antagonists, is technically incorrect.) Atropine is the cholinolytic drug of choice and should be given intramuscularly or preferably intravenously as soon as possible after poisoning. Early administration is

Table 45.2 Summary of signs and symptoms of nerve agent poisoning

Organ (and main receptor)		Signs or symptoms
Smooth muscle (muscarinic)	Iris	Miosis[†]
	Gastrointestinal tract	Abdominal cramps, diarrhoea, involuntary defecation
	Bladder	Involuntary micturition
	Heart	Bradycardia[†]
Glands (muscarinic)	Nasal mucosa	Rhinorrhoea
	Bronchial mucosa	Bronchorrhoea
	Sweat	Hyperhidrosis
	Lachrymal	Lachrymation
Skeletal muscle (nicotinic)		Weakness, fasciculations
Central nervous system (nicotinic and muscarinic)		Anxiety, headache, confusion, convulsions, respiratory depression, respiratory arrest

[†] These effects may occasionally be replaced with paradoxical effects resulting from nicotinic stimulation within the autonomic ganglia (sympathetic response), resulting in mydriasis and tachycardia.

critical as the severity of signs and symptoms may progress rapidly. However, the excessive use of atropine should be avoided as the consequential drying of bronchial secretions may render them difficult to remove, large doses of atropine may induce arrhythmias (particularly in the case of myocardial hypoxia due to respiratory failure) and bladder dysfunction may necessitate transurethral catheterization.

Being a muscarinic antagonist, atropine has no effect on the nicotinic receptors of the neuromuscular junction and so cannot relieve paralysis of the respiratory and skeletal muscles. Therefore, oximes such as pralidoxime and obidoxime (Toxogonin) are used to reactivate AChE and so reverse paralysis. However, the effectiveness of reactivation is dependent on the oxime administered and the actual toxic agent. For example, pralidoxime is relatively ineffective compared with obidoxime for the treatment of tabun (GA) exposure. However, as discussed earlier, it is unlikely that the precise identity of the causative agent will be known at the start of an incident, so the selection of the most efficacious oxime is, at least during the initial stages of an incident, unlikely to be an option.

Pralidoxime methanesulphonate (pralidoxime mesylate or P2S) is currently the oxime of choice and should be administered via the intramuscular or intravenous route as soon as possible after the onset of signs and symptoms of nerve agent exposure. Adverse effects of oximes include headache, disturbances of vision and muscular weakness, so care should be taken to monitor the patient's condition before and after administration to permit differentiation between the signs of deepening nerve agent intoxication and the side-effects of therapy.

Nerve agent poisoning may be complicated by convulsions, the control of which using benzodiazepines (such as diazepam) has been shown to enhance the likelihood of survival.[29,30]

Skin-damaging (blistering or vesicating) agents

Vesicant compounds were first introduced to the battlefield during World War I. Mustard gas was particularly effective, with 14 000 British casualties being produced during the first 3 months of its use and 120 000 by the end of the war.[31] Although effective in producing casualties, it carried only a low lethality (approximately 2 per cent). Other agents of this genre include phosgene oxime ('nettle gas'), T-2 mycotoxin, nitrogen mustards and lewisite (also known as the 'dew of death' on account of its systemic toxicity). This section will concentrate on the effects of sulphur mustard.

Sulphur mustard is widely known as 'mustard gas'. This is an inappropriate term as the compound is a liquid at room temperature (with a freezing point of around 14 °C) and gives off a vapour resembling mustard, garlic or leeks as a result of impurities. When prepared as a pure product, the smell of mustard can be described as 'sweet and agreeable'. Sulphur mustard (military designation 'H') has often been referred to as HS (HunStoff) or more commonly 'HD' (specifically pertaining to the distilled product).

Sulphur mustard is poorly miscible with water, and this, in combination with its low freezing point, leads to a lengthy persistence of the compound in cooler environments, particularly if protected from the wind and rain. Sulphur mustard vapour passes quickly through normal clothing (including leather), although most modern protective clothing is relatively impermeable. In the liquid state, sulphur mustard passes quickly through ordinary surgical gloves, so heavy gloves (made of butyl rubber or neoprene) should be worn when decontaminating casualties.

Sulphur mustard is toxic via ingestion and exposure of the skin, lung and eyes. In comparison with the nerve agents, sulphur mustard is not generally considered to be a lethal agent. Its intended effect on the battlefield is to disable rather than kill and, on a weight-for-weight basis, sulphur mustard can be considered equipotent to nerve agents in this respect.

The actual mechanism of action of sulphur mustard is largely unknown, although the subsequent dermal, ocular and pulmonary lesions have been well defined.[32-34] The effects of mustard on target organs vary according dose and physical state (i.e. liquid or vapour). However, the following organ-specific generalizations can be made.

Skin effects following exposure to mustard vapour become apparent after a latent period of 1–24 hours with the onset of erythema. The latent period is inversely proportional to dose: high concentrations have a short latency period and vice versa. If sufficient exposure has occurred, blisters will subsequently appear after 2–18 hours. Again, the duration of the latency period is dose dependent, and it may take several days for these lesions to develop fully. Above a threshold dose of approximately $10\,\mu g/cm^2$, exposure to undiluted liquid mustard will invariably result in blister formation, and significant contamination may result in a 'doughnut blister' comprising a central area of necrotic tissue surrounded by a ring of blister(s). The affected skin subsequently undergoes necrosis with the formation of an eschar, from around 3 days after exposure, which may then either slough or enter a cycle of sloughing and eschar formation for several weeks. Altered pigmentation (hyper- or hypopigmentation) has been reported, which may persist for months to years after exposure.

The eyes are the most sensitive target organ and, as with the skin, may be subject to an asymptomatic latent period prior to the onset of injury. In general, the ocular latency period is shorter than for dermal lesions. Following exposure to vapour, initial signs may include conjunctivitis and blepharospasm, sometimes accompanied by photophobia. More substantial exposure may cause corneal damage resulting in oedema and cloudiness of vision, which may start to improve after 7 days. Exposure to higher doses may result in permanent scarring between the iris and lens. Ocular contamination with liquid mustard will invariably cause severe damage, with corneal perforation, opacification and deep scarring, possibly leading to permanent blindness.

The pulmonary effects of mustard are largely confined to the conducting airways, with damage being particularly marked in the larger airways. At higher doses, severe damage to the submucosa and other layers of the airway wall may occur. In the deeper lung, damage is usually less marked, although severe exposure can produce haemorrhagic pulmonary oedema.

In addition to the eyes, respiratory system and skin, exposure to significant quantities of sulphur mustard may lead to systemic effects, most notably aplastic anaemia due to damage to the bone marrow.[35] In mustard gas casualties, the peripheral white cell count has been observed to begin to fall on about the fourth day after exposure (following an initial post-exposure rise).

There is no specific therapy for sulphur mustard gas, and no antidote has been demonstrated to be clinically effective in removing mustard from the body. Despite this, appropriate treatment can ameliorate the more severe effects and prevent opportunistic infection.

Large blisters should be subject to aseptic aspiration. It has been erroneously assumed that blister fluid contains free mustard and so may represent a significant hazard to medical staff. This is incorrect,[36] as is also the case for lewisite blisters. Following aspiration, blisters should be covered with sterile dry dressings. Silver sulfadiazine cream (Flamazine) has been widely used and is useful in preventing secondary infection. For deeper (full-thickness) burns, skin grafting should be considered as this may increase the rate of healing. Recent studies have demonstrated that physical removal of necrotic tissue from partial-thickness burns may significantly enhance healing rates.[37,38]

The current treatment for eye exposure includes daily saline irrigations, the application of petroleum jelly to the follicular margins to prevent sticking and antibacterial (e.g. chloramphenicol) eye drops to prevent infection. Mydriatics (e.g. hyoscine drops) have been used to prevent irido-lenticular adhesions and to reduce pain caused by spasm of the ciliary muscle. It has been suggested that if eye pain is particularly severe, local anaesthetic drops (such as amethocaine hydrochloride) be applied, although expert ophthalmological opinion should be sought before commencing local anaesthetic or corticosteroid treatment. Antioxidant drops (potassium ascorbate 10 per cent and sodium citrate 10 per cent, alternately) have also been recommended. Sunglasses can be used to alleviate photophobia. Most importantly, constant reassurance that blindness will not be produced should be given where deemed appropriate, with advice that recovery will occur (albeit slowly).

Antibiotic cover is recommended if the respiratory effects are more than very mild. Codeine linctus is of value in preventing coughing at night. Betamethasone has been claimed to be of benefit for enhanced regeneration of the airway epithelium,[39] although no clinical trials of glucocorticoids in sulphur mustard injuries of the respiratory tract have been reported. Very severe respiratory damage may demand intensive care, and respiratory physicians and anaesthetists should be consulted if evidence of deteriorating respiratory function appears.

Lung-damaging agents (pulmonary oedemogens)

During World War I, the chemical warfare compounds with the highest lethality were those which induced pulmonary oedema, such as chlorine and phosgene. Approximately 85 per cent of deaths resulting from exposure to chemical warfare compounds during World War I were caused by phosgene.[40] In a civilian context, chlorine and phosgene are of particular concern as they are widely used in industry. The possibility of a terrorist organization releasing a large quantity of chlorine needs careful consideration: chlorine was effective when released from cylinders in World War I, and similar activities have recently been conducted by insurgents in Iraq.

Phosgene is rapidly dispersed by the wind. However, it may linger in low-lying areas such as cellars, tunnels and hollows as it is heavier than air. The skin is impermeable to phosgene, so the primary route of absorption is the lung. Systemic effects are unlikely to occur as its reactivity is such that hydrolysis (to hydrochloric acid, carbon dioxide and water) is complete before penetration of the epithelial lining of the lungs can occur.[41]

The exact mechanism of action of phosgene remains obscure but is likely to involve free radical formation, a decline in intracellular cyclic AMP with an increase in capillary permeability and an associated decrease in tissue glutathione levels leading to activation of transcription factors for genes controlling the production of inflammatory mediators.[42] The outcome is a permeability-induced pulmonary oedema (as opposed to a hydrostatic pulmonary oedema).

Some have described eye irritation, coughing, lachrymation, choking and a feeling of tightness of the chest as early signs and symptoms of phosgene exposure. However, observations during World War I have indicated that the absence of such effects does not preclude serious or potentially fatal exposure. Phosgene is particularly insidious as inhalation of a lethal dose of the compound can be followed by a symptomless latent period varying (according to dose) from 30 minutes to 1 day.[43] During this latent period, it is notoriously difficult to distinguish between mild or severe exposure, and a lethal, florid pulmonary oedema can be provoked following physical exertion.[31] Therefore, if phosgene exposure is suspected, absolute bed rest for at least 24 hours is strongly advocated even in the absence of any signs or symptoms.

Following the latent period, dyspnoea, painful cough and cyanosis may rapidly appear. Increasing quantities of (initially whitish but later pink) fluid are expectorated, with a marked efflux of fluid (the 'champignon d'écume') sometimes appearing immediately prior to death. The cause of death is usually cardiac failure and circulatory collapse caused by hypoxia.

In the first instance, patients reporting a putative exposure to phosgene should, as mentioned above, be confined to bed for at least 24 hours. The management of phosgene poisoning is concerned primarily with pulmonary oedema. There is no specific antidote of any proven value. Steroids, antibiotics, bronchodilators, respiratory stimulants and cardiac stimulants have all been suggested, although none has received universal support. However, it is generally agreed that supplementary oxygen be administered. As in all cases of permeability pulmonary oedema, the administration of intravenous fluids should be approached with great caution.

SUMMARY

The deliberate release of hazardous materials to cause adverse health effects is commonly perceived as a modern-day problem, although such activities are woven into the fabric of human history. Although there are a vast number of materials that potentially exhibit the requisite chemical, biological or radioactive properties such as to pose a serious risk to public health, good preparation, the provision of a generic response and appropriate medical countermeasures should effectively mitigate the extent of a terrorist incident.

REFERENCES

◆ = Major review article

1. Oser BL. Toxicology then and now. *Regul Toxicol Pharmacol* 1987; **7**: 427–43.
2. Philippe G, Angenot L. Recent developments in the field of arrow and dart poisons. *J Ethnopharmacol* 2005; **100**: 85–91.
3. Murray PR, Baron EJ, Pfaller MA, Tenover FC, Yolken RH, eds. *Manual of Clinical Microbiology*, 7th edn. Washington, DC: American Society for Microbiology, 1996.
4. Baron S, ed. *Medical Microbiology*, 4th edn. Galveston, TX: University of Texas Medical Branch, 1996.
5. International Atomic Energy Agency. *Generic Procedures for Medical Response During a Nuclear or Radiological Emergency*. New York: International Atomic Energy Agency and World Health Organization, 2005.
6. Roberts G, Maynard RL. Responding to chemical terrorism: operational planning and decontamination. In: Marrs TC, Maynard RL, Sidell FR, eds. *Chemical Warfare Agents: Toxicology and Treatment*. Chichester: Wiley, 2008: 175–90.
7. Chilcott RP, Dalton CH, Hill I *et al*. In vivo skin absorption and distribution of the nerve agent VX (O-ethyl-S-[2(diisopropylamino)ethyl] methylphosphonothioate) in the domestic white pig. *Hum Exp Toxicol* 2005; **24**: 347–52.
8. Chilcott RP, Dalton CH, Hill I *et al*. Evaluation of a barrier cream against the chemical warfare agent VX using the domestic white pig. *Basic Clin Pharmacol Toxicol* 2005; **97**: 35–58.
9. Chilcott RP, Jenner J, Carrick W, Hotchkiss SA, Rice P. Human skin absorption of Bis-2-(chloroethyl)sulphide (sulphur mustard) in vitro. *J Appl Toxicol* 2000; **20**: 349–55.
10. Hattersley IJ, Jenner J, Dalton C, Chilcott RP, Graham JS. The skin reservoir of sulphur mustard. *Toxicol In Vitro* 2008; **22**: 1539–46.
11. Logan TP, Graham JS, Martin JL, Zallnick JE, Jakubowski EM, Braue EH. Detection and measurement of sulfur mustard offgassing from the weanling pig following exposure to saturated sulfur mustard vapor. *J Appl Toxicol* 2000; **20**(Suppl. 1): S199–204.
12. Chilcott RP, Jenner J, Hotchkiss SA, Rice P. In vitro skin absorption and decontamination of sulphur mustard: comparison of human and pig-ear skin. *J Appl Toxicol* 2001; **21**: 279–83.

13. Smith HW, Clowes GHA, Marshall EK. On dichloroethylsulfide (mustard gas). IV: The mechanism of absorption by the skin. *J Pharmacol Exp Ther* 1919; **13**: 1–30.

14. Chilcott RP. Dermal aspects of chemical warfare agents. In: Marrs TC, Maynard RL, Sidell FR, eds. *Chemical Warfare Agents: Toxicology and Treatment*, 2nd edn. Chichester: Wiley, 2008: 409–22.

15. Ohbu S, Yamashina A, Takasu N et al. Sarin poisoning on Tokyo subway. *South Med J* 1997; **90**: 587–93.

16. Rodgers JC. Chemical incident planning: a review of the literature. *Accid Emerg Nurs* 1998; **6**: 155–9.

17. Hankin SM, Keatings J, Ramsay CN. *Report on an Evaluation of the Scottish CBRN & Hazmat Decontamination Algorithm (SCHDA)*. Glasgow: Health Protection Scotland, 2008.

18. Clarke SF, Chilcott RP, Wilson JC, Kamanyire R, Baker DJ, Hallett A. Decontamination of multiple casualties who are chemically contaminated: a challenge for acute hospitals. *Prehosp Disaster Med* 2008; **23**: 175–81.

♦19. Marrs TC, Maynard RL, Sidell FR. *Chemical Warfare Agents: Toxicology and Treatment*, 2nd edn. Chichester: Wiley, 2008.

20. Sidell FR, Takafuji ET, Franz DR. *Medical Aspects of Chemical and Biological Warfare*. Bethesda, MD: Office of the Surgeon General Department of the Army, United States of America, 1997.

21. Tammelin LE. Dialkoxy-phosphorylcholines, alkoxy-methyl-phosphorylthiocholines and analagous choline esters. *Acta Chem Scand* 1957; **11**: 1340–9.

22. Fuortes LJ, Ayebo AD, Kross BC. Cholinesterase-inhibiting insecticide toxicity. *Am Fam Phys* 1993; **47**: 1613–20.

23. Goel A, Aggarwal P. Pesticide poisoning. *Natl Med J India* 2007; **20**: 182–91.

24. Masuda N, Takatsu M, Morinari H, Ozawa T. Sarin poisoning in Tokyo subway. *Lancet* 1995; **345**: 1446.

25. Nozaki H, Aikawa N, Fujishima S et al. A case of VX poisoning and the difference from sarin. *Lancet* 1995; **346**: 698–9.

26. Chilcott RP, Dalton CH, Hill I, Davidson CM, Blohm KL, Hamilton MG. Clinical manifestations of VX poisoning following percutaneous exposure in the domestic white pig. *Hum Exp Toxicol* 2003; **22**: 255–61.

27. Jimmerson VR, Shih TM, Mailman RB. Variability in soman toxicity in the rat: correlation with biochemical and behavioral measures. *Toxicology* 1989; **57**: 241–54.

28. Willems JL. Clinical management of mustard gas casualties. *Ann Med Milit Belg* 1989; **3**: S1–61.

29. Lipp JA. Effect of diazepam upon soman-induced seizure activity and convulsions. *Electroencephalogr Clin Neurophysiol* 1972; **32**: 557–60.

30. Lipp JA. Effect of benzodiazepine derivatives on soman-induced seizure activity and convulsions in the monkey. *Arch Int Pharmacodyn Ther* 1973; **202**: 244–51.

31. MacPherson WG, Herringham WP, Elliott TR, Balfour A (eds). *History of the Great War Based on Official Documents*. Vol. II: *Medical Services. Diseases of the War*. London: HMSO, 1923.

32. Ireland MM. *Medical Aspects Of Mustard Gas Warfare*. Medical Department of the United States in the World War, Volume XIV. Washington, DC: Medical Department of the United States, 1926.

33. Mann I. An experimental and clinical study of the reaction of the anterior segment of the eye to chemical injury, with special reference to chemical warfare agents. *Br J Opthalmol* 1948; Monograph Supplement XIII.

34. Warthin AS, Weller CV. *The Medical Aspects of Mustard Gas Poisoning*. London: Henry Kimpton, 1919.

35. Smith RP. Toxic responses of the blood. In: Klaasen CD, Amdur MO, Doull J, eds. *Casarett and Doull's Toxicology: The Basic Science of Poisons*. London: Macmillan, 1986: 223–44.

36. Sulzberger MB, Katz JH. The absence of skin irritants in the contents of vesicles. *US Navy Med Bull* 1943; **41**: 1258–62.

37. Evison D, Brown RF, Rice P. The treatment of sulphur mustard burns with laser debridement. *J Plast Reconstr Aesthet Surg* 2006; **59**: 1087–93.

38. Rice P, Brown RF, Lam DG, Chilcott RP, Bennett NJ. Dermabrasion – a novel concept in the surgical management of sulphur mustard injuries. *Burns* 2000; **26**: 34–40.

39. Calvet JH, Coste A, Levame M, Harf A, Macquin-Mavier I, Escudier E. Airway epithelial damage induced by sulfur mustard in guinea pigs, effects of glucocorticoids. *Hum Exp Toxicol* 1996; **15**: 964–71.

40. HMSO. *Medical Manual of Defence Against Chemical Agents*. London: HMSO, 1972.

41. Nash T, Pattle RE. The absorption of phosgene by aqueous solutions and its relation to toxicity. *Ann Occup Hyg* 1971; **14**: 227–33.

42. Maynard RL, Chilcott RP. Toxicology of chemical warfare agents. In: Ballantyne B, Marrs TC, Syversen T, eds. *General and Applied Toxicology*, 3rd edn. Chichester: Wiley, 2009: 2876–911.

43. Vedder EB. *The Medical Aspects of Chemical Warfare*. Baltimore: Williams & Wilkins, 1925.

44. Heptonstall J, Gent N. *CBRN Incidents: Clinical Management and Health Protection*. London: Health Protection Agency, 2006.

46

Management of chemical incidents

VIRGINIA MURRAY

Society as a whole is extremely dependent upon chemicals. They are used daily in food production and preservation, water sanitation, housing, housekeeping and household equipment, transportation and health care.[1] This dependence is supported by a vigorous chemical industry, with distribution by a transport infrastructure of railway and road haulage, sea and air cargo. The continuing rapid growth and globalization of the chemicals industry means that incidents involving the inadvertent release of chemicals will almost inevitably continue to be a problem.

Chemical incidents are not infrequent and may occur as very rapidly obvious releases, such as chemical spills, fires and explosions, or as less immediately apparent events such as the contamination of a product or land contamination. Incidents can occur accidentally or deliberately. Some chemical incidents may have an impact beyond their original location, in some cases crossing national borders. For example, in north-west Romania, cyanide was released from a gold mine into the local river system, leading to fish deaths in three countries.[2] Chemical incidents that lead to human exposure present an important public health challenge both nationally and globally.

Since chemical incidents are so varied in nature they are difficult to define. As a result several definitions are used:

- The Health Protection Agency (HPA), UK, defines them as all incidents representing 'an acute event in which there is, or could be, exposure of the public to chemical substances which cause, or have the potential to cause, ill health'. All incidents with an off-site impact, as well as on-site incidents where members of the public are affected, are included in this definition and, for the purposes of the definition, hospital staff and emergency services personnel should be regarded as members of the public.[3]

- The South West London Health Protection Unit plan defines a chemical incident in two ways: 'An acute event in which there is, or could be, exposure of the public to chemical substances which cause, or have the potential to cause, ill-health' or 'Individuals suffering from a similar illness, which might be due to such event.'

- The International Programme on Chemical Safety (a joint activity of World Health Organization, the International Labour Organization and the United Nations Environment Programme) defines chemical incidents as incidents that, in actual or potential exposure of the public to a chemical substance or its hazardous by-products, caused, or had the potential to cause, ill-health. Incidents that occurred on industrial premises and only resulted in exposure to employees were excluded.[4]

Table 46.1 lists some recent incidents resulting from explosions, fires, spills, leaks and other incidents of note (described as 'big bang' events); Table 46.2 provides some examples of recent incidents where clinical illness indicated that a chemical incident had occurred (often described as 'rising tide' events).

Every day in Britain, serious chemical incidents occur that threaten people's health, and the UK Health Protection Agency provides authoritative scientific and medical advice to the National Health Service and other bodies about the known health effects of chemicals, poisons and other environmental hazards.[5] Of the 1978 incidents recorded in

Table 46.1 Examples of some recent acute chemical incidents of note

Type of incident	Summary of event
Explosions and fires	
Buncefield explosion and fire, UK,[19] December 11th, 2005	In the early hours of Sunday December 11th, 2005, a number of explosions occurred at Buncefield Oil Storage Depot, Hemel Hempstead, Hertfordshire, UK. At least one of the initial explosions was of massive proportions, and there was a large fire, which engulfed a high proportion of the site. Over 40 people were injured, with no fatalities. Significant damage occurred to both commercial and residential properties in the vicinity, and a large area around the site was evacuated on emergency service advice. The fire burned for several days, destroying most of the site and emitting large clouds of black smoke into the atmosphere that travelled over the south of England and towards Europe
Enschede, Netherlands,[20] May 13th, 2000	A fire broke out within the SE Fireworks depot in the eastern Dutch city of Enschede on May 13th, 2000. The fire caused a massive explosion, killing 22 people and injuring over 900. Around 1500 homes were damaged or destroyed, and 1250 people were left homeless. The cost of the damage was estimated to be more than half a billion Euros. Emergency services from all around the area, including Germany, assisted at the scene
Toulouse, France,[21] September 21st, 2001	At 10.15 am on September 21st, 2001, a huge explosion occurred at the AZF (Azote de France) fertilizer factory, located 3 km (2 miles) from the centre of the city of Toulouse in France, the AZF factory being located next to a phosgene plant. The explosion shattered shop and car windows and tore doors from their hinges in the city centre. Over 500 houses became uninhabitable. At least 29 people were killed, and thousands were injured
Danvers, Massachusetts,[22] November 22nd, 2006	A massive chemical explosion occurred at a factory in Danvers, Massachusetts in the early morning of November 22nd, 2006. The factory, which produced solvent-based commercial printing inks, was destroyed, and more than 100 homes and businesses up to 1 mile away were damaged, some beyond repair. As of early May 2007, over 50 families were still unable to return to their homes. No one was killed in the incident, but 10 members of the local community were injured. It was noted that the water run-off from the water used by firefighters had left a purple sheen on the river. Tests carried out by the US Environmental Protection Agency following the incident showed low levels of the solvent toluene
Spills	
Cataguases, Brazil, March 29th, 2003	The accident occurred on March 29th, 2003 at the site of the Cataguases de Papel Ltda, a paper and pulp company in Cataguases, Minas Gerais state, about 125 miles (200 km) north of Rio de Janeiro. A reservoir used to store chemical residues burst, dumping 1.2 billion litres of toxic waste, including caustic soda, into the rivers Pompa and Paraiba do Sul in south-eastern Brazil. Dead fish floated belly up in the rivers, and people in the affected areas lined up for water from trucks. Fishing and irrigation were banned. Swimming at some beaches where the poisoned rivers met the sea was also banned. More than 20 towns in Minas Gerais state were affected by the spill. Campos, a large coastal city north of Rio de Janeiro with an estimated population of 400 000 people, had shut its water supply and irrigation channels, leaving the all the population without water
Erika, France,[23] December 12th, 1999	Erika, the 25-year-old vessel chartered by French oil company Total-Fina, foundered along France's Breton coastline, spilling 12 000 tons of heavy oil and precipitating the worst ornithological disaster in history, in which 300 000 birds were killed, with 100 km of coast polluted. The spill had major economic effects on fishing, oyster-farming and tourism
Baia Mare, Romania,[23] January 31st, 2000	A poorly designed tailings dam at a Romanian gold mine ruptured and, over the course of 4 days, released water contaminated with cyanide, a leaching agent used to extract the gold, into the Someş River, a tributary of the Szamos, Tisza and Danube rivers. The cyanide reached levels of over 700 times normal concentrations and caused a major fish kill. The contaminated water flowed into Hungary and Yugoslavia in the Szamos and Tisza rivers and back into Romania in the Danube
Others	
Garbage Slide in Manila, Phillipines,[24] July 11th, 2000	On July 11th, 2000, strong rains caused the collapse of the enormous garbage heap in northern Manila where hundreds of scavengers had built their houses. The slide and subsequent fire claimed the lives of at least 193 people, with hundreds more still missing. It was feared that run-off from the dump had contaminated the nearby La Mesa reservoir, the main source of drinking water for Manila's 10 million residents. This disaster highlighted the city's inadequate solid waste management programme, which allows open landfills to become hills of decomposing rubbish
Shanxi province, China,[25] September 8th, 2008	The collapse of a waste product reservoir at an illegal mine during rainfall led to a mudslide several metres high that buried a market, several homes and a three-storey building. At least 254 people died, and 35 were injured

Table 46.2 Examples of some recent 'rising tide' chemical incidents of note

Type of incident	Summary of event
Global product contamination,[26,27] US, Spain, Croatia, Italy, Germany, Taiwan and Colombia January 1998 to October 15th, 2001	The US Food and Drug Administration investigated reports of over 50 patient deaths worldwide, including four in the USA, that might have been caused by dialyzers made by Baxter Healthcare Corporation, US. Baxter voluntarily recalled the dialyzers in mid-October after reports of deaths associated with its product in kidney dialysis patients in Spain, Croatia, Italy, Germany, Taiwan, Colombia and the USA. Most of the dialysis patients who died experienced shortness of breath, chest tightness, cardiac arrest or stroke symptoms within hours of being dialyzed. A perfluorohydrocarbon-based performance fluid used in a manufacturing step played a role in the deaths of these patients
Global product contamination,[28] China, Taiwan, Singapore, Vietnam, USA, UK and other countries 2007–09	It was reported that more than 294 000 children in China were affected by adulterated formula food. Over 50 000 were hospitalized, and at least six died. There were also reports of children in other parts of Asia – such as Taiwan, Singapore and Vietnam – being affected. Those who became ill had ingested melamine-contaminated powdered infant formula, some 22 brands being implicated. In the wake of this discovery, the contaminated formula was taken off the market. Other products were also reported to be potentially at risk, including animal feed
Possible dietary supplement contamination,[29] USA, 1989	In the summer and autumn of 1989, an epidemic outbreak of eosinophilia-myalgia syndrome (EMS) occurred in the USA. This illness is associated with the use of dietary supplements containing L-tryptophan. In all, more than 1500 cases of EMS, including at least 37 deaths, were reported to the national Centers for Disease Control and Prevention, although the true incidence of the disorder is thought to be much higher. In certain epidemiological studies, more than 95 per cent of cases of EMS were traced to L-tryptophan supplied by Showa Denko KK of Japan. However, many people who consumed Showa Denko L-tryptophan did not develop EMS, and cases of EMS and a related disease, eosinophilic fasciitis, occurred prior to and after the 1989 epidemic. EMS and related disorders are also reported to be associated with exposure to L-5-hydroxytryptophan, which is not made in the same manner as L-tryptophan (e.g. via fermentation processes). Based on these observations, the US Food and Drug Administration concluded that other brands of L-tryptophan, or L-tryptophan itself, regardless of the levels or presence of impurities, could not be eliminated as causal or contributing to the development of EMS. The serious nature of this disease necessitated that caution be exercised
'Toxic Oil Syndrome' Spain,[30] May 1981	The outbreak of the condition eventually called Toxic Oil Syndrome (TOS) in Madrid and north-western Spain in May 1981 was unique because of its size (20 000 individuals being affected, with over 300 dying within a few months and a few thousand invalids), the novelty of the clinical condition and the complexity of its aetiology. A cause has not been finally identified. The illness is currently described as a multisystem disease initiated by a non-necrotizing endothelial injury, with an immune mechanism underlying its inception and/or evolution. Clinically, it started as a varying combination of fever, rash, lung and pleural effusions, myalgias, paraesthesias and eosinophilia: in a sizeable proportion of survivors, it evolved to lung hypertension, cachexia, contractures and scleroderma

2006 and 2007, 74 per cent (1456) were classified as actual, 18 per cent (368) as potential and 8 per cent (154) as for information. Up to 27 970 people were estimated to have been exposed, with 6220 reporting symptoms. More than 1000 people were exposed in each of six separate events (five of which involved contamination of water). Twenty per cent (396) of chemical incidents resulted in the evacuation of nearby populations during 2006 and 2007.[3]

As with all chemical, biological and radiological incidents and extreme weather events, it is important to consider a series of measures that cover prevention, preparedness, response and recovery (Figure 46.1). All countries have their own governmental arrangements for incident management.

UK arrangements are summarized in the UK Civil Contingencies Act and accompanying non-legislative measures, which deliver a single framework for civil protection in the UK that is capable of meeting the challenges of the twenty-first century. The Act is separated into two substantive parts: (1) local arrangements for civil protection, and (2) emergency powers.[6] Further work on the Civil Contingencies Act Enhancement Programme has been underway in 2009.[7] From this, the UK Resilience website describes integrated emergency management as comprising six related activities – anticipation, assessment, prevention, preparation, response and recovery – and acts a focus for all developments in these areas.[8]

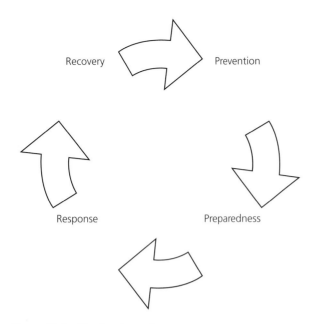

Figure 46.1 The disaster cycle.

In summary, the UK central government arrangements for responding to an emergency set out a concept of operation's states that includes the following areas:

- *Preparedness*: All those individuals and organizations that might have to respond to emergencies should be properly prepared, including having clarity of roles and responsibilities.
- *Continuity*: Response to emergencies should be grounded in the existing functions of organizations and familiar ways of working, albeit delivered at a greater tempo, on a larger scale and in more testing circumstances.
- *Subsidiarity*: Decisions should be taken at the lowest appropriate level, with coordination at the highest necessary level. Local responders should be the building block of response on any scale.
- *Direction*: Clarity of purpose should be delivered through a strategic aim and supporting objectives that are agreed and understood by all involved, to prioritize and focus the response.
- *Integration*: Effective coordination should be exercised between and within organizations and tiers of response, as well as assuring timely access to appropriate guidance and appropriate support for the local or regional level.
- *Communication*: Good two-way communication is critical to an effective response. Reliable information must be passed correctly and without delay among those who need to know, including the public.
- *Cooperation*: Positive engagement based on mutual trust and understanding will facilitate information sharing and deliver effective solutions to issues arising.
- *Anticipation*: Risk identification and analysis is needed of potential direct and indirect developments to anticipate and thus manage the consequences.

CHEMICAL INCIDENT MANAGEMENT

With more than 40 million chemical substances known to man,[9] of which some 60 000–70 000 are in regular use, and with many new chemical substances entering the marketplace each month, the provision of adequate toxicological information during a chemical incident may be difficult. In many chemical incidents, it may be very difficult to identify the chemicals released. Indeed, adequate risk assessment data may be limited as one of the main difficulties of dealing with a chemical incident is obtaining rapid information on the identity of the chemical or mix of chemicals involved and their health hazards.

Chemical incident management requires multiagency (including fire, police, ambulance, healthcare and many other agencies and organizations) and multidisciplinary skills and expertise, including those provided by clinicians and nurses as well as public health, health protection, toxicological, environmental science, environmental epidemiology and risk assessment professionals. It is probably simplest to describe management in terms of the pre-event phase, the acute phase, the post-acute phase and the post-event phase.

THE PRE-EVENT PHASE

The pre-event phase involves planning, training and exercises.

Planning

The management of any incident can proceed effectively only if there has been adequate planning in advance of an incident being identified. All agencies must agree on what their roles and responsibilities will be. They also need to agree the route and mechanisms by which individual agencies will be notified of an incident.

Training

Once the roles and responsibilities of the various agencies have been identified, each agency must ask itself whether it has the resources and expertise to fulfil its obligations. Within the health setting, this will entail identifying which healthcare and health protection staff may be involved in incident management and then identifying (and satisfying) their training needs. Such training assessment should not be restricted to medical staff but must include all staff included in on-call rotas.

Exercises

The key to effective incident management is good teamwork. This can develop only when team members are confident with one another. Such confidence grows with experience gained through being involved in the management of real events or in exercises. Exercises are essential for building confidence in individuals and in the team, and can also identify areas where existing plans are inadequate.

THE ACUTE PHASE

This section focuses on public health protection and on some of the clinical management issues likely to be encountered. The primary objectives of the health response to chemical incidents are:

- to conduct a risk assessment to determine the potential impact of the incident on the health of the local population;
- to communicate with other organizations involved in the response to the incident, with colleagues within the healthcare system and with the public;
- to take action to prevent or minimize the adverse health impact of the incident;
- to ensure that healthcare resources are provided as required.

In summary, health practitioners may have direct responsibility for the actions that need to be taken to prevent or minimize any adverse health impacts or/and may just need to satisfy themselves that the appropriate agency is carrying out the necessary action. Again, this underlines the need for agencies to collaborate in responding to chemical incidents. The information required or type of actions to be taken within the three primary objectives in the health response to chemical incidents include the following:

- Risk assessment to determine the severity of the incident, which requires information about the chemical, the incident source and location, the population exposure and any likely adverse health effects and information on procedures for chemical containment. In addition, information is needed on concentrations and movements of chemicals into the environment and thus on the potential for transfer to people.
- Communication with the other agencies and organizations and with the public, by contacting and alerting other responders and maintaining contact (knowing the roles and responsibilities of each organization involved) and by alerting and advising the local population.
- Health actions to prevent or minimize harm, which include forming an incident control team or attending other forms of multiagency fora, assisting in providing advice on the prevention and minimization of population exposure and environmental contamination, and ensuring that secondary contamination does not occur, possibly by recommending the decontamination of casualties.

Risk assessment

Clearly, the management of an incident cannot begin until the incident has been detected, notified and confirmed by relevant agencies and organizations. It is crucial that incidents are detected as early as possible, while there is still time for preventive action to minimize harm. Chemical incidents can be detected in a number of ways including:

- reporting of a chemical incident as it takes place (via the frontline responders such as police, fire and ambulance or the media);
- observation of adverse health effects acutely (such as the occurrence of respiratory irritation) or chronically (such as an increased incidence of cancer);
- observation by taste or odour, or routine environmental sampling of chemical contamination of air, water or land;
- observation of ecological effects on fauna and flora, such as dead fish in water, or dead or adversely affected birds or plant life.

To be able to meet these objectives of the acute-phase response, health practitioners will need to gather information about various aspects of the incident. Some of this information will be directly available; other information will require liaison with other health professionals and agencies involved in the management of the incident. As new information becomes available, the risk assessment will need to be reviewed. Initial data required include:

- where the incident has occurred and in what type of location (road, motorway, factory, residential area, etc.);
- what has actually happened – the 'nature' of the incident (fire, road traffic accident, explosion, leak, etc.);
- when the incident started, and whether it is continuing, getting worse or getting better;
- what chemicals are or may be involved, and what quantities are being or have been released into the environment;
- whether the release is being contained locally close to the site of release or whether residential and other areas are likely to be affected;
- whether there are casualties on site, and if so, what their symptoms are, how many are affected, and whether they are being managed locally or transferred to hospitals or other healthcare facilities;
- whether there are casualties among the surrounding population, and if so, what their symptoms are, how many are affected, and whether they are being managed locally, in hospitals or in other healthcare facilities.

Decisions including, for example, the need for sheltering or evacuation may be taken using these data.

The initial risk assessment is frequently the most difficult task, and the subsequent management of the incident will often rest on this decision. For the public health practitioner, the key question is: 'Does this incident pose a risk to the health of the surrounding population?' Risk can be direct – from chemical contaminants passing through air, food or water to the surrounding population – or indirect – for example by chemically contaminated individuals arriving at hospital and contaminating the hospital environment. It can be very difficult to make this initial risk assessment, particularly for someone not used to handling chemical incidents. Information about an incident should be collected systematically using the basic concept used in chemical/environmental risk assessment: the source–pathway–receptor concept (Figure 46.2).[10]

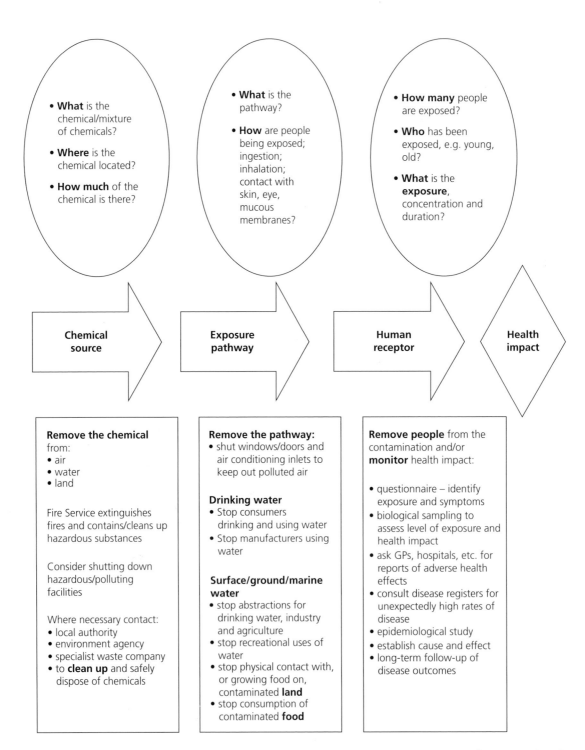

Figure 46.2 The source–pathway–receptor concept in chemical incident response. GP, general practitioner. (Reproduced from Eagles, Goodfellow, Welch and Murray,[10] with permission.)

Three inputs are essential for the risk assessment process:

1 a good description of the incident;
2 the experience and training of the staff from the agency or organization making the initial and ongoing risk assessments;
3 support from experienced expert chemical incident professionals who are skilled in medical toxicology, environmental science, epidemiology, communication and other relevant sciences such as atmospheric dispersion modelling.

Communication is a vital aspect of the public health response to a chemical incident. The response to chemical incidents requires multiagency involvement, and effective communication links with all the other organizations involved is necessary to ensure that:

- health professionals have the most up-to-date information about the incident to enable them to make an accurate risk assessment and take appropriate action;
- public health objectives as well as clinical management issues are understood and supported by all the organizations involved.

Initial response

If the initial risk assessment indicates a risk to the public's health, whether actual or potential, action is required. This will involve immediate care, clinical support and health protection support and coordination in addition to working with other, perhaps many other, agencies and organizations in a coordinated and timely manner. The following information provides a summary of some of the issues pertinent to chemical incident management for clinical support and public health support.

CLINICAL RESPONSE

The main issues of clinical management can be summarized as command, safety and medical and scientific expert support.[11] Effective command is one of the main aims of management: contaminated casualties should be managed as close to the scene as feasible without compromising patient care or putting responders at undue risk. This minimizes the potential spread of contamination while also allowing early resuscitation and clinical care. Toxicological information is vital, and support must be provided by experts to facilitate the provision of effective care.

Triage

The triage of the casualties is an essential preliminary to treatment. Triage facilitates the work of responders so that resources can be directed towards the patients most in need and also those most susceptible to help. Consequently,

in the setting of a mass casualty incident, triage may appear to direct treatment priorities away from the most severely ill and nearly dead patients. This may initially be counterintuitive to some personnel but is critically important if clinical resources are to be applied optimally. Three broad triage categories for chemically contaminated casualties should be used:

- P1 – requires resuscitation *during decontamination* in a stretcher facility;
- P2 – treatment may be delayed until *after decontamination* in a stretcher facility;
- P3 – minor injuries; the individual may walk unaided to an *ambulant decontamination* facility;
- P4 – expectant, *palliative care* only. In a chemical incident, a P4 triage decision can only be made if a non-breathing patient is intubated and ventilated given that almost all chemical injuries can be treated this way. Thus, a P4 triage grading is only likely if there are associated major injuries from trauma or blast.

Decontamination

Although a satisfactory evidence base for the effectiveness of decontamination and its complex processes is not yet available, it is currently considered to be a first step in the management of casualties. Decontamination means the removal of all potentially contaminated clothing, and washing of the patient to remove any residual contamination from the skin and hair. It is important to identify contaminated 'dirty' areas and uncontaminated 'clean' areas. Ideally, these should be separate, and there should be a monitoring of the flow of individuals between the two areas in order to reduce cross-contamination.

Decontamination prior to the transfer to hospital of casualties is the optimal method but is not always possible. This can be due to adverse weather conditions or lack of equipment, training or facilities. Disposed-of clothing should be put in sealed, labelled, double-thickness clear bags in order to prevent further exposure or secondary contamination, as well as for medicolegal or forensic purposes.

Resuscitation

Airway and ventilation management should begin as early as possible, particularly for P1 patents during decontamination, given the potential chemical effects on the respiratory system as a target. Resuscitation should be provided using established clinical methods and guidelines. Resuscitation may have to proceed concomitantly with decontamination. Thus, resuscitation personnel should be aware of the potential for self-contamination via skin or mucosal contact and should use appropriate personal protective clothing. Safety is of vital importance in order to prevent any additional casualties.

Treatment

The preliminary part of treatment of any contaminated victim is to remove the patient from any ongoing exposure to the chemicals or toxins if this has not already been done. This simple manoeuvre significantly reduces the hazard to the casualty. Treatment then consists of general supportive care along with any available specific measures for individual toxicants. Attention to the airway, oxygenation, deciding whether the patient is capable of breathing spontaneously or whether assisted ventilation is needed, intravenous access and hydration are mandatory. The treatment of other concomitant medical conditions and injuries and action to reduce the risk of hypothermia are also essential. A low threshold for seeking expert advice or mobilizing trained mobile medical teams should be maintained. Specific antidotes should be made available if required, for example atropine and pralidoxime for organophosphate exposures.

Biological samples

The collection of appropriate biological samples at an early stage is invaluable in order to confirm exposure and determine the degree of absorption of toxic chemicals.

Transfer to healthcare facilities

There is a delicate balance to be struck between the early transfer of casualties to hospital and treatment of casualties at the scene. The latter may lead to delays in patients being transferred to hospital, whereas the former may delay instituting early decontamination and treatment. These issues are open to judgement and often depend on individual circumstances, for example the number and severity of contaminated casualties, the location of the incident, the weather conditions, the distance away from appropriate medical facilities and the resources available at the scene.

Vehicles taking casualties to hospital should take a route that does not pass through contaminated areas or plumes. Vehicles used to transport contaminated casualties should be separated from other vehicles and used only for the incident. Likewise, all equipment and devices used during the incident should be kept together in order to facilitate comprehensive decontamination at the end of the incident. Experience has shown that there can be secondary contamination from the later use of contaminated equipment, clothing or vehicles.

Healthcare management

The management of chemical incident casualties at healthcare facilities requires clinical and nursing skills to understand immediate and delayed health risks such as the risk of developing delayed pulmonary oedema following exposure to a respiratory irritant such as phosgene. Close links with expert toxicological support and public health command structures to support the use of healthcare facilities and follow-up is required. Psychological support may be required for those dealing with the incident and with casualties, but routine 'counselling' should not be provided.[12]

PUBLIC HEALTH/HEALTH PROTECTION RESPONSE

Health protection and public health response professionals act as the interface between clinical healthcare and the overall management of a chemical incident. It is they who will attend the operational, tactical or strategic incident meetings or, in the UK, the Science and Technical Advice Cell[13] or perhaps the Cabinet Office Briefing Rooms[14] as required (Figure 46.3). It is they who, with toxicological and other experts, will contribute to many decisions including sheltering and evacuation and the calling in of an incident control team if required.

Shelter or evacuation?

In the event of a serious chemical incident where the public may be exposed to smoke from a fire or to chemicals released into the air, two main options exist for protecting the public – sheltering and evacuation. The prevailing expert view, based largely on experimental and modelling studies, is that sheltering is the better option.

A study comparing the health outcomes in sheltered and evacuated populations after a chemical fire suggested that there are health advantages in people sheltering rather than evacuating.[15] The study examined the response to a fire that started in a factory manufacturing plastic goods in south-west England. The factory was situated on an industrial estate adjoining a large residential area. The initial response of the emergency services was to begin evacuating residents from their homes to a nearby leisure centre. This decision was subsequently reviewed, and residents were advised to stay inside their homes, i.e. to shelter. The resultant partial evacuation offered a rare opportunity to compare the relative health benefits offered by these two modes of intervention.

A postal questionnaire survey was carried out among residents in the affected area and compared the health outcomes among the people evacuated (one-third) and those who sheltered in their homes (two-thirds). The survey showed that evacuation did not confer any additional health benefit over sheltering. If anything, evacuated residents seemed to have more ill-health effects soon after the incident than sheltered residents, although the difference did not seem to persist beyond 2 weeks. Although the study has its limitations, it is a comparative study based on a real incident. The results reinforce the prevailing expert view that favours sheltering over evacuation as a response to protect populations exposed to chemical air pollution incidents. It is consistent with UK policy.

Incident control team

The purpose of the incident control team is to improve communication between the various agencies involved in the management of a chemical incident in order to:

- provide a coordinated management response to the incident;

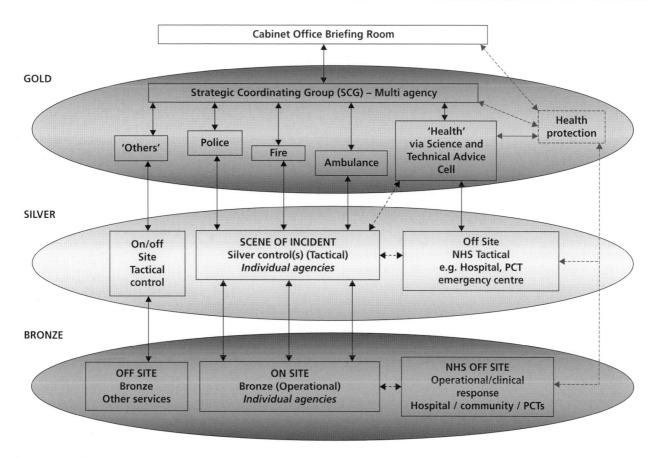

Figure 46.3 Command and control. NHS, National Health Service; PCT, primary care trust.

- pool information and resources;
- understand the needs of other organizations and the impact of the incident;
- share the responsibility for decision-making;
- provide authoritative statements to colleagues and the media.

Several agencies are likely to be represented on the incident control team. Each agency will have its own priorities and responsibilities, some of which may not be immediately consistent with the need to protect the health of the surrounding population. The incident control team has several responsibilities:

- undertaking and updating the assessment of risk to the general public: risk assessments must be made locally, taking into account advice from experts on the spread of toxic chemical(s) in the environment and knowledge of the local population;
- determining what advice should be given to the emergency and health services and to the public on how to manage suspected illness;
- determining the most appropriate advice to give the public on how they can avoid exposure, including information on recovery from contamination.[16]

Information allowing the population at risk to be estimated can come from (1) reports of casualties requiring hospital attention or of those suffering from adverse health effects in the community, and (2) information about the chemical(s) released and the areas affected, and predictions about possible dispersion of released substances.

It is easier to identify the area and the total population at risk if information is presented in map form, either on paper or electronically (i.e. via a geographical information system). For example, an Ordnance Survey map of the general area could serve as a base map, and overlays could be added to show the distribution of reported cases of adverse health effects, complaints about air or water quality, or results from environmental sampling. Also, the estimated areas of atmospheric plumes or land area covered by a spill could be shown. Another use is in a drinking water incident where an overlay map showing the different sections of the water supply network would be useful.

From information on the population at risk and the initial risk assessment, the public should be advised whether there is a risk to their health, and if so, what they should do. Considerable thought must be given to what key messages need to be relayed to the public and to the most appropriate ways of getting them across.

In any major incident, there are likely to be agencies that may need or may wish to be informed about the incident. Information needs will vary from agency to agency. Clearly, local hospitals will need to know about potential numbers of casualties, the signs and symptoms casualties may be experiencing and how casualties should be managed. Hospitals that may be directly affected by the incident will need to know whether they should take action to protect their own staff and patients. General practitioners may also need to be contacted and given advice on the diagnosis and management of suspected cases, and on whether they would be required to notify public health agencies of possible cases. In addition to local healthcare providers, national and regional health agencies, such as the relevant equivalent of the UK Department of Health and other agencies such as the Health Protection Agency, will need to be informed so that they can fulfil their public health obligations.

The key to good incident management is flexibility – being able to increase and decrease the resources committed to an incident and being able to configure those resources in response to changing demands.

Documentation

The response to chemical incidents needs to be well documented. Details must be recorded of the incident, of actions taken and of the decisions made – including justification for the decisions and details of the information on which they were based. The absence of information in specific areas should also be recorded. All documentation should be timed and dated in order to:

- allow an easy transfer of management to other personnel in the event of a lengthy incident;
- allow an efficient response to requests for information from enforcement agencies or, during an inquiry, for information about how the incident was managed (responders should be aware that incident notes may be removed without warning by the police if a public inquiry is announced);
- provide information that can be used to improve the management of future incidents and to disseminate lessons learnt from the present one;
- provide retrospective evidence for the justification of decisions based on the information available at the time (decisions may, of course, be changed in the light of further information, and evidence of the reasoning behind any decisions made may be of particular value in a public inquiry).

THE ONGOING RESPONSE

In many ways, the ongoing response is a refinement of the first stage of incident management. More information is obtained, and the incident becomes better described. Risks are reassessed, and the need for further emergency service,

health service and protective action is considered. The main difference between the early and late phases is that, as time passes, decisions are more likely to be shared

Post-incident recovery and support may require a monitoring of occupational exposure. This should be carried out by occupational medical services and should be available to all responders as needed. This is a requirement if there is evidence of damage to personal protective clothing, penetration and/or permeation of contaminant through personal protective clothing or if there are clinical signs of exposure, and will depend on the chemical involved.

THE POST-ACUTE PHASE

The post-acute phase starts as soon as the primary incident has been brought under control. The key issue to be addressed is whether there are likely to be any ongoing health effects in the exposed population, and if so, ensuring the provision of appropriate healthcare. With appropriate expert toxicological, environmental science and epidemiological advice as required, a definitive risk assessment should be developed. Once this information is available, it can be fed into healthcare planning activities. The exact exposure will frequently be unclear and the health effects uncertain. It is in such circumstances that the need for epidemiological surveillance and other studies will arise.

THE POST-INCIDENT PHASE

In the closing stages of an incident, it is important that a comprehensive summary of the incident be compiled, including details of the actions taken by the various organizations involved. A post-incident report:

- provides a record of the incident for easy future reference;
- disseminates lessons learnt, thus helping to improve the management of future incidents;
- systematically records information for use in any subsequent legal action or if required for official reports.

After every incident, it is important to identify what worked well and also what improvements could be made. After most large incidents, a 'wash-up' meeting is organized. At such a meeting, the response of the emergency and other services is reviewed to determine whether it was adequate and appropriate. It may be appropriate and useful to conduct a full post-incident audit to ensure that action is taken to improve emergency plans and the future management of events, and also to identify any preventive action to avoid the same incident or similar incidents recurring.

One function of the post-incident review may be to determine any long-term resource implications, via, for example, follow-up health studies or long-term environmental monitoring programmes. Adequate staffing and financial resources will need to be allocated for these activities.

Post-event learning is an essential aspect of chemical incident management. Because significant chemical incidents occur on an infrequent basis, it is particularly important to document any lessons learnt from managing such incidents. Changes to plans and procedures should be made and recorded; this is important because different incidents are likely to be dealt with by different teams. Lessons learnt in managing an incident have value for others working in the field. Wherever possible, incidents should be written up and published for the wider public health community.

An example of where this debriefing process and incident report has been used is documented in the record of an incident involving the spontaneous combustion of coal.[17] This chemical incident released a wide range of airborne pollutants that would, in high concentrations, have been hazardous to health. Little is known about how the effects on health change in relation to the release of multiple substances. Although the resultant health effects reported were few, the coordinated response by local authorities and health authorities highlighted the advantage of a multidisciplinary approach. Public health departments needed to be aware of chemical hazards within their districts. Prompt environmental monitoring and exposure measurement needed to be arranged as this was crucial to making an appropriate response. It was considered that updated information was needed from private companies and public bodies to allow improved risk registers to be compiled.

CONCLUSION

Many chemical incidents have occurred since the 1950s around the world. For many incidents, management has been complex and difficult. Many incidents have been reviewed in depth to increase the understanding of the process required for prevention, preparedness, response and recovery, and an understanding of the issues associated with the management of incidents is growing. Prevention by planning to reduce risks, be they from chemicals, factory location or controls, is key in the long term. Preparedness requires multidisciplinary, multiagency working in terms of planning, training and exercises. Response requires the rapid identification of an incident with effective coordinated clinical and health protection responses and collaboration with partners. Recovery to normal requires a post-incident phase, which is vital to identify lessons and to implement effective change. Chemical incident management is therefore an emerging field.

Many sources of information are available on the Internet, such as the dedicated site for Chemicals & Poisons on the HPA website,[5] and more are in development, including the Public Health Response to Chemical Incident Emergencies (CIE) Toolkit, a collaborative project involving partners from across Europe,[18] and a UK Recovery Handbook for Chemical Incidents, a collaboration across UK government partners and stakeholders.[31] This remains an active field where, although much has been done, much more needs to be learned and shared both with fellow professionals and with the public who may be at risk.

REFERENCES

1. Health Protection Agency. Chemical Incident Management. Available from: http://www.hpa.org.uk/webw/HPAweb&Page&HPAwebAutoListName/Page/1158313435037?p=1158313435037 (accessed August 16, 2009).

2. United Nations Environment Programme, Office for the Coordination of Humanitarian Affairs. Cyanide Spill at Baia Mare Romania: Before, During and After. Report of UNEP/OCHA Assessment Mission. Available from: http://www.rec.org/REC/Publications/CyanideSpill/ENGCyanide.pdf (accessed November 25, 2009).

3. Health Protection Agency. Chemical Incidents Surveillance Review: January 2006 – December 2007. Available from: http://www.hpa.org.uk/web/HPAwebFile/HPAweb_C/1211184033548 (accessed August 16, 2009).

4. Olowokure B, Pooransingh S, Tempowski J, Palmer S Meredith T. Global surveillance for chemical incidents of international public health concern. *Bull World Health Organ* 2005; **83**: 928–35.

5. Health Protection Agency. Chemicals & Poisons. Available from: http://www.hpa.org.uk/webw/HPAweb&Page&HPAwebContentAreaLanding/Page/1153386734384?p=1153386734384 (accessed August 16, 2009).

6. Office of Public Sector Information. Civil Contingencies Act 2004. Available from: http://www.opsi.gov.uk/acts/acts2004/ukpga_20040036_en_1 (accessed August 16, 2009).

7. UK Resilience. Civil Contingencies Act Enhancement Programme. Available from: http://www.cabinetoffice.gov.uk/ukresilience/news/ccact_enhancement_programe.aspx (accessed November 25, 2009).

8. UK Cabinet Office. Welcome to UK Resilience. Available from http://www.cabinetoffice.gov.uk/resilience.aspx (accessed November 25, 2009).

9. American Chemical Society, Chemical Abstract Service. CAS Registers 40 Millionth Substance. Available from http://www.cas.org/newsevents/connections/derivative.html (accessed August 16, 2009).

10. Eagles E, Goodfellow F, Welch F, Murray V. *The Environment and Public Health*. Internal publication. London: Chemical Incident Response Service, 2002.

11. Crawford IWF, Mackway-Jones K, Russell DR, Carley SD. Planning for chemical incidents by implementing a Delphi based consensus study. *Emerg Med J* 2004; **21**: 20–3.

12. Rose S, Bisson J, Wessely SA. Systematic review of single-session psychological interventions ('debriefing') following trauma. *Psychother Psychosom* 2003; **72**: 176–84.

13. UK Cabinet Office. UK Resilience Provision of Scientific and Technical Advice to Strategic Co-Ordinating Groups During a Major Incident. Available from: http://www.cabinetoffice.gov.uk/ukresilience/news/stac_guidance.aspx (accessed November 25, 2009).

14. UK Cabinet Office. Working Together To Protect Britain's People. The Security Challenges Facing the UK Are Increasingly Complex and Unpredictable, Ranging from Disease to Cyber Warfare. Supporting the Prime Minister and Cabinet. Available from: http://www.cabinetoffice.gov.uk/reports/annualreport/dept2008/html/working_together.aspx (accessed November 25, 2009).

15. Kinra S, Lewendon G, Nelder R et al. Evacuation decisions in a chemical air pollution incident: cross-sectional survey. Br Med J 2005; **330**: 1471–4.

16. UK Cabinet Office. UK Resilience Recovery Guidance – Environmental Issues. Environmental Pollution and Decontamination. Available from: http://www.cabinetoffice.gov.uk/ukresilience/response/recovery_guidance/environmental_issues/poll (accessed November 25, 2009).

17. Freudenstein U, Crowley D, Welch F. Chemical incident management: gaseous emissions from a stockpile of coal. Public Health 2000; **114**: 41–4.

18. Health Protection Agency. The Public Health Response to Chemical Incident Emergencies Toolkit (CIE Toolkit). Available from: http://www.hpa.org.uk/webw/HPAweb&HPAwebStandard/HPAweb_C/1217574164393?p=1194947302241 (accessed August 16, 2009).

19. Health and Safety Executive, Buncefield Investigation Homepage. Available from: http://www.buncefieldinvestigation.gov.uk/index.htm (accessed August 16, 2009).

20. The Netherlands Ministry of Housing, Spatial Planning and the Environment. A Brief History of National External Safety Policy in The Netherlands. January 2006. Available in: http://www2.vrom.nl/docs/internationaal/External%20Safety%20Directory.pdf (accessed November 25, 2009).

21. United Nations Environment Programme, Division of Technology, Industry, and Economics, Sustainable Consumption & Production Branch. Ammonium Nitrate Explosion in Toulouse – France 21 September 2001. Available from: http://www.unep.fr/scp/sp/disaster/casestudies/france/ (accessed August 16, 2009).

22. US Chemical Safety Board. CSB Issues Report of Massive 2006 Blast in Danvers, Massachusetts. Available from http://www.fireengineering.com/display_article/328579/25/none/none/GOVMT/CSB-issues-report-on-massive-2006-blast-in-Danvers,-Massachusett (accessed August 16, 2009).

23. United Nations Environment Programme, Division of Technology, Industry, and Economics, Sustainable Consumption & Production Branch. Transport. Available from: http://www.unep.fr/scp/sp/disaster/technological.htm (accessed August 16, 2009).

24. United Nations Environment Programme, Division of Technology, Industry, and Economics, Sustainable Consumption & Production Branch. Ports and Sea Transport Disasters. Available from: http://www.unep.fr/scp/sp/disaster/transport.htm (accessed November 25, 2009).

25. World Information Service on Energy. WISE Uranium Project Chronology of Major Tailings Dam Failures. Available from: http://www.wise-uranium.org/mdaf.html (accessed August 16, 2009).

26. US Food and Drug Administration, Centre for Devises and Radiation Health. FDA Investigating Role of Baxter's Recalled Dialyzers in Kidney Dialysis Patient Deaths. Available from: http://www.fda.gov/MedicalDevices/Safety/RecallsCorrectionsRemovals/ListofRecalls/ucm065000.htm (accessed November 25, 2009).

27. Ferriman A. Baxter identifies processing fluid as possible cause of deaths. Br Med J 2001; **323**: 1088.

28. Ingelfinger JR. Melamine and the global implications of food contamination. N Engl J Med 2008; **359**: 2745–8.

29. US Food and Drug Administration, Center for Food Safety and Applied Nutrition. Office of Nutritional Products, Labeling, and Dietary Supplements. Information Paper on L-Tryptophan and 5-Hydroxy-L-tryptophan. February 2001. Available from: http://vm.cfsan.fda.gov/~dms/ds-tryp1.html (accessed August 16, 2009).

30. Terracini B. The limits of epidemiology and the Spanish Toxic Oil Syndrome. Int J Epidemiol 2004; **33**: 443–4.

31. Galea A, Brook N, Baker D, Dobney A, Mobbs S, Murray V. A UK Recovery Handbook for Chemical Incidents. HPA Chemical Hazards and Poisons Report. January 2010; 16: 61. Available at: http://www.hpa.org.uk/web/HPAwebFile/HPAweb_C/1263812796194 (accessed 6 March 2010).

SECTION **H**

Diseases influenced by climate

Heat and cold

WILLIAM R. KEATINGE

HEAT

Excess deaths in hot weather vary greatly from year to year. Britain, for example, has mild summers, but short spells of unusually hot weather can double the death rate for a few days (Figure 47.1).[1] Annual heat-related deaths usually number around 800, but the figure reached 4651 in the unusually hot summer of 1976. The great majority of these deaths occurred in people aged 75 or older who were living ordinary lives at home and not taking part in any unusual activity. Heat-related mortality is often as high in cool as in warm countries.[2,3] For example, it is higher in the cool summers of Finland than the warmer summers of London.

Daily data are essential to determine both heat-related and the cold-related mortality. Cold-related mortality has often been measured as excess mortality in the winter months compared with either the average mortality throughout the year or mortality in the summer months, but this ignores heat-related deaths. Such a calculation would indicate no cold-related deaths if those deaths in winter were high but heat-related deaths in summer were equally high. The true picture would be that there were many deaths from both heat and cold.

Daily mortalities show that mortality in temperate countries is usually lowest at around 18 °C (64 °F). By determining this temperature of minimum mortality in each region and using it as a baseline, total daily deaths in excess of the baseline on warmer days of the year gives the number of heat-related deaths in the region.[2,3] Daily deaths in excess of this baseline on colder days of the year give the number of cold-related deaths. Using weekly or monthly mortalities rather than daily mortalities in this way would underestimate both temperature-related mortalities, because the week or month of minimum mortality would include some days that

were hotter and some that were colder than the average for that week or month. Average mortality in that week or month would not be the true minimum, because it would

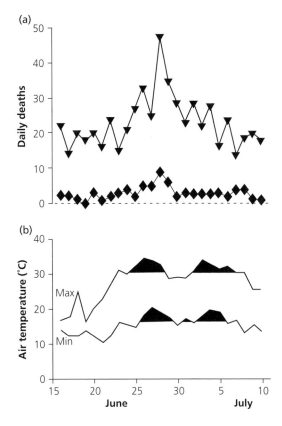

Figure 47.1 Daily deaths from coronary (inverted triangles) and cerebral thrombosis (diamonds) during a heatwave in London (a). Temperatures shown in (b). (Adapted from Keatinge *et al.*,[5] with permission.)

Professor Bill Keatinge contributed this chapter for the book. He died in 2008. The text has been left as he finished it.

include some heat-related deaths on hotter days and cold-related deaths on colder days of the week or month.

Many heat-related deaths in the summers of temperate countries are caused by the normal operation of internal mechanisms of the body that resist any change in body temperature, rather than by the changes in body temperature themselves. Coronary and cerebral thromboses cause many of the deaths in heatwaves.[4,5] The reason underlying this is that both water and salt are lost in sweat. This makes the blood more concentrated. The resulting increases in red blood cell count, platelet count and plasma cholesterol level (Table 47.1) do not matter much in young people with healthy arteries, but in elderly people with atheromatous arteries they increase the risk of an arterial thrombus forming.

Drinking water would then restore normal blood composition. The fact that salt as well as water is lost in sweat means that there is in practice little change in the concentration of salt in the blood, and little sensation of thirst. Volunteers exposed to air at 41 °C (106 °F) for 6 hours lost 1.83 kg of almost isotonic salt and water as they sweated in a hot chamber, but they did not feel thirsty or drink even though water was freely available. The problem is particularly serious in people who are not acclimatized to heat as they lose more salt in sweat. It is only when they have a meal, and take in their normal amount of salt with it, that they feel thirsty and restore their blood volume to normal by drinking water. As people exposed to heat stress often do not feel hungry, they are liable to eat nothing until evening. This means that, in hot weather, they need advice to eat normal meals and drink water with them, particularly if they have little experience of heat stress. This intake of salt and water will correct the loss of salt and water, shortening the period of risk from thrombosis.

Patients with severe chronic respiratory disease are particularly prone to increased mortality in hot weather. This may be because they often have a degree of heart failure. Heart failure makes it difficult to increase the blood flow to the skin, and therefore to increase heat loss from the body as its temperature rises.

Global warming is now well underway. Future risks from heat exposure during global warming depend not only on the degree of that warming, but also on how rapidly and how effectively people adjust to it. In cold countries, heat-related mortality starts at a lower temperature, and then rises more steeply with any further rise in temperature, than it does in hot countries (Figure 47.2). An analysis of British data shows that, from 1971 to 2003, summer temperature rose significantly by 1.4 °C (35 °F) in south-east England. It also tended to rise in other parts of Britain. However, increasing tolerance to heat prevented any overall rise in heat-related mortality from the hotter summers. People apparently learnt to control heat stress rapidly enough to prevent the hotter summers from increasing the average annual heat-related mortality.

However, global warming will inevitably expose people in each region to an occasional heatwave more severe than any they have previously encountered. The duration as well as intensity of heatwaves is important, as daily mortality during them increases progressively during a succession of

Table 47.1 Blood changes during exposure to heat and cold

	Before	Change during the first hour	Change during 6 hours
Heat			
Viscosity (mPas)	3.8 ± 0.1	$+ 0.2 \pm 0.1$*	$+ 0.8 \pm 0.1$***
Red cell count ($\times 10^{12}$/L)	4.50 ± 0.11	$+ 0.09 \pm 0.03$*	$+ 0.40 \pm 0.06$***
Platelet count ($\times 10^9$/L)	268 ± 17	$+ 38 \pm 9$**	$+ 56 \pm 13$**
Cholesterol (mmol/L in plasma)	4.15 ± 0.22	$+ 0.018 \pm 0.08$	$+ 0.059 \pm 0.14$**
Cold			
Viscosity (mPas)	3.4 ± 0.3	$+ 0.4 \pm 0.1$*	$+ 0.7 \pm 0.1$***
Red cell count ($\times 10^{12}$/L)	4.65 ± 0.23	$+ 0.11 \pm 0.06$	$+ 0.35 \pm 0.07$**
Platelet count ($\times 10^9$/L)	291 ± 27	$- 10 \pm 4$	$+ 23 \pm 9$*
Cholesterol (mmol/L in plasma)	5.19 ± 0.28	$+ 0.08 \pm 0.05$	$+ 0.41 \pm 0.09$**

None of these variables rose significantly during control experiments in thermoneutral conditions. Heat exposure was in air at 41 °C (106 °F), cold exposure was in air at 24 °C (75 °F), with light clothing and rapidly moving air. Blood viscosity was measured at a shear rate of 230/s.
Change from initial value: *$P < 0.05$, ** $P < 0.01$, *** $P < 0.001$.
Data from Keatinge et al.[5,10]

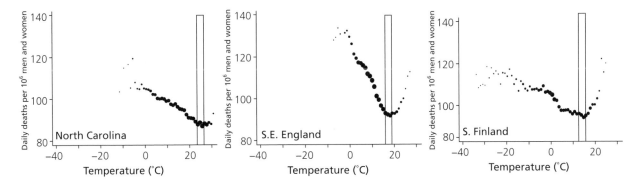

Figure 47.2 Mortality in relation to daily temperature in a hot, temperate and cold country. Pooled data at age 55+. The areas of the circles are proportional to number of days at that temperature. (Adapted from Donaldson et al.,[3] with permission.)

days at the same high level. Elderly people in a population unprepared for heat stress can suffer heavy mortality when an unusually severe heatwave strikes a region.

The most dramatic recent example was the French heatwave of 2003. In this, temperatures in central France rose to around 28 °C every day for 10 days and caused more than 14 000 deaths. Further south, temperatures were often higher, but people were accustomed to them and they caused fewer deaths. Heat-related mortalities may be even higher in some tropical regions where poverty prevents people protecting themselves from the heat, although factors such as seasonal deaths from exposure to parasites and a lack of reliable daily data for deaths often make the assessment of heat-related deaths difficult in such cases. If the rate of warming in Britain continues at the same rate as it has since 2003, the risk of a heatwave in Britain close to the severity and duration of the French heat wave of 2003 is as high as 25 per cent.

Preventing a future heatwave from causing deaths on a similar scale sounds simple, as air-conditioning can keep buildings cool. Air-conditioning has in fact greatly reduced heat-related mortality in the USA, but it consumes a great deal of electrical energy, and fuel burnt to generate the energy in turn accelerates global warming. The dangers of continued global warming are numerous. They include the flooding of coastal districts, and fertile regions becoming deserts. These changes are so serious that the need to take all reasonable steps to reduce them is becoming widely accepted.

Strategies used in summer by people in southern Europe can often keep buildings cool without air-conditioning. Shutters, or other shade outside windows, can prevent sunshine entering buildings and causing a greenhouse heating of the interior. Failing that, thick indoor curtains can reduce such heating, albeit less completely. New buildings need to be designed to resist rapid warming on hot days. Too often, they are built with great expanses of glass and with no way to screen these from sunshine. They can then look dramatic but heat up rapidly on a hot, sunny day. Heavy structural material in a building can retard the daily rise in temperature by absorbing heat, but new buildings are often lightly

constructed compared with older ones. Adequate roof insulation is also important to prevent heat entering through the roof when sunshine heats it.

The management of both buildings and personal lifestyles can make a major contribution to keeping cool in hot weather. In the early morning, windows should be opened and ventilation started. Windows should be closed only when the outside temperature feels warmer than the indoor temperature. It is important to give reminders to the public at the start of summer to check that windows can be opened and that electric fans are available to increase ventilation. There must, of course, always be enough air exchange through ventilators or a slightly open window to provide fresh air for anyone in the room and remove humidity and carbon dioxide. Light clothing should be worn. Exercise can increase the body's heat production as much as 10-fold, so restricting physical work to the early morning and the evening is important to reduce heat stress. People in southern Europe commonly do this and take a siesta during the hottest time of the day.

Increased blood flow to the skin normally sheds unwanted body heat to the surroundings, but if the surrounding temperature rises to near body temperature, evaporative cooling is also needed to prevent the body overheating. For this to be effective, people need both to sweat and to evaporate the sweat. Some medical drugs, particularly psychoactive drugs, suppress sweating. Water can be sprinkled on the clothing of people taking these, or failing to sweat for any other reason, to replace the function of sweat. Air movement by a fan helps evaporation, but humid air can hamper it.

Crowded rooms are therefore particularly difficult to keep cool in hot weather, as the heat and water vapour given off by the occupants adds to both the heat and the humidity of the room. Some air-conditioning will then be needed. Elderly and other vulnerable people in crowded accommodation are at particular risk of heat stroke, but crowded offices without air-conditioning can simply make people too uncomfortable to work effectively in hot weather. The best solution is to have air-conditioning available in such places, as well as taking the simpler measures to cool buildings. Air-conditioning can then be used as a back-up if the simpler methods to maintain a tolerable indoor temperature fail.

Air pollution by ozone increases on sunny days and has been blamed for up to half of the mortality seen during heatwaves. It does sometimes trigger asthma, and perhaps other health problems, but after allowance for heat stress due to sunshine, and to acclimatization as summer progresses, any increase in mortality due to ozone has proved hard to identify.[6]

Heat stress is not the only threat to health in hot, sunny weather. Sunburn is caused by ultraviolet radiation rather than heat, but hot weather tempts people to shed clothes and expose their skin to the sun. High altitude and snow or water all increase the intensity of ultraviolet radiation from the sun, since less ultraviolet is filtered out by the atmosphere at high altitude, and radiation reflected from snow or water can double the exposure. Suncreams giving low protection are then often insufficient, and suncreams giving high protection may themselves damage the skin. The safest way to prevent sunburn is to allow only short exposures of skin to the sun, and otherwise cover it up with light clothing.

Global warming tends to spread tropical diseases to cooler climates. These diseases are mostly transmitted by insects and can be prevented by attacking these. Malaria was endemic throughout much of Europe in the Middle Ages. It died out in Britain when swamps that harboured the larvae of the mosquitoes that carried malaria were drained. In recent times, insecticides, which kill these larvae, provide another effective weapon for controlling malaria. The use of such measures should be able to control any spread of mosquito-borne infections to current temperate regions.

In earlier times, food poisoning by bacteria and viruses caused high summer mortality even in temperate regions such as Europe, until better hygiene and refrigeration controlled it. Parasitic diseases such as schistosomiasis still cause deaths in some tropical countries, but these too can be prevented, usually by avoiding exposure to the parasites. In the case of schistosomiasis, this means not immersing the feet or other parts of the body in water that is liable to contain the parasites. Such measures need to be kept under review as global warming proceeds.

Treatment of heat stress

Immediate cooling is essential for anyone whose body temperature rises to or above 41 °C. A denaturation of body proteins can rapidly cause death if the body's core temperature reaches 43–44 °C (109–111 °F). A cool bath or shower at home provides a very simple and effective method of cooling, but this needs to be started at once, otherwise the rise in body temperature can damage the body tissues even if it does not cause death. The cerebellum is particularly sensitive, and damage to it by heat can result in a lasting impairment of muscular coordination if the patient survives.

People seriously dehydrated by prolonged heat stress without access to water also benefit from intravenous saline and glucose. The loss of salt and water in the sweat can otherwise cause circulatory failure, with cessation of sweating, a hot dry skin, and a rapid rise of body core temperature to a lethal level if the victim stays in a hot environment.

COLD

Cold air

Of all environmental hazards, cold weather probably causes most ill-health and death worldwide. In the early 1980s, the media headlined stories that a hundred thousand elderly people in Britain chilled to death in their homes every year. It was assumed that they died of simple hypothermia, with severe cold stress causing the body temperature to fall to a level at which the heart and brain stopped working.

There were indeed around a hundred thousand more deaths in winter than would be expected if mortality stayed at summer level throughout the year. However, few of the excess deaths in winter were ever certified as being due to hypothermia. Death certificates indicated coronary and cerebral thrombosis (heart attacks and strokes) as the cause of most of them, with respiratory illness causing the majority of the rest. It was suggested that those death certificates were wrong. That was possible, as ordinary clinical thermometers did not register temperatures below 35 °C (95 °F), the lower limit of normal body temperature; therefore, they would not pick up a dangerously low body temperature. Doctors might then mistakenly attribute deaths that were really due to hypothermia to a common cause of death such as a heart attack.

However, measurements of body temperature of patients admitted to hospitals in London, using special low-reading thermometers, showed very few patients with a low body temperature.[7] Most of the excess winter deaths were due to heart attacks and strokes, as reported on the death certificates, but it was not obvious how cold weather was causing these.

The increase in blood pressure caused by exposure to cold might cause a few immediate deaths from heart failure. It could also cause progressive damage to arteries that would increase the rate of heart attacks and strokes after many days or weeks. An analysis of the winter deaths showed that they did not fit either of those patterns. A statistical analysis of deaths had been complicated by air pollution associated with cold spells in winter. Severe smogs used to cause considerable mortality – one in 1952 causing 4000 deaths in London – but since then air pollution in London and other Western cities had greatly reduced. Pollutants such as particulate matter with a diameter less than 10 μm (PM_{10}) particles and sulphur dioxide gas still sometimes trigger asthma, but the number of deaths from air pollutants is now too low to interfere with the analysis of deaths associated with cold weather. These analyses show deaths from arterial thrombosis increasing within a day or two of cold weather, and then falling (Figure 47.3).[8,9] Any explanation of the deaths would have to be consistent with this time course.

Experiments on volunteers[10] have shown changes in blood composition during exposure to cold, which can explain this pattern of deaths and the fact that they occur mainly in the elderly. The changes are part of the body's normal adjustment to mild cold. The cutaneous vasoconstriction induced by cold exposure conserves body heat by shutting down blood flow to the skin, preventing the blood flow from transferring heat from the body core to the skin. However, this also shifts blood volume out of the skin and into central organs such as the heart and liver. This overload of central blood volume is corrected by the kidneys excreting salt and water, and by salt and water filtering out of the blood and into the interstitial space.

That deals with the surplus volume, but the loss of salt and water from the blood increases the concentrations of factors that promote clotting – blood viscosity and red cell and platelet count, as well as plasma fibrinogen and cholesterol. This might not matter if protein C, the factor that opposes intravascular clotting, also increases to a similar degree. However, protein C is a small molecule that can diffuse out of the circulation into the extracellular space, so that its plasma concentration changes little.[11] The increases in thrombogenic factors do little harm to young people whose arteries are in good condition, but they are dangerous to the elderly. The risk of clots forming in the atheromatous arteries of elderly people increases when the blood becomes concentrated due to cold, as it does from sweating during heat stress, increasing the probability of deaths from coronary and cerebral thrombosis.

Respiratory illness causes most of the remaining excess deaths in winter. General exposure to cold, like other stress, suppresses the body's immune responses by increasing the production of steroids. This impairs the response to infection, including influenza and pneumonia. It was important to know whether this, or local cooling of the airways from breathing very cold air, caused the respiratory deaths after cold weather, as exercise outdoors in cold air will have opposite effects on these. Exercise produces heat that can prevent general chilling but causes deep breathing that increases airway cooling. The local cooling is substantial and is sufficient to cause pain in much of the airway during exercise in air temperatures near to or below −20°C (−4°F).

The airway cooling does have some harmful effects. Deep breathing of very cold air during exercise can cause temporary asthma in long-distance skiers. It may also account for chronic bronchitis that occurs, even in non-smokers, in the extreme cold of eastern Siberia. There is

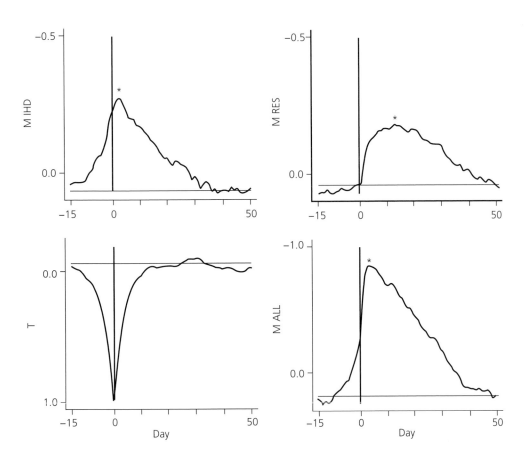

Figure 47.3 Time course of the increase in deaths in relation to cold days in winter (at mean daily temperatures of 0–15°C): a time series analysis of increases in deaths from ischaemic heart disease (IHD), respiratory disease (RES) and all causes (ALL), and of daily temperature (T,°C), in relation to a day 1°C colder than average. *Peak mortalities all differ from average ($P < 0.001$). M, mortality. (Adapted from Donaldson and Keatinge,[9] with permission.)

also evidence that local cooling of the airways by breathing cold air at less extreme temperatures worsens upper respiratory infections, which could progress to pneumonia, particularly in elderly people.

However, these effects of airway cooling cause far fewer of the excess winter deaths than general body chilling does. This was one of the conclusions from the Eurowinter survey, funded by the European Union. The survey covered eight regions of Europe, from the Arctic regions of Finland to the Mediterranean cities of southern Europe.[12] People in cold countries such as Finland were more physically active when outdoors in cold weather, but both respiratory and all-cause mortality increased less steeply with fall in temperature than they did in people in warmer countries such as Greece. Any harm from the deep breathing of cold air was outweighed by a benefit from the heat produced by exercise. Respiratory infections cause some deaths directly, but cause others by increasing plasma fibrinogen levels, with a resulting increase in arterial thrombosis.[13]

Winter deaths in all regions of Europe surveyed started to rise as soon as the outdoor temperature fell enough to cause mild discomfort, rather than when it reached levels low enough to overwhelm the body's defences. This fitted the other evidence that ordinary adjustments to mild cold, rather than hypothermia, caused the excess deaths. The amount of winter mortality in each region depended on how effectively people protected themselves from cold indoors as well as outdoors. People in countries with severe winters were more conscious of the dangers and took far more care to keep warm.

The most striking illustration came when the survey was extended to Siberia. Russian data are complicated by large numbers of alcohol-related deaths, but the coldest city in the world, Yakutsk in eastern Siberia, had no increase in deaths in winter. People there wore massive fur clothing outdoors in cold weather, and they kept their homes warm. This prevented any increase in deaths as outdoor temperatures fell as low as $-48\,°C$ ($-54\,°F$). In contrast, deaths rose more steeply in London than in any other city covered by the surveys. London had mild winters, but there was a British tradition that cold was good for you. This meant, for example, that bedroom windows were generally left open at night. English travellers even remarked how unhealthy life must be in the USA, where central heating kept houses warm in winter.

Direct evidence that outdoor exposure to cold could cause winter deaths independently of cold houses came from a study of elderly people who lived in fully heated housing provided by a housing association.[14] These people kept warm indoors but spent a considerable time outdoors, and talks with them showed that they spent a lot of the day outdoors, often waiting for buses, and without enough clothing to keep them warm. Deaths among these residents rose as much as those of other elderly people in winter.

During the following years, heating and insulation in British homes was improved, partly by government action and organizations such as Age Concern. This was useful but dealt with only indoor exposure to cold. Media reports on the research included the importance of elderly people keeping warm outdoors as well, by exercise and by warm clothing with windproofs if it was windy and waterproofs if it was wet. One government minister, Edwina Currie, briefly took up the need for outdoor protection, but left office shortly afterwards. Official action in Britain remained focused on warm houses. Probably for this reason, excess winter deaths fell only slowly, to 20 000–30 000 by the year 2000.

Density of occupation of housing is also important but received much less attention than heating and insulation. A dwelling with one person living in it needs as much heating as a whole family living in the same place. People can cut down greatly on their heating costs if they move to a smaller place when their children leave home, or if their partner dies.

The decision to move to a smaller home is often difficult. Elderly people can worry about the disruption of moving to a smaller place, even if it is in the same area where they can remain close to their friends. The solution is often to move before poor health makes it difficult. Once done, the rewards go beyond lower heating bills. On a personal level, a smaller home is easier to look after, particularly if it is on a single floor and particularly if the person becomes disabled. On a wider level, the lower energy requirements of a smaller home reduce the carbon dioxide emissions that cause global warming. As concern about the consequences of global warming increases, the need to assess the benefits of high occupation density against concerns about confined space in homes will grow. It will not be easy to strike the balance, but for many people, some downsizing of the space per person can be welcome once they have given it serious thought.

Sudden infant death syndrome, 'cot death', is more common in winter. This, paradoxically, seems to be due to overheating. It is believed to be caused by parents worrying that the infant may be cold, and overheating it by excessive bed clothes in a well-heated house. If the house is warm, above $19\,°C$ ($66\,°F$), the infant will need no more clothing than normal, but a parent who has just come in from the cold will still feel cold and may assume that the infant is cold too. Putting more bed clothes on an infant who has not been out into the cold can then cause dangerous overheating. An awareness of this, and also of the importance of placing infants on their back to sleep, has greatly reduced the number of cot deaths.

Cold water

Immersion in water removes most of the external insulation normally provided by air, greatly accelerating heat loss. Deaths at sea were routinely attributed to drowning until near the end of World War II. It was only then that a committee chaired by Admiral Talbot reported that over

30 000 men in the British Royal Navy had died in the water during the war. Lifebelts or lifejackets, and later Carley floats, were available to prevent simple drowning for anyone unable to swim. Hypothermia caused most of the deaths, either directly or by making the victims unconscious so that they drowned despite having the flotation equipment.[15] Deaths from the sinking of large ships are fewer in peacetime, but disasters such as the loss of the *Laconia* and the *Estonia* cause mass deaths from time to time in both war and peace.

When ships are sinking, they often list, preventing lifeboats on the high side of the ship being launched. Damage to and the jamming or mishandling of equipment also often prevents successful launching. This has often forced people to enter the water. Ships now carry inflatable rafts, which can be launched more reliably than lifeboats. They are fitted with canopies, but people often need to spend time in the water before reaching a raft. Hypothermia can then make it difficult to board the raft, and many have died of cold while in the water or after boarding. Personal protection from cold during immersion is still important.

Large-scale immersion trials on volunteers have shown that people can do a great deal to slow their rate of body cooling in the water.[16] Even non-waterproof thick clothing can more than halve the rate of body cooling in cold water. It is also better to float still than to swim about, as swimming in cold water generally increases heat loss more than it increases heat production. In very cold seawater, it is important to protect all immersed skin, as seawater freezes at $-1.9\,^{\circ}C$ ($29\,^{\circ}F$), while human tissues freeze at $-0.53\,^{\circ}C$ ($31\,^{\circ}F$). This means that fingers, for example, can freeze within a few minutes in liquid sea water at its freezing point, greatly reducing the victim's chances of survival. Shipwreck victims can therefore improve their chances of surviving if they put on a lifejacket and dress warmly, including mittens or gloves, before entering the water, and then float still in a lifejacket rather than swim about while waiting for rescue.

People's body build greatly affects their heat loss in water. Cold immersion is almost the only situation (except lack of food) where it is useful to be fat. Most of the external insulation that is usually provided by air is lost on immersion in cold water. Once blood flow to the skin shuts down in the cold, the layer of fat under the skin provides internal insulation, and body heat loss depends on how thick this is. Shipwrecks do not give people time to put on fat, but people who happen to have a thick layer of subcutaneous fat have a huge advantage over those who do not. A fat person can stabilize his or her body temperature at a safe level for many hours in water at $12\,^{\circ}C$ ($54\,^{\circ}F$), whereas a thin one can die in water at $24\,^{\circ}C$ ($75\,^{\circ}F$).

Children generally cool more quickly than adults in cold water. This is partly because they usually have less fat to provide insulation, and partly because their small size gives them a smaller body mass to produce heat in relation to body surface area, from which heat is lost. Women generally have thicker subcutaneous fat than men and have it more evenly distributed. In particular, they have thicker limb fat, which can be scanty in men, even those with thick subcutaneous fat over their abdomen. The practical message is that children need priority in rescue from cold water, and that women often do well as long-distance swimmers.

Water temperatures below $12\,^{\circ}C$ can cause even people with plenty of subcutaneous fat to cool. The fat only provides effective insulation while the blood flow through it to the skin is stopped. Blood flow in the skin often returns in long immersions in water below about $12\,^{\circ}C$. The reason is that when the temperature of the skin drops below this level, blood vessels in the skin become paralysed by cold and gradually relax. As blood flow returns to the skin, carrying heat through the subcutaneous fat to the skin, heat loss from the body to the water rises. Consequently, even fat people generally cool down rapidly within an hour of the start of immersion in water at $5\,^{\circ}C$ ($41\,^{\circ}F$).

The exceptions have been fat people who are acclimatized to the cold. Adaptation to cold appears to improve the ability of blood vessels to resist cold paralysis, and this can allow people with enough fat to stabilize their body temperature at a safe level for many hours in water down to $5\,^{\circ}C$. At such water temperatures, clothing retards body heat loss much more than its insulating effect would suggest. Although ordinary thick clothing only increases skin temperature by a few degrees, this is often enough to prevent or greatly reduce cold paralysis of the blood vessels in very cold water.

Even without thick clothing, fat people who are acclimatized to the cold can, exceptionally, not only survive, but even benefit from swimming about while waiting for rescue from water below about $12\,^{\circ}C$. Immersion of limbs in water at or below $12\,^{\circ}C$ for around 3 hours otherwise causes an unpleasant condition called immersion injury. This is a degeneration of nerve and muscle that can cause lifelong pain and disability in the limbs, usually the legs. It is caused directly by a low temperature of the tissue, and not indirectly through anoxia from low blood flow. Fat people acclimatized to the cold have swum for hours in such water without getting this injury. The reason is presumably that the high blood flow and high heat production in limb muscle during swimming keep the limb warm enough to prevent cold injury.

Fat can keep people afloat, as well as keeping them warm. Fat is buoyant, whereas the rest of the body is not. That means that a fat person can float without swimming, while a thin person sinks. This is important after accidents to small boats, which take a steady toll of deaths in cold water. They usually happen close enough to shore for people who can swim to expect to reach it without difficulty. In practice, many people who do try to swim ashore in very cold water never reach it but drown suddenly on the way. One reason for that is that the sudden cooling of the skin by the cold water causes a immediate intense reflex intake of breath, followed by gasping and difficulty in breathing, in people who are not acclimatized to the cold.[16] This lasts several minutes and can cause panic.

Another reason is that the viscosity, or stickiness, of water increases at low temperature, so that swimming in water near freezing point is like swimming in dilute treacle. Together with the breathing disturbance, this can cause rapid exhaustion and drowning. Although thin, fit young people can get exhausted and drown very rapidly when swimming clothed in water near freezing point, older and less fit, but fatter and more buoyant, people can keep swimming for many minutes. The practical message is that even people who are very confident of their swimming ability should always wear a buoyancy aid when taking out a small boat on cold water. A wetsuit is particularly useful, providing both buoyancy and protection from hypothermia.

'Dry drowning', in which little fluid is found in the lungs of people who have died suddenly in water, was often attributed to reflex vagal arrest of the heart. There was, however, little evidence that the inhalation of water could in fact cause such arrest for the 10–20 minutes needed to cause death, and later evidence has attributed most of these cases to water being inhaled into the lungs but then being rapidly absorbed into the circulation. Other cases of 'dry drowning' were due to laryngeal spasm, with little water ever reaching the lungs. Sudden death in cold water can occasionally be explained only by the large rises in arterial blood pressure caused by the cold, which can trigger ventricular fibrillation of the heart without any inhalation of water.[17]

The main need for swimmers and scuba-divers is to be aware of the risk of hypothermia, and of the fact that it often shows itself as confusion and exhaustion. Long-distance swimmers have died when urged to continue swimming after this has happened. For scuba-divers, the main risk is that distress from body cooling can induce them to come to the surface more rapidly than is recommended, putting them at risk of decompression sickness. Wetsuits worn by divers protect against the cold, but their insulation is provided by air bubbles in their rubber fabric, and at depth these bubbles are compressed, removing most of the insulation. It is important to restrict the depth and duration of dives in very cold water in order to allow time for decompression at a safe rate. Milder degrees of hypothermia cause a loss of short-term memory and slow reasoning down. This has been a serious hazard to deep-water divers servicing undersea oil installations, but has largely disappeared with a better control of warm water supplied to the diving suit.

Treatment of hypothermia

Hypothermia should be suspected in people rescued after prolonged exposure to cold air or water. It can be confirmed by finding a rectal or oesophageal temperature below 35 °C, or excluded by finding either these temperatures or a sublingual or ear (external auditory meatus) temperature above 35 °C. A low sublingual or ear temperature in cold surroundings, or within an hour of rescue from these, does not prove hypothermia, as local cooling can depress these temperatures well below cardiac temperature.

If hypothermia is found, the patient should be kept lying flat. Prolonged hypothermia can cause dehydration due to a renal loss of salt and water, and this can lead to brain damage from a lack of blood to the head if the patient sits or stands upright for long. For people rescued from cold water, rewarming should be started by a warm bath if one is available within 30 minutes of rescue; without this, heat loss from the body core to cold peripheral tissues can reduce cardiac temperature to a lethal level during this time. To avoid scalds, the water must not be so hot as to be painful when tested by a rescuer dipping an elbow into it. Adrenaline should not be given, as it frequently precipitates ventricular fibrillation during hypothermia.

People who have become hypothermic from exposure to cold air should be put on a stretcher and insulated to stop further heat loss until they are brought into the warm. Rewarming is then best done by air at or a little above 37 °C (99 °F). It will be more effective without thick clothing or a reflective space blanket, which simply retards the transfer of heat from warm air into the patient. Active rewarming should be stopped once body core temperature rises above 35 °C. If the haemoglobin level is found to be above normal as body temperature rises, intravenous saline can help to correct the haemoconcentration and restore blood volume.

It is important to check for a carotid pulse and take an ECG as soon as possible in people who appear to rescuers to be dead from hypothermia. Pulse rate and respiration are abnormally slow in hypothermia, and contraction of the arteries often makes it impossible to feel the peripheral pulses. Victims of hypothermia in this state will often recover if simply brought into a warm room and allowed to rewarm slowly. When someone is found collapsed in the cold, it is essential to start treatment at once, giving priority to this over investigation of the circumstances. A particular concern is that people developing severe hypothermia sometimes experience not only confusion but a paradoxical sensation of warmth, which leads them to shed clothing before collapsing and losing consciousness. This has led rescuers to assume mistakenly that they are the victim of assault, and to delay rescue while the details of the supposed crime scene are investigated.

Even if the patient has already developed cardiac arrest or ventricular fibrillation before rescue, he or she may still be revivable. The brain can survive a cessation of blood flow for longer in hypothermia than at normal body temperature. This has allowed people in hypothermia, usually children who have fallen through the ice, to be revived after 60 minutes of circulatory arrest, although some degree of brain damage must be expected if the arrest has lasted for more than about 30 minutes. Most of the successful resuscitations from circulatory arrest in hypothermia have used extracorporeal circulation to restore circulation at once, as well as to rewarm the patient.

Frostbite is a major complication in people who have been exposed to air many degrees below freezing point and is obvious from the hard, white skin. It is important not to cause mechanical damage to frozen limbs by bending them. Small areas of frostbite, such as fingers and toes, are now treated by rapid rewarming in water no warmer than 40 °C (104 °F). This minimizes local circulatory obstruction, when capillary damage from freezing lets plasma escape and allows red cells to sludge and block blood flow in the capillaries, with subsequent ischaemic injury to the tissue. However, if a large portion of a limb is frozen, rapid thawing can be dangerous by releasing enough potassium from its tissues to cause cardiac arrest. Such patients are best treated by thawing the limbs in hospital under full biochemical control.

REFERENCES

1. Macfarlane A, Waller RE. Short term increases in mortality during heatwaves. *Nature* 1976; **264**: 434–6.
2. Keatinge WR, Donaldson GC, Cordioli E *et al*. Heat related mortality in warm and cold regions of Europe, observational study. *BMJ* 2000; **321**: 670–3.
3. Donaldson GC, Keatinge WR, Nayha S. Changes in summer temperature and heat related mortality since 1971 in North Carolina, South Finland and Southeast England. *Environ Res* 2003; **91**: 1–7.
4. Heyer HE, Teng C, Barris W. Increased frequency of myocardial infarction during the summer months in a warm climate. *Am Heart J* 1953 ; **45**: 741–55.
5. Keatinge WR, Coleshaw SRK, Easton JC, Cotter F, Mattock MB, Chelliah R. Increased platelet and red cell counts, blood viscosity and plasma cholesterol level during heat stress, and mortality from coronary and cerebral thromboses. *Am J Med* 1986; **81**: 795–800.
6. Keatinge WR, Donaldson GC. Heat acclimatisation and sunshine cause false indications of mortality due to ozone. *Environ Res* 2006; **100**: 670–3.
7. Woodhouse PR, Coleshaw SRK, Keatinge WR. Factors associated with hypothermia in a group of inner city hospitals. *Lancet* 1989; **2**: 1201–3.
8. Bull GM, Morton J. Environment, temperature and death rates. *Age Ageing* 1978; **7**: 210–14.
9. Donaldson GC, Keatinge WR. Early increases in ischaemic heart disease mortality dissociated from, and later changes associated with, respiratory mortality, after cold weather in south east England. *J Epidemiol Commun Health* 1997; **51**: 643–8.
10. Keatinge WR, Coleshaw SRK, Cotter F, Mattock M, Murphy M, Chelliah R. Increases in platelet and red cell counts, blood viscosity, and arterial pressure during mild surface cooling: Factors in mortality from coronary and cerebral thrombosis in winter. *BMJ* 1984; **289**: 1405–8.
11. Neild PJ, Syndercombe-Court D, Keatinge WR, Donaldson GC, Mattock M, Caunce M. Cold-induced increases in erythrocyte count, plasma cholesterol and plasma fibrinogen of elderly people without a comparable rise in protein C or factor X. *Clin Sci* 1994; **86**: 43–8.
12. Eurowinter Group: Keatinge WR, Donaldson GC, Bucher K *et al*. Cold exposure and winter mortality from ischaemic heart disease, cerebrovascular disease, respiratory disease, and all causes in warm and cold regions of Europe. *Lancet* 1997; **349**: 1341–6.
13. Woodhouse PR, Khaw K-T, Plummer M, Foley A, Meade TW. Seasonal variations in plasma fibrinogen and factor VII activity in the elderly: Winter infections and death from cardiovascular disease. *Lancet* 1994; **343**: 435–9.
14. Keatinge WR. Seasonal mortality among elderly people with unrestricted home heating. *BMJ* 1986; **293**: 732–3.
15. McCance RA, Ungley CC, Crosfill JWL, Widdowson EM. *The Hazards to Men in Ships Lost at Sea, 1939–1944*. Special Report Series No. 291. London: Medical Research Council, 1956.
16. Keatinge WR. *Survival in Cold Water. The Physiology and Treatment of Immersion Hypothermia and of Drowning*. Oxford: Blackwell Scientific Publications, 1969.
17. Keatinge WR, Hayward MG. Sudden death in cold water and ventricular arrhythmia. *J Forensic Sci* 1981; **26**: 459–61.

48

Global climate change

SARI KOVATS, ANTHONY J. McMICHAEL

Global climate change, caused by the accumulation of greenhouse gases in the lower atmosphere as a consequence of human activity (Box 48.1), is a remarkable and fundamental source of risks to human health – 'remarkable' because the risk is of a scale and type not previously encountered by human species; 'fundamental' because the risks mostly arise from changes to various biophysical and ecological systems and processes that make up the life-support systems of this planet.

The risks to health are many and varied. Some climate and weather factors act directly and predictably – such as the health effects of heatwaves, or the physical and mental consequences of floods and storms. Other health effects are mediated by disturbances of natural processes; for example, various temperature-sensitive biological processes are involved in infectious disease transmission. Climate is ultimately the determinant of food and water availability, but access is in most populations determined by social and economic factors. Many impacts of climate change may occur more diffusely, by increasing poverty. At the high end of future climate projections, rapid rates of warming may result in social and economic disruption, leading to a displacement of marginal populations and, potentially, to increased tensions and conflict. These more indirect impacts of climate change are likely to be more significant for health in the long term if climate change is not mitigated, but it is inherently more difficult to study or predict the health effects.

> ## BOX 48.1: The Causes of Global Climate Change
>
> The world's climate is changing. Over the past half-century, Earth's average temperature has changed to an extent and at a pace that clearly differ from the historically observed character of natural background variations in world climate. Globally, the rate of warming over the last 50 years (0.13 °C per decade) is nearly twice that of the last 100 years. The global mean temperature increase from the period 1850–1899 to 2001–2005 has been 0.76 °C. In Europe, the warming trend has been +0.90 °C for the period 1901–2005.
>
> The Fourth Assessment Report of the Intergovernmental Panel on Climate Change (IPCC) concluded, from changes in a range of geophysical parameters, that most of the warming since 1950 has been due to human actions. The human-induced 'greenhouse' capture of additional outward-bound radiative energy is now measurably changing global climate patterns. The Technical Summary of the IPCC Working Group I (2007) provides excellent information on the basic mechanism of climate change, as well as on past trends and future projections.[6] The global atmospheric concentration of carbon dioxide (the main greenhouse gas) increased from a pre-industrial value of 280 parts per million (ppm) to 379 ppm in 2005 – and is now approaching 390 ppm. This concentration far exceeds the natural range (estimated from ice cores) over the last 650 000 years (180–300 ppm).

Climate change mostly does not affect health on its own – that is, as a separate, single, exposure. It is one of the emerging set of global environmental changes that are occurring in response to the now-excessive pressures by the human population on this planet, Earth. The UN Environment Programme's report *Global Environmental Outlook 2007*, in its review of the current state and future prospects of Earth's environmental and ecological systems,[1] has emphasized that social stability and human well-being, health and survival, are at increasing risk from systemic environmental changes. The report documented worrying negative trends in the world's fertile soils, freshwater supplies, coastal and reef ecosystems, fish stocks, concentrations of human-activated nitrogen (mostly from nitrogenous fertilizers and fossil fuel combustion), ocean acidity and numbers and stocks of species.[2,3] All these changes pose risks to population health.[4,5]

Much of the public and political discussion about climate change has been preoccupied with risks to economic growth, physical infrastructure and iconic species. Impacts on health are, rather belatedly, now gaining more attention and contributing to the wider climate policy debates.[7,8] Climate change endangers the physical and ecological systems upon which biological functioning and health depend; it jeopardizes the sustainability of Earth's life-support systems, hence its fundamental relevance to the rationale for urgent and radical mitigation action. Meanwhile, it is important that 'adaptation' policies are established to limit the risk to health in the near term. Climate change requires us to develop new approaches for both research and policy.

There are six main research tasks in relation to climate change and health (Figure 48.1), which refer to three different time domains:

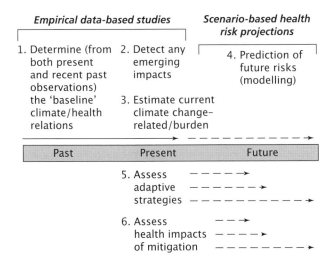

Figure 48.1 The six research tasks in relation to climate change and health.

- *present*: learning, from observational studies, about the sensitivity of health outcomes to variations in climate and weather exposures;
- *recent past*: the detection and attribution of changes in population health due to observed anthropogenic climate change;
- *future*: scenario-based assessments of future health burdens, to estimate how climate change will affect health over the coming decades, with, in addition, monitoring and evaluation of the health consequences of adaptation strategies and mitigation actions.

Scientific reports during the first decade of the twenty-first century have indicated that the change in global climate is occurring more quickly than was predicted by climate science in the 1990s.[9,10] The Fourth Assessment Report of the Intergovernmental Panel on Climate Change (IPCC)[6] concluded in 2007 that climate change had already begun to affect many physical and biotic systems.[11,12] Long-term drying is already emerging in southern and western Africa, southern Europe, India and Australia.[6] There is also very good evidence that heatwaves are increasing in frequency and intensity, in conjunction with a decline in the frequency of very cold days.[13] Other extreme weather events may also have increased in frequency or intensity, although that aspect of climate change is more complex.[14]

CLIMATE, WEATHER AND CLIMATE CHANGE EXPOSURES

It is important to distinguish between climate change and climate variability. *Climate change* is defined as a statistically significant departure from either the prior mean state of the climate or its variability, and persisting for an extended period (typically decades or longer).[6] Climate change may be due to natural internal processes within the climate system, or to external forcings. The latter includes anthropogenic changes in the composition of the atmosphere and changes in land use. In this chapter, we will use the term 'climate change' to mean anthropogenic climate change caused by fossil fuel-burning and other human activities.

Climate variability can be expressed in various temporal scales (by day, season or year) and is an inherent characteristic of climate, whether or not the climate system is subject to change. 'Weather' is the state of the atmosphere at a given time and place in terms of temperature, moisture, wind velocity and barometric pressure variables. In simple terms: climate is what you expect, weather is what you get.

For observational studies, climate exposures can be described in three broad temporal categories:

- long-term changes in mean temperature and other climate norms (e.g. anthropogenic climate change);

- climate variability about norms over periods ranging from a few years to several decades, including:
  - shifts in the frequency/probability distributions of climate variables;
  - recurring climate phenomena such as the El Niño-Southern Oscillation (ENSO);
- isolated extreme events, either simple extremes (temperature/precipitation extremes) or complex events (tropical cyclones, floods and droughts).

These types of exposure are not independent of one another. A shift in the mean of a climate variable will entail a non-linear change in the frequency of extreme events, defined according to fixed criteria.[15]

There has been long-standing interest in how weather and climate affect human health. There is a long history of observations about some climates and seasons having more benefits to health than others. In 400 BC, Hippocrates advised people who wished to investigate medicine properly, to 'first consider the seasons of the year, and the effects each of them produces'.[16] Seasonal patterns are apparent in death rates[17] and in many infectious diseases, such as influenza, malaria and salmonellosis. It has, however, only relatively recently been recognized that large-scale changes in climate patterns and conditions over time also affect the health of populations.

These large-scale patterns provide a useful analogue for thinking about the future impacts of climate change.[18] The most famous is the ENSO. Others include the North Atlantic Oscillation that affects weather in Europe, and the Quasi-Biennial Oscillation that affects weather in Australia. The ENSO is a strong determinant of *interannual* variability in South America, Australia and East Africa. There is good evidence that, in certain locations, the ENSO influences certain infectious diseases, such as malaria and cholera.[19,20] The changes in precipitation are the principle mechanism by which El Niño affects mosquito-borne disease. Individual El Niño events, however, should not be confused with long-term climate change – although climate change itself is anticipated to affect the frequency and/or intensity of El Niño (and La Niña) events in the future.[6]

METHODS FOR ESTIMATING THE CURRENT IMPACT OF WEATHER AND CLIMATE ON HEALTH

Bioclimatology is the study of the effects of climate on living things – and because almost every aspect of climate and weather has some effect on living organisms, this covers a wide range of health effects. Some health issues have been researched more than others, particularly the influence of weather and climate on arthropods that act as vectors, parasites or hosts for plant, animal and human diseases. The direct effect of weather and climate on physiological processes in healthy humans and their

responses has also been studied. The influence of microclimates in dwellings and urban centres on human health is now an emerging area of interest as well.

Research on the potential health impacts of climate change, however, needs to be informed by the observed effects of weather and climate on human disease outcomes, primarily using epidemiological methods.[21] There are four main types of observational studies relevant for climate change and health:

- the health impacts of individual extreme events (heatwaves, floods, storms and droughts);
- spatial studies, in which climate is an explanatory variable in the distribution of the health outcome (or a related outcome such as disease vector);
- temporal studies of changes in climate-related health outcomes:
  - short-term (daily or weekly) changes in meteorological parameters;
  - interannual climate variability;
  - longer term (decadal) changes in the context of detecting early effects of climate change (see below);
- experimental laboratory and field studies of biological phenomena likely to mediate some of the health effects of climate change, for example studies on vectors, pathogens or plant biology.

Empirical studies of the effects of weather or climate on health outcomes provide the evidence base for understanding future risks, assessing whether actual (climate change) impacts have occurred, and developing intervention strategies. As with all epidemiological studies, it is important that information on potential confounders is included in the analysis. Cross-sectional studies are particularly subject to confounding, as non-climate determinants are significant when comparing between populations with different climate exposures, and there are few robust studies of this type. Time series studies of short-term (daily or weekly) associations require adjustment for season and trend to avoid spurious associations. Meteorological observations are relatively easy to obtain and of good quality. It is important to use the appropriate observed meteorological data for the population of interest. Finally, there should be a plausible biological explanation for any association between weather parameters and disease outcome. Table 48.1 summarizes the current state of knowledge regarding the impacts of weather on health outcomes.

The number of published observational studies of weather and climate effects is increasing as interest in climate change grows. Many time series studies have been published that quantify the mortality effects of temperature in diverse populations. Unlike other environmental exposures, the impact of ambient temperature appears to be population specific. This is discussed in more detail in Chapter 47 on heat and cold. Chapter 32 discusses water-borne disease transmission,

Table 48.1 Summary of current knowledge on the impacts of weather on health outcomes

Category of health outcome	Known effects of weather and climate variability
Heat stress	• Deaths from cardiorespiratory disease increase with high and low temperatures • Heat-related illness and death due to heatwaves
Air pollution-related mortality and morbidity	• Weather affects air pollutant concentrations • Weather affects the distribution, seasonality and production of aeroallergens
Health impacts of weather disasters	• Floods, landslides and windstorms cause direct effects (deaths and injuries) and indirect effects (infectious disease, loss of food supplies and long-term psychological morbidity)
Mosquito-borne diseases, tick-borne diseases (e.g. malaria and Dengue fever)	• Higher temperatures reduce the development time of pathogens in vectors and increase potential transmission to humans • Vector species require specific climatic conditions (temperature and humidity) to be sufficiently abundant to maintain transmission
Water-/food-borne diseases	• The survival of important bacterial pathogens is related to temperature • Extreme rainfall can affect the transport of disease organisms into the water supply. Outbreaks of water-borne disease have been associated with contamination caused by heavy rainfall and flooding, associated with inadequate sanitation • Increases in drought conditions may affect water availability and water quality (chemical and microbiological load) due to extreme low flows

Adapted from Kovats and Akhtar,[33] with permission.

which can also be affected by extreme weather events such as heavy rainfall.[22]

METHODS FOR ESTIMATING THE FUTURE IMPACT OF CLIMATE CHANGE ON HEALTH

Global climate change is a distinctive and as yet unfamiliar type of environmental health hazard. In particular, it has a global scale (as all populations will be affected in some way) and is characterized by the long time period over which the climate change process and its full environmental and human impacts will unfold. Due to the long latency of greenhouse gases in the atmosphere, there is an important immediate need to identify and estimate global and regional health impacts in order to inform policy-making directed at reducing climate change emissions. The planet is already committed to a certain amount of climate change due to past emissions. The remainder of this chapter will focus on the likely health impacts of climate change and the methods used to assess them.

Most climate change impacts, adaptation and vulnerability assessments use a scenario-driven approach in order to take into account the uncertainty about future climates and the future world in which those climates will be experienced.[23] Scenarios are a plausible and often simplified description of how the future may develop, based on a coherent and internally consistent set of assumptions about the driving forces and key relationships. They provide an important tool for estimating the potential impact of climate change on specific health outcomes (Box 48.2).

Climate scenarios are plausible representations of future climate that have been constructed for use in investigating the potential impacts of climate change.

Climate scenarios are generally derived from the output of global or regional climate models. National climate scenarios have been specifically constructed for national impact assessments.[24] A range of methods are used to downscale the coarse-resolution output of the climate models to provide appropriate climate information at the local scale. The first generation of climate change scenarios described changes in average conditions, but the latest scenarios now include estimates of changes in the magnitude and occurrence of extreme weather events, as well as probabilistic projections.

As nearly all aspects of our natural, physical and social environments will change in the future, it is important that those changes are reflected in the scenarios used in climate impact studies. In practice, however, only population growth and economic growth (in gross domestic product per capita) have been quantified and routinely included in climate impact studies. Some examples of scenario-based assessments of future heat-related mortality due to climate change are listed in Table 48.2. These studies use climate scenarios to estimate the future changes in local temperature exposure, and some (but not all) use population scenarios to estimate the future total population and/or the proportion of older age groups who are much more susceptible to heat-related mortality. A limitation of these studies is that they must make assumptions about how future populations will respond to exposure to high temperatures, including the rate of acclimatization.

Several countries have undertaken national assessments of the impacts of climate change on health, including the UK,[26] Portugal,[27] Australia and New Zealand[28] and Canada.[29] As with other sectors affected by climate change, the focus of the assessments has shifted from science-based questions to more policy-related ones.

BOX 48.2: Advantages and disadvantages of scenarios in impact studies

Scenarios are useful because they:
- *articulate key considerations and assumptions*: scenarios can help to imagine a range of possible futures if we follow a key set of assumptions and considerations;
- *blend quantitative and qualitative knowledge*: scenarios are powerful frameworks for using both data and model-produced output in combination with qualitative knowledge elements;
- *identify constraints and dilemmas*: exploring the future often yields indications for constraints in future developments and dilemmas for strategic choices to be made;
- *expand our thinking beyond the conventional paradigm*: exploring future possibilities that go beyond our conventional thinking may result in surprising and innovative insights.

There are disadvantages in using scenarios:
- *lack of diversity*: scenarios are often developed from a narrow, disciplinary-based perspective, resulting in a limited set of standard economic, technological and environmental assumptions;
- *extrapolations of current trends*: many scenarios have a 'business-as-usual' character, assuming that current conditions will continue for decades;
- *inconsistency*: sets of assumptions made for different sectors, regions or issues are often not consistent with each other;
- *lack of transparency*: key assumptions and underlying implicit judgements and preferences are not made explicit. For example, it may not be clear which factors or processes are exogenous or endogenous, and to what extent societal processes are autonomous or influenced by concrete policies.

Adapted from Martens and Hilderink,[25] with permission.

Table 48.2   Examples of scenario-based assessments of the health impacts of climate change: heat-related mortality

Area	Health effect	Model	Climate scenario; time slices	Main results	Reference
Lisbon, Portugal	Heat-related mortality	Empirical-statistical model derived from observed summer mortality	PROMES and HadRM2. 2020s, 2050s, 2080s	Increase in heat-related mortality from a baseline of 5.4–6.0 deaths/100 000 to 5.8–15.1 deaths/100 000 by the 2020s, 7.3–35.9 deaths/100 000 by the 2050s and 19.5–248.4 deaths/100 000 by the 2080s	[65]
Four cities in California, USA (Los Angeles, Sacramento, Fresno, Shasta Dam)	Annual number of heatwave days, length of heatwave season and heat-related mortality	Empirical-statistical model derived from observed summer mortality	PCM and HadCM3 driven by SRES B1 and A1FI emission scenarios. *2030s, 2080s	Increase in the annual number of days classified as heatwave conditions. By 2080s, in Los Angeles, the number of heatwave days increases fourfold under B1 and 6 to eightfold under A1FI. The annual number of heat-related deaths in Los Angeles increases from about 165 in the 1990s to 319–1182 under different scenarios	[66]
Australian capital cities	Heat-related mortality in people older than 65 years	Empirical-statistical model derived from observed daily mortality	CSIRO Mk2, ECHAM4 and HadCM2 driven by A2 and B2 emission scenarios and a stabilization scenario at 450 ppm in 2100	Increase in temperature-attributable death rates from 82/100 000 across all cities under the current climate to 246/100 000 in 2100; death rates decrease with the implementation of policies to mitigate greenhouse gases	[28]
Europe 50 × 50 km grid	Heat-attributable mortality (all-cause)	Statistical model based on region-specific exposure-response functions	SRES–A2 and B2 (PRUDENCE RCM scenarios)	By 2020s, an approximated increase of 25 000 heat deaths per year, assuming acclimatization	[67]

ppm, parts per million.

Many anticipated effects of climate change are not disease specific but address broader determinants of health that are not readily quantified, such as poverty, displacement and access to food or water.[30] A review of climate change impact assessments found that the literature is heavily biased towards quantitative assessments within the prescribed scenarios for easily measured (and costed) outcomes (Figure 48.2).[31] There has been less work on non-market-based outcomes such as health and ecological impacts. Furthermore, the issue of surprises or fundamental systems changes caused by climate change has been poorly addressed in the health risks assessment domain, since there is, at this stage, a lack of tools and methods to use.

CURRENT STATE OF KNOWLEDGE ABOUT HEALTH EFFECTS OF CLIMATE CHANGE

The many impacts of climate change on human health can be visualized using the three main causal pathways shown in Figure 48.3.[32] These pathways span the immediate and direct effects of climate events, from changes in biophysical and ecological processes, to the spectrum of adverse effects on social stability and well-being and mental health that result from the impoverishment of communities and groups.

Some benefits to population health from climate change are likely to also occur. For example, some parts of the world may become too dry for mosquitoes (and therefore to sustain endemic mosquito-borne infections). Winters will become milder, and thus climate warming will reduce the mortality associated with cold in mid-to-high latitude countries.

The 'direct' health effects (see path 1 in Figure 48.3) include altered risks of mortality and morbidity from an increased risk of exposure to environmental heat (and heatwaves), the respiratory health consequences of changes in exposures to air pollutants and aeroallergens, and the health consequences of extreme weather events (windstorms or floods). Intensified rainfall, with flooding, can overwhelm urban wastewater and sewer systems.[33] There is general agreement among researchers that, as climate change progresses, the more 'indirect' effects on health are likely to constitute a greater population health burden than the 'direct' effects. In this, the risks of malnutrition and altered patterns of infectious diseases would be paramount.

The key global assessment for the impact of climate change on health is the IPCC Assessment report.[34] The Fourth Assessment Report was published in 2007, and the Fifth Assessment Report is expected to be published in approximately 2013. The global assessments inform the importance of the issue of health impacts, and also reinforce arguments for mitigation. The assessment relies on only the peer-reviewed literature, which is currently limited and inevitably biased towards impacts in high-income countries.

Infectious disease

An indirect effect on health is that of changes in the patterns of infectious disease occurrence, particularly the faeco-oral type of infection (via food, water or flies and associated with a lack of hygiene) and vector-borne infectious diseases (e.g. malaria, Dengue fever and leishmaniasis).

Climatic conditions affect the rates of transmission of many food-borne and water-borne diseases, reflecting the

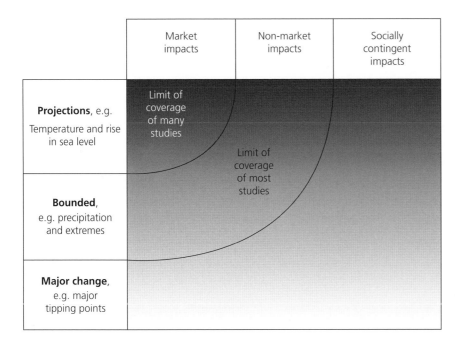

Figure 48.2 The coverage of existing climate change impact studies (all sectors). (Modified from Watkiss and Downing,[31] with permission.)

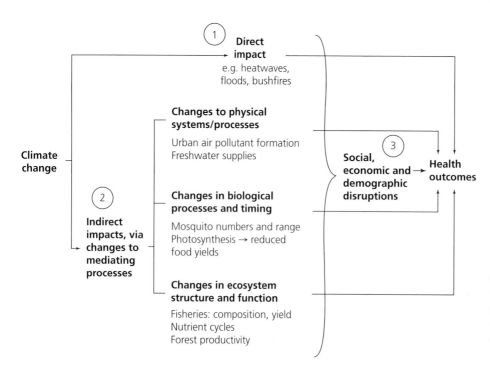

Figure 48.3 The main pathways by which climate change affects human health. Note the progression – from category 1 (relatively simple and direct), through category 2 (changes to complex environmental and ecological systems) to category 3 (health risks from the social–economic–demographic consequences of climatic – environmental disturbances).

fact that many are caused by bacteria that multiply more quickly at higher temperatures. Food poisoning is known to peak in the warmer months. Simple monotonic associations have been shown between environmental temperature and salmonellosis notifications in Europe[35] and Australia.[36] In contrast, infection by *Campylobacter* displays a much weaker relationship to temperature, although it has a strong seasonality. Studies have shown that short-term increases in diarrhoeal diseases in Peru[37] and Fiji[38] are associated with hot weather. On a global scale, arid areas have a higher incidence of diarrhoeal morbidity compared with areas with other climates.[39]

The survival of cholera in the environment is sensitive to temperature, salinity and other abiotic factors. It is now well established that the cholera vibrio proliferates in warmer water in lakes, estuaries and coastal waters, especially in association with algal blooms.[40] Cholera is primarily transmitted via the faeco-oral route and is associated with a lack of access to safe water and sanitation, and to poor hygiene. Thus, cholera transmission is increased either when conditions are dry and the microbial contamination of surface water is therefore concentrated, or when flooding causes a displacement of people and the overflow of sewage and latrines. Large-scale climate patterns such as ENSO have been shown to affect cholera transmission in Bangladesh.[41]

The arthropods (insects and ticks) that transmit vector-borne infectious diseases are typically very sensitive to climatic conditions. Both the development and replication of the pathogen in the vector organism proceed more quickly at higher temperatures. The abundance and distribution of vector species is also determined by the availability of breeding sites, where they are dependent on vegetation, and rainfall patterns,

as well as the control measures that are in place. Chapters 37–42 of this volume describe in more detail the environmental (including climatic) determinants of the vectors of infectious disease.

Uncertainties remain about how the transmission of many of these infectious diseases responds to variations in climate conditions. Nevertheless, it is an important task to attempt to estimate the likely future pattern of risk of transmission under a range of climate scenarios – which must incorporate a range of assumptions about the capacity of countries to control the disease in the future. To date, most of the scenario-based modelling of future changes in infectious disease risks has focused on mapping the changing distribution of only the vectors (e.g. the tick vectors of Lyme disease in Canada[42]) or changes in the (geographical) population at risk of malaria[43,44] and schistosomiasis (for which water snails are the intermediate host).[45] Such studies suggest that the seasonality of potential transmission of malaria will change, leading to an increased number of person–months at risk.

Broadly speaking, the malaria assessments indicate that (if nothing else changes) climate change will expand the range in highland regions and restrict the range in arid and semi-arid regions in Africa.[46–48] Decreases in rainfall are likely to reduce the transmission of malaria in many regions, although this benefit may be undermined by the increasing use of irrigation or dams. The potential for expansion in the African highlands is a cause for concern because the region is densely populated.[20,48] Future impact studies will need to incorporate the important non-climate determinants of infectious diseases, such as future land-use change, as well as changes in the distribution and abundance of vectors.

Extreme weather and disasters

It is likely that the most obvious effects of climate change on human health will be from an increase in the frequency and intensity of extreme weather events, such as heatwaves, floods and storms.

Heat is a natural hazard, and much is known about the effects of high temperatures on the human body. Heatwaves can have significant impacts on health and present a challenge for public health and civil protection services.[49] As one of the most certain impacts of future anthropogenic climate change will be an increase in heatwaves in many populations, it is very likely that that the future burden of heat-related mortality will increase.

The 'excess mortality' attributed to a heatwave event is apparent as the short-term increase in the numbers of deaths, a peak in mortality similar to that seen for very severe pollution episodes. The number of deaths does, however, depend upon the definition of the heat episode. Reviews have shown that the total impact of a heat event will be dependent on a number of factors including the heatwave magnitude, timing in the season, population experience of heatwave events and public health response options.[50] In the long term, as the climate changes, populations are likely to be become less sensitive to temperature extremes due to improvements in the underlying health of the population.[51,52] Conversely, populations are ageing, and the number of elderly people susceptible to temperature extremes will increase.

Floods are the most frequent cause of weather disaster and are associated with a range of impacts on health.[53] The effect of climate change on future river-flooding is complex. A rise in sea level is likely to increase coastal flooding in areas where increasing the coastal defences is difficult or unaffordable.[54] Droughts are also projected to increase with climate change and may affect health particularly in poor rural populations, where local food supplies are affected. Climate change will adversely affect both physical and psychological health whenever a loss of livelihoods, a displacement of the population and economic disruption occur. Such disruptions may occur because of multiple impacts on a vulnerable population, including rising sea levels, agro-ecosystem decline and freshwater shortages.

DETECTION AND ATTRIBUTION OF HEALTH EFFECTS TO OBSERVED CLIMATE CHANGE

There is now good evidence that the recent observed climate change has affected many biological and ecological phenomena.[11] The evidence has been categorized in four ways:[55]

- *effects on physiology*: the metabolic or development rates of animals, and plant processes;

- *effects on distribution*: the response to shifts in mean temperature and precipitation conditions;
- *effects on phenology*: the timing of life-cycle events, for example the budding of flowers or egg-laying;
- *adaptation*: as species with short generation times and rapid population growth rates may undergo some microevolution.

In contrast to those non-human biological and ecological phenomena, human health is often well buffered by culture, behaviour and healthcare. The causal climate change 'signal' is thus blunted or otherwise hidden. For example, the transmission of a vector-borne disease such as malaria is determined by a range of environmental and social factors, particularly local vector control measures. Similarly, if climate change affects local grain yields, humans (unlike polar bears that are no longer able to catch their prey because of the receding ice floes) can trade or switch to other crops. Thus, the detection and attribution to climate change of changes in human health outcomes poses a complex challenge to researchers and public health policy-makers.

Recent scientific papers indicate an emerging influence of climate change on infectious disease patterns, although none yet meets the formal criteria stipulated by the IPCC for attribution to anthropogenic forcing of the climate system.[11] There is some evidence for a northwards extension of the tick vector for tick-borne encephalitis over the past two decades in Sweden[56,57] and possibly in Canada,[42] but there is no evidence of a concomitant increase in the disease itself. The resurgence of highland malaria in parts of eastern and southern Africa is consistent with local warming,[58] but also with many other factors known to have contributed to the resurgence of the disease (e.g. drug resistance and population movement).[59]

An observation that recent climate change has been associated with changes in vectors or infectious disease itself does not, of itself, prove a causative relationship, since it is not usually possible to exclude all possible alternative explanations for any such change in disease patterns.[59] The most direct evidence would be a trend in disease over many years that is significantly correlated with a change in climate after adjusting for correlations with other potential driving mechanisms. However, this level of clarity of evidence will be difficult to achieve for human health impacts,[60] especially those mediated by climate-induced changes in complex natural systems. Inference will be further strengthened by congruent observations in other, similar, populations and locations.

The health event most associated with observed climate change is probably the 2003 heatwave that affected most of Western Europe and caused approximately 35 000 deaths. It is, in general, not appropriate to attribute single events to anthropogenic climate change. The appropriate question is to ask to what extent the underlying distribution of the climate or weather parameter has been changed due to climate change. For example, probabilistic methods were used to estimate that climate change had approximately doubled the likelihood of the 2003 event.[61] For individual outbreaks of an infectious disease, the causes are extremely complex, and it would be unwise to attribute such single events to global climate change. For example, an oyster-related outbreak caused by *Vibrio parahaemolyticus* in Alaska has been attributed to an increase in mean coastal water temperatures. In particular, it has been suggested that the outbreak was triggered by the exceedence of a critical temperature threshold for the first time throughout the oyster harvest season.[62] Attribution aside, such studies are important for highlighting the mechanisms by which climate variability is a determinant of current disease.

VULNERABILITY TO CLIMATE CHANGE

Vulnerability to climate change will vary between and within populations. Subpopulations that are most vulnerable to the health impacts of climate change depend on the region of interest, the health outcome and population characteristics, including human, institutional, social and economic capacity, the distribution of income and the provision of medical care and health protections. The populations most vulnerable to climate change include slum-dwellers and homeless people in large urban areas, particularly those in coastal low-lying areas, and populations living in water-stressed regions and highly dependent on natural resources. However, as shown during Hurricane Katrina and the 2003 extreme heatwave in Europe, developed countries may not be prepared to cope with the projected increase in the intensity and frequency of extreme weather events.

In Australia, for example, groups vulnerable to climate change include:[63]

- those living in regions where climate-sensitive infectious diseases may tend to spread;
- rural (especially farming) communities in southern and eastern Australia (exposed to long-term drying conditions);
- older and frailer individuals, especially in relation to heatwaves;
- coastal communities living in current and potential cyclone risk zones;
- remote indigenous communities facing heat, drying, water shortages and a loss of their traditional food species.

The health sector thinks in terms of prevention, which is analogous to adaptation.[64] Given that some climate change will occur, countries need to ensure that climate change does not cause additional problems for health. Indeed, some countries are already developing adaptation strategies. Adaptation interventions can take many forms, depending on the scale (global, regional or local), the type

of health risk, the time frame and the resources available. This has implications for the ways in which intervention options are selected and how they are evaluated. These issues are discussed in more detail in the Chapter 49.

CONCLUSION

The climate is already changing. Additional climate change over the coming few decades is unavoidable because of the already accrued emissions in the atmosphere, with their full 'forcing' effect as yet unrealized. This warming commitment will be very greatly supplemented by the effect of future worldwide emissions, leading to potential very high projections of future warming.

The prospect of human-induced climate change is casting a long shadow over the prospects for future human health. Indeed, there is emerging evidence of adverse effects already occurring. The immediate and consequent health impacts of extreme weather events are relatively easily identified. In the longer term, however, a greater health hazard for much of the world's population will arise from shifts in environmental, ecological and living conditions. Impaired crop yields, disrupted fisheries, altered patterns of infectious disease and the diverse health consequences of economic hardship will account for much of the burden of disease and premature death attributable to climate change.

Climate change endangers Earth's life-support systems. These are the systems that we, the human species, necessarily depend upon – even though, from our detached and mostly urban vantage point, we may only hazily appreciate that dependency. There is little point in pursuing policies to ensure future economic growth if, at the same time or subsequently, population health status and life expectancies fall. Viewed in anthropocentric terms, sustaining human well-being, health and survival must be the real 'bottom line' of the rationale for averting climate change and for achieving a sustainable way of living on this planet.

REFERENCES

● = Key primary paper

1. United Nations Environment Programme. *Global Environmental Outlook 2007: GEO-4.* Nairobi: UNEP, 2007.
2. Butler CD, Corvalan CF, Koren HS. Human health, well-being, and global ecological scenarios. *Ecosystems* 2005; 8: 153–62.
3. Corvalan C, Hales S, McMichael AJ (2005) Ecosystems and Human Well-being: Health Synthesis. A Report to the Millennium Ecocystem Asssessment. Available from: http://www.millenniumassessment.org/documents/document.357.aspx.pdf (accessed November 26, 2009).

4. Earth System Science Partnership. *Global Environmental Change and Human Health: Science Plan and Implementation Strategy*. ESSP Report No. 4. Paris: ESSP, 2006.

5. McMichael AJ. *Planetary Overload: Global Environmental Change and the Health of the Human Species*. Cambridge: Cambridge University Press, 1993.

6. Panel on Climate Change. *Climate Change 2007: The Physical Science Basis. Contribution of Working Group I to the Fourth Assessment Report of the Intergovernmental Panel on Climate Change*. Cambridge: Cambridge University Press, 2007.

7. Costello A, Abbas M, Allen A *et al*. Managing the health effects of climate change. *Lancet* 2009; **373**: 1693–733.

8. Haines A, McMichael AJ, Smith KR *et al*. Public health benefits of strategies to reduce greenhouse gas emissions: Overview and implications for policy-makers. *Lancet* 2009 (in press). DOI: doi:10.1016/S0140-6736(09)61759-1.

9. Rahmstorf S, Cazenave A, Church JA *et al*. Recent climate observations compared to projections. *Microb Ecol* 2007; **316**: 709.

10. Steffensen JP, Andersen KK, Bigler M, Clausen HB, Dahl-Jensen D, Fischer H. High-resolution Greenland ice core data show abrupt climate change happens in few years. *Microb Ecol* 2008; **321**: 680–4.

11. Rosenzweig C, Karoly DJ, Vicarelli M *et al*. Attributing physical and biological impacts to anthropogenic climate change. *Nature* 2008; **453**: 353–7.

●12. Parry ML, Canziani OF, Palutikof JP, van der Linden PJ, Hanson C (eds). *Climate Change 2007: Impacts, Adaptation and Vulnerability. Contribution of Working Group II to the Fourth Assessment Report of the Intergovernmental Panel on Climate Change*. Cambridge: Cambridge University Press, 2007.

13. Alexander LV, Zhang X, Peterson TC *et al*. Global observed changes in daily climate extremes of temperature and precipitation. *J Geophys Res* 2007; **D05109**: 1–22.

14. Emanuel K. Increasing destructiveness of tropical cyclones over the past 30 years. *Nature* 2005; **436**: 686–8.

15. Katz RW, Brown BG. Extreme events in a changing climate: Variability is more important than averages. *Clim Change* 1992; **21**:289–302.

16. Hippocrates. *On Airs, Waters and Places*. Whitefish, MT: Kessinger Publishing, 2004.

17. Sakamoto-Momiyama M. *Seasonality in Human Mortality*. Tokyo: University of Tokyo Press, 1977.

18. Hales S, Edwards S, Kovats RS. Impacts on health of climate extremes. In: McMichael AJ, Campbell-Lendrum D, Ebi KL, Corvalan C, Scheraga JS, Woodward A (eds) *Climate Change and Human Health: Risks and Responses* (pp. 79–96). Geneva: World Health Organization, 2003.

●19. Kovats RS, Bouma MJ, Hajat S, Worrall E, Haines A. El Nino and health. *Lancet* 2003; **362**: 1481–9.

20. Pascual M, Bouma MJ. Do rising temperatures matter? *Ecology* 2009; **90**: 906–12.

21. McMichael AJ. The health of persons, populations, and planets: epidemiology comes full circle. *Epidemiology* 1995; **6**: 633–6.

22. Nichols G, Lane C, Asgari N, Verlander NQ, Charlett A. Rainfall and outbreaks of drinking water related disease in England and Wales. *J Water Health* 2009; **7**: 1–8.

23. Carter TR, Jones RN, Lu X *et al*. New assessment methods and the characterisation of future conditions. In: Parry ML, Canziani OF, Palutikof JP, van der Linden PJ, Hanson C (eds) *Climate Change 2007: Impacts, Adaptation and Vulnerability. Contribution of Working Group II to the Fourth Assessment Report of the Intergovernmental Panel on Climate Change* (pp. 133–71). Cambridge: Cambridge University Press, 2007.

24. Hulme M, Dessai S. Negotiating future climates for public policy: A critical assessment of the development of climate scenarios for the UK. *Environ Sci Policy* 2008; **11**: 54–70.

25. Martens P, Hilderink HB. Human health in transition: Towards more disease or sustained health? In: Martens P, Rotmans J (eds) *Transitions in a Globalising World* (pp. 61–84). Lisse: Swets & Zeitlinger, 2001.

26. Department of Health/Health Protection Agency. *Health Effects of Climate Change in the UK 2008: An update of the Department of Health Report 2001/2002*. London: Department of Health/Health Protection Agency, 2008.

27. Casimiro E, Calheiros JM. Human health. In: Santos FD, Forbes K, Moita R (eds) *Climate Change in Portugal: Scenarios, Impacts, and Adaptation Measures – SIAM Project* (pp. 241–300). Lisbon: Gradiva, 2002.

28. McMichael AJ, Woodruff RE, Whetton P *et al*. *Human Health and Climate Change in Oceania: Risk Assessment 2002*. Canberra: Commonwealth of Australia, Department of Health and Ageing, 2003.

29. Health Canada. *Human Health in a Changing Climate: A Canadian Assessment of Vulnerabilities and Adaptive Capacity*. Ottawa: Health Canada, 2008.

30. Woodward A, Hales S, Weinstein P. Climate change and human health in the Asia Pacific region: Who will be the most vulnerable? *Clim Res* 1998; **11**: 31–8.

31. Watkiss P, Downing TE. The social cost of carbon: valuation estimates and their use in UK policy. *Integr Assess* 2008; **8**(1).

●32. World Health Organization. *Climate Change and Human Health: Risks and Responses*. Geneva: WHO, 2003.

33. Kovats RS, Akhtar R. Climate, climate change and health in Asian cities. *Environ Urban* 2008; **20**: 165–75.

34. Confalonieri U, Menne B, Akhtar R *et al*. Human health. In: Parry ML, Canziani OF, Palutikof JP, van der Linden PJ, Hanson C (eds) *Climate Change 2007: Impacts, Adaptation and Vulnerability. Contribution of Working Group II to the Fourth Assessment Report of the Intergovernmental Panel on Climate Change*. Cambridge: Cambridge University Press, 2007.

35. Kovats RS, Edwards S, Hajat S, Armstrong B, Ebi KL, Menne B. The effect of temperature on food poisoning: Time series analysis in 10 European countries. *Epidemiol Infect* 2004; **132**: 443–53.

36. D'Souza RM, Becker N, Hall G, Moodie KB. Does ambient temperature affect foodborne disease? *Epidemiology* 2004; **15**: 86–92.

37. Checkley W, Epstein LD, Gilman RH *et al*. Effects of El Nino and ambient temperature on hospital admissions for diarrhoeal diseases in Peruvian children. *Lancet* 2000; **355**: 442–50.

38. Singh RBK, Hales S, deWet N, Raj R, Hearnden M, Weinstein P. The influence of climate variation and change on diarrhoeal disease in the Pacific Islands. *Env Health Pers* 2001; **109**: 155–9.

39. Lloyd S, Kovats RS, Armstrong B. Global cross-sectional study of the association between diarrhoea morbidity, weather and climate. *Clim Res* 2007; **34**: 119–27.

40. Alam M, Hasan NA, Sadique A *et al*. Seasonal cholera caused by *Vibrio cholerae* serogroups O1 and O139 in the coastal aquatic environment of Bangladesh. *Appl Environ Microbiol* 2006; **72**: 4096–104.

41. Pascual M, Bouma MJ, Dobson AP. Cholera and climate: Revisiting the quantitative evidence. *Microbes Infect* 2002; **4**: 237–46.

42. Ogden NH, Maarouf A, Barker IK *et al*. Climate change and the potential for range expansion of the Lyme disease vector *Ixodes scapularis* in Canada. *Int J Parasitol* 2006; **36**: 63–70.

43. Tanser FC, Sharp B, Le Sueur D. Potential effect of climate change on malaria transmission in Africa. *Lancet* 2003; **362**: 1792–8.

44. Tanser FC, Sharp B, Le Sueur D. Potential effect of climate change on malaria transmission in Africa. *Lancet* 2003; **362**: 1792–8.

45. Yang GJ, Vounatsou P, Zhou XN, Tanner M, Utzinger J. A potential impact of climate change and water resource development on the transmission of *Schistosoma japonicum* in China. *Parasitologia* 2005; **47**: 127–35.

46. Tanser FC, Sharp B. Global climate change and malaria. *Lancet Infect Dis* 2005; **5**: 256–7.

47. Thomas CJ, Davies G, Dunn CE. Mixed picture for changes in stable malaria distribution with future climate in Africa. *Trends Parasitol* 2004; **20**: 216–20.

48. Lafferty KD. The ecology of climate change and infectious diseases. *Ecology* 2009; **90**: 888–90.

49. Kovats RS, Hajat S. Heat stress and public health: A critical review. *Annu Rev Public Health* 2008; **29**: 41–55.

50. Koppe C, Jendritzky G, Kovats RS, Menne B. *Heatwaves: Impacts and Responses.* Copenhagen: World Health Organization, 2003.

51. Carson C, Hajat S, Armstrong B, Wilkinson P. Declining vulnerability to temperature-related mortality in London over the twentieth century. *Am J Epidemiol* 2006; **164**: 77–84.

52. Donaldson GC, Keatinge WR, Nayha S. Changes in summer temperature and heat-related mortality since 1971 in North Carolina, South Finland, and Southeast England. *Environ Res* 2003; **91**: 1–7.

53. Ahern MJ, Kovats RS. Health impacts of floods. In: Few R, Matthies F (eds) *Flood Hazards and Health: Responding to Present and Future Risks* (pp. 28–53). London: EarthScan; 2006.

54. Nicholls RJ, Wong PP, Burkett VR *et al*. Coastal systems and low-lying areas. In: Parry ML, Canziani OF, Palutikof JP, van der Linden PJ, Hanson CE (eds) *Climate Change 2007: Impacts, Adaptation and Vulnerability. Contribution of Working Group II to the Fourth Assessment Report of the Intergovernmental Panel on Climate Change* (pp. 315–56). Cambridge: Cambridge University Press, 2007.

55. Hughes L. Biological consequences of global warming: is the signal already here? *Tree* 2000; **15**: 56–61.

56. Lindgren E. Climate and tick-borne encephalitis in Sweden. *Conserv Ecol* 1998; **2**: 5–7.

57. Lindgren E, Talleklint L, Polfeldt T. Impact of climatic change on the northern latitude limit and population density of the disease-transmitting European tick, *Ixodes ricinus*. Env Health Pers 2000; **108**: 119–23.

58. Pascual M, Ahumada JA, Chaves LF, Rodo X, Bouma MJ. Malaria resurgence in East African highlands: Temperature trends revisited. *Proc Natl Acad Sci USA* 2006; **103**: 5829–34.

59. Kovats RS, Campbell-Lendrum D, McMichael AJ, Woodward A, Cox J. Early effects of climate change: Do they include changes in vector borne diseases? *Philos Trans R Soc Lond B* 2001; **356**: 1057–68.

60. Randolph SE. Perspectives on climate change impacts on infectious diseases. *Ecology* 2009; **90**: 927–31.

61. Stott PA, Stone DA, Allen MR. Human contribution to the European heatwave of 2003. *Nature* 2004; **432**: 610–14.

62. McLaughlin J, DePaula A, Bopp CA *et al*. Outbreak of *Vibrio parahaemolyticus* gastroenteritis associated with Alaskan oysters. *N Engl J Med* 2006; **353**: 1463–70.

63. Woodruff RE, Hales S, Butler CD, McMichael AJ. *Climate Change and Health Impacts in Australia*: Effects of Dramatic CO_2 Emission Reductions. Report for the Australia Conservation Foundation and the Australian Medical Association. Canberra: Australian National University, 2006.

64. Ebi KL, Smith JB, Burton I. *Integration of Public Health with Adaptation to Climate Change: Lessons Learned and New Directions.* Lisse: Taylor & Francis Group, 2005.

65. Dessai SR. Heat stress mortality in Lisbon. II: An assessment of the impacts of climate change. *Int J Biometeorol* 2003; **48**: 37–44.

66. Hayhoe K, Cayan D, Field CB *et al*. Emissions pathways, climate change, and impacts on California. *Proc Natl Acad Sci USA* 2004; **101**: 12422–7.

67. Ciscar JC (ed.) Climate Change Impacts in Europe. Final Report of the PESETA Research Project. 24093 EN. Available from: http://peseta.jrc.ec.europa.eu (accessed November 25, 2009).

49

Adaptation to climate change

GIOVANNI LEONARDI

The recognition that climate change, as an environmental hazard operating on a global scale, poses a unique challenge to human societies is being accompanied by a growing awareness that this threat is non-linear and potentially irreversible, and that proposed actions may have wide-ranging practical and ethical implications.[1] Responses to climate change have been classified according to whether they aim to reduce emissions of greenhouse gases (mitigation) or reduce the impacts of ongoing and expected climate change on human communities (adaptation). Effective mitigation benefits not only human systems, but also all natural systems.[2] However, the distinction is not always easy to apply in practice as mitigation and adaptation do not occur independently: when one is implemented, the other can be affected in both or either of favourable and adverse ways.[3] Decisions on adaptation and mitigation are taken at different governance levels, and inter-relationships exist within and across each level.

It is not yet possible to answer the question of whether or not investment in adaptation would buy time for mitigation. In public health terms, the mitigation of climate change is a prerequisite of avoiding the widening of health inequities globally. However, adaptive responses to climate change, while necessary, are a less sure way to reduce health inequities, since self-interested adaptation by those populations with most resources might well increase the health gap.[4] Some actions can help to foster both adaptation and mitigation, for example sustainable agricultural systems, soil and water conservation measures

involving planting trees that then absorb greenhouse gases, and renewable energy initiatives.

Some have suggested that when interventions affect the hardware of human organization (energy systems, buildings and transport systems), they will be most effective when they are designed to achieve both mitigation and adaptation.[5] In this context, the term 'mainstreaming' describes the integration of policies and measures that integrate climate change into development planning and ongoing sector-based decision-making. The benefit of mainstreaming is to ensure the sustainability of investments and to reduce the sensitivity of development activities to current and future climatic conditions.[6] Although this approach seems reasonable, this chapter will focus on an overview of strategies for adapting to climate change, including those which have not been designed with mitigation as an additional aim. It should be remembered that although adaptation action has become an unavoidable and indispensable complement to mitigation action, it is certainly not an alternative to reducing greenhouse gas emissions.[7]

Are these questions too difficult to answer, and is our capacity for effective action too small? Perhaps not. The main theme of this chapter is the idea of 'resilience'. Resilience has been defined as the state's capacity to absorb sudden shocks, to adapt to longer term changes in socioeconomic conditions and to resolve societal disputes sustainably without catastrophic breakdown. The opposite is 'brittleness'.[5] It has been argued that a rush towards greater efficiency has made our civilization brittle and vulnerable. The model strategy for increasing resilience is to increase redundancy and reduce unnecessary complexity – to maintain 'slack' in the system.[5] Managing climate change risk means being prepared for scenarios we know are unlikely to happen but would be disastrous if they did occur. We do this when we take out insurance: we are prepared for our house burning down and for our house *not* burning down.

AREAS FOR ACTION ON ADAPTATION

Climate change, an environmental health hazard of unprecedented scale and complexity, requires health practitioners to develop new ways of thinking, communicating and acting.[8] It necessitates thinking in terms of a sustained time frame, and it needs a systems approach beyond the current boundaries of the health sciences and health sector. Communicating the risks posed by climate change requires messages that motivate constructive engagement rather than indifference, fear or despair. Actions that address climate change should offer a range of health, environmental and social benefits.[8]

An encouraging observation is that the prerequisites for effective public health action are analogous to the determinants of adaptive capacity; therefore, the long history of public health managing external environmental and other threats can be applied to adaptation to climate change.[9] An awareness of the specific sources of variability and uncertainty, and of the need to conduct a formal evaluation of any interventions proposed, will be key to the design of successful actions.

The framework of primary, secondary and tertiary prevention may be useful for bringing health and other sectors together:

- *Primary prevention* includes health promotion and requires action on the determinants of health to prevent disease occurring.
- *Secondary prevention* is essentially the early detection of disease, accompanied by appropriate intervention, such as health promotion or treatment.
- *Tertiary prevention* aims to reduce the impact of the disease and promote quality of life through active rehabilitation.

In this framework, actions to adapt to climate change may be considered to be secondary or tertiary prevention, whereas actions to limit climate change (mitigation) could be described as primary prevention.

The World Health Organization (WHO) has proposed an agenda for research on climate change and public health.[10] It has recommended five research areas, listed here with comments on their relevance to public health services.

Recommendation 1: Interactions of climate change with other health determinants and trends

The implication of this for public health services is that they should strive to identify effective measures to strengthen public health systems in order to address several environmental health risks, integrating adaptation to climate change with factors such as economic development, energy management, urbanization, the conservation of water, soil and other natural capital resources that support human life and welfare, social impacts and access to care.

Recommendation 2: Direct and indirect effects of climate change

This proposal is a reminder that the immediate effects of disease vector distribution, heatwaves, drought events and flooding, for example, should be addressed by public health services with due consideration of the long-term trends on factors underlying these hazards. These include the management of water resources and their indirect consequences on drought and flood trends, as well as related human conflicts. Hostility between human population groups could be reduced by an explicit collaborative management of access to natural resources. Health practitioners have enormous experience in liaising with numerous stakeholders when promoting change to services.

Recommendation 3: Comparing the effectiveness of short-term interventions

Short-term interventions by the health services or others can be monitored using public health methods. For the results to be applicable without delay, both the proposed interventions and evaluation methods would benefit from a vigorous exchange of information and coordination between service providers and researchers when designing and interpreting evaluation programmes. Possible comparisons are between countries, such as heatwave plans in different European countries. By highlighting the value of approaches in different contexts, international comparisons may provide information of relevance to countries where evaluatory research is not feasible.

Recommendation 4: Assessing the health impact of policies from non-health sectors

There are benefits to health from climate mitigation interventions in non-health sectors as well, and further evidence on joint benefits is required. Public health services at a national and regional level will need to assess the health impact of policy decisions made by non-health sectors addressing climate change, a task not as difficult as it may sound provided the relevant non-health sector is willing to address this in collaboration with public health agencies.

Recommendation 5: Strengthening public health systems to address the health effects of climate change

General public health skills are the foundation of effective interventions to address climate change, just as with any other challenge to health. While researchers work to document the most effective means of implementing integrated strategies that reduce threats to climate change, public health service providers can include adaptation to climate change in their mandate.

BASIC PUBLIC HEALTH FUNCTIONS IN RELATION TO CLIMATE CHANGE

The main public health functions required include the following:[11,12]

- Document and communicate the actual health risks. National and (appropriate) subnational formal health risk assessments could be carried out to identify the main health risks, their likely chronology and the vulnerable subpopulations.
- Anticipate the 'pressure points' where health impacts are most likely to appear, and ensure that there is a good, continuing, health-outcome surveillance in place.
- Develop methods of causal attribution, such that the public and policy-makers can be advised on the plausible likely contribution of climate change to the impacts of otherwise 'natural' events (e.g. Hurricane Katrina, Europe's 2003 heatwave and the ongoing droughts in several continents). This also requires appropriate handling and communication of the complex issue of uncertainty.
- Develop rationally targeted prevention (adaptive) strategies. Accrue experience and knowledge about the options for reducing risk. Evaluate these for specified populations/communities in terms of an averted disease/death/disability burden and in terms of their costs and benefits.
- Commit to a systematic updating of scenario-based (future) health risk assessments. This will assist the public's and policy-makers' understanding of the likely future risks to health in response to future social and economic change.

The topic of adaptation, or 'rationally targetted prevention', is mainly addressed by the fourth of these five public health functions. This chapter focuses on this function and outlines some of the suggestions that have been made concerning adaptation to climate change and its health consequences. In particular, the text outlines several adaptive strategies, including the overall role of health agencies, specific activities in relation to extreme events and longer term plans, and the role of municipalities.

ROLE OF HEALTH AGENCIES IN ADAPTATION

There are four groups of adaptations that may be considered specifically by health systems:[13]

- the modification of existing prevention strategies: responses to climate change affect all systems of human organization, so they are likely to be more effective if integrated into the day-to-day management of all sectors that could affect human health;
- the translation of policies and knowledge from other countries;
- the restoration of surveillance, maintenance and prevention programmes that have been weakened or abandoned due to financial considerations;
- the development of new policies to address new threats.

At a time when the resources for supporting adaptation strategies may be scarce, and the time available for developing and implementing these strategies is also scarce, we must share with the utmost openness all experience and knowledge about the available options. For the same reasons, it is also extremely desirable that any intervention should be accompanied by arrangements for its own evaluation, so that lessons learnt can be rapidly learned and convincingly disseminated.

Health responses to climate change need to be based on the essential public health services.[14] Strengthening existing public health approaches involves:

- public education;
- preventive programmes;
- the surveillance of disease;
- the forecasting of future health risks.

This needs to be complemented by activities that extend beyond the health sector:[12]

- early warning systems;
- neighbourhood support schemes;
- climate-proofed housing design;
- urban planning;
- water catchment;
- farming practices;
- disaster preparedness.

HEALTH SYSTEMS TO SUPPORT THE MANAGEMENT OF EXTREME EVENTS

Enhanced disaster response preparedness

According to the United Nations International Strategy for Disaster Reduction (UN ISDR), a disaster is a serious disruption of the functioning of a community or a society involving widespread human, material, economic or environmental losses and impacts, which exceeds the ability of the affected community or society to cope using its own resources.[15]

Disasters are increasing in both number and severity. International institutional frameworks to reduce disasters are being strengthened under UN supervision.[16] The UN ISDR has produced recommendations[17] relevant at international and national levels:

- Make adaptation to climate change a fundamental pillar of any post-Kyoto agreement.
- Ensure that disaster risk reduction and climate risk management are core elements of adaptation to climate change.
- Establish mechanisms to provide sufficient funding for adaptation to climate change and risk reduction, especially to protect the most vulnerable.
- Take immediate action to implement adaptation to climate change and risk reduction in vulnerable countries in the next 3 years.

At the World Conference on Disaster Reduction in Japan in 2005, an agreement was reached by participating countries on a 'Framework for Action 2005–2015: Building the Resilience of Nations and Communities to Disasters'. This Hyogo Framework for Action identified five priorities for action that formed the basis of national platforms for disaster reduction:[18]

1. Ensure that disaster risk reduction is a national and a local priority with a strong institutional basis for implementation.
2. Identify, assess and monitor disaster risks, and enhance early warning.
3. Use knowledge, innovation and education to build a culture of safety and resilience at all levels.
4. Reduce the underlying risk factors.
5. Strengthen disaster preparedness for effective response at all levels.

At national and local level, guidance has been prepared by several agencies for specific natural hazards and related extreme events. Good overviews are available of such specific guidance in relation to health impacts,[19] highlighting the fragmentary nature of the evidence and systems available when considered across the several hazards expected. Work is in progress to improve this

situation rapidly. Resilience in response to any specific hazard can be enhanced by linking specific lessons with existing civil protection systems.

Sudden impact disasters can be seen as a continuous time sequence of five different phases,[20] each phase lasting from seconds to months or years, and each merging into the other:

- the non-disaster or inter-disaster phase;
- the pre-disaster or warning phase;
- the impact phase;
- the emergency phase (also called the relief or isolation phase);
- the reconstruction or rehabilitation phase.

Vulnerability reduction programmes can be identified for all the types of extreme weather event expected to increased in frequency and severity with climate change, and will reduce susceptibility and increase resilience.[21] Health security aspects of climate change were recognized by the WHO,[22] and national security aspects of environmental crises have also been identified. A convergence of objectives between health and civil protection activities could lead to fruitful developments in intervention design, implementation and evaluation.

The next section provides a brief overview of evidence for interventions in relation to adaptation to specific hazards.

HEATWAVES

Climate change will increase the frequency and the intensity of heatwaves, and a range of measures, including improvements to housing, the management of chronic diseases and institutional care of the elderly and the vulnerable, will need to be developed to reduce the health impacts.[23] Following the European heatwave of 2003, several projects have been conducted to estimate health impacts, factors affecting the vulnerability of populations and physical infrastructure, and to outline a framework for preparedness and response. This effort has resulted in the production of guidance for the introduction and development of heat-health action plans[24] and links to national plans. The principles identified are as follows:

- Use existing systems and link to general emergency response arrangements.
- Adopt a long-term approach (mitigation actions and adaptation of the built environment).
- Be broad (a multiagency approach).
- Communicate effectively.
- Ensure that responses to heatwaves do not exacerbate the problem of climate change.
- Evaluate (because if plans and their implementation are not evaluated, they will not improve).

The WHO identified the following core elements for a successful implementation of heat-health action plans:[24]

- the agreement of a lead national body;
- accurate and timely alert systems;
- a heat-related health information plan;
- a reduction in indoor heat exposure (medium- and short-term strategies);
- particular care for vulnerable population groups;
- preparedness of the health- and social care system;
- long-term urban planning;
- real-time surveillance and evaluation.

FIRES

Fire incidents are expected to increase, in particular in the Mediterranean, with increased drought risk. The smoke produced by big vegetation fire incidents, such as those which have occurred in southern Europe, South East Asia and other areas, poses not only threats, but also challenges for improving air-quality monitoring in emergency situations, for enhancing personal protection and for developing advanced early warning systems. Coping with all issues of vegetation fire smoke is not a specialized issue: it is both a core disaster discipline and a key methodology that can be applied to other disasters and threats.

Areas of significant interest regarding vegetation fire smoke are the chemistry of the forest fire smoke, the medical and toxicological effects of smoke, the exposure limits set by international organizations, air-quality monitoring near the flame-front, personal protective equipment, the cross-border transfer of smoke and crisis management.

Several pilot projects in relation to the impact of fire have been developed, aiming to identify high-risk areas, establish effective solutions to control and reduce the spread of fires, and restore affected areas. This information could and should be made available systematically through health and civil protection systems and also as an alert to hospitals in terms of the potential flow of patients.

Crisis management of forest fire smoke is important because smoke not only affects the population in the vicinity of the fire, but also impacts on populations who live further away from the fire. A number of questions need to be answered:

- Are there any evacuation criteria for coping with the short-term health impacts of forest fire smoke?
- Are there any methods or tools for coping with the cross-border impact of vegetation fire smoke?
- What are the evacuation procedures?
- Do operational emergency plans include coping with forest fire smoke?
- Is there a need to develop special guidelines and emergency plans for coping with vegetation fire smoke?

DROUGHTS

The provision of sufficient storage capacity for growing water demands and increasing climate variability is one of the main concerns for water managers in the coming decades, requiring a careful management of groundwater.[25] A spatial analysis could reveal the degree of threat of progressive drought and the threat to related ecological security.[26] An analysis of fluctuations in groundwater and the vegetation dependent on it, in relation to each other and to wider factors, is important for managing water and predicting vegetation responses.[27]

Virtual water (also known as embedded water, embodied water or hidden water) refers, in the context of trade, to the water used in the production of a good or service. For instance, it takes on average $1300\,m^3$ of water to produce one metric tonne of wheat. The virtual water trade concept has been proposed to help thinking about water scarcity and management and as a potential solution for water-short countries.[28] In particular, some eastern European countries, the Mediterranean, Africa and Asia will be facing an increasing frequency of drought. The biggest impacts are likely to be on water shortage – with negative impacts on agriculture with a potential risk of migration. The reuse of waste water and desalinization in coastal areas are among the possible remedial actions, although these may in principle carry some risks related to human health, for example algae and endocrine-disrupting chemicals.

WINDSTORMS

The most common effects on humans from windstorms are road traffic accidents (overturning vehicles or collisions with fallen trees) and individual accidents (being blown over or struck by flying debris or masonry). Building failure represents a less significant, but still important, impact on human life (falling chimneys etc.).[29] Possible public health actions cover the range from preparedness and mitigation to pre-disaster communication, evacuation, and during-disaster advice, surveillance and reconstruction.

FLOODS

Floods have the greatest damage potential of all natural disasters worldwide and affect the greatest number of people. On a global basis, there is evidence that the number of people affected, and the economic damages resulting from flooding, are rising at an alarming rate. Society must move from the current paradigm of a post-disaster response: the current event–disaster cycle must be broken. More than ever, there is a need for decision-makers to adopt holistic approaches for flood disaster management.[30]

Interventions before, during and after floods can reduce short- and long-term health impacts. Hospitals, ambulances, retirement homes, schools and kindergartens in flood-prone areas are at risk, and the evacuation of patients and vulnerable groups might present a further risk. Crop-growing areas may require specific protection.[31] The impact of floods on regional security, economics, health and political stability is more difficult to measure and quantify. If predictions of increased flooding under future climate change are correct, flooding is an issue that health agencies and civil protection agencies have to address by coordinated planning and action, and by cooperation in preparedness and response.

Specific features of river floods and sea floods have been identified, leading to a range of planning, response and prevention strategies, including non-structural flood-management policies.[32] The tsunami risk in Europe should be considered as well and requires specific approaches.[33] Health effects can be prevented by a greater emphasis on disaster preparedness and strategies for risk reduction before a flood occurs. This requires a cross-sector approach and includes targetted information being distributed to the most vulnerable populations in advance.

Specific lessons learned from flooding events include the need:[34]

- for adequate housing and planning;
- to review all flood risk, including surface water and groundwater;
- to review flood defence and drainage infrastructure;
- to prepare advanced warnings;
- to strengthen social networks to access information;
- to estimate the health impacts of structural and non-structural defence mechanisms;
- to prepare and test evacuation plans;
- to establish long-term disease surveillance;
- to review property insurance;
- to modernize flood risk legislation.

Early warning systems

Early warning is the provision of timely and effective information, through identified institutions, that allows individuals exposed to a hazard to take action to avoid or reduce their risk and prepare for effective response.[15] Early warning systems include a chain of actions, namely:

- understanding and mapping the hazard;
- monitoring and forecasting impending events;
- processing and disseminating understandable warnings to political authorities and the population;
- undertaking appropriate and timely actions in response to the warnings.

To be effective, early warning systems for natural hazards need to have not only a sound scientific and technical basis, but also a strong focus on the people exposed to risk. They also need a systems approach that incorporates all of the relevant factors in that risk, whether arising from the natural hazards or social vulnerabilities, or from short-term or long-term processes.[16]

Public health measures include health promotion and heatwave warning systems (although the effectiveness of acute measures in response to heatwaves has not yet been formally evaluated).

Civil protection and community alerts

It has been suggested that civil defence and civil protection are distinct forms of societal response to disasters, the former having an emphasis on central control as in anti-terrorism measures, and the latter being a more democratic form of crisis management involving more sectors of society.[35] Civil defence is a progenitor of civil protection. In an epoch of global terrorism and an increased frequency and severity of natural disasters, the two must co-exist. The maintenance or restoration of law and order may be fundamental to civil defence, but civil protection is based on the encouragement of social solidarity rather than the repression of antisocial tendencies.[36]

Civil protection requires members of the public to assume progressively more responsibility for their own safety and security. This involves a responsibility of health and civil protection agencies to ensure that they understand the risks of disaster and have the means to face up to them. Traditional, indigenous and social coping mechanisms need to be reinforced wherever appropriate.[37]

Practical actions include community alerts for fragile older persons, the development of scenarios when alerts become applicable, buddy systems, liaison arrangements with public agencies, local action groups for upgrading flooding defences and so on. Technological support may be available (alerts via mobile phone message to carers, and satellite networks). Support for the design and evaluation of such community activity may be available through local public health and civil protection departments and could help their development and widespread implementation.

HEALTH SYSTEMS TO SUPPORT MEDIUM- AND LONG-TERM ADAPTATION

Weather, climate and water influence virtually all human activities, so almost every sector of the economy – health, energy, transport, food security, management of water, tourism – needs meteorological and hydrological services. The World Meteorological Organization has issued guidance on how weather-, climate- and water-related information can contribute to the socioeconomic development of nations – especially those of the developing world – and the well-being of their populations.[38] Climatologists have collaborated with public health specialists to highlight the role of biometeorology as a key discipline that can enable public health responses to climate change.[39]

Three areas where health practitioners would be able to contribute are surveillance systems, adaptation of the built environment, and food and water supplementation systems. These are described in the following sections.

Surveillance systems

Most surveillance efforts have been devoted to infectious diseases, and this may not need to change. The advantage of retaining a focus on infections is that the current systems would continue to be used, thereby putting climate-focused surveillance on a solid foundation.

Many new studies have demonstrated significant associations between climate variability and infectious disease transmission (see Chapter 48) and have specifically highlighted the potential for developing climate-based early warning systems. To date, however, only limited experience of full operational applications has been gained. For some diseases, such as malaria and Rift Valley fever, early warnings based on climatic conditions are beginning to be used in selected locations to alert ministries of health to the potential for an increased risk of outbreaks and to improve epidemic preparedness; coverage is, however, patchy.[40] A close collaboration of infectious disease surveillance experts with epidemiologists experienced in climate-related analysis would help to extend, improve and evaluate such systems in the context of early detection of climate-related trends.

However, a key change for providing surveillance interpretation relevant to climate change adaptation would be to reframe some of the infectious disease surveillance systems so that they can be used as elements of a wider 'environmental public health' surveillance framework. A proposed framework for conducting environmental public health surveillance involves data from three points in the process by which an agent in the environment produces an adverse outcome on health status: hazards, exposures and outcomes.[41] Within this framework, it would become easier to define and use surveillance systems for the detection of shifts in infectious disease patterns in relation to climatic changes; in addition, public health agencies would be able to recognize the value of existing systems.

Adaptation of the built environment

If a broad definition of 'built environment' is adopted, as comprising all the manmade components of people's surroundings distinct from the natural environment, this encompasses transport infrastructure and managed green spaces as well as buildings.[42] For each category, built environment strategies to address climate change have been defined, and expected impacts on quality of life and health co-benefits have been described. These settings range from small-scale to global connecting systems, and they afford several opportunities to benefit health by addressing climate change.

Urban settlements, especially cities, need to be adapted in two ways: first, changing and designing settlements that contribute less to the causes of climate change (e.g. building energy-efficient and green housing); and second, adapting settlements to be climate resilient and to be able to cope with the increasing risks of climate change.[43] The design of sustainable cities is an ongoing effort aimed at improving or maintaining quality of life in the face of a multitude of constraints, of which climate change is only one, but it has already led to a multitude of at least partially successful innovations.[44]

Enhancing food and water security and supplementation

The Food and Agriculture Organization defines food security as a 'situation that exists when all people, at all times, have physical, social, and economic access to sufficient, safe, and nutritious food that meets their dietary needs and food preferences for an active and healthy life'.[45] As described in Chapter 48, the availability of, stability of, access to and utilization of food supplies may be affected as a consequence of climate change.[46]

There is an immense diversity of agricultural practices because of the range of climate and other environmental variables – cultural, institutional and economic factors, as well as their interactions.[47] This means that there is a correspondingly large array of possible adaptation options. Many defining features of livelihoods on dry lands in Africa and elsewhere can be regarded in principle as adaptive strategies to climate variability,[48] for example:

- allocating farm labour across the seasons in ways that follow unpredictable rainfall variations: 'negotiating the rain';
- making use of biodiversity in cultivated crops and wild plants;
- increasing the integration of livestock into farming systems;
- working land harder in terms of labour input per hectare;
- diversifying livelihoods;
- the on-farm storage of food and feed;
- the late planting of vegetable crops when cereals fail because of drought.

Many planning frameworks for adaptation have been developed in the last decade. It has been suggested that involving stakeholders from project inception is critical to the successful implementation of such frameworks.[47] Other possible roles for the health practitioner are in linking physical activity to local opportunities for food growing in gardens and allotments;[49] supporting plans for every health organization to minimize wastage at the buying stage; and working in partnership with suppliers to lower the carbon impact of all aspects of procuring and promoting sustainable food throughout their business.[50]

Food supplementation systems have been developed largely for areas within developing countries where droughts have caused widespread famine. However, in many countries, including developed ones, the effect of threats to food security may result in increases in food prices. Food supplementation may be required following any disaster, including those linked to climate change.

The availability of fresh water is changing in relation to climate warming, as mentioned in Chapter 48. At the same time, changes in land use are also affecting the availability of water resources. These combined effects have consequences not restricted to estimates of future flood risk, water supply and water quality, but extending to the capacity of engineers to analyse water systems. Therefore, planners will need to adapt the concepts and tools used to analyse water resources so that water infrastructure, channel modifications and drainage works can be adapted. Such a framework for managing water resources is required urgently as it is crucial for human adaptation to climate change.[51]

The temporary suspension of drinking water supply is not uncommon during extreme natural events. Paradoxically, this may occur not only during regular or occasional drought periods, but also during floods. During the 2007 floods in the UK, the affected population lacked access to drinking water for several days, and alternative supplies of drinking water were provided by water companies. Public health agencies have a role in setting the minimum amount of drinking water required by categories of individuals in affected populations.[52]

PUBLIC HEALTH AS A FUNCTION OF THE LOCAL AUTHORITY (MUNICIPALITY)

The key role of careful energy management in ensuring the transition to sustainable food production, housing and transport has been highlighted.[5] Municipalities need to mitigate *and* adapt, and use the energy available to them in order to achieve the integration of these two goals. This requires the prioritization of their efforts in four areas: overall planning, infrastructure, facilities and emergency preparedness.[5] Overall planning includes provisions with regard to population density, transport, vegetation and landscaping, and disease or pests that affect humans, plants and livestock.

The infrastructure requires effort to respond to the changing risk of unmet water demands, to floods and droughts, as well as to energy provision and sewers. Facilities that should be considered as a priority include schools, elderly residential and nursing homes, hospitals, parks and recreation facilities. Emergency preparedness at municipality level would cover plans for flood, drought, heatwaves and blackouts. The overall message is that, to effectively manage a transition to an adapted municipality, there is a need to be creative, to challenge standard operational procedures, to work with civil society and to plan long.

THE ROLE OF HEALTH PROFESSIONALS

Although it is clear that there are many important roles for health professionals in motivating and contributing to designing local responses to possible disasters associated with extreme weather events, there remains a question about the adequacy of a purely local response to climate change, a threat to public health that has a global and pervasive nature. Even a sound public health approach focused on prevention, one recognizing that anticipatory and precautionary adaptation is more effective and less costly than last-minute emergency adaptation, may be insufficient.[53]

A historical perspective highlights the concrete possibility that we face a third revolution in human history, after the early shift from hunter-gatherer to agrarian societies and the major industrial revolution that followed this. New circumstances might require a new way of thinking about health, a recognition that our way of life will change radically and that public health methods also will have to change – to include new methods such as scenario-planning and a radical synthesis of knowledge from disparate disciplines such as philosophy and economics, along with the more familiar public health sciences.[54]

CONCLUSION

Adaptation to climate change is likely to reduce the impact on health in two ways: changes in the role of public health agencies and individual clinicians with regard to their role in extreme weather events, surveillance and infectious disease; and modifications in non-health sectors, i.e. food production, transport and buildings.

Overall, the public health community can promote increased resilience of their community as the practical task of achieving adaptation to climate change. However, as the climate crisis is a global crisis, the adaptive response for public health has to be at more than local level, and it also has to be consistent with a strategic response. In this sense, the design and evaluation of interventions aimed at adapting health systems to the consequences of climate change will also direct and support individuals and communities along a sustainability transition. There is no contradiction between these two levels of adaptive response, and only by pursuing both at the same time can public health be supported.

REFERENCES

● = Key primary paper
◆ = Major review article

1. Patz JA, Gibbs HK, Foley JA *et al.* Climate change and global health: Quantifying a growing ethical crisis. *EcoHealth* 2007; **4**: 397–405.

2. Semenza JC, Hall DE, Wilson DJ *et al.* Public perception of climate change: Voluntary mitigation and barriers to behaviour change. *Am J Prev Med* 2008; **35**: 479–87.

◆3. Klein RJT, Huq S, Denton F *et al.* Inter-relationships between adaptation and mitigation. In: Parry ML, Canziani OF, Palutikof JP *et al.* (eds) *Climate Change 2007: Impacts, Adaptation and Vulnerability, Contribution of Working Group II to the Fourth Assessment Report of the Intergovernmental Panel on Climate Change.* Cambridge: Cambridge University Press, 2007: 745–77.

4. Friel S, Marmot M, McMichael AJ *et al.* Global health equity and climate stabilisation: A common agenda. *Lancet* 2008; **372**: 1677–83.

5. Homer-Dixon T. *The Upside of Down: Catastrophe, Creativity and the Renewal of Civilisation.* London: Souvenir Press, 2007.

6. Klein RJT, Schipper EL, Dessai S. Integrating mitigation and adaptation into climate and development policy: Three research questions. *Environ Sci Policy* 2005; **8**: 579–88.

7. EU Commission. Adapting to Climate Change in Europe – Options for EU action. Green Paper from the Commission to the Council, the European Parliament, the European Economic and Social Committee and the Committee of the Regions, SEC(2007) 849. Available from: http://ec.europa.eu/environment/climat/adaptation/index_en.htm (accessed December 5, 2008).

8. Frumkin H, McMichael AJ. Climate change and public health: Thinking, communicating, acting. *Am J Prev Med* 2008; **35**: 403–10.

9. Ebi KL, Smith JB, Burton I. *Integration of Public Health with Adaptation to Climate Change. Lessons Learned and New Directions.* London: Taylor & Francis, 2005.

10. World Health Organization. Protecting Health from Climate Change: Global Research Priorities. Available from: www.who.int/entity/phe/news/madrid_report_661_final_lowres.pdf (accessed November 25, 2009).

11. Kovats RS, Hajat S. Heat stress and public health: A critical review. *Annu Rev Public Health* 2008; **29**: 41.

12. McMichael AJ, Nyong A, Corvalan C. Global environmental change and health: Impacts, inequalities, and the health sector. *BMJ* 2008; **336**: 191–4.

13. Ebi KL, Smith J, Burton I, Scheraga J. Some lessons learned from public health on the process of adaptation. *Mitig Adapt Strateg Glob Change* 2006; **11**: 607–620.

14. Frumkin H, Hess J, Luber G *et al.* Climate change: The public health response. *Am J Public Health* 2008; **98**, 435–45. Also available from: http://www.louisvilleky.gov/NR/rdonlyres/4EB6612D-5274-48AD-9D85-74FBBC3D4860/0/ClimateChangeThePublicHealthResponse.pdf (accessed November 25, 2009).

15. International Strategy for Disaster Reduction. Defining a Few Key Terms. 2009. Available from: http://www.unisdr.org/eng/media-room/facts-sheets/fs-Defining-a-few-key-terms.htm (accessed November 25, 2009).

●16. Basher R. Global early warning systems for natural hazards: Systematic and people-centred. *Philos Transact A Math Phys Eng Sci* 2006; **364**: 2167–82.

17. International Strategy for Disaster Reduction. Climate Change and Disaster Risks. ISDR Recommendations for Action Now and Post-Kyoto. Available from: http://www.unisdr.org/eng/risk-reduction/climate-change/docs/ISDR%20recommendations%20for%20COP-13.pdf (accessed November 25, 2009).

18. International Strategy for Disaster Reduction. Hyogo Framework for Action 2005–2015: Building the Resilience of Nations and Communities to Disasters (HFA). Available from: http://www.unisdr.org/eng/hfa/hfa.htm (accessed November 25, 2009).

19. Menne B, Ebi K. *Climate Change and Adaptation Strategies for Human Health.* Darmstadt: Steinkopff Verlag, 2005.

20. Noji EK. *The Public Health Consequences of Disasters.* New York: Oxford University Press, 1997.

21. Keim ME. Building human resilience: The role of public health preparedness and response as an adaptation to climate change. *Am J Prev Med* 2008; **35**: 508–16.

22. World Health Organization. Protecting Health from Climate Change – World Health Day 2008. Available from: http://www.who.int/world-health-day/toolkit/report_web.pdf (accessed November 25, 2009).

23. Kovats RS, Hajat S. Heat stress and public health: A critical review. *Annu Rev Public Health* 2008; **29**: 41.

◆24. Matthies F, Bickler G, Cardenosa Marin N, Hales S (eds). Heat-health Action Plans: Guidance. Available from: http://www.euro.who.int/Document/E91347.pdf (accessed November 25, 2009).

25. Tuinhof A, Olsthoorn T, Heederik JP, de Vries J. Groundwater storage and water security: Making better use of our largest reservoir. *Water Sci Technol* 2005; **51**: 141–8.

26. Jiao Y, Xiao D. Spatial neighboring characteristics among patch types in oasis and its ecological security. *Ying Yong Sheng Tai Xue Bao* 2004; **15**: 31–5.

27. Naumburg E, Mata-Gonzalez R, Hunter RG *et al.* Phreatophytic vegetation and groundwater fluctuations: A review of current research and application of ecosystem response modeling with an emphasis on great basin vegetation. *Environ Manage* 2005; **35**: 726–40.

28. Lundqvist J, Furuyashiki K. Workshop 7 (synthesis): Role and governance implications of virtual water trade. *Water Sci Technol* 2004; **49**: 199–201.

29. Baker C, Lee B. Guidance on Windstorms for the Public Health Workforce. Chemical Hazards and Poisons Report Issue 49. Available from: http://www.hpa.org.uk/web/HPAwebFile/HPAweb_C/1222068844046 (accessed February 11, 2009).

30. United Nations. Guidelines for Reducing Flood Losses. Available from: http://www.unisdr.org/eng/library/isdr-publication/flood-guidelines/Guidelines-for-reducing-floods-losses.pdf (accessed November 25, 2009).

31. Casteel MJ, Sobsey MD, Mueller JP. Fecal contamination of agricultural soils before and after hurricane-associated flooding in North Carolina. *J Environ Sci Health A Tox Hazard Subst Environ Eng* 2006; **41**: 173–84.

32. Poff NL. Ecological response to and management of increased flooding caused by climate change. *Philos Transact A Math Phys Eng Sci* 2002; **360**: 1497–510.

33. Emerson N, Pesigan A, Sarana L *et al*. Panel 2.7: First 30 days: Organizing rapid responses. *Prehosp Disaster Med* 2005; **20**: 420–2.

◆34. Menne B, Apfel F, Kovats S, Racioppi F (eds). *Protecting Health in Europe from Climate Change*. Geneva: World Health Organization, Regional Office for Europe, 2008.

35. Alexander, D. From civil defence to civil protection – and back again. *Disaster Prev Manage* 2002; **11**: 209–13.

36. Alexander D. Understanding Katrina, Perspectives from the Social Sciences. Symbolic and Practical Interpretations of the Hurricane Katrina Disaster in New Orleans. Available from: http://understandingkatrina.ssrc.org/Alexander (accessed November 25, 2009).

37. Kirschenbaum, A. *Chaos, Organization, and Disaster Management*. New York: Marcel Dekker, 2004.

38. World Meteorological Organization. Weather, Climate, Water and Sustainable Development. Available from: http://www.eird.org/isdr-biblio/PDF/Weather%20Climate%20Water.pdf (accessed November 25, 2009).

39. Ebi KL, Burton I, McGregor G. *Biometeorology for Adaptation to Climate Variability and Change*. Berlin: Springer, 2008.

40. Kuhn K, Campbell-Lendrum D, Haines A *et al*. Using Climate To Predict Infectious Disease Epidemics. Available from: http://www.eird.org/isdr-biblio/PDF/Using%20climate%20to%20predict.pdf (accessed November 25, 2009).

41. Thacker SB, Stroup DF, Parrish RG, Anderson HA. Surveillance in environmental public health: Issues, systems, and sources. *Am J Public Health* 1996; **86**: 633–8.

◆42. Younger M, Morrow-Almeida HR, Vindigni SM, Dannenberg AL. The built environment, climate change, and health: Opportunities and co-benefits. *Am J Prev Med* 2008; **35**: 517–26.

43. Costello A, Abbas M, Allen A *et al*. Managing the health effects of climate change. *Lancet* 2009; **373**: 1693–733.

44. Brown LR. Designing sustainable cities. In: *Plan B 2.0 Rescuing a Planet Under Stress and a Civilization in Trouble*. New York: W.W. Norton & Co, 2006.

45. Food and Agriculture Organization. *The State of Food Insecurity in the World 2001*. Rome: FAO, 2002.

46. Schmidhuber J, Tubiello FN. Global food security under climate change. *Proc Natl Acad Sci USA* 2007; **104**: 19703–8.

47. Howden SM, Soussana JF, Tubiello FN *et al*. Adapting agriculture to climate change. *Proc Natl Acad Sci USA* 2007; **104**: 19691–6.

48. Morton JF. The impact of climate change on smallholder and subsistence agriculture. *Proc Natl Acad Sci USA* 2007; **104**: 19680–5.

49. Transition Town Totnes. Community Food and Wellbeing Garden. Available from: http://www.totnes.transitionnetwork.org/taxonomy/term/116 (accessed February 11, 2009).

50. National Health Service Sustainable Development Unit. Saving Carbon, Improving Health: NHS Carbon Reduction Strategy for England. Available from: http://www.sdu.nhs.uk/page.php?area_id=2 (accessed November 25, 2009).

51. Milly PCD, Betancourt J, Falkenmark M, Hirsch *et al*. Stationarity is dead: Whither water management? *Science* 2008; **319**: 573–4.

52. Pitt M. Learning Lessons from the 2007 Floods, UK Cabinet Office, 2008. Available at http://archive.cabinetoffice.gov.uk/pittreview/thepittreview.html (accessed February, 11 2009).

53. Woodruff RE, McMichael AJ, Hales S. Action on climate change: No time to delay. *Med J Aust* 2006; **184**: 539–40.

●54. Hanlon P, Carlisle S. Do we face a third revolution in human history? If so, how will public health respond? *J Public Health* 2008; **30**: 355–61.

SECTION ▮

Pressure

50

The hyperbaric environment

JOHN A.S. ROSS

INTRODUCTION

This chapter is intended as an overview of an extremely complex and interactive subject and addresses only the major issues without going into any real detail. Its main objective is to describe the hyperbaric environment in relation to human exposure and its major hazards rather than to consider medical issues in detail. There are five categories of exposure to the hyperbaric environment:

1. caisson or compressed air workers who operate in pressurized workings designed to prevent the ingress of water;
2. patients who need to be compressed either to receive hyperbaric oxygen or to be treated for decompression illness;
3. people who look after these patients in a pressurized chamber;
4. underwater divers who descend to work in the water and return to the surface after each work period;
5. underwater divers who live at the pressure of the underwater workplace and commute to work in a pressurized diving bell.

Two environments must be considered: that of a gas-filled, pressurized container and that underwater. Pressure is described in kilopascals (kPa), 100 kPa being equivalent to 1 bar (approximately 1 atmosphere), 10 m of seawater (msw) or 750 mmHg. The SI standard atmosphere (101.3 kPa, 760 mmHg) is not used.

THE PRESSURIZED ENVIRONMENT

There are three fundamental issues that typify exposure to pressure for humans. These are the compression and

decompression of gas-filled spaces in the body, exposure to gases at high pressure and the effects of hydrostatic pressure itself.

Compression and decompression of gas filled body cavities

The body contains several structures that normally contain free gas. These include the intestines, the lung, the middle ear and the nasal sinuses. With compression, the volume of a fixed mass of gas reduces in direct proportion to the pressure applied. Structures that can be distorted, such as the intestines, reduce in volume. Structures that cannot be compressed, such as the middle ear and nasal sinuses, require communication to the ambient environment so that gas can enter and maintain their volume.

For the ear, this is done through the Eustachian tube, and for the sinuses gas enters via their ostia in the nasal cavity. If these passages are blocked in any way, a negative pressure develops in the space. In the outer ear, if the external meatus is blocked by wax or occluded by a tight-fitting hood, there can be distortion of the tympanic membrane outwards with oedema and haemorrhage. In the middle ear, if the Eustachian tube is blocked the tympanic membrane is pushed inwards and traumatized, with inevitable perforation if compression is continued. In the sinuses, negative pressure is compensated by mucosal oedema formation and haemorrhage. In both instances, the victim experiences considerable pain, which normally encourages a return to normal ambient pressure.

The lung is an intermediate organ in this respect as, if gas is breathed during compression, volume is maintained by normal respiration. Alternatively, if a breath-hold dive is undertaken, the pulmonary gas space is compressed, with distortion of the chest wall, rising of the diaphragm as the abdominal contents move towards the head and, as pressure increases further, collapse of the compressible airways and alveoli with the potential for negative pressure-induced pulmonary oedema and haemorrhage. So the breath-hold diver runs the risk not only of drowning, but also of being unable to inflate a collapsed lung on the surface by spontaneous effort.[1] Accordingly, for both reasons, it is advisable to have equipment immediately available for positive-pressure ventilation of the lungs at the surface.

During decompression, or ascent in the water, gas expansion occurs. Again, this causes few problems in the distensible gut, although very rapid decompression has been associated with intestinal and gastric perforation. Blockage of the Eustachian tube while at pressure so that the middle ear cannot decompress is unusual but, if it happens, tympanic rupture is very likely. Blockage of the sinuses is more common and is, when it happens, potentially the most painful event in the victim's life, with the potential for subcutaneous or intracerebral bony rupture of the sinus. Causes for these events might include hay fever medication that wears off during an exposure to pressure or an upper respiratory tract infection.

Should gas be trapped in the lung or airway during decompression, the results may be catastrophic. Gas expansion has the potential to rupture the alveolar septum and airway walls. This can happen with a pressure change of as little as 10–11 kPa (0.1–0.2 bar), a pressure equivalent to a water depth of just 1 m.[2] For a mild event, there may just an episode of restrosternal chest pain with some cough as the lung tissue is stretched. Rupture of the pulmonary tissue may lead to gas tracking into the pleural space to cause pneumothorax, into the mediastinum to cause pneumomediastinum, or into the abdominal cavity to cause pneumoperitoneum.

Gas tracking into the pulmonary vein enters the cerebral and coronary circulations. The clinical signs are those of a cerebrovascular event or stroke, and the victim can also sustain a myocardial infarction. Causes of these events are concomitant pulmonary pathology such as infection, the bronchoconstriction of asthma or a pulmonary anatomical abnormality such as bullae, which are usually in the lung apices, and breath-holding during decompression. The problem is an important cause of accidental death in divers and has been reviewed.[3] As in the gut, very rapid decompression can lead to similar problems with no underlying pathology.

Exposure to gases at high pressure

GAS DENSITY

As gas is compressed, it becomes more dense in direct proportion to the ambient pressure, and as gas density increases, so does resistance to breathing. The critical velocity of air falls, giving rise to more turbulent flow within the airways. Gas flow under conditions of turbulence becomes proportional to the square root of the driving pressure, or, in other words, the pressure driving gas across the area of turbulent flow becomes proportional to the square of gas flow. The work of breathing is increased, and maximum breathing capacity is limited.

As a consequence, it has been observed that the maximum voluntary ventilation (MVV; the maximum exhaled breathing volume in 15 seconds × 4 in L/min body temperature and pressure saturated) is approximately proportional to the reciprocal of the square root of gas density.[4] At an absolute pressure of about 400 kPa, MVV is limited to about one-half of its surface value at a pressure of 100 kPa. Maximum ventilation during exercise is between 70 and 75 per cent MVV, and under experimental conditions in an air-filled chamber, heavy work was poorly tolerated and associated with marked carbon dioxide retention at 300 and 600 kPa absolute.[5] Heavy work at atmospheric pressure is normally associated with hypocapnia due to ventilation–perfusion mismatch, but hypercapnia is the rule at increased pressure owing to hypoventilation.

RAISED PARTIAL PRESSURE AND GAS PHARMACOLOGY

The partial pressures of the constituents of air increase in direct proportion to pressure. Accordingly, for example, at a pressure of 400 kPa, the worker is breathing 81 kPa oxygen and 316 kPa nitrogen.

Hyperoxia

An increased partial pressure of oxygen increases oxidant-related stress in the lung. An inhaled partial pressure of oxygen of 30 kPa causes an increase of albumin flux across the alveolar–capillary membrane in man,[6] and 50 kPa causes an increase in alveolar–capillary permeability and the number of alveolar neutrophils.[7] Breathing 79–89, 101 and 202 kPa oxygen, symptoms of pulmonary oxygen poisoning occurred at 6, 4 and 3 hours respectively.[8] At higher levels, symptoms come on sooner, but the clinical picture can be interrupted by the onset of central nervous system toxicity. Symptoms start as a dry tickling sensation on inspiration and progress to retrosternal chest pain with a feeling of tightness worse on inspiration and with a dry cough that becomes increasingly persistent. Severe poisoning is associated with dyspnoea first on exercise and then at rest.

Inhalation of 100 kPa oxygen is fatal in animal models, where increasing permeability of the pulmonary endothelium can be demonstrated, with an increasing diffusion barrier to oxygen that leads to hypoxia and interstitial pulmonary oedema. The breakdown of alveolar epithelial permeability occurs late in the development of pulmonary oxygen poisoning, but it leads to alveolar flooding with a protein-rich transudate and systemic hypoxia leading to death. Lower levels of exposure in animal models can give rise to pulmonary fibrosis, but the initial insult is caused by a chemical pneumonitis that is reversible. Oxygen exposure is associated with a progressive reduction in pulmonary vital capacity that, once the onset of symptoms occurs, takes some days to resolve, although symptomatic relief occurs soon after the withdrawal of hyperoxic exposure.

During pressure chamber exposures, at shorter and higher partial pressures than cause the onset of symptomatic pulmonary oxygen toxicity, oxygen shows proconvulsive and frankly convulsive effects.[9,10] Subconvulsive manifestations show the full gamut of an epileptic prodromal period. The convulsion, however, may occur without warning and has all the manifestations of a grand mal event with tonic, clonic and post-ictal phases. Levels of oxygen exposure below those that cause frank oxygen toxicity but close to the daily tolerable dose are associated with a chronic fatigue syndrome typified by tiredness and non-specific symptoms that can present as a flu-like illness and absence from work. The topic has been subjected to general review.[11]

Inert gas narcosis

High partial pressures of nitrogen cause subanaesthetic effects termed nitrogen or inert gas narcosis, and these are first manifest at about 400 kPa in air or a partial pressure of about 316 kPa of the gas. The mode of action is similar to other general anaesthetic agents such as xenon, and the anaesthetic potency of nitrogen is placed on a ranking of inert gas narcosis that ranges from xenon through argon, nitrogen and hydrogen to neon and helium, the latter demonstrating their activity only at pressures disguised by the high density of neon with its respiratory effects and the action of high hydrostatic pressure for helium.

The early stages of nitrogen narcosis may be typified by euphoria in inexperienced subjects. With experience and training this may be suppressed, but there is an underlying progressive deterioration in cognitive function with an early loss of planning capabilities and an early inability to deal with novel situations.[12] Few divers are able to work effectively at pressures in air greater than 700 kPa. Trained behaviours may be relatively well retained, however, and acclimatized divers have performed useful tasks breathing air at 1000 kPa, although this is considered a hazardous and extreme activity.[13] Memory is affected and events during exposure may be forgotten. There is an accompanying reduction in manual dexterity.[14] The problem of inert gas narcosis, together with the respiratory effect of high gas density, has led to a statutory pressure restriction of 600 kPa for the use of compressed air in diving. At higher pressures, nitrogen is replaced with a much less narcotic and less dense inert gas, which is almost universally helium.

Raised partial pressure and inert gas uptake and excretion

While exposure to increasing partial pressures of inert gas may lead to narcosis during compression and at pressure, a further problem develops due to inert gas uptake.

At atmospheric pressure, the amount of nitrogen dissolved in the blood and body tissues is at equilibrium and depends upon the solubility of and partial pressure of nitrogen in each tissue. As a rough guide, a young 75 kg male body contains 1.0 L of nitrogen dissolved in body tissues, excluding the gas spaces of the lungs.[15] The underlying relationship is:

$$\text{Mass of gas dissolved} \approx \text{Gas solubility} \times \text{Partial pressure of the gas}$$

As atmospheric pressure is increased, so is the partial pressure of nitrogen, and the amount of nitrogen dissolved in the tissues increases in direct proportion. So, at equilibrium at twice atmospheric pressure, the 75 kg male body will contain 2.0 L of dissolved nitrogen. The dynamics of gas uptake can be modelled as wash-in phenomena for each tissue. The underlying relationship here is:

$$\text{Inert gas uptake} \approx \text{Tissue blood flow} \times \text{Gas solubility in tissue} \times \text{Arterio-venous partial pressure difference}$$

The speed of gas uptake can be described in terms of half-life, with this being approximately 60 minutes for the whole body for nitrogen. Such considerations are, however, powerfully influenced by tissue blood flow and conditions altering it normally, such as exercise, or abnormally, such as cold and hypovolaemia.

Inert gas uptake is considered unimportant during compression or any stay in pressure. During decompression, however, the relationship is reversed:

$$\text{Inert gas excretion} \approx \text{Tissue blood flow} \times \text{Gas solubility in blood} \times \text{Veno-arterial partial pressure difference}$$

Within this relationship, if the rate of gas removal is insufficient, the partial pressure of inert gas in a tissue can exceed atmospheric pressure, so called supersaturation. In this condition, bubbles can form, particularly where pressure is reduced, such as in areas of blood flow turbulence, in areas where there are shearing forces, in muscles for example, and round joints and tendons. Once bubbles form, they provide an alternative route for the excretion of gases from tissues and can grow and persist for some time. The presence of free bubbles either in tissue or in the bloodstream may lead to decompression illness.[16] Local effects of bubbles are musculoskeletal pain predominantly associated with joints, and peripheral nerve dysfunction, commonly in spinal cord roots, with paraesthesiae or dysaesthesiae with localized pareses.

Bubbles in the venous return from the tissues are common during decompression,[17] and their occurrence is related to the amount of inert gas taken up (the degree of pressure and the time spent there) and the speed of decompression. In common with iatrogenic injection of air into the veins, these bubbles lodge in the pulmonary capillary circulation, where, in moderation, they seem to cause no overt harm as the lung acts as a filter. It is possible, however, for bubbles to bypass the pulmonary filter in either of two ways: transpulmonary shunting and intracardiac right-to-left shunting. The first of these is not thought to be a major risk factor as yet, but the second is regarded as important since the retrospectively determined presence of a patent foramen ovale is positively associated with neurological, spinal cord, vestibular and cutaneous decompression illness.[18–20] Small right-to-left shunts are though to carry a low risk, but large defects are important. The presence of a patent foramen ovale doubles the risk of decompression illness.[21]

Furthermore, systemic embolization to the lungs raises right heart pressure and this can precipitate the opening of a patent foramen ovale, with particle injection into the left atrium and systemic embolization. Other causes of a raised right heart pressure, such as coughing or performing a Valsalva manoeuvre (during middle ear pressure equalization, for example) might also be important.

Decompression is also a risk factor for aseptic bone necrosis occurring in the shaft and juxta-articular areas of the long bones (dysbaric bone necrosis). There is a strong positive association between decompression illness and bone necrosis. Both conditions depend upon the degree and duration of exposure to increased ambient pressure, and although the precise aetiology remains to be established, the two conditions are likely to share causative factors; this has been reviewed.[22] The majority of lesions seen are in long bone shafts and are held to be of no long-term health consequences. Juxta-articular lesions are clinically important if they cause collapse of the articular surface leading to painful arthritis of the joint involved, usually the hip or shoulder.

In order to avoid decompression illness or bone necrosis, decompression is performed over a time period sufficient to avoid undue supersaturation, and this may be prolonged. The calculation of decompression timetables is beyond the scope of this chapter, and the reader is referred to the specialist literature.

Raised hydrostatic pressure

The introduction of helium made human compression to high pressure feasible. It soon became clear, however, that rapid compression to pressures of 1500 kPa induced peripheral tremor and loss of manipulative ability.[23] For a short time, this condition was referred to as helium narcosis, but it became apparent that the tremor was not associated with cognitive impairment. Further work, largely in animals but also to a significant extent in man, indicated that the tremor was indicative of a proconvulsant action of hydrostatic pressure itself.

Increased hydrostatic pressure leads to a condition termed the high-pressure nervous syndrome (HPNS). The

initial sign is an increase of physiological tremor peripherally. As the pressure is increased, the tremor spreads centrally and myoclonic jerking occurs, with other non-specific symptoms such as dizziness, epigastric discomfort, nausea and stomach cramps with impaired cerebral capacity and sleep disturbances. There have been sporadic individual reports of visual and auditory hallucinations. Electroencephalography indicates a move of dominant frequency from the alpha into the theta and delta bands, and spindling with occasional spike and wave events may be seen. Further compression, in animal models, can lead to seizures and death.

The HPNS reverses on decompression, and although there is clearly cause for concern, there has been no convincing demonstration of persisting organic pathology in man after the dive. The underlying mechanism is thought to lie in a pressure-induced decreased release of the inhibitory amino acids gamma-aminobutyrate and glutamate, with increased sensitivity of excitatory N-methyl D-aspartate receptors.[24] Psychotic episodes have been noted at high pressure in mixtures of exotic gases, however, and these have been attributed a physicochemical aetiology based on cell membrane compression by hydrostatic pressure, and membrane expansion as the inert gas dissolves in plasma membrane lipids.[25]

The HPNS limits the pressure to which man can go, and although compression to 7200 kPa has been achieved using the inert gas narcosis properties of hydrogen to suppress the syndrome, the highest routine operational diving pressure is in the order of 3000 kPa.[26]

Caisson workers

Compressed air can be used to keep water out of underground or underwater civil engineering workings, for example in the construction of tunnels and bridge foundations. A pressureproof container of some kind, the caisson, is placed over the workings and ventilated with air at a pressure sufficient to exclude water.

In the past, gangs of men worked for prolonged shifts in the pressurized workings, and the major concerns were industrial accident and decompression illness. One early account reports 3692 cases of 'compressed air illness' with 20 associated deaths in 10 000 workers occurring over a period of 557 days in the construction of railway tunnels under the East River in New York.[27] The rate of decompression illness in compressed air workers remained high in the UK and, in the 1980s and into the 1990s, it was not unusual for 25 per cent of workers on a contract to be affected. Improved practice and surveillance has, however, improved the situation,[28] and the introduction of oxygen breathing during decompression has improved safety internationally[29] and was introduced as a statutory requirement in the UK during 2003.

As might be expected from the high level of decompression illness, dysbaric osteonecrosis was also common in compressed air workers, and in 1980 the Medical Research Council Decompression Sickness Panel reported that 17.6 per cent of a sample of 2534 workers had definite bone lesions.[30] The improvements in practice introduced since then that have reduced the incidence of decompression illness are expected also to have reduced the risk of dysbaric bone necrosis.

The use of manual labour in caissons is now kept to a minimum for economic reasons, but the blades of tunnel-boring machines still must be changed manually. As tunnelling techniques have improved, higher caisson pressures have been used, and saturation diving techniques have been used to provide safe working conditions for tunnellers.[31]

Hyperbaric patients

Recompression and the administration of 100 per cent oxygen at increased ambient pressure (hyperbaric oxygen treatment) is the standard treatment for decompression sickness and diving-related arterial gas embolism. Hyperbaric oxygen also reverses the tissue hypoxia caused by carbon monoxide poisoning and might improve long-term outcomes in this condition. A number of other conditions might also respond to this treatment, notably post-radiotherapy tissue damage.[32] Hyperbaric oxygen is also used in the treatment of a plethora of other conditions without any real justification.

Generally, hyperbaric oxygen treatment has a low side-effect profile. Minor degrees of otic barotrauma of little clinical significance are relatively common in patients who are not divers. Patients at the pressures used for the treatment of decompression illness and carbon monoxide poisoning are at risk of central nervous system oxygen toxicity and convulsions. For this reason, patients should not be left unattended, although there is full recovery in otherwise well people. Cases of decompression illness requiring prolonged hyperbaric treatment are at risk of pulmonary oxygen poisoning, and when this occurs, the partial pressure of oxygen must be reduced, after which full recovery takes place over a number of days.

The major risk to patients, however, is fire in the hyperbaric chamber. The chamber is an enclosed space from which rapid escape is difficult and in some cases not possible. The ignition temperature is lowered and the rate at which materials burn is increased in compressed air (21 per cent oxygen). The likelihood of a fire being initiated is more probable than at atmospheric pressure, and contamination of the chamber atmosphere with the oxygen used in treatment dramatically increases this hazard. The risk is controlled by keeping the use of combustible material to a minimum, controlling the percentage of ambient oxygen in the chamber to 23 per cent or less, limiting sources of ignition such as static electricity discharges and using low-powered electrical devices that are protected against overheating.

This subject has been reviewed,[33] and although there have been several chamber fires with fatalities since the publication of this review, its conclusions remain valid. From 1923 to 1996, there were 77 fatalities due to chamber fires in 35 incidents, 25 of which were in therapeutic hyperbaric oxygen systems. Prior to 1980, fires were mostly caused by electrical ignition, but since that date the cause has usually been a prohibited, high-risk item taken into the chamber either by a patient or an attendant. Examples of these have been liquid petroleum lighters, children's toys and catalytic hand-warmers. Fatalities have occurred in chambers with more than 28 per cent oxygen and containing a lot of combustible materials. To the author's knowledge, there have been no fires in hyperbaric chambers in the UK.

Unwell people may require a range of services for patient care support, including for electronic monitoring, artificial ventilation of the lungs and control of intravenous infusion. The equipment necessary should be compatible with exposure to increased ambient pressure, should not be adversely affected by increasing gas density and should not pose a fire hazard. The market for such equipment for hyperbaric use is small, and manufacturers do not certify their products for such use. Accordingly, it is the responsibility of each individual hyperbaric medicine unit to test and certify equipment for use in its chamber.[34] These considerations extend to implanted equipment, but most pacemakers are tested for pressure resistance by the manufacturers, who realize that many of their satisfied customers are recreational divers.

Hyperbaric therapy attendants

Hyperbaric chamber attendants are in theory at risk of the hazards encountered in compressed air working. Apart from decompression illness occurring in sensitive individuals,[35] however, problems relating to the hyperbaric environments are unusual.[36] The risks to health encountered by such workers are more those of the healthcare environment and include hazards such as manual handling, sharps injury and control of infection. This latter is complicated by the incompatibility of alcohol-based cleaning or decontamination products with the hyperbaric environment as they constitute a significant fire hazard.

Hyperbaric therapy attendants work in an atmosphere of compressed air at pressures up to 600 kPa. Nitrogen narcosis impairs cognitive ability and may render individuals overconfident. Clinical judgement may therefore be impaired, and it is important for attendants to be aware of this. Decisions about patient management in the chamber are best performed by staff outside the chamber and only implemented by the hyperbaric attendant. If compression to more than 300 kPa is required, this should ideally be done using helium and oxygen and the hazard of nitrogen narcosis avoided.

THE UNDERWATER ENVIRONMENT

Immersion

Underwater diving while breathing compressed air is the most common method by which humans are exposed to pressure for any length of time. This has cardiovascular and respiratory effects equivalent to head-out immersion in water that are unrelated to the ambient pressure and have recently been reviewed.[37,38]

Immersion in thermally neutral (34 °C) water compresses the peripheral circulation, reducing the peripheral pooling of blood and increasing central blood volume. Cardiac output rises with increased stroke volume, and peripheral vascular resistance falls so that blood pressure remains unchanged. Atrial distension releases atrial natriuretic peptide, which cause diuresis, natriuresis and vasodilatation with a reduction in plasma renin activity. The degree of diuresis is attenuated by physical fitness, but it does persist throughout immersion exposures of 12 hours.

Diuresis is also markedly affected by the temperature of the water. Exposure to cold water causes sympathetic stimulation, raised plasma noradrenaline (norepinephrine) levels and vasoconstriction. This amplifies the effect of immersion in increasing central blood volume and increases diuresis. Immersion in water at 14 °C for 1 hour can double urine output from approximately 2 L up to 4 L in young male subjects.[39] Increased water temperature seems to have the opposite effect, causing a fall in peripheral vascular resistance and reversing natriuresis. Water above the thermally neutral temperature is poorly tolerated by man, however, and carries a significant risk of hyperthermia when sweating can give rise to hypovolaemia and electrolyte disturbances.

Immersion can therefore clearly give rise to significant fluid balance problems for divers. Most importantly, while relative fluid balance remains normal during the dive as a diuresis progressively reduces central blood volume, the diver may, on coming out of the water, be dehydrated. The response to dehydration of peripheral and splanchnic vasoconstriction can reduce inert gas excretion, and the peripheral vasoconstriction associated with exposure to cold has the same effect. After a dive, both factors increase the risk of decompression sickness.

An immersion-induced increase in pulmonary blood flow leads to a rise in pulmonary blood volume that reduces vital capacity and increases residual volume. The chest wall is compressed hydrostatically, and this increases the work of breathing and leads to negative-pressure breathing. The hydrostatic pressure difference between the breathing equipment and the airway can also alter static lung loading, which may be positive or negative depending on the nature of the equipment and the posture of the diver.[38]

In water, most people float and, for the diver, further buoyancy is added by the diving suit, so that weights are needed to enable any descent and to move around underwater. A free-swimming diver is essentially weightless, and limb movement is impeded by the water. These factors render the use of tools, particularly those requiring a degree of force, awkward and inefficient. Movement through the water is impeded by drag, which is dependent on the velocity of water flowing round the body, and divers are very vulnerable to currents. A 0.5 knot current puts considerable demands on a swimmer, and a 1 knot current can stop any forward progress. Cold water can add to the difficulty of using tools by reducing manual dexterity and sensitivity.

Hypothermia reduces cognitive function and the mechanical efficiency of movement, and the ability to work is further reduced by an impaired exercise capability. This is largely due to the greater work of breathing associated with increased gas density at depth and the effect of breathing equipment in increasing static chest loading and resistance to breathing.[40] The effect is compounded by reduced lung volume following from increased central blood volume, although this effect does wear off with the duration of immersion due to diuresis.

The overall effect is a tendency for the diver to hypoventilate and retain carbon dioxide. Hypoxia is not an issue as the partial pressure of oxygen increases with depth. Hypercapnia can lead to impaired cognitive function due to acidosis and is proconvulsant, leading to an increased risk of hyperoxic convulsions. Carbon dioxide retention causes an indirect release of adrenaline and noradrenaline into the circulation. Circulatory responses to these increased levels of circulating catecholamines may impair thermal homeostasis and inert gas excretion, thus increasing the risk of decompression sickness.

Human vision is impaired underwater.[41] If in contact with water, the eye loses the ability to focus as the refractive index of the eye is similar to that of water (1.33). This problem is overcome by wearing a facemask or goggles, but these limit the field of vision and distort vision since there is refraction at the window of the mask and objects appear larger and closer than they actually are. Water absorbs light and, even when it is clean, only about 20 per cent of light penetrates to a depth of 10 m; very little light penetrates to 90 m. This light attenuation is accompanied by colour distortion since different wavelengths of light are absorbed to varying degrees, with red and orange light being absorbed the most.

A further factor limiting vision is particle suspension in water. Turbulent water over a muddy bottom can lead to zero-visibility conditions. At depth, where artificial light is required, the back-scattering of light from particles in the water also impedes vision. The scattering and absorption of light by particles also evens out differences in light intensity, and the diver may lose track of the surface, which further complicates orientation. The sensation of weightlessness in the water can add to the disorientation, particularly in conditions of low visibility; in extreme cases, the diver may lose track of the surface.

Hearing is also affected by immersion, and hearing in divers has been the subject of a recent comprehensive review.[42] Although sound travels more quickly and is transmitted better in water than in air, contact of the eardrum with water damps down human hearing. In addition, since sound in water is transmitted relatively freely through the human body, hearing by bone conduction is more important in water than it is in air. At low frequencies, tympanic hearing dominates, and bone conduction is greater for higher frequencies.

Audiometry with a wet ear shows peak hearing at about 800 Hz, while for airborne sound peak sensitivity is at about 4 kHz. At peak sensitivity, underwater hearing is 35–40 dB less sensitive than in air. The wet ear is therefore protected and is most sensitive to noise-induced damage at 800 Hz. The risk of underwater noise-induced hearing loss can be assessed by the use of an underwater noise weighting scale. If the diver's ears are kept dry, however, as within a hood or helmet, airborne noise assessment methods are more appropriate. Divers are considered at risk of hearing loss,[43] and the greatest risk to hearing for them is noise. Noise sources include nearby vessels, the breathing equipment and the use of tools, particularly powered tools such as water jets, drill or hammers. These latter also carry the risk of hand–arm vibration syndrome.

Underwater diving

SURFACE-ORIENTED DIVING

The diver descends to the underwater worksite and returns to the surface after a time dictated by the duration of the job but, more importantly, by the need for a safe decompression avoiding decompression illness. A variety of methods of supplying breathable gas are used.

Usually, a hose from the surface supplies the breathing equipment, and the diver carries only a small cylinder of compressed breathing mixture for use in an emergency. The hose can carry a cable for communications, with the diver wearing an oral–nasal mask through which he or she can talk to the dive supervisor. Commercial divers frequently work unaccompanied, but there is a statutory requirement for another, the standby diver, to be immediately ready to go into the water in the event of an emergency.

Other types of equipment are used for different diving tasks, and various types of self-contained underwater breathing equipment are available; these, however, carry the disadvantages of limited gas supply, difficult or absent communications and the possibility of losing touch with the dive supervisor or boat. The entrapment of free-swimming divers in enclosed spaces, such as are found in wrecks, is an important hazard complicated by low visibility and disorientation.

Thermal protection is provided by either a wetsuit, which traps a layer of water between the suit and the skin, or a dry suit, in which the diver is isolated from the water. Wetsuits are generally made of neoprene foam that loses its insulating property with depth of water as the gas in the suit is compressed and offers no protection against contaminants in the water or at the dive site. Dry suits trap an insulating layer of gas against the diver's body and, with an appropriate undergarment, the thermal protection offered is very effective. With compression, the layer of gas is reduced and is topped up, generally from the diver's breathable gas supply. With decompression, the gas layer expands and should be vented so that buoyancy is controlled.

Dry suits are the preferred option in the UK and have the benefit of providing protection against contaminated waters. They do require, however, a degree of maintenance, and training in buoyancy control is essential. Loss of dry suit buoyancy control is associated with about a third of recreational diving accidents in Scotland, and these accidents generally occur on the first day of a diving holiday or after a spell during which the equipment has not been used. Another factor in such accidents is the deployment of a surface marker buoy by the diver prior to ascent as a warning to surface craft. Entanglement in the buoy line can take the diver to the surface. The use of a buoyancy compensator, an inflatable and deflatable waistcoat, further complicates buoyancy control for the inexperienced diver.

Divers performing long shallow dives may use hot-water suits for thermal comfort. These are more normally used by saturation divers and are described in the relevant section below.

Decompression

The major risks in surface-orientated diving are related to decompression, with its accompanying dangers of gas embolism, decompression illness and dysbaric osteonecrosis. The risk of the latter two have been much reduced by the application of statutory limits to the duration and depth of air diving in the UK[44] and probably by the now widespread use of diving computers carried by the diver. These measure depth and time and give continuous information on the safety of the decompression schedule being used.

The number of divers working in the North Sea was documented for the years 2000–03,[45] and during this time the incidence of decompression illness in this population, calculated from the number of cases notified by industry to the Health and Safety Executive, varied between 13 and 41 cases per 100 working years. The current prevalence of dysbaric osteonecrosis among divers in the UK is unknown, but a systematic study of the condition by the Medical Research Council Decompression Sickness Panel indicated that 4.0 per cent of a sample of 4980 UK divers had some form of dysbaric osteonecrosis; juxta-articular lesions were seen in 1.2 per cent, with these changes progressing to articular damage in 0.2 per cent.[46] A subsequent review of some 7000 divers confirmed this prevalence of clinically relevant joint damage.

The use of oxygen or an oxygen-enriched gas mixture is another method used to either reduce the risk of decompression illness or extend the safe duration of a dive, and, at depths from about 10 m, 100 per cent oxygen can be breathed to speed up inert gas excretion. One hundred per cent oxygen is also used by military divers in rebreather diving apparatus, in which the exhaled gas passes through a carbon dioxide-absorbing chemical filter and oxygen is added to maintain the volume of gas in the circuit.

Oxygen toxicity convulsions

The use of raised partial pressures of oxygen raises the problems of oxygen toxicity. Practically speaking, three syndromes are seen: pulmonary oxygen toxicity, grand mal epileptic seizures with their prodromal symptomatology (central nervous system oxygen toxicity) and a generalized fatigue syndrome. Pulmonary oxygen toxicity is not thought to pose a significant problem for surface-orientated diving as exposures are generally too short for a clinical effect to be seen.

Central nervous system oxygen toxicity is of the greatest concern for the diver using oxygen-enriched mixtures. It was first systematically described by Donald in Royal Navy covert exercise divers using 100 per cent oxygen in rebreather diving equipment,[9,47,48] and the effect has been briefly reviewed.[10] There is substantial intra- and interindividual variability in central nervous system sensitivity to breathing hyperbaric oxygen. Broadly speaking, the higher the oxygen partial pressure breathed, the quicker is the onset of symptoms. Operationally, in a dry pressure chamber, convulsive manifestations are seen at oxygen partial pressures of 280 kPa and above even when periods of exposure are limited to 20 minutes during the treatment of decompression illness. In the water, however, divers are very much more sensitive, and convulsions have been reported from partial pressures as low as 130 kPa. The reasons for this difference are unclear but have been attributed to carbon dioxide retention and exercise. The potential for immersion to alter cerebral blood flow may be another contributory factor.

Tolerance levels for oxygen are illustrated by the time limits applied by the US Navy for 100 per cent oxygen breathing during shallow diving (Table 50.1). Nevertheless, oxygen-related convulsion do occur, in which case the survival of the victim depends upon rescue by fellow divers to the surface.

The use of high partial pressures of oxygen mixed with inert gas at greater depth is more hazardous since rescue to the surface may not be possible, and oxygen partial pressures of 130 kPa and less are advisable. If a mouthpiece is used, a convulsion leads to its loss soon after the diver loses consciousness, and drowning ensues. Even with assistance, this situation is difficult to retrieve. For this reason, an oral–nasal mask strapped to the diver's head is advisable, allowing, as it does, survival during and after the fit.

Oxygen enrichment of the diver's breathing gas has clear advantages related to a reduced uptake of inert gas

Table 50.1   Single depth oxygen exposure limits

Depth (metres seawater)	Partial pressure oxygen (kPa)	Permissible duration (minutes)
7.6	176	240
9.1	191	80
10.1	206	25
10.2	221	15
15.2	252	10

Adapted from NAVSEA SS521-AG-PRO-01 US Navy Diving Manual, revision 6, 2008.

and the ability to reduce decompression time or increase the time available for work under water. It has proved possible to calculate the maximum daily dose of oxygen that a diver can tolerate without central nervous system or pulmonary effects.[8,11] If this dose is repeatedly used by divers from day to day, however, a further manifestation of oxygen toxicity appears. This is intense fatigue leading to disability, probably relating to the high level of oxidative stress.[49] This effect is also seen in some patients receiving multiple hyperbaric oxygen treatment sessions.

Carbon dioxide intoxication

Surface-orientated divers are at risk of carbon dioxide retention during exercise due to the respiratory effects of immersion and the increased work of breathing caused by breathing equipment and increased gas density.[38] Divers using closed or semi-closed breathing equipment run the further risk of failure of carbon dioxide absorption in the breathing equipment. While carbon dioxide retention at atmospheric pressure is associated with hypoxia, this is usually not the case at pressures where the partial pressure of oxygen is elevated, and in rebreather equipment, a fixed elevated partial pressure of oxygen is automatically maintained.

The early symptoms of carbon dioxide retention are hyperventilation, anxiety, tachycardia and flushing. There is increased release of noradrenaline and adrenaline into the circulation, and the resulting stimulation of the cardiovascular system leads to impaired thermal homeostasis and increased tissue blood flow with increased risks of hypothermia and decompression illness. At arterial partial pressures up to about 12.7 kPa, consciousness is largely unaffected, but above this level there is progressive loss of cerebral function until a state typical of surgical anaesthesia supervenes at a partial pressure of about 26.8 kPa in normoxic animal models.[50] At higher levels, there is an increase in muscle tone with cortical seizure activity and a progressive reduction in central nervous system cellular activity due to acidosis.

The disturbance of cognitive function associated with normoxic or hyperoxic hypercapnia is such that the victim may not be aware of the seriousness of the situation until it is too late to get to safety. Under conditions of immersion, the anxiety experienced may amount to outright panic.

Hypoxia

While hypoxia is the norm in breath-hold diving, it is unusual during other diving techniques unless there is failure of the gas supply or breathing equipment. In commercial surface-supplied diving, the diver should have an emergency reserve of breathing gas, and all free-swimming divers can carry back-up breathing gas regulators. If, however, breathing gas is lost at depth, the diver must ascend to the surface as rapidly as possible. The risk of decompression illness is clear but of secondary importance since that of hypoxia is paramount. This hypoxic risk is magnified as the diver approaches the surface since the alveolar oxygen partial pressure falls as pressure reduces in the same manner as it increased during compression. It is not uncommon for a diver losing the gas supply at depth to be unconscious and cyanosed on the surface but to revive rapidly after the appropriate resuscitative procedures have been carried out by the surface crew. The free-swimming diver is most at risk here, while the surface-supplied diver can be both located and helped to the surface by the diving umbilical.

Technical diving

Recent years have seen the development of the surface diving method referred to as technical diving, particularly in the recreational diver sector. Here, helium is used to reduce gas density and inert gas narcosis, and control of the oxygen partial pressure is used to reduce decompression time. Depths of more than 100 m can be achieved. The standard breathing gas, however, tends to be a helium and air mixture, and at some depth, the diver will encounter the same problems of inert gas narcosis and respiratory restriction that limits the use of air at, however, much greater depth and so posing a much greater hazard.

SATURATION DIVING

In the commercial sector, diving to greater than 50 msw, and often less, especially in support of the offshore oil and gas industry, is achieved by the use of saturation diving techniques. Here, the inert gas nitrogen is replaced with helium, and oxygen levels are controlled to levels that can tolerated for extended periods of time. Teams of divers are compressed in complexes of large chambers, usually on board a diving support vessel, in which they stay for up to 28 days in UK waters. The pressure chambers are held at the approximate pressure of the underwater workplace, and divers commute in diving bells at pressure to and from the worksite at the beginning and end of their shift. In this way, round-the-clock underwater work is possible and the dangers of decompression are largely avoided.

The practice of saturation diving involves a number of specific environmental challenges, which are the helium environment, oxygen exposure, isolation and the possibility of environmental contamination. In addition, divers are exposed to workplace factors during their shift such as exposure to noise and vibration and the risk of industrial accidents on the sea bed or elsewhere.

Helium is approximately five times less dense than nitrogen, and its use compensates for the increase in resistance to breathing with compression. In this respect, a depth of 300 msw breathing helium and oxygen is approximately equivalent to 50 msw breathing air. In addition, over the pressure range for which it is used, helium has no narcotic properties. On the other hand, helium distorts speech and alters thermal equilibrium.

There is speech distortion even in air with increasing pressure in air, and the voice becomes more nasal with a non-linear shift of the higher formant frequencies.[51] Further distortion is caused by the use of helium. All may be familiar with the comical character of squeaky 'helium speech' at atmospheric pressure. This is caused by a change in the resonating characteristics of the larynx, oropharynx, nose and sinuses. There is a non-linear shift of formant frequencies to the right, and the energy associated with fricative sounds shifts upward in frequency. At increased pressure, distortion increases as the proportion of oxygen in the breathing mixture falls while maintaining the same partial pressure. The process is incompletely understood, and divers may adjust their voice at pressure to make it more comprehensible. Certainly, helium speech in divers equilibrated in a chamber at 100–140 msw depth is comprehensible.

THERMAL BALANCE

Helium has a higher thermal conductivity than air and conducts heat to and from the body more efficiently (Table 50.2). Heat loss by convection is also directly proportional to gas density. As a result, the range of temperature providing thermal comfort in a helium–oxygen atmosphere is narrow, at 29–31 °C at pressures of 720–2070 kPa, in comparison to 20–30 °C in air at atmospheric pressure for a lightly clad person.[52] Thermal homeostasis is disrupted in a helium–oxygen environment, and the diver becomes effectively poikilothermic.

Problems of thermal balance accompany the saturation diver into the water. Water temperature is typically 4–6 °C in the North Sea, and with a shift in the water lasting about 6 hours, passive thermal insulation is inadequate. In addition, as gas density increases so does obligatory heat loss from the respiratory tract. With a breathing mixture of helium and oxygen, during light activity at 2070 kPa, respiratory heat loss approaches metabolic heat production. Accordingly, an active heating system is used. Water is heated on the surface and pumped down the umbilical into the diver's suit, where it is distributed over the skin surface by a system of perforated tubes escaping via the wrist and ankle openings. The hot water flow is controlled to a comfortable level by the diver.

Initial concerns regarding the efficacy of this system[53] have not been sustained by more detailed investigation,[54]

Table 50.2   Physical characteristics of air and 40 kPa oxygen in helium at different pressures

	Equivalent depth (metres seawater)	Density (kg/m³)	Thermal conductivity (W/m per °C)	Specific heat (kJ/kg per °C)
Air 100 kPa	0	1.15	0.027	1.052
Air 200 kPa	10	2.30		
Air 600 kPa	20	6.90		1.064
Helium 60 kPa, oxygen 40 kPa	0	0.603	0.116	0.833
Helium 960 kPa, oxygen 40 kPa	90	2.023	0.150	1.200
Helium 1960 kPa, oxygen 40 kPa	190	3.586	0.153	1.221
Helium 3960 kPa, oxygen 40 kPa	390	6.675	0.154	1.231

Adapted from Flook,[52] with permission.

and it is widely used throughout the industry. The diving suit used is, however, open to ambient water at the wrists and ankles, and the hot water is taken out of the sea beside the diving vessel. As a result, these suits do not protect against environmental contamination. For example, there are reports of jellyfish being picked up in the hot water inlet and pumped through to the suit, much to the diver's discomfort.

There are also reports of lesions at the ankle called drilling mud burns. These latter have been reported by as many as 19 per cent of divers at some time in their career[55] and are a contact dermatitis. The standard wetsuit allows water ingress, and this is a particular problem with the lower limbs. Contact with contaminated bottom mud can cause an acute dermatitis due to allergy to the mud components, with diesel, tall oil and synthetic olefins being identified as allergens or irritants in one short study.[56] Sensitivity to polyamines and related chemicals in drilling mud has also been identified.[57] These lesions can be quite extensive, but there seems to be little realization that they are a dermatitis and, accordingly, reportable under the UK Reporting of Injuries Diseases and Dangerous Occurrence Regulations 1995. Exposure of the skin to hydrocarbons raises the strong possibility of dermal uptake, but this risk has not yet been considered in the context of commercial diving.

Underwater diving exposes the diver to higher than normal partial pressures of oxygen. During surface-orientated diving, if central nervous system toxicity is avoided, the duration of exposure is usually insufficient to have any important consequences. In saturation diving, however, the diver is exposed to a raised oxygen partial pressure throughout the dive.

At stable pressure, the oxygen partial pressure in the living chamber is kept between 30 and 40 kPa and is raised to about 50 kPa during the prolonged decompression period. During excursions from the living chambers to the underwater worksite, the partial pressure of oxygen is commonly 70 kPa. This level of oxygen exposure is not associated with obvious side-effects. In man, however, as

discussed earlier, exposure to these levels of oxygen increases the albumin concentration and number of inflammatory cells in bronchoalveolar lavage fluid.[6,7] This may indicate a pulmonary response to oxidant stress rather than an overt pathological process.

Nevertheless, there is an underlying level of concern regarding the use of high partial pressures of oxygen in saturation diving. Where an increased partial pressure of oxygen is used to reduce decompression times, the practice can be defended. Increased oxygen exposure at stable pressure, however, has little underlying supportive logic.

Isolation

Saturation diving is carried out on continental shelves. Although the dive site may be close to shore, it is more commonly some hundreds of miles from port. Geographical isolation is compounded by temporal isolation occasioned by the need for a safe decompression. A typical decompression time for return to surface after a saturation dive to 100 msw is 3 days and 14 hours but longer if the team adopts the common practice of stopping the decompression overnight. Dive team members are further isolated from their colleagues on the surface by the metal containment of the pressure chambers and difficulties of vocal and visual communication. There are two major consequences of this degree of isolation, one practical and the other completely unresearched.

Men living in saturation diving systems are at risk of traumatic injury as a result of accidents and also of intercurrent illness. The complete spectrum of human ailment has been witnessed in these systems since their inception in the 1970s, from an epidemic of Bornholm disease to major blast injury and traumatic amputation. It is not possible to deliver the standard of care available in advanced mainland hospitals within a saturation diving habitat. For a while in the North Sea, the concept of transfer of the unwell diver in a small transportable pressure chamber to a hospital-based hyperbaric system was explored. The system was, however, used only once, and many of the problems described persist in a hospital-based hyperbaric unit. In practice, injured or unwell saturation divers offshore have been treated and stabilized in the diving system before transfer to hospital after decompression. This situation remains a constant cause for concern.

During saturation, divers work a shift system and are isolated from any normal day/night cycle. They are active during their shift but are otherwise asleep or, when awake, largely inactive. During the days spent in decompression to the surface, there is little reason for them to move from their bunks in the chamber. Common complaints in divers after the end of a saturation dive are fatigue and irritability that has been likened to jet lag. It is likely that saturation divers experience a considerable degree of chronobiological dislocation, and this may have knock-on effects on accident causation and into the post-dive period.

Environmental contamination

The atmosphere in the saturation chamber complex is recycled through a gas-conditioning plant that controls temperature, oxygen, carbon dioxide and humidity. Atmospheric contaminants in the system can be removed by activated charcoals or molecular sieve material. Gaseous contaminants, however, such as carbon monoxide, hydrogen and argon, can be removed only by flushing the system with fresh gas. Recirculation rather than ventilation is used for economic and logistical reasons as helium is expensive and the dive support vessel can only carry a certain amount of fresh gas. Any material coming into contact with the gas mixture breathed by the diver can off-gas (i.e. emit a noxious gas) and cause contamination. Two questionnaire surveys reported that 34–35 per cent of divers reported exposure to contaminated gases during their career.[58,59]

There are many possible sources of contamination.[59] In the system of pressure chambers, two-part epoxy paints are used to finish the inside surfaces and, during curing, off-gas high levels of compounds such as ethylbenzene and xylene. Although the fabrics used in chamber coverings and upholstery have proved to be problem-free, the same may not be the case for cushioning material in seating and mattresses. Traditionally, pressure chambers have been made entirely from steel. Recently, however, there has been a move to finish the inside of the chamber in more attractive and easily cleaned synthetic materials. The materials themselves and the glues and sealants necessary for their use can all cause problems, and their employment requires careful assessment and atmospheric monitoring. Cleaning agents are another cause of contamination and are used for general chamber hygiene and for cleaning breathing equipment for use in oxygen.

These sources of contamination and the enclosed nature of saturation diving have led to occupational exposure limits being developed for hyperbaric conditions. The most important factor in generating these limits has been the duration of potential exposure, which is, rather than the 8 hours of a conventional work shift, up to 28 days with currently accepted diving practice. This been dealt with by taking the acceptable time-weighted average

Table 50.3 Anaesthetizing and convulsant doses of common petrochemicals in rats[61–63]

Agent	Anaesthetizing dose (kPa)	Convulsant dose (kPa)
Ethane	159	
Propane	94	
Butane	34.5	
Pentane	12.7	
Hexane	4.67	
Heptane	1.98	
Octane	1.7	
Cyclohexane	4.2	2.2 (seizure)
Benzene	1.01	0.74 (jerking)
Toluene	0.45	0.3 (hyperactivity)
m- and p-Xylene	0.145	0.09 (tremors, p-xylene)

occupational exposure limit over 8 hours divided by 5.0 as acceptable over a saturation dive.[60] This arbitrary approach produces exposure levels for carbon monoxide below current air quality standards, and permissible benzene exposures 200 times the current UK air quality target. There clearly remains a requirement to consider contaminants on an individual basis.

Although exposure to gas contaminants in the living chambers is an important consideration, divers are at greater short-term risk from petrochemical exposure during the working shift. Oilfield diving may involve work in areas heavily contaminated with petrochemicals in the vicinity of an operating well. The diving bell atmosphere is heated, and carbon dioxide and oxygen levels are controlled. There is no gas purification system, however, and contaminants can be removed only by flushing, with a requirement for the divers to use respiratory protective equipment if they are able.

Petrochemicals in the water can evaporate into the atmosphere of the diving bell and thus contaminate the living chamber atmosphere when the bell returns to the system. The possibility of dermal exposure has already been mentioned, and work in contaminated water deposits quantities of petrochemical on the divers' suits and equipment. Ambient temperature in the water is below the boiling point of liquid crudes and condensates. These can adhere to the diver's equipment in the water, and rapidly evaporate if they are taken into the bell. The partial pressure of gaseous hydrocarbon generated by such events can be very high. In this context, the petrochemicals involved have important narcotic and convulsive properties (Table 50.3) and predispose to cardiac dysrhythmias. There have been fatalities associated with such accidents, and monitors have been developed to detect hydrocarbons in the bell. This equipment is, however, designed to detect narcotic levels of fume only and not levels of contamination that breach occupational exposure limits.

Welding is another source of workplace contamination for divers. Underwater pipeline welding may be carried out in a gas-filled habitat that encloses the structure to be worked on. Divers travel to the welding habitat by diving bell and, once inside, breath chamber atmosphere using standard personal protective equipment as required. The techniques used are manual metal arc and tungsten inert gas welding of carbon steel.

As the weld is constructed, each layer is cleaned and shaped using high-speed grinding equipment. Although local extraction is used to remove welding fume from the habitat with a control of gaseous contamination from the welding arc, less attention is paid to fume extraction during grinding; as a result, very high levels of nanoparticulate dust can be generated with a mean particle diameter in the region of 22 nm. Dust collected during hyperbaric welding operations has been found to be pro-oxidant in a synthetic respiratory tract lining fluid, and at the lowest concentration tested (5 µg/mL), it had significant inflammatory properties that exceeded those of crystalline quartz and a nickel-containing welding fume.[64] These effects might be modulated by the hyperbaric environment. Raised oxygen partial pressure may amplify any oxidant stress induced by the inhalation of fume, and the toxicity of some metals may be potentiated by hydrostatic pressure.[65]

Most hyperbaric welding is done using manual metal arc welding. Tungsten inert gas welding is also used, albeit to a lesser extent, and argon is used as the shielding gas. The argon released remains in the welding habitat and can only be removed by flushing the chamber atmosphere. Argon is 10 times denser than helium and is about 50 per cent more potent as a narcotic agent than nitrogen.[66] A partial pressure of 200 kPa is considered safe, but during operational welding the argon level in the habitat is kept below 100 kPa in order to avoid narcosis and respiratory restriction. At shallow depths, lower levels are necessary in order to avoid dilutional hypoxia. Argon, however, tends to pool below the weld, and dangerously high localized levels are possible.

Saturation divers are prone to skin infections, notably by *Pseudomonas aeruginosa*.[67] The source of infection is probably seawater at the worksite and seawater used in the hot-water suit worn while working underwater. Inadequate filtration of desalinated water has been identified as a further source of contamination in the saturation diving pressure chamber complex.[68]

SUMMARY

The hyperbaric environment is complex and affects human physiology in a complex and interactive manner. It is possible, however, for humans to operate safely in this environment with an understanding of the physical and physiological limitations that it imposes. Despite this, exposure to harmful agents remains a concern, as does the management of intercurrent illness in saturation diving.

REFERENCES

● = Key primary paper
◆ = Major review article

◆1 Lindholm P, Lundgren CEG. The physiology and pathophysiology of human breath-hold diving. *J Appl Physiol* 2009; **106**: 284–92.
●2 Malhotra MS, Wright HC. The effects of a raised intrapulmonary pressure on the lungs of fresh unchilled cadavers. *J Pathol Bacteriol* 1961; **82**: 198–202.
3. Godden D, Currie G, Denison D et al. British Thoracic Society guidelines on respiratory aspects of fitness for diving. *Thorax* 2003; **58**: 3–13.
4. Wood WB. Ventilatory dynamics under hyperbaric states. In: Lambertsen CJ, Greenbaum LJ Jr (eds) *Proceedings of the 2nd Symposium of Underwater Physiology.* Publication 1181. Washington DC: National Academy of Sciences/National Research Council, 1963: 108–13.
5. Fagreus L, Linnarsson D. Maximal voluntary and exercise ventilation at high ambient air pressure. *Forsvarmedicin* 1973; **9**: 275–8.
6. Griffith DE, Holden WE, Morris JF, Min LK, Krishnamurthy GT. Effects of common therapeutic concentrations of oxygen on lung clearance of 99mTc DTPA and bronchoalveolar lavage albumin concentration. *Am Rev Resp Dis* 1986; **13**: 233–7.
7. Griffith DE, Garcia JGN, James HL, Callahan KS, Iriana S, Holiday D. Hyperoxic exposure in humans effects of 50 percent oxygen on alveolar macrophage leukotriene B4 synthesis. *Chest* 1992; **101**: 392–7.
◆8. Clark JM, Lambertsen CJ. Pulmonary oxygen toxicity: A review. *Phar Rev* 1971; **23**: 37–133.
9. Donald K. *Oxygen and the Diver.* Hanley Swan, Worcestershire: The Spa/Kenneth Donald, 1999.
10. Bitterman N. CNS oxygen toxicity. *Undersea Hyperb Med* 2004; **31**: 63–72.
11. Clark JM, Thom SR. Oxygen under pressure. In: Brubakk AO, Neuman TS (eds) *Bennett and Elliott's Physiology and Medicine of Diving.* Edinburgh: Saunders, 2003: 358–418.
12. Behnke AR, Thompson RM, Motley EP. The psychological effects from breathing air at 4 atmospheres pressure. *Am J Physiol* 1935; **112**: 554–58.
13. Adolfson J. Deterioration of mental and motor functions in hyperbaric air. *Scand J Psychol* 1965; **6**: 26–31.
●14. Case EM, Haldane JBS. Human physiology under high pressure. *J Hyg* 1941; **41**: 225–49.
15. Behnke AR, Willmon TL. Gaseous nitrogen and helium elimination from the body during rest and exercise. *Am J Physiol* 1940; **131**: 619–26.
16. Francis TJR, Mitchell SJ. Pathophysiology of decompression illness. In: Brubakk AO, Neuman TS (eds) *Bennett and Elliott's Physiology and Medicine of Diving.* Edinburgh: Saunders, 2003: 530–56.
17. Bakovic D, Glavas D, Palada I et al. High-grade bubbles in left and right heart in an asymptomatic diver at rest after surfacing. *Aviat Space Environ Med* 2008; **79**: 626–8.

●18. Wilmshurst P, Bryson P. Relationship between the clinical features of neurological decompression illness and its causes. *Clin Sci* 2000; **99**: 65–75.

19. Gempp E, Blatteau JE, Stephant E, Louge P. Relation between right-to-left shunts and spinal cord decompression sickness in divers. *Int J Sports Med* 2009; **30**: 150–3.

20. Mitchell SJ. Doolette DJ. Selective vulnerability of the inner ear to decompression sickness in divers with right-to-left shunt: The role of tissue gas supersaturation. *J Appl Physiol* 2009; **106**: 298–301.

21. Bove AA. Risk of decompression sickness with patent foramen ovale. *Undersea Hyperb Med* 1998; **25**: 175–8.

◆22. Jones JP, Neuman TS. Dysbaric osteonecrosis. In: Brubakk AO, Neuman TS (eds) *Bennett and Elliott's Physiology and Medicine of Diving*. Edinburgh: Saunders, 2003: 659–79.

23. Bennett PB. *Psychometric Impairment in Men Breathing Oxygen–Helium at Increased Pressures*. RN Personnel Research Committee, Underwater Physiology Subcommittee, Report No. 251. London: Medical Research Council, 1965.

24. Daniels S. Cellular and neurophysiological effects of high ambient pressure. In: Hope A, Risberg J (eds) *Long-term Health Effects of Diving*. Bergen: NUI AS, 2006: 229–40.

25. Abraini JH. Evidence for inert gas narcosis mechanisms in the occurrence of psychotic like episodes at pressure environment. *Neuroreport* 1995; **6**: 2435–9.

26. Brubakk AO. Deep diving in Brazil. In: Hope A, Risberg J (eds) *Long-term Health Effects of Diving*. Bergen: NUI AS, 2006: 124–34.

●27. Keays FL. Compressed air illness with a report of 3,692 cases. *Dept Med Publ Cornell Univ Med Coll* 1908; **2**: 1–55.

28. Colvin AP. *Human Factors in Decompression Sickness in Compressed Air Workers in the United Kingdom 1986–2000*. HSE Report No. 171. Sudbury: HSE Books, 2003: 3–36.

29. Kindwall EP. Compressed air tunneling and caisson work decompression procedures: Development, problems, and solutions. *Undersea Hyperb Med* 1997; **4**: 337–45.

30. McCallum RI, Harrison JAB. Dysbaric osteonecrosis: Aseptic necrosis of bone. In: Bennet PB, Elliott DH (eds) *The Physiology and Medicine of Diving*. London: WB Saunders, 1993: 563–84.

31. Vellinga TP, Sterk W, de Boer AG, van der Beek AJ, Verhoeven AC, van Dijk FJ. Doppler ultrasound surveillance in deep tunneling compressed-air work with Trimix breathing: Bounce dive technique compared to saturation-excursion technique. *Undersea Hyperb Med* 2008; **35**: 407–16.

32. Ritchie K, Baxter S, Macpherson K, Mandawa L, Macintosh H, Wilson S. *The Clinical and Cost Effectiveness of Hyperbaric Therapy*. HTA Programme Systematic Review No. 2. Edinburgh: NHS Quality Improvement Scotland, 2008.

●33. Sheffield PJ, Desautels DA. Hyperbaric and hypobaric chamber fires: A 73 year analysis. *Undersea Hyperb Med* 1997; **24**: 153–64.

34. Burman F, Sheffield R, Possey K. Decision process to assess medical equipment for hyperbaric use. *Undersea Hyperb Med* 2009; **36**: 137–44.

35. Risberg J, Englund M, Aanderud L, Eftedal O, Flook V, Thorsen E. Venous gas embolism in chamber attendants after hyperbaric exposure. *Undersea Hyperb Med* 2004; **31**: 417–29.

36. Cooper PD, Van den Brook C, Smart D. Hyperbaric chamber safety II: 14-year health review of multiplace chamber attendants. *Diving Hyperb Med* 2009; **39**: 71–87.

◆37. Epstein M. Renal effects of head out water immersion in humans: A 15 year update. *Physiol Rev* 1992; **72**: 563–621.

38. Pendergast DR, Lundgren CEG. The underwater environment: Cardiopulmonary, thermal and energetic demands. *J Appl Physiol* 2009; **106**: 276–83.

39. Sramek P, Simeckova M, Jansky L, Savlikova J, Vybiral S. Human physiological responses to immersion into water of different temperatures. *Eur J Appl Physiol* 2000; **81**: 436–42.

◆40. Moon RE, Cherry AD, Stolp BW, Camporesi EM. Pulmonary gas exchange in diving. *J Appl Physiol* 2009; **106**: 668–77.

41. Shilling CW, Werts MF, Schandelmeier NR (eds). *The Underwater Handbook*. New York: Plenum Press, 1976: 271–99.

42. Anthony G, Wright NA, Evans MA. Review of diver noise exposure. *Underwater Technol* 2010 March (in press).

43. Ross JAS, Macdiarmid JI, Dick FD, Watt SJ. Hearing symptoms and audiometry in professional divers and offshore workers. *Occup Med (Lond)* 2010; **60**: 36–42.

44. Health and Safety Executive. *Exposure Limits for Air Diving Operations*. DVIS5 C20. Sudbury: HSE Books, 1998.

45. Logan CW. *Experience and Employment Profile of North Sea Diving Personnel: Profile for the Years 2000–2003*. IMCA D 038. London: International Marine Contractors Association, 2005.

46. Medical Research Council Decompression Sickness Central Registry and Radiological Panel. Aseptic bone necrosis in commercial dives. *Lancet* 1981; **2**: 384–8.

●47. Donald K. Oxygen poisoning in man. Part 1. *Br Med J* 1947; May 17: 667–72.

●48. Donald K. Oxygen poisoning in man. Part 2. *British Medical Journal* 1947; May 24: 712–16.

49. Sterk W, Schrier LM. Effects of intermittent exposure to hyperoxia in operational diving. In: Ornhagen H (ed.) *Diving and Hyperbaric Medicine. Proceedings of the X1 Annual Scientific Meeting of the European Undersea Biomedical Society*. FOA Report C50021-HI. Stockholm: National Research Defence Institute, 1985: 123–31.

◆50. Prys-Roberts C. Hypercapnia. In: Gray TC, Nunn JF, Utting JE (eds) *General Anaesthesia*, 4th edn, Vol. 1. London: Butterworths, 1980: 435–60.

51. Lucks Mendel L, Walton JH, Hamill DW, Pelton JD. Use of speech production repair strategies to improve diver communication. *Undersea Hyperb Med* 2003; **30**: 313–20.

◆52. Flook V. Physics and physiology in the hyperbaric environment. *Clin Phys Physiol Meas* 1987; **8**: 197–230.

53. Keatinge WR, Hayward MG, McIver NKI. Hypothermia during saturation diving in the North Sea. *Br Med J* 1980; February 2: 291.

54. Mekjavic IB, Golden FStC, Eglin M, Tipton MJ. Thermal status of saturation divers during operational dives in the North Sea. *Undersea Hyperb Med* 2001; **28**: 149–55.

55. Macdiarmid JI, Ross JAS, Taylor CL *et al.* *Co-ordinated Investigation into the Possible Long Term Health Effects of Diving at Work. Examination of the Long Term Health Impact of Diving: The ELTHI Diving Study.* Research Report No. 230. Sunbury: HSE Books, 2004.

56. Ormerod AD, Dwyer CM, Goodfield MJ. Novel causes of contact dermatitis from offshore oil-based drilling muds. *Contact Derm* 1998; **39**: 262–3.

57. Ormerod AD, Wakeel RA, Mann TA, Main RA, Aldridge RD. Polyamine sensitization in offshore workers handling drilling muds. *Contact Derm* 1989; **21**: 326–9.

58. Lossius PA, Anderson PA, Holand B, Høilund AP, Nicolaysen G. *Pionerdykkerne I nordsjøen. [Pioneer divers in the North Sea.]* Oslo: Norges offentlige utredninger [Norway's Public Reports], 2003: **5.**

59. Flook V. Off-gassing of volatile hydrocarbons in hyperbaric environments. *Underwater Technol* 2009; **28**: 57–66.

60. Health and Safety Executive. *Occupational Exposure Limits for Hyperbaric Conditions: Hazard Assessment Document EH75/2.* Sudbury: HSE Books, 2000.

61. Liu J, Laster MJ, Taheri S, Eger II El, Koblin DD, Halsey MJ. Is there a cutoff in anesthetic potency for the normal alkanes? *Anesth Analg* 1993; **77**: 12–18.

62. Fang Z, Sonner J, Laster MJ *et al.* Anaesthetic and convulsant properties of aromatic compounds and cycloalkanes: Implications for mechanisms of narcosis. *Anesth Analg* 1996: **83**: 1097–104.

63. Fang Z, Ionescu P, Chortfoff BS *et al.* Anaesthetic potencies of n-alkanols: Results of additivity and solubility studies suggest a mechanism of action similar to that for conventional inhaled anesthetics. *Anesth Analg* 1997; **84**: 1042–8.

64. Ross JAS, Semple S, Duffin R, Kelly F, Feldmann J, Raab A. Characterisation of fume from hyperbaric welding operations. *J Phys* 2009: Conf Ser 151 2009 012042.

65. Syversen T, Jenssen J. High hydrostatic pressure potentiation of the toxic effects of chromate in cell culture. *Undersea Biomed Res* 1987; **14**: 11–19.

66. Behnke AR, Yarbrough OD. Respiratory resistance, oil-water solubility, and mental effects of argon compared with helium and nitrogen. *Am J Physiol* 1939; **126**: 409–15.

67. Alcock SR. Acute otitis externa in divers in the North Sea. A microbiological investigation of seven saturation dives. *J Hyg (Camb)* 1977; **78**: 395–409.

68. Ahlen C, Mandal LH, Iversen OJ. An in-field demonstration of the true relationship between skin infections and their sources in occupational diving systems in the North Sea. *Ann Occup Hyg* 2003; **47**: 227–33.

51

Air travel and altitude

YVONNE NUSSBAUMER-OCHSNER AND KONRAD E. BLOCH

OVERVIEW

Air flight and high-altitude medicine have increasingly gained general interest for a number of reasons. Globally, professional and recreational air traffic has increased enormously, and the number of passengers with pre-existing health problems has also grown. More people pursue professional work and leisure activities in mountain areas, and there are growing permanent settlements at altitudes above 2500 m. As the population ages, the proportion of people with pre-existing morbidity engaging in recreational activities (skiing, mountaineering, etc.) and air travel is also likely to rise. This chapter reviews the normal physiological adaptation to hypobaric hypoxia and the potential adverse health effects of air travel and high-altitude sojourns in healthy subjects and patients with pre-existing diseases, along with their prevention and treatment.

The atmosphere

The relative composition of the air is similar all over the world and at all altitudes. The major components are: nitrogen (78 per cent), oxygen (21 per cent) and small quantities of argon, carbon dioxide and other trace gases. The main problem humans face at altitude is the reduced barometric pressure, leading to lower inspired (Pio_2) and arterial (Pao_2) partial pressures of oxygen. When air is inhaled, it is warmed and saturated with water vapour. The partial pressure of water vapour at body temperature (37 °C) is 47 mmHg. The Pio_2 at sea level is therefore 149 mmHg, i.e. 0.21 times the barometric pressure minus the water vapour pressure, or $0.21 \times (760-47) = 149$ mmHg (Figure 51.1).

Most of the undesirable effects of high altitude are due to hypoxia. The low barometric pressure itself during a sojourn at altitude generally has no relevant consequences, but it may become important during air travel if decompression is very rapid, such as in the case of sudden loss of cabin pressure in an aeroplane cruising at high altitude.

According to Boyle's law, the pressure (P) of a given mass of gas is inversely proportional to its volume (V), or $P \times V =$ constant, at a constant temperature (i.e. 37 °C body temperature). With increasing altitude, barometric

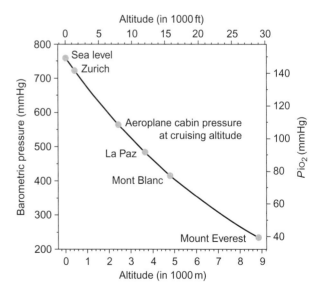

Figure 51.1 Relationship between altitude, barometric pressure and inspired partial pressure of oxygen (Pio_2) at sea level and at different locations. The cabin pressure in commercial aeroplanes at cruising altitude is around 570 mmHg, corresponding to a terrestrial altitude of 2438 m (8000 ft).

pressure falls, resulting in an enlargement of air spaces within the body such as the middle ear, the paranasal sinuses, the intestines and trapped air in poorly ventilated areas of diseased lungs.

Physiological response to reduced barometric pressure

Exposure to hypobaric hypoxia at high altitude or during air travel triggers normal physiological responses termed acclimatization, which mitigate the effects of hypoxia. Adaptation to hypoxia and altitude depends on the rate and degree of the hypoxic and hypobaric stress. For example, the effect of a sudden loss of cabin pressure on an aircraft pilot at 6500 m differs markedly from that seen in a mountaineer acclimatized for several days to the same altitude. Whereas the pilot might lose consciousness within a few minutes in addition to suffering from severe barotrauma, the healthy and physically fit mountaineer might feel perfectly well and even continue his climb to higher altitudes.

RESPIRATORY ACCLIMATIZATION

Acclimatization to altitude starts within seconds after exposure and continues over several days and weeks. One of the first and most important mechanisms of acclimatization is an increase in ventilation mediated by hypoxic stimulation of the peripheral chemoreceptors, especially in the carotid body.[1] Hyperventilation improves arterial oxygenation but may reduce the arterial partial pressure of carbon dioxide ($Paco_2$) below a critical threshold (the apnoeic threshold) so that ventilation ceases until the $Paco_2$ rises again due to metabolic activity. The

resulting crescendo–decrescendo breathing pattern of tachypnoea–hyperpnoea alternating with bradypnoea–hypopnoea and central apnoeas is called periodic breathing.

Periodic breathing at altitude most commonly occurs at rest and during sleep when cortical drives to breathe diminish. Although it disturbs sleep quality, it seems not to play an independent role in the pathogenesis of acute mountain sickness (AMS).[2] Children show less nocturnal periodic breathing at high altitude compared with adults due to a lower carbon dioxide apnoea threshold (and therefore a greater CO_2 reserve), a reduced carbon dioxide sensitivity below eupnoea and a shorter circulation time (Figure 51.2).[3] At altitude, vital capacity is reduced[4] due to impaired respiratory muscle strength,[5] while maximal expiratory air flow is less reduced because of the reduced air density. Recent studies using specialized techniques have revealed mild changes in pulmonary function in climbers ascending to high altitude suggesting premature closure of the peripheral airways and reduced diffusing capacity possibly related to subclinical interstitial fluid accumulation.[4]

CARDIOVASCULAR ACCLIMATIZATION

The normal cardiovascular response to hypoxaemia is an increase in heart rate and cardiac output to maintain adequate oxygen delivery. Hypoxia is a strong stimulus for pulmonary arterial vasoconstriction and increases pulmonary vascular resistance and pulmonary artery pressure at high altitude. The increased afterload in the pulmonary circulation can as a result strain the right ventricle. Excessive and heterogeneous hypoxic pulmonary vasoconstriction may contribute to the pathogenesis of high-altitude pulmonary oedema (HAPE).

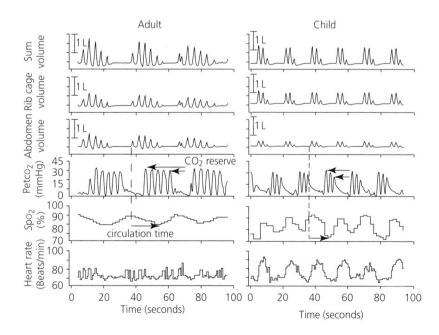

Figure 51.2 Breathing pattern recorded by inductance plethysmography in an adult man and an 11-year-old child at 3450 m (11 320 ft, bariatric pressure 497 mmHg) reveals a characteristic waxing and waning of ventilation, high-altitude periodic breathing associated with oscillations of heart rate and arterial oxygen saturation. Petco$_2$, expiratory pressure of carbon dioxide; Spo$_2$, oxygen saturation as measured by pulse oximetry. (Adapted from Kohler et al.,[3] with permission.)

ACCLIMATIZATION OF OTHER ORGAN SYSTEMS

The acclimatization to hypoxia involves nearly all organ systems, including the blood, muscles, and endocrine and renal systems. The time frame of the changes varies from seconds to a few minutes to weeks.[6]

AIR TRAVEL

More than 1 billion people throughout the world currently travel on commercial aircraft each year,[7] but few are aware that altered atmospheric conditions in an aircraft cabin might affect their well-being and health.

Changes in cabin pressure

Commercial aircraft cruise at altitudes from 10 000 ft (3048 m) up to 60 000 ft (18 288 m).[8] To avoid the adverse effects of hypobaric conditions on crew and passengers, the cabin is pressurized to a minimum of about 565 mmHg, corresponding to a terrestrial altitude of around 8000 ft (2438 m), which is adequate for healthy individuals.[9] Higher pressurization would increase financial costs since it would require a greater structural stability and weight of the aircraft, and hence higher fuel consumption. The P_{IO_2} of passengers is about 14.4 kPa (108 mmHg or 0.21 × [560−47] mmHg), i.e. 28 per cent lower than at sea level and equivalent to breathing a 15 per cent oxygen–air mixture at sea level (normobaric hypoxia), see Figure 51.3. P_{aO_2} during air travel is decreased to 7.0–8.5 kPa (53–64 mmHg), but arterial oxygen saturation decreases little (by about 4 per cent[10]) as the change in P_{aO_2} occurs at the flat portion of the oxyhaemoglobin dissociation curve. Air travel in an unpressurized cabin at altitudes greater than 10 000 ft (3048 m) requires the use of supplemental oxygen to avoid oxygen desaturation.[11]

Adverse health effects of air travel

BAROTRAUMA OF THE EAR

Incidence and pathology

Injury related to inappropriate pressure equalization is called barotrauma. Dysfunction of the Eustachian tube with inadequate middle ear ventilation is the most frequently encountered medical disorder associated with air travel, affecting about 5 per cent of adult and 25 per cent of paediatric passengers.[12,13] During aeroplane ascent, when the cabin pressure decreases, air in the middle ear decompresses passively through the Eustachian tube to the nasopharynx. On descent, cabin pressure increases, whereas pressure within the middle ear initially remains at the lower cruising pressure. To equilibrate the middle ear with the cabin pressure, passengers must periodically open their Eustachian tube by swallowing or by performing a Valsalva

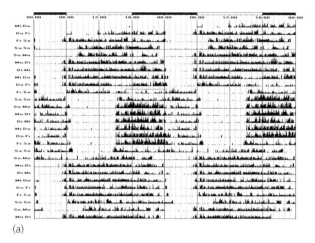

(a)

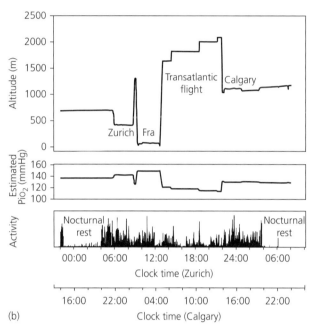

(b)

Figure 51.3 (a) Activity was continuously recorded by a wrist accelerometer along with a barometric pressure sensor in a traveller for 9 days before a trip from Zurich (Switzerland) to Calgary (Canada), during his stay in Canada, and after his return. The activity and rest periods (low activity periods correspond to sleep) are plotted on consecutive lines for each 48 h period (double plot). They reveal a clear change in the circadian rhythm associated with the change in time zone of 8 hours during the stay in Canada and vice versa after return to Zurich. (b) Barometric pressure, estimated inspiratory P_{O_2} and activity recorded during the transatlantic flight from Zurich to Calgary with a stop-over in Frankfurt (Fra). Cabin pressure was stepwise decreased during the transatlantic flight to a maximal terrestrial altitude equivalent of 2100 m.

manoeuvre. For those with concurrent nasal congestion caused by colds or allergy, or for infants and children, the task may be impossible. As the pressure differential increases, stretching of the tympanic membrane may cause pain. The feeling of a blocked ear, hearing loss and vertigo may occur due to bleeding into the tympanic membrane and rupture of the round or oval window membranes.

Management

The best measure against barotrauma is to avoid flying during periods of an upper respiratory tract infection or congested nose. If this is not feasible, nasal decongestants or antihistamines prior to flight may be used, and Valsalva manoeuvres should be repeatedly performed during descent.

ACUTE MOUNTAIN SICKNESS

At the cabin pressure of commercial aircraft, overt AMS rarely occurs, even during long-distance flights. Nevertheless, certain symptoms that are also present in AMS, such as malaise, fatigue and sleep disturbance, are common during air travel but mostly caused by uncomfortable seating, noise and other external factors rather than by hypoxia (Figure 51.4).[9]

MOTION SICKNESS

Motion sickness is triggered by stimulation of the vestibular system and proprioceptive sensors of the body during rapid movement of the aircraft in turbulence, creating conflicting neurological signals. Symptoms consist of nausea, vomiting, pallor and sweating. For passengers susceptible to motion sickness, prophylactic anticholinergic and antihistaminergic medications (scopolamine or antihistamines) are available over the counter.

VENOUS THROMBOEMBOLISM

Incidence and pathology

'Economy-class syndrome' refers to discomfort during and after long-distance flight in narrow aeroplane seats and includes an association between air travel and venous thromboembolism (VTE). However, VTE does not solely occur in economy-class passengers but is generally well known in those who sit for long periods in aeroplanes, buses and cars. The absolute risk for a symptomatic VTE within 8 weeks after a flight of over 4 hours has been estimated at 1 per 4600 passengers.[14] This corresponds to an incidence rate of 3.2 per 1000 person–years compared with 1.0 per 1000 person–years in individuals not exposed to air travel. The incidence of VTE is very low when the flight time is less than 4 hours but progressively increases with longer duration flights. Well-established factors such as clotting disorders, hormone therapy and recent surgery predispose to VTE during long-haul air travel.[15]

Management

In otherwise healthy travellers without known risk factors for VTE, there is no need for specific prophylaxis other than changing position and moving the legs from time to time, assuring appropriate fluid intake and avoiding excessive amounts of caffeine and alcohol during flight (Table 51.1). Elastic stockings seem to be effective in preventing VTE

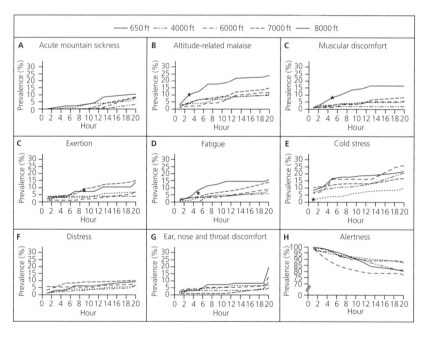

Figure 51.4   Passenger discomfort during a simulated long-distance flight at various cabin pressures (corresponding to terrestrial altitudes of 650–8000 ft) was evaluated with the Environmental Symptoms Questionnaire. The criterion of acute mountain sickness was met in 7.4 per cent of 502 passengers but was independent of cabin pressure. Arterial oxygen saturation was reduced by 4 per cent at 7000–8000 ft, and this contributed to an increased frequency of discomfort reported by passengers. Altitude-related malaise, muscular discomfort, exertion, fatigue and cold stress were significantly related to altitudes. A star on a line denotes a significant difference of a symptom at that altitude compared with all other altitudes from the time marked by the star until the end of the flight. A star between two lines denotes a significant difference of these two altitudes compared with all other altitudes from the time denoted by the star to the end of the flight. (Adapted from Muhm *et al.*, with permission.[9])

Table 51.1 Recommendations for prophylaxis in deep venous thromboembolism (VTE) during long-distance flights (duration more than 6 hours)

Risk factors	Recommendations
No known risk factors	No specific prophylactic measures
Low-to-medium risk factors*	Wearing of elastic stockings
High risk factors[†]	Low-molecular-weight heparin prophylaxis

All risk classes: changing position, moving legs from time to time, assuring appropriate fluid intake, avoiding excessive amounts of caffeine and alcohol during flight

*Age >40 years, obesity, active inflammation, recent minor surgery (within last 3 days), varicose veins, hormone therapy (including oral contraception), polycythaemia, pregnancy/postnatal, lower limb paralysis, recent lower limb trauma (within 6 weeks).

[†] Previous VTE, known coagulation disorders, severe obesity, neoplastic diseases within the previous 2 years, recent major surgery (within 6 weeks), large varicous veins, family history of VTE.
Adapted from Medical Guidelines for Airline Travel.[11]

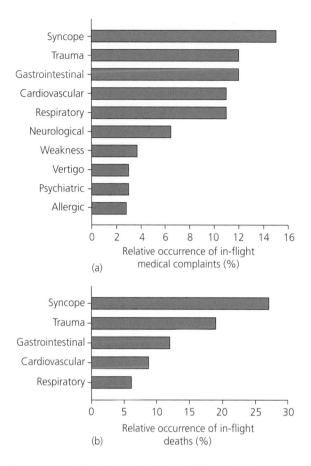

Figure 51.5 Relative distribution of in-flight medical complaints (a) and of fatal events (b) of air passengers. There were 22.6 events in 1 million passengers. Of these, 7.6 per cent required a diversion, and approximately one death occurred in 10 million passengers. (Data from Delaune et al.[25])

during long-distance flights in low-to-medium-risk subjects.[16–18] In patients with previous thrombosis and other high-risk conditions for VTE (i.e. coagulation disorders, severe obesity, limitation of mobility due to bone or joint problems, recent neoplastic disease, recent surgery and varicose veins), low-molecular-weight heparin prophylaxis is recommended before flights lasting more than 6 hours (e.g. subcutaneous enoxaparin 1000 IU/10 kg of body weight 2–4 hours before departure).[7,16] Aspirin has been recommended for VTE prophylaxis in intermediate-risk air passengers[7] but has been less effective than low-molecular-weight heparin in certain studies.[19]

INFECTIONS

Related to the relatively small volume in which passengers travel during a flight, there is a greater risk of transmitting infections. There are case reports on the person-to-person transmission of tuberculosis, influenza, measles, smallpox, cholera and enteritis.[20–22] Vectors for malaria, yellow fever and dengue have also been identified on aircraft.

INCIDENCE OF IN-FLIGHT HEALTH EVENTS

Assessing in-flight medical risk is difficult because there are no established reporting requirements.[23,24] One study revealed one in-flight medical incident per 44 212 passengers (22.6 per million passengers), or one in every 378 flights.[25] A total of 7.9 per cent of the in-flight events required a diversion, resulting in 210 diversions per million flights. Most in-flight medical events are not serious, vasovagal episodes being the most common (Figure 51.5). Death is rare, at 0.1 cases per million flight passengers.[25] Diverting an aircraft from its scheduled

destination entails high costs and challenging logistics so the Federal Aviation Administration requires all commercial aeroplanes with more than 30 seats to carry an emergency medical kit. Many airlines carry an automatic external defibrillator.

JET LAG

Incidence and physiology

Travel across time zones leads to a mismatch (asynchrony) between the activity of internal rhythm-generating systems and the local time cues ('Zeitgebers') – the so-called jet lag syndrome. Typical symptoms are daytime sleepiness and an inability to fall asleep at night (after an eastward flight) or early awakening (after a westward flight).

Management

Travellers should try to synchronize their circadian rhythm with the local time by exposing themselves to sunlight and engaging in physical activities during the daytime. To improve the symptoms of jet lag and accelerate adaptation to a new time zone during eastward travel, melatonin may be prescribed 30 minutes before the target bedtime at the destination, in a dose of 0.5 mg.[26] Melatonin is naturally released by the pineal gland in the evening and induces sleep; it is suppressed by light exposure. The use of melatonin should be considered in travellers crossing more than five time zones in whom jet lag syndrome would seriously interfere with their planned activities.

Air travel with a pre-existing medical condition

Little is known about the potential risk of flying for patients with pre-existing diseases.[7,27]

Passengers with a medical condition that could lead to problems during flight require an incapacitated passengers handling advice (INCAD) and a Medical Information Sheet (MEDIF) for the air carrier. These documents describe health status, the nature of the incapacity, any special arrangements required at the airport and/or during flight, required medications including supplemental oxygen, and the need for special seats, wheelchairs or stretchers.

AIR TRAVEL DURING PREGNANCY

In uncomplicated pregnancy, flying is not harmful to the mother and her fetus if additional risk factors are excluded. Most airlines allow pregnant women to fly up to the 35th or 36th week of gestation.[28] Air travel is not recommended during pregnancy for women who have either medical or obstetric complications. These include patients at risk of premature delivery (prior history, cervical incompetence or multiple gestations), conditions that lower placental reserve (intrauterine growth retardation) and women who are at increased risk (pre-eclampsia and placenta praevia).

As in the non-pregnant state, the decrease in cabin pressure leads to a decrease in Pao_2.[29] The $Paco_2$ remains unchanged, indicating that flying does not further augment the existing hyperventilation in pregnancy. During flight, maternal heart rate and blood pressure increase while fetal heart rate usually remains within normal limits.

AIR TRAVEL IN PATIENTS WITH RESPIRATORY DISEASE

When assessing patients with respiratory disease who are planning air travel, careful consideration must be given to their overall condition, the type and functional severity of their pulmonary disorder, the anticipated duration of the flight and their prior flight tolerance. The British Thoracic Society recommends a pre-flight assessment in patients with respiratory disease prior to air travel[7] by history and physical examination, spirometry, a 50 metre walk test and pulse oximetry. In persons with a resting sea level oxygen saturation of between 92 and 95 per cent and with additional risk factors, further evaluation is recommended (Table 51.2). Recommendations on the use of in-flight oxygen are listed in Table 51.3.

Air travel with obstructive lung disease

Chronic obstructive pulmonary disease (COPD) and asthma are both common, and many patients with these diseases are exposed to altitude during vacations or when flying. Patients with more than mild COPD and a low arterial oxygen saturation at sea level (<92 per cent) are susceptible to the unfavourable effects of altitude because of their limited ability to increase ventilation, reduced

Table 51.2   Pre-flight evaluation in patients with lung disease

Patients with following pulmonary diseases should be screened:

- Severe chronic obstructive pulmonary disease or asthma
- Severe restrictive pulmonary diseases (respiratory muscle diseases or chest wall disorders)
- Cystic fibrosis
- Hospital discharge for acute respiratory illness within the previous 6 weeks
- Recent pneumothorax
- Pulmonary tuberculosis
- Pre-existing lung disease requiring oxygen or ventilator support
- Risk or history of previous venous thromboembolism
- History of intolerance of air travel
- Co-morbidity with other conditions worsened by hypoxia (coronary artery disease or cerebrovascular disease)

Hypoxic challenge testing is recommended for patients with resting sea level oximetry between 92% and 95% and additional pulmonary risk factors. Additional pulmonary risk factors include: hypercapnia; forced expiratory volume in 1 second less than 50% predicted; lung cancer; restrictive lung disease involving the parenchyma (fibrosis), the chest wall (kyphoscoliosis) or the respiratory muscles; ventilator support; cerebrovascular or cardiac disease; discharge for an exacerbation of chronic lung or cardiac disease within the previous 6 weeks

Adapted from the British Thoracic Society Guidelines,[7] with permission.

Table 51.3   Recommendations for in-flight oxygen in patients with lung disease

Screening result	Recommendations
Sea level Spo_2 >95%	Oxygen not required
Sea level Spo_2 92–95% and no risk factors	Oxygen not required
Sea level Spo_2 92–95% and additional risk factors*	Perform hypoxic challenge testing
Sea level Spo_2 <92%	In-flight oxygen
Requires long-term supplemental oxygen at sea level	Increase flow during air travel

Spo_2, oxygen saturation as measured by pulse oximetry.
*See Table 51.2.
Adapted from the British Thoracic Society Guidelines,[7] with permission.

muscle strength, impaired gas exchange and pulmonary hypertension. Whether emphysematous bullae increase the risk of a pneumothorax due to volume expansion at reduced cabin pressure is not clear.

Management

Patients with COPD with a forced expiratory volume in 1 second less than 50 per cent of that predicted or an arterial oxygen saturation of less than 95 per cent and additional risk factors should be assessed prior to air travel to determine whether they need supplemental oxygen, by predicting the Pao_2 at cruising altitude by either hypoxic challenge or the use of prediction equations. However, the contribution of such assessment to preventing in-flight medical events has not been evaluated.[30] One prediction equation estimates Pao_2 during air travel as:

$$Pao_2alt = (0.519 \times Pao_2SL) + (11.85 \times FEV_1) - 1.76$$

where Pao_2alt is the Pao_2 at altitude and Pao_2SL is the Pao_2 at sea level.[31]

The recommended Pao_2 to be maintained during flight is 6.7–7.3 kPa.[32,33] This range is arbitrary but seems reasonable because, below these values, pulmonary artery pressure rises excessively and oxygen saturation falls more rapidly in the steep portion of the oxyhaemoglobin dissociation curve. Patients with a predicted Pao_2 of less than 7.3 kPa at altitude should travel with supplemental oxygen.

Patients with bronchial asthma should be stable before flying long distance and carry appropriate relief and maintenance medication in their hand luggage.

Air travel after thoracic surgery or pneumothorax

A pneumothorax is an absolute contraindication to air travel because of the risk of a tension pneumothorax. Guidelines of the Aerospace Medical Association state that after the successful drainage of a pneumothorax or uncomplicated thoracic surgery patients should be safe to fly after 2 or 3 weeks.[33] The British Thoracic Society recommends a 6 week delay after resolution of a pneumothorax before travel – patients with radiologically confirmed resolution should be able to fly after a 7 day wait.[7] After definitive surgical intervention, patients should be allowed to fly once they have recovered from the effects of surgery.

Air travel in chronic respiratory failure

There are no data on the potential risk of air travel in patients with chronic respiratory failure due to neuromuscular disease such as muscular dystrophy or chest wall deformity (kyphoscoliosis). Recommendations therefore rely on pre-flight evaluation by spirometry, respiratory muscle tests, arterial blood gas analysis and the judgment of an experienced clinician.

BOX 51.1: Muscular dystrophy and flying

The problem

A 24-year-old patient with Duchenne muscular dystrophy plans a trip from Switzerland to the USA (a flight duration of about 7 hours). He is tetraparetic and wheelchair dependent and requires nocturnal non-invasive positive-pressure ventilation for alveolar hypoventilation. His vital capacity is 12 per cent of that predicted, but his arterial blood gases are normal.

Potential risks

Diminished diaphragmatic strength impairs an adequate increase in ventilation in response to hypoxia: hypoxaemia and hypercapnia may occur during flight. Hypoxaemia may worsen during physical exertion, on lying flat or when sleeping.

Management

The effects of hypoxic exposure are evaluated while the patient spends 6 hours up a nearby mountain, altitude 2473 m (bariatric pressure 571 mmHg, similar to the cabin pressure in commercial aeroplanes). At predefined intervals, he breathes ambient air, uses supplemental oxygen and uses his ventilator in turn. An analysis of an activity log and pulse oximetry (Figure 51.6) suggests that supplemental oxygen at a rate of 2 L per minute will maintain appropriate oxygenation during flight. The medical officer of the airline approves the transport of the patient under a nurse's supervision. The trip is successfully completed, no adverse events occurring. Pulse oximetry during the flight confirms an oxygen saturation of more than 90 per cent at all times.

AIR TRAVEL WITH CARDIOVASCULAR DISEASE

Incidence and pathophysiology

The mild tachycardia induced by exposure to hypoxia during flight, excitement and physical exertion during travel increases myocardial oxygen demand and represents a risk of cardiac decompensation for patients with a limited cardiac reserve.[34] Although the overall incidence of cardiac in-flight complaints is relatively low, i.e. an estimated 2–10 per million passengers, cardiac events and chest pain account for a major proportion of in-flight medical complaints (11–51 per cent) and are the major cause of diversions (27 per cent) and in-flight death (6 of 7 deaths in 100.7 million passengers) (see Figure 51.5).[25] Some cardiovascular conditions thought to represent a particular risk for complications during flight are listed in Table 51.4. Affected patients should refrain from commercial flight.[33,35]

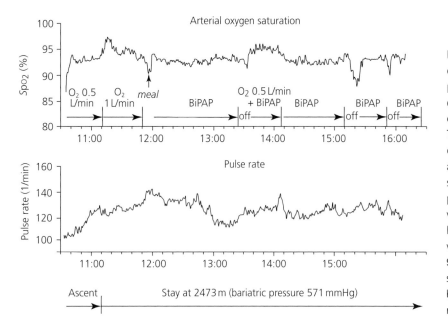

Figure 51.6 Time course of arterial oxygen saturation and pulse rate in a patient with Duchenne muscular dystrophy during a stay up a mountain to simulate conditions during a long-distance flight. The barometric pressure was similar to that encountered in an aeroplane at cruising altitude (571 mmHg). The patient spent some time on nasal oxygen and on bi-level positive airway pressure (BiPAP) mask ventilation with a portable ventilator. During periods without oxygen or assisted ventilation, the oxygen saturation fell below 90 per cent. Note the oscillations of oxygen saturation and pulse rate due to periodic breathing. SpO_2, oxygen saturation as measured by pulse oximetry.

Management

Patients with recent myocardial infarction should not fly until they are in stable condition and able to perform their usual physical activities. Patients should not fly until at least 2–3 weeks after an uncomplicated myocardial infarction.[33,36] Exercise testing may help to identify myocardial ischaemia. Patients should carry their medication in their hand luggage. The physician should provide the patient with a complete list of medication and a medical report including a copy of a recent electrocardiogram and a pacemaker card if applicable. The use of supplemental oxygen is advisable in patients with cardiac failure if the PaO_2 is less than 70 mmHg (9.3 kPa) and if there is pulmonary hypertension.

TRAVEL TO HIGH ALTITUDE

Whereas high mountain areas had previously been accessible only to healthy and well-trained mountaineers, the construction of roads, trains and cable cars has made these regions easily accessible even to those unaware of the potential hazards of a high-altitude sojourn. This has led to an increase in the prevalence and variety of high-altitude-related health problems.

High-altitude-related illness

ACUTE MOUNTAIN SICKNESS AND HIGH-ALTITUDE CEREBRAL OEDEMA

Incidence and diagnosis

Acute mountain sickness is the most common altitude-related illness. It occurs in both genders and at all ages, the

---

BOX 51.2: Flying with cardiovascular disease

The problem

A 69-year-old man, on treatment for hypertension, booked a flight of 8 hours' duration to a holiday destination. One week before his scheduled departure, he consulted his physician because of occasional left-sided chest pain on exertion for 4 weeks. His blood pressure was 185/105 mmHg.

Potential risks

There was uncontrolled hypertension and possible coronary artery disease with recent-onset angina. The patient was at risk of suffering from potentially serious myocardial ischaemia if exposed to the stress of travel and mild hypoxaemia during flight.

Management

The patient was advised to cancel his flight and postpone his vacation until further evaluation of the chest pain was complete and optimal treatment established. The physician confirmed that the patient was medically unfit to fly, and the patient's travel insurer reimbursed expenses related to cancellation of the travel arrangements.

---

incidence depending on the ascent rate and the altitude reached. The incidence of AMS is 9–40 per cent at altitudes up to 3000 m and increases up to 68 per cent above 4000 m.[37,38]

Acute mountain sickness is a non-specific syndrome consisting of headache, gastrointestinal symptoms (anorexia, nausea and vomiting), insomnia, fatigue and

Table 51.4 Cardiovascular conditions that are contraindications to commercial air flight

Uncomplicated myocardial infarction within 2–3 weeks
Complicated myocardial infarction within 6 weeks
Unstable angina
Severe, decompensated congestive heart failure
Uncontrolled hypertension
Coronary artery bypass graft within 10–14 days
Cerebrovascular accident within 2 weeks
Uncontrolled arrhythmia
Eisenmenger's syndrome
Severe, symptomatic valvular heart disease

Adapted from Medical Guidelines for Air Travel,[33] with permission.

dizziness in an unacclimatized person who has recently arrived at an altitude above 2500 m. The Lake Louise Consensus Group requires headache as the cardinal symptom along with at least one other symptom occurring in the setting of acute altitude exposure to make the diagnosis of AMS (Table 51.5). Symptoms are quantified either using the Lake Louise score or the Environmental Symptoms Questionnaire cerebral score (AMS-c score). In severe AMS, subjects are no longer able to pursue their usual activities. There is no physiological measurement that predicts individual susceptibility.

Symptoms of AMS occur within 6–12 hours after ascent to high altitude and generally improve without treatment within 24–48 hours. Acute mountain sickness can progress to life-threatening high-altitude cerebral oedema. This is characterized by ataxia, altered consciousness, somnolence and bizarre behaviour, and can progress to coma and death due to brain herniation.

Pathophysiology

The exact pathophysiological mechanisms leading to AMS/high-altitude cerebral oedema are not understood, but the primary trigger is hypobaric hypoxia, which induces various neurohumoral and haemodynamic responses. Patients with a low hypoxic ventilatory drive are more likely to suffer from AMS.[39,40] Fluid maldistribution due to an oversecretion of aldosterone and antidiuretic hormone, as observed in unacclimatized travellers at high altitude, may lead to an increase in cerebral blood flow.[41] Due to impaired hypoxic autoregulation, increased blood flow results in augmented capillary pressure, causing fluid leakage into the brain.[38]

Prevention

Prevention consists of graded ascent and sufficient time for acclimatization. Once an altitude of 3000 m has been reached, an ascent rate not exceeding 300 m per 24 hours has been suggested, albeit on limited scientific evidence. One randomized controlled trial at extreme altitude (7545 m at Muztagh Ata, China) demonstrated that a few

more days of acclimatization will contribute to a lower incidence of AMS and a greater success of reaching the top without AMS.[42] Some mountaineers believe that the recommended ascent rate is too slow and that a faster ascent is feasible as long as the sleeping altitude is kept low.

In special situations, pharmacological prophylaxis is warranted. Acetazolamide (Diamox) is the preferred drug, taken in a dose of 125–250 mg twice daily starting the day before ascent.[43] Acetazolamide is a carbonic anhydrase inhibitor that causes bicarbonate diuresis and acidifies the blood, thereby stimulating ventilation and improving oxygenation. Dexamethasone in a dose of 4 mg given every 12 hours is also an effective AMS prophylaxis, potentially superior to acetazolamide.[44–46] A combination of the two may be more effective than either drug alone.[47]

Treatment

Descent and oxygen are generally advisable treatments for any altitude-related illness, but descent is not always possible and oxygen may be impractical to carry. Depending on the severity of the AMS, a stepwise procedure is recommended: mild forms of AMS respond well to analgesics (e.g. non-steroidal anti-inflammatory drugs). If symptoms cannot be controlled, standard medication is acetazolamide. This decreases periodic breathing, restores sleep quality and may reduce excessive pulmonary arterial pressure at high altitude. The dose of acetazolamide is 250 mg twice daily.[43] Side-effects include paraesthesia, polyuria and altered taste.

In severe AMS and in high-altitude cerebral oedema, dexamethasone is life-saving, especially in combination with acetazolamide. In cases of high-altitude cerebral oedema, dexamethasone is given in a dose of 8 mg initially (intravenously or orally), followed by 4 mg every 6 hours.[48,49] Supplemental oxygen if available and immediate descent are essential.

HIGH-ALTITUDE PULMONARY OEDEMA

Pathophysiology and diagnosis

High-altitude pulmonary oedema is a non-cardiogenic and, initially, non-inflammatory high-permeability pulmonary oedema. Hypoxia induces unevenly distributed pulmonary vasoconstriction and pulmonary hypertension. The overperfusion of lung areas not protected by hypoxic vasoconstriction leads to capillary stress with fluid leakage into the interstitium and alveoli.[50] Decreased function of the sodium channel on the alveolar epithelial cells and of the Na/K-ATPase pumps that maintain alveolar fluid clearance further promotes HAPE.[51,52]

HAPE affects previously healthy individuals. Individual susceptibility, physical exertion and a fast ascent rate are predisposing factors.[53] HAPE is rare below 3500 m but occurs in about 2–4 per cent of mountaineers at 4559 m within 2–5 days of ascent.[54] The clinical picture consists of dyspnoea with minimal activity, decreased exercise

Table 51.5 Lake Louise Acute Mountain Sickness (AMS) Scoring System

A Self-report questionnaire

Symptom		Scoring
1	Headache	0 No headache 1 Mild headache 2 Moderate headache 3 Severe headache, incapacitating
2	Gastrointestinal symptoms	0 No gastrointestinal symptoms 1 Poor appetite or nausea 2 Moderate nausea or vomiting 3 Severe nausea and vomiting, incapacitating
3	Fatigue and/or weakness	0 Not tired or weak 1 Mild fatigue or weakness 2 Moderate fatigue or weakness 3 Severe fatigue or weakness, incapacitating
4	Dizziness or lightheadedness	0 Not dizzy 1 Mild dizziness 2 Moderate dizziness 3 Severe dizziness, incapacitating
5	Difficulty sleeping	0 Slept as well as usual 1 Did not sleep as well as usual 2 Woke many times, poor night's sleep 3 Could not sleep at all

B Clinical assessment

Sign		Scoring
6	Changed mental status	0 No change in mental status 1 Lethargy or lassitude 2 Disorientated or confused 3 Stupor or semi-consciousness 4 Coma
7	Ataxia (heel-to-toe walking)	0 No ataxia 1 Manoeuvres to maintain balance 2 Steps off line 3 Falls down 4 Cannot stand
8	Peripheral oedema	0 No peripheral oedema 1 Peripheral oedema at one location 2 Peripheral oedema at two or more locations

C Functional score

9	Overall, if you had any symptoms, how did they affect your activity?	0 No reduction in activity 1 Mild reduction in activity 2 Moderate reduction in activity 3 Severe reduction in activity (e.g. bed rest)

The Lake Louise AMS Scoring System tries to quantify the severity of disease by scoring typical symptoms of AMS. The sum of the responses to questions 1–5 is calculated and a score >3 points on the AMS Self-reported Questionnaire in the presence of headache – while at an altitude over 2500 m – constitutes AMS. If the results of the Self-reported Questionnaire and the clinical assessment are summed, the criterion for AMS is >4 points.

tolerance, cough and chest tightness with tachypnoea, tachycardia, crackles on auscultation, cyanosis and a mildly elevated body temperature.[55] HAPE typically develops during the night as hypoxia-induced hyperventilation is less pronounced during sleep.

Prevention

The main measure to prevent HAPE is a slow ascent. In patients with a history of HAPE, 20 mg slow-release nifedipine every 8 hours can prevent HAPE.[56] Dexamethasone and phosphodiesterase-5 inhibitors such as sildenafil or tadalafil can also lower pulmonary artery pressure and prevent HAPE.[57,58]

Treatment

Definitive treatment consists of descent and oxygen where available. Oxygen relieves hypoxia and reduces pulmonary artery pressure.[56] While waiting for evacuation, nifedipine 10–20 mg, depending on blood pressure, can be given to lower the pulmonary artery pressure.[59] Whether other pulmonary vasodilators such as sildenafil are useful in the treatment of HAPE requires further study.[60] If descent is impossible and oxygen not available, a portable inflatable hyperbaric bag may be life-saving. Concomitant AMS or high-altitude cerebral oedema requires dexamethasone. Diuretics have no place in the treatment of HAPE as mountaineers are often volume depleted and diuretics risk further volume depletion and possible thromboembolism due to haemoconcentration.[56]

COLD INJURIES – HYPOTHERMIA AND FROSTBITE

Life-threatening deep hypothermia with coma and cardiac arrest is potentially reversible under cardiac resuscitation and sufficient core rewarming.

Local frostbite is not life-threatening but has often mutilating effects potentially requiring amputation. Protection by wearing adequate clothing is usually effective, but cold can become a serious problem when unexpected cold exposure occurs. When tissue freezes, frostbite occurs, typically affecting the fingers, toes, nose and ear tips. The extremity first becomes numb, appearing pale but soft to touch. Once tissue freezes, the skin appears waxy white and is hard on touch.

On-site care involves the removal of non-adherent wet clothing, but rubbing affected areas worsens tissue damage. Rapid rewarming in warm water at 40–42 °C for 15–30 minutes is mandatory and may minimize tissue loss.[61] After rewarming, the difference between superficial and deep frostbite can be established:[62] superficial frostbite affects the skin and subcutaneous tissues; deep frostbite also affects the bones, joints and tendons. After rewarming in superficial frostbite, clear blisters form, whereas with deep frostbite the skin shows haemorrhagic blisters. Favourable prognostic factors include retained

sensation, normal skin colour and clear fluid in the blisters. A four-level classification scheme for severity of frostbite injuries was proposed by Cauchy et al. based on the presentation of the initial lesions, a bone scan and the blister presentation.[63] The classification predicts prognosis and helps in guiding the timing and need for amputation.

CHRONIC MOUNTAIN SICKNESS AND HIGH-ALTITUDE PULMONARY HYPERTENSION

Chronic mountain sickness (CMS) occurs in natives or long-time residents living at an altitude above 2500 m, typically in the Andes, North America and to a lesser extent the Himalayas and Tibet. Chronic hypoxia leads to erythrocytosis (haemoglobin concentration $\geq$19 g/dL for females and $\geq$21 g/dL for males[64]) due to stimulated erythropoietin secretion and pulmonary arterial hypertension, which may lead to right heart failure. The mechanisms leading to CMS are not fully understood. Compared with those without CMS, residents with CMS have a blunted hypoxic ventilatory response and more pronounced hypoventilation during sleep, with lower oxygen saturations.

Symptoms consist of headache, dizziness, fatigue, dyspnoea, cough and exercise intolerance that improves on descent to low altitude. In high-altitude pulmonary hypertension, dyspnoea, cough and exercise intolerance appear.

High-altitude travel in patients with pre-existing disease

HIGH-ALTITUDE TRAVEL WITH OBSTRUCTIVE LUNG DISEASE

Asthma

In an evaluation of 5835 adventure travellers, 3.5 per cent reported having asthma, 2.5 per cent were climbing to high altitude, and a considerable proportion had serious exacerbations during travel, in some cases life-threatening (Figure 51.7).[65] The risk of an asthma attack during travel was increased in subjects with uncontrolled asthma before departure, longer travelling periods and a high level of physical activity. Exacerbations occur despite the known improvement in bronchial hyperresponsiveness at altitude.[66,67]

Management

Travellers should continue their usual medication for asthma control and be instructed in the use of rescue medication. The nose and mouth should be protected adequately against wind and cold, and strenuous exercise should be avoided. Patients with poorly controlled and severe asthma should be cautioned against travelling to high altitude.

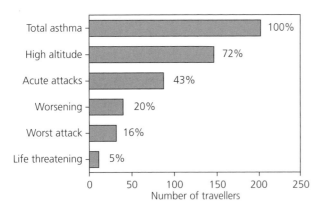

Figure 51.7 In an evaluation of 5835 adventure travellers, 3.5% declared suffering from asthma. Of these 225 travellers (100%) nearly 3 out of 4 (72%) were climbing to high altitude and a considerable proportion had serious exacerbations with acute attacks during travel that were the worst they had ever experienced and were even life threatening in some (data from [65]).

Chronic obstructive pulmonary disease

In patients with moderate-to-severe COPD, exercise capacity may be limited at altitude due to their inability to increase ventilation appropriately in response to a reduced partial pressure of oxygen and because of impaired diffusion and pulmonary hypertension. Studies on altitude tolerance in COPD are scant, and recommendations are therefore based on common sense and expert opinion. The effect of an altitude exposure and the need for supplemental oxygen may be evaluated as described above for pre-flight assessment. If hypoxaemia is already present at low altitude, supplemental oxygen should be used at an adjusted flow rate during altitude travel to maintain an arterial oxygen saturation of over 90 per cent. Patients should continue their regular medication and carry rescue medication for exacerbations.

HIGH-ALTITUDE TRAVEL WITH RESTRICTIVE LUNG DISEASE

Patients with restrictive lung disease may become more hypoxaemic at altitude, particularly if their diffusing capacity is impaired, as in interstitial lung disease. Advice as for COPD should be based on baseline physiology. Administration of supplemental oxygen might be required,[68] and rescue medication including an antibiotic in case of a respiratory infection should be readily available.

HIGH-ALTITUDE SOJOURN WITH OBSTRUCTIVE SLEEP APNOEA SYNDROME

Case reports of obstructive sleep apnoea (OSA) suggest that sleep-related breathing disturbances may switch from obstructive to central sleep apnoea at altitude. In a

---

BOX 51.3: Altitude sojourn in chronic obstructive pulmonary disease (COPD)

The problem

A 75-year-old patient with severe COPD lives at an altitude of 490 m and uses long-term oxygen therapy at a rate of 2 L per minute. He plans to spend a weekend in a mountain resort at 1650 m. He asks for advice on potential hazards and necessary precautions.

Potential risks

Estimated barometric pressure at 1650 m is 623 mmHg (see Figure 51.1), inspired partial pressure of oxygen (Pio_2) is therefore $(623 - 47) \times 0.21 = 121$ mmHg, i.e. 14 per cent lower than the corresponding value of 140 mmHg at 490 m. The physical stress of travel and the reduced Pio_2 at altitude expose the patient to a risk of significant oxygen desaturation and excessive pulmonary hypertension, severe breathlessness and limited exercise capacity.

Management

The patient's history reveals well-controlled hypertension, and he is in good general condition. Spirometry shows a vital capacity of 80 per cent predicted and a forced expiratory volume in 1 second that is 41 per cent of that predicted. Arterial blood gas analysis on room air shows: pH 7.42, $Paco_2$ 4.3 kPa, Pao_2 7.1 kPa and an arterial oxygen saturation of 90 per cent. The patient is able to climb a flight of stairs with only moderate dyspnoea. He is counselled to use liquid oxygen at the rate of 3 L per minute during travel and his stay at altitude, and to order replacement liquid oxygen from the local provider at the mountain resort. He is also advised to abstain from smoking, to carry and use his inhalers as usual and to carry prednisolone and antibiotics for any exacerbation of his COPD.

---

randomized controlled cross-over study, OSA patients living below 500 m showed pronounced reductions in arterial oxygen saturation due predominantly to frequent central apnoeas in addition to obstructive apnoeas during the night after ascent to altitudes of 1860 and 2590 m.[69] The daytime vigilance of these patients was reduced at 2590 m compared with low altitude (490 m). Which treatment for OSA at altitude is most effective – continuous positive airway pressure, acetazolamide as for high-altitude periodic breathing[70] or both combined – is currently not known. At present, the advice is to continue with continuous positive airway pressure if travelling to altitude.

HIGH-ALTITUDE TRAVEL WITH CARDIOVASCULAR DISEASE

The recommendations for patients with cardiovascular disease regarding travel at altitude correspond to those for air travel. Patients with recent myocardial infarction or severe congestive heart failure should not travel to high altitude. If these travellers have no choice, apart from maintaining their usual medication, supplemental oxygen should be considered and strenuous exercise avoided.

CONCLUSION

Subjects visiting high altitude and undertaking air travel are both exposed to hypobaric hypoxia. Depending on the duration and extent of hypoxic exposure, the body may adapt considerably to the altered environmental conditions, largely by increasing ventilation and heart rate. During prolonged flights and altitude sojourns, additional acclimatization mechanisms take place. However, in patients with pre-existing medical conditions, the limited capacity for physiological adaptation may expose them to the risk of suffering from the symptoms and complications of altitude exposure and air travel. A careful pre-travel evaluation and preparations to ensure medical care during travel will help to reduce unfavourable consequences.

REFERENCES

● = Key primary paper
◆ = Major review article

1. Weir EK, Lopez-Barneo J, Buckler KJ, Archer SL. Acute oxygen-sensing mechanisms. *N Engl J Med* 2005; **353**: 2042–55.
2. Erba P, Anastasi S, Senn O, Maggiorirni M, Bloch KE. Acute mountain sickness is related to nocturnal hypoxemia but not to hypoventilation. *Eur Respir J* 2004; **24**: 303–8.
3. Kohler M, Kriemler S, Handke E, Brunner-Larocca H, Zehnder M, Bloch KE. Children at high altitude have less nocturnal periodic breathing than adults. *Eur Respir J* 2008; **32**: 189–97.
4. Senn O, Clarenbach CF, Fischler M *et al*. Do changes in lung function predict high-altitude pulmonary edema at an early stage? *Med Sci Sports Exerc* 2006; **38**: 1565–70.
5. Deboeck G, Moraine JJ, Naeije R. Respiratory muscle strength may explain hypoxia-induced decrease in vital capacity. *Med Sci Sports Exerc* 2005; **37**: 754–8.
◆6. Ward MP, Milledge JS, West JB. *High Altitude Medicine and Physiology*, 3rd edn. London: Arnold, 2000.
●7. British Thoracic Society Standards of Care Committee. Managing passengers with respiratory disease planning air travel: British Thoracic Society recommendations. *Thorax* 2002; **57**: 289–304.
8. Cottreli JJ. Altitude exposures during aircraft flight. Flying higher. *Chest* 1988; **93**: 81–4.
9. Muhm JM, Rock PB, McMullin DL *et al*. Effect of aircraft-cabin altitude on passenger discomfort. *N Engl J Med* 2007; **357**: 18–27.
10. Schacke G, Scutaru C, Groneberg DA. Effect of aircraft-cabin altitude on passenger discomfort. *N Engl J Med* 2007; **357**: 1445–6.
●11. Aerospace Medical Association Medical Guidelines. Task Force Medical Guidelines for Airline Travel, 2nd edn. *Aviat Space Environ Med* 2003; **74**(5 Suppl.): A1–19.
12. Brown TP. Middle ear symptoms while flying. Ways to prevent a severe outcome. *Postgrad Med J* 1994; **96**: 135–7, 141–2.
13. Stangerup SE, Tjernstrom O, Harcourt J, Klokker M, Stokholm J. Barotitis in children after aviation; prevalence and treatment with Otovent. *J Laryngol Otol* 1996; **110**: 625–8.
14. Kuipers S, Cannegieter SC, Middeldorp S, Robyn L, Buller HR, Rosendaal FR. The absolute risk of venous thrombosis after air travel: a cohort study of 8,755 employees of international organisations. *PLoS Med* 2007; **4**: e290.
15. Schwarz T, Siegert G, Oettler W *et al*. Venous thrombosis after long-haul flights. *Arch Intern Med* 2003; **163**: 2759–64.
16. Cesarone MR, Belcaro G, Nicolaides AN *et al*. Venous thrombosis from air travel: the LONFLIT3 study – prevention with aspirin vs low-molecular-weight heparin (LMWH) in high-risk subjects: a randomized trial. *Angiology* 2002; **53**: 1–6.
17. Belcaro G, Geroulakos G, Nicolaides AN, Myers KA, Winford M. Venous thromboembolism from air travel: the LONFLIT study. *Angiology* 2001; **52**: 369–74.
18. Philbrick JT, Shumate R, Siadaty MS, Becker DM. Air travel and venous thromboembolism: a systematic review. *J Gen Intern Med* 2007; **22**: 107–14.
19. Cesarone MR, Belcaro G, Nicolaides AN *et al*. Venous thrombosis from air travel: the LONFLIT3 study – prevention with aspirin vs low-molecular-weight heparin (LMWH) in high-risk subjects: a randomized trial. *Angiology* 2002; **53**: 1–6.
20. Centers for Disease Control and Prevention. Exposure of passengers and flight crew to *Mycobacterium tuberculosis* on commercial aircraft, 1992–1995. *Morb Mortal Wkly Rep* 1995; **44**: 137–40.
21. Moser MR, Bender TR, Margolis HS, Noble GR, Kendal AP, Ritter DG. An outbreak of influenza aboard a commercial airliner. *Am J Epidemiol* 1979; **110**: 1–6.
22. Amler RW, Bloch AB, Orenstein WA, Bart KJ, Turner PM Jr, Hinman AR. Imported measles in the United States. *JAMA* 1982; **248**: 2129–33.
23. Speizer C, Rennie CJ III, Breton H. Prevalence of in-flight medical emergencies on commercial airlines. *Ann Emerg Med* 1989; **18**: 26–9.
24. Cummins RO, Schubach JA. Frequency and types of medical emergencies among commercial air travelers. *JAMA* 1989; **261**: 1295–9.

25. Delaune EF III, Lucas RH, Illig P. In-flight medical events and aircraft diversions: one airline's experience. *Aviat Space Environ Med* 2003; **74**: 62–8.

26. Sack RL, Auckley D, Auger RR et al. Circadian rhythm sleep disorders. Part I: Basic principles, shift work and jet lag disorders. An American Academy of Sleep Medicine review. *Sleep* 2007; **30**: 1460–83.

●27. Luks AM, Swenson ER. Travel to high altitude with pre-existing lung disease. *Eur Respir J* 2007; **29**: 770–92.

28. American College of Obstetricians and Gynecologists, Committee on Obstetric Practice. ACOG committee opinion. Air travel during pregnancy. *Int J Gynaecol Obstet* 2002; **76**: 338–9.

29. Huch R, Baumann H, Fallenstein F, Schneider KT, Holdener F, Huch A. Physiologic changes in pregnant women and their fetuses during jet air travel. *Am J Obstet Gynecol* 1986; **154**: 996–1000.

30. Martin SE, Bradley JM, Buick JB, Bradbury I, Elborn JS. Flight assessment in patients with respiratory disease: Hypoxic challenge testing vs. predictive equations. *QJM* 2007; **100**: 361–7.

31. Dillard TA, Berg BW, Rajagopal KR, Dooley JW, Mehm WJ. Hypoxemia during air travel in patients with chronic obstructive pulmonary disease. *Ann Intern Med* 1989; **111**: 362–7.

32. Celli BR, MacNee W; committee members. Standards for the diagnosis and treatment of patients with COPD: a summary of the ATS/ERS position paper. *Eur Respir J* 2004; **23**: 932–46.

●33. Medical Guidelines for Air Travel. Aerospace Medical Association, Air Transport Medicine Committee, Alexandria, Va. *Aviat Space Environ Med* 1996; **67**(10 Suppl.): B1–16.

34. Gullette EC, Blumenthal JA, Babyak M et al. Effects of mental stress on myocardial ischemia during daily life. *JAMA* 1997; **277**: 1521–6.

35. Possick SE, Barry M. Evaluation and management of the cardiovascular patient embarking on air travel. *Ann Intern Med* 2004; **141**: 148–54.

●36. Gendreau MA, DeJohn C. Responding to medical events during commercial airline flights. *N Engl J Med* 2002; **346**: 1067–73.

37. Maggiorini M, Muller A, Hofstetter D, Bartsch P, Oelz O. Assessment of acute mountain sickness by different score protocols in the Swiss Alps. *Aviat Space Environ Med* 1998; **69**: 1186–92.

38. Basnyat B, Subedi D, Sleggs J et al. Disoriented and ataxic pilgrims: an epidemiological study of acute mountain sickness and high-altitude cerebral edema at a sacred lake at 4300 m in the Nepal Himalayas. *Wilderness Environ Med* 2000; **11**: 89–93.

39. Moore LG, Harrison GL, McCullough RE et al. Low acute hypoxic ventilatory response and hypoxic depression in acute altitude sickness. *J Appl Physiol* 1986; **60**: 1407–12.

40. Hackett PH, Rennie D. Rales, peripheral edema, retinal hemorrhage and acute mountain sickness. *Am J Med* 1979; **67**: 214–18.

41. Bartsch P, Maggiorini M, Schobersberger W et al. Enhanced exercise-induced rise of aldosterone and vasopressin preceding mountain sickness. *J Appl Physiol* 1991; **71**: 136–43.

42. Bloch KE. Effect of ascent protocol on acute mountain sickness and success at Muztagh Ata. *High Alt Med Biol* 2009; **10**: 25–32.

43. Grissom CK, Roach RC, Sarnquist FH, Hackett PH. Acetazolamide in the treatment of acute mountain sickness: clinical efficacy and effect on gas exchange. *Ann Intern Med* 1992; **116**: 461–5.

44. Johnson TS, Rock PB, Fulco CS, Trad LA, Spark RF, Maher JT. Prevention of acute mountain sickness by dexamethasone. *N Engl J Med* 1984; **310**: 683–86.

45. Ellsworth AJ, Meyer EF, Larson EB. Acetazolamide or dexamethasone use versus placebo to prevent acute mountain sickness on Mount Rainier. *West J Med* 1991; **154**: 289–93.

46. Rock PB, Johnson TS, Larsen RF, Fulco CS, Trad LA, Cymerman A. Dexamethasone as prophylaxis for acute mountain sickness. Effect of dose level. *Chest* 1989; **95**: 568–73.

47. Bernhard WN, Schalick LM, Delaney PA, Bernhard TM, Barnas GM. Acetazolamide plus low-dose dexamethasone is better than acetazolamide alone to ameliorate symptoms of acute mountain sickness. *Aviat Space Environ Med* 1998; **69**: 883–6.

48. Ferrazzini G, Maggiorini M, Kriemler S, Bartsch P, Oelz O. Successful treatment of acute mountain sickness with dexamethasone. *Br Med J (Clin Res Ed)* 1987; **294**: 1380–2.

49. Hackett PH, Roach RC, Wood RA et al. Dexamethasone for prevention and treatment of acute mountain sickness. *Aviat Space Environ Med* 1988; **59**: 950–4.

50. Hultgren HN. High-altitude pulmonary edema: current concepts. *Annu Rev Med* 1996; **47**: 267–84.

51. Sartori C, Allemann Y, Duplain H et al. Salmeterol for the prevention of high-altitude pulmonary edema. *N Engl J Med* 2002; **346**: 1631–6.

52. Hummler E, Barker P, Gatzy J et al. Early death due to defective neonatal lung liquid clearance in alpha-ENaC-deficient mice. *Nat Genet* 1996; **12**: 325–8.

53. Bartsch P, Maggiorini M, Ritter M, Noti C, Vock P, Oelz O. Prevention of high-altitude pulmonary edema by nifedipine. *N Engl J Med* 1991; **325**: 1284–9.

54. Bartsch P, Mairbaurl H, Maggiorini M, Swenson ER. Physiological aspects of high-altitude pulmonary edema. *J Appl Physiol* 2005; **98**: 1101–10.

55. Maggiorini M, Bartsch P, Oelz O. Association between raised body temperature and acute mountain sickness: Cross sectional study. *BMJ* 1997; **315**: 403–4.

56. Oelz O, Maggiorini M, Ritter M et al. Nifedipine for high altitude pulmonary oedema. *Lancet* 1989; **2**: 1241–4.

57. Maggiorini M, Brunner-La Rocca HP, Peth S et al. Both tadalafil and dexamethasone may reduce the incidence of high-altitude pulmonary edema: a randomized trial. *Ann Intern Med* 2006; **145**: 497–506.

58. Anand IS, Prasad BA, Chugh SS *et al.* Effects of inhaled nitric oxide and oxygen in high-altitude pulmonary edema. *Circulation* 1998; **98**: 2441–5.

59. Hackett PH, Roach RC, Hartig GS, Greene ER, Levine BD. The effect of vasodilators on pulmonary hemodynamics in high altitude pulmonary edema: a comparison. *Int J Sports Med* 1992; **13**(Suppl. 1): S68–71.

60. Zhao L, Mason NA, Morrell NW *et al.* Sildenafil inhibits hypoxia-induced pulmonary hypertension. *Circulation* 2001; **104**: 424–8.

61. Britt LD, Dascombe WH, Rodriguez A. New horizons in management of hypothermia and frostbite injury. *Surg Clin North Am* 1991; **71**: 345–70.

62. Vogel JE, Dellon AL. Frostbite injuries of the hand. *Clin Plast Surg* 1989; **16**: 565–76.

63. Cauchy E, Chetaille E, Marchand V, Marsigny B. Retrospective study of 70 cases of severe frostbite lesions: a proposed new classification scheme. *Wilderness Environ Med* 2001; **12**: 248–55.

64. Leon-Velarde F, Maggiorini M, Reeves JT *et al.* Consensus statement on chronic and subacute high altitude diseases. *High Alt Med Biol* 2005; **6**: 147–57.

65. Golan Y, Onn A, Villa Y *et al.* Asthma in adventure travelers: a prospective study evaluating the occurrence and risk factors for acute exacerbations. *Arch Intern Med* 2002; **162**: 2421–6.

66. Spieksma FT, Zuidema P, Leupen MJ. High altitude and house-dust mites. *Br Med J* 1971; **1**: 82–4.

67. Vervloet D, Penaud A, Razzouk H *et al.* Altitude and house dust mites. *J Allergy Clin Immunol* 1982; **69**: 290–6.

68. Seccombe LM, Kelly PT, Wong CK, Rogers PG, Lim S, Peters MJ. Effect of simulated commercial flight on oxygenation in patients with interstitial lung disease and chronic obstructive pulmonary disease. *Thorax* 2004; **59**: 966–70.

69. Nussbaumer Y, Schuepfer N, Ulrich S, Bloch KE. Exacerbation of sleep apnoea due to frequent central events in patients with the obstructive sleep apnoea syndrome at altitude. A randomized trial. *Thorax* 2010 (in press).

70. Fischer R, Lang SM, Leitl M, Thiere M, Steiner U, Huber RM. Theophylline and acetazolamide reduce sleep-disordered breathing at high altitude. *Eur Respir J* 2004; **23**: 47–52.

SECTION J

Land

52

Contaminated land and health

ANDREW KIBBLE, DAVID RUSSELL

Formed at the interface between the atmosphere and the earth's crust, soil is a complicated and variable medium made up of a complex of mineral and organic solids, aqueous and gaseous voids and a considerable microbial biomass. Soil is inherently heterogeneous because of the wide range of rock types and other environmental factors that influence soil formation (climate, cover, time, etc.). All soils contain humus, the polymerized organic matter formed by the decomposition of dead vegetation. This normally makes up between 0.1 per cent and 1 per cent of the soil but can be as much as 70 per cent in peaty soils. Soils also contain variable quantities of primary minerals from the parent material or from ice or waterborne deposits, together with secondary minerals such as hydrated metallic oxides. The latter with humus forms the colloidal fraction that can give soil a sorptive property, which is important in understanding pollutant fate and behaviour.

Soil is integral to human well-being. Many essential nutrients and trace elements are obtained principally through our diet, and the main source of these elements is often from soil and underlying rock material.[1] It is well established that low concentrations or the unavailability of trace elements in soil can result in dietary deficiencies. For example, serious health effects have been reported in communities living on land with low selenium, such as areas of China, Eastern Siberia and Finland, where selenium deficiency causes endemic Keshan disease, a potentially fatal form of cardiomyopathy.[2,3]

Soils can also present a toxicological or physical risk to health. Soils rich in heavy metals such as cadmium and lead can have measurable and often severe effects on local populations, especially where the contaminant transfers into the food chain. Although many chemicals and pathogens can occur naturally in concentrations high enough to present a public health risk, for example exposure in soils to the bacterium *Clostridium tetani*, which can cause tetanus, anthropogenic activities are the main sources of significance in the environment.

It is generally accepted that most soil in the developed world is contaminated to one degree or another as a result of industrial activity and natural sources, and because of the global distribution of many chemicals (e.g. dioxins and polychlorinated biphenyls). Individual sites can often have a long history of use, which may have left a mixture of contaminants in a variety of soil and ground types, while many areas can have naturally elevated levels of certain substances (e.g. arsenic and radon). Where land has become contaminated, it may present a risk to humans, the wider environment and property. Furthermore, contamination may affect not just the current use of the land, but also any future redevelopment. Actual or perceived contamination may contribute to the long-term dereliction of sites and increase pressure to develop greenfield sites.

KEY CONTAMINANTS

Land may be polluted by a wide range of harmful substances, and it can be extremely difficult to identify possible contaminants. Many researchers have suggested a number of contaminants or groups of contaminants that may be key indicators of contaminated land (Table 52.1). While identifying such key contaminants has many merits, particularly when it comes to developing health-based, predefined environmental criteria, it must be emphasized that any investigation of contaminated land must not rely

Table 52.1 Key soil contaminants in the UK

Inorganic contaminants	Organic contaminants
Metals	**Aromatic hydrocarbons**
Barium	Benzene
Beryllium	Chlorophenols
Cadmium	Ethylbenzene
Chromium	Phenol
Copper	Toluene
Lead	o-Xylene
Mercury	Polycyclic aromatic hydrocarbons
Nickel	
Vanadium	**Chlorinated aliphatic**
Zinc	**hydrocarbons**
	Chloroform
Semi-metals and	Carbon tetrachloride
non-metals	Vinyl chloride
Arsenic	1,2-Dichloroethane
Boron	1,1,1-Trichloroethane
Selenium	Trichloroethene
Sulphur	Tetrachloroethene
	Hexachlorobuta-1,3-diene
Inorganic chemicals	Hexachlorocyclohexanes
Cyanide (complex)	Dieldrin
Cyanide (free)	
Nitrate	**Chlorinated aromatic**
Sulphate	**hydrocarbons**
Sulphide	Chlorobenzenes
	Chlorotoluenes
Other	Pentachlorophenol
Asbestos	Polychlorinated biphenyls
pH (acidity/alkalinity)	Dioxins and furans
Acetone	
Oil/fuel hydrocarbons	**Organometallics**
	Organolead compounds
	Organotin compounds

solely on these key indicators. Many sites may contain substances not covered within these key contaminants. A knowledge of the site history and the chemicals used will help to identify potential contaminants. Industry profiles[4] are available which provide information on the processes, materials and wastes associated with specific industries, and these can be used to identify potential contaminants.

HOW DO POLLUTANTS BEHAVE IN SOILS?

A detailed discussion on how pollutants behave in soil is outside the scope of this chapter, but it is important to briefly understand some key concepts that can help to describe pollutant behaviour and availability. Unlike true fluid media such as water or air, pollutants in soil tend not to disperse or dilute quickly. This can result in discrete pockets of pollution (also known as 'hotspots').

Furthermore, since soils contain solid, liquid and vapour phases, the partitioning of a pollutant into one or more of these phases will govern the behaviour, and ultimately the environmental and potential public health impact, of that pollutant.

The behaviour of pollutants in soils is governed by a complex interacting series of oxidation/reduction (redox), absorption, precipitation and desorption processes. Soils can absorb or release pollutants depending on the types of mineral particle present, the presence of organic matter, the soil pH, the redox potential and moisture. Where contaminants absorb onto soil surfaces, they become less mobile and leachable, and thereby less potentially bioavailable (Box 52.1 and Figure 52.1). Compounds that form weak bonds with soil and organic matter will be more mobile and bioavailable. For example, phenol compounds are highly mobile in soil because of their low tendency to absorb and can leach into ground or surface water. Furthermore, their volatility can result in volatilization and a risk of vapour inhalation from the soil.

Soil pH can be an important parameter controlling the absorption and release of charged (ionic) compounds. The charge on these surfaces is pH dependent, with absorption typically increasing with increasing pH. Heavy metals are typically most mobile in acidic soils, which can result in plant uptake or the contamination of drinking water supplies as a result of soil leaching.[6,7] For example, arsenic compounds are usually bound to insoluble iron and aluminium oxycompounds within the soil and are consequently relatively immobile and generally unavailable for plant uptake. In acidic soils, these iron- and aluminium-binding species become more soluble, releasing arsenic and making it more bioavailable. For organic contaminants such as polycyclic aromatic hydrocarbons (PAHs) and total petroleum hydrocarbons, their hydrophobic/lipophilic properties favour adsorption onto and into soil organic matter.[7]

As a result of its absorptive properties, soil can provide a sink for many pollutants that might otherwise

---

BOX 52.1: Bioavailability and bioaccessibility

- Bioaccessibility is the degree to which a chemical is released from the soil into solution and thereby becomes available for absorption when that soil is ingested and undergoes digestion
- This is typically assessed using an in vitro test that simulates the dissolution of contaminants in a simulated gastrointestinal environment that may subsequently be absorbed
- Bioavailability is the degree to which a substance is absorbed and becomes available to the target tissue (without first becoming metabolized)
- Figure 52.1 illustrates the relationship between exposure, bioavailability and bioaccessibility

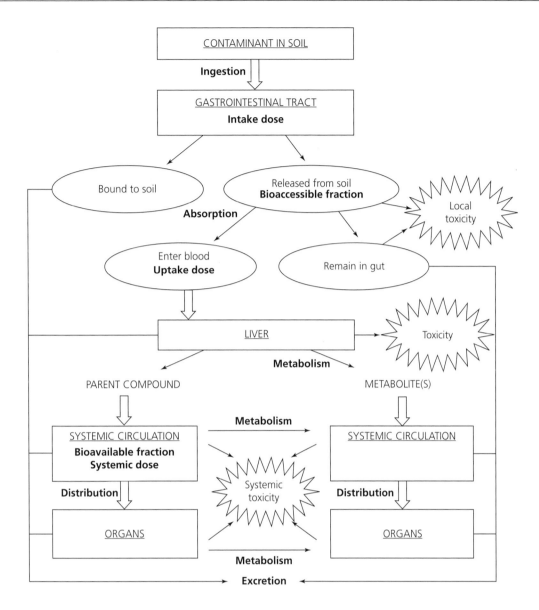

Figure 52.1 Graphical representation of the oral route of exposure, illustrating the difference between bioavailability and bioaccessibility. (Reproduced from Environment Agency,[5] with permission.)

enter surface or groundwater or return to the atmosphere. Sediments and soils can have a high storage capacity for heavy metals. Many form extremely strong bonds within the soil matrix and may remain in the same location for decades. Since heavy metal complexes do not degrade quickly and are often relatively immobile, they will tend to accumulate in soil over time as their rate of input into the environment will usually exceed their rate of removal. Similarly PAHs derived from combustion processes are strongly absorbed to soil organic matter.[8] Soil is a major 'sink' for PAHs, particularly in urban areas where concentrations may outweigh rural sites by a factor of more than 10.[9]

Such physicochemical properties can reduce bioavailability, with a growing body of evidence that the availability of chemicals in soil is less than in other environmental media and can be highly variable. Therefore,

any change in soil chemistry that reduces the capability of the soil matrix to absorb contaminants can have significant public health consequences. The application of lime is often employed to increase soil pH and so reduce the bioavailability of heavy metals.

The high variability in bioavailability of substances in soil will greatly influence the risk to health and can make risk assessments difficult. Whereas most risk assessments assume 100 per cent bioavailability, studies in monkeys exposed to arsenic in household dust and soil report a relative bioavailability of only 10–30 per cent.[10]

EXPOSURE

The principal routes of exposure to soil are shown in Box 52.2.

BOX 52.2: Potential exposure pathways to soil contaminants

Dermal
- Direct contact with soil

Ingestion
- Ingestion of water
- Ingestion of soil
- Ingestion of homegrown vegetables, fruits and crops
- Ingestion of homegrown dairy products and meats

Inhalation
- Inhalation of vapours (indoors and outdoors)
- Inhalation of dust
- Inhalation of particles (indoors and outdoors)

Ingestion

For residential areas, the ingestion of soil is perhaps the most important exposure pathway. Soil may be ingested directly, either as the result of deliberate ingestion or from accidental hand-to-mouth ingestion. Those at greatest risk tend to be young children of age 2 years or less who may deliberately put soil in their mouths; in older children, such mouthing behaviour declines with age.

People who have frequent contact with soil, such as gardeners, tend to ingest more soil, and behaviours that involve frequent hand-to-mouth contact, such as smoking, can also lead to higher soil ingestion rates. Particles of soil may also be ingested attached to food items, and poorly washed food may contain significant quantities of soil. Very fine grains of soil may become embedded in plant tissues and may not be removed by washing, preparation or cooking. Soil can adhere to plant surfaces either through 'soil splash' or through harvest practices.[11] Exposure to soil may also occur indoors. A significant proportion of indoor dust originates from outdoor soil through foot-tracking or other transport mechanisms.[12] In some cases, exposure to soil in house dust is as important as the direct ingestion of soil.[13]

A number of studies have been undertaken to estimate such exposure. Mass-balance studies using trace elements as markers suggest that soil ingestion rates in children vary considerably, with reports of 13 mg or less per day to over 200 mg per day depending on the study and whether the children participated in outdoor activities.[14–16] Geophagia, the deliberate consumption of earth, clay or soil, is not uncommon in some cultures, such as in the southern USA and Africa, and may result in the consumption of large quantities.[17]

Plant uptake

There are several mechanisms by which plants can take up soil contaminants, including via the root system, uptake of

particulate material deposited on the plant surface, and uptake of vapours and gases by the leaf pores. Uptake rates for soil contaminants will vary between plant species and as a result of soil geology and the physicochemical properties of the pollutant.

For many contaminants, such as heavy metals, root uptake is the predominant mechanism. The availability of the contaminant for uptake will depend on the chemical form of the metal, the soil type, the soil pH and the presence of organic matter. Contaminants that bind strongly into the matrix of soils are less available than those which do not bond or form weaker bonds. Once taken up, the rate of transport of the contaminant to the edible portion of the plant is important, as is the contaminant's half-life and the potential for the contaminant to bioaccumulate in the food chain.

Exposure to soil contaminants via the food chain has been well documented and can be a very important route of exposure where locally grown crops are a major contributor to the total diet. A statistically significant relationship between urinary cadmium levels and cadmium in soil and crops has been reported in people growing and consuming their own vegetables.[18]

Contact

Although we may be exposed to soil contaminants by direct skin contact, the skin acts as a barrier to dermal absorption and will prevent many chemicals penetrating the skin and being absorbed into the bloodstream. The rate and amount of percutaneous absorption of a chemical is very complex and depends on numerous factors including the timing, frequency and duration of the contact event, the physiological characteristics of the skin (e.g. skin thickness), the physicochemical nature of the chemical (e.g. lipophilicity) and the behaviour of the chemical in soil.[19] Because many contaminants become absorbed into the soil matrix, the potential for percutaneous absorption and subsequent systemic toxicity is greatly reduced.

Lipophilic substances and those which are most bioavailable clearly have the greatest potential for percutaneous absorption into the bloodstream. Dermal exposure is perhaps greatest with organic compounds such as phenols and pesticides, whereas for inorganic substances (e.g. metals), dermal contact is typically a very minor route of exposure.

Inhalation

Dusts rich in contaminated soil, or vapours and gases released by soil contaminants, are potential exposure pathways. Soil-derived atmospheric dust can be a source of airborne pollution in areas where past activities have contaminated the soil.[20] Gases released from the land can present a hazard to human health, especially when they migrate into confined spaces. Indeed, for many volatile organics, vapour ingress into properties may be a very important route of exposure.

RISK ASSESSMENT

Extent of contamination

Two-thirds of the world's population live in an urban environment, with this figure predicted to increase significantly further in the next 30 years. In the UK, government policy dictates that 60 per cent of new housing be built on previously used 'brownfield' sites, a proportion of which is likely to be contaminated. As a result, there is significant potential for exposure to potentially contaminated land sites.

It is extremely difficult to make accurate estimates of the extent of contaminated land in the UK or other developed countries. Since land is typically already in use, the true nature of the underlying soil may not be fully described until the land has been fully investigated and assessed, usually during planned redevelopment. In England and Wales, the Environment Agency has estimated that there may be 300 000 hectares of industrial land that may require assessment.[21]

Over the last decade, most countries have developed systems to identify and map potentially contaminated sites, usually based on understanding the causes of contamination. As such systems have developed, so the reported number of contaminated sites has steadily increased. For example, the development of local inventories in the Netherlands increased the estimated number of suspected contaminated sites requiring clean-up from 2000 in 1982 to 350 000 in 2002.[22]

As soil pollution is widespread, the remediation of all sites is not economically viable. Accordingly, in many countries, decisions about the redevelopment of contaminated land are risk-based. In this way, resources are targetted towards priority areas and take account of cost–benefit analysis as well as health concerns. Contaminated land policy in most developed countries is therefore associated with managing the risk, setting a series of generic societal objectives, whereas scientific input is based upon risk assessment and undertakes a technical evaluation of the risk in a specific scenario, with specific end points, such as health end points or the impact upon an ecological system.

What is contaminated land?

It is important to appreciate that the presence of chemicals or other substances does not mean that the land will be classified as contaminated. Many countries have strict legal definitions of what is meant by contaminated land. In the UK, contaminated land is defined by Part 2A of the Environmental Protection Act 1990 as 'Any land which appears to the local authority in whose authority it is situated to be in such a condition, by reason of substances in, or under land that significant harm is being caused or there is significant possibility of such harm being caused'.

In this context, *significant harm* includes such health effects as death, disease, serious injury, genetic mutation, birth defects and reproductive effects. However, since it may be extremely difficult to demonstrate causality between exposure and health effect, the Act also recognizes *significant possibility of significant harm* (often termed SPOSH). Within this legal framework, contaminated land is therefore defined by the potential or actual health effects of exposure as opposed to the concentration of contaminant(s) in the soil. Implicit in this definition is a need to determine whether significant exposure is occurring through viable source–pathway–receptor (SPR) linkages (Box 52.3). Risk assessment is thus needed to establish or refute completed SPR linkages. In the UK, as in many other countries, this is undertaken in a tiered manner.

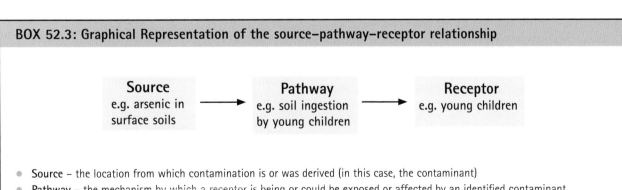

BOX 52.3: Graphical Representation of the source–pathway–receptor relationship

Source
e.g. arsenic in surface soils → **Pathway**
e.g. soil ingestion by young children → **Receptor**
e.g. young children

- **Source** – the location from which contamination is or was derived (in this case, the contaminant)
- **Pathway** – the mechanism by which a receptor is being or could be exposed or affected by an identified contaminant
- **Receptor** – that which may be adversely affected by the contaminant(s)

Investigating and assessing contaminated land

In the UK, the first step of any investigation is to carry out a preliminary desk-top investigation, its principal output being the establishment of an initial *conceptual model* and preliminary risk assessment. This requires an exploration of historical records and other sources of information, consultation and site reconnaissance. The conceptual model refers to the identification of potential contaminants and their distribution, likely environmental media contaminated and the presence of receptors, including buildings, ecological systems or organisms forming part of that system – property in the form of crops, buildings, livestock, wild and domestic animals as well as human beings. This forms the basis of establishing the SPR linkages.

Without all three components being present – i.e. individuals or communities being or to be exposed (receptors), a contaminant or contaminants (source) and a medium through which exposure can occur (e.g. air, water, soil or food; the pathway) – there cannot be a risk to human heath. The basic concept of a conceptual model is to correctly identify the potential receptors, contaminants and pathways and therefore enable the determination of whether there is a potential risk to human health. This is a crucial step, as if the SPR linkages are not valid or do not accurately represent the site, the extent of exposure may be underestimated and the risk may be greater than believed.

If appropriate, field investigation should be undertaken to support the preliminary risk assessment and to further characterize the initial conceptual model. In the exploratory phase, analytical confirmation of the presence of contamination may be required, whereas the main investigation phase has as its principal aim the accurate representation and analysis of the contaminants and their concentration and distribution in environmental media. This may require a consideration of hydrogeological aspects, surface and groundwater migration, determination of the presence of abstraction points, and ascertaining the likely exposure of crops and implications for air quality. It is therefore essential that any analyses undertaken are representative, adhere to established pre-analytical requirements and are analysed by accredited laboratories. This is vitally important as the subsequent risk assessment is predicated upon the quality of the data produced. Each tier of a contaminated land investigation essentially has a similar structure, the basic components of which are illustrated in Box 52.4.

Assessing significant possibility of significant harm (SPOSH)

Assessing significant possibility of significant harm is usually based on computer models or complex algorithms

---

> ### BOX 52.4: A typical tiered contaminated land investigation
>
> **Hazard identification** – establishing contaminant sources
> **Hazard assessment** – analysing the potential for unacceptable risk (what pathways and receptors could be present, what pollutant linkages could result and what the effects could be)
> **Risk estimation** – predicting the magnitude and probability of the possible consequences (what degree of harm or pollution might result, to what receptors and how likely is it) that may arise as a result of the hazard
> **Risk evaluation** – deciding whether the risk is unacceptable

that attempt to describe exposure from SPR relationships. Exposure is then assessed and compared against established health criterion values (HCVs). Exposures that are predicted to be less than a given HCV are considered to pose an acceptable or minimal risk and no further action is required. If, however, exposure is deemed to exceed a given HCV, further action may be required. This may involve further investigation and the site may be determined as contaminated, with a subsequent requirement to manage the risk through remediation, restriction of access or the construction of barriers to break SPR linkages and thus prevent exposure. Figure 52.2 illustrates how HCVs are typically derived for both threshold chemicals and non-threshold (genotoxic) carcinogens.

The risk to health

Much concern has focused on reported associations with adverse reproductive outcomes and various cancers. These serious diseases are relatively rare, and the evidence of a link with environmental pollution such as contaminated land is often inconsistent or contradictory. Such concerns can, however, arouse great public concern. Furthermore, negative perceptions of the environment can have an impact on general physical and mental health. For example, property blight as a result of actual or even perceived contamination can cause financial hardship, stress and anxiety, which can have a major effect on health.

Most epidemiological studies have focused on populations living on or near landfill sites. In the UK and many other countries, a wide range of waste materials has been deposited in landfill sites, including known hazardous chemicals, and exposure to releases from landfills is certainly plausible (e.g. inhalation, contaminated topsoil or polluted water sources). It has been estimated that, in the UK, approximately 80 per cent of British people live within 2 km of a closed or active landfill site.[23]

There have been a number of reviews of published epidemiological evidence, particularly around possible

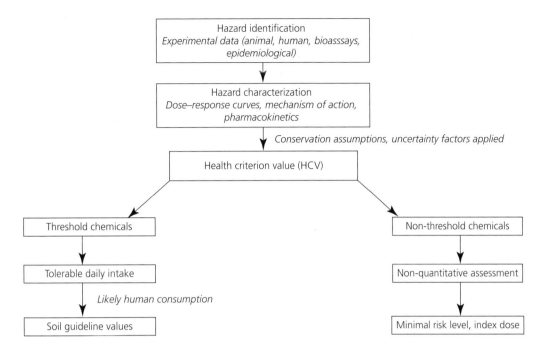

Figure 52.2 Overview of the derivation of health criterion values for exposure to contaminants in soil. Adapted with permission from Environment Agency.

associations with an increased risk of adverse birth outcomes. Vrijheid conducted a systematic review of epidemiological studies around landfill sites and concluded that there might be a risk of adverse birth outcomes associated with living near certain types of landfill site, specifically those containing hazardous materials.[24]

Other reviews suggest, however, that the evidence is not yet convincing. Kibble and Saunders[25] noted that that the published literature was inconsistent but that there was some potential evidence of health effects, particularly associated with reproductive health and self-reported symptoms. Redfearn and Roberts[26] concluded that published research was inconsistent and that only low birth weight could be considered as a plausible health effect. A detailed review by Defra[27] in the UK of the environmental and health effects surrounding the management of municipal solid waste (including landfills) concluded that although there was some evidence to indicate that birth defects occurred slightly more often in children born to mothers living close to landfill sites, it was not possible to say whether the landfills caused or contributed to this apparent excess.

The Small Area Health Statistics Unit (SAHSU) has undertaken the largest study of landfills and birth outcomes in the UK.[23] Potentially exposed populations within a 2 km radius circle of all known landfill sites operational between 1982 and 1997 were examined.[23,28] Residence near landfills was estimated to result in a small increased risk of giving birth to a baby with a congenital malformation. For all anomalies combined, the relative risk (adjusted for confounders) was 1.01 (99 per cent confidence interval 1.005–1.023). The study also analysed the risk before and after the landfill sites opened and found that risks were significantly higher after opening for low birth weight and stillbirth, but for many other anomalies risks were higher prior to site opening, suggesting that other risk factors might be important.

The evidence of a link with cancer is currently less convincing. Few studies show statistically significant excesses, and published reviews of the literature agree that there is currently no consistent evidence of a link between landfill sites and cancer.[24–27] The large SAHSU study also examined the incidence of childhood and adult leukaemias, hepatobiliary cancers and cancers of bladder and brain. No excess risk for those living within 2 km of a landfill site for each of the cancer types studied was found.[23] The UK government's independent expert advisory Committee on Toxicity of Chemicals in Food, Consumer Products and the Environment considered the outcomes of this large study and concluded that it was inappropriate to draw firm conclusions on the possible health effects of landfill sites.[29]

Current evidence, therefore, does not support a strong link between ill-health and landfill sites. Where associations are reported, they tend to centre on possible reproductive effects such as congenital malformations or low birth weight, and the better quality studies tend to show either small or no effects. The methods used in such studies currently contain some inherent limitations. Many studies are compromised by a lack of objective exposure data because they fail to quantify potential exposure pathways, and there are also issues surrounding case ascertainment, bias, confounding and multiple testing. As a result, it is generally considered that the evidence of an association with adverse birth outcomes or cancer is inconclusive, but more work is clearly needed to better understand the risk.

There can, however, be little doubt that where exposure occurs, contaminated land can present a serious risk to health. High levels of lead in soil have been long known to present a serious risk to health.[13,30–34] Lead-contaminated soil has had a significant impact on health in communities around the Bunker Hill Superfund Site, Idaho, USA, where many decades of industry have left large areas of land contaminated with lead. A survey in 1983 showed a clear association between high blood lead levels and children living in contaminated residential areas, even among children born after the local lead smelter had closed.[12] The removal or covering of contaminated soil in the most affected communities in Bunker Hill has served to reduce both blood lead levels and also lead levels in household dust.[35,36]

In Jamaica, the backyard smelting of lead has resulted in extremely high lead levels in soils and indoor dust, leading to elevated blood lead levels and children presenting with lead encephalopathy.[31] Severe chronic exposure to lead was exacerbated by a significant history of pica and chronic nutritional anaemia. Several studies have also shown that seasonal increases in children's blood lead levels relate, in part, to exposure via activity with summer days of outdoor play and open windows and doors leading to an increased exposure to contaminated soils.[33,37,38]

Exposure to cadmium-contaminated soil has also been shown to cause health problems. Cadmium is particularly toxic to the kidney and can also lead to a poor absorption of calcium, which is required for healthy bones. Studies of Japanese communities living in the Jinzu Valley river basin have shown renal induced tubular injury and severe skeletal deformities and osteoporosis due to chronic cadmium poisoning, locally termed 'itai-itai' disease.[39,40] In this case, exposure occurred primarily via the contamination of locally grown rice grown in soil heavily polluted with cadmium as a result of nearby mining activities. A particular subset of the population was most affected, namely post-menopausal women prone to developing osteoporosis and other calcium-related disorders. Malnutrition was also another influencing factor in this condition.

Environmental exposure to cadmium from polluted soil has been reported in other countries, and many researchers report associations between exposure and mortality. Environmental exposure to cadmium in areas of North-East Belgium with a history of smelting has been associated with total and non-cardiovascular disease and mortality, as well as with also renal dysfunction.[41,42] Again, historical land contamination was identified as an ongoing source of exposure.

CONCLUSION

We are only just beginning to fully understand how contaminated land can influence health. We are all exposed to pollutants in soil via a number of different ways, and in some circumstances exposure may be sufficient to cause ill-health. However, our understanding of such exposure pathways and the way pollutants behave in the soil environment is relatively poor, and consequently many health studies struggle to quantify the extent of exposure. Current epidemiological evidence of a link between health and contaminated land is inconsistent and certainly not complete. As our understanding of contaminated land increases, so the link with health will become better defined.

REFERENCES

● = Key primary paper

◆ = Major review article

●1. Oliver MA. Soil and human health: A review. *Eur J Soil Sci* 1997; **48**: 573–92.

● 2. Li GS, Wang F, Kang D, Li C. Keshan disease: An endemic cardiomyopathy in China. *Hum Pathol* 1985; **16**: 602–9.

●3. Yang GQ, Chen JS, Wen Zm *et al*. The role of selenium in Keshan disease. *Adv Nutr Res* 1984; **6**: 203–31.

4. Industry Profiles for the UK. Available from: http://www. environment-agency.gov.uk/research/planning/33708.aspx (accessed November 26, 2009).

◆5. Environment Agency. *Human Health Toxicological Assessment of Contaminants in Soil*. Science Report SC050021/SR2. Bristol: Environment Agency, 2008.

◆6. Alloway BJ, Ayres DC. *Chemical Principles of Environmental Pollution*. London: Blackie, 1993.

◆7. Alloway BJ. Soil processes and the behaviour of heavy metals. In: Alloway BJ (ed.) *Heavy Metals in Soils* (pp. 11–37). London: Springer, 1995.

●8. Wilcke W. Polycyclic aromatic hydrocarbons (PAHs) in soil – a review. *J Plant Nutr Soil Sci* 2000; **163**: 229–48.

●9. Wild SR, Jones KC. Polynuclear aromatic hydrocarbons in the United Kingdom environment: A preliminary source inventory and budget. *Environ Pollut* 1995; **88**: 91–108.

●10. Freeman GB, Schoof RA, Ruby MV *et al*. Bioavailability of arsenic in soil and house dust impacted by smelter activities following oral administration to cynomolgus monkeys. *Fundam Appl Toxicol* 1995; **28**: 215–22.

◆11. Sheppard SC. Soil and human health: a review. *Environ Geochem Health* 1995; **14**: 113–20.

●12. Paustenbach DJ, Finley BL, Long TF. The critical role of house dust in understanding the hazards posed by contaminated soils. *Int J Toxicol* 1997; **16**: 339–62.

●13. Von Linden I, Spalinger S, Petroysan V, von Braun M. Assessing remedial effectiveness through the blood lead:soil/dust lead relationship at the Bunker Hill Superfund Site in the Silver Valley of Idaho. *Sci Total Environ* 2003; **303**: 139–70.

●14. Davis S, Waller P, Buschbom MA *et al*. Quantitative estimates of soil ingestion in normal children between the ages of 2 and 7 years: Population-based estimates using aluminum, silicon, and titanium as soil tracer elements. *Arch Environ Health* 1990; **45**: 112–22.

●15. van Wijnen JH, Clausing P, Brunekreef B. Estimated soil ingestion by children. *Environ Res* 1990; **51**: 147–62.

●16. Stanek EJ III, Calbrese EJ. Daily estimates of soil ingestion in children. *Environ Health Perspect* 1995; **103**: 276–85.

●17. Reid RM. Cultural and medical perspectives on geophagia. *Med Anthropol* 1992; **13**: 337–51.

●18. Hellströom L, Elinder CG, Dahlberg B *et al*. Cadmium and end-stage renal disease. *Am J Kidney Dis* 2001; **38**: 1001–8.

19. United States Environmental Protection Agency. *Summary Report for the Workshop on Issues Associated with Dermal Exposure and Uptake*. EPA/630/R-00/003, 2000. US Environmental Protection Agency, Risk Assessment Forum, Washington, DC. Available from: http://www.epa.gov/osa/raf/publications/pdfs/SUMDERMALDEC21.PDF (accessed November 18, 2009).

●20. Harrison RM, Yin J, Mark D *et al*. Studies of the coarse particle (2.5–10 μm) component in UK urban atmospheres. *Atmos Environ* 2001; **35**: 3367–79.

◆21. Environment Agency. *Indicators for Land Contamination*. Science Report SC030039/SR. Bristol: Environment Agency, 2005.

22. Environmental Data Compendium. Number of Soil Pollution Sites in the Netherlands, 1982–2002. Available from: http://www.mnp.nl/mnc/i-en-0258.html (accessed November 18, 2009).

◆23. Elliott P, Morris S, Briggs D *et al*. *Birth Outcomes and Selected Cancers in Populations Living Near Landfill Sites. Report to the Department of Health*. Imperial College London: Department of Epidemiology and Public Health, Small Area Health Statistics Unit, 2001.

◆24. Vrijheid M. Health effects of residence near hazardous waste landfill sites: A review of epidemiologic literature. *Environ Health Perspect* 2000; **108**(Suppl. 1): 101–12.

◆25. Kibble AJ, Saunders PJ. Contaminated land and the link with health. In: Harrison RM (ed.) *Assessment and Reclamation of Contaminated Land* (pp. 65–84). Issues in Environmental Science and Technology, Issue No. 16. Cambridge: Royal Society of Chemistry, 2001.

◆26. Redfearn A, Roberts D. Health effects and landfill sites. In: Harrison RM, Hester RE (eds.) *Environmental and Health Impact of Solid Waste Management Activities* (pp. 103–40). Cambridge: Royal Society of Chemistry, 2002.

◆27. Enviros, University of Birmingham, Defra. *Review of Environmental and Health Effects of Waste Management: Municipal Solid Waste and Similar Wastes*. London: Defra, 2004.

●28. Elliott P, Briggs D, Morris S *et al*. Risk of adverse birth outcomes in populations living near landfill sites. *Br Med J* 2001; **323**: 363–8.

29. Committee on Toxicity. *COT Statement (Non Food) on the Study by the Small Area Health Statistics Unit (SAHSU) on Health Outcomes in Populations Living Around Landfill Sites – August 2001*. COT/2001/04. London: Department of Health, 2001. Available from: http://cot.food.gov.uk/cotstatements/cotstatementsyrs/cotstatements2001/sahsulandfill (accessed November 18, 2009).

●30. Baghurst PA, Tong SL, McMichael AJ *et al*. Determinants of blood lead concentrations to age 5 years in a birth cohort study of children living in the lead smelting city of Port Pirie and surrounding areas. *Arch Environ Health* 1992; **47**: 203–10.

●31. Lalor G, Rattray R, Vutchkov M *et al*. Blood lead levels in Jamaican school children. *Sci Total Environ* 2001; **269**: 171–81.

●32. Schell LM, Denham M, Stark AD *et al*. Relationship between blood lead concentration and dietary intakes of infants from 3 to 12 months of age. *Environ Res* 2004; **96**: 264–73.

●33. Maynard E, Thomas R, Simon D *et al*. An evaluation of recent blood lead levels in Port Pirie, South Australia. *Sci Total Environ* 2003; **303**: 25–33.

●34. Laidlaw MAS, Mielke HW, Filippelli GM *et al*. Seasonality and children's blood lead levels: Developing a predictive model using climatic variables and blood lead data from Indianapolis, Indiana, Syracuse, New York, and New Orleans, Louisiana (USA). *Environ Health Perspect* 2005; **113**: 793–800.

●35. Sheldrake S, Stifelman M. A case study of lead contamination cleanup effectiveness at Bunker Hill. *Sci Total Environ* 2003; **303**: 105–23.

●36. Von Lindern IH, Spalinger SM, Ber BN *et al*. The influence of soil remediation on lead in house dust. *Sci Total Environ* 2003; **303**: 59–78.

●37. Yin LM, Rhoads GG, Lioy PJ. Seasonal influences on childhood lead exposure. *Environ Health Perspect* 2000; **108**: 177–82.

●38. Kemp FW, Neti PVSV, Howell RW *et al*. Elevated blood lead concentrations and vitamin D deficiency in winter and summer in young urban children. *Environ Health Perspect* 2007; **115**: 630–5.

●39. Nogawa K, Kobayashi E, Okubo Y *et al*. Environmental cadmium exposure, adverse effects and preventive measures in Japan. *BioMetals* 2004; **17**: 581–7.

◆40. Jarup L. Hazards of heavy metal contamination. *Br Med Bull* 2003; **68**: 167–82.

●41. Staessen JA, Lauwerys RR, Ide G *et al*. Renal function and historical environmental cadmium pollution from zinc smelters. *Lancet* 1994; **343**: 1523–7.

●42. Nawrot TS, van Hecke E, Lutgarde T *et al*. Cadmium-related mortality and long-term secular trends in the cadmium body burden of an environmentally exposed population. *Environ Health Perspect* 2008; **116**: 1620–8.

53

Disposal of diseased animals

SIMON POLLARD

OVERVIEW

In the developed world, animal carcase disposal has become a highly controlled process with detailed legislative requirements relating to biosecurity, chemical exposure, carcase destruction and the disposal of treatment residues. Well-structured operational guidance documents have been drafted by governments that set out procedures and responsibilities for carcase disposal. This contrasts markedly with the situation in developing countries, where these procedures are rarely in place, and exposures to dangerous pathogens, carcase contents, by-products and residues are frequently uncontrolled, posing the potential for animal and human disease transmission.

The underpinning philosophy[1] for animal disposal has remained relatively unchanged for decades – diseased animals should be culled humanely, and carcases disposed of quickly, safely and responsibly, away from populations and water courses. Individuals involved in the practice should pay particular attention to their personal safety, and storage or transportation facilities should be contained and disinfected. The scale of such disposals has, however, altered in recent years, and mass culls and disposal operations are now commonplace.

The key risks from animal disposals are ones of onward infection, physical injury or chemical exposure to operational staff and members of the public in close proximity to disposal operations; of infection to other animals close by when the disease agent is persisting in the environment; and to the wider environment, especially the long-term pollution of groundwaters. Open and accurate communication on disposal practices and the management of risk to all those concerned is essential. Importantly, carcase disposal is properly conceptualized as a multistage

'process', presenting opportunities for exposure to pathogens, chemicals and other hazardous agents along its length. Modern, risk-based controls[2] focus on intervening to reduce these exposures at critical points as early and effectively as possible.

DISPOSAL AS A PROCESS

When diseased animals die, are killed through natural disasters or to prevent suffering (welfare culls), or when they are culled to reduce the spread of infectious disease, arrangements have to be made for carcase disposal. Historically, for individual or small numbers of animals (fewer than five), disposal at the farm or holding was appropriate, with a basic set of controls. Typically, carcases were buried on-farm in clay-lined pits, away from people and surface or groundwaters, with approximately 1 m of clay cover to prevent scavenging.

However, concerns since the 1990s over the impact of disposal practices on environmental quality, especially the potential impact of persistent chemicals and biological agents on human, animal and environmental health, have resulted in a reappraisal of carcase disposal options.[3] This has especially been the case for the types of mass disposal required in response to exotic animal disease outbreaks, where thousands, tens of thousands and, in the extreme, millions of animals may be culled, with their carcases requiring disposal.[4] For example, the UK Foot and Mouth outbreaks in 1967, 2001 and 2007 resulted in the slaughter, for disease control purposes, of 442 000, more than 4 000 000 and 2160 animals, respectively.

In these circumstances, public health practitioners may find themselves dealing with a range of medical, environmental and animal health risks including the psychological distress caused to animal owners and operational field staff,[5] the occupational or public health impacts of culling, disinfection and disposal, and the environmental impacts of disposal, including the potential transmission of viable pathogens and hazardous chemicals at some distance from operational sites of disposal. This chapter deals with the occupational, public and environmental health impacts associated with the disposal of animal carcases.

With the exception of isolated, single animal deaths, modern carcase disposal in developed countries is a multistage process[6] initiated by the collection of fallen stock or the culling of live stock (e.g. birds, pigs, sheep, cattle or pigs), with the subsequent disinfection of carcases, their transport to localized collection points and the potential off-site transport to waste-processing[7] (e.g. incineration, rendering or mass burial) facilities. Clearly, the movement and transport of animals, some weighing in excess of half a tonne, brings with it a series of occupational hazards for front-line workers and contractors, with the potential for falls from height (loading and off-loading), transport accidents, manual handling injuries (lifting specialist and heavy equipment), chemical exposures (the use of gassing agents and undiluted disinfectants) and acquired infections.

The occupational precautions promoted by the UK Health and Safety Executive for workers disposing of carcases affected with bovine spongiform encephalopathy are applicable to all carcase disposal operations. Workers should:

- cover cuts and abrasions with waterproof dressings before work starts;
- wear protective clothing, including gloves;
- avoid cuts and puncture wounds during work;
- use eye protection if there is a risk of splashing;
- wash their hands before eating, drinking and smoking;
- wash down contaminated areas with detergent and water;
- rinse protective clothing free of debris after use and wash with water and detergent.

Ensuring biosecurity and environmental protection objectives is also critical. Certain viruses are persistent in the environment once released, notably foot and mouth virus (reportedly up to 28 days in soil in the autumn), and carcases also produce large volumes of blood, urine, faeces and milk that may contain disease agents and other pathogens of concern.

Typically, in the event of the need for off-site disposal, carcases are loaded into specialist leak-proof vehicles and transported to a disposal facility by a predetermined route. Loads are usually covered and escorted to ensure that the vehicle does not develop a leak. At the disposal facility, carcases are disposed of under supervision. Following the initial removal of the carcases from the site of discovery, all litter, equipment and areas occupied by the affected animals are sprayed down with an approved disinfectant and left to dry. Thorough cleansing and disinfection of the premises involves removing the litter and other organic material, and a full wash-down, followed by degreasing and the application of an approved disinfectant at a recommended dilution. Restocking can commence after a recognized delay (such as 21 days) following full cleansing and disinfection.

The early stages of carcase disposal are common, irrespective of the waste technology employed later in the process to destroy or dispose of the carcase. Here, differences mainly arise in the extent to which waste-processing alters the viability and containment of hazardous agents, their relative destruction and the generation of post-treatment waste residues (e.g. ash, or meat and bone meal) requiring onward disposal. The overall carcase disposal 'process chain' has five key stages: (1) disinfection and collection; (2) transport; (3) pre-processing; (4) processing; and (5) dealing with residues that can be further described:

- Disinfection and collection:
  - containment *in situ*;
  - destruction at source;
  - gathering carcases to local storage;
  - contained storage of gathered carcases;
  - containment during local processing;
  - destruction during local processing.
- Transport:
  - transport to facility.
- Pre-processing:
  - containment prior to processing.
- Processing:
  - containment during off-site processing;
  - destruction during processing.
- Dealing with residues:
  - containment of residuals;
  - destruction of residuals.

Carcase disposal cannot be performed without risks to people, animal health and the environment. Such risks extend beyond the disease-causing agent to include all hazards associated with a carcase, its by-products and the associated infrastructure of disposal – detergents, disinfectants, wastes from disinfection, veterinary medicines, other animal-borne pathogens and amenity hazards such as odour and noise. Managing the risks from a multistage process and from a multitude of potential hazards becomes an exercise in identifying the key opportunities for exposure to the significant hazards of concern, and then devising practical preventive practices and interventions at critical points of control in order to minimize risk.[2]

A risk-informed approach[8] to carcase disposal is distinct from one solely and narrowly concerned with an optimal waste technology for carcase destruction. Instead, by virtue of risk assessments at varying levels of sophistication, it correctly considers the whole process and seeks to identify where exposures are likely to be most significant along the process chain.[6] These become priorities for risk management through sound contingency-planning[9] and the communication of operation advice to field staff.

A wide range of hazards is posed during carcase disposal.[8] Assessing the risk of harm from these hazards during disposal requires information on the relative potency of the hazard, its likely exposure point concentration or the magnitude of exposure, the relative availability of exposure pathways and the sensitivity and vulnerability of individual receptors (Figure 53.1).

Individual countries have lists of chemicals used and specific agents of concern, and the circumstances of disposal play a large part in determining which hazards are likely to be of most interest. By illustration, Table 53.1 provides a candidate list of potentially significant hazards posed by carcase disposal operations in the UK as they relate to four exotic animal diseases – avian influenza, Newcastle disease, foot and mouth virus and classical swine fever. The table represents hazardous agents: (1) believed to pose potentially significant risks to human health, animal health or the environment; *and* (2) that are capable of evading destruction; *and* (3) that are also capable of presenting in sufficient doses to be of potential

concern. The toxicology of these individual hazardous agents is covered elsewhere.[10]

A risk-based approach to carcase disposal distinguishes between potential hazards and those actually realized and posing ongoing consequences for public and animal health and the environment. An assessment of the 2001 UK foot and mouth disease outbreak provides some detail on the extent to which potential hazards may be realized as

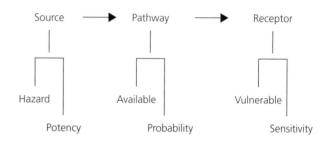

Figure 53.1 Decisions on carcase disposal should be risk-informed. The significance of risks is determined by the potency of a hazard, by the probability of accessing available exposure pathways and by the sensitivity of receptors vulnerable to exposures. Without exposure pathways connecting the source of a hazard to a receptor, exposure cannot occur and risks cannot be realized.

Table 53.1 Significant hazards associated with carcase disposal

Biological agents	Chemical agents	Amenity, nuisance impacts
Foot and mouth disease	Ammonia, ammoniacal nitrogen and nitrates	Odour
Classical swine fever	Detergents (including phosphates and linear	Noise
Newcastle disease virus	alkylbenzenesulphonate-surfactants)	Derived products (litters, slurry
Salmonella spp.	Disinfectants (formaldehyde, phenols, hypochlorite, peroxide,	and manures)
Bioaerosols (*Actinomycetes* and	quaternary ammonium salts, FAM-30 and Virkon S)	Milk/treated milk (also
Aspergillus spp.)	Biochemical oxygen demand	biochemical oxygen demand)
Influenza (H5, H7)	Veterinary medicines (in carcase; e.g. pesticides, antibacterials,	Smoke
Influenza (other A strains)	coccidiostats and barbiturates)	Ash
Campylobacter spp.	Methane	Waste treatment/waste water
Coxiella burnetii (Q-fever)	Nitrogen oxides	treatment residues (e.g.
African swine fever	Particulates	alkaline hydrolysis residues,
Bovine spongiform	Polynuclear aromatic hydrocarbons	waste waters, sludges and
encephalopathy (prion)	Sulphur oxides	residual farm wastes)
Cryptosporidium spp.	Kerosene and other accelerants (e.g. FeeDol)	Organic fertilizers and
Scrapie	Breakdown products (e.g. pesticide residues and metabolites)	soil-improvers
Swine vesicular disease	Heavy metals (lead, arsenic)	
	Dissolved organic carbon and total organic carbon	
	Extremes of pH	
	Benzene, toluene, ethylbenzenes and xylenes	
	Wood resins and chemicals in wood preservatives (e.g.	
	pentachlorophenol and chromated copper arsenate)	
	Dioxins, furans, polychlorinated biphenyls	
	Insecticides (permethrins and organophosphates)	

experienced during a national disease outbreak. The prevailing view following this large outbreak has been that environmental impacts have been minor (Figure 53.2).[7]

This said, among the specific environmental (as opposed to economic or sectoral) impacts reported part-way through the outbreak[11], and requiring effective management, were:

- a large number (approximately 200) of *reported* water pollution incidents from the surface run-off of blood and carcase fluids early on in the crisis, when slaughter rates outstripped disposal capacity, although few of these resulted in *significant* water pollution (in the region of only three high-category pollution incidents from slurry spill and disinfectant run-off);
- the generation of large quantities of ash from constructed animal pyres (typically 15 tonne ash per 300 tonne pyre), requiring onward containment and disposal;
- the generation of very high-strength initial leachate (>75 000–100 000 mg/L chemical oxygen demand; >500–2000 mg/L total nitrogen; 400–3000 mg/L potassium[12]) at landfills taking animal carcases;
- a high prevalence of odour complaints in the proximity of mass burial sites during disposal operations (300 for one large burial site);
- localized, short-term deteriorations in local air quality during pyre-burning.[13,14]

WASTE MANAGEMENT

The scale of carcase disposals during large disease outbreaks or natural disasters frequently overwhelms the available waste-management infrastructure in countries managing these events.[2] As an example, since 1997 in Asia alone, over 200 million chickens and ducks have been killed by the highly pathogenic avian influenza virus H5N1, or culled in efforts to contain the disease. For individual outbreaks, in 2004, the Ministry of Agriculture, Food and Fisheries in British Columbia, Canada, incinerated and composted around 17 million culled birds following an outbreak of the H7N3 avian influenza virus. Similar disposals, adopting a range of waste technologies, have been required in the USA, Hong Kong, Italy (1999–2001; H7N1 avian influenza; approximately 13 million birds), the Netherlands, Belgium and Germany, Hungary and most recently the UK (2006; low pathogenic H7N3; around 49 000 poultry incinerated and rendered; February 2007; highly pathogenic H5N1; in the region of 159 000 turkeys rendered).

The selection of carcase disposal options in these outbreaks has been based on the scale of the requirement, the available waste technology capacity and the logistics of disposal, rather than on any prior analysis of exposures to public and animal health and to the environment. On-farm burial, on-farm pyres, rendering, high-temperature

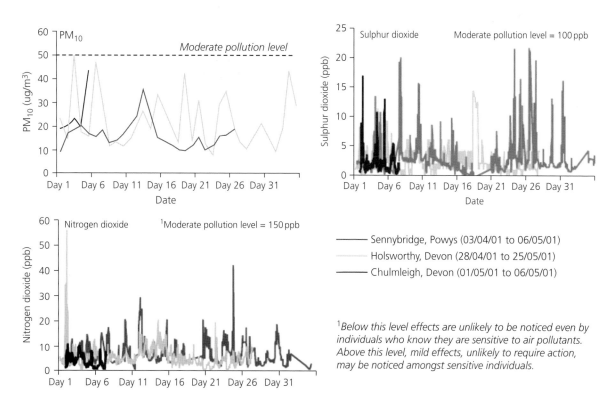

Figure 53.2 Local air quality in the vicinity of pyres used for carcase disposal during the 2001 UK foot and mouth outbreak. PM$_{10}$, particles with a diameter of 10 μm or less; ppb, parts per billion. (Adapted from Environment Agency,[11] with permission.)

incineration, mass burial, landfill and composting have all been employed at various stages. In contrast, many responses in developing countries have historically adopted uncontrolled disposal without apparent reference to the risks across the full process chain.

In an attempt to bring a formality of approach to decisions on disposal, some jurisdictions have promoted a hierarchy of disposal strategies[7,8] that, while keeping a broad range of technological options open (Table 53.2), seeks to set preferences for certain technologies over others. The relative attractions and disadvantages of carcase disposal technologies are discussed by Hickman et al.[4] and Scudamore et al.[7] In brief, carcase destruction in licensed, engineered process facilities is preferred over controlled burial in landfill, pyre-burning or on-farm burial, where little process control or containment is assured. A recent assessment of opportunities for pathogenic and chemical exposure[2] during carcase disposal lends additional weight for a hierarchy of disposal[8] and reinforces afresh the necessity for quick and effective action at the outbreak premises, where the principal opportunities for exposure, and thus risk management, exist.[15]

ASSESSING AND MANAGING EXPOSURES

Decisions on carcase disposal should be made by reference to national contingency plan objectives (biosecurity), and they should also address issues of cost and regulatory

Table 53.2 A revised disposal hierarchy for carcase disposal in the event of exotic animal disease outbreaks

Disposal option*	Statement of preference
Alkaline hydrolysis, atmospheric rendering, Biogas, composting (in vessel), controlled incineration, co-combustion in cement kilns, gasification, mobile incineration and pressure rendering	These are the preferred options
Air curtain incinerator, composting (Windrow), mass burial and permitted landfill	These are secondary options
Mass pyre and on-farm pyre	These are possible options, but not recommended
Anaerobic digestion (pits), on-farm burial and do nothing	These are generally undesirable options

*Options listed within each of the four categories are not presented in any order of preference.

Adapted from Pollard et al.,[2] with permission.

compliance. Governments should not be concerned solely with either the cheapest or the safest disposal option at any cost, but rather with developing a hierarchy of responses. This will be specific to the disease, the country where disposal occurs and the specific conditions of the outbreak, and, even with comprehensive contingency arrangements in place, decision-makers may need to be prepared to make use of the least preferred options.[3]

The lessons from past events point to the need for well-organized and well-communicated contingency plans[9] for exotic animal disease outbreaks, specific attention to logistical issues during the early stages[16] and long-term monitoring programmes, especially where mass burials have been employed.[17] The management of outbreaks involving a large number of animals has brought attention to the broader range of hazards involved (see Table 53.1), and especially to pathogenic agents beyond the zoonotic agent of immediate concern.[18]

Disposal practices during recent outbreaks have also been informed by qualitative and quantitative exposure assessments (Table 53.3). The multiple barrier concept[6] of exposure is valuable in conceptualizing where efforts should best be concentrated to avoid onward exposures. Occupational, biosecurity and environmental protection controls act as barriers to onward infection. Opportunities for exposure occur where these barriers are absent or not effectively maintained (Figure 53.3). In these circumstances, exposure pathways become highly available and are accessible to hazardous agents released during disposal operations, illustrated for a range of waste technology process chains in Figure 53.4.

Although the likelihood of environmentally mediated harm to public health from carcase disposal is deemed negligible, the protection of groundwater and surface waters remains a priority (Figure 53.5).[12,19] The availability of these exposure pathways as potential routes for the transmission of disease to humans is driven, in part, by the possibility of agents bypassing water treatment processes that might otherwise deactivate or remove pathogens.[19]

Australia has produced a series of regularly updated practical response plans for managing emergency animal disease incidents. The operational procedures manual for carcase disposals (2007)[20] includes a multiattribute technique for selecting disposal options, with operator safety, community concerns, international acceptance, transport availability, legislative requirements, industry standards, cost-effectiveness and speed of resolution as key decision attributes. Within the manual, a strong emphasis is placed on understanding the survivability and persistence of the exotic disease agent within the environment in order to inform decisions on animal health biosecurity.

In support, a comprehensive review of the persistence of disease agents is provided by Williams (2003).[21] Essential as this is to controlling onward infections of exotic disease among animals, other host pathogens such

Table 53.3 Qualitative exposure assessment template for public health hazards from carcase disposal options

| Disposal option A – assessment of public health risks | | | | | | | | | |
| Conceptual model | | | Risk assessment | | | | | Risk management/ residual risk | |
Hazard	Pathway	Receptor	Probability	Consequence	Size of risk	Justification	Key factors	Risk management	Residual risk
What is the hazard?	*What is the exposure route?*	*What receptor is exposed?*	*How likely is exposure? (H/M/L)*	*How severe are the effects (H/M/L)?*	*How big is the risk (H/M/L)?*	*What is this judgement based on?*	*What factors affect the level of risk?*	*How can the risk be managed?*	*What level of risk remains?*
Carbon monoxide	Release from pyres into air	Nearby residents	L	L	L	Significant quantities of carbon monoxide release are unlikely	Distance to houses	Ensure that pyres are not built near houses	L

H, high; M, medium; L, low.
Adapted from Department of Health,[8] with permission.

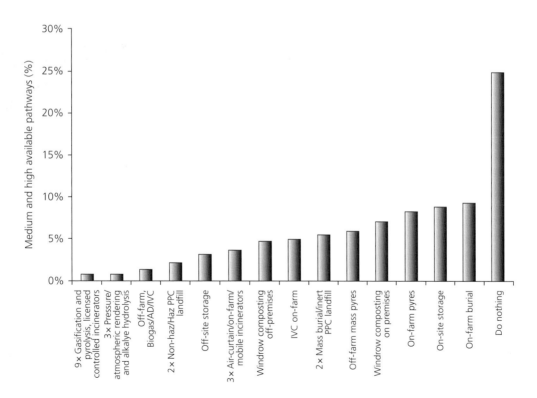

Figure 53.3 Percentage contribution of medium- and high-availability exposure pathways to total exposure associated with carcase disposal options (animal, human and environmental receptors).
AD, anaerobic digestion; Haz, hazardous waste; IVC, in-vessel composting; PPC, pollution, prevention and control regulated. Numbers denote the number of technology configurations in each class. For example nine types of processing facility fit the Gasification and pyrolysis class.

as *Campylobacter* spp., *Salmonella* spp., *Cryptosporidium*, *Escherichia coli* O157 and *Giardia* may prove equally if not more important hazards for other receptors (public health and environment), especially where the exotic disease agent dies with its host or is short-lived in the environment.

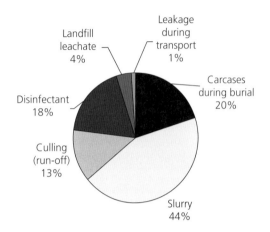

Figure 53.4   Sources of surface water pollution during the 2001 UK foot and mouth outbreak. (Adapted from Environment Agency,[11] with permission.)

SUMMARY

Governments that are in a heightened state of preparedness to manage animal disease outbreaks have undertaken generic analyses of carcase disposal options[3] so that decisions on their suitability are risk-informed; they have a developed capability for site-specific risk assessments[12] so that local environmental settings and exposures during actual disposals are accounted for; and they have made operational arrangements for the coordination of expert advice[18] from health departments, health agencies, veterinary officials, environment agencies, emergency planners, researchers and local operational partners, so that risk management is sensitive to real conditions 'on the ground' when decisions are required.[22] Flexible, adaptive management is required for emergency situations, informed by the range of risks associated with individual disposal strategies. Although outbreaks inevitably focus on the animal disease of concern, carcase disposal involves many more physical, chemical and biological hazards and the potential for psychological distress. An overemphasis on either a single zoonotic agent or individual waste-treatment technology may detract attention from the most potent agent of concern and so a systems-based analysis of exposure is vital.

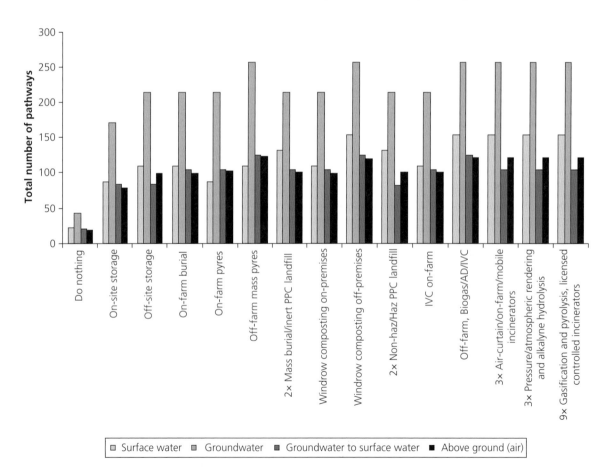

Figure 53.5   Relative importance of exposure pathways to overall exposure (all receptors). AD, anaerobic digestion; Haz, hazardous waste; IVC, in-vessel composting; PPC, pollution, prevention and control regulated. Numbers denote the number of technology configurations in each class. For example nine types of processing facility fit the Gasification and pyrolysis class.

REFERENCES

● = Key primary paper
◆ = Major review article

1. Anon. News and comment. Recommendations of the BSAVA working party on carcase disposal. *J Small Animal Pract* 1982; **23**:183–4.

●2. Pollard SJT, Hickman GAW, Irving P *et al.* Exposure assessment of carcase disposal options in the event of a notifiable exotic animal disease – methodology and application to avian influenza virus. *Environ Sci Technol* 2008; **42**: 3145–54.

◆3. National Agricultural Biosecurity Center. *Carcass Disposal: A Comprehensive Review. Report Prepared for the United States Department of Agriculture, Animal and Plant Health Inspection Service, National Agriculture Biosecurity Centre.* Manhattan, KS: Kansas State University, 2004.

●4. Hickman G, Hughes N. Carcase disposal: a major problem of the 2001 FMD outbreak. *State Vet J* 2002; **12**: 27–32.

5. Ellis DB. Carcass Disposal Issues in Recent Disasters, Accepted Methods and Suggested Plan to Mitigate Future Events. MBA thesis, Texas State University, 2001.

6. Department for Food, Environment and Rural Affairs. *A Risk-based Review of Carcass Disposal Options in the Event of a Notifiable Exotic Animal Disease – Methodology and Application to Avian Influenza*, Version 0.9. Prepared by Cranfield University for the State Veterinary Service, Contingency Planning Division, Contingency Plans and Disposals Branch. London: Defra, 2007.

●7. Scudamore JM, Trevelyan GM, Tas MV, Varley EM, Hickman GAW. Carcass disposal: lessons from Great Britain following the foot and mouth disease outbreaks of 2001. *Rev Sci Tech Off Int Epiz* 2002; **21**: 775–87.

8. Department of Health. *A Rapid Qualitative Assessment of Possible Risks to Public Health from Current Foot and Mouth Disposal Options. Main Report June 2001.* London: TSO, 2001.

9. Department for Environment, Food and Rural Affairs. Defra's Framework Response Plan for Exotic Animal Diseases (for Foot and Mouth Disease, Avian Influenza, Newcastle Disease, Classical Swine Fever, African Swine Fever and Swine Vesicular Disease). Presented to Parliament Pursuant to s14A of the Animal Health Act, 2002, v1.0, December 2006, Defra, London, 128pp. Available from: http://www.defra.gov.uk/animalh/diseases/control/contingency/exotic.htm (accessed June 2009).

10. Sullivan JB Jr, Kriger GR. *Hazardous Materials Toxicology. Clinical Principles of Environmental Health.* Baltimore: Williams & Wilkins, 1992.

◆11. Environment Agency. *The Environmental Impact of the Foot and Mouth Disease Outbreak: An Interim Assessment.* Bristol: Environment Agency, 2001.

12. Marsland PA, Smith JWN, Young CP. *Foot and Mouth Disease Epidemic. Disposal of Culled Stock by Burial: Guidance and Reference Data for the Protection of Controlled Waters.* NGWCLC report NC/02/04/01. Bristol: Environment Agency/WRc, 2003.

13. Lowles I, Hill R, Auld V, Stewart H, Colhoun C. Monitoring the pollution from a pyre used to destroy animal carcasses during the outbreak of foot and mouth disease in Cumbria, United Kingdom. *Atmos Environ* 2002; **36**: 2901–5.

14. Department of Health. *Foot and Mouth. Effects on Health of Emissions from Pyres Used for Disposal of Animals.* London: Department of Health/DETR/Food Standards Agency/Environment Agency/AEA Technology, 2001.

15. World Organization for Animal Health. *Terrestrial Animal Health Code (2006).* Paris: World Organization for Animal Health, 2006.

16. de Klerk PF. Carcass disposal: lessons from the Netherlands after the foot and mouth disease outbreak of 2001. *Rev Sci Tech Off Int Epiz* 2002; **21**: 789–96.

17. Annells DH, Williams GH, Coulton R, McKelvey P, Tas M. FMD burial site leachate disposal – a technical and commercial appraisal. Proceedings of the Aqua Enviro Management of Wastewater Conference, Edinburgh, 15–17 April, 2002. Part 2, pp. 245–58.

18. Environment Agency. *Avian Influenza Reference Guide,* Version 1.0. Bristol: Environment Agency, 2006.

19. DNV Technica. *Overview of Risks from BSE via Environmental Pathways for the Environment Agency.* Report C7243. London: DNV Technica, 1997.

◆20. Primary Industries Ministerial Council. *Australian Veterinary Emergency Plan. AUSVETPLAN. Operational Procedures Manual.* Disposal version 3.0. Canberra: Commonwealth of Australia, 2007.

◆21. Scott Williams Consulting Pty Ltd. *Persistence of Disease Agents in Carcases and Animal Products.* Report for Animal Health Australia, revised version. Deakin, ACT: Animal Health Australia/ Scott Williams Consulting Pty Ltd, 2003.

22. Texas Animal Health Commission. *Appendix 3.6.5. General Guidelines for the Disposal of Carcasses.* Austin, TX: Texas Animal Health Commission, 2005.

OTHER RESOURCES

- The US Department of Agriculture maintains a bibliography of papers and reports on the disposal of dead production animals at: http://www.nal.usda.gov/awic/pubs/carcass.htm
- National websites providing coordinated advice on carcase disposal are available for the UK at http://www.defra.gov.uk, for Australia at http://www.animalhealthaustralia.com.au and for the USA at http://www.aphis.usda.gov
- Key international web sites also maintain valuable information on carcase disposal:
  - European Commission's standing committee on the food chain and animal health: http://ec.europa.eu/food/committees/regulatory/scfcah/animal_health/index_en.htm
  - World Organisation for Animal Health: http://www.oie.int/eng/en_index.htm

Radiant energy

54

Radiofrequency radiation

DAVID COGGON

The radiofrequency (RF) band of the electromagnetic spectrum covers frequencies ranging from 3 kHz to 300 GHz, corresponding to wavelengths from 100 km down to 1 mm. Some RF electromagnetic fields are generated by sources in outer space, a natural phenomenon that is exploited by radiotelescopes. However, most of the RF fields to which we are exposed come from anthropogenic sources that have been developed largely over the past century. In particular, during the past two decades, there has been a rapid growth in the use of technology based on RF radiation for mobile telecommunications.

This development presents a challenge in the assessment and management of risk. If there are health hazards from the new technology, it is important that they be identified, characterized and controlled at the earliest opportunity. Otherwise, there is a danger that a substantial number of people could be harmed. On the other hand, an overprecautionary regulatory approach could be costly in lost opportunities for economic growth and improved standards of living. Moreover, in some circumstances, it could also have adverse consequences for health. For example, mobile phones have been used to summon help in emergency situations more rapidly than would otherwise have been possible.

This chapter describes the main sources of exposure to RF fields; the ways in which exposures can be characterized, quantified and measured; how RF fields can or might produce biological effects; and the types of evidence from in vitro, animal and human studies that bear on risk assessment for RF technology. The evidence base on the biological effects of RF fields is large, wide-ranging and continually evolving, and is not reviewed in detail here. Readers seeking a more detailed account should refer to authoritative systematic reviews such as those published by the Expert Panel of the Royal Society of Canada,[1] the Independent Expert Group on Mobile Phones,[2] the Health Council of the Netherlands,[3] the Advisory Group on Non-ionising Radiation[4] and the International Commission on Non-Ionizing Radiation Protection.[5]

SOURCES OF EXPOSURE

As indicated above, the RF fields to which we are exposed arise largely from manmade sources. The main uses of RF fields are for telecommunications and heating. Specific applications include: radio and television broadcasting; mobile (cell) phones; cordless phones; wireless local area networks (WiFi); other wireless communication between mobile devices (Bluetooth); satellite links (e.g. for radiolocation and radionavigation); electronic article surveillance and RF identification; radar; RF welding; induction heating; diathermy; and microwave ovens. Each of these technologies exploits particular bands of the RF spectrum. For the purposes of telecommunication, the radiation is modulated by the superimposition of lower-frequency signals, representing, for example, a spoken message. In addition, the RF radiation used in radar and in some forms of telecommunication is pulsed.

CHARACTERIZATION, QUANTIFICATION AND MEASUREMENT OF EXPOSURES

Electric and magnetic fields can be characterized in terms of their strength, their direction and the frequencies with which they vary over time. They can be measured externally to biological organisms, but their effects on tissues will depend on the internal fields that are generated thorough interaction between the organism and the external field.

External fields

The properties of RF electromagnetic fields alter with the distance from their source. At distances of more than a few wavelengths (the far-field region), electric and magnetic fields are at right angles to each other, are in phase and have a simple quantitative interrelation. In this circumstance, the strength of the fields can conveniently be quantified in terms of the radiated power density (measured in W/m^2), which is the product of the electric and magnetic fields. Power density normally falls off rapidly with distance from the source. Closer to the source, in the near-field region, the field structure is more complex, and power density is not a meaningful summary measure. Instead, electric and magnetic fields (measured in V/m and A/m) must be separately specified.

Instruments are available that can measure RF electric and magnetic fields (either in a single direction or in three orthogonal directions) in specified frequency ranges at a chosen location. In addition, body-mounted sensing instruments have now been developed that sample and log field measurements at repeated short intervals, thus providing information about external exposures over time at the point on the surface of the body where the instrument is located.

Table 54.1 gives some examples of typical field strengths or power densities produced by common sources of RF fields. It should be noted that public exposures from mobile phone base stations (masts) are orders of magnitude lower than those from mobile phone handsets.

Internal fields

At frequencies less than 100 kHz (as are used for some applications in radiolocation, electronic article surveillance and induction heating), the index of internal dose most closely related to biological effects is the electric field strength in the tissue. At higher frequencies, however, the most relevant measure of dose is the specific (energy) absorption rate, which is related to the square of the electric field strength in the tissue.

The electric field strengths and specific absorption rate in tissues that are produced by an external field can be estimated by numerical calculation or from experiments in which small measuring probes are inserted into models of the relevant body parts (phantoms), which contain fluids with electrical properties similar to the average value for exposed tissues. As frequency increases, the absorption of energy becomes increasingly confined to the surface layers of the body, and above 30 GHz it is largely limited to the skin.

INTERACTION WITH BIOLOGICAL TISSUES

The only well-established mechanism by which RF fields cause biological effects is through the rise in temperature that occurs when energy is absorbed from an oscillating electric field. The heat is produced through resistance to the currents that are generated when the fields cause the movement of ions and other charged objects. Thermal effects of this type are the basis for current regulatory limits on exposure to RF fields in the UK and many other countries. There has, however, been much speculation over whether biological effects might occur at levels of exposure insufficient to cause significant heating.

Higher frequency electromagnetic radiation such as X-rays and gamma rays can cause direct damage to DNA, leading to mutations and an increased risk of cancer.

Table 54.1 Typical field strengths and power densities produced by common sources of radiofrequency fields

Exposure scenario	Typical exposure
Public exposure to electronic article surveillance midway between panels when entering or leaving premises	Up to 20 A/m
Occupational exposure at 50 m from an AM broadcast mast	450 V/m
Public exposure at 1500 m from a 300 kW FM radio mast	4 V/m
Maximum public exposure at ground level from a high power 1 MW television transmitter mast	3 V/m
2.2 cm from a 2 W GSM mobile phone handset	400 V/m, 0.8 A/m
Public exposure at 50 m from a GSM mobile phone base station operating at a maximum of 50 W per channel	1 mW/m^2 (0.6 V/m, 1.6 mA/m)
50 cm from a microwave oven leaking at the British Standards Institute emission limit	0.5 W/m^2
Public exposure at 3 m from a 100 mW speed check radar	$<2.5 W/m^2$

GSM, global system for mobile communication.

However, RF radiation is non-ionizing, and its energy quanta (up to 1.2 MeV) are much smaller than those needed to break even the weakest chemical bonds in DNA. Thus, it seems unlikely that RF radiation could damage DNA directly.

Other mechanisms of non-thermal biological interaction that have been proposed include: induction of the resonant movement of charged ions in cells; an effect on the attraction between cells because they become electrically polarized in the applied field; an effect on the non-linear electrical properties of cell membranes; an effect on the folding of proteins; the demodulation of signals by tissues so that they are subject to lower frequency fields (e.g. at the frequency with which a transmission is pulsed); and an effect on chemical reactions through a mechanism involving radical ion pairs.[2,4] However, each of these hypotheses has theoretical weaknesses, and none is supported by consistent experimental evidence. Thus, there is no clear biophysical pointer to specific types of biological effects that might be produced by RF fields at levels of exposure insufficient to cause significant heating of the tissues.

STUDIES IN VITRO AND IN WHOLE ANIMALS

The potential biological effects of RF fields have been intensively investigated, particularly since the advent of mobile phone technology. Much of this research has been carried out in vitro (e.g. in isolated cells, cell or tissue cultures, or slices of living brain) and in whole animals, with a particular focus on possible non-thermal effects. A wide range of potential effects have been studied (Boxes 54.1 and 54.2).

The interpretation of findings is complicated by the variety of experimental systems that have been employed, many of which are not standardized. In addition, the exposures tested have differed in their intensity, frequency

---

> **BOX 54.1: Biological outcomes for which possible effects of radiofrequency fields have been studied in vitro**
>
> - Movement of ions across cell membranes
> - Calcium efflux from brain tissue
> - Excitability of neurones
> - Release of neurotransmitters
> - Ornithine decarboxylase activity in cells
> - Gene expression in cells
> - Cell transformation and proliferation
> - Mutation of DNA
> - Chromosomal aberrations
> - Sister chromatid exchanges
> - Formation of micronuclei
> - Other DNA damage (e.g. by comet assay)
> - Enzyme activity

> **BOX 54.2: Biological outcomes for which possible effects of radiofrequency fields have been studied in whole animals**
>
> - Integrity of the blood–brain barrier
> - Release of neurotransmitters
> - Electroencephalography
> - Thermoregulatory behaviour
> - Other aspects of behaviour
> - Learning and memory
> - Secretion of melatonin
> - Cataract formation and other changes in the eye
> - Gene expression (e.g. for heat-shock protein)
> - Mutation of DNA
> - DNA damage
> - Cancer incidence
> - Promotion of cancers induced by known genotoxic carcinogens
> - Immune responses
> - Longevity and general physical condition
> - Reproduction and development
> - Cardiovascular function

---

and modulation. In some cases, it is difficult to determine from published reports exactly what exposure was applied, and whether or not it could have produced significant heating of the target cells or tissues. Thus, where studies have generated apparently conflicting results, it may be unclear whether the discrepancy is attributable to differences in the exposure that was tested, differences in the experimental method or chance variation.

Systematic reviews have found that the overall evidence for non-thermal biological effects of RF fields is inconsistent.[2,4] Where apparent effects have been observed, they have typically been small, making them difficult to discriminate from random background variation. Moreover, attempts to replicate positive findings have generally been unsuccessful. There is still substantial uncertainty about some of the effects investigated, but the available body of evidence suggests that RF fields at levels insufficient to raise temperature are not genotoxic and do not initiate or promote cancer in animals. Thus, while new evidence continues to emerge, there are currently no well-established biological effects of RF fields at exposure levels that do not cause significant heating of the tissues.

STUDIES IN HUMANS

Research on human subjects provides the other major source of information on the potential health risks from RF fields. Both experimental and observational methods have been used.

Experimental studies

Experimental studies have been used to investigate possible short-term effects of RF fields, including the induction of symptoms and changes in neurophysiological outcomes such as cognitive function and patterns of brain activity on an electroencephalogram. The exposures studied have generally been designed to mimic those from mobile phones or mobile phone base stations. A particular focus has been the phenomenon of 'electrical hypersensitivity', in which a minority of susceptible people experience symptoms such as headache, fatigue and giddiness when they are near to electrical equipment and sources of RF fields.

As yet, experimental studies have not clearly demonstrated any effects of RF fields at levels of exposure insufficient to cause significant heating of tissues. A few positive findings have been reported from individual investigations, but these have not been independently replicated and may have occurred simply by chance. The balance of evidence from experiments in which 'blinded' participants have been randomly assigned to real or sham RF exposures and asked to report symptoms and sensations indicates that neither normal nor 'electrosensitive' subjects can detect exposure, and that symptoms in electrosensitive people are determined by perceived rather than actual exposure. This suggests that electrical hypersensitivity occurs through psychological mechanisms rather than a direct noxious effect of RF fields.

Observational epidemiology

Epidemiological studies have explored the relationship of RF fields to a wide range of health outcomes (Box 54.3). Most investigations have focused on possible longer term effects of exposure. In addition, cross-sectional surveys have been used to assess the prevalence of electrical hypersensitivity in various populations.

Box 54.4 lists the main sources of exposure that have been investigated epidemiologically. Many earlier studies looked at relatively high occupational exposures from sources such as radio and radar transmitters and short-wave diathermy. More recently, however, the main emphasis has been on exposures related to mobile phone technology, from either handsets or base stations. With regard to exposure from handsets, particular attention has been given to possible risks of brain cancer, meningioma, acoustic neuroma and carcinoma of the parotid gland, since these tumours occur in the tissues that are closest to the handset antenna, and are therefore the most heavily exposed.

There is good evidence from observations in humans that heat injury can occur from unusually high exposures to RF fields, for example as a consequence of failed protective interlocks on microwave ovens. In addition, a

---

BOX 54.3: Health outcomes that have been investigated in epidemiological studies

- Brain tumours
- Acoustic neuroma
- Parotid gland tumours
- Uveal melanoma
- Testicular cancer
- Leukaemia
- Lymphoma
- Male and female sexual function and fertility
- Spontaneous abortion
- Birth outcome and congenital malformations
- Cataract
- Functional disturbances of the nervous and cardiovascular systems (headache, fatigue, irritability, loss of appetite, sleepiness, sweating, difficulty with concentration and memory, depression, emotional instability, bradycardia, tachycardia, hypertension and abnormalities of cardiac conduction)
- Haematological abnormalities

BOX 54.4: Sources of exposure that have been investigated in epidemiological studies

- Radio and radar antennas
- Microwave ovens
- Radiofrequency sealers
- Plastic welding machines
- Diathermy used in physiotherapy
- Mobile phone base stations
- Mobile phone handsets

---

phenomenon known as 'microwave hearing', characterized by the perception of buzzing, clicking or popping sounds, is a well-established effect of exposure to pulse-modulated RF radiation at levels in excess of $4\,\text{W/m}^2$ with frequencies in the range from $200\,\text{MHz}$ to $6.5\,\text{GHz}$. This arises through the thermoelastic expansion and contraction of soft tissues in the head, and is not thought to have any long-term consequences.

Otherwise, epidemiological studies have not clearly indicated any adverse effects of RF fields. Where positive results have been reported, they have been inconsistent between studies, in some cases possibly because of biases in the methods of investigation. In particular, a number of case–control studies have indicated an increased risk of brain cancer on the side of the head on which subjects report that they normally hold a mobile phone. However, the same studies have tended to find a reduced risk of brain tumours on the side opposite to that on which the phone is reported to be held. This suggests a bias from differential recall. Many people will not always hold a phone on the same side of the head, and those who do not may preferentially report that they have used a mobile phone on a particular side if they know that they have developed a tumour on that side.

There are limits, however, to the reassurance of safety that can be drawn from the absence of epidemiological evidence for long-term health hazards from mobile phones and other sources of RF fields. One major constraint is the accuracy with which exposures can be characterized and quantified, particularly in retrospective studies. For example, studies of illness and disease in relation to radio and radar transmitters have often used the distance of residence from the transmitter as an index of exposure. However, exposures do not always fall off as a simple function of distance from the source. Moreover, people differ in the proportion of their time that they spend at home, and when elsewhere, their exposures may be quite different.

Studies of exposures from mobile phones are often limited by the accuracy with which participants can recall their frequency and duration of phone usage. Furthermore, even if usage could be accurately ascertained (e.g. through the use of mobile phone operators' billing records), difficulties would remain in assessing other factors that modify the exposures of relevant tissues, such as the exact position of the phone's antenna, and the power with which it transmits (which will vary according to distance from the base station with which it is communicating). Further challenges arise in assessing exposure to other possible sources of RF fields such as cordless phones and WiFi, which must also be taken into account.

Another limitation of the current evidence base is that adverse effects might in some way depend on the specific frequency and modulation of RF fields. Thus, an absence of detectable hazard from, say, television transmitters would not necessarily imply that mobile phone emissions were safe. Frequency bands and signal characteristics have changed in each successive generation of mobile phones, and if there were a delayed effect specific to the latest generation (e.g. a risk of cancer following a long induction period), this would not be apparent in the epidemiological studies carried out to date because too short a period has elapsed since the phones came into use. There is currently no known or strongly suspected mechanism whereby biological tissues could demodulate RF fields so that they were sensitive to fields with specific signal characteristics. The possibility cannot, however, be confidently ruled out.

OVERVIEW

Overall, therefore, current evidence provides no strong pointers to adverse health effects of RF fields other than those mediated through the heating of tissues. Uncertainties remain, however, particularly in relation to possible longer term effects of fields produced by the newest radiocommunication devices, which use different frequencies and patterns of modulation from earlier technology. Given the widespread and still growing use of such devices, this is an indication for continued research and vigilance.

REFERENCES

◆ = Major review article

◆1. Royal Society of Canada Expert Panel Report. *A Review of the Potential Health Risks of Radiofrequency Fields from Wireless Telecommunication Devices. An Expert Panel Report Prepared at the Request of The Royal Society of Canada for Health Canada.* Publication No. RSC/EPR 99-1. Ottawa: Royal Society of Canada, 1999.

◆2. Independent Expert Group on Mobile Phones. *Mobile Phones and Health.* Chilton: NRPB, 2000.

◆3. Health Council of the Netherlands. *Mobile Telephones: An Evaluation of Health Effects.* Publication No. 2002/01E. The Hague: Health Council of the Netherlands, 2002.

◆4. Advisory Group on Non-ionising Radiation. Health effects from radiofrequency electromagnetic fields. *Documents of the NRPB* 2003; **14**(2).

◆5. International Commission for Non-Ionizing Radiation Protection Standing Committee on Epidemiology: Ahlbom A, Green A, Kheifets L, Savitz D, Swerdlow A. Epidemiology of health effects of radiofrequency exposure. *Environ Health Perspect* 2004; **112**: 1741-54.

55

Power-frequency electric and magnetic fields

LEEKA KHEIFETS, JOHN SWANSON

HISTORICAL OVERVIEW

Human beings, in common with all other forms of life on this planet, have evolved in the presence of static electric and magnetic fields (EMFs; the earth's static magnetic field, and static electric fields produced in the atmosphere). There are also very low levels of alternating fields at some frequencies as a result of natural processes. However, significant exposure to alternating EMFs has arisen only over the last century and a half, starting with the first public electricity supplies in the 1880s, and has risen since as the use of electricity has become more widespread.

The most obvious danger of electricity, electrocution, has been familiar through all this time. Although in the early days of electricity, fear of the unknown led to some concern about other health effects, there was no serious scientific concern about health risks other than electrocution until the 1960s, when suggestions emerged from Russia of lethargy, impotence, insomnia and similar symptoms in substation workers. However, the real start of the present ongoing scientific concern was in 1979, with the publication of an epidemiological study[1] linking childhood cancer to proximity to electricity distribution and transmission facilities.

Since then, further epidemiological studies finding associations between various measures of exposure to power-frequency magnetic fields and childhood cancer, in particular childhood leukaemia, have established this as a genuine scientific concern. Other epidemiological studies have looked at a wide range of other health effects in relation to magnetic and electric fields, sometimes finding associations and sometimes not, but without the same consistency as exists for childhood leukaemia and magnetic

fields. Laboratory studies have not supported a link between exposure to power-frequency EMFs and disease.

In the public arena, concern about EMFs is often associated with concern about the facilities that produce them and often surfaces as opposition to overhead power lines. The early epidemiological studies on EMFs are now considered methodologically weak, and it is probably fair to conclude that the initial scientific effort devoted to EMFs was a response to public rather than to scientific concern. However, later studies have been better conducted, and the EMF issue now stands as an unresolved public health issue (albeit probably one with a limited public health impact) that merits further research to resolve it.

INTRODUCTION TO EXTREMELY-LOW-FREQUENCY EMFS

A 'field' is a concept used to express the influence that an electric charge has on other charges in its vicinity. Fields exist wherever electricity is used, following well established laws of physics; it is not possible to use or to transmit electricity without producing EMFs.

At power frequencies (50 or 60 Hz depending on the country) the two fields, electric and magnetic, are essentially separate entities. Electric fields are produced by voltages and are independent of the current; magnetic fields depend on current and are independent of voltage. Both fall with distance from the source. In practical electrical circuits, where there has to be a 'go' and a 'return', both fields also depend on the physical separation of the component conductors. A key difference is that electric

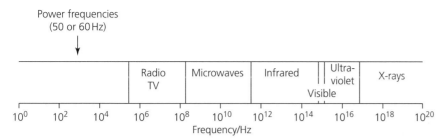

Figure 55.1 The electromagnetic spectrum.

fields are perturbed by conducting objects; in particular, the electric field produced by a source outside a home is largely screened inside the home by the building structure. Magnetic fields are perturbed very little by normal building materials or by human beings.

Power-frequency EMFs are part of the continuous electromagnetic spectrum (Figure 55.1), but the properties of fields are highly dependent on the frequency. At radio frequencies and above, including the frequencies used by cellular communications, the two fields are coupled together and propagate through space as radiation. The established way in which such fields interact with the body is by causing heating. Power-frequency fields, in the 'extremely-low-frequency' or ELF range, with frequencies millions or hundreds of millions times lower, have very different properties. The radiofrequency and power-frequency EMF issues should be regarded as separate issues (see Chapter 54).

In addition, at even lower frequencies, are static fields, notably the earth's magnetic field. Power-frequency magnetic fields are usually substantially smaller than the earth's static field and can therefore be regarded as a ripple superimposed on top of it. For any biological effect that depended on the total field, the result, averaged over times longer than a single cycle, would, to first order, be due just to the earth's field; the alternating field could have at most only a second-order effect. But any biological effect that depended specifically on the alternating component would, of course, not be affected by the earth's field.

EXPOSURES

Sources of exposure

The most common source of magnetic field in homes, present wherever there is an electricity supply, is the low-voltage distribution wiring carrying electricity to the home. The field is sometimes dominated by currents in the wiring within the home. Most countries wire their distribution systems in a way that results in the 'go' and 'return' currents in each circuit not being exactly equal; there is an out-of-balance current, and it is principally these out-of-balance currents, usually called 'net' or 'ground' currents, that produce the field. This 'background' field is present over the whole volume of every home and does not greatly depend on whether the distribution wiring is overhead or underground.

In addition to the background field, there are localized areas of higher magnetic field produced by domestic electrical appliances when they are operating, usually falling to background levels within a metre or so of the appliance.

Magnetic fields are also produced by high-voltage transmission lines. Fields from such lines typically fall to background levels within 100 m or less. Only a small fraction of homes are this close to such lines, but for homes which are, the high-voltage power line becomes the principal source of the magnetic field inside the home.

Electric fields from sources outside the home are less significant inside the home because of screening by the building materials, so electric fields in homes come mainly from internal sources, such as house wiring and appliances, and tend to be more variable over the area of the home than magnetic fields.

Levels of exposure

Magnetic fields are measured in teslas (T) or the more practical unit microteslas (μT or millionth of tesla). Electric fields are measured in volts per metre (V/m) or kilovolts per metre (kV/m).

The 'exposure' of a person to magnetic fields is usually expressed as the time-average of the field. The field from domestic appliances is experienced only when a person is quite close to them, and in most cases, exposure is therefore of short duration. Therefore, although appliances usually provide the highest instantaneous exposure of an individual to power-frequency fields over the course of a day, time-average exposure from them is limited, being estimated variously as 50 per cent or less of total time-average exposure. However, mobile phones (which produce ELF as well as radiofrequency fields) and computers are increasingly used for long periods close to the body by children and may now contribute more to time-weighted average exposure.

For adults at work, occupational exposure is significant, but other than occupational exposure, and particularly for young children, exposure outside the home tends not to be a major source. Most studies of environmental exposure therefore focus on the field in the home. In most countries, the distribution across homes of the average field in each home forms a log-normal distribution, which is best described by the geometric mean. For those countries where information is available, the geometric mean can be as low as 0.01 μT in some European countries,

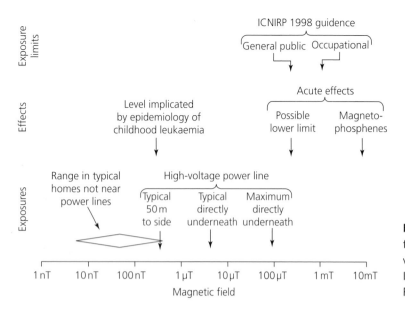

Figure 55.2 Comparison of levels of magnetic field, produced by various sources, needed to produce various effects in the body, and set as exposure limits. ICNIRP, International Commission on Non-Ionizing Radiation Protection.

up to perhaps $0.1\,\mu T$ in parts of the USA. In individual homes close to power lines, fields can reach several microteslas. The different levels in different countries can be understood in terms of different wiring practices and electricity consumption.[2,3]

Epidemiological studies, discussed later, have implicated long-term average fields of greater than 0.3 or $0.4\,\mu T$ in homes as being associated with an increased risk of childhood leukaemia. The fraction of such homes in the population is a key parameter. This varies from 0.4 per cent in the UK to 5 per cent in North America.[2,3] These various field levels are summarized in Figure 55.2.

ACUTE EFFECTS

Acute effects on the body

The principal established biological effect of these fields is that they induce electric fields and therefore also currents in the body.[4] The effect that is usually the first to be noticed is described by the term magnetophosphenes, a flickering sensation in the periphery of vision that can also be produced by pressure on the eyeball, by mechanical shock or by a direct application of weak electric currents to the head. It is produced by currents induced in the retina, and the threshold current density for the induction of magnetophosphenes is approximately $50\,mV/m$ or $10\,mA/m^2$ at 20 Hz, with the threshold for 50 or 60 Hz currents being higher.

This is a fairly subtle effect, and is not usually regarded as harmful in itself but as evidence of effects on neural tissue and therefore of potential harm from other effects. Actual harm or clearly undesirable effects, such as muscle stimulation, are manifest only at higher fields, typically above $1\,A/m^2$. On the other hand, induced fields may theoretically be able to affect networks of interconnected neurones at lower levels than are required to produce

magnetophosphenes, although this has not been experimentally demonstrated.

In addition, electric fields can produce direct effects on the body through causing body hairs to vibrate, and indirectly through inducing charge. When a person and a conducting object touch, one grounded but the other isolated and therefore with a charge induced on it, the charge is transferred as a small discharge or 'microshock'. Because it is concentrated on a small area of the skin, it can be painful, but it is not usually regarded as harmful. Thresholds for these acute effects of electric fields vary across individuals, but are typically 5–$10\,kV/m$ for direct perception and a few kV/m, depending on the size of the object touched, for microshocks.[5]

Effects on implanted medical devices

The most common implanted medical device is the pacemaker, but other devices include defibrillators, cochlear implants and neurostimulators. Electric and magnetic fields can cause interference usually through the sensing electrodes. The sensitivity of these devices depends on manufacturer and design, and in some cases even varies between units of the same issue. The threshold for magnetic field interference appears to be in the range of 200–$1200\,\mu T$, and for electric field interference above 1.5–$2\,kV/m$.[6] Pacemakers with bipolar sensing leads, which are now more common, are less sensitive than this, and interference is rare in practice.[7]

Exposure limits

The acute effects on the body described above are well established, and exposure limits have therefore been set to protect against them. A few countries have developed their own exposure limits, but increasing use is being made of the limits published by the International Commission on Non-Ionizing Radiation Protection (ICNIRP).[8] These protect against induced currents by setting a basic restriction for public exposure on the induced current density in the central nervous system of $2\,mA/m^2$. Numerical modelling[9–11] suggests that this corresponds to a uniform, unperturbed external field of roughly $360\,\mu T$ and $9\,kV/m$ (see Figure 55.2). Normal design considerations, for example for power lines, mean that most environmental exposures comply with these levels, even in countries where it is not a requirement, although the highest-voltage power lines can exceed $9\,kV/m$ in rare circumstances.

CHRONIC EFFECTS

Reviews of chronic effects

In addition to these established acute effects, there are suggestions of chronic effects, principally epidemiological evidence that magnetic fields are associated with an increased risk of childhood leukaemia. The evidence has been reviewed by several authoritative bodies, and we summarize it here to give an overview before discussing the evidence in more detail. The ICNIRP[8] does not regard the evidence as strong enough to form the basis for exposure limits. Consistent with this, the International Agency for Research on Cancer (IARC) classified magnetic fields as 'possibly carcinogenic' (group 2B carcinogen) in 2001,[12] and the World Health Organization (WHO) reaffirmed this classification in 2005.[3] The classification is based on 'limited' evidence in humans and 'inadequate' evidence in animals; the 'limited' evidence in humans was provided by epidemiological studies of childhood leukaemia.

The reviews by the IARC[12] and WHO[3] provide comprehensive coverage of the scientific literature. We do not attempt to give detailed references for each possible health effect we consider here, but instead refer readers to these reviews.

Strands of evidence

The evidence for chronic effects of EMFs is almost entirely epidemiological, and accordingly much of the remainder of this chapter is devoted to this evidence. However, we will first briefly consider the main other strands of evidence.

OVERVIEW OF LABORATORY EVIDENCE

Laboratory work has essentially failed to find any reliable and reproducible evidence of the effects of magnetic fields at environmental levels on biological systems, either in vivo or in vitro.

It is estimated that many hundreds of studies have now been published. Most of these have been negative. A number have, however, reported positive findings, which

has led to attempted but failed replications. As a result, positive findings in EMF studies are treated with scepticism: replication by independent laboratories is regarded as essential. This has led to the general conclusion that robust evidence for effects remains lacking.

Specifically, a number of large-scale, well-conducted animal studies have examined EMFs as a possible carcinogen. These studies[3,12] include several long-term animal carcinogenicity studies of the type widely used to assess risks to humans. Some of these assays involved both sexes, two different species and a large number of animals. Animals were studied over the course of their lifetimes for survival and clinical signs of neoplasia, and detailed post mortem examinations were undertaken. Nearly all these studies found no suggestion of an increased incidence of cancer.

In addition to studies of spontaneous tumour development, numerous assays have evaluated EMFs as a promoter or co-promoter of carcinogenesis in animal models. Animals in these studies were genetically modified to be predisposed to cancer and/or were treated with a known initiator or a complete carcinogen, such as ionizing radiation or a carcinogenic chemical. The animals were then exposed to EMFs over a period of months. These studies have also been largely negative. It should be noted, however, that a good animal model of childhood leukaemia is lacking.[3,12]

OVERVIEW OF MECHANISMS

If there is a biological effect of environmental-level EMFs, it must be mediated through a physical interaction between the field and a biological system. This has been explored through theoretical investigations, in particular testing whether any proposed mechanism could produce an effect large enough to be detectable above the changes to biological systems that occur all the time naturally, for example as a result of random thermal motion of molecules. No such mechanism has been identified; the mechanisms that come closest are the induction of currents, and the effects of magnetic fields on magnetite particles or on the spin of free radicals.[13]

Introduction to the epidemiology of EMFs

For children, it is reasonable to approximate total exposure to the background field in the home. Accordingly, this is what most epidemiological studies of children have measured. Some have additionally investigated exposure in schools, but without significant effects on the findings. Some have separately assessed exposure from individual appliances, but with limited accuracy. A few studies have attempted to measure actual personal exposure with meters, but issues of the child's behaviour changing with age and particularly following diagnosis and treatment mean that these are usually regarded as prone to bias. Accordingly, epidemiological evidence for children almost entirely concerns exposure to background fields in homes. For largely practical reasons, most epidemiological studies of children have investigated the home occupied at the time of diagnosis of the disease, for example cancer, with only a few investigating previous homes or the home at birth.

For adults, there are some occupations that result in exposures larger than residential exposures, and most epidemiological studies in adults have focused on occupational rather than residential exposure. A smaller number of studies of adults have looked at residential exposure, and fewer still combine the two to estimate total exposure. As a result, almost all evidence concerning EMFs and disease in adults relates to occupational rather than environmental exposure and is not covered here in any detail.

Epidemiological evidence on childhood leukaemia

The disease for which the evidence of a link with EMFs is strongest, and also the disease which has been most investigated, is childhood leukaemia. With over 20 studies having been reported, it is possible to focus on only the methodologically better studies. These are characterized by better exposure assessments, in particular having either measurements of the field in the home extending for 24 hours or longer, or a reasonably reliable calculation of the field from external sources. Nine such studies were pooled in an analysis by Ahlbom et al. in 2000.[14] A different pooled analysis that included all available studies regardless of quality found similar results.[15] Subsequent studies[16,17] have found similar results. The results from the key studies are summarized in Table 55.1.

These pooled analyses find an association between elevated magnetic fields and childhood leukaemia. This finding has often been presented in terms of an elevated relative risk in the highest exposure category (in Ahlbom et al.'s pooled analysis,[14] 2.00 [95 per cent confidence interval 1.27–3.13] for field in the home >0.4 μT; in Greenland et al.'s analysis,[15] 1.7 for a field >0.3 μT), with no elevation of risk in the lower exposure categories. However, the data could also be seen as compatible with a progressive increase in risk.

The association is remarkably consistent across studies. Not only has it been reported in many countries, but it is also found in studies with two different designs. One involves research workers entering homes to measure the fields. This approach is subject to selection and

Table 55.1   Result from key epidemiological studies (listed in reference [14]) of magnetic fields and childhood leukaemia, relative risks (confidence intervals)

Study	0.1–<0.2 μT	0.2–<0.4 μT	≥0.4 μT	≥0.4 μT Observed	Expected
Measurement studies					
Canada	1.29 (0.84–1.99)	1.39 (0.78–2.48)	1.55 (0.65–3.68)	13	10.3
Germany	1.24 (0.58–2.62	1.67 (0.48–5.83)	2.00 (0.26–15.17)	2	0.9
New Zealand	0.67 (0.20–2.20)	4 cases/0 controls	0 cases/0 controls	0	0
UK	0.84 (0.57–1.24)	0.98 (0.50–1.93)	1.00 (0.30–3.37)	4	4.4
USA	1.11 (0.81–1.53)	1.01 (0.65–1.57)	3.44 (1.24–9.54)	17	4.7
Calculated field studies					
Denmark	2.68 (0.24–30.45)	0 cases/8 controls	2 cases/0 controls	2	0
Finland	0 cases/19 controls	4.11 (0.48–35.1)	6.21 (0.68–56.9)	1	0.2
Norway	1.75 (0.65–4.72)	1.06 (0.21–5.22)	0 cases/10 controls	0	2.7
Sweden	1.75 (0.48–6.37)	0.57 (0.07–4.65)	3.74 (1.23–11.37)	5	1.5
Summary					
Measurement studies	1.05 (0.86–1.28)	1.15 (0.85–1.54)	1.87 (1.10–3.18)	36	20.1
Calculated field studies	1.58 (0.77–3.25)	0.79 (0.27–2.28)	2.13 (0.93–4.88)	8	4.4
All studies	1.08 (0.89–1.31)	1.11 (0.84–1.47)	2.00 (1.27–3.13)	44	24.2
Key studies subsequent to those in reference [14]					
Germany[16,24]	1.10 (0.75–1.60)	1.58 (0.74–3.36)	2.48 (0.70–8.86)	5	
Japan[17]	0.91 (0.50–1.63)	1.12 (0.53–2.36)	2.56 (0.76–8.58)	6	

Total leukaemia. Relative risks (95 per cent confidence interval in parentheses) by exposure level with adjustment for age, sex and socioeconomic status (measurement studies) and East/West in Germany. Reference level: <0.1 μT. Observed and expected case numbers ≥0.4 μT, with expected numbers given by modelling probability of membership of each exposure category based on distribution of controls including co-variates.
Based on Table 3, Ahlbom et al.,[14] with permission.

participation bias but captures all sources of residential exposure. The other involves calculation of the fields in homes resulting from proximity to high-voltage power lines outside homes, with no subject participation. This approach is less (if at all) subject to bias, but the exposure assessment is more limited (where the power line produces a high field, the calculated field is usually a good measure of the total field in the home, but as the field reduces, the power-line field becomes a less good predictor of the total field).

Exposure to magnetic fields in homes is related to socioeconomic status, so participation bias could potentially affect the results of some studies, particularly those which require entry into the home to measure fields and require the subjects' consent. In addition, whereas some studies have selected controls from population or health-service registers that should be practically complete and therefore free from bias, others have selected controls from insurance registers or by a random dialling of telephone numbers, both of which often introduce bias. The operation of bias so as to elevate the risk ratio has been demonstrated in at least one study: reanalysis (using, perforce, a simpler exposure assessment that did not require subject consent) including some subjects who declined to participate in the original study reduced the relative risk.[18]

The remaining question is whether the amount of bias present is enough to account for the risk found. Theoretical analyses suggest that bias would have to be quite large to explain the existing findings. In addition, bias does not appear able to explain the results of studies that selected controls from population registers and did not require subject participation; the results from only such studies, although statistically weaker than the total evidence, still show an elevation for childhood leukaemia.[19]

The majority of studies have been conducted in countries similar in terms of electrical practice and socioeconomic development: in Europe and in North America. Such evidence as there is from other parts of the world (e.g. from Japan[17]) is supportive, but there is no reliable evidence from developing countries. No confounding has been identified (and theoretical analyses indicate that any confounding factor would have to be both a large risk factor in itself and highly associated with magnetic fields to explain the results found). In particular, although it is likely that there is an association between exposure to magnetic fields and socioeconomic status, adjusting for the latter does not seem to affect the results of the studies.

Proximity to power lines and hence exposure to the fields they produce is associated both with other physical factors produced by power lines and with socioeconomic factors. It is possible, but not established, that one of these factors could act as a confounding factor in studies specifically of power lines. A specific suggestion is that ionization of the air by the high electric fields close to high-voltage power lines ('corona ions') may increase the risk of some health effects by interacting with airborne pollutants,[20] although modelling suggests that any such effect would not be quantitatively significant.[21] Attention has been focused on this possibility by a recent study that found a similar increase in risk to other studies close to the power lines, but also found that the increased risk extended too far to be explicable in terms of magnetic fields.[22] Another suggestion is that magnetic fields are associated with small voltages on house plumbing systems, which could cause small currents to flow through the bone marrow of children, for example during bathing.[23] This suggestion also remains quantitatively speculative.

A number of subsidiary issues have been investigated but without any clear answer emerging, primarily because the number of subjects in the studies is too low. Such issues include whether the increased risk is associated with any specific subtype of leukaemia, whether the aetiologically relevant period for exposure is close to diagnosis or some other period, and whether time-weighted average exposure (implicitly or explicitly used in most studies) is the correct metric of the field. A suggestion that the risk is specific to exposure at night-time has not been sustained.[24]

There is some preliminary suggestion that magnetic field exposure may be related to prognosis as well as to incidence,[25,26] but this has not been fully investigated. Some studies have investigated childhood leukaemia as a possible consequence of parental exposure but with no consistent results.

If magnetic fields do cause childhood leukaemia, the increase in average exposure consequent upon increased electricity use should have led to an increase in childhood leukaemia rates, although this could be masked by changes in other risk factors. The rate of childhood leukaemia is indeed increasing in Western countries, but the correlation between exposure and leukaemia rates has too much statistical uncertainty to allow any meaningful conclusion. Viewed over the whole of the twentieth century, however, the major increases in leukaemia rate (the first half of the century) and electricity consumption (the second half of the century) came at different times, arguing against a link.[27]

The preceding discussion has related to magnetic fields. Seven studies have looked at electric fields, with a variety of exposure assessment techniques, and almost uniformly null results.[28]

Evidence on other health effects

OTHER CHILDHOOD CANCERS

There are no other childhood cancers for which the same volume of studies exists as for childhood leukaemia, and no similarly coherent pattern of results has emerged.

For central nervous system/brain tumours, there have been around a dozen studies, of which perhaps six are of a comparable quality to the studies of leukaemia included in the pooled analysis. These studies suggest there may be a slightly elevated risk in the highest exposure category, but this is based on small numbers, and the estimate of increased risk is very imprecise.[29] Some studies have found elevated risks for all cancers combined, but where other cancers have been investigated as a separate group, generally no increase has been found.

ADULT LEUKAEMIA AND BRAIN TUMOURS

Of the studies specifically related to environmental as opposed to occupational exposure, five studies of adult leukaemia have consistently failed to find elevated risks, and four studies of brain cancer were likewise generally negative, albeit with isolated findings of a risk in specific subtypes.

The vast bulk of evidence on these cancers, however, comes from occupational studies, where there are around 50 studies each. The results are, however, inconsistent. While meta-analysis[30] shows statistically significant risk ratios of 1.2 or less, the small risks, the inconsistencies between studies, the failure of more recent studies to strengthen the observed association and the lack of an exposure–response relationship argue against magnetic fields being responsible for the observed excess risk.

OTHER ADULT CANCERS

Early studies of breast cancer produced mixed results. However, more recent studies, generally larger and carefully conducted, have generally been negative, and overall, the epidemiological evidence does not now indicate an association with breast cancer.

There are no particular suggestions of a link to any other adult cancers.

REPRODUCTIVE DISORDERS

There is little evidence of developmental malformations in children (or of subsequent leukaemia risk in children) as a result of parental exposure, or evidence of teratogenic effects in animals.

Two studies of miscarriage in California[31,32] found an association not with average exposure, but with the mother's peak exposure to magnetic fields during the pregnancy. This result has been treated with caution as, first, peak exposure generally comes from a close approach to domestic appliances and is therefore strongly related to lifestyle factors, including the level of activity during pregnancy, and second, there are problems with measuring this aspect of exposure.

CARDIOVASCULAR DISEASE

Laboratory investigations, although inconsistent, have suggested that certain electric and magnetic field combinations may produce small (<10 per cent change from the mean) cardiovascular effects, in particular changes in heart rate variability. This led to the hypothesis that an exposure to magnetic fields might be associated with arrhythmia-related disease and myocardial infarction but not with atherosclerosis and chronic coronary heart disease. An initial epidemiological study[33] found an overall reduction in cardiovascular mortality among utility workers compared with the general population, with no increase in risk of atherosclerosis and chronic coronary heart disease, but with an increased risk of acute myocardial infarction, thus fitting the hypothesis. Subsequent epidemiological studies have not found this effect, and there is doubt as to the validity of the information on cause of death in the earlier study. Overall, the evidence speaks against an aetiological relation between EMF exposure and cardiovascular disease.[34]

NEURODEGENERATIVE DISEASE

It has been hypothesized that exposure to ELF fields is associated with several neurodegenerative diseases.[3,12] This hypothesis is based mainly on the results of studies of occupational exposures. For Parkinson's disease and multiple sclerosis, the number of studies has been small, and there is no evidence for an association with these diseases. For Alzheimer's disease and amyotrophic lateral sclerosis, more studies have been published. Some of these reports suggest that people employed in electrical occupations might have an increased risk of amyotrophic lateral sclerosis. So far, no biological mechanism has been established that can explain this association, and it is often considered that it could have arisen because of confounders related to electrical occupations, such as electric shocks.[3] One study[35] has implicated residence close to power lines in mortality from Alzheimer's disease.

DEPRESSION AND SUICIDE

There have been over 15 epidemiological studies of depression or suicide, with highly inconsistent results. Some of the early and positive studies were methodologically weak, but there are also some positive findings among better, more recent studies. Overall, it is very difficult to draw conclusions from this literature.[3,5,12]

ELECTROSENSITIVITY

Reports of sensitivity to electric and magnetic fields first appeared in the late 1970s when computers and display screens became part of the modern office. More recently, sensitivity to the presence of electricity generally has been reported. Symptoms include eye strain, fatigue, headache, difficulty in concentrating, dizziness, nausea, disturbances in sleep patterns, stress and some dermatological problems.

Double-blind, controlled laboratory studies including provocation studies have not found consistent associations between actual exposures and either symptoms or biochemical measures. Although the symptoms are undoubtedly real and sometimes disabling, they appear to be unrelated to exposure to EMFs.[36]

PUBLIC HEALTH BURDEN

If magnetic fields do cause childhood leukaemia, an estimate can be made of the number of attributable cases. This depends on various parameters, for example the percentage of homes in different countries exposed at different field levels, and also requires assumptions, particularly in the form of the exposure–response relationship. Attributable cases would be reduced if the relative risk found in epidemiological studies were larger than the true value because of bias, or increased if the relative risk were lower than the true value because of exposure misclassification.

Estimates range from a fraction of a percentage point in a low-exposure country such as the UK to about 8 per cent in a high-exposure area such as in North America. Thus, magnetic fields would appear not to constitute a major public health issue even if they are causally linked with leukaemia.[37,38] If, however, attributable numbers are also calculated from the weaker epidemiological evidence for association with diseases other than childhood leukaemia, the total rises considerably as some of these are common diseases.

CONCLUSION

Electric and magnetic fields are present in the environment as an inevitable consequence of the use of electricity by society. They induce currents in the body that can, at high levels, cause nerve stimulation. The field levels required to produce these effects are, however, rarely experienced in the environment.

Magnetic fields are classified by the IARC and WHO as 'possibly carcinogenic to humans', the key effect being childhood leukaemia. The evidence in favour of this classification is almost entirely epidemiological. Weighing against causation are the absence of robust experimental evidence of carcinogenicity despite thousands of experiments, the absence of a plausible biophysical mechanism, and the likelihood that some degree of bias is present in at least some of the epidemiological studies. Weighing in favour of causation are the consistency of the epidemiological studies and the failure to find alternative explanations. The evidence for magnetic fields causing any diseases other than childhood leukaemia is significantly weaker than that relating to childhood leukaemia. Although it seems unlikely that exposure to magnetic fields constitutes a major threat to public health, there are unresolved scientific questions that deserve further study.

DISCLAIMER

J.S. worked on this chapter with the permission of National Grid, but the views expressed are the authors' alone and not necessarily those of National Grid.

REFERENCES

● = Key primary paper
◆ = Major review article

●1. Wertheimer N, Leeper E. Electrical wiring configurations and childhood cancer. *Am J Epidemiol* 1979; **109**: 273–84.

2. Swanson J, Kaune WT. Comparison of residential power-frequency magnetic fields away from appliances in different countries. *Bioelectromagnetics* 1999; **20**: 244–54.

◆3. World Health Organization. *Extremely Low Frequency Fields*. Environmental Health Criteria Monograph, Vol. 238. Geneva: WHO, 2007.

4. Reilly JP. Neuroelectric mechanisms applied to low frequency electric and magnetic field exposure guidelines. Part I: Sinusoidal waveforms. *Health Phys* 2002; **83**: 341–55.

5. Reilly JP. Electric and magnetic field coupling from high voltage AC power transmission lines – classification of short-term effects on people. *IEEE Trans Pwr Apparat Sys* 1978; **PAS-97**(6): 2243–52.

6. Sastre A, Kavet R. *Susceptibility of Implanted Pacemakers and Defibrillators to Interference by Power-Frequency Electric and Magnetic Fields. EPRI TR-108893 – Final Report.* 1997. Palo Alto, CA: Electric Power Research Institute.

7. Trigano A, Blandeau O, Souques M et al. Clinical study of interference with cardiac pacemakers by a magnetic field at power line frequencies. *J Am Coll Cardiol* 2005; **45**: 896–900.

●8. International Commission on Non-Ionizing Radiation Protection. Guidelines for limiting exposure to time-varying electric, magnetic, and electromagnetic fields (up to 300 GHz). *Health Physics* 1998; **19**: 1–19.

9. Dimbylow PJ. Current densities in a 2mm resolution anatomically realistic model of the body induced by low frequency electric fields. *Phys Med Biol* 2000; **45**: 1013–22.

10. Dimbylow PJ. Induced current densities from low-frequency magnetic fields in a 2mm resolution, anatomically realistic model of the body. *Phys Med Biol* 1998; **43**: 221–30.

11. Dimbylow PJ. Development of the female voxel phantom, NAOMI, and its application to calculations of induced current densities and electric fields from applied low frequency magnetic and electric fields. *Phys Med Biol* 2005; **50**: 1047–70.

◆12. International Agency for Research on Cancer. *Non-ionizing Radiation.* Part 1: *Static and Extremely low-Frequency (ELF) Electric and Magnetic Fields.* Monographs on the Evaluation of Carcinogenic Risks to Humans, Vol. 80. Geneva: World Health Organization, 2002.

◆13. Swanson J, Kheifets L. Biophysical mechanisms: a component in the weight of evidence for health effects of power-frequency electric and magnetic fields. *Radiat Res* 2006; **165**: 470–8.

●14. Ahlbom A, Day N, Feychting M *et al.* A pooled analysis of magnetic fields and childhood leukaemia. *Br J Cancer* 2000; **83**: 692–8.

●15. Greenland S, Sheppard A, Kaune T, Poole C, Kelsh MA. A pooled analysis of magnetic fields, wire codes, and childhood leukemia. *Epidemiology* 2000; **11**: 624–34.

16. Schuz J, Grigat JP, Brinkmann K, Michaelis J. Residential magnetic fields as a risk factor for childhood acute leukaemia: results from a German population-based case-control study. *Int J Cancer* 2001; **91**: 728–35.

17. Kabuto M, Nitta H, Yamamoto S *et al.* Childhood leukemia and magnetic fields in Japan: a case-control study of childhood leukemia and residential power-frequency magnetic fields in Japan. *Int J Cancer* 2006; **119**: 643–50.

18. Hatch EE, Kleinerman RA, Linet MS *et al.* Do confounding or selection factors of residential wiring codes and magnetic fields distort findings of electromagnetic fields studies? *Epidemiology* 2000; **11**: 189–98.

19. Mezei G, Kheifets L. Selection bias and its implications for case-control studies: A case study of magnetic field exposure and childhood leukaemia. *Int J Epidemiol* 2006; **35**: 397–406.

20. Fews AP, Henshaw DL, Wilding RJ, Keitch PA. Corona ions from powerlines and increased exposure to pollutant aerosols. *Int J Radiat Biol* 1999; **75**: 1523–31.

21. Advisory Group on Non-Ionising Radiation. *Particle Deposition in the Vicinity of Power Lines and Possible Effects on Health.* Documents of the NRPB, Vol. 15, No 1. Chilton: National Radiological Protection Board, 2004.

22. Draper G, Vincent T, Kroll ME, Swanson J. Childhood cancer in relation to distance from high voltage power lines in England and Wales: A case-control study. *BMJ* 2005; **330**: 1290.

23. Kavet R, Zaffanella LE, Daigle JP, Ebi KL. The possible role of contact current in cancer risk associated with residential magnetic fields. *Bioelectromagnetics* 2000; **21**: 538–53.

24. Schuz J, Svendsen AL, Linet MS *et al.* Nighttime exposure to electromagnetic fields and childhood leukemia: an extended pooled analysis. *Am J Epidemiol* 2007; **166**: 263–9.

25. Foliart DE, Pollock BH, Mezei G *et al.* Magnetic field exposure and long-term survival among children with leukaemia. *Br J Cancer* 2006; **94**: 161–4.

26. Svendsen AL, Weihkopf T, Kaatsch P, Schuz J. Exposure to magnetic fields and survival after diagnosis of childhood leukemia: A German cohort study. *Cancer Epidemiol Biomarkers Prev* 2007; **16**: 1167–71.

27. Kheifets L, Swanson J, Greenland S. Childhood leukemia, electric and magnetic fields, and temporal trends. *Bioelectromagnetics* 2006; **27**: 545–52.

28. Kheifets L, Renew D, Sias G, Swanson J. Extremely law frequency electric fields and cancer: Assessing evidence. *Bioeletromagnetics* 2010; **31**(2), 89–101.

29. Mezei G, Gadallah M, Kheifets L. Residential magnetic field exposure and childhood brain cancer: A meta-analysis. *Epidemiology* 2008; **19**: 424–30.

●30. Kheifets L, Monroe J, Vergara X *et al.* Occupational electromagnetic fields and leukemia and brain cancer: An update to two meta-analyses. *J Occup Environ Med* 2008; **50**: 677–88.

31. Lee GM, Neutra RR, Hristova L *et al.* A nested case-control study of residential and personal magnetic field measures and miscarriages. *Epidemiology* 2002; **13**: 21–31.

32. Li DK, Odouli R, Wi S *et al.* A population-based prospective cohort study of personal exposure to magnetic fields during pregnancy and the risk of miscarriage. *Epidemiology* 2002; **13**: 9–20.

33. Savitz DA, Liao D, Sastre A *et al.* Magnetic field exposure and cardiovascular disease mortality among electric utility workers. *Am J Epidemiol* 1999; **149**: 135–42.

34. Kheifets L, Ahlbom A, Johansen C *et al.* Extremely low-frequency magnetic fields and heart disease. *Scand J Work Environ Health* 2007; **33**: 5–12.

35. Huss A, Spoerri A, Egger M, Roosli M. Residence near power lines and mortality from neurodegenerative diseases: Longitudinal study of the Swiss population. *Am J Epidemiol* 2009; **169**: 167–75.

◆36. Rubin GJ, Das MJ, Wessely S. Electromagnetic hypersensitivity: A systematic review of provocation studies. *Psychosom Med* 2005; **67**: 224–32.

37. Greenland S, Kheifets L. Leukemia attributable to residential magnetic fields: results from analyses allowing for study biases. *Risk Anal* 2006; **26**: 471–82.

38. Kheifets L, Afifi AA, Shimkhada R. Public health impact of extremely low-frequency electromagnetic fields. *Environ Health Perspect* 2006; **114**: 1532–7.

56

Radon: health effects of environmental exposures

GERALD M. KENDALL

Radon is a natural radioactive gas that occurs widely in the environment. Over recent decades, it has been recognized that, for most people, radon is much the most important radioactive hazard to which they are exposed.[1,2] The origins of radon are exotic and fascinating.[3] The universe as formed by the Big Bang consisted almost exclusively of the light elements hydrogen and helium. Stars formed from this material and generated the energy to shine by converting them into heavier elements. When massive stars have exhausted their nuclear fuel, they die in supernova explosions in which heavy elements such as uranium and thorium are formed. These form part of the interstellar dust from which new stars and solar systems, including our own, are formed.

The isotopes of uranium and thorium found on earth have extremely long half-lives, but they eventually undergo radioactive decay. The products of these decays are themselves radioactive and decay further until they become stable isotopes of lead. Most of the nuclides in the decay chains of uranium and thorium are isotopes of solid elements, but some are isotopes of the inert gas radon. There are several isotopes of radon, but the longest lived of these, radon-222, with a half-life of about 4 days, is normally the most important, and we will concentrate attention on it here.

Because radon is chemically inert, it exists as single atoms rather than as chemical compounds. This means that it is a gas which will tend to escape into the atmosphere from the solid material in which it was formed, for example rocks and soils. If radon gas is breathed in, most will be exhaled before it decays. However, radon that decays in the atmosphere produces isotopes of solid elements that are themselves radioactive. These decay products are not gases and attach themselves to natural aerosol particles in the atmosphere. If these aerosols are breathed in, most of them are trapped in the airways (see the next section of the chapter). It is the decay products, rather than the radon gas, that normally deliver most of the radiation dose. However, 'radon' is used as convenient shorthand to cover both the gas and its short-lived decay products.

Concentrations of radon in the open air are generally low, but high levels can build up in confined spaces such as caves and mines, as well as in some buildings. Radon inhaled in such places can give rise to high radiation doses to the lung, resulting in lung cancer. The first observation of a harmful effect of radiation was of lung cancer in certain groups of miners from central Europe (see below). However, most human exposure to radon occurs environmentally rather than occupationally, and for the most part in houses.

The average concentration of radon in UK homes is about $20\,Bq/m^3$; that is, in each second, 20 radon atoms undergo radioactive decay in each cubic metre of room air. In the outside air, the concentration is typically about $4\,Bq/m^3$. If radon concentrations in a home exceed $200\,Bq/m^3$, it is recommended that action should be taken to reduce the level. However, radon policy is under review,[4] and this Action Level may be reduced. In the control of radon exposures, a distinction is made between 'exposures' to radon and 'doses' from radon. In this chapter, 'exposures' is used in a general sense. Radon levels in other countries are often higher than they are in the UK.[5]

Among environmental exposures to radiation, for example cosmic rays or routine discharges from the nuclear fuel cycle, direct epidemiological investigation is not usually practicable because the number of induced cancers is too small to be detected against the natural background incidence. Risks must be estimated using calculations of the radiation doses likely to be incurred combined with risk per unit dose factors derived from epidemiological studies of other populations. Radon is exceptional in that an excess of lung cancer can be seen in epidemiological studies of populations exposed at normal environmental levels.

In this chapter, we will consider the radiation doses from radon to various organs and tissues of the body, and the epidemiological evidence that cancer is indeed induced. We will then review the environmental levels of radon as found in the UK. Fuller and more detailed reviews of the levels and risks of radon exposure have been carried out by a number of authorities, including

- the United Nations Scientific Committee on the Effects of Atomic Radiation;[1,2,5]
- the Sixth Committee on Biological Effects of Ionizing Radiation (BEIR VI) of the National Research Council in the USA;[6]
- the International Agency for Research on Cancer.[7,8]
- the Advisory Group on Ionising Radiation (AGIR) of the Health Protection Agency;[9]
- the World Health Organization.[10]

These authorities should be consulted for more detail.

RADIATION DOSES FROM RADON

As described above, radon is a gas that escapes into the atmosphere from the matrix in which it is formed. If it is breathed in, most will be exhaled before it decays. However, radon that decays in the atmosphere produces radioactive isotopes of solid elements. These decay products attach themselves to natural aerosol particles in the atmosphere. If these aerosols are breathed in, a high proportion of them are trapped in the airways. There are clearance mechanisms to remove such deposited material, but radon decay products have short half-lives (less than half an hour), and most will decay before they are removed from the respiratory tract. It is these decay products which normally deliver most of the radiation dose.

Most of the energy released in the radioactive decay of radon and its decay products is in the form of alpha particles. These have short ranges of 50–100 μm and therefore irradiate only the cells close to where they decay. However, there is dense ionization, and therefore great cell damage, along the tracks of the alpha particles. A crucial question is the location of the sensitive cells in which cancers are induced relative to the place where the radioactive decay takes place. It is thought that, for many cancers, the groups of sensitive cells are small, and there is some uncertainty in their location relative to that of the radon decay products. This means that there is corresponding uncertainty in the doses that the sensitive cells receive. Nevertheless, the

question is important for a wide variety of radionuclides, and it has received a good deal of attention.

Models have been developed to allow the calculation of doses to a wide variety of organs and tissues, and these have been described in publications from the International Commission on Radiological Protection.[11–14] There are two parts to the models. First, there is a biokinetic part in which movement of the nuclides round the body is considered, taking into account the rates at which transfers from one organ to another occur, elimination from the body and the rate of radioactive decay. This leads to a numerical estimate of the number of radioactive decays that occur in each 'source organ'. In the second part of the models, the absorption of energy in each 'target tissue' from all the decays in the source organs is estimated. These lead directly to estimates of doses to the organs. More details of the estimation of radiation doses from internal emitters are in Chapter 30.

Calculations of doses from radon gas and from radon decay products have been undertaken.[15–18] Table 56.1 shows the calculated doses from the decay products of radon (Rn) at the average concentration found in the UK. Because most of the radioactive decays take place in the respiratory tract and because most of the energy is released in the form of short-ranged alpha particles, doses to the lung and associated tissues are much larger than those to other body organs. Among the other organs, those with a relatively high fat content tend to have somewhat higher doses. This is because of the influence of radon gas, which is preferentially soluble in fat.

One of the important factors in deciding the pattern of doses from radon decay products is the rate at which they escape from the respiratory tract to the rest of the body. There are three standard models,[13] known as type F, type

Table 56.1 Summary of rounded annual doses (μSv) to the organs and tissues of an adult from inhaling air containing radon decay products in equilibrium with radon gas at the UK average concentration of 20 Bq/m³

Organ or tissue	Annual dose (μSv)
Lung	3600
Extrathoracic airways	4500
Kidney	520
Bone surfaces	150
Red bone marrow	30
Liver	40
Other organs and tissues	10–20
Effective dose	530

Type F kinetics are assumed for the decay products. The equilibrium factor between radon gas and decay products is taken to be 0.41. The effective dose is a weighted sum of organ doses designed to give a measure of the radiation detriment to the body as a whole. It may be regarded as a kind of average dose.
After Kendall et al. (2005).[16,17]

M and type S, standing for fast, moderate and slow clearance. The calculations shown in the table are for type F. Although the position is not totally clear, there are also arguments that would suggest that type M (or some intermediate) is appropriate. If type M had been adopted, the doses to the respiratory tract would have been even more dominant than those given in the table. However, even with the conservative assumption on which the table is based, the message is clear. The doses to the lung and the extrathoracic part of the respiratory tract (the nose, pharynx and larynx), are an order of magnitude greater than those to any other body organ. If the – arguably more realistic – assumption of type M kinetics had been made the difference would have been more than two orders of magnitude.

The clear implication is that, although radon and its decay products may induce cancers in other organs, it is the respiratory tract that is at greatest risk. Epidemiological studies support the conclusions drawn from the dose calculations.

EVIDENCE ON THE RISKS OF RADON EXPOSURE

In the section above, we showed that arguments based on the calculation of doses to different body organs indicated that radon and its decay products might pose a risk of lung cancer. In this section, we consider more direct evidence on this question. Evidence on the carcinogenic effects of radiation exposure can come from a variety of sources:

- directly, in epidemiological studies of exposed populations;
- from laboratory studies involving animals;
- by extrapolation from the general body of knowledge about radiobiology and the mechanisms of radiation damage in tissues.

The first of these is the most direct and reliable. In the case of radon, although not for most other environmental radiation exposures, there is considerable epidemiological evidence, and this is the main topic of this section. However, the other sources of evidence are outlined briefly here.

Laboratory studies

The data from animal studies were historically important in understanding the radon hazard, but evidence from epidemiological studies of human beings has largely superseded them. Laboratory studies involved carefully measured exposures and allowed investigation of the possible effects of potential co-carcinogens, in particular tobacco smoke.[19–21] Nevertheless, many of these studies

were conducted at radon concentrations higher than those of interest in a domestic context. Moreover, differences are observed between different animal species and strains. This makes it particularly difficult to extrapolate to humans.

Radiobiology and mechanistic considerations

Even for carcinogens for which the epidemiological evidence is very strong, there is inevitably a region where exposures are too low for the risk to be distinguished from the natural background figures. Mechanistic considerations are used to decide how to extrapolate the observed risk down to the lowest exposures.[22] In the case of radiation-induced cancer, it is generally assumed that the risk falls off linearly with dose, with no threshold below which the risk is zero. This is certainly not regarded as an exact rule, applicable in all circumstances. Rather it is a working hypothesis that is reasonably robust and perhaps more likely to err on the side of conservatism.

Epidemiological studies of radon and lung cancer

Much the most direct evidence on the risks of radon exposure comes from epidemiological studies on human populations. Three broad types of epidemiological study have been undertaken:

- case–control studies of exposure to individuals within their homes;
- cohort studies of miners exposed occupationally;
- geographical correlation (or ecological) studies linking mean radon concentrations in areas of various sizes with the mean cancer rates in those areas.

A general problem in studies of radon and lung cancer is that cigarette-smoking is overwhelmingly the dominant cause of lung cancer. Very careful allowance must be made for the effects of smoking in the analysis, particularly since the two carcinogens may interact in a way that is not understood and that must be determined from the data. This is a particular problem for ecological studies, which do not have information relating to individuals. Ecological studies face severe methodological difficulties[23,24] and are less reliable than cohort or case–control studies that include individual measurements of radon in homes and individual smoking histories. Ecological studies are discussed in more detail in other reviews,[6,9] and we will not consider them further here.

CASE–CONTROL STUDIES OF RADON AND LUNG CANCER

In the context of environmental exposures to radon, studies of the effects of radon in homes provide the most direct evidence on risks. These studies are usually of case–control design and include measurements of radon concentrations in the homes of cases and controls, as well as also information about smoking.

A number of well-designed case–control studies have been published, and these have provided strong support for the idea that radon causes lung cancer. However, increased statistical power is obtained by combining them. This can be done either by combining the published results of each of the studies in a meta-analysis or by combining the data on all the individuals in a pooled analysis. A difficulty with the meta-analyses is that the various studies differ from one another in the details of the methods used in the analysis. Pooled analyses are able to apply a uniform metric for radon exposures and for the effect of smoking. For these reasons, we focus on the evidence from pooled analyses of individual data in assessing the risks of lung cancer associated with residential radon exposure.

Three main pooled analyses based on individual data have been undertaken: of European studies,[25,26] of North American studies[27,28] and of Chinese studies.[29] The risk estimates from these studies are reported in terms of the percentage increase in the risk of lung cancer per 100 Bq/m^3 increase in radon exposure without any variation with time since exposure or age at exposure.

A very important question in the interpretation of these domestic studies concerns the reliability and interpretation of the radon measurements. Radon concentrations vary greatly with time, and short-term measurements will inevitably carry a considerable uncertainty. To overcome these difficulties, the case–control studies discussed here used measurements over periods of several months in as many as possible of the homes in which study participants had lived.

But there is another more subtle question that must be considered when interpreting the radon measurements. Successive long-term radon measurements in a home are found to vary considerably, reflecting principally the year-to-year variations in the radon concentration. The distribution of measured radon concentrations is highly skewed and is found to be approximately log-normal. The play of chance then means that radon concentrations that are measured to be in the high end of the distribution are likely to be too high. Radon concentrations in the low end of the distribution may have a high error in relative terms, but the absolute error will be small (a 30 per cent error in a measurement of 1000 Bq/m^3 is 300 Bq/m^3; in a measurement of 20 Bq/m^3, it is only 6 Bq/m^3).

Analyses based on measured radon concentrations, rather than on the true long-term average radon concentration for each home, will underestimate the risk of lung cancer unless special methods of analysis are employed to take the random variation into account. These special methods of analysis effectively convert the basis of the estimate from measured radon concentrations to estimated true long-term average radon concentrations.

Of the published studies, only the European pooling study has so far made this correction.

The European pooling study

This study included data from 13 European studies of residential radon and lung cancer. Results were published by Darby et al. in 2005.[25,26] A total of more than 7000 lung cancer cases and over 14 000 controls were included. The study examined the effect on lung cancer risk of exposures to radon during the 30-year period ending 5 years prior to the diagnosis of lung cancer. Darby et al. used very fine stratification to allow for the effect of smoking. They also made a detailed correction for random uncertainties in the measurement of radon concentrations.

The European pooling study showed a clear association between increasing exposure to radon and lung cancer. There was no significant variation between the level of risk estimated for the component studies, and the results were not dominated by any single study. The risk appeared to be approximately linear with no evidence for a threshold below which there was no risk. The results suggested that, if a threshold value exists, it cannot be higher than 150 Bq/m^3.

Furthermore, the investigators found a statistically significant association between radon levels and lung cancer even when analysis was restricted to people in homes with concentrations below 200 Bq/m^3 ($P = 0.04$). When individuals with measured radon levels of 100–199 Bq/m^3 were compared with those with measured radon levels below 100 Bq/m^3, their risk of lung cancer was increased by 20 per cent (95 per cent confidence interval [CI] 3–30 per cent; $P = 0.01$). The proportionate increase in risk per 100 Bq/m^3 did not vary significantly with age, sex or smoking status.

When the analysis was conducted in terms of measured radon concentrations, it was estimated that the risk of lung cancer increased by 8 per cent per 100 Bq/m^3 increase in mean measured radon concentration (95 per cent CI 3–16 per cent). When the analysis was repeated in terms of true long-term average radon concentrations, i.e. with the correction for measurement error reported above, the final estimated risk was higher, at 16 per cent (95 per cent CI 5–31 per cent).

Radon measurements were available for an average of 23 years of the 30-year period of interest. Where measurements had not been possible, estimated values were used in the construction of the mean measured radon exposure for an individual, based on the mean measured value in all the residences for individuals in the control group in the local area. Darby et al. examined the way in which risk estimates varied with the number of homes that the individuals taking part in the study had occupied during the 30-year period of interest, and also with the proportion of the 30-year period for which measurements were available. There was no evidence that risk estimates differed between those with complete and incomplete radon exposure histories. This was in contrast to the other pooled analyses.

The North American pooling study

Krewski and co-workers[27,28] published a pooling that involved 3662 cases and 4966 controls from seven studies in the USA and Canada. The reference period considered was the 25-year period ending 5 years before the diagnosis of lung cancer, slightly shorter than in the European pooling. In this analysis, there was also detailed allowance for smoking, but it was less finely stratified than that used in the European pooling.

When compared with individuals whose mean measured radon concentrations were less than 25 Bq/m³, individuals with higher mean measured radon concentrations had increased risks of lung cancer, but for no individual category was the increase statistically significant. When analysed for any trend with increasing radon concentration, the increase in risk per 100 Bq/m³ measured radon concentration was 11 per cent (95 per cent CI 0–28 per cent). There was no significant heterogeneity between the levels of risk estimated for the component studies, and the risk estimate did not change substantially when any of the studies was excluded from the analysis.

Krewski *et al.* also considered analyses restricted to subgroups for whom radon exposure histories were more complete. For those individuals for whom monitoring data were available for at least 20 years out of the 25-year exposure-time window, the increase in risk per 100 Bq/m³ measured radon was 21 per cent (95 per cent CI 3–50 per cent). A similar result was obtained by restricting attention to those who had lived in only one or two houses. As discussed below, the authors regarded these analyses as giving better risk estimates than the unrestricted analyses. There was no significant variation in the estimated increase in risk per 100 Bq/m³ with smoking status, sex, age or educational level.

The Chinese pooling study

Lubin and co-workers[29] published a study that involved 1050 cases and 1996 controls from two studies in two areas in China, Gansu and Shenyang; the first of these studies was much the larger. As with the North American pooling, a 25-year reference period was considered, ending 5 years before diagnosis. Four smoking categories were considered in the analysis.

For the pooled data, the increase in risk per 100 Bq/m³ was 13.3 per cent (95 per cent CI 1–36 per cent). This positive slope was chiefly due to the Gansu data, although the results of the two component studies were compatible with each other. For subjects resident in only one home for the whole of the 25-year reference period, the increase in risk per 100 Bq/m³ measured radon was 32 per cent (95 per cent CI 7–91 per cent).

As with the European and North American pooling, there was no significant difference between the risk estimates calculated for the different smoking categories.

The risk estimate was higher in analyses restricted to those study subjects who had provided information on confounders themselves compared with those where it had been obtained from a surrogate.

EPIDEMIOLOGICAL STUDIES OF MINERS

High radon levels can build up in mines, and the high levels of fatal lung disease resulting from these exposures were noted in the sixteenth century.[30] A good review of the history of our understanding of the radon risk is in Publication 65 from the International Commission on Radiological Protection.[12] Epidemiological studies of miners were important in establishing the link between radon exposure and lung cancer.[6]

Uranium is the parent of radon and, as might be expected, uranium mines are particularly liable to high radon levels, although other mines can also be affected. In the case of uranium mining, a particular factor was the intense demand for uranium in the aftermath of World War II. This led both to large numbers of miners being employed and also to a tendency for safety measures to take second place to production. Historically, the evidence on radon risks from miner studies was very important, and they still have the potential to provide important information on questions such as the variation of risk with time since exposure. However, there are difficulties in extrapolating the results of miner studies to estimate the risks of radon exposures in the home. These are discussed below.

A further complication is that analyses of miner data have often been conducted using 'working levels' (WLs) and 'working level months' (WLMs) as a measure of exposure. A WL is equivalent to a radon concentration of about 3700 Bq/m³ of radon if all the radon decay products are in equilibrium with radon gas. In practice, in homes, the concentration of radon decay products is well below that of the gas, and a WL is typically equivalent to perhaps 7500 Bq/m³ radon. A WLM is defined as exposure to 1 WL for a working month of 170 hours.

A major review of the miner data was published in 1999 by the BEIR VI Committee of the National Academy of Sciences in the USA.[6] The BEIR VI Committee considered 11 major studies, covering a total of over 60 000 male miners, among whom over 2500 deaths from lung cancer had occurred.

The BEIR VI Committee modelled the excess relative risk (ERR) using expressions that took account of attained age and of exposure rate:

$$ERR = \beta\, w^\star\, \Phi_{age}\, \gamma_z$$

Here β represents the slope of the exposure–risk relationship, and $w^\star$ is the weighted radon exposure given by:

$$w^\star = w_{5-14} + \theta_{15-24}\, w_{15-24} + \theta_{25+}\, w_{25+}$$

where w_{5-14} is the radon exposure 5–14 years previously, etc., θ represents the weighting factors (in practice less than one), Φ_{age} is a parameter that allows the ERR to vary with age, and γ_z is a parameter that allows for variations with exposure rate.

In fact, two models were used, differing in the γ parameter, which varied either with duration of exposure or with mean concentration (the 'exposure–age–duration' and 'exposure–age–concentration' models).

However, the BEIR VI models are complex and ERRs are hard to compare with the results from the domestic studies. A more informative risk estimate was given by Darby et al.,[26] who estimated that, for miners exposed at less than 0.5 WL, risks were in the range 19–30 per cent per $100\,Bq/m^3$.

Despite the power of the miner studies, there are some problems in extrapolating the results to domestic circumstances. Exposures in mines were usually much higher than in homes, and miners were typically exposed relatively briefly (for only a few years) rather than over decades. This means that the question of extrapolation of the risks from high exposures to those typical of domestic exposure must be considered. Conversely, it makes it much easier for miner studies to investigate the way in which risks vary with time since exposure to radon.

The way in which radon decay products deposit in the lungs, and therefore the radiation doses that result, depends on the nature of the aerosols to which the decay products are attached. These are complex matters,[6] but there is no doubt that circumstances differ between homes and mines. It is possible to use modelling studies to try to allow for these differences, but substantial uncertainties remain. Many of the miners may in addition have been exposed to other carcinogens such as arsenic. As noted above, it is also important to take account of smoking in estimating the induction of lung cancer by radon, and smoking data were limited or absent in many of the miner cohorts.

The residential studies use measurements of radon concentrations in the homes of the individual cases and controls. However, it is inevitable that these measurements were nearly always made many years after the lung cancer was diagnosed. The miner studies generally rely on estimates of individual exposures made from radon measurements in various areas of the mine. These measurements were often patchy. However, the exposure estimates for the miner studies were based on contemporary measurements.

Most importantly, the published analyses of the miner cohorts have not considered the uncertainties in the measurements of miner exposures and their effect on the resulting risk estimates.

Summary of the risks of radon exposure

A response to the public health risk from radon depends on as complete an understanding as possible of the quantitative nature of the risk. How big is the risk to individuals of different kinds (e.g. adults and children) at different levels of exposure? Although it is always easy to pose questions that have no certain answers, in the case of radon we have direct evidence which is better than that for any other environmental radioactive hazard. The two main bodies of evidence, described above, are the case–control studies of domestic exposures – particularly the pooling of these studies – and the studies of occupational exposures of miners. Clearly, the former are more directly informative in terms of public health risk.

THE OVERALL MAGNITUDE OF THE RISK

The risk estimates from the domestic case-control studies are reported in terms of the percentage increase in the risk of lung cancer per $100\,Bq/m^3$ increase in radon exposure over a period of 25 or 30 years. The estimates reported by the three major domestic pooling studies were as follows:

- European pooling: 8 per cent (95 per cent CI 3–16) per $100\,Bq/m^3$;
- North American pooling: 11 per cent (95 per cent CI 0–28) per $100\,Bq/m^3$;
- Chinese pooling: 13 per cent (95 per cent CI 1–36) per $100\,Bq/m^3$.

All the studies also considered subsets of the data for individuals for whom measurements were more complete or who had lived in only one or two houses:

- European pooling: 9 per cent (95 per cent CI 3–18) per $100\,Bq/m^3$;
- North American pooling: 18 per cent (95 per cent CI 0–43) per $100\,Bq/m^3$;
- Chinese pooling: 32 per cent (95 per cent CI 7–91) per $100\,Bq/m^3$.

In the case of the North American and Chinese poolings, these restricted analyses thus resulted in higher risk estimates than did the basic analysis. The authors argued that these restricted analyses gave more reliable risk estimates. This was on the basis that exposure estimates based on measurements in the houses in question are better than those which include imputed values, and that it is easier to make reliable estimates of exposure for individuals who have lived in few houses.

As described above, estimates based on measured radon concentration will underestimate the true risks associated with residential radon, due to the year-to-year random variation in radon concentrations in a home. The only pooling study that has carried out a detailed analysis of the risks of residential radon based on true long-term average, as opposed to measured, radon concentrations, is the European pooling study. In this study, the estimate based on true long-term average concentrations was double the estimate based on measured radon concentrations, i.e. 16 per cent (95 per cent CI 5–31 per cent).

In addition, the European pooling investigators noted a number of factors that could not be included in the analysis of the pooling studies:

- There would have been errors in the assignment of individuals to smoking categories.
- There are likely to have been variations in the radon concentration between the different rooms in a home.
- In some countries, there may have been systematic changes in the radon concentrations over the last few decades, due to increased energy efficiency.
- There may also be some element of risk resulting from exposure to radon concentration outside the 25 or 30 year exposure-time window considered.

The overall effect of these factors is likely to mean that the true effect of radon might be somewhat higher than those reported.

Estimates of the ERR at $100 \, Bq/m^3$ from the pooled residential studies are broadly consistent with those based on the miner data. Darby et al.[26] report that, for miners exposed at less than 0.5 WL (i.e. to radon concentrations no higher than a few thousand Bq/m^3) risks were in the range 19–30 per cent per $100 \, Bq/m^3$. The higher estimate related to miners with lower total exposures (those below 50 WLM).

The best single estimate of the ERR at $100 \, Bq/m^3$ is probably that derived from the European pooling with the correction for measurement uncertainties. This 16 per cent per $100 \, Bq/m^3$ increase in true long-term average radon concentration in the home is based on a 30-year exposure period. However, the European investigators noted a number of reasons to believe that the true risk might be higher, and other pooling studies also provide evidence in this direction. On balance, the evidence does indeed suggest that the true risk is higher, but it is hard to provide a reliable numerical estimate.

THE SHAPE OF THE EXPOSURE–RESPONSE RELATIONSHIP

A very important question is the shape of the exposure–response curve at low exposures. Is it linear, or are low exposures either more or less dangerous that might be expected on the basis of a simple linear extrapolation of the risks observed at higher doses? In particular, is there a threshold below which exposure to radon has no deleterious effects at all? There will always be a low-dose area where direct epidemiological evidence is lacking, and there have been a number of suggestions that simple linear extrapolation into this region is overcautious, for example Becker (1999).[31] The publication of the pooling studies pushes back the frontier at which epidemiology provides evidence.

The pooling studies suggest that the risk is approximately linear, with no evidence for a threshold below which there is no risk. In particular, the European pooling suggested that, if a threshold value exists, it cannot be higher than $150 \, Bq/m^3$. Furthermore, there was a statistically significant association between radon levels and lung cancer even when the analysis was restricted to people in homes with concentrations below $200 \, Bq/m^3$. The risk of lung cancer in individuals with measured radon levels of $100–199 \, Bq/m^3$ was 20 per cent above those with a measured radon below $100 \, Bq/m^3$. The BEIR VI Committee[6] and AGIR[9] recommended that the radon risk should be taken to be linear with dose, without a threshold. This is the usual assumption in radiation protection.[22]

RISKS IN MEN AND IN WOMEN

In the pooling studies, there was no evidence for different risks in men and women. There were no female miners, so the occupational studies provide no information on this point.

RISKS TO INDIVIDUALS OF DIFFERENT AGES

Lung cancer is predominantly a disease of middle and old age. The domestic case–control studies do not provide any information on the risks of exposure to radon at young ages and provide no evidence for a relative risk that varies with age. The miner studies find that the relative risk declines after age 50. This is a question on which more data would be very valuable.

RISKS IN SMOKERS AND NON-SMOKERS

Lung cancer is much very much more common in cigarette-smokers than in non-smokers. The risks of radon exposure might act independently of the smoking risk so that the two hazards added together. In this case, the absolute risk in smokers would be the same as in non-smokers. Alternatively, the radon risk might multiply the underlying lung cancer risk so that the relative risk was the same for the two groups. In this case, the absolute risk to smokers would be much higher than to non-smokers because the underlying risk to the former would be much greater. The truth might of course lie somewhere between these absolute and relative risk models, and in fact the evidence suggests that the risks are closer to multiplicative than additive. The risk to recent ex-smokers is thought to be similar to that in current smokers, while the risk to long-term ex-smokers tends towards that in never smokers.

The pooled domestic case–control studies do not show a difference between the relative risk per unit exposure in smokers and non-smokers; however, the statistical uncertainties are significant. The miner studies suggest that the relative risks in non-smokers are substantially larger than in smokers. The underlying risk in smokers is much higher than in non-smokers. If the same relative risk applies to the two groups, radon-induced lung cancer will be rare in non-smokers. If a higher relative risk applies to non-smokers, this may not be the case.

EXPOSURE TO RADON IN DWELLINGS

Mechanisms and levels

As we have seen, radon derives ultimately from uranium in rocks, soils and building materials. In practice in the UK, most of the radon indoors is contributed by uranium in the ground underneath the building rather than from building materials. There are two stages in the build-up of radon in houses: the transfer of radon to air in the soil beneath the house, and the transfer of soil gas into houses.[32,33] Concentrations of radon in soil gas are ultimately determined by geology. However, the processes involved are complicated. High levels of radon are more likely to be found in soil gas if the local rocks and soils contain high concentrations of uranium.

However, the ease with which radon can escape from the matrix where it is formed can be even more important. Usually, the radon comes from the ground within a few metres of the building, but if the ground is particularly permeable or fissured, it may come from a greater distance. If the underlying rock is overlaid with clay, radon is unlikely to be able to escape to the surface as it could if the covering were of a more porous material. Granite tends to have high levels of uranium and, in consequence, radon levels are high in some granite areas, particularly if the granite is weathered or fractured as in south-west England. However, high radon levels are not found in all granite areas and, conversely, high radon levels can also be found elsewhere, for example on limestones, sandstones and some other geologies.

The transport of radon from soil gas to room air is also complex. It depends on the details of construction of the house (particularly on cracks or openings in the floor) and on the way it is occupied (e.g. the temperature relative to outdoors and the ventilation). In most houses, there is an underpressure relative to the air outside. The result is that the building draws in outside air, typically at the rate of one air change an hour. Most of this inflow comes through doors and windows, but perhaps 1 per cent or so comes from the ground. In an average house, this amounts to a couple of cubic metres of soil gas entering the house each hour. It is this pressure-driven flow rather than diffusion which is responsible for most of the radon entering houses.

The radon concentration in a building depends on the rate of entry of the radon and the rate at which it is removed by ventilation. Increasing the ventilation rate will not, however, always decrease the radon concentration. This is because ventilation rate and underpressure are related, and some ways of increasing ventilation, such as the use of extractor fans or opening upstairs windows, can also increase the underpressure.

The factors described above vary greatly from one dwelling to another and lead to large differences in radon concentrations. The building regulations applied to the construction of the house could also have a major influence. In addition, the underpressure and ventilation rate vary with time in all buildings. Underpressure tends to be highest in cold weather and at night because the difference in temperature between indoors and outdoors is greatest. At these times, ventilation routes such as windows and doors are generally closed, so a higher proportion of the air drawn in by underpressure comes from the soil, thus increasing radon concentrations.

The mean radon concentration in UK dwellings has been estimated to be about $20\,Bq/m^3$.[34] It was found that the distribution of radon concentrations is skewed with a long tail and is closely approximated by a log-normal distribution. As expected from the skewness of the log-normal distribution, the median radon level was lower, at around $10\,Bq/m^3$. On the basis of the log-normal distribution, about 500 000 houses (just over 2 per cent of the total housing stock) were predicted to have radon levels above $100\,Bq/m^3$, about 100 000 houses to exceed the UK radon Action Level of $200\,Bq/m^3$ and around 3000 to exceed $1000\,Bq/m^3$. These estimates are not precise. An informal assessment of the uncertainty was ± 30 per cent.

Large numbers of measurements of radon levels have been made in houses in the UK (Table 56.2). These both

Table 56.2 Summary of radon measurements in UK dwellings

	Housing stock	Number of radon measurements	Average radon concentration (Bq/m³)	Number at or above the Action Level (200 Bq/m³)
England	22 316 000	456 500	21	51 100
Scotland	2 442 000	18 400	16	370
Wales	1 335 000	16 800	20	1 780
Northern Ireland	744 000	22 900	19	1 150
Totals	26 837 000	514 600	20	54 400

Data as at April 2008, provided by the Radiation Protection Division of the Health Protection Agency.

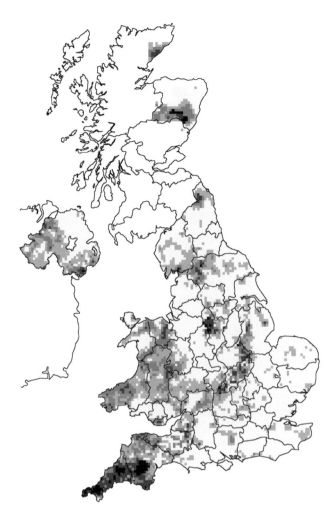

Figure 56.1 Map of the UK showing the percentage of homes with seasonally adjusted measurements about 200 Bq/m³, the current UK Action Level for radon. (Reproduced from Health Protection Agency,[4] with permission.)

indicate specific houses where remedial measures may be needed and also allow radon maps to be developed. As might be expected, there is a considerable variation in radon level from one part of the country to another. Figure 56.1 shows a map of radon levels in the UK. The map is based on the results of many measurements in homes; more recently, these data have been combined with geological information to provide more detailed maps,[35] but as yet these cover only England and Wales.

It can be seen that the highest concentrations are in granite areas of the south-west peninsula, but that elevated levels are also found elsewhere, for example on the limestone of the Derbyshire Dales. Greater detail in the mapping is possible in the high-radon areas where more measurements have been made. Nevertheless, it must be remembered that radon levels are variable and that maps indicate only where high levels are likely. Adjacent and apparently similar houses can have radon levels that differ by an order of magnitude, and the actual levels in a house can be determined only by direct measurement.

Control of domestic exposures to radon in the UK

Controls on domestic exposure to radon have been in place in the UK since the 1980s.[3] It is recommended that action should be taken to reduce long-term radon concentrations in those homes where an 'Action Level' was exceeded. This Action Level was set at 200 Bq/m³ in 1990. Emphasis was placed on reducing radon levels as far as possible, and not just on edging below the Action Level. A radon 'Affected Area' is a part of the country where radon concentrations in 1 per cent or more of existing dwellings are expected to exceed the Action Level. It was expected that anti-radon programmes would initially be concentrated within radon Affected Areas.

Building regulations[36–39] specify anti-radon measures to be incorporated in new buildin   gs in parts of the country where there is a risk of high radon levels. These measures will have the effect of reducing mean radon levels in new homes and thus reducing the collective radon exposure of the population. It is, however, important to realize that this will be in the long term and that no practicable anti-radon programme can offer a short-term way of reducing the main part of the population exposure, which occurs in the large number of existing houses with low-to-medium radon concentrations.

Radon policy develops with time, and the development of the UK radon programme has been described by Kendall *et al.* (2005).[17] Radon programmes in other countries are broadly similar.[40,41] The publication of the pooling of radon case–control studies (see above) has provided new evidence on radon risks that is likely to lead to a review of radon policy. Another input to this review is likely to be health economics. A recent analysis by Gray *et al.*[42] provides strong evidence that radon preventive measures would be cost-effective much more widely than they have been applied in the past, and the Health Protection Agency has already recommended that they should be incorporated in all new houses.[4] One may also speculate that it will be hard to continue with an Action Level of 200 Bq/m³ when harm has been demonstrated down to 150 Bq/m³ or below. WHO has recently advocated a Reference (Action) Level of 100 Bq/m³ or, if this is impractical in the country in question, a level no higher than 300 Bq/m³.[10] The International Commission on Radiological Protection has also recommended a reference level no higher than 300 Bq/m³.[43]

PRACTICAL CONTROL OF RADON LEVELS IN NEW BUILDINGS

An effective seal to the ground can cheaply and easily be incorporated as the floor of a new building is being constructed. The measures required for protection against moisture, for example the inclusion of an impermeable membrane in the foundations of the building, can be adapted to provide basic protection from radon. In areas where radon levels are particularly high, extra protection can be built into new houses. As well as the membrane, a ventilated sub-floor void or a radon sump can be installed. A radon sump is a small cavity under the floor slab, which can have an electric fan sucking air connected to it. In the case of the sump, the electric fan would generally not be fitted until testing had demonstrated a high radon level. More details can be found in publications of the Building Research Establishment.[36]

PRACTICAL CONTROLS OF RADON LEVELS IN EXISTING BUILDINGS

Incorporating radon remedial measures into an existing building is less easy than including preventive measures during construction. In particular, sealing the floor of an existing building will often not be a cost-effective option. Nevertheless, radon remedial measures are not technically difficult and are not expensive compared with many other building works. If the building has a solid floor, a radon sump connected to a fan will generally substantially lower indoor radon levels. This reduces or reverses the normal underpressure in the building with respect to the soil gas and results in very much less radon being sucked through the small imperfections in the floor slab. Radon levels can also be reduced by improving the ventilation under suspended floors and by various other means.[44]

SUMMARY

Calculations suggest that radon gives the largest component of the radiation dose incurred by the average UK citizen. Epidemiological studies of human populations provide overwhelming evidence that radon is acting as a cause of lung cancer in the general population at concentrations found in some ordinary homes. Furthermore, the risk can be quantified over a large range of radon concentrations. In particular, there is substantial evidence of a risk even below $200\,Bq/m^3$, the level at which action is currently advocated in the UK and in many other countries.

Radon in homes has been recognized as a problem for over 30 years. In the UK, government has funded measurement campaigns in high-radon areas to alert those householders who may be at risk. Building regulations have been laid down to help prevent high radon levels in new buildings. Reducing radon concentrations in existing buildings is less easy than incorporating anti-radon measures as the house is being built, but useful reductions can normally be obtained at modest cost. Nevertheless, in the light of new information on radon risks, policies on the control of radon are under review.[3,4]

REFERENCES

1. United Nations Scientific Committee on the Effect of Atomic Radiation. *Ionising Radiation: Sources and Biological Effects. UNSCEAR Report 1982. Report to the General Assembly.* New York: United Nations, 1982.
2. United Nations. *Sources and Effects of Ionizing Radiation. United Nations Scientific Committee on the Effects of Atomic Radiation. 1993 Report to the General Assembly with scientific annexes.* New York: United Nations, 1993.
3. Kendall GM, Green BMR, Miles JCH, Dixon DW. The development of the UK radon programme. *J Radiol Prot* 2005; **25**: 475–92.
4. Health Protection Agency. *HPA Advice On Radon Protective Measures In New Buildings.* London: HPA, 2008.
5. United Nations Scientific Committee on the Effects of Atomic Radiation. *Sources and Effects of Ionising Radiation.* New York: United Nations, 2006.
6. Sixth Committee on Biological Effects of Ionising Radiation. *The Health Effects of Exposure to Indoor Radon.* Washington: United States National Academy of Sciences, National Research Council, National Academy Press, 1999.
7. International Agency for Research on Cancer. Man-made mineral fibres and radon. *IARC Monogr Eval Carcinog Risks Hum* 1988; **43**.
8. International Agency for Research on Cancer. Ionizing radiation. Part 2: some internally deposited radionuclides. Views and expert opinions of an IARC Working Group on the Evaluation of Carcinogenic Risks to Humans. Lyon, 14–21 June 2000. *IARC Monogr Eval Carcinog Risks Hum* 2001; **78**: 1–559.
9. Health Protection Agency. *Radon and Public Health: Report of the independent Advisory Group on Ionising Radiation.* Documents of the Health Protection Agency, Radiation, Chemical and Environmental Hazards Division. RCE-11, HPA, June 2009. ISBN: 978-0-85951-644-0.
10. World Health Organization. *WHO Handbook on Indoor Radon: A public health perspective.* Zeeb H, Shannoun F (eds). World Health Organization 2009. ISBN: 978 92 4 154767 3.
11. International Commission on Radiological Protection. *Age-Dependent Doses to Members of the Public from Intake of Radionuclides.* Part 1. ICRP Publication No. 56. Report No. 20. Oxford: Elsevier, 1990.
12. International Commission on Radiological Protection. *Protection Against Radon-222 at Home and at Work.* ICRP Publication No. 65. Report No. 23. Oxford: Pergamon, 1994.
13. International Commission on Radiological Protection. *Human Respiratory Tract Model for Radiological Protection.* ICRP Publication No. 66. Report No. 24. Oxford: Pergamon, 1995.
14. International Commission on Radiological Protection. *Age-dependent Doses to Members of the Public from Intake of Radionuclides.* Part 5: *Compilation of Ingestion and Inhalation Dose Coefficients.* ICRP Publication 72. Report No. 26. Oxford: Pergamon Press, 1999.
15. Richardson RB, Eatough JP, Henshaw DL. Dose to red bone marrow from natural radon and thoron exposure. *Br J Radiol* 1991; **64**: 608–24.
16. Kendall GM, Smith TJ. Doses to organs and tissues from radon and its decay products. *J Radiol Prot* 2002; **22**: 389–406.

17. Kendall GM, Smith TJ. Doses from radon and its decay products to children. *J Radiol Prot* 2005; **25**: 241–56.

18. Khursheed A. Doses to systemic tissues from radon gas. *Radiat Prot Dosimetry* 2000; **88**: 171–81.

19. Cross FT, Monchaux G. Risk assessment of radon health effects from experimental animal studies. A joint review of PNNL (USA) and CEACOGEMA (France) data. In: Inaba J, Yonehara H, Doi M (eds) *Indoor Radon Exposure and its Health Consequences. Quest for the True Story of Environmental Radon and Lung Cancer.* Tokyo: Kodansha Scientific, 1999: 85–105.

20. Monchaux G, Morlier JP, Morin M *et al.* Carcinogenic and cocarcinogenic effects of radon and radon daughters in rats. *Environ Health Perspect* 1994; **102**: 64–73.

21. Collier CG, Strong JC, Humphreys JA *et al.* Carcinogenicity of radon/radon decay product inhalation in rats – effect of dose, dose rate and unattached fraction. *Int J Radiat Biol* 2005; **81**: 631–47.

22. International Commission on Radiological Protection. *Recommendations of the ICRP.* ICRP Publication No. 103. Report No. 37. Oxford: Elsevier, 2008.

23. Greenland S. Ecologic versus individual-level sources of bias in ecologic estimates of contextual health effects. *Int J Epidemiol* 2001; **30**: 1343–50.

24. Lubin JH. The potential for bias in Cohen's ecological analysis of lung cancer and residential radon. *J Radiol Prot* 2002; **22**: 141–8.

25. Darby S, Hill D, Auvinen A *et al.* Radon in homes and risk of lung cancer: collaborative analysis of individual data from 13 European case-control studies. *BMJ Clin Res Ed* 2005; **330**: 223–7.

26. Darby S, Hill D, Deo H *et al.* Residential radon and lung cancer – detailed results of a collaborative analysis of individual data on 7148 persons with lung cancer and 14,208 persons without lung cancer from 13 epidemiologic studies in Europe. *Scand J Work Environ Health* 2006; **32**: 1–83.

27. Krewski D, Lubin JH, Zielinski JM *et al.* Residential radon and risk of lung cancer: a combined analysis of 7 North American case-control studies. *Epidemiology* 2005; **16**: 137–45.

28. Krewski D, Lubin JH, Zielinski JM *et al.* A combined analysis of North American case-control studies of residential radon and lung cancer. *J Toxicol Environ Health A* 2006; **69**: 533–97.

29. Lubin JH, Wang ZY, Boice JD *et al.* Risk of lung cancer and residential radon in China: pooled results of two studies. *Int J Cancer* 2004; **109**: 132–7.

30. Agricola G. *De Re Metallica.* New York: Dover Publications, 1950.

31. Becker K. Dangerous indoor radon? *Radiat Prot Dosimetry* 1999; **83**: 345–6.

32. National Radiological Protection Board. *Health Risks from Radon. A joint Publication with the Faculty of Public Health Medicine and the Chartered Institute of Environmental Health.* Chilton, UK: NRPB, 2000.

33. Kendall GM, Miles JCH, Cliff KD *et al. Exposure to Radon in UK Dwellings.* Report No. NRPB-R272. Chilton, Oxon: NRPB Publications, 1994.

34. Wrixon AD, Green BMR, Lomas PR *et al. Natural Radiation Exposure in UK Dwellings.* Report No. NRPB-R190. Chilton, Oxon: NRPB Publications, 1998.

35. Miles JCH, Appleton JD, Rees DM *et al. Indicative Atlas of Radon in England and Wales.* Report No. HPA-RPD-033. Chilton, Oxon: Health Protection Agency, 2007.

36. Building Research Establishment. *Radon: Guidance on Protective Measures for New Dwellings.* Report No. BR 211. Garston: BRE, 1991.

37. Building Research Establishment. *Radon: Guidance on Protective Measures for New Buildings.* Report No. BR 211. Garston: BRE, 2007.

38. Building Research Establishment. *Radon: Guidance on Protective Measures for New Dwellings in Scotland.* Report No. BR376. East Kilbride: BRE, 1999.

39. Building Research Establishment. *Radon: Guidance on Protective Measures for New Dwellings in Northern Ireland.* Report No. BR413. East Kilbride: Building BRE, 2001.

40. Åkerblom G. *Radon Legislation and National Guidelines.* SSI Report No. 99:18. Stockholm: Swedish Radiation Protection Agency (SSI), 1999.

41. Synnott H, Fenton D. *An Evaluation of Radon Reference Levels and Radon Measurement Techniques and Protocols in European Countries.* Radiological Protection Institute of Ireland Report, for ERRICCA2 (European Radon Research and Industry Collaborative Concerted Action) European Commission Contract FIRI-CT-2001–20142. Dublin: Radiological Protection Institute of Ireland, 2005.

42. Gray A, Read S, McGale P, Darby S. Lung cancer deaths from indoor radon and the cost effectiveness and potential of policies to reduce them. *BMJ Clin Res Ed.* 2009; **338**: a3110.

43. International Commission on Radiological Protection. *ICRP Statement on Radon 2009.* Approved by the International Commission on Radiological Protection November 2009. Downloadable from http://www.icrp.org/icrp_radon.asp (accessed March 2010).

44. Building Research Establishment. *Surveying Dwellings with High Indoor Radon Levels: A BRE Guide to Radon Remedial Measures in Existing Dwellings.* Report No. BR 250. Garston: BRE, 1993.

Noise

ANDY MOORHOUSE

Many experts consider noise to be a quality-of-life issue rather than strictly a health concern. Nevertheless, environmental noise is increasingly being considered under the banner of health. This is not surprising if we take a broad definition of health: a state of complete physical, mental and social well-being might be considered to be free from annoyance due to noise. But there is more to it than this; recent research has linked noise exposure to more mainstream health risk factors, in particular to cardiovascular disease.

Several categories of noise can be defined: occupational noise, which occurs exclusively in the workplace; neighbourhood noise, which includes noise from neighbours and other people nearby; and environmental noise, which here will be taken to include noise from transportation, including surface transport (road and rail), air and sea transport, as well that from industry. The World Health Organization (WHO)[1] defines 'community noise' as noise emitted from all sources except the workplace; it thus consists of environmental and neighbourhood noise as defined above. This chapter is primarily concerned with environmental noise, although occupational noise is briefly mentioned in order to provide some context. Environmental vibration is also briefly mentioned since it is closely related to noise and the two are often considered together.

Undoubtedly the most influential source of guidance on environmental noise and health is the WHO guidelines for community noise[1] (which is sometimes dated 1999 and sometimes 2000). The guidelines list possible adverse health effects of noise:

- noise-induced hearing impairment;
- interference with speech communication;
- sleep disturbance;
- cardiovascular and physiological effects;
- mental health effects;

- the effects of noise on performance;
- the effects of noise on residential behaviour and annoyance.

In this chapter, we review the main topics from this list, citing the main studies that have appeared since the WHO guidelines were published. Most attention is devoted to annoyance, sleep disturbance and cardiovascular disease since these are the effects of environmental noise for which the most advanced knowledge exists. First, however, we introduce some basic concepts required for interpreting environmental noise data.

QUANTIFYING SOUND EXPOSURE

It is first necessary to draw a clear distinction between the objective nature of 'sound' and the subjective nature of 'noise'. Sound is simply a vibration transmitted through the air as a wave. Most sound, like natural sounds, speech and music, is either neutral or beneficial in its effects. Sound only becomes noise when it becomes unwanted or contributes to some harmful effect such as annoyance. A useful definition of noise is therefore 'unwanted sound', implying that it is unwanted by someone for some reason. Therefore, 'noise' depends not just on the physical aspects of the sound itself, but also on the human reaction to it, which brings into play a raft of complex psychological and other factors. In practice, this distinction is often blurred, and the terms 'sound' and 'noise' are commonly used interchangeably. For professionals working in the field, however, it is essential to differentiate between the physical and the subjective aspects of noise. In the remainder of this section, we will discuss the (objective) measurement of sound.

Environmental noise indicators

That sound is measured in decibels, abbreviated dB, is common knowledge. However, it is important to be aware that a number of different indicators based on dB are in common use that cannot necessarily be compared. It is thus essential to be clear which indicator is being used before any conclusions can be drawn from the results of measurements. Environmental sound is a highly complex, multidimensional phenomenon that varies with time, has varying frequency content, occurs at different times of day and has a wide range of other distinguishing characteristics. The aim of environmental sound indicators is to distil this complex phenomenon into a single number representative of sound exposure, and, not surprisingly, there are several ways in which this can be done.

Considering first the question of frequency content, common experience tells us that music consists not only of rhythm but also melody, comprising sound at different pitches. Frequency is closely related to the concept of musical pitch, so, for example, we might describe high- or low-pitched sounds that would contain predominantly high or low frequencies. The frequency variation in environmental sounds is conveniently taken into account by using an 'A' weighting filter during measurement. The A-weighting is applied to mimic the frequency response of the human ear, so that the contributions of sounds at frequencies to which we have lower sensitivity are attenuated (reduced), and

those to which we are most sensitive are emphasized. For example, very high-frequency sounds, audible to bats but not humans, would not register on an A-weighted measurement. When A-weighting has been applied, as is nearly always the case when dealing with environmental sound, the symbol A occurs in the indicator subscript.

The question of how to account for the time variation of environmental sound is somewhat more complicated, and several different approaches are in use. The most common approach is to use the 'equivalent continuous' sound level $L_{Aeq,T}$, effectively the average level over the time period T. The upper case 'L' denotes 'level' and indicates a decibel quantity. An alternative is to use a maximum level, L_{Amax}, occurring during the measurement period (this should be measured using a 'fast' time constant on the sound level meter). L_{Aeq} is found to correlate with general annoyance, whereas L_{Amax} captures the single noisiest event, which might be important in sleep disturbance.

Statistical measures are also sometimes used, notably the level exceeded for 10 per cent or 90 per cent of the measurement period, referred to as L_{A10} and L_{A90} respectively. The 24 hour indicator L_{den} (day–evening-night level) additionally takes into account the time of day at which the sound occurs: the sound levels measured during the evening and night are increased by 5 and 10 dB, respectively, to account for the fact that disturbance is more likely during these periods. The most common noise indicators are summarized in Table 57.1.

Table 57.1   Summary of environmental noise indicators

Indicator	Use	Description
$L_{Aeq,T}$	As a general descriptor of environmental sound exposure	The equivalent continuous sound pressure level, i.e. the sound pressure level of a hypothetical constant sound containing the same energy as the actual sound whose level may vary over the measurement period. It can be helpful to think of it as an average level. The measurement period, T, must be stated, so for example we have $L_{Aeq,16\ hour}$
L_{day} $L_{evening}$ L_{night}	Noise-mapping	Day, evening and night levels. These are similar to $L_{Aeq,T}$ for the following time periods: • Day – 07:00–19:00 hours • Evening – 19:00–23:00 hours • Night – 23:00–07:00 hours However, these are long-term averages, i.e. determined over all the day/evening/night periods of the year
L_{den}	'Noise'-mapping	Day–evening-night level. This is similar to an $L_{Aeq,20\ hour}$, but sound occurring during the evening and night is given a 'penalty' of 5 dB and 10 dB respectively
L_{A90}	As an indicator of the steady background sound level	The sound level exceeded for 90% of the measurement period. Broadly speaking, this corresponds to the steady background sound level*
L_{A10}	Sometimes used to assess traffic noise	The sound level exceeded for 10% of the measurement period. This is an indicator of the higher levels occurring during the measurement period*
L_{AE}	To quantify sound events, like pass-by sound from trains	Sound exposure level. The sound pressure level of a hypothetical sound that, if maintained constant for 1 second, would contain the same energy as the actual sound over the measurement period (which may be longer or shorter than 1 second). It does not correspond to a level actually experienced by a listener but is mostly used for calculation purposes

*Generally, any percentage value could be used. These descriptors are known generically as 'percentile' levels.

Sounds with identical $L_{Aeq,T}$ may, however, differ considerably in their capacity to cause annoyance or disturbance because of the character of the sounds. This is recognized in British Standard 4142, where a correction of 5 dB is added to a measured $L_{Aeq,T}$ from an industrial source if the sound 'contains a distinguishable, discrete, continuous note (whine, hiss, screech, hum, etc.)', if it 'contains distinct impulses (bangs, clicks, clatters, or thumps)' or if it is 'irregular enough to attract attention'. The fact that the judgement is made on a purely subjective basis is, in a sense, an acknowledgement that we are not currently able to account for the complex experience of hearing sounds in a single indicator in a reliable, objective manner. Nevertheless, the indicators summarized in Table 57.1 are likely to remain important for the foreseeable future.

Measurement uncertainty

An appreciation of the uncertainty inherent in measured sound levels is useful when interpreting measured data. Sound level meters cannot generally measure more accurately than the nearest 0.5 dB, whereas considerably larger variance could occur in field measurements due to weather, microphone positioning, the effect of the operator and several other factors. The paramount importance of proper calibration should also be mentioned here: many measurement standards require full, traceable calibration every 12 or 24 months, together with a field calibration on site before and after measurement.

Sound sources and receivers

Environmental noise indicators as described above define the noise at a given receiver location (which should always be specified); for example, we may quote the $L_{Aeq,T}$ outside a dwelling or at 10 m from the edge of a motorway. As such, they characterize the noise 'immission', or the noise 'coming in' to the location. However, when dealing with noise sources, we talk of the noise 'emission', or the noise 'going out' from the source.

Two basic approaches are used to characterize the emission of sound sources: the first is to specify the immission at a standard receiver location, an example of which is for road vehicle pass-by noise that is specified in terms of sound levels at a receiver location 7.5 m from the closest point. Alternatively, sound sources are characterized by their sound power level (given the symbol L_{WA}, W denoting power). Sound power level quantifies the total sound energy emitted per second from the source and is independent of the location of the source. It is important to appreciate that *sound power levels*, which characterize a source, are not directly comparable to *sound pressure levels*, which apply at a given receiver location. This is a common cause of confusion since both use the decibel scale. Sound power levels are used in the 'Outdoor Equipment Directive'[2]

as a means of labelling, and setting limits for outdoor equipment, as will be discussed later. Thus, sound power levels provide legislators with a useful tool for controlling many of the sources of environmental sound. There are various sources of guidance should the reader require a further explanation of these concepts.[3,4]

Comparing noise levels

As with other senses, the sensation produced by a sound stimulus is related to the logarithm of the intensity of the stimulus (Weber–Fechner law). In *objective* terms, a 3 dB increase or decrease in sound level corresponds to a doubling or halving of the sound energy, and an increase or decrease of 10 dB corresponds to a 10-fold increase in sound energy. However, in *subjective* terms, most people associate an increase or decrease in sound level of about 10 dB with a perceptual doubling or halving of loudness; a 3 dB increase or decrease in the level of a sound is often quoted as the smallest change likely to be noticed by most people. These rules of thumb are summarized in Table 57.2. There are important implications here regarding the cost and effectiveness of noise control: in order to provide a halving of loudness in perceptual terms, a 10-fold decrease in sound energy is required, i.e. a reduction to one-tenth of its original value. A further halving requires a further 10-fold decrease, so a reduction to one-hundredth of its original value.

It can be seen that statements like 'new legislation will reduce road noise by half' are unclear or misleading – this could mean 3 dB or 10 dB depending on whether a subjective or an objective basis is assumed. Instead, the comparison should be made in decibels, for example '3 dB greater than', '10 dB less than', etc., and if necessary an interpretation can be given as to what this means in perceptual terms, for example 'a reduction of 10 dB, which would be perceived as approximately a halving of loudness'.

Table 57.2 Rules of thumb for changes in level of steady sounds

Increase of 10 dB	Objectively	10-fold increase in sound energy
	Subjectively	Doubling of loudness
Increase of 3 dB	Objectively	Doubling of sound energy
	Subjectively	Just noticeable difference (see text)
Decrease of 10 dB	Objectively	10-fold decrease in sound energy
	Subjectively	Halving of loudness
Decrease of 3 dB	Objectively	Halving of sound energy
	Subjectively	Just noticeable difference (see text)

A further note of caution is that the rules of thumb for perception apply to changes in the level of the sound when all other factors remain constant (frequency content, time structure and character of the sound). Consider the common example where the $L_{Aeq,T}$ (the average sound level) changes due to an increase or decrease in the number of noise events, such as vehicle movements. If the change in the L_{Aeq} were small, say 2 dB, Table 57.2 might be taken as an indication that it would not be noticed; however, if individual events were distinguishable, for example air overflights or train pass-bys, the time structure of the sound before and after the change would be quite different, so the rule of thumb cannot be safely applied. But if individual events were indistinguishable (e.g. noise from a distant busy road), it could be assumed that only the level of the sound would change, in which case the rule of thumb would be valid.

MEASURING THE EFFECTS OF NOISE

As seen in the previous section, quantifying sound exposure is more complex than it may at first appear. In this section, we consider the question of how to quantify the effects of noise on people, or how they respond to noise, which is arguably even more difficult. Measurement of the human response to noise is needed to examine both the extent of noise impact and the likely effectiveness of measures taken to mitigate noise.

A fundamental idea, underpinning much research and practice in the field of environmental noise, is that there exists a relationship between the (objective) noise exposure and the (subjective) response. Such relationships are described as dose–response relationships (also sometimes called dose–effect, exposure–effect and other variations). These usually take the form of a graphical or mathematical relationship between the dose and response measures, some examples of which are given later. In order to derive such relationships, it is clear that compatible measurements of both dose (see the previous section) and response (this section) are required.

Various 'instruments' have been developed to measure response to noise and are usually specific to the adverse effect being considered. For example, community reaction surveys are used to quantify annoyance, electroencephalogram (EEG) and actigram responses may be used to evaluate sleep disturbance, and measurements of hearing loss have been used to evaluate the risk of hearing damage from occupational noise exposure. Further variations include surveys of complaints, used to quantify the adverse effects of noise on a community, school examination results, used to investigate the effect of noise on children's learning, and cost analyses such as an evaluation of the (hypothetical) willingness to pay to mitigate noise nuisance. Investigations can be conducted in the field or in laboratory settings.

Attitudes of populations to noise can be investigated using large-scale social surveys. One example is the Noise Attitude Survey carried out in the UK around 1990 and again around 2000.[5] This consisted of a questionnaire survey of around 5000 people around the UK asking which noise sources people could hear and whether they were adversely affected. The results provide a valuable record of attitudes to noise nationally, and furthermore, by comparing the results of the two surveys, changes in attitudes over the intervening decade can be monitored.

Responses to noise can be presented in various ways, for example the number of people affected, the percentage of the population affected, the area affected, etc. It is currently common practice to assess annoyance according to the percentage of the population 'highly annoyed, bothered or disturbed', although this is only one of many possible measures.

Dose–response relationships should generally be treated with some caution since there tends to be a wide scatter in any measurement of subjective response, including those from social surveys. This point is illustrated in Figure 57.1, taken from a study by Fields and Walker that has become widely accepted as the definitive study of annoyance caused by noise from trains.[6] The measure of response used was the 'summed annoyance index', which is plotted against $L_{Aeq,24\ hour}$. Note that, for a given sound level, the response of individual subjects may vary significantly, some subjects reporting high annoyance and others very low annoyance. Alternatively, the sound levels recorded for any given response measure vary by more than 30 dB, which can be interpreted in terms of the rules of thumb given in the previous section. Despite the scatter, Fields and Walker were able to derive a meaningful dose–response relationship, but it should be clear that this can only provide a general trend for a population and that the response of particular individuals may vary significantly from the trend. It follows that surveys based on a small sample or on a sample living in a particular area may not extend to the wider population.

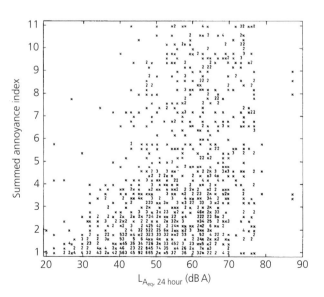

Figure 57.1 Average responses to railway noise at different levels. (Adapted from Fields and Walker,[6] with permission from Elsevier.)

The fact that there is inherently a degree of scatter in any dose–response relationship has important implications for determining acceptable limits for noise. In effect, one must decide what proportion of the population should be protected and set the limits accordingly. Setting the limit too high may leave too many people unsatisfied, but too low a limit might carry severe cost penalties for the reasons described in the previous section. In any case, there is still likely to be a proportion of people, however small, left with the impression that they are not properly protected.

A further method of gauging the adverse impact of noise is through surveys of complaints. In the UK, the Chartered Institute of Environmental Health compiles annual statistics of formal complaints to local authorities. For various reasons, however, it is far more difficult to extract reliable trends from such data than it might first appear. For example, the number of complaints may be significantly affected by the existence or otherwise of a complaint-recording mechanism and the extent to which it is known about by potential complainants. The number of complaints may also vary due to factors not related to noise, for example with the amount of publicity surrounding a particular issue.

Since the publication of the WHO guidelines in 2000, there have been important developments in the European Union (EU). The Environmental Noise Directive[7] requires all Member States to generate maps of the L_{den} and L_{night} caused by transportation noise sources. These indicators were selected because of their correlation with annoyance and sleep disturbance, respectively. It should be noted that such maps indicate objective levels of sound, but by combining these with dose–response relationships, the results can be presented in terms of the percentage of people highly annoyed and sleep disturbed.

EFFECTS OF NOISE ON HEALTH

In this section, we will discuss the effects of noise on health, but first we will consider the possible mechanisms by which such effects may occur. There is no doubt that exposure to noise at high levels can cause physiological damage to the hearing system (see 'Noise-induced hearing impairment', below). However, in this chapter, we are primarily concerned with environmental sound for which the levels of noise at the ear are considerably lower, of the order of approximately 30–60 dBA (the units dBA indicating A-weighted decibels, as described above). Physiological damage is not expected at these levels.

The amount of physical power in sound is considerably less than is often appreciated. To illustrate this, if we take a sound level of 57 dBA, which is the average external daytime level in the UK, the sound intensity is only $0.5\,\mu W/m^2$, or half a millionth of a Watt per square metre. If we take the average body as having a surface area of slightly more than 1 square metre, the acoustic power incident on the body at 57 dBA will be of the order of one

micro-Watt, i.e. one millionth of a Watt, only a small fraction of which will actually enter the body in the form of vibration. To put this in context, the intensity of strong sunlight is about $1\,kW/m^2$, and the power of a typical beating heart in an adult is of the order of 1 W. It is therefore evident that the acoustic power associated with environmental sound is extremely small compared with that of everyday occurrences and normal body processes.

This conclusion may at first appear to contradict everyday experience since we often experience sounds as being 'powerful'. The apparent contradiction can be partly explained by the extraordinary sensitivity of the ear. We may also speculate that the experience of power is essentially emotional rather than physical, and that there is perhaps a role played by association: for example, although the physical energy in the sound of a bulldozer is small, the sound is associated with the considerable physical power of the machine itself.

It is clear that more subtle mechanisms must play a role if noise is to affect non-auditory aspects of health at the levels found in environmental noise. A plausible explanation has been found in the stress hypothesis: the function of the stress mechanism is to prepare the organism to cope with a demanding stressor (linked to the fight or flight response). Any resulting arousal of the sympathetic and endocrine system is then associated with changes in physiological functions and the metabolism of the organism, including blood pressure and a range of other factors, which in the long term may increase the risk of disease. In this model, stress does not necessarily follow on from annoyance and could conceivably arise at low noise levels.[8]

In the WHO guidelines,[1] guideline values are given as a basis for preventing some of the health effects considered. Table 57.3 reproduces the table of values from these guidelines that has been highly influential worldwide. Some of these values are discussed in the following subsections.

Noise-induced hearing impairment

Exposure to noise levels of more than around 80 dBA for a few hours a day can lead to a progressive loss of hearing. Noise-induced hearing loss is the most prevalent irreversible occupational hazard worldwide.[1] Although sufferers will generally still be able to hear, their ability to understand speech will be reduced, and this can become a significant social handicap, which is taken seriously by health authorities worldwide. Damage can also result from individual noise events if the level is sufficiently high, which normally occurs only in the case of explosions or firearms. Noise-induced hearing loss does not occur at levels below $L_{Aeq,24\,hour}$ of 70 dB(A).[9] Exposure above these levels may occur in occupational settings, but there may be risks in other situations too, such as with amplified music (including headphone use) or in certain leisure activities such as shooting and motor sports.[10]

Table 57.3 Guideline values for community noise in specific environments

Specific environment	Critical health effect(s)	L_{Aeq} (dB)	Time base (hours)	L_{Amax} fast (dB)
Outdoor living area	Serious annoyance, daytime and evening	55	16	–
	Moderate annoyance, daytime and evening	55	16	–
Dwelling, indoors	Speech intelligibility and moderate annoyance, daytime and evening	35	16	50
Inside bedrooms	Sleep disturbance, night-time	30	8	45
Outside bedrooms	Sleep disturbance, window open (outdoor values)	45	8	60
School class rooms and pre-schools, indoors	Speech intelligibility, disturbance of information extraction, message communication	35	during class	–
Pre-school Bedrooms, indoors	Sleep disturbance	30	sleeping-time	45
School, playground outdoor	Annoyance (external source)	55	during play	–
Hospital, ward rooms, indoors	Sleep disturbance, night-time	30	8	40
	Sleep disturbance, daytime and evenings	30	16	–
Hospital, treatment rooms, indoors	Interference with rest and recovery	#1	–	–
Industrial, commercial, shopping and traffic areas, indoors and outdoors	Hearing impairment	70	24	110
Ceremonies, festivals and entertaiment events	Hearing impairment (patrons:<5 times/year)	100	4	110
Public addresses, indoors and outdoors	Hearing impairment	85	1	110
Music through headphones/earphones	Hearing impairment (free-field value)	85 #4	1	110
Impulse sounds from toys, fireworks and firearms	Hearing impairment (adults)	–	–	140 #2
	Hearing impairment (children)	–	–	120 #2
Outdoors in parkland and conservation areas	Disruption of tranquillity	#3	–	–

#1: As low as possible.
#2: Peak sound pressure (not L_{Amax}, fast), measured 100 mm from the ear.
#3: Existing quiet outdoor areas should be preserved and the ratio of intruding noise to natural background sound should be kept low.
#4: Under headphones, adapted to free-field values.
Adapted from World Health Organization,[1] with permission.

Noise and annoyance

Annoyance triggered by noise is a common experience, although what precisely is meant by annoyance may vary widely. In the WHO guidelines, annoyance is defined as 'a feeling of displeasure associated with any agent or condition, known or believed by an individual or group to adversely affect them'.[1] It is, however, acknowledged that a range of other negative feelings may arise from noise exposure, encompassing anger, disappointment, dissatisfaction, withdrawal, helplessness, depression, anxiety, distraction, agitation and exhaustion.[1]

As described above, annoyance is most commonly measured by community surveys, i.e. on a subjective, self-reporting basis. Interference with tasks, such as reading or watching television, can also be measured, and it might be thought that such an approach might provide a more objective basis for the assessment of annoyance, although this turns out not to be the case.[1] Task interference is

therefore usually treated as a separate category. The difficulties of defining annoyance have to some extent been circumvented by the introduction of a standard form of questionnaire:[11] annoyance effectively then becomes defined by the way it is measured.[12] It should, however, be noted that, although the standard approach has been adopted by the noise community, this does not imply that there is a complete consensus on all points.

Annoyance triggered by noise is widespread. As an example, a survey of a representative sample of the population in the UK in 1999 found road traffic to be the most commonly reported source of noise, heard by 84 per cent of respondents, with 40 per cent of respondents being to some extent 'bothered, annoyed or disturbed' by it.[5] Overall, survey results suggest that although the majority of the population do not consider themselves to be significantly bothered by noise, a significant minority are affected, and many of these people consider some of the effects to be seriously damaging to their overall quality of life.

One of the first dose–response curves was derived by Schultz in 1978[13] by combining the results of 11 surveys of community response to noise from road, rail and air transport to produce a single curve showing the relationship between sound level and annoyance. The Schultz curve, as this has become known, has been periodically updated as the results of new surveys become available: Figure 57.2 shows the original Schultz (1978) curve, together with updated curves from 1991[14] and 1994[15] (from van Kempen et al.[16]).

The WHO recommends that the average noise level in dwellings during the day should be below 35 dB $L_{Aeq,16\,hour}$

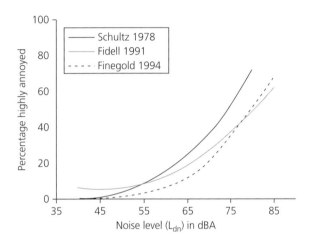

Figure 57.2 Comparison of the Schultz, Fidell and Finegold versions of the Schultz curve. (Adapted from van Kempen et al.,[16] with permission.)

to prevent annoyance.[1] Furthermore, to protect the majority of people from being seriously annoyed during the daytime, the sound pressure level on balconies, terraces and outdoor living areas should not exceed 55 dB L_{Aeq} for a steady, continuous noise, and 50 dB L_{Aeq} to prevent moderate annoyance. The guidelines are given in terms of L_{Aeq} as averaged sound levels have been found to give good correlation with reported annoyance.[1] It is also pointed out that, in some situations, lower limits may be required, in particular where the sound contains a high proportion of low-frequency sound and where perceptible vibration accompanies the noise.

The adoption of the Environmental Noise Directive[7] and noise-mapping in Europe has gone hand in hand with the investigation and adoption of dose–response relationships for annoyance and sleep disturbance. In 2002, the EU published a position paper on dose–response relationships for annoyance from transportation noise[17] (see also reference 18). The preferred indicator of annoyance in the population is given as the percentage of persons annoyed or highly annoyed. The paper goes on to present dose–response curves giving the percentage of people annoyed and highly annoyed as a function of L_{den} for different noise sources (road, rail and air traffic); some of these are reproduced in Figure 57.3 (also published in reference 19). Note that L_{den} is measured outside and the reduction in sound level from outside to inside is typically 15 dB when bedroom windows are open. The L_{den} at which the curves start is therefore broadly consistent with the WHO guideline value of 30 dB L_{Aeq} for inside bedrooms (see the next section). Note that there are significant differences between the curves for the different sources:

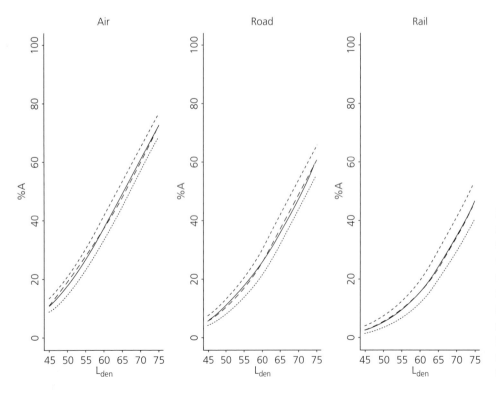

Figure 57.3 The percentage annoyed persons (%A) as a function of the noise exposure of the dwelling (L_{den}). The solid lines are the estimated curves, and the dashed lines are polynomial approximations. The figure also shows the 95 percent confidence intervals (dotted lines). (Adapted from European Communities,[17] with permission.)

according to the curves, for the same L_{den}, aircraft noise annoys more people than road traffic noise, and railway noise causes the least annoyance.

It is proposed in the position paper that the dose–response curves may facilitate the elimination of noise 'black spots', the preservation and extension of quiet areas (white areas), and an improvement in the acoustical quality of residential areas with intermediate noise levels (grey areas). These curves should not be taken to apply to local situations, to local sources such as helicopters, or to assessing the short-term effects of a change in noise climate.

Noise and sleep disturbance

Proper sleep is a prerequisite for good health, and common experience tells us that sleep can be disturbed by noise. The effects of noise on sleep have therefore been widely studied. However, there is still much that is not understood, some of the evidence is not consistent or is even contradictory, and deriving reliable dose–response relationships has proved difficult.[12] Self-reported sleep disturbance is quite widespread: in a review carried out in the Netherlands, the number of adults who reported to be highly sleep disturbed due to night-time traffic noise was reported to be between one hundred thousand and one million.[20] The number disturbed by road traffic noise was between two and four times as large as that from rail and aircraft, and noise from neighbours, air traffic and recreation was also reported. The report concludes that, by affecting sleep, night-time traffic noise is one of the most important effects exerted by the physical environment on health.

Sleep is more complex than it may first appear, and it is well known that various stages occur during sleep; in particular, rapid eye movement (REM) sleep can be distinguished from non-REM sleep and slow-wave sleep (SWS). The effects of noise are also complex. A recent EU position paper on night-time noise, compiled by a panel of experts,[21] distinguishes three stages in the development of effects, depending on the time frame. Instantaneous effects are said to comprise a release of stress hormones, a change in blood pressure, a change in heart rate, vasoconstriction, the onset of motility (movement), a change in sleep stage and awakening. Effects during and after one night of exposure include increased sleep latency (time getting to sleep), increased average motility, altered duration of the REM/SWS stages, sleep structure fragmentation, increased cortisol in the blood, increased (nor)adrenaline ([nor] epinephrine)/dopamine and altered mood and performance the next day. Long-term effects are listed as self-reported (chronic) sleep disturbance, a chronic increase in motility, an increased use of sleeping pills, and an increased risk of hypertension and myocardial infarction. Consistent with the stress hypothesis, an important first stage of effects appears to be arousal, itself a complex phenomenon that is not fully understood.[22]

Thus, a complex picture emerges of the effects of noise, which partly explains the difficulty in establishing dose–response relationships.

These different factors suggest a range of methods to assess the effects of sleep disturbance. A range of measurement methods is possible, including surveys of self-reported disturbance, surveys of drug use, EEG responses, measurements of heart rate, blood pressure and actimetry.[23] Actimeters are wrist-worn devices that monitor movements that can be analysed to assess the duration of the sleep period, sleep onset time and wake-up time.[22] Field and laboratory studies have been conducted, and experimental studies in controlled environments, including in the laboratory, have generally provided the strongest basis for our understanding.[1]

However, laboratory study results cannot be relied upon to predict effects in domestic environments. In part, this is due to habituation, which cannot be fully reproduced in controlled environments. It is clear that habituation to night-time noise does occur to some extent, although perhaps not completely, especially for heart rate. Interestingly, physiological or behavioural measurements often show lower responses than are obtained from subjective reports. This may in part be due to awakenings being wrongly attributed to noise, and a report by a committee of UK experts has concluded that self-report is not a good indicator of objective sleep disturbance. However, the extent to which people *feel* they are disturbed, or otherwise, by noise in their sleep is clearly of some importance even if it does not relate well to actual sleep disturbance.[12]

In their guidance document,[1] the WHO provided guideline values for night-time noise exposure:

- L_{Amax} of 45 dB;
- L_{Aeq} of 30 dB.

The L_{Aeq} should be taken over the period of sleep, normally taken to be 8 hours. Note that two limits are given: L_{Amax} corresponds to the single noisiest event during the period of sleep, which is said to be important for arousal and therefore for instantaneous effects; and L_{Aeq} is effectively the average level over the sleep period, which correlates more with long-term effects.[22] The guideline values are based on the lowest levels at which physiologically measured disturbance has been observed and are considered by some to be conservative. Nevertheless, they have been highly influential and have been widely adopted. The WHO also recommends that special attention be given to noise sources in an environment with a low background noise level, environments where a combination of noise and vibrations are produced, and sources with low-frequency components.[1]

It should be noted that the WHO limits are for sound levels inside bedrooms: external levels may be estimated by assuming a 15 dB reduction for an open window. The corresponding external levels would therefore be

L_{Amax} 60 dB and L_{Aeq} 45 dB. Although this rule of thumb is expected to be quite reliable if windows actually are open, this will, however, often not be the case. If windows are closed, a greater reduction from inside to outside would be expected, which is more difficult to estimate and subject to greater variation since it will depend on the types of window, how well sealed they are, etc.

Since the publication of the WHO guidelines,[1] there has been considerable progress. The 2004 EU position paper[21] gives a more comprehensive set of dose–response relationships, relating to the number of awakenings, the onset of motility, self-reported sleep disturbance, any chronic increase of motility and the increased risk of hypertension.

A relationship is given for number of awakenings in terms of the L_{AE} (which effectively quantifies the sound energy at the receiver in a noise event such as an aircraft flyover). Figure 57.4 shows a similar relationship between the predicted number of awakenings and the external night-time noise level L_{night}; hence it is based on an average over the night rather than on a level for individual events. Because L_{night} is defined as an external level and the event-based relationship for awakening is based on internal levels, it was necessary in deriving Figure 57.4 to adjust for the reduction of sound from outside to inside. The EU used a similar approach to that described above, except that they adopted a reduction of 21 dB rather than 15 dB, based on the assumption that the window would be closed for a proportion of the year. The WHO guideline value of 30 dB internal L_{Aeq} would therefore correspond to 51 dB outside. It can be seen from Figure 57.4 that this corresponds approximately to the onset of awakenings. In this respect, therefore, the WHO and EU criteria are seen to be consistent. Figure 57.5 shows the relationship between the probability of aircraft-induced motility and the L_{Amax} inside the bedroom.

As with other dose–response relationships for noise, the above relationships and thresholds should be treated

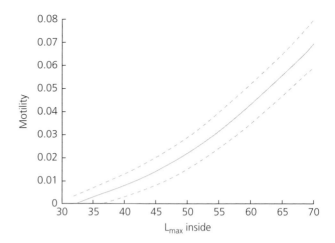

Figure 57.5 Probability of (aircraft) noise-induced motility at the 15 second interval in which the indoor maximum sound level occurs (solid line) and the 95 per cent confidence interval (dotted lines), as a function of L_{Amax} inside the bedroom. (Adapted from European Commission Working Group,[21] with permission; see also Passchier-Vermeer et al.[24])

with some caution. First, considerable variation would be expected between individuals subject to the same exposure. Additionally, some of the evidence is conflicting: a more recent WHO publication argues for considerably lower night-time noise guidelines than have previously been suggested.[25] A final note of caution concerns the strength of the cause-and-effect relationship: although dose–response relationships are becoming well established, it should be remembered that the WHO estimates that 80–90 per cent of awakenings in noisy environments are caused by factors other than noise,[1] and a committee of experts in the UK has concluded that there is only a weak association between outdoor noise levels and sleep disturbance.[12]

Cardiovascular and physiological effects

Associations between noise and cardiovascular risk factors were discussed by Berglund et al. in the 2000 WHO guidelines,[1] although at that time no dose–response relationships existed. There has been considerable activity in the field since then, as evidenced in reviews by Babisch,[8,26,27] van Kempen et al.[28] and the Health Council of the Netherlands.[20]

Acute exposure to noise is known from laboratory studies on animals to cause physiological activation including increases in heart rate and blood pressure. The physiological response to short-term exposure tends to be short-lived, but the effects of long-term exposure are less certain. There is also evidence from many studies conducted in occupational settings where individuals exposed to continuous sound levels of 85 dBA or greater over the long

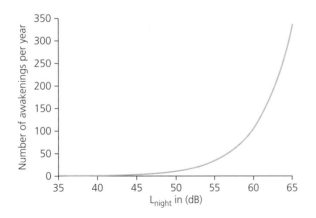

Figure 57.4 Worst case prediction of aircraft noise induced behavioural awakenings. (Adapted from European Commission Working Group,[21] with permission.)

term tend to have higher blood pressure than those not exposed. There are often other factors that could raise blood pressure in such settings, such as risk of injury, and it has also been shown that the effects are worse for workers performing complex tasks.[12] Nevertheless, we are concerned in this chapter with whether such effects could occur with the much lower noise levels found in environmental noise.

Some evidence appeared in the 1970s, when Knipschild reported that, in areas with more aircraft noise around Schiphol Airport in Amsterdam, more people were under medical treatment for heart trouble and hypertension, had a higher usage of cardiovascular drugs and demonstrated higher blood pressures.[29] The effects could not be explained by age, sex, smoking habits, height/weight or socioeconomic differences. Until recently, however, there was little evidence to support these findings.

In a review of a wide range of surveys from Europe, the Soviet Union, the USA and Australia in 2000, Babisch found a mixed picture with some inconsistent evidence.[26] Overall, he found 'no epidemiological evidence' of a relationship between noise exposure and mean blood pressure in adults, although increases were consistently found in children. He also found 'little evidence' of hypertension and 'some evidence' of increased risk of ischaemic heart disease in subjects living in areas where outdoor noise levels exceeded 65–70 dB(A). This review was updated in 2006,[27] by which time the results of more studies of road traffic and aircraft noise had become available. Here, Babisch reported increased evidence of an association between community noise and ischaemic heart disease. However, for subjects living in areas with a daytime average sound pressure level of less than 60 dB(A), there was not much indication of a risk.

The recent large-scale, European-funded Hypertension and Exposure to Noise Near Airports (HYENA) study investigated hypertension using blood pressure measurements.[30,31] The team studied 4861 subjects, half men, who had lived near one of the six major European airports for at least 5 years. After correcting for confounding factors such as country, age, body mass index, alcohol intake, education and exercise, some statistically significant exposure–response relationships were found between noise exposure and risk of hypertension. For night-time aircraft noise ($L_{Aeq,8\ hour}$), as shown in Table 57.4, a 10 dB increase in exposure was associated with an odds ratio of 1.14 (95 per cent confidence interval [CI] 1.01–1.29). Similar results were reported for road traffic noise, although here the result was more significant for men than women. However, no corresponding significant relationship was found for daytime noise exposure to aircraft noise ($L_{Aeq,16\ hour}$). Jarup et al.'s paper concluded that the increased risk of hypertension in relation to aircraft and road traffic noise near airports may contribute to the burden of cardiovascular disease, hypertension being an important risk factor for myocardial infarction and stroke.[26]

Table 57.4 The odds ratios (95% confidence intervals) of hypertension related to aircraft and road traffic noise using continuous variables, showing the risk per 10 dB increase in noise exposure

Variable	Odds ratio (95% confidence interval)	P-value
$L_{Aeq,216\ hour}$ aircraft	0.928 (0.829–1.038)	0.190
L_{night} aircraft	1.141 (1.012–1.286)	0.031
$L_{Aeq,24\ hour}$ road traffic	1.097 (1.003–1.201)	0.044

All noise indicators were included in the model, which was adjusted for country, age, sex, body mass index, alcohol intake, education and exercise.
Adapted from Jarup et al.,[30] with permission).

As the results from an increasing number of surveys become available, and through an increasing use of meta-analysis, some dose–response relationships have begun to emerge.[8,16,28] These have in turn led to estimates of the number of people at risk: Kempen et al.,[14] Babisch[8] and Berry[32] have all estimated the number of early deaths related to the effects of noise, although Kempen et al. concede that epidemiological evidence for an association between noise and cardiovascular disease is limited. The number of people affected is small, and the findings are the subject of ongoing debate. Nevertheless, these estimates may well have an impact on the way in which noise is viewed.

Effect of noise on children's cognition

The effects of noise on children's cognition were noted in the WHO guidelines under the heading of performance,[1] although no noise level guidelines were given. Since then, Hygge et al. have completed a study of 326 children (mean age 10.4 years) in Munich before and after the closing of the old airport and the opening of a new one.[33] They found that long-term memory and reading were impaired in the noise group at the new airport and improved in the formerly noise-exposed group at the old airport. Short-term memory also improved in the latter group after the old airport had been closed, and speech perception was impaired in the newly noise-exposed group near the new airport.

Further studies include the international Road Traffic and Aircraft Noise Exposure and Children's Cognition and Health (RANCH) project,[34] which concluded that a chronic environmental stressor (aircraft noise) could impair cognitive development, specifically reading comprehension, in children. However, the same effects were not observed for road traffic noise, where, if anything, episodic memory showed better performance in high road traffic noise areas. Shield and Dockrell also found external noise to be associated with a significant negative impact upon performance in standardized tests in school children in the UK.[35]

Low-frequency noise and vibration

It is stressed several times in the WHO guidelines that special attention should be paid to situations where the noise contains significant low-frequency components or is accompanied by perceptible vibration.[1] There is no evidence that low-frequency noise (usually taken to include noise in the frequency range 10–200 Hz) at environmental levels has a direct physiological effect on the body.[12,36,37] However, low-frequency noise is considered sufficiently important that specific legislation and guidelines have been adopted in Germany, Denmark, Sweden, the Netherlands, Poland, the UK, Japan and Australia.[36]

The effects of vibration on health can be classed as annoyance, hand–arm vibration (associated with the use of power tools) and whole-body vibration (associated mostly with transportation). Whereas the latter two categories are acknowledged to cause physiological damage, only annoyance is of concern at the levels encountered in the environment. The reader is referred to Griffin's comprehensive handbook for further information.[38]

NOISE CONTROL

At the beginning of this chapter, we discussed the measurement and quantification of sound by various noise indicators. We then went on to discuss possible health effects and dose–response relationships that, if sufficiently developed, might serve as a basis for setting targets for noise at receiver locations. In cases where existing or predicted noise levels exceed target levels, it is necessary to consider noise reduction or control. In this section, we present the possible approaches to noise control and try to give the reader a feel for the amount of attenuation possible from various common measures.

A useful framework within which to consider noise control options is the source–paths–receiver model.

'Receiver' and 'source' have already been defined, and the term 'paths' refers to any paths for transmission of sound between the two. There may be options for noise control at source, in the transmission path or at the receiver. The preferred order of treatment is source first, paths second and receiver as a last resort.

Options for noise control at source can be classified as administrative or engineering. Administrative options include restrictions on hours of operation, rerouting of traffic or speed limits and specification of noise limits for vehicles, plant or equipment. Rules of thumb for estimating the noise reduction achievable from reducing exposure time and the number of noise events are given in Table 57.5. An important example of the use of limits is the use of vehicle pass-by noise limits. Here, the method of measurement has been agreed internationally, but individual countries are free to set their own noise limits.

A further significant example of the use of noise limits is the European Outdoor Equipment Directive,[2] which applies to a wide range of more than 50 types of outdoor equipment including, for example, lawnmowers, refuse collection vehicles, dozers, concrete-breakers and even bottle banks and mobile waste containers. Equipment not meeting specified noise emission limits is prohibited from sale in the EU; the legislators have thereby indirectly encouraged manufacturers to establish programmes of noise control by engineering design. Thus, it is hoped that noise limits eventually cascade down into practical engineering. The redesign of equipment for low noise can require advanced skills and know-how if it is to be cost effective, but the commercial drivers created by noise limits have provided sufficient incentive for manufacturers in several industrial sectors, including automotive and aerospace engineering.

An effective method of noise reduction in the transmission path is to increase the distance between the source and receiver: a doubling of distance will give a 3 dB reduction from a line source (like a road or railway) and a

Table 57.5 Attenuation from common noise control measures

Measure	Situation	Noise reduction
Increase in distance	Point source (individual vehicle or machine)	6 dB reduction per doubling of distance
Increase in distance	Line source (road, rail)	3 dB reduction per doubling of distance
Barrier*	Source just visible over barrier	5 dB
Barrier*	Source completely hidden	Typically 10 dB reduction, but may vary from 5 dB to around 20 dB
Windows	From outside to inside through an open window	Reduction of 15 dB
Time reduction	Sound levels that are predominantly steady	3 dB reduction in L_{Aeq} from halving the time of exposure
		1 dB reduction in L_{Aeq} from a 20% decrease in exposure time
		Little or no reduction in L_{Amax} or L_{AE}
Reduction in number of noise events	Noise due to individual events, e.g. vehicle or aircraft pass-bys	3 dB reduction in L_{Ae} from halving the number of events
		1 dB reduction in L_{Aeq} from a 20% decrease in events
		Little or no reduction in L_{Amax} or L_{AE}

*Includes solid screens, earth berms and bunds.

6 dB reduction from a point source (Table 57.5). Noise control in the transmission path also refers to methods for blocking or absorbing sound between the source and the receiver. The most commonly used example is acoustic screening, which usually takes the form of fences, walls or earth mounds (the term 'noise barriers' often being used). Buildings can also be used as screens, for example by using commercial or retail buildings to shield residential properties or parks from major noise sources.

It is important that the screens, or barriers, are without gaps and holes so that sound does not pass directly through them, and they must be sufficiently long to prevent sound transmission round the ends. Typical noise reductions from barriers are given in Table 57.5. Barriers and screens work by deflecting sound from the receiver rather than removing the sound energy entirely, and may in rare cases simply move a problem to another location rather than solving it. Furthermore, reducing noise transmission by one path may reveal another significant transmission path. For these reasons, noise control at source is preferred over noise control along the transmission path.

Noise control at the receiver includes personal hearing protection, whether worn at work or at night in bed. We might also include improvements in façade sound insulation in this category (Table 57.5). Although control at the receiver may sometimes seem the most cost-effective solution, it is usually considered to be a last resort because it contravenes the 'polluter pays' principle.[1]

CONCLUSION

It is clear that the effect of noise on health is an active area of research and that many new results are appearing all the time. At current state of development, dose–response relationships relating to annoyance and sleep disturbance are becoming widely accepted. Regarding cardiovascular risks, there are signs of the emergence of a similar approach, although this is more controversial. On the one hand, the risk factors are relatively small and, as might be expected in studies of this type, there remains inconsistency and uncertainty within the body of evidence as a whole. Many in the environmental noise community are concerned that these small, and to some extent uncertain, risks do not detract attention from more widespread effects of noise as discussed in this chapter. On the other hand, evidence for effects of noise on physical health has been welcomed by many. At least part of the reason is the widely held view that noise has not been given the attention it deserves in policy and that evidence of 'real' health effects will help to move noise issues up the political agenda.

A final comment concerns our attitude to sound in the environment, which, if the preceding pages are any guide, is couched mainly in negative terms, noise being defined as unwanted sound. Some researchers are now exploring a new paradigm that takes a more positive view of sound in the environment.[39] The approach recognizes that many people (69 per cent in a UK survey[5]) are satisfied with their sound environment, or 'soundscape', and that while some sounds are perceived as 'noise', many sounds are pleasing and enriching. Researchers in the field of soundscapes aim to encourage integration of positive sounds into design and to foster a more positive attitude to sound in the environment.

REFERENCES

● = Key primary paper
◆ = Major review article

◆1. Berglund B, Lindvall T, Schwela D (eds), for the World Health Organization. *Guidelines for Community Noise.* Geneva: WHO, 2000.
2. European Commission. *Directive 2000/14/EC of the European Parliament and the Council of 8 May 2000 on the Approximation of the Laws of the Member States Relating to the Noise Emission in the Environment by Equipment for Use Outdoors.* Brussels: European Commission, 2000.
3. Bies DA, Hansen CH. *Engineering Noise Control: Theory and Practice*, 3rd edn. London: Spon Press, 2003.
4. The Environment Agency (2002) IPPC H3 Horizontal Noise Guidance. Part 2: Noise Assessment and Control. Available from: http://www.environment-agency.gov.uk (accessed November 2009).
5. Grimwood CJ, Skinner CJ, Raw G. *The UK National Noise Attitude Survey 1999/2000.* Noise Forum Conference, May 20th, 2002. London: Chartered Institute of Environmental Health, 2002.
6. Fields JM, Walker JG. The response to railway noise in residential areas in Great Britain. *J Sound Vib* 1982; **85**: 177–255.
7. European Commission. *Directive 2002/49/EC, 25 June 2002 Relating to the Assessment and Management of Environmental Noise.* Brussels: European Commission, 2002.
◆8. Babisch W. *Transportation Noise and Cardiovascular Risk. Review and Synthesis of Epidemiological Studies. Dose-Effect Curve and Risk Estimation.* Berlin: Federal Environmental Agency, 2006.
9. International Standards Organisation. *Acoustics – Determination of Occupational Noise Exposure and Estimation of Noise-Induced Hearing Impairment.* ISO Standard 1999. Geneva: ISO, 1990.
10. World Health Organization. *Prevention of Noise-induced Hearing Loss. Report of an Informal Consultation Held at the World Health Organization, Geneva on 28–30 October 1997.* Strategies for Prevention of Deafness and Hearing Impairment No. 3. Geneva: WHO, 1997.
11. International Standards Organisation. *Acoustics – Assessment of Noise Annoyance by Means of Social and Socio-acoustic Surveys.* ISO/TS 15666:2003. Geneva: ISO, 2003.

12. Department of Health. *Environmental Noise and Health in the UK. Draft for Comment, published on Behalf of an Ad Hoc Expert Group on Noise and Health.* London: HPA, 2009.

●13. Schultz TJ. Synthesis of social surveys on noise annoyance. *J Acoust Soc Am* 1978; **64**: 377–405.

14. Fidell S, Barber DS, Schultz TJ. Updating a dosage–effect relationship for the prevalence of annoyance due to general transportation noise. *J Acoust Soc Am* 1991; **89**: 221-33.

15. Finegold LS, Harris S, von de Gierke H. Community annoyance and sleep disturbance: Updated criteria for assessing the impacts of general transportation noise on people. *Noise Control Eng J* 1994; **42**: 25-30.

◆16. van Kempen EEMM, Staatsen B, van Kamp I. *Selection and Evaluation of Exposure–Effect Relationships for Health Impact Assessment in the Field of Noise and Health.* RIVM Report No. 630400001/2005. Bilthoven: Dutch National Institute for Public Health and the Environment, 2005.

●17. European Communities. *Position Paper on Dose Response Relationships Between Transportation Noise and Annoyance.* Luxembourg: Office for Official Publications of the European Communities, 2002.

●18. Miedema HME, Vos H. Exposure response functions for transportation noise. *J Acoust Soc Am* 1998; **104**: 3432–45.

19. Miedema HME, Oudshoorn CGM. Annoyance from transportation noise: Relationships with exposure metrics Ldn and Lden and their confidence intervals. *Environ Health Perspect* 2001; **109**, 409-16.

◆20. Health Council of the Netherlands. *The Influence of Night-time Noise on Sleep and Health.* Publication No. 2004/14E. The Hague: Health Council of the Netherlands, 2004.

●21. European Commission Working Group on Health and Socio-Economic Aspects 2004. *Position Paper on Dose–Effect Relationships for Night Time Noise.* Brussels: European Commission.

◆22. Miedema HME, Passchier-Vermeer W, Vos H. *Elements for a Position Paper on Night-Time Transportation Noise and Sleep Disturbance.* Delft: TNO Inro, 2003.

23. Basner M, Buess H, Elmenhorst D *et al. Effects of Nocturnal Aircraft Noise.* FB 2004-07/E. Cologne: DLR-Institut für Luft- und Raumfahrtmedizin, 2004.

24. Passchier-Vermeer W, Vos H, Steenbekkers JHM, van der Ploeg FD, Groothuis-Oudshoorn K. *Sleep Disturbance and Aircraft Noise Exposure.* Leiden: TNO-PG, 2002.

25. World Health Organization. *Night Noise Guidelines (NNGL) for Europe. Final Implementation Report.* Geneva: WHO, 2007.

◆26. Babisch W. Traffic noise and cardiovascular disease: Epidemiological review and synthesis. *Noise Health* 2000; **2**: 9–32.

◆27. Babisch W. Transportation noise and cardiovascular risk: Updated review and synthesis of epidemiological studies indicate that the evidence has increased. *Noise Health* 2006; **8**: 1–29.

28. van Kempen EE, Kruize H, Boshuizen HC, Ameling CB, Staatsen BA, de Hollander AE. The association between noise exposure and blood pressure and ischaemic heart disease: A meta-analysis. *Environ Health Perspect* 2002; **110**: 307-17.

29. Knipschild PV. Medical effects of aircraft noise: Community cardiovascular survey. *Int Arch Occup Environ Health* 1977; **40**: 185–90.

30. Jarup L, Babisch W, Houthuijs D *et al.* Hypertension and Exposure to Noise near Airports – the HYENA study. *Environ Health Perspect* 2008; **116**: 329-33.

31. Haralabidis AS, Dimakopoulou K, Vigna-Taglianti F *et al.*, for the HYENA Consortium. Acute effects of night-time noise exposure on blood pressure in populations living near airports. *Eur Heart J* 2009; doi:10.1093/eurheartj/ehn013.

32. Berry BF. *Effect of Noise on Physical Health Risk in London. Report on Phase 2 – Estimates of the Numbers of People at Risk.* BEL Technical Report BEL 2008-002. Version 2.0. Shepperton, Surrey: BEL, 2008.

33. Hygge S, Evans GW, Bullinger M. A prospective study of some effects of aircraft noise on cognitive performance in schoolchildren. *Psychol Sci* 2002; **13**: 469–74.

34. Stansfeld SA, Berglund B, Clark C *et al.* Aircraft and road traffic noise and children's cognition and health: A cross-national study. *Lancet* 2005; **365**: 1942-9.

35. Shield BM, Dockrell JE. The effects of environmental and classroom noise on the academic attainments of primary school children. *J Acoust Soc Am* 2008; **123**: 133-44.

◆36. Leventhall HG, Benton S, Pelmear P. *A Review of Published Research on Low Frequency Noise and its Effects.* Project Report. London: Defra, 2003.

37. Hansen CH (ed.). *The Effects of Low Frequency Noise and Vibration on People.* Essex: Multi-Science Publishing, 2007.

38. Griffin MJ. *Handbook of Human Vibration.* London: Academic Press, 1990.

39. Schafer RM. *Soundscape. Our Sonic Environment and the Tuning of the World.* Rochester, VT: Destiny Books, 1994.

Genetic, environmental and infectious causes of cancer

58

Environmental carcinogenesis

DAVID H. PHILLIPS, STAN VENITT

CANCER CAUSATION, MECHANISMS AND PREVENTION

In the global population in 2002, there were 10.9 million new cases of cancer, 6.7 million deaths from cancer and 24.6 million people alive with cancer. The risks of developing cancer vary greatly between different countries and cultures, and change with time and with migration, suggesting that most cancer is caused by environmental exposures or 'lifestyle', rather than by inherited susceptibility.[1] Here we discuss those cancers which are thought to be caused by environmental exposures rather than by lifestyle. Lifestyle factors, such as tobacco smoking, consuming alcohol, sunbathing, the use of herbal remedies and choice of diet are largely within the control of individuals and could be said to be voluntary. Exposure to environmental carcinogens tends to be beyond the control of individuals and not usually constrained by personal choice.

In this chapter, we summarize a variety of agents or exposures known to be associated with a range of human cancers. There are additional exposures to which populations are subjected that are not strictly environmental, but arise as a by-product of processes or activities that generate carcinogens which are released into the environment. Environmental tobacco smoke ('passive smoking') is a notable example. The contamination of food with carcinogens can occur via several routes. For example, polycyclic aromatic hydrocarbons (PAHs), carcinogenic heterocyclic amines and acrylamide can be produced by particular ways of cooking, especially at high temperature.[2–4] Food may contain carcinogenic mycotoxins such as aflatoxin resulting from the fungal contamination

of staple foods such as cereals and pulses. Domestic cooking or heating with inadequate ventilation may cause pollution of the indoor air with carcinogens generated from the combustion of solid fuel or from food during cooking. Emissions from factories of pollutants in air, soil or water may expose neighbouring communities to carcinogens.

Identifying environmental carcinogens raises the hope of preventing cancer in populations exposed to them. Given the large scale of the global burden of cancer now and for the foreseeable future, the prevention of cancer, rather than its cure, is more likely to succeed in alleviating this major public health problem. Vaccination, improvements in diet, living conditions, education and sanitation, and the provision of clean drinking water have already led to extraordinary reductions in mortality from infectious diseases in rich, industrialized countries, where cancer and heart disease are now the leading causes of death. It is likely that cancer mortality could also be decreased dramatically by improvements in public health based on a knowledge of those factors which diminish the risk of cancer and those which enhance it. Examples of action already taken to prevent cancer or limit exposure to environmental carcinogens include the bans imposed on smoking in public places in countries such as the UK and France, the provision in Chile of drinking water treated to remove arsenic, the immunization of populations against hepatitis B, and the reduction of aflatoxin levels in food in order to reduce or prevent liver cancer.

Understanding the way in which carcinogens provoke the changes that lead to cancer may well inform methods for reducing or preventing cancer. The last few decades have seen a vast increase in our knowledge of the mechanisms of carcinogenesis, and it is now accepted that human cancer develops in a series of steps, that it originates in single cells and that mutational events play a central role in carcinogenesis. In this 'somatic mutation' model of cancer, it is proposed that a single cell acquires a mutation in a regulatory gene that confers a selective growth advantage over its normal neighbours. This single cell divides to produce a clone of mutant offspring. The mutant clone expands by further cell divisions, and one of its cells acquires a mutation in a second regulatory gene, thereby producing a clone carrying mutations in two regulatory genes. A cell in this doubly mutant clone then acquires an advantageous mutation in a third regulatory gene, and produces a clone that is even more aberrant in its capacity for autonomous growth. This process of selective 'clonal evolution' continues until a clone appears that has accumulated enough mutant genes to enable it to express the full malignant phenotype. Most cancers that have been examined are clonal in composition, and their cells carry mutations in growth-regulatory genes or have lost such genes. This supports the theory that clonal evolution driven by somatic mutation and Darwinian selection is a crucial mechanism in carcinogenesis.[5,6]

This mechanism is well supported by a wealth of evidence from a variety of different experimental and epidemiological methods, but cannot of itself explain the multifactorial nature of most human cancer, especially the strong effects of diet[7] and obesity[8] on human cancer, and the effects of the genetic disposition to a susceptibility or resistance to given cancers that is seen in individuals and in ethnic groups. Genetic studies of inherited cancer susceptibility using linkage analysis have revealed several highly penetrant, but relatively rare, 'cancer genes' of large effect,[5] and the recent development of genome-wide association scans has disclosed a growing list of polymorphic gene loci that confer a moderate or low but significant risk of cancer, at various sites, to substantial subgroups of populations.[9,10] Similar techniques are being applied to the elucidation of the 'cancer genome', whereby the genetic signature of a given type of cancer is assembled by identifying mutated genes consistently associated with that tumour type.[9,11,12] To what extent these new discoveries will unravel the complex interaction between voluntary exposures due to 'lifestyle' (e.g. diet, obesity, tobacco and alcohol), environmental carcinogens and genetic susceptibility to cancer remains to be seen. The establishment of a number of large 'biobanks', whereby future population-based studies of diseases, including cancer, will be feasible, offers the promise of unravelling hitherto unrecognized environmental and genetic risk factors for human ailments.

What follows are examples of environmental chemicals for which there is evidence (of varying strengths) of their involvement in the aetiology of human cancer. In some cases, these chemicals have been found to have been the cause of occupational cancer, and their wider distribution in the environment is at the very least cause for concern,

even if the risk to the general population remains to be quantified.

ARSENIC IN DRINKING WATER

It has been known for many decades that arsenic and arsenic compounds could cause cancer when used medicinally on the skin of patients treated with Fowler's solution, and occupationally in the lungs of mining and smelting workers exposed by inhalation.[13] It is, however, now recognized that *environmental* exposure to inorganic arsenic in drinking water poses a high risk of cancer to very large populations in many parts of the world,[14] and it is perhaps the best documented and most important example of a purely environmental carcinogen. Inorganic arsenic in drinking water is classified as carcinogenic to humans (group 1) by the International Agency for Research on Cancer (IARC), and it causes cancer of the urinary bladder, lung and skin; there is also limited evidence for an increased risk of kidney cancer.[15] The IARC monograph[15] provides a comprehensive review of the chemistry of, occurrence of and exposure to arsenic in drinking water, as well as a detailed account of its metabolism, genotoxicity and the evidence for its human carcinogenicity.

The mechanism by which arsenic exerts its carcinogenic effects is not understood, although several different mechanisms have been suggested, including the induction of oxidative stress, diminished DNA repair, altered DNA methylation patterns, enhancement of cell proliferation and suppression of p53-mediated pathways.[16] Arsenic is genotoxic; elevated frequencies of micronuclei, chromosomal aberrations and aneuploidy have been detected in the peripheral lymphocytes or urothelial cells, or both, of people exposed to arsenic. Thus, in humans it is a chromosomal mutagen (an agent that induces mutations involving more than one gene, typically large deletions or rearrangements). These effects have also been observed in mammalian cells treated in vitro, but arsenic does not induce point mutations in mammalian cells or bacteria in vitro.

Table 58.1 shows where and how many people are exposed to concentrations of arsenic in drinking water that exceed the current World Health Organization guideline value of $10 \, \mu g/L$,[17] a limit now in force in many developed countries, including the European Union[18] and the USA.[19] Many millions of people are at risk, and those at highest risk live in areas such as Bangladesh and parts of China where drinking water comes from local wells and where the treatment of water to reduce arsenic levels is problematic. For example, in Bangladesh, 10 million local hand-pumped tube wells were installed, over several decades, to replace pathogen-contaminated surface water sources.[20] Unfortunately 30–90 per cent of such wells in many villages produce water that contains arsenic at levels higher than the already high national standard of $50 \, \mu g/L$, placing over 130 million Bangladeshis at high risk of

Table 58.1   Regions of the world with naturally elevated levels of arsenic in groundwater

Country/region	Affected area (km²)	Potentially exposed population	Arsenic concentration (μg/L)
Bangladesh	118 849	≈3 × 10⁷	<0.5–2500
India/West Bengal	38 865	6 × 10⁶	<10–3200
China/Taiwan	4000	≈10⁵	10–1820
China/Xinjang, Shanxi	38 000		40–750
Thailand	100	1.5 × 10⁴	1–>5000
Mongolia/Inner Mongolia	4300	≈10⁵	1–2400
Argentina/Chaco-Pampean Plain	106	2 × 10⁶	<1–7550
Northern Chile/Antofagasta	35 000	5 × 10⁵	100–1000
Bolivia		5 × 10⁴	
Mexico	32 000	4 × 10⁵	8–620
Germany/Bavaria	2500		<10–150
Hungary, Romania/Danube Basin	110 000	4 × 10⁵	
Spain		>5 × 10⁴	<1–100
Greece		1.5 × 10⁵	
Ghana		1.5 × 10⁵	<1–175
Canada/Moira Lake, Ontario	100		50–3000
Canada/British Columbia	50		0.5–580
USA/Arizona	200 000		<1300
USA/California	5000		<1–2600
USA/Nevada	1300		<2600

Adapted from International Agency for Research on Cancer,[15] with permission.

arsenic-related diseases, including cancer. It is estimated that arsenic in drinking water doubles the lifetime mortality risk from liver, bladder and lung cancers (229.6 versus 103.5 per 100 000) in Bangladesh.[20] Because the arsenic-related cancers have a latency of 20–30 years, the full effects of this public health disaster have yet to be realized. In the meantime, various methods of reducing or preventing the arsenic contamination of drinking water in Bangladesh are under consideration.[21]

That reducing arsenic levels in public water supplies can affect mortality from arsenic-related cancers has been demonstrated in an ecological study in Chile encompassing exposure over 50 years.[22] Before 1958, municipally supplied drinking water in the second most northerly administrative region of Chile (Region II), centred on Antofagasta (Chile's second largest city), contained about 90 μg/L arsenic. This already high concentration rose to an average of 870 μg/L when, in 1958, the water supply was augmented with river water containing very high levels of arsenic. In 1971, water treatment plants were installed, and by 1990, arsenic levels fell to about 40 μg/L.

This natural experiment in chemical carcinogenesis in a population of over 400 000 people allowed the investigators to study time trends in the development of arsenic-related cancers, comparing Region II with another part of Chile (Region V) where water is not contaminated with arsenic. They found that lung and bladder cancer mortality rate ratios (RRs) for Region II compared with Region V started

to increase about 10 years after high arsenic exposures began and continued to rise until peaking between 1986 and 1997 (Figure 58.1). The peak lung cancer mortality RRs were 3.61 (95 per cent confidence interval [CI] 3.13–4.16) for men and 3.26 (95 per cent CI 2.50–4.23) for women. The peak bladder cancer RRs were 6.10 (95 per cent CI 3.97–9.39) for men and 13.8 (95 per cent CI 7.74–24.5) for women. Combined lung and bladder cancer mortality rates in Region II were highest in the period 1992–94, with mortality rates of 153 and 50 per 100 000 men and women, respectively, in Region II compared with 54 and 19 per 100 000 in Region V. The long latency is striking: mortality from lung and bladder cancers remained high until the late 1990s, even though major decreases in arsenic exposure had occurred more than 25 years earlier.

Another study of this population examined the effect of arsenic exposure in early life on long-term mortality.[23] The authors compared mortality rates in Antofagasta between 1989 and 2000 with those of the rest of Chile, in subjects who were born during or just before the peak exposure period and who were 30–49 years of age at the time of death. For the birth cohort born just before the high-exposure period (1950–1957) and exposed in early childhood, the standardized mortality ratio (SMR) for lung cancer was 7.0 (95 per cent CI 5.4–8). For those born during the high-exposure period (1958–70) with probable exposure in utero and in early childhood, the standardized

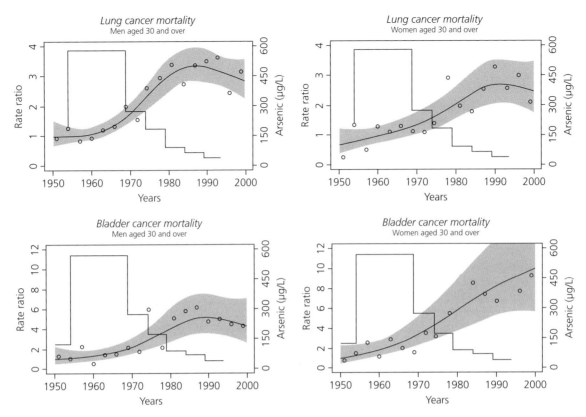

Figure 58.1 Lung and bladder cancer mortality rate ratios comparing Region II with Region V in Chile for men and women aged 30 and above, separately, as estimated by Poisson regression with smoothing. The shading represents the 95 per cent confidence bands. The circles represent the mortality rate ratios plotted at the midpoint of each successive 3-year period. Histograms of the population-weighted average arsenic water concentrations for Region II, from 1950 to 1994 in 5-year increments, are also presented (vertical axes at right). (Adapted from Marshall et al.[22] with permission.)

mortality rate for lung cancer was 6.1 (95 per cent CI 3.5–9.9). These findings suggest that exposure to arsenic in drinking water during early childhood or in utero greatly increases subsequent mortality in young adults from both malignant and non-malignant lung disease. The authors of this study state that the magnitude of the effects of arsenic exposure in utero and in early childhood on lung cancer is far greater than that reported for ionizing radiation or tobacco smoke.

That arsenic in drinking water causes cancers of the skin, bladder and lung is beyond doubt; the evidence for other sites (e.g. kidney and liver) is less persuasive and requires further analytical studies. Moreover, with many large populations chronically exposed to arsenic levels above the World Health Organization guideline of 10 µg/L, the full scale of the carcinogenic effects of arsenic on the human population has still to be evaluated.[14]

AFLATOXINS AND VIRAL HEPATITIS

Mycotoxins are a group of secondary fungal metabolites of diverse chemical structure that can induce a variety of toxic manifestations, including carcinogenicity, when ingested. Aflatoxins are a group of mycotoxins (B_1, B_2, G_1,

G_2 and M_1) produced by several species of the mould fungus *Aspergillus*. *Aspergillus flavus* and *A. parasiticus* are the most common and overwhelmingly account for the contamination of feed and food crops throughout the world. The occurrence, chemistry, toxicology and carcinogenicity of aflatoxins have been reviewed in great detail.[24]

The contamination of feed and food crops with aflatoxins occurs mainly in tropical countries with warm humid climates (favourable to mould growth) and is less common in temperate climates. The predominant crops affected are peanuts, maize, cottonseed and, to a lesser extent, certain spices. Human exposure to aflatoxins at levels of nanograms to micrograms per day occurs mainly by the consumption of maize and peanuts. Aflatoxins can form in crops before or immediately after harvesting by the infection of plants and developing nuts or seeds, or during storage under conditions that favour mould growth. Improving storage conditions is easier than preventing infection during crop growth and explains the continuing difficulty of eliminating aflatoxins from these important crops.

Human exposure to aflatoxins is associated with a high risk of hepatocellular carcinoma, one of the most frequent and fatal cancers worldwide. Hepatocellular carcinoma is endemic in China, Taiwan, Korea and sub-Saharan Africa (with an incidence between 20 and 100 cases per 100 000) but is far less common in 'developed' areas such as Western Europe and the USA (10 cases per 100 000).[25,26] The exact role of aflatoxins in human liver carcinogenesis is not fully understood because hepatocellular carcinoma is also closely associated with chronic infection with hepatitis B and hepatitis C, and the precise way in which these viruses interact with aflatoxins to induce hepatocellular carcinoma has still to be revealed. Nevertheless it can be stated that the combination of aflatoxin + hepatitis B/hepatitis C accounts for more than 75 per cent of the 200 000 cases of hepatocellular carcinoma in sub-Saharan Africa every year.[26]

Of the different forms of aflatoxin, B_1 (AFB_1) is the most widely studied and the most potent. It is a powerful carcinogen in a variety of species, causing hepatocellular (sometimes cholangiocellular) carcinoma in rats, hamsters, salmon, trout, ducks, tree shrews and monkeys. AFB_1 is a potent mutagen, inducing point mutations and chromosomal anomalies in a variety of experimental systems employing different target organisms, and in human somatic tissues such as peripheral lymphocytes from AFB_1-exposed individuals. It is metabolized to a reactive form that binds covalently to DNA bases and to proteins to form DNA and protein adducts, which can be detected in the liver and body fluids of exposed individuals and which can be used as biomarkers of exposure.[27]

AFB_1 exposure can also leave a molecular footprint in the form of a highly specific mutation in the p53 gene (*TP53*) in human liver tumours. *TP53* is a tumour suppressor gene whose phosphoprotein gene product plays a central role in normal cell division, in differentiation and development, and in maintaining genomic stability.[5] Somatic mutation at specific sites in *TP53* is common in a variety of human cancers, allowing the assembly of 'mutation spectra' for many tumour types. The linkage of mutation spectra with different environmental exposures may offer clues to the causal relationships between a particular exposure and a given cancer.[28] In areas (e.g. China and Africa) where aflatoxin exposure, chronic hepatitis B/hepatitis C infection and hepatocellular carcinoma are common, a specific point mutation of *TP53* (GC to TA transversion at the third position of codon 249[ser]) in liver tumours is also common.[24] This mutation has also been detected in DNA from the serum of patients with hepatocellular carcinoma, suggesting that it could be a biomarker of exposure to AFB_1 and possibly an indicator of early disease.[25]

The combination of aflatoxin, hepatitis B and hepatitis C has been predicted to increase, in the next 40–50 years, the incidence of hepatocellular carcinoma in sub-Saharan Africa to higher levels than are currently seen for any form of cancer in 'developed' countries.[26] A safe and effective hepatitis B vaccine has been available for at least 25 years, and there are proven means for reducing aflatoxin exposure. Current knowledge should be sufficient to curb a widespread cancer epidemic before it reaches an unprecedented

magnitude. A series of actions that could achieve this aim has been proposed,[26] including the following:

- the development of sustainable childhood vaccination strategies;
- a reduction in exposure to aflatoxin;
- understanding the spread of hepatitis C virus;
- developing the registration, early detection and treatment of hepatocellular carcinoma.

MESOTHELIOMA FROM ASBESTOS AND RELATED FIBRES

Mesothelioma has been recognized since the 1960s as being caused by the inhalation of asbestos fibres. Since then, many thousands of industrial workers exposed to asbestos have succumbed to the disease, often after very long latent periods (up to 40 years). Of the main types of asbestos, crocidolite (blue asbestos) is the most hazardous, followed by amosite (brown asbestos). Chrysotile (white asbestos) is, by comparison, much less harmful.[29]

Inhaled asbestos fibres move from the lung to the pleural cavity where they induce tumours that originate from mesothelial cells. Asbestos exposure also increases synergistically the risk of lung cancer among tobacco smokers.[28] More than 85 per cent of cases of mesothelioma occur in people with a documented exposure to asbestos, but virtually all inhabitants of industrial societies have measurable levels of asbestos fibres in their lungs. How many of the non-occupational cases may also be due to asbestos is unclear, but a number of studies have shown an increased mortality and incidence of mesothelioma among the family members of asbestos workers, as a result of 'household exposure'.[30]

There is no other validated cause of mesothelioma, although a number of other agents have been considered that may act in concert with asbestos, including simian polyoma virus 40 (SV40). Human infection with SV40 occurred in the late 1950s and early 1960s through contaminated polio vaccines, which were grown in kidney cell cultures derived from the kidney tissue of rhesus macaques. These monkeys are frequently infected with SV40, although the virus is harmless to them.

The association between SV40 infection and human mesothelioma is controversial. Some researchers support a link, while others do not. On the one hand, mechanistic studies show that SV40 and asbestos can act together in human cells in culture and in experimental animals to produce tumours or tumour-like biological effects at much lower levels than are produced by either agent acting alone.[31,32] This lends credence to the view that exposure to SV40 could put someone exposed to asbestos at greater risk than someone not infected. One recent epidemiological study found that asbestos-exposed individuals who were infected with SV40 were at higher risk of developing mesothelioma than those not infected.[33] On the other hand, the evidence that SV40 DNA sequences were found in a high proportion of patients with mesothelioma has been seriously called into question, and the majority of more recent studies have not replicated the finding.[34] At present, opinion is divided on the involvement of SV40 in the aetiology of mesothelioma.[35]

A very remarkable epidemic of mesothelioma has been documented in three small villages in the region of Cappadocia in central Turkey, where it is responsible for over 50 per cent of deaths.[36] The probable cause is exposure to erionite, a fibrous zeolite mineral present in the local stone used in building construction, the dust of which contaminates the air and houses in these villages. In experimental studies, erionite is a more potent carcinogen than crocidolite.[37] Largely on the basis of the Cappadocia epidemic and on supporting animal studies, erionite has been classified by the IARC as a human carcinogen.[38] Yet within these villages there are some houses and families in which mesothelioma does not occur, even though they are also exposed to erionite, and a neighbouring village, where erionite is also found, has had few if any cases. Moreover, erionite exposure elsewhere in the world (e.g. in the USA) has not been linked to malignant mesothelioma.[39] Pedigree studies in Cappadocia now suggest that there is a genetic predisposition component to the disease epidemic, which combines with the environmental exposure to render some individuals, but not others, highly susceptible.[39] Although it may at present be a daunting task to identify the gene(s) responsible for this susceptibility, its eventual identification, given the small size of the cohort at risk, may shed light on host factors that influence susceptibility to the more numerous and widespread cases of mesothelioma caused by the inhalation of asbestos.

POLYCYCLIC AROMATIC HYDROCARBONS

The generation of PAHs during the incomplete combustion of organic matter renders this class of compounds ubiquitous in the environment, where they are highly persistent owing to their chemical stability and inertness.

Many PAHs, but particularly those with 4–6 fused benzo rings, are carcinogenic.[40] They are metabolized in mammalian cells to reactive intermediates that bind covalently to DNA and thereby initiate the carcinogenic process. This complex family of organic chemicals was first identified in the first half of the twentieth century as the carcinogenic components of such occupational carcinogens as soot, coal tar and creosote, and they are also the probable cause of occupational lung cancer in a number of heavy industries, including coke production, iron- and steel-founding, and aluminium production, where atmospheric concentrations of PAHs are high. Workers in such industries have significantly increased levels of DNA damage, in the form of PAH–DNA adducts, than unexposed controls.[27]

The presence of PAHs in tobacco smoke, and the similarity between the mutational signature induced in experimental systems by benzo[a]pyrene, a key PAH, and the mutation spectrum in the TP53 gene in lung tumours from smokers provides molecular evidence for the causal role of PAHs in tobacco-induced lung cancer: when benzo[a]pyrene diol epoxide, the metabolically activated form of benzo[a]pyrene, reacted with the TP53 gene, it was found that codons 157, 248 and 273 were preferentially modified, which correlated with the sites most frequently mutated in smokers' lung tumours.[41]

There is widespread occurrence of PAHs in the atmosphere, particularly in urban and industrialized environments as a result of automobile emissions, coal-fired power stations and other polluting sources of fossil fuel combustion. Their presence in soil, water and food is also well documented. As a result of the widespread exposure of the general population to carcinogenic PAHs, there is concern about their possible impact on human cancer, although it is difficult to quantify how great a risk they pose. Nevertheless, comparisons of mortality between urban and rural populations have attributed at least some of the differences to air quality, of which PAH concentrations are thought to be a contributing factor.[42]

A recent analysis of tobacco-smoking and solid-fuel use in China calculated that the continuation of these activities, both of which generate carcinogenic PAHs, at present levels between 2003 and 2033 would result in 65 million deaths from chronic obstructive pulmonary disease and 18 million deaths from lung cancer;[43] 82 per cent of these chronic obstructive pulmonary disease deaths and 75 per cent of the lung cancer deaths would be attributable to smoking and solid-fuel use. However, a gradual cessation of both by 2033 could avoid about a third of the deaths from each disease.[43]

There has been speculation for many years about the environmental cause(s) of oesophageal cancer in geographical areas of the world where the incidence of the disease is abnormally high.[44] These include the 'Asian belt', stretching from European Russia and Turkey in the west to eastern areas of China in the east, where the disease is largely confined to Mongol and Turkic ethnic groups (this being evidence suggestive of a genetic susceptibility factor within the region). There are also several other provinces of China with very high rates (e.g. Henan), an area of South America encompassing Southern Brazil, Uruguay and north-eastern Argentina, and areas of Southern Africa that include the Transkei, Zimbabwe, western Kenya and southern Malawi.[45]

The major causes of oesophageal cancer worldwide are alcohol and tobacco-smoking, although these factors appear to be of lesser importance in many high-risk regions.[45] Dietary exposure to nitrosamines (e.g. consumed in alcohol in north-western France), in some cases possibly combined with nutritional deficiencies, has also been implicated. More recently, it has been found that a high consumption of PAHs occurs in areas where there is high incidence of oesophageal cancer in China, northern Iran and South America. The high levels of PAHs in Henan and Iran have been suggested to be a consequence of cooking methods and food storage,[46,47] both subject to contamination from coal smoke, while in South America the custom of drinking very hot *mate* has been found to be a source of exposure to high levels of PAHs through the infusion of yerba mate leaves that have been dried and processed using burning wood, gas or oil.[48]

Thus, although exposure to carcinogenic PAHs may not be the sole factor, it is one that appears to be common to at least three areas where there is a high incidence of oesophageal cancer. Human biomonitoring studies also provide evidence of a higher exposure to PAHs in these populations, as indicated by the levels of PAH metabolites in urine[49,50] and by the presence of PAH–DNA adducts in oesophageal tissue.[51]

ENDEMIC NEPHROPATHY AND ASSOCIATED UROTHELIAL CANCER

Balkan endemic nephropathy (BEN) is prevalent in distinct regions of Croatia, Serbia, Bosnia, Romania and Bulgaria. The condition is estimated to affect around 25 000 people, with a further 100 000 thought to be at risk. The disease has been recognized for around 50 years, and during that time its spatial distribution, in certain rural locations along tributaries of the River Danube (Figure 58.2), has remained remarkably constant, to the extent of characterizing 'BEN villages' and 'non-BEN villages', and even to the extent of there being BEN-affected households in close proximity to disease-free ones.

The disease, which has a long incubation period, affecting adults but never children, develops into end-stage renal failure and the frequent development of upper urinary tract cancer. Although the occurrence of a disease with such a distinctive geographical distribution strongly suggests that the causative factor is an environmental one, the search for the culprit has so far proved inconclusive. Nevertheless, three distinct candidates have emerged, although none, as yet, can entirely account for the spatial distribution of the disease. (It should be noted that although BEN afflicts some families but not others, it is not a genetic disorder in the sense that it does not follow a pattern of Mendelian inheritance, and it is not confined to any particular ethnic groups.)

One possible causative factor is the contamination of groundwater with organic chemicals leached from Pliocene lignite. Shallow deposits of this low-grade coal

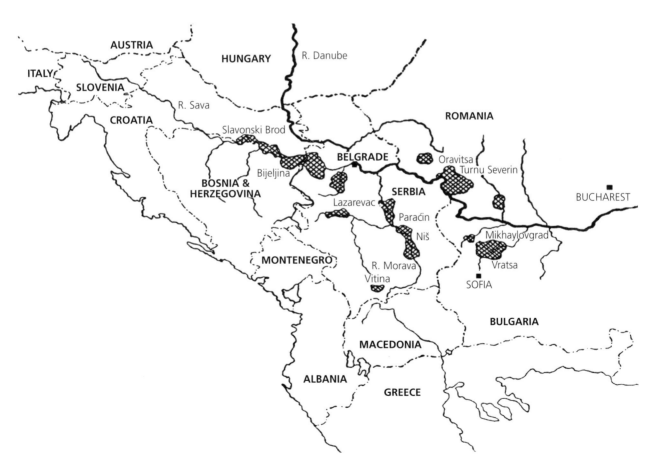

Figure 58.2 Map of the Balkans in south-eastern Europe. The shaded areas indicate regions where Balkan endemic nephropathy occurs. (From Stefanovic and Radovanovic,[63] with permission.)

have been reported to contaminate wells in endemic areas to a greater extent than in non-endemic areas. Even though some reports have described the chemicals as toxic and carcinogenic, their exact nature remains ill-defined,[52] although they have been reported to include PAHs.[53] Nevertheless, there is no obvious mechanistic link between PAHs and nephrotoxicity or urothelial cancer.

Another agent suspected of involvement in BEN is ochratoxin A. This fungal metabolite, produced by moulds of the *Aspergillus* and *Penicillium* genera, is nephrotoxic and carcinogenic, and there are similarities between BEN and porcine nephropathy, for which the cause has been demonstrated to be the contamination of animal feed with ochratoxin A.[54] Although the mycotoxin has been found to be a contaminant of foodstuffs such as cereals and grain in the Balkans, the extent to which human exposure differs between BEN and non-BEN areas is not clear.[55] From experimental studies, there is controversy over whether ochratoxin A is a genotoxic or a non-genotoxic carcinogen, and whether it interacts directly with DNA in mammalian cells to form DNA adducts,[56] or indirectly to cause oxidative damage to DNA.[57] Such uncertainties make it difficult to obtain molecular evidence for the involvement of ochratoxin A in the aetiology of BEN.

The third candidate is aristolochic acid, a nephrotoxin produced by the plant *Aristolochia clematitis*, which grows wild in wheat fields in the Balkan region. Its seeds have been found to contaminate wheat grain used to make bread.[54] It remains to be established, however, how widespread the contamination of wheat flour is or whether exposure to aristolochic acid could occur by other means (e.g. uptake from the soil by other plants), and also whether exposure levels are significantly different between BEN and non-BEN regions.[55]

New light has, however, been shed on the aetiology of this disease by the occurrence in the 1990s of an outbreak of renal failure among patients at a slimming clinic in Belgium. It was discovered that *Aristolochia fangchi* had been accidentally included in a herbal slimming concoction instead of another plant (*Stephania tetrandra*), apparently because they have very similar names in traditional Chinese medicine (guang fang-ji and han fang-ji, respectively). Within months of the resulting ingestion of high doses of aristolochic acid (contributed by the *Aristolochia* in the formulation), renal failure developed in about 5 per cent of individuals, and this was followed by the rapid onset of urothelial cancer in about half of these affected individuals.

Aristolochic acid is a genotoxic carcinogen[58] that forms DNA adducts in exposed tissues.[59] The analysis of urothelial DNA from such patients has shown clearly the presence of aristolochic acid–DNA adducts, thereby strongly implicating aristolochic acid as the aetiological agent.[59] The condition, initially termed Chinese herbs nephropathy, is now more commonly referred to as

aristolochic acid nephropathy (AAN) as a consequence of this evidence. Aristolochic acid is still present in marketed herbal products despite a call for a worldwide ban, and AAN may be a worldwide problem.[60] The pathology of AAN is remarkably similar to that of BEN.

Evidence has recently been presented for the presence of aristolochic acid–DNA adducts in BEN patients.[61,62] An analysis of *TP53* mutations in BEN tumours and in one aristolochic acid nephropathy tumour has shown a preponderance of AT to TA point mutations.[61,62] Aristolochic acid forms DNA adducts mainly with adenine bases in DNA, and AT to TA transversions are the predominant mutation induced by aristolochic acid in experimental systems.[62] This compelling evidence of the detection of aristolochic acid DNA adducts and the characterization of *TP53* mutations in patients with urothelial cancer associated with BEN represents a definitive molecular insight into the causation of this disease.

Whether aristolochic acid is the sole environmental causative agent for BEN, whether different agents may be solely or partially responsible for its occurrence in different regions of the Balkans, or indeed whether two or more agents act in concert remains to be determined. Even if the disease turns out to be multifactorial, the elimination of only one environmental agent may be sufficient to control the disease.

REFERENCES

● = Key primary paper

◆ = Major review article

◆1. Parkin DM, Bray F, Ferlay J, Pisani P. Global cancer statistics, 2002. *CA Cancer J Clin* 2005; **55**: 74–108.

◆2. Phillips DH. Polycyclic aromatic hydrocarbons in the diet. *Mutat Res* 1999; **443**: 139–47.

●3. Martinez ME, Jacobs ET, Ashbeck EL *et al*. Meat intake, preparation methods, mutagens and colorectal adenoma recurrence. *Carcinogenesis* 2007; **28**: 2019–27.

◆4. Felton JS, Knize MG. A meat and potato war: implications for cancer etiology. *Carcinogenesis* 2006; **27**: 2367–70.

◆5. Venitt S. Biological mechanisms and biomarkers. In: Baxter PJ, Adams PH, Aw T-C, Cockcroft A, Harrington JM (eds) *Hunter's Diseases of Occupations*, 9th edn. London: Arnold, 2000: 741–89.

◆6. Greaves M. Cancer causation: the Darwinian downside of past success? *Lancet Oncol* 2002; **3**: 244–51.

◆7. American Institute for Cancer Research. *Food, Nutrition, Physical Activity, and the Prevention of Cancer: A Global Perspective*. Washington, DC: American Institute for Cancer Research, 2007.

◆8. Renehan AG, Tyson M, Egger M *et al*. Body-mass index and incidence of cancer: a systematic review and meta-analysis of prospective observational studies. *Lancet* 2008; **371**: 569–78.

●9. Campbell PJ, Stephens PJ, Pleasance ED *et al*. Identification of somatically acquired rearrangements in cancer using genome-wide massively parallel paired-end sequencing. *Nat Genet* 2008; **40**: 722–9.

●10. Tenesa A, Farrington SM, Prendergast JG *et al*. Genome-wide association scan identifies a colorectal cancer susceptibility locus on 11q23 and replicates risk loci at 8q24 and 18q21. *Nat Genet* 2008; **40**: 631–7.

●11. Greenman C, Stephens P, Smith R *et al*. Patterns of somatic mutation in human cancer genomes. *Nature* 2007; **446**: 153–8.

●12. Massion PP, Zou Y, Chen H *et al*. Smoking-related genomic signatures in non-small cell lung cancer. *Am J Respir Crit Care Med* 2008; **178**: 1164–72.

◆13. International Agency for Research on Cancer. Arsenic and arsenic compounds. In: *IARC Monographs on the Evaluation of Carcinogenic Risk of Chemicals to Humans*. Vol. 23: *Some Metals and Metallic Compounds*. Lyon: IARC, 1980: 39–143.

◆14. Lubin JH, Beane Freeman LE, Cantor KP. Inorganic arsenic in drinking water: an evolving public health concern. *J Natl Cancer Inst* 2007; **99**: 906–7.

◆15. International Agency for Research on Cancer. Arsenic in drinking water. In: *IARC Monographs on the Evaluation of Carcinogenic Risk of Chemicals to Humans*. Vol. 84: *Some Drinking-water Disinfectants and Contaminants, Including Arsenic*. Lyon: IARC, 2004: 39–267.

◆16. Beyersmann D, Hartwig A. Carcinogenic metal compounds: recent insight into molecular and cellular mechanisms. *Arch Toxicol* 2008; **82**: 493–512.

◆17. World Health Organization. *Guidelines for Drinking-water Quality*, First Addendum, 3rd edn. Vol. 1: *Recommendations*. Geneva: WHO, 2006.

◆18. Council Directive 98/83/EC of 3 November 1998 on the quality of water intended for human consumption; Regulation (EC) No 1882/2003 of the European Parliament and of the Council of 29 September 2003 L 284 1 31.10.2003.

19. United States Environmental Protection Agency. National Primary Drinking Water Regulations; Arsenic and Clarifications to Compliance and New Source Contaminants Monitoring. Available from: http://www.epa.gov/fedrgstr/EPA-WATER/2001/January/Day-22/w1668.htm (accessed November, 2009).

◆20. Chen Y, Ahsan H. Cancer burden from arsenic in drinking water in Bangladesh. *Am J Public Health* 2004; **94**: 741–4.

◆21. Ng JC, Moore MR. Arsenic in drinking water: a natural killer in Bangladesh and beyond. *Med J Aust* 2005; **183**: 562–3.

●22. Marshall G, Ferreccio C, Yuan Y *et al*. Fifty-year study of lung and bladder cancer mortality in Chile related to arsenic in drinking water. *J Natl Cancer Inst* 2007; **99**: 920–8.

●23. Smith AH, Marshall G, Yuan Y *et al*. Increased mortality from lung cancer and bronchiectasis in young adults after exposure to arsenic in utero and in early childhood. *Environ Health Perspect* 2006; **114**: 1293–6.

◆24. International Agency for Research on Cancer. Aflatoxins. In: *IARC Monographs on the Evaluation of Carcinogenic*

Risk of Chemicals to Humans. Vol. 82: *Some Traditional Herbal Medicines, Some Mycotoxins, Naphthalene and Styrene*. Lyon: IARC, 2002: 169–300.

◆25. Hussain SP, Schwank J, Staib F *et al*. TP53 mutations and hepatocellular carcinoma: insights into the etiology and pathogenesis of liver cancer. *Oncogene* 2007; **26**: 2166–76.

◆26. Hainaut P, Boyle P. Curbing the liver cancer epidemic in Africa. *Lancet* 2008; **371**: 367–8.

◆27. Phillips DH. DNA adducts as markers of exposure and risk. *Mutat Res* 2005; **577**: 284–92.

◆28. Olivier M, Petitjean A, Marcel V *et al*. Recent advances in p53 research: an interdisciplinary perspective. *Cancer Gene Ther* 2009; **16**: 1–12.

◆29. International Agency for Research on Cancer. Asbestos. In: *IARC Monographs on the Evaluation of Carcinogenic Risks to Humans. Overall Evaluations of Carcinogenicity: An Updating of IARC Monographs Volumes 1 to 42*. Lyon: IARC, 1987: 106–16.

●30. Ferrante D, Bertolotti M, Todesco A *et al*. Cancer mortality and incidence of mesothelioma in a cohort of wives of asbestos workers in Casale Monferrato, Italy. *Environ Health Perspect* 2007; **115**: 1401–5.

●31. Kroczynska B, Cutrone R, Bocchetta M *et al*. Crocidolite asbestos and SV40 are cocarcinogens in human mesothelial cells and in causing mesothelioma in hamsters. *Proc Natl Acad Sci USA* 2006; **103**: 14128–33.

●32. Bocchetta M, Di Resta I, Powers A *et al*. Human mesothelial cells are unusually susceptible to simian virus 40-mediated transformation and asbestos cocarcinogenicity. *Proc Natl Acad Sci USA* 2000; **97**: 10214–19.

●33. Cristaudo A, Foddis R, Vivaldi A *et al*. SV40 enhances the risk of malignant mesothelioma among people exposed to asbestos: a molecular epidemiologic case-control study. *Cancer Res* 2005; **65**: 3049–52.

◆34. Shah KV. SV40 and human cancer: a review of recent data. *Int J Cancer* 2007; **120**: 215–23.

◆35. Carbone M, Albelda SM, Broaddus VC *et al*. Eighth international mesothelioma interest group. *Oncogene* 2007; **26**: 6959–67.

◆36. Carbone M, Emri S, Dogan AU *et al*. A mesothelioma epidemic in Cappadocia: scientific developments and unexpected social outcomes. *Nat Rev Cancer* 2007; **7**: 147–54.

●37. Wagner JC, Skidmore JW, Hill RJ, Griffiths DM. Erionite exposure and mesotheliomas in rats. *Br J Cancer* 1985; **51**: 727–30.

◆38. International Agency for Research on Cancer. Erionite. In: *IARC Monographs on the Evaluation of the Carcinogenic Risk of Chemicals to Humans*. Vol. 42: *Silica and Some Silicates*. Lyon: IARC, 1987: 225–39.

●39. Dogan AU, Baris YI, Dogan M *et al*. Genetic predisposition to fiber carcinogenesis causes a mesothelioma epidemic in Turkey. *Cancer Res* 2006; **66**: 5063–8.

◆40. Luch A (ed.). *The Carcinogenic Effects of Polycyclic Aromatic Hydrocarbons*. Singapore: Imperial College Press, 2005.

●41. Denissenko MF, Pao A, Tang M, Pfeifer GP. Preferential formation of benzo[a]pyrene adducts at lung cancer mutational hotspots in P53. *Science* 1996; **274**: 430–2.

◆42. Ravindra, Mittal AK, Van Grieken R. Health risk assessment of urban suspended particulate matter with special reference to polycyclic aromatic hydrocarbons: a review. *Rev Environ Health* 2001; **16**: 169–89.

●43. Lin HH, Murray M, Cohen T *et al.* Effects of smoking and solid-fuel use on COPD, lung cancer, and tuberculosis in China: a time-based, multiple risk factor, modelling study. *Lancet* 2008; **372**: 1473–83.

◆44. Yang CS. Research on esophageal cancer in China: a review. *Cancer Res* 1980; **40**: 2633–44.

◆45. Higginson J, Muir CS, Muñoz N. Esophagus. In: *Human Cancer: Epidemiology and Environmental Causes. Cambridge Monographs on Cancer Research.* Cambridge: Cambridge University Press, 1992: 263–72.

●46. Roth MJ, Strickland KL, Wang GQ *et al.* High levels of carcinogenic polycyclic aromatic hydrocarbons present within food from Linxian, China may contribute to that region's high incidence of oesophageal cancer. *Eur J Cancer* 1998; **34**: 757–8.

●47. Hakami R, Mohtadinia J, Etemadi A *et al.* Dietary intake of benzo(a)pyrene and risk of esophageal cancer in North of Iran. *Nutr Cancer* 2008; **60**: 216–21.

●48. Kamangar F, Schantz MM, Abnet CC *et al.* High levels of carcinogenic polycyclic aromatic hydrocarbons in mate drinks. *Cancer Epidemiol Biomarkers Prev* 2008; **17**: 1262–8.

●49. Kamangar F, Strickland PT, Pourshams A *et al.* High exposure to polycyclic aromatic hydrocarbons may contribute to high risk of esophageal cancer in northeastern Iran. *Anticancer Res* 2005; **25**: 425–8.

●50. Fagundes RB, Abnet CC, Strickland PT *et al.* Higher urine 1-hydroxy pyrene glucuronide (1-OHPG) is associated with tobacco smoke exposure and drinking mate in healthy subjects from Rio Grande do Sul, Brazil. *BMC Cancer* 2006; **6**: 139.

●51. van Gijssel HE, Divi RL, Olivero OA *et al.* Semiquantitation of polycyclic aromatic hydrocarbon-DNA adducts in human esophagus by immunohistochemistry and the automated cellular imaging system. *Cancer Epidemiol Biomarkers Prev* 2002; **11**: 1622–9.

◆52. Voice TC, Long DT, Radovanovic Z *et al.* Critical evaluation of environmental exposure agents suspected in the etiology of Balkan endemic nephropathy. *Int J Occup Environ Health* 2006; **12**: 369–76.

◆53. Voice TC, McElmurry SP, Long DT *et al.* Evaluation of the hypothesis that Balkan endemic nephropathy is caused by drinking water exposure to contaminants leaching from Pliocene coal deposits. *J Expo Sci Environ Epidemiol* 2006; **16**: 515–24.

◆54. Bamias G, Boletis J. Balkan nephropathy: evolution of our knowledge. *Am J Kidney Dis* 2008; **52**: 606–16.

◆55. Long DT, Voice TC. Role of exposure analysis in solving the mystery of Balkan endemic nephropathy. *Croat Med J* 2007; **48**: 300–11.

●56. Pfohl-Leszkowicz A, Castegnaro M. Further arguments in favour of direct covalent binding of ochratoxin A (OTA) after metabolic biotransformation. *Food Addit Contam* 2005; **22**(Suppl. 1): 75–87.

●57. Schilter B, Marin-Kuan M, Delatour T *et al.* Ochratoxin A: potential epigenetic mechanisms of toxicity and carcinogenicity. *Food Addit Contam* 2005; **22**(Suppl. 1): 88–93.

◆58. International Agency for Research on Cancer. *Aristolochia* species and aristolochic acids. In: *IARC Monographs on the Evaluation of Carcinogenic Risk of Chemicals to Humans.* Vol. 82: *Some Traditional Herbal Medicines, Some Mycotoxins, Naphthalene and Styrene.* Lyon: IARC, 2002: 69–129.

◆59. Arlt VM, Stiborova M, Schmeiser HH. Aristolochic acid as a probable human cancer hazard in herbal remedies: a review. *Mutagenesis* 2002; **17**: 265–77.

◆60. Debelle FD, Vanherweghem JL, Nortier JL. Aristolochic acid nephropathy: a worldwide problem. *Kidney Int* 2008; **74**: 158–69.

●61. Grollman AP, Shibutani S, Moriya M *et al.* Aristolochic acid and the etiology of endemic (Balkan) nephropathy. *Proc Natl Acad Sci USA* 2007; **104**: 12129–34.

◆62. Arlt VM, Stiborova M, Brocke JV *et al.* Aristolochic acid mutagenesis: molecular clues to the aetiology of Balkan endemic nephropathy-associated urothelial cancer. *Carcinogenesis* 2007; **28**: 2253–61.

◆63. Stefanovic V, Radovanovic Z. Balkan endemic nephropathy and associated urothelial cancer. *Nat Clin Pract Urol* 2008; **5**: 105–12.

PART 4

ENVIRONMENT AND THE PEOPLE

59

Is this patient suffering as a result of an environmental exposure?

WARE G. KUSCHNER, PAUL D. BLANC

GENERAL CONSIDERATIONS – FRAMING THE QUESTION

The goal of this chapter is to provide an approach to addressing the question: 'Is this patient suffering as a result of an environmental exposure?' That is, in the clinical context of a one-on-one assessment, is the medical finding at hand attributable to an environmental effect? Even this restatement begs a number of questions. Is this 'medical finding' meant to be a constellation of symptoms, a laboratory abnormality, a functional impairment, a syndrome or a known disease process? Does 'attributable' mean in whole or in part, and to what degree of certainty? Finally, what does 'environmental exposure' mean for the purposes of this exercise? Is this both the ambient and the indoor environment? Does this include exposures through air pollution, water contamination and even the food chain?

As the variety of exposures covered in detail elsewhere in this book makes clear, environmental exposures and the adverse effects associated with them span a very wide range of possible pathologies. Thus, it stands to reason that there is no simple algorithmic strategy that, for all or even most patients, will answer the question of whether an environmental exposure explains the clinical presentation being considered. Nonetheless, a targeted medical history combined with selected clinical data can provide insights

that help the clinician better assess the potential relationship between a suspect environmental exposure and a specific adverse health effect. As a matter of practice, addressing the question of environmental aetiology in a 'real-world' clinical setting can be viewed as a two-step process:

- suspecting that an illness may be attributable, at least in part, to an environmental exposure;
- gathering information to support or refute the hypothesis that a patient's environment is indeed causing or contributing to the patient's morbidity.

This chapter provides a conceptual framework for recognizing the possibility that an environmental exposure is affecting a patient's health as well as a practical, systematic approach to exploring this question.

EXPOSURE–EFFECT RELATIONSHIPS: DRAWING ON EPIDEMIOLOGICAL MODELS

Environmental exposure cause–effect relationships may be readily apparent and verifiable in some circumstances. In other settings, concerns about the potential role of an environmental exposure as a cause of an adverse health effect may only be resolved after a process of diligent scrutiny and analysis.

The British biostatistician Sir Austin Bradford Hill established a set of guidelines to determine the strength of the association between an exposure postulated to be harmful and its postulated effect.[1] See p. 5–6 and p.38 for more detail. Although the 'Bradford Hill criteria' are more commonly applied to answer epidemiological questions of causation,[2] a review of the criteria may be helpful in informing assessments of individuals with potentially significant exposure histories.

The clinician may consider each of the following criteria in addressing the possibility that a patient is suffering as a result of an environmental exposure:

- Strength and association: Is there a strong relationship between repeated exposures and the effect within individuals or groups?
- Consistency: Has the exposure–response relationship under consideration been demonstrated in other individuals?
- Specificity: Is the health effect plausibly attributable to only a single putative exposure?
- Temporality: Did the exposure precede development of the condition?
- Dose–response relationship: Do repeated exposures of varying intensity produce repeated effects of severity that correlate with the exposure dose?
- Biological plausibility: Does the relationship make sense with the accepted understanding of pathological processes?
- Biological coherence: Is the relationship consistent with what is already known about either the exposure or the effect?
- Experimental evidence: Have any animal or human studies demonstrated that putative exposure is causally linked with the effect?
- Analogy: Is the exposure–response relationship similar to other established causal connections?

A consideration of Bradford-Hill's epidemiological criteria for causation can be helpful in determining whether a patient is suffering as a result of an environmental exposure. But, as we will show below, population-based approaches have limitations as well as strengths when one attempts to apply these precepts in the individual clinical context.

ATTRIBUTION AND CAUSALITY IN THE INDIVIDUAL CONTEXT

The patient who complains of the abrupt onset of headache, nausea and confusion while operating an internal combustion engine-powered generator inside a small closed garage may immediately be suspected of having carbon monoxide poisoning. Measurement of the blood carboxyhaemoglobin concentration serves to confirm clinically significant exposure that, in turn, guides appropriate acute care. In this case, several elements facilitate a diagnosis:

- The history and clinical findings are typical of carbon monoxide exposure.
- A test is available that confirms exposure to the toxicant and provides an assessment of the magnitude of exposure through biological monitoring.
- There is a body of literature that has defined the correlation (dose–response) between the biomarker of exposure – carboxyhaemoglobin concentration – and clinical effects attributable to such intoxication.
- The biological mechanism of effect and rationale for treatment is well understood.
- The temporal relationship between the exposure and the response is tight, facilitating prompt evaluation of the patient and the rapid acquisition of conclusive data to prove the causal relationship.

These elements are certainly compatible with, but are not identical to, the epidemiological guidelines for causality. Furthermore, in other circumstances where conclusions about the role of an environmental exposure are elusive and may ultimately never be possible to establish with causal certainty at the individual level, the rigid application of a population-based approach does not provide a practical basis for one-on-one assessment. For instance, a patient with bronchogenic carcinoma may report multiple exposures each of which could be casually related to lung cancer, including elevated radon exposure in the home confirmed through home testing, long term co-habitation with a heavy smoker, and prior low-intensity direct cigarette exposure as an active smoker. It would be impossible to 'prove' whether either of the continuing environmental exposures (i.e. radon and second-hand smoke) or the patient's distant primary cigarette-smoking practice 'caused' the disease, although the magnitude of the relative risks associated with each factor might be compared with one another to draw probabilistic inferences.

Notwithstanding the challenges of addressing the question of causation, the patient or a referring clinician may seek an 'explanation' for suffering, seek the best possible answer to the question of causation, and want to know how the aetiology may impact on management strategies. Moreover, the clinician may be required to take a broad view in considering possible relationships between environmental exposures and a wide spectrum of adverse health conditions. We intentionally use the term 'adverse health effect' instead of limiting this solely to 'illness', 'disease' or 'injury' in order to be inclusive in addressing the kinds of end points the clinician may face in dealing with environmental attribution.

In many scenarios, the medical-scientific assessment of causality may be inconclusive and unsatisfying. For example, exposure to vapours, fumes or gases may be associated with irritant effects in some individuals, complaints of headache in others or even subjective changes in cognition in others, and these are all common and non-specific symptoms rather than a discrete syndrome. Moreover, the relative frequency of such various complaints, compared with those who have not been exposed, may not yield a high ratio, that is, the excess may be modest (e.g. a relative risk of 1.25), and it may be difficult or impossible to classify those studied in groups, let alone an individual case, according to the degree of exposure in a way that clearly generates dose–response increments. In addition, the association in question may have been observed in some studies but not in others, an inconsistency that is often the case when it is difficult to define a group of heterogeneous exposures with precision. Thus, in environmental exposure assessments at the population level, many of the classic causal associations (specific effect, strong association, dose response or reproducibility) may not have been met.

RELATIVE RISK, ATTRIBUTABLE RISK, AND LATENCY AT THE INDIVIDUAL LEVEL

The attribution of an environmental aetiology at the individual level faces challenges that extend beyond the Bradford Hill guidelines. This is most clearly the case in terms of relative and attributable risk, epidemiological constructs that are also relevant in this clinical context. To return to the example of second-hand smoke exposure, the epidemiological evidence does support a causal association with lung cancer, even though the excess risk is modest (that is less, approximately 1.4). Stated in terms of attributable risk, the excess proportion of disease would be 29 per cent in a group uniformly exposed to second-hand smoke. Although we do not typically translate this into individual risk, one could say, for a single patient with lung cancer and such a history of environmental exposure, that there is a 29 per cent (40 in 140) likelihood that the disease was indeed due to that cause.

Most environmental factors do not achieve a level of relative risk exceeding 2.0. Such strong associations (which are more typical of high-level occupational exposures) do allow the clinician, in the individual patient context, to conclude that the exposure at hand is more likely than not to be casually associated with the adverse effect in question. This is because, past a relative risk threshold of 2.0, the attributable risk given a documented exposure is greater than 50 per cent. In many medico-legal situations, more-likely-than-not (i.e. > 50 per cent likelihood, or the balance of probabilities) defines causality. In practice, this dichotomization still leaves many clinicians extremely uncomfortable, given that cut-offs for diagnostic 'certainty', even if probabilistic by nature, are usually quite a bit higher.

The opposite scenario is also true. The assignment of a likely causal or contributing role to an environmental exposure may override an otherwise modest attributable risk derived from classical epidemiological estimations. For example, in the same second-hand smoke scenario, the source of exposure may have been growing up with two parents who were both heavy smokers while living upstairs from a smoky tavern, and then presenting with bronchogenic carcinoma as a lifetime non-smoker at age 35. In that scenario, a causal attribution on the individual level may indeed be warranted, despite the less than 50 per cent attributable risk estimate noted previously, since the individual exposure of the case in question far exceeds the presumed central tendency (average) of those studied at the group level.

Temporal patterns of exposure and response may also weigh heavily in attribution assessments. In diseases where a long latency between exposure and disease is necessary, potential exposure to an environmental carcinogen only within the last 5 or even 10 years clearly makes a causal association highly unlikely. In contrast, a tightly linked temporal association, where this is biologically plausible, strongly supports causality. The most clear-cut scenario for this is an exposure rechallenge with the recrudescence of an adverse effect, for example in an herbal-associated hepatitis.

SPECIAL DIAGNOSTIC SUBSETS: PATHOGNOMONIC PROCESSES, OCCUPATIONAL DISEASES AND PSYCHOLOGICAL DISORDERS

Certain pathophysiological processes are by definition 'environmental,' at least in the broadest sense of the term. The case scenario of carbon monoxide intoxication previously presented falls within this category. Heavy metal poisoning and the pneumoconioses are other examples of such conditions. Using 'environmental' to encompass a wider range of exposures, many infectious diseases can also be viewed as inherently attributable to exposures spread by air or water contamination or, in other scenarios, by an animal vector.

In such cases, determining whether a patient suffers from an environmental exposure does not concern the diagnosis of a specific condition or identifying its 'cause' (presuming that the specific heavy metal or microbial pathogen has already been confirmed by testing), but rather pinpointing, if possible, the source of the exposure. This undertaking may be an obvious and immediate public health priority (e.g. identifying the source of infection in an index case of cholera), may be relegated to a role of secondary clinical importance (e.g. finding the source of asbestos exposure in a non-occupational case of mesothelioma) or ignored altogether (e.g. pinpointing a possible point-source of allergen exposure in allergic aspergillosis). No matter what level of priority is placed on this process, the systematic environmental assessment in pathognomonic conditions should, however, be targeted to the practices and co-factors known to be linked to the specific exposure in question.

This often begins with ascertaining whether the exposure of concern occurred due to an occupational or a non-occupational pathway, as alluded to above in relation to asbestos-caused mesothelioma. The occupational/non-occupational dichotomy is driven in large part by the largely separate social insurance schemes that cover these two aetiologies in many countries. Conceptually, the approach to assessment of exposure is not fundamentally different, although it is safe to generalize that occupational exposures are generally higher than those from environmental sources, and occupational disease is, by definition, limited to those who have a history of employment at some point. It should also be recognized that the dividing line between occupation and avocation, and salaried and unsalaried employment, are not so clear cut. This is particularly true for women's work in the home.[3] Nonetheless, classic occupational injury and illness and its clinical diagnosis presents a topic far beyond the scope of this chapter and will not be considered further here.

Psychological factors may play an important role in influencing how some environmental exposures are experienced and, in turn, their potential for producing an adverse health effect. For example, certain individuals reproducibly experience a discrete constellation of physical signs and symptom manifestations (e.g. nausea, tachycardia and diaphoresis) in response to specific environmental stimuli. If the stimulus is standing in front of a large audience, the response is commonly known as 'stage fright.' Other environmental triggers for similar responses may be diagnosed appropriately as a form of panic disorder, but if the purported trigger is exotic or hazardous for other reasons, an environmentally related toxic mechanism may be wrongly suspected or invoked. One unifying construct that has been applied to a number of these is 'odour-triggered' panic disorder.[4] When symptoms are reported by multiple individuals, such as occurs in the well-described syndrome of 'mass psychogenic illness', the likelihood of an environmental misattribution rises even higher.[5] Post-traumatic stress disorder, which can occur after an environmental event (e.g. toxic gas release from an industrial or transportation event), is also a psychological illness that can be confused with a potentially toxicant-mediated syndrome.

Although we recognize that such psychological disorders can be associated with substantial morbidity, they are nonetheless beyond the purview of this chapter. But it is important that the clinician consider this subset of 'environmental' psychological disorders in the differential diagnosis where appropriate while, at the same time, avoiding the invocation of a somatoform disorder as a 'default' label for any symptom complex not easily explained, yet where environmental factors may indeed be playing a role.

TAKING A CLINICAL ENVIRONMENTAL HEALTH HISTORY

The first step in determining whether the patient is suffering as a result of an environmental exposure is, as was emphasized at the outset, to entertain the possibility that the patient's environment indeed may be a factor. Such concerns may originate from the patient who offers a hypothesis on the cause of the problem, or from the clinician whose experience and training may lead to the suspicion of a link between the environment and an adverse health condition.

The patient may volunteer the history of an abrupt onset of coughing and respiratory distress immediately after a household cleaning product-mixing misadventure. In this case, the history offered by the patient provides ample information about both cause and effect. Although it may be of some use for the clinician to learn additional details about the products that produced the irritant injury (e.g. hypochlorite bleach mixed with an acid tile-cleaning product), the evidence of causation has been easily obtained and the health consequences of the exposure have been readily defined by the patient's description, allowing the clinician to focus immediately on delineating the severity of impairment (i.e. through pulmonary function testing) and initiating treatment as indicated.

In contrast, a patient who presents with various non-specific systemic complaints and also reports ill-health in family members with an onset tied to increased wood-burning at home has linked a general exposure (wood-burning) and the onset of symptoms, but has not pinpointed a specific factor or contaminant in the wood causing such illness. An astute clinician may be able to take that information and, through follow-up questioning, determine that the patient has been burning wood from old decking that had been made of chromated copper arsenate pressure-treated wood to protect the structure from rotting. This might prompt the measurement of urine arsenic concentration and lead to a diagnosis of arsenic intoxication.

On other occasions, the patient may have no insight whatsoever into the aetiology. A patient who presents with nausea and is found to be in acute hepatic failure after eating vegetables provided by a friend whose hobbies include wild mushroom-hunting, may be correctly diagnosed with *Amanita* poisoning only after an extensive medical history that includes the consideration of a range of toxicants as potential aetiological factors.

Once the possibility of an environmental factor has been considered and appears to be plausible, the clinician will probably need more historical information to investigate this suspicion further. In many clinical settings, both occupational and environmental factors can be subsumed under a broader designation of toxic exposures. Recent guidelines for taking an exposure history have summarized history domains with the mnemonic 'CH²OPD²': community, home, hobbies, occupation, personal habits, diet and drugs.[6]

For the purpose of this discussion, we will focus on exposure in the home and community environments encountered through the respiratory tract, by ingestion and through skin contact. The US Agency for Toxic Substances and Disease Registry (ATSDR) has specified that an environmental history should explore the location of the house, the house water supply and changes in air quality. The ATSDR also recommends queries about the patient's proximity to industrial complexes and hazardous waste sites resulting in the contamination of air, water or soil. Additionally, the ATSDR cites hobbies as potential sources of toxicant exposure, for example model-building, pottery-making, photography, silkscreen-printing, gardening, stained-glass-making and wood-working.[7]

In general, assessments of the home and community environments should consider exposures that may be encountered through the respiratory tract, by ingestion and through skin contact.[8–11] It is relevant to consider a variety of exposure sources including:

- home heating and ventilation;
- renovation work and 'handyman' projects;
- household cleaning products;
- fabrics and carpeting;
- indoor sources of mould;
- second-hand smoke;
- water quality and sanitation;
- pets, both common and 'exotic';
- hobbies, amateur pursuits and avocations;
- nearby community sources.

SPECIFIC EXPOSURES FOR TARGETTED ASSESSMENT

Home heating, cooking and ventilation

In developing nations, biomass fuels are widely used indoors for cooking and heating and increase the risk of chronic obstructive lung disease and associated respiratory symptoms. Wood-burning fireplaces that provide inadequate ventilation may produce elevated ambient concentrations of particulates and carbon monoxide.[12] The improper use of non-stick cookware (e.g. an empty pan heated to a very high temperature when inadvertently left on a stove) can cause a flu-like illness (i.e. polymer fume fever) or, with higher temperatures, acute lung injury.[13]

Environmental history questions may include: 'How is your home heated and ventilated?', 'Can you describe to me how you cook your food?' and 'Have there been any recent cooking or heating mishaps?'

Renovation work and 'handyman' projects

Home renovation may result in exposure to a variety of toxicants. The risks of hazardous exposure are especially relevant if the patient is engaged in do-it-yourself renovation. Relevant exposures include paint additives,[14] fibreglass insulation,[15] waterproofing and caulking sprays, and aerosolized caulking sprays.[16] Environmental history questions may include: 'Have you had recent renovation

work done in your home?' If the answer is yes, 'Who did the work?', 'What work was done?', 'What supplies were used?' (e.g. paints with biocides, insulation materials, two-part polymers or adhesives), 'Were any of the materials obtained through industrial as opposed to routine consumer sources?', 'Was any special rental equipment used, such as pressure guns, welding tools, torches, or grinders?' and 'Was there dust, fume or mist visible in your home?'

Household cleaning products

The use of bleach, ammonia and other volatile agents in high concentration, either alone or especially in combination, can produce toxic vapours.[17] The use of these agents in confined spaces may be especially hazardous. Skin and respiratory tract irritation, cough and irritant-induced asthma may be attributable to misadventures with cleaning products. Questions should ascertain how, where and when the products are used and may include: 'What agents did you use?' and 'Did you mix more than one product or use products sequentially on the same surface?'

Fabrics, furniture and carpets

New carpets and furniture can release noxious odours, and fabrics such as rugs and curtains may have a role in the development of allergies, asthma and non-specific effects such as headache and cough.[18] Questions should explore whether there are new fabrics and carpets in the home and where they are located, and elicit details about the materials from which they are made, including: 'Have you any new furnishings and, if so, are there any special smells from them?' and 'Any new carpets and, if so, were they glued down?' In addition, ascertaining whether any waterproofing aerosols have been used is appropriate if respiratory tract injury is suspected.

Indoor sources of mould

A spectrum of effects has been linked with mould exposure, including pulmonary diseases and neuronal-psychiatric effects.[19, 20] Water damage in the home increases the risk of mould contamination. An environmental history should include questions about leaks, faulty drainage, poor ventilation, burst pipes and flooding, including: 'Is there any dry wall construction that has been damaged?' and 'Have you any carpeting on a concrete floor (e.g. in the basement) that has been wet or flooded?'

Second-hand smoke

Childhood infections, coughs and other cardiopulmonary disorders have been linked to second-hand smoke exposure.[21] Although it is challenging to attribute a new health problem to chronic second-hand smoke exposure, any cigarette smoke exposure should be viewed as concerning and as a potential threat to a patient's well-being. Simple questions include: 'Do you live with a smoker?' and 'Is cigarette-smoking allowed indoors where you live?'

Pets, both common and exotic

Susceptible individuals may suffer from allergic rhinitis, dermatitis and asthma when exposed to cats.[22] Pulmonary disorders, including extrinsic allergic alveolitis, may develop in bird fanciers.[23] Accordingly, questions about pets in the home may be useful. Bear in mind, however, that the patient may not consider the creatures in question 'pets', so the generic question 'Do you keep any pets?' may have to be qualified to include fish, reptiles, exotic creatures and so forth.

Hobbies and avocations

A variety of recreational or avocational activities – pursuits that are engaged in for pleasure and are not work related – often described as 'hobbies' are associated with exposure to potentially hazardous toxicants. Pigments used in painting, glazes employed in ceramics, and photographic emulsion salts have the potential to cause metal-related respiratory tract toxicity. Health effects include lead poisoning and metal-associated sensitization leading to asthma or rhinitis. Fibre-based crafts that involve the handling of raw textile materials, especially silk, are associated with respiratory allergic sensitization. Jewellery-making has been linked to solder flux (colophony, also known as rosin) exposure, a known cause of asthma. Wood-working may cause airway irritation, metal-working may cause metal fume fever, and glass-etching has been linked with asthma.[24]

Beyond such crafts, other leisure pursuits may include gardening (with exposure to allergens or pesticides), athletics and sports (with physical injury and other risks) or even pursuits involving collectables. It is advisable to address this heterogeneous area in the most open-ended way possible, for example: 'Do you have any hobbies, avocations or other regular amateur or leisure pursuits?'

Water quality and sanitation

While high-quality municipal water and sanitation systems represent great public health achievements in most developed societies, some communities may have problems with groundwater contamination and sewage management. A history of recurrent diarrhoeal illnesses in multiple family members, especially in rural communities, should prompt questions about the source of water and sewage management, but other problems may be more insidious, such as nitrate contamination (a cause of methaemoglobinaemia), heavy metal contamination (especially arsenic) and petrochemical groundwater 'migration'. Key questions can include: 'Does your household water come from a municipal grid?' and 'If you have well water, how deep is the well and who tests the water quality?'

Community exposures

Extreme examples of environmental threats to health include major industrial accidents resulting in the release of toxicants into neighbouring communities. The Union Carbide disaster in Bhopal, India, in 1984 resulted in the deaths of at least 3000 and perhaps as many as 20 000 individuals due to methyl isocyanate gas. The Chernobyl nuclear reactor disaster in the former Soviet Union resulted in an estimated 4000 excess cancer cases in the most highly exposed neighbouring communities. Less dramatic threats to health may also result from water and air contamination from industrial sources. The identification of clusters of health conditions in communities neighbouring an industrial complex should raise questions about the possibility of airborne and waterborne industrial contaminants.

Agricultural sources of environmental exposures, especially animal confinement buildings, may be relevant in rural communities.[25] Proximity to busy harbours and highways that serve as trucking corridors may result in exposure to high concentrations of diesel exhaust particulates that have been linked with a spectrum of adverse cardiopulmonary effects.[26, 27]

Unfortunately, these scenarios do not lend themselves very well to 'generic' screening questions. In the case of follow-up after a conflagration, questions often focus on distance from the epicentre of the event, the duration of exposure and illness among those in the same area at the same time.

MANAGEMENT CONSIDERATIONS

The answer to the question 'Is this patient suffering as a result of an environmental exposure?' is very often 'possibly'. Although both clinician and patient would probably prefer greater certainty, it may not be possible to determine with certitude that the patient's problem is caused by exposure 'x'. How, then, should the patient be managed in the face of diagnostic uncertainty? Important determinants of patient management include both the strength of the association between an exposure and its effect and the severity of the effect itself. Additional considerations will inevitably include the costs and complexity of management and the societal-legal implications of attributing an environmental exposure to a health problem.

For example, when a very strong and likely causal relationship between exposure and illness can be demonstrated, management may be apparent and uncontroversial, irrespective of the burden of treatment. A relevant scenario would be that of a child with developmental abnormalities diagnosed with lead intoxication whose home is contaminated with lead-based paint. Proper management demands that either the child be removed from further exposure or the home undergo lead abatement.

In cases where an exposure is considered, with less confidence, as a 'possible' cause of harm, management may also be apparent and uncontroversial if minimally burdensome. For example, if a new cleaning product is considered as a potential cause of dermatitis, or a new rug in a home is considered to be a possible cause of exacerbation of asthma, it is reasonable that exposure avoidance measures be enacted. In these cases, even if the evidence linking the exposure to the putative problem is modest or slight, the burden of a trial of avoidance therapy is minimal (e.g. cessation of use of the cleaning product or removal of the rug) and may prove to be both diagnostic and therapeutic.

In other circumstances, establishing causation may be difficult, complicated by legal, economic and social factors, and abatement strategies may be burdensome. For example, if a patient presents with worsening asthma and an ambient environmental trigger is suspected, efforts to mitigate continuing exposure may be burdensome (e.g. relocating to another living place) or challenged by other stakeholders (e.g. for a reduction in sulphur dioxide emission from an upwind cement factory). In such circumstances, efforts do what is 'right' for both the patient (beyond standard asthma treatment) and even the patient's community (presuming that there may be others with asthma as well) may fall well outside the standard clinical arena. Although a more complete discussion of medical and social justice is beyond the remit of this chapter, clinicians should recognize that such considerations may become relevant in the course of addressing questions of causation in and management of individual patients.

SUMMARY

In summary, the first step to answering the question 'Is this patient suffering as a result of an environmental exposure?' is to determine whether it is even an appropriate question to raise. Clinical circumstances, including a patient's complaints, should inform the clinician of the reasonableness of considering an environmental exposure as a cause of a health condition. Once this is viewed as plausible, answering the question may be uncomplicated or quite challenging. A complete medical history that includes a targetted environmental exposure history is the first step

to answering the question. The clinician's consideration of a putative environmental exposure–response relationship can be informed by a review of the Bradford Hill guidelines for causation. Relevant testing to assess for evidence of environmental toxicant exposure or effect may facilitate diagnosis. Finally, the clinician's education, training and experience, combined with targetted reviews of the scientific literature, are essential factors in addressing questions of environmental causation.

REFERENCES

● = Key primary paper

◆ = Major review article

●1. Hill AB. The environment and disease: association or causation? *Proc R Soc Med* 1965; **58**: 295–300.

◆2. Kundi M. Causality and the interpretation of epidemiologic evidence. *Environ Health Perspect* 2006; **114**: 969–74.

3. Blanc PD. The role of household exposure in lung disease among women. *Eur Respir Mon* 2003; **25**: 118–30.

4. Shusterman D. Review of the upper airway, including olfaction, as mediator of symptoms. *Environ Health Perspect* 2002; **4**: 649–53.

5. Jones TF, Craig AS, Hoy D *et al.* Mass psychogenic illness attributed to toxic exposure at a high school. *N Engl J Med* 2000; **342**: 96–100.

◆6. Marshall L, Weir E, Abelsohn, Sanborn MD. Identifying and managing adverse environmental health effects. Part 1: Taking an exposure history. *CMA J* 2002; **166**: 1049–55.

◆7. US Agency for Toxic Substances and Disease Registry. Taking an Exposure History: What Is Included in the Environmental History (Part 3) of an Exposure History Form? Available from: http://www.atsdr.cdc.gov/csem/exphistory/ehenvironmental_history.html (accessed November 4, 2009).

◆8. Blanc PD. Taking a targeted environmental respiratory history. American College of Chest Physicians: Pulmonary and Critical Care Update 2007; Vol. 21. Available at: http://www.chestnet.org/education/online/pccu/vol21/lessons11_12/index.php (accessed November 4, 2009).

9. Goldman RH, Peters JM. The occupational and environmental health history. *JAMA* 1981; **246**: 2831–6.

10. Kilpatrick N, Frumkin H, Trowbridge J *et al.* The environmental history in pediatric practice: a study of pediatricians' attitudes, beliefs, and practices. *Environ Health Perspect* 2002; **110**: 823–7.

11. Marshall L, Weir E, Abelsohn A *et al.* Identifying and managing adverse environmental health effects. Part 1: Taking an exposure history. *CMAJ* 2002; **166**: 1049–55.

◆12. Naeher LP, Brauer M, Lipsett M *et al.* Woodsmoke health effects: a review. *Inhal Toxicol* 2007; **19**: 67–106.

13. Son M, Maruyama E, Shindo Y *et al.* Case of polymer fume fever with interstitial pneumonia caused by inhalation of

polytetrafluoroethylene (Teflon). *Chudoku Kenkyu* 2006;
19: 279–82.

14. Wieslander G, Norback D, Edling C. Occupational exposure to water based paint and symptoms from the skin and eyes. *Occup Environ Med* 1994; **51**:181–6.

15. Maxim LD, Eastes W, Hadley JG *et al*. Fiber glass and rock/slag wool exposure of professional and do-it-yourself installers. *Regul Toxicol Pharmacol* 2003; **37**: 28–44.

16. Herrick RF, McClean MD, Meeker JD *et al*. An unrecognized source of PCB contamination in schools and other buildings. *Environ Health Perspect* 2004; **112**: 1051–3.

17. Sawalha AF. Storage and utilization patterns of cleaning products in the home: toxicity implications. *Accid Anal Preven* 2007; **39**: 1186–91.

18. Mendell MJ. Indoor residential chemical emissions as risk factors for respiratory and allergic effects in children: a review. *Indoor Air* 2007; **17**: 259–77.

19. Sahakian NM, Park JH, Cox-Ganser JM. Dampness and mold in the indoor environment: implications for asthma. *Immunol Allergy Clin North Am* 2008; **28**: 485–505.

◆20. Fung F, Hughson WG. The fundamentals of mold-related illness: when to suspect the environment is making a patient sick. *Postgrad Med* 2008; **120**: 80–4.

21. Eisner MD, Wang Y, Haight TJ *et al*. Secondhand smoke exposure, pulmonary function, and cardiovascular mortality. *Ann Epidemiol* 2007; **17**: 364–73.

22. Takkouche B, Gonzalez-Barcala FJ, Etminan M *et al*. Exposure to furry pets and the risk of asthma and allergic rhinitis: a meta-analysis. *Allergy* 2008; **63**: 857–64.

23. Morell F, Roger A, Reyes L *et al*. Bird fancier's lung: a series of 86 patients. *Medicine (Baltimore)* 2008; **87**: 110.

24. Blanc PD. Hobby pursuits. In: Tarlo S, Cullinan P (eds) *Environmental and Occupational Lung Disease*. Wiley, 2009 (in press).

25. Iversen M, Kirychuk S, Drost H *et al*. Human health effects of dust exposure in animal confinement buildings. *J Agric Saf Health* 2000; **6**: 283–8.

◆26. Brook RD. Cardiovascular effects of air pollution. *Clin Sci (Lond)* 2008; **115**: 175–87.

◆27. Chen TM, Gokhale J, Shofer S *et al*. Outdoor air pollution: particulate matter health effects. *Am J Med Sci* 2007; **333**: 235–43.

60

Public perception of risk

SARAH DAMERY

OVERVIEW

The understanding and management of risk has received much attention in recent years, and it has been suggested that risk is the primary issue of concern that occupies our modern societies.[1] Debates about risk embody tensions between expert assessments of risk on the one hand, and public perceptions of risk on the other. Technological, health and environmental issues span scientific, economic and political interests and concerns, and encompass a multitude of conflicting interests and values. Many risks involve an interplay between expert assessments, public perceptions and risk management priorities. It has been argued that understanding how members of the public perceive risk is fundamental if risks are to be managed effectively – particularly in the case of risks to human health, which may create situations where there is a requirement for public compliance with risk management policies, often taking the form of behavioural change (to prevent the spread of infectious disease, for example).

Making sense of the ways in which members of the public perceive risk has, however, been notoriously difficult, and many attempts to formalize or categorize risk perceptions have been unsuccessful. This is largely because of an unhelpful conceptual dichotomy typically drawn between 'experts' and 'the public' in which the primacy of scientific expertise and its rationality and objectivity, in contrast to the supposed irrationality and subjectivity of public understandings, is seen as paramount.[2,3] Here, members of the public are characterized as lacking the ability to view risk objectively, primarily because they do not have the necessary information on which such risk assessments can be based. Because of this, it is often argued that public risk perceptions must be shaped by expert inputs in order to ensure that the public have the 'correct' perceptions of risk.

More recent ways of thinking about the expert–public relationship, drawing on cognitive psychology, sociology and other disciplines, have argued that the distinction between experts and the public is unhelpful, not least because scientific and technical assessments of risk may themselves be uncertain and subject to ignorance or indeterminacy. In addition, for many risk issues, members of the public can be experts in their own right.[4–6] So, although the 'expert' may know more than the 'public' about the generalities and mechanisms of risk-related processes, applying this knowledge in reality is always limited by the difficulty of understanding the myriad context-specific influences that may operate for any given risk. In contrast to these generalized processes, members of the public may possess locally embedded knowledge that experts may not have, even if this knowledge is largely qualitative. These conceptualizations suggest that risk is essentially socially constructed, as are all resulting risk perceptions.[7]

This chapter will first outline traditional conceptions of risk, arguing that the scientific assessment of risk in the field of the environment and human health is often characterized by extreme uncertainty. Second, successive attempts to categorize public risk perceptions will be outlined, including the cognitive psychology 'psychometric' approach of Paul Slovic and colleagues,[8] Mary Douglas's alternative cultural theory approach,[9,10] and Kasperson et al.'s social amplification of risk framework.[11] Third, more recent ideas about how we might understand risk and public perception will be introduced, which argue that the distinction between experts and the public is no longer helpful, and that public perceptions of risk can have their own rationality, which is not necessarily inferior to expert assessment, but which is crucially dependent on issues such as trust in the credibility of information sources about risks, or in the competence of the institutions managing them.[12–14] This chapter takes a deliberately theoretical rather than empirical approach, so that it might provide a useful context for understanding some of the factors relating to specific environmentally induced risks to human health that form the earlier chapters of this volume.

THE PROBLEM WITH RISK

Risk has traditionally been conceived as a technical or numerical phenomenon. The Royal Society posited a clear distinction between objective and perceived risk, arguing that it was possible to measure risk exactly through statistical means using probability assessment. As a result, risk was defined as 'the probability that a particular adverse event occurs during a stated period of time, or results from a particular challenge. As a probability in the sense of statistical risk, risk obeys all the formal laws of combining probabilities' (p. 16 in reference [15]). Later work lamented the public 'misunderstanding' of risk, and called for a broader public understanding of the role of science and scientific expertise in assessing risks of all types, and an improvement in the ability of the public to engage with ideas of risk and uncertainty.[2]

It was further stated that there exists a gap between what is scientific (and can therefore be measured) and the ways in which public opinion gauges risk.[3] Because of this, remedial approaches were suggested based on better informing these ignorant publics in order to correct their misperceptions and convert them to the correct, objective view of 'real' risks as defined by scientific and technical expertise.[16] This approach has been referred to as the 'information deficit' paradigm, which typically assumes that if the determinants of public risk perceptions can be uncovered, the 'gap' between expert and public knowledge about risk can be filled by the provision of appropriately worded information, by educational initiatives or through the implementation of sound measures designed to bring about behavioural change.

In the case of the environment and health (as broadly defined), the objective measurement of risk is, however, itself highly problematic and is often subject to extensive scientific uncertainty or indeterminacy.[12,13] Risks may arise through multiple pathways and have synergistic effects, posing difficulties for the surveillance and monitoring of diseases and agents; hazard, risk and exposure assessments are compromised by problems associated with establishing robust dose–response relationships and thresholds of harm, and some risks may arise from specific point sources, whereas others are highly diffuse. There may also be large spatial differences between sources and impacts, and a temporal lag between cause and effect. Added to this, the framing of risk issues, and even the choice of those issues which are considered

worthy of investigation and those which are not, may be fundamentally important.[17, 18]

In many cases, decisions about risk may be influenced to a large extent by the values of the involved experts.[19] An extensive body of work exists on the 'sociology of scientific knowledge', in which it is argued that, far from science being rational, objective and value-free, social factors play a significant role in determining the knowledge produced.[20–24] It has also been argued that we have moved from an era of 'normal science',[25] in which scientists worked to incrementally accumulate detail in accordance with an established broad theory, and where the underlying assumptions of that theory remained unchallenged, into an era of 'post-normal science'. Under a post-normal scientific paradigm, we face 'hard' decisions about environmental and human health risks for which the necessary scientific inputs will be irredeemably 'soft', uncertain, contested and characterized by extreme complexity.[26] In this sense, many health risks are 'trans-scientific',[27] in that although they can be stated in scientific terms, they are in principle beyond the practical capacity of science to address. Unfortunately, these difficulties in establishing objective assessments of risk have all too often been ignored or downplayed, with scientific and technical expertise portrayed instead as robust and sound.

'MEASURING' PUBLIC PERCEPTIONS OF RISK

In the 1970s and 80s, research into uncovering and explaining public risk perceptions was extensively undertaken. In broad terms, this research hoped that by better understanding public risk perceptions, we could:

- improve methods of eliciting public opinions about risk;
- provide a basis for understanding and anticipating public responses to risks and hazards;
- improve the communication of risk information between the public, technical experts and policy-makers.[8,28]

These ideas have had surprising longevity in the field of risk perception research, despite displaying a number of flaws that have only recently been fully articulated in the academic risk literature.

The 'psychometric' approach

This body of work was based on advances in cognitive behavioural and social psychology.[8] Starr had initially drawn attention to the fact that whether or not members of the public were prepared to tolerate a given risk was linked to the extent to which it was voluntary or involuntary, whether the impacts affected society at large or were individualized, and whether or not individuals had had past experience of dealing with the risk in question.[29] All of these factors were argued to determine public risk perceptions and affect individual decision-making. Psychometric research drew attention to the importance of the qualitative aspects of various risks, working on the assumption that any observed differences between expert and public risk understandings were due to erroneous perceptions held on the part of the public. In this view, perceived risk was argued to be a distorted view of actual risk, shaped by ignorance, prior beliefs and an inability on the part of members of the public to understand concepts of probability, along with the influence of personal experiences, which are inherently subjective.

Much psychometric work studied personality typologies in order to understand why people misperceived 'real' risks, and to uncover the factors accounting for the observed deviations. Work was based on large-scale questionnaires designed to measure individual risk perceptions and judgements about the risks associated with different hazards or health issues. Individuals were asked to rate the importance of different risks, which were then analysed using scaling techniques and multivariate statistics. Perhaps the best-known representation of these findings is the two-dimensional scatter diagram created by Paul Slovic and colleagues.[8,28] In this diagram, using factor analysis, public attitudes towards a wide variety of hazards are plotted on two axes, labelled 'unknown' risk, and 'dread' risk. The resulting display of points is commonly interpreted as meaning that the public would like a stricter control of risks that are less familiar and more frightening (such as chemical leaks and nuclear reactor accidents) and are less concerned about more familiar risks (such as tobacco or alcohol use). Public perceptions were thus thought to exaggerate the unknown, even though statistics based on mortality rates or financial costs revealed that many familiar risks are more frequent, and more costly, than some unfamiliar ones.[14]

However, the psychometric approach received a great deal of criticism. Although the scatter diagrams plotted perceptions of the risk of different hazards graphically and allowed comparisons to be drawn between them, it became obvious that this was only revealing part of the overall picture. The use of rating scales as the main method of obtaining information about individual risk perceptions had a framing effect on the answers people could give. There was also no easy way in which small-scale psychometric studies conducted with specific social or demographic groups could be extrapolated to the wider population, so it remained difficult to incorporate public perceptions of risk into broader risk management policy. More fundamentally, it was argued[30] that the psychometric approach focused too much on the ways in which the general public thought about risk rather than on how management institutions and policy-makers performed the same function.

Cultural theory

The cultural theory approach, developed by Mary Douglas and colleagues in the 1980s, grew out of a dissatisfaction with the limitations of psychometric research and its ignorance of the cultural basis of people's risk understandings and perceptions: 'psychometricians [have] isolated the cultural factors and treated them as another variable in an experimentally derived technical framework...[rather than] explore the cultural underpinnings of risk perception' (p. 8 in reference [31]). In arguing that the psychometric approach simply studied *what* people perceive as risky rather than *why* they hold such perceptions, Douglas challenged the risk perception literature by suggesting that individual perceptions must be studied *culturally* as part of a network of social and institutional relations that constrain or enable social behaviour.[9] All risks were argued to be social constructs, with individual and societal perceptions acting as cultural filters through which people made sense of the information available to them.[32]

Others have similarly argued that perceptions are the outcome of processes operating at both the individual and societal levels, such that risk perception is determined on the one hand by individuals' own private understandings, accumulated over time through experience, and on the other hand by wider opinions and interaction as a member of a social milieu.[33] Put more simply, people's risk perceptions are shaped by their opinion about a given risk, their interpretation of communications they may receive about it and, importantly, friends, family and other social networks that they are part of.

Because risk perceptions are individually and culturally referenced, Douglas argued that there could be no single 'correct' risk perception. Instead, risks are selected from a universe of risk choices, and the selection is the result of social influences.[9,10] Each individual has their own 'portfolio' of risks that they are concerned about; each individual highlights some risks and downplays others.[34] This suggests that underlying social value systems are likely to have as strong an influence on public risk perception as the 'measured' physical properties of risks, hazards or events.[35]

In order to make sense of this, cultural theorists employed 'grid and group' risk analysis, related first to the extent to which people are governed by social groups in the way they live their lives, and second, to the extent to which social interaction is governed by rules. Perceptions of risk were argued to vary according to four cultural biases or 'world views': individualist, fatalist, hierarchist and egalitarian. Each of these world views was seen as defining which dangers should be accepted and avoided, how risks should be distributed, how serious risks were considered to be, and who should be blamed when things went wrong.[36,37] Each variable was measured as high or low on a pair of orthogonal axes, generating four visions of social life, each with its own characteristic views of the world and approaches to risk. The theory was that if the predominant cultural bias of an individual can be quantified at any given time, it should be possible to predict what hazards that individual will perceive as risky, i.e. who fears what and *why*.

However, as was the case with the psychometric approach, cultural theory has been criticized, primarily because in attempting to link risk perceptions to particular cultural biases and world views, it offers an essentially static 'snapshot' of what is in reality dynamically constructed. More recent research has argued that risk perceptions are constantly being modified in the light of new information.[14] Moreover, interpretation plays a central role in the social construction of risk. This is glossed over by the cultural theory approach, as is the possibility that an individual could have more than one cultural bias depending on the particular risk in question.[38]

The social amplification of risk framework

Further to the psychometric and cultural theory approaches to the study of individual and societal risk perceptions, a third model emerged in the 1980s and 90s which tried to advance risk perception research beyond the impasse it had reached. This model, developed by Kasperson et al.,[11] became known as the social amplification of risk framework (SARF). SARF tried to integrate the technical analysis of risk and the cultural, social and individual response structures shaping the public acceptance of risk as a means of explaining why apparently minor hazards or risks that experts see as having a relatively low statistical chance of occurring can become a focus of social concern (risk amplification), while other potentially more serious events with a greater probability of happening receive comparatively little public attention (risk attenuation). SARF was based primarily on communications theory, in which the media in particular was seen as an important source of risk information, along with the symbols and imagery with which events and hazards were portrayed to the public.[39,40]

However, SARF also received criticism, centred around the simplicity of the mechanisms put forward by its proponents to explain risk amplification and risk attenuation, which focused on what was essentially a simplistic model of the public's uptake of media information. Although on the surface offering an attractive argument about the ways in which risk understandings are developed and the reasons for this, research into the social amplification of risk has also been argued to be too mechanistic, and ignorant of the social construction of risk.

MORE RECENT APPROACHES TO PUBLIC RISK PERCEPTION

The approaches to understanding public risk perceptions outlined above generally founder on their construction of the underlying problem. Successive research approaches since the 1970s have taken the view that the goal of risk perception research was to identify the factors accounting for deviations between actual (as measured by experts) and perceived risk, with the assumption that if these factors could be uncovered and the reasons for the public misperception of expert risk assessments found, the gap

between the experts and the public could be closed by the judicious use of public education and information provision to correct public misunderstandings. However, more recent qualitative social and political analyses of risk perception question the validity of this dichotomy in the first place, suggesting instead that all perceptions of risk, whether expert or lay, represent partial or selective views of risky events or hazards.[41]

Following this, technical, economic and psychological approaches to studying environmental risk have increasingly been rejected in favour of cultural and sociological approaches.[6,14,42] Sociological approaches in particular have been influenced heavily by Ulrich Beck's claim that we now live in a 'risk society', where risk is an inescapable and underlying factor for all of us, at all times.[1,43] Alongside Beck's risk society theory, more recent research on environmental risk and uncertainty has recast the notion of public understandings and risk conceptualizations in several important ways. The first of these concerns the public assessment of risk, which, as previously discussed, has traditionally been seen as ignorant and irrational. Commentators such as Wynne argue instead that public risk assessments, far from being ignorant, have their own rationality, which may differ from that of the 'experts', but is not necessarily inferior to theirs.[13] As such, members of the public can play an important role not only in criticizing expert knowledge, but also in generating their own forms of knowledge and understanding.[44] In this sense, citizen knowledge can in certain cases be *at least as* robust and well informed as that of experts. Of course, it is important to stress that the recognition that members of the public can be well informed about environmental and health risks in certain contexts does *not* mean that citizen knowledge is necessarily better than scientific and expert knowledge. Instead, the recognition of public rationality demonstrates that a whole *array* of rationalities for conceptualizing and understanding risk may exist.

These ideas about public risk understandings and perceptions demonstrate the problems associated with a reliance on expert, top-down information transfer based on constructions of environmental and health risks that may not be shared by those towards whom they are directed.[30] Members of the public may not understand the complexities of risk research, but it has been argued that public understandings of, and responses to, risks may be 'rationally based in judgements of the behaviour and trustworthiness of expert institutions'.[13] Therefore, in many cases, it is *trust* that is the key to understanding public risk perceptions,[45] rather than information, as is often assumed.[46,47]

Trust

A key assumption is that the public have an inherent trust in science and scientific expertise, and that a wider exposure to scientific thinking will lead to greater acceptance of, and support for, scientific and technical expertise in relation to the environment and human health.[48] The widely observed lack of public dissent to scientific reassurance about health risks is often equated with public acceptance.[13,49–51] However, researchers have explained this lack of dissent by ascribing it not to an inherent trust in scientific and technical expertise, but to the failure of science to address public concerns. Members of the public, particularly those living in more economically deprived localities, are often resigned to dependency on particular institutions with no perceived power to alter them for the better.[1,4]

Perception and behaviour

It is often assumed that a better understanding of science will lead to better decisions being made by members of the public. This is particularly so in relation to health risk, as the management of such risks often relies on the public being willing to change their behaviour in the way they are expected to. This relates to the assumption that if the gap between expert and public knowledge is bridged with the appropriate information, this will lead to people making a clearer link between policy and action, becoming more virtuous and adopting more positive behaviours, particularly in relation to health.[52,53] However, as Blake argues,[54] several obstacles mediate the relationship between individuals, knowledge, perceptions and risk-related action:

- those pertaining to individuality (largely cognitive);
- those linked with responsibility (i.e. the evaluation of one's personal role in relation to a particular issue);
- practicality (i.e. the ability to act).

The combination of these obstacles in different contexts creates a discontinuity between people becoming concerned about a particular issue and going a step further and turning that concern into meaningful action.

CONCLUSION

It may be that understanding the determinants of public perceptions of risk is an unattainable goal, since it is likely that the same risk will be perceived differently by any two individuals due to issues related to sociodemographic, experiential and contextual factors, irrespective of any 'objective' or statistical assessment of a given risk that may exist. This social construction of risk largely explains the failure of successive paradigms of risk perception research in being able to formalize and predict public perceptions of, and reactions to, specific risks, particularly as the goal of these approaches – that of delivering information designed to bridge the gap between 'expert' and 'public' perceptions – is itself flawed. More recent ways of considering risk have stressed the ephemeral nature of risk and the way in which it is perceived by different groups, and that the distinction between experts and the public is not necessarily a helpful one, particularly in the face of the multidimensional nature of many risks. Added to this, the notion that there exists robust and objective scientific knowledge about risks relating to the environment and human health has been shown to be problematic, given the difficulty in establishing dose–response pathways and determining the exposures and cause-and-effect relationships associated with most risks in this field. Both 'expert' and 'public' perceptions are beset by uncertainty and indeterminacy.

REFERENCES

● = Key primary paper

◆ = Major review article

●1. Beck U. *Risk Society: Towards a New Modernity*. London: Sage, 1992.

2. Royal Society. *The Public Understanding of Science*. London: Royal Society, 1985.

3. Royal Society. *Risk Analysis, Perception and Management: Report of a Royal Society Study Group*. London: Royal Society, 1992.

4. Irwin A. *Citizen Science: A Study of People, Expertise and Sustainable Development*. London: Routledge, 1995.

5. Irwin A, Wynne B (eds). *Misunderstanding Science? The Public Reconstruction of Science and Technology*. Cambridge: Cambridge University Press, 1996.

◆6. Lash S, Szerszynski B, Wynne B (eds). *Risk, Environment and Modernity: Towards a New Ecology*. London: Sage, 1996.

7. Lupton D. *Risk*. London: Routledge, 1999.

8. Slovic P, Fischoff B, Lichtenstein S. *The Assessment and Perception of Risk*. London: Royal Society, 1981.

9. Douglas M. *Risk Acceptability According to the Social Sciences*. London: Routledge, 1986.

10. Douglas M. *Dominant Rationality and Risk Perception*. Sheffield: Political Economy Research Centre, 1994.

●11. Kasperson RE, Renn O, Slovic P. Social amplification of risk: a conceptual framework. *Risk Anal* 1988; **8**: 177–87.

●12. Wynne B. Uncertainty and environmental learning: reconceiving science and policy in the preventive paradigm. *Glob Environ Change* 1992; **2**: 111–27.

13. Wynne B. May the sheep safely graze? A reflexive view of the expert-lay knowledge divide. In: Lask S, Szerszynski B, Wynne B (eds) *Risk, Environment and Modernity: Towards a New Ecology*. London: Sage, 1996: 44–83.

●14. Adams J. *Risk*. London: Sage, 1995.

15. Royal Society. *Risk Assessment: A Study Group Report*. London: Royal Society, 1983.

16. Owens S. Engaging the public: information and deliberation in environmental policy. *Environ Plan A* 2000; **32**: 1141–8.

17. Hajer M. *The Politics of Environmental Discourse: Ecological Modernisation and the Policy Process*. Oxford: Clarendon, 1995.

18. Weale A. *The New Politics of Pollution*. Manchester: Manchester University Press, 1992.

19. Rowe G, Horlick-Jones T, Walls J, Pidgeon N. Difficulties in evaluating public engagement initiatives: reflections on an evaluation of the UK GM Nation? Public debate about transgenic crops. *Public Underst Sci* 2005; **14**: 331–52.

20. Jasanoff S. The songlines of risk. *Environ Values* 1999; **8**: 135–52.

21. Jasanoff S, Markle GE, Petersen JC, Pinch T (eds). *Handbook of Science and Technology Studies*. London: Sage, 2002.

22. Latour B. *Science in Action: How To Follow Scientists and Engineers Through Society*. Cambridge, MA: Harvard University Press, 1987.

23. Latour B. *We Have Never Been Modern*. Cambridge, MA: Harvard University Press, 1993.

24. Woolgar S. *Science: The Very Idea*. Chichester: Ellis Horwood, 1988.

25. Kuhn TS. *The Structure of Scientific Revolutions*. Chicago: University of Chicago Press, 1962.

26. Ravetz JR, Funtowicz SO. Uncertainty and quality in science for policy. *EPA J* 1989; **15**: 21–2.

27. Weinberg A. Science and trans-science. *Minerva* **10**: 209–22.

●28. Slovic P, Fischoff B, Lichtenstein S. Why study risk perception? *Risk Anal* 1982; **2**: 83–93.

29. Starr C. Social benefit versus technical risk. *Science* 1969; **165**: 1232–8.

30. Jasanoff S. The political science of risk perception. *Reliab Eng Syst Saf* 1998; **59**: 91–9.

31. Plough A, Krimsky S. The emergence of risk communication studies: social and political context. *Sci Technol Human Values* 1987; **12**(3): 4–10.

32. Fessenden-Raden J, Fitchen JM, Heath JS. Providing risk information in communities: factors influencing what is heard and accepted. *Sci Technol Human Values* 1987; **12**(3): 94–101.

33. Macgill S. Risk perception and the public: insights from research around Sellafield. In: Brown J (ed.) *Environmental Threats: Perception, Analysis and Management*. London: Belhaven, 1989: 48–66.

34. Johnson BB, Covello V (eds). *The Social and Cultural Construction of Risk*. Dordrecht: Kluwer Academic, 1987.

●35. Douglas M, Wildavsky A. *Risk and Culture: An Essay on the Selection of Technical and Environmental Dangers*. Berkeley, CA: University of California Press, 1982.

36. Bostrom A, Morgan MG, Fischoff B, Smuts T. What do people know about global climate change? Mental models. *Risk Anal* 1994; **14**: 959–70.

37. Pidgeon N, Beattie J. The psychology of risk and uncertainty. In: Calow P (ed.) *Handbook of Environmental Risk Assessment and Management*. Oxford: Blackwell Science, 1997: 289–318.

38. Horlick-Jones T. Meaning and contextualisation in risk assessment. *Reliab Eng Syst Saf* 1998; **59**: 79–89.

●39. Petts J, Horlick-Jones T, Murdock G. *Social Amplification of Risk: The Media and the Public*. London: HMSO, 2001.

◆40. Pidgeon N. Risk communication and the social amplification of risk: theory, evidence and policy implications. *Risk Decis Policy* 1999; **4**: 145–59.

41. Demeritt D. The construction of global warming and the politics of science. *Ann Assoc Am Geogr* 2001; **91**: 307–37.

42. Bennett P. Governing environmental risk: regulation, insurance and moral economy. *Prog Hum Geogr* 1999; **23**: 189–208.

43. Beck U. *Ecological Politics in an Age of Risk*. Cambridge: Polity Press, 1995.

44. O'Connor M. Dialog and debate in a post-normal practice of science: a reflection. *Futures* 1999; **31**: 671–87.

45. O'Neill J. Value pluralism, incommensurability and institutions. In: Foster J (ed.) *Valuing Nature*. London: Routledge, 1997: 75–88.

46. Bickerstaff K, Walker G. Clearing the smog? Public responses to air quality information. *Local Environ* 1999; **4**: 279–84.

47. Hinchcliffe S. 'Helping the Earth Begins at Home': the social construction of socio-environmental responsibilities. *Glob Environ Change* 1996; **6**: 53–62.

48. Szerszynski B, Lash S, Wynne B. Ecology, realism and the social sciences. In: Lash S, Szerszynski B, Wynne B (eds) *Risk, Environment and Modernity: Towards a New Ecology*. London: Sage, 1996: 1–26.

49. Irwin A, Wynne B. Conclusions. In: Irwin A, Wynne B (eds) *Misunderstanding Science? The Public Reconstruction of Science and Technology*. Cambridge: Cambridge University Press, 1996: 213–21.

50. Slovic P. Beyond numbers: a broader perspective on risk perception and risk communication. In: Mayo DG, Hollander RD (eds) *Acceptable Evidence: Science and Values in Risk Management*. Oxford: Oxford University Press, 1991: 48–65.

◆51. Slovic P. Perceptions of risk: reflections on the psychometric paradigm. In: Krimsky S, Golding D (eds) *Social Theories of Risk*. Westport: Praeger, 1992: 117–52.

52. Eden S. Public participation in environmental policy: considering scientific, counter-scientific and non-scientific contributions. *Public Underst Sci* 1996; **5**: 183–204.

53. Yearley S. Making systematic sense of public discontents with expert knowledge: two analytical approaches and a case study. *Public Underst Sci* 2000; **9**: 105–22.

54. Blake J. Overcoming the 'value–action gap' in environmental policy: tensions between national policy and local experience. *Local Environ* 1999; **4**: 259–78.

Environmental law

FRANCIS McMANUS

Although there were laws that related to various forms of environmental pollution before the nineteenth century, it was during that century when the foundations of modern environmental law were laid. The Industrial Revolution forced many of those who were employed in the country to work in factories that were situated in towns. This caused a rapid expansion of industrial towns as a consequence. An unbearable strain was placed on the housing stock. Furthermore, in order to accommodate this rapid influx of population, landlords, many of whom were also employers, either subdivided their houses or erected jerry-built property for the purpose.

The living conditions of the working classes were, in the main, grossly insanitary (for a graphic account of the state of Edinburgh during the first half of the nineteenth century, see reference [1]). It was not uncommon to find more than one family sharing a poorly lit, poorly ventilated room in a house that also lacked a water supply and a water closet. Indeed, the census enumerator's notes on the 1861 Census indicate that 10 Irish people occupied a house that comprised one room situated at 33 Cables Wynd in Leith. In another house situated in Laurie's Close, nine Irish people occupied a one-roomed house. The rapid expansion of industrial towns during the Victorian era resulted not only in high-density housing, but also in new factories being situated in such close proximity to houses that it was inevitable that those who lived in the houses would be affected by the smoke and fumes belching from the factories. Planning controls did not exist to regulate such a problem.

Pollution control was a general problem in urban Britain. Wohl argues that the remarkable growth of industry in the nineteenth century was simply too rapid and widespread to result in anything other than urban pollution.[2] As a general rule, local authorities were reluctant to take formal action against polluters, and the prosecution of offenders was used only as a last resort. The problem of smoke pollution in urban Britain was so great, and the unwillingness of local authorities to take remedial action so pronounced, that smoke suppression societies had been set up by 1843 in such towns as Manchester and Leeds.[3]

Pollution from chemical works was also a major environmental problem. This prompted the passing of the Alkali Etc. Works Regulation Act 1863, which was originally confined to regulating alkali works, the largest chemical industry. The Act also allowed central government to appoint an inspectorate to regulate such works. The Alkali Inspectorate that was appointed under the Act was the first pollution inspectorate in the world.[4] The Act was a success and was amended in due course to allow other chemical processes to be regulated. The number of works and processes over which the inspectors had control rapidly expanded. In 1864, there were 84 alkali works that were registered under the Act. By the end of the century, 1000 works and 1500 processes were registered.[5]

The rapid growth of towns also placed a great strain on public utilities such as water supply and drainage. The water companies or municipal authorities, which were responsible for public water supply, were simply inclined to provide enough water to meet the immediate needs of the area that was served. The result of this so-called 'droplet' method of water supply was a general shortage of water. Edinburgh provides a good example of such a parsimonious approach to water supply. In effect, the Edinburgh Water Company systematically and gradually moved westwards across the Pentlands and appropriated springs there between 1826 and 1863 to meet the immediate needs of the rapidly expanding population of Edinburgh and district. Glasgow was unique as far as the UK was concerned in that it harnessed the water from Loch Katrine in 1859 to, in effect, provide a limitless supply of water. This bore more heavily on the poor, who often had to queue at public wells for their water. The middle classes tended to have cisterns that could therefore store water during the periods when the mains supply was cut off.

As far as municipal drainage was concerned, the outstanding problem was simply the lack of public sewers and drains. This state of affairs prevented the installation of water closets in buildings. Another direct consequence of there being an insufficient number of sewers was the universal practice of using watercourses as sewers to convey both industrial and domestic effluent to the sea. In 1876, the state of Britain's watercourses prompted Parliament to pass the Rivers Pollution Prevention Act, which remained the principal water pollution statute for almost 80 years. However, it took many years for the Act to be implemented.

Victorian society was under constant threat of infectious disease. Diseases such as typhus, typhoid, smallpox, scarlet fever, dysentery and measles were endemic and occurred cyclically. However, cholera was the most feared disease during the nineteenth century.[2] Although we all know now that cholera is carried from person to person by the faeco-oral route, it was widely believed during the first half of the nineteenth century that smell, especially smell from organic material, spread cholera. Those who adhered to this miasmatic theory of transmission of disease were known as miasmatists. The opposing theory for the transmission of disease was the contagion theory. The adherents to this theory believed that disease, including cholera, was spread from person to person by physical contact. However, until germs were discovered by the sterling work of Pasteur, Lister, Koch and their followers, the contagionists lacked credibility in that there were no theoretical foundations to which their beliefs could attach. The contagion theory simply did not work.

Although the miasmatic theory of transmission of disease had its critics, the miasmatists were certainly in the majority. The miasmatic theory reached its zenith in the late 1840s. Therefore, any legislation during this period that was aimed at addressing the cholera threat had, *per force*, to strike at the cause of the disease, that is to say, environmental odours that emanated from waste, excremental and putrefacient material, which were the most common sources of odour. The government therefore passed a series of statutes (namely the Public Health Act 1848 and the Nuisance Removal Acts 1846, 1848, 1849 and 1856) that placed heavy reliance on the concept of nuisance as an instrument of environmental control.

The cholera-based legislation that was passed during the Victorian era reflected not only government policy, but, importantly, also public values about the deleterious effect that the environment could have on human health. Environmental laws that have stood the test of time have largely been driven and shaped by the government's accurate perception of public values concerning various forms of pollution and their harmful effect on human health. Indeed, the Royal Commission on Environmental Pollution has recognized that, when setting environmental standards, decisions must be informed by an understanding of people's values.[6]

On the recommendation of a Sanitary Commission, Parliament passed the Public Health Act in 1875. This Act laid the basis for all subsequent legislation in the field. The Act consolidated over 100 statutes and remained in existence, amended by further Acts in 1907 and 1935, until it was replaced by the Public Health Act 1936.[4]

As far as Scotland was concerned, the most important statute dealing with public health in the Victorian era was undoubtedly the Public Health (Scotland) Act 1897, which was modelled on the English Public Health Act 1875. The 1897 Act made provision for a whole host of matters that impinged on the general environment as well as human health, including the removal of nuisances, offensive trades, unsound food, the provision of hospitals, the prevention of epidemic diseases and the provision of sewers, drains and water supply.[7] However, the most important feature of the 1897 Act was that its provisions were mandatory as opposed to permissive; for example, local authorities were placed under a mandatory duty to remove nuisances, whereas under the Public Health (Scotland) Act 1867, local authorities simply had the power to remove nuisances. Indeed, it was only after the provisions of the 1897 Act became implemented that Scotland really began to catch up with England as far as public health was concerned. However, Scotland was by then a long way behind.[8]

By way of conclusion, by the end of the nineteenth century, the foundations of modern environmental law had been firmly laid. Indeed, there were no fundamental changes in the substantive law or environmental policy until after World War II.[7]

We will now briefly discuss how the law developed.

THE EUROPEAN COMMUNITY

Any discussion of environmental law would be incomplete without a mention of the role of the European Union (EU). As originally enacted, the Treaty of Rome 1957 made no mention of environmental policy. The main catalyst that brought about a fundamental change in philosophy and approach to matters was the 1972 United Nations Conference on the Environment at Stockholm. This conference highlighted the global concern over damage that was being inflicted on the world and its ecosystems. Later in the same year, the European Community Summit meeting in Paris recognized that the continuing encouragement of economic growth would require improvements in the quality of life.

The Commission was therefore directed to formulate the first formal statement on European Community environmental policy. This addressed the overall aim of preventing, or greatly reducing, air pollution. After the general policy had been enunciated, it was deemed appropriate to formulate an action programme for the 4-year period from 1973 to 1976. The First Action Programme laid down the Commission's plans to deal with pollution of the atmosphere, water and land, especially waste management. The programme also dealt with the protection of natural habitats and wildlife.

The First Action Programme was followed by a Second, Third, Fourth, Fifth and Sixth Programme.[9–16] The Fifth Action Programme spanned the period 1993–2000. It placed emphasis on the principle of sustainable development. It favoured less emphasis being placed on prescriptive legislation and more on economic instruments. The Sixth Action Programme covers the period from 2002 to 2012. Combating climate change is given particular emphasis, as is nature and biodiversity, health and the quality of life, the use of natural resources and waste. The Programme also emphasizes the need for existing environmental laws to be better enforced by Member States and for public access to environmental information.

As stated above, the Treaty of Rome did not make special provision for the environment. When the Community later came to develop an environmental policy in the early 1970s, in response to both the obvious damage that was occurring to the environment and also to the public demand for action, the Community had to seek 'creative' solutions to the problem of there being no constitutional basis on which to promulgate environmental laws.[17] This situation was remedied by the Single European Act 1986, by which it was recognized that environmental policy was an established part of the Treaty. As far as environmental matters are concerned, the most important subsequent amendments to the Treaty of Rome were made by the Treaty of Maastricht in 1992 and the Treaty of Amsterdam in 1997. The Treaty (Article 174(2), as amended) sets out the principles on which European environment policy is based. These are:

- the high level of protection principle;
- the precautionary principle;
- the prevention principle;
- the source principle;
- the polluter pays principle.

High level of protection

The Treaty provides that Community policy on the environment is required to aim at a high level of protection over the environment. The principle of a high level of protection has been described as one of the most important substantive principles of European environment policy.[18]

The precautionary principle

The precautionary principle simply means that if a certain activity may have a detrimental effect on the environment but incontrovertible scientific or technical evidence to that effect is lacking, it is, nonetheless, preferable to take the necessary prophylactic action rather than run the risk of harm occurring. Professor Jans cites that a good example of the precautionary principle can be found in Directive 98/81 on the use of genetically modified microorganisms. Article 5(4) of the Directive states that where there is doubt as to the appropriate classification of genetically modified microorganisms, the more stringent protective measures need to be applied unless sufficient evidence, in agreement with the competent authority, justifies the application of less stringent measures.[18]

The prevention principle

Traditionally, UK environmental control legislation has tended to allow regulatory bodies to take remedial action only after an adverse state of affairs has come into existence. For example, the nuisance removal provisions of the Nuisance Removal Acts, the Public Health Acts and currently the Environmental Protection Act 1990 (EPA) simply gave local authorities power to serve abatement notices after the nuisance had come into existence. In contradistinction, the 'prevention principle' is based on the philosophy that prevention is better than cure. One should, therefore, prevent damage occurring in the first place.

The source principle

The source principle requires that environmental damage should be rectified at source. According to this principle, damage to the environment should be addressed at source as opposed to using 'end-of pipe' technology. The source principle also implies a preference for emission standards rather than environmental quality standards.[18] However, Professor Kramer has observed that the source principle simply represents wishful thinking. He argues that if the environmental damage that accrues from cars in the form of air pollution, noise and waste generation were required to be dealt with at source, this would mean that cars would have to be abolished, or perhaps the price of fuel increased to reduce the use of cars.[19]

The polluter pays principle

Under the polluter pays principle, which has been engrained in European Community environmental policy since the 1970s, the polluter should be made to pay for the damage that he inflicts on the environment. For example, a person who runs an activity that pollutes the environment should pay a fee for a permit to run the activity in question and allow it to be effectively regulated.

NOISE POLLUTION

Noise has been a perennial environmental problem in the UK since the Industrial Revolution. The problem of noisy neighbours and neighbourhood noise remains a major social phenomenon and continues to present local authorities with one of their most exacting and demanding challenges.[20] A recent survey that was carried out on behalf of the National Society for Clean Air and Environmental Protection[21] found that, as far as Britain as a whole was concerned, the most common sources of noise disturbance were children (16 per cent), cars/motorbikes (15 per cent) and shouting/arguments (15 per cent).

Generally speaking, noise, unlike certain other forms of pollution, has tended not to be an emotive subject in the eyes of the general public. Individuals tend to take an interest in the subject only if personally affected by noise. In the development of environmental law, noise control is, indeed, the Cinderella.[22] The lowly status accorded to noise is no doubt due to the very nature of the pollutant. Noise is, of course, invisible. Furthermore, it leaves no residue, and therefore has no fall-out factor as is associated with other pollutants.

Noise almost seems to have been tacitly accepted by society as the inevitable consequence of modern life.[23] Of significance is the fact that, as a whole, the public have failed to recognize the important fact that noise is potentially harmful to human health. There was no national legislation that dealt with noise until 1960, when effective pressure group action (in effect, a one-man pressure group, the Noise Abatement Society, in the form of the late John Connell)[24] managed to secure the passing by Parliament of the Noise Abatement Act 1960. Noise pollution can either be dealt with by action under the common law by way of the law of nuisance, or under various statutes that arm local authorities, in the main, with power to deal with various forms of noise pollution.

The most important common law control over noise is the law of nuisance. The law of nuisance was until 1960 the main form of control in relation to noise pollution. It still continues to be invoked by those who are affected by noise, but less frequently because of the advent of a plethora of statutory controls over noise. A wide variety of noise sources have been held to constitute a nuisance at common law. The list includes noise from printworks,[25] building works,[26] singing,[27] cattle,[28] an unruly family,[29] power boats,[30] a military tattoo,[31] religious services (in one case 'loud and strident singing, yelling, frenzied praying, stamping of feet, clapping of hands, groaning etc.'[32]) and fetes.[33] The law of nuisance in terms of noise control is, however, a crude instrument indeed, with the outcome of any particular case being uncertain.

As far as the statutory control of noise is concerned, the most important is the EPA, which places a duty on a local authority to abate statutory nuisances occurring within its area. Essentially, the EPA (Section 80) places a duty on a local authority to serve an abatement notice on the person who is responsible for the nuisance. Subject to certain defences, it is made an offence to fail to comply with the abatement notice. The statutory nuisance removal provisions of the EPA have generated a plethora of complicated case law, with the outcome of a particular case depending on somewhat fine distinctions; much case law has indeed centred on how detailed and specific the abatement notice needs to be in order to be valid.[34]

An attempt to break away from nuisance-based law was made by the Noise Act 1996, which covers England and Wales and Northern Ireland, the Act having been introduced into Parliament as a Private Member's Bill. Essentially, the Noise Act gives local authorities additional powers to deal with night-time noise (defined in Section 2(6) of the Act as the period beginning at 11 pm and ending with the following 7 am).

By way of overview, the Noise Act (Section 3) allows a warning notice to be served on a person who is responsible for noise (or, as Section 3(6) stipulates, the licensee in relation to licensed premises) that exceeds the permitted level, that is to say, a predetermined level that has been set by central government, currently 35 dB(A). It is made an offence for a person on whom a warning notice has been served to exceed the permitted level of noise without reasonable excuse. The Noise Act (Section 4(2)) stipulates that a person guilty of an offence under that section is liable on summary conviction to a fine not exceeding level 3 (currently £1000) on the standard scale (as set by Section 4(3)).

One of the undesirable features of the nuisance removal provisions of the EPA and its predecessors (for example, the nuisance removal provisions contained in the Public Health Acts 1875 and 1936 as far as England and Wales is concerned, and the nuisance removal provisions in the Public Health (Scotland) Act 1897 as far as Scotland is concerned) is the time taken between the nuisance coming into existence and the author of the nuisance being punished by the courts. An important feature of the Noise Act is that it allows fixed penalty notices to be served on the relevant person if the relevant officer has reason to believe that the person either is committing or has just committed an offence (Section 8(1), with the penalty set by Section 8A being £100 unless the local authority has set a different amount).

The EU is becoming more interested in environmental noise in recent years. One of the most important pieces of legislation that the EU has passed is Directive 2002/49/EC, the objective of which is to establish a common EU framework for both the assessment and the management of exposure to environmental noise. Member States are required to prepare noise maps, the purpose of which is to ascertain the extent of noise pollution in the relevant area and then prepare action plans to deal with the problem.

AIR POLLUTION

The London smog disaster of 1952 made clear the fact that air pollution had a pronounced effect on human health, and the Beaver Committee was established in order to investigate the problem. The Committee's report[35] was almost entirely accepted by the government, and the recommendations were incorporated in the Clean Air Act 1956 (now the 1993 Act), which really instituted a completely new regime as far as the control of air pollution was concerned. In summary, the Act makes it an offence to emit dark smoke from a chimney of any building. The Act makes further provision for reducing pollution from furnaces *inter alia* by regulating the capacity of furnaces to produce smoke, grit and dust. Furthermore, chimney heights are regulated in order to ensure that they are of a sufficient height to disperse effluvium.

It was beyond doubt that domestic premises which were heavily dependent on bituminous fuels as a source of heat were partly responsible for the London smog disaster. The status quo was not an option. Something had to be done quickly to remedy the situation. So-called command and control legislation would need to be employed to secure the necessary improvements. It was also equally clear that the requisite legislative measures would have to interfere with individual liberty. The Englishman's castle, replete with its traditional fireplace and chimney, was no longer to be sacrosanct from state intervention.

In the last analysis, the government opted for the concept of smoke control areas. In essence, the 1956 Act (now contained in Part 3 of the Clean Air Act 1993) empowered local authorities to set up such areas. After such an area came into existence, it was an offence, subject to certain defences, for the occupier of premises to emit smoke from the chimney of a building to which the relevant order related, on pain of penalty (under Section 18 of the Clean Air Act 1993, a local authority is given discretion over which classes of building the relevant smoke control order should apply to).

The concept of smoke control areas was embraced with great enthusiasm by local authorities in the UK. The 1960s and 70s witnessed large areas of urban Britain being designated as smoke control areas. Without doubt, the effect of the smoke control area policy had a profound beneficial effect on the external environment.

As far as pollution from industry was concerned, there was prior to 1990 a single medium approach to the regulation of pollution from industry. That is to say, the relevant enforcement authority simply had the statutory power to regulate one form of pollution from industry. For example, the Alkali Inspectorate, and its successors, were solely charged with the responsibility of regulating the impact of the relevant factory on the atmosphere. No account could therefore be taken of the effect of the relevant regulatory controls on the general environment. For example, if the Alkali Inspectorate required a factory owner to install a grit arrestment plant in order to reduce the amount of effluvium from the premises, the upshot of which was that the effluent from the plant was stored in settling tanks that discharged into a nearby stream, the regulation of that discharge would fall to another enforcing authority in terms of a completely separate legal regime.

A fundamental change to air pollution control in the UK came in the form of the EPA, which adopted a more holistic approach to the regulation of pollution. The Act introduces the concept of integrated pollution control. It was the intention of the Act to make industries that posed a substantial threat to the environment in general to be subject to integrated pollution control and also to be subject to central government control, and industries that simply possessed the capacity to pollute the air to be subject to local authority pollution control.

The EPA gives central government the power to make regulations that specify the nature of processes which fall to be regulated under the Act. The Environmental Protection (Prescribed Processes and Substances) Regulations 1991 designate a variety of processes that require to be authorized for the purposes of the Act. The regulations divide the various processes into two categories, namely Part A and Part B processes. Part A processes are processes that are subject to integrated pollution control. Part B processes are subject to local air pollution control. As at December 2008 in England, Part A processes are subject to regulation by the Environment Agency, whereas Part B processes are regulated by local authorities. However, in Scotland both Part A and Part B processes are regulated by the Scottish Environment Protection Agency (SEPA). Essentially, it is made an offence, *inter alia*, for anyone to carry on a prescribed process unless that process has been authorized by the relevant enforcing authority and also that the process is conducted in accordance with the conditions that the relevant enforcing authority has seen fit to impose (Section 23).

The regime under the EPA will be phased out by that under the Pollution Prevention and Control Act 1999, which introduces the concept of integrated pollution prevention and control. The Act has been 'fleshed out' by detailed regulations (the Pollution Prevention and Control (England and Wales) Regulations 2000 for England and Wales, and the Pollution Prevention and Control (Scotland) Regulations 2000 for Scotland).

The purpose of the Act is to implement EC Directive 96/61, which takes a more holistic approach to protecting the environment from emissions from industrial activities. For example, the Directive requires Member States, in granting the requisite permit, to consider not only emissions, but also waste minimization, noise and vibration, and the conservation of resources. The Directive requires Member States to ensure that, in operating installations, preventive measures are taken against pollution through the use of 'best available techniques', which is similar to the concept of best available techniques not entailing excessive cost in the EPA regime. The concept of best available techniques has been described as being at the heart of the integrated pollution prevention and control system.[36] Important changes in the new regime include the regulation of activities from installations rather than processes. The definition of an installation is wider than that for a process under the EPA regime.

As far as general air quality is concerned, Part IV of the Environment Act 1995 places a duty on central government to prepare an air quality strategy for Great Britain. The strategy was produced in 1997 but has been revised and updated over the years, the most recent version being published in 2007.[37] The strategy sets out a framework of standards and objectives relating to the pollutants of most concern (10 'priority pollutants', namely, ammonia, sulphur dioxide, particulate matter (PM_{10}), nitrogen dioxide, carbon monoxide, lead, benzene, 3-butadiene, tropospheric ozone and polycyclic aromatic hydrocarbons being identified), with the aim of reducing air pollution problems throughout the year.

The Act (Section 82) imposes a duty on local authorities to cause a review to be conducted of the quality of the air within the local authority's area in order to ascertain whether the air quality standards and objectives that are contained in the strategy are being, or will be, achieved within a given period (the relevant period being set by the Air Quality (England) Regulations 2000, as amended). If it appears that the air quality standards and objectives are not being achieved, or are not likely to be achieved, within the relevant period, the local authority is required, under the Environment Act 1995 (Sections 83 and 84) to designate the area an air quality management area and prepare an appropriate action plan in order to remedy the situation.

The EU has been active in the field of ambient air quality. In 1996, a Framework Directive (96/62/EC) on air quality assessment and management was agreed, which identifies a number of atmospheric pollutants. The Directive will be 'fleshed out' as it were by Daughter Directives that will set appropriate target and limit values (e.g. Directive 99/30/EC, which relates to limit values for sulphur dioxide, nitrogen dioxide and other oxides of nitrogen, particulate matter and lead). The Directives are transposed and implemented in the UK by regulations such as the Air Quality Standards Regulations 2007 and the Air Quality Standards (Scotland) Regulations 2007.

Finally, no discussion on the subject of air pollution would be complete without mention of climate change. Both the UK government and the Scottish Executive are committed to reducing the emissions of Kyoto Protocol greenhouse gases. The Climate Change Act 2008 sets up a framework for the UK to achieve its long-term goal of reducing carbon dioxide emissions. The main thrust of the Act is to set emissions reduction targets and a system of carbon budgeting, that is, the total amount of carbon emissions that are allowed in a given period. The Act also makes provision for the creation of an independent advisory body, the Committee on Climate Change, to advise the government and devolved administrations on how to reduce carbon emissions. In addition, the Scottish Parliament has recently passed the Climate Change (Scotland) Act 2009.

WASTE AND CONTAMINATED LAND

Waste

Until 1974, the law relating to the control of waste on land was mainly, but not exclusively, based on the provisions of public health legislation (the Public Health Act 1875, which was repealed by the Public Health Act 1936, and the Public Health (Scotland) Act, which was repealed in 2009 by the Public Health etc. (Scotland) Act 2008), which essentially made it a criminal offence for anyone to unlawfully dump waste on land, and also armed local authorities with the power to remove such waste. In addition, the legislation placed a legal responsibility on local authorities to collect and dispose of municipal waste.

The Control of Pollution Act 1974 radically reformed the legal regime relating to waste. One of the most important changes brought about by the Act was the provision that one needed a licence from the relevant enforcement authority in order to lawfully dispose of waste in the UK. The Act originally placed a duty on local authorities to issue licences, but the responsibility for issuing disposal licences was then transferred to the Environment Agency and, for Scotland, the SEPA. In addition, planning permission to develop land in order to accommodate a landfill site has also been required since 1947 with the passing of the Town and County Planning Act of that year.

However, the waste management regime that was introduced by the Control of Pollution Act 1974 was relatively short-lived, and Part II of the EPA introduced important changes to the licensing system pertaining to the waste management licensing system (much of the substantive law relating to waste management licensing being contained in the Waste Management Licensing Regulations 1994, as amended) and the local framework for waste regulation and disposal.[38] Perhaps one of the most innovative provisions of EPA was the introduction of the concept of the duty of care in relation to individuals who import, produce, carry, keep, treat or otherwise dispose of controlled waste (Section 34). The intention of EPA is to place a statutory responsibility on all those who deal with controlled waste from its very creation to its ultimate disposal to prevent environmental harm accruing from the waste.

One of the most controversial and indeed most litigated topics concerning the subject of waste is the fundamental question: 'What is waste?' The original definition of waste as contained in the EPA and the Waste Management Regulations 1994 has been amended in order to take account of EC Directives (75/442/EEC and 91/156/EEC, replaced by a new codified version in the form of Directive 2006/12/EC). The practical effect of such a change has made this area of the law highly complicated and in urgent need of reform. Indeed, the concept of waste has proved to be particularly difficult to define with any certainty.[36]

There are additional controls in relation to forms of waste that present a greater threat to the environment and/or human health. The Hazardous Waste (England and Wales) Regulations 2005 regulate the management of particularly hazardous waste and impose additional controls to those which exist under the EPA. Separate controls exist for Scotland (see the Special Waste Regulations 1996, as amended).

Contaminated land

Contaminated land may arise from a number of activities. One category comprises the intentional deposit of material on land. Examples of this are landfill sites, tips, lagoons for industrial effluent, deposits of dredgings, 'made ground' and filled dock basins, as well as the deposit of sewage sludge or other materials on agricultural land. Another category is contamination arising incidentally in the course of an industrial activity, including spillages and leaks of materials from storage tanks and drums, escapes of materials such as dust and liquids in the course of the activity itself, and contamination resulting from the deposition of airborne particulate matter.[39]

There are a number of Acts and regulations that make provision for contaminated land. However, the most important regime that deals with contaminated land is found in Part IIA of the EPA, which was introduced by the Environment Act 1995. The EPA is supplemented by detailed regulations (the Contaminated Land (England) Regulations 2006 and the Contaminated Land (Scotland) Regulations 2000, as amended). The expression 'contaminated land' is defined in Section 78A(2) of the EPA as any land that appears to the local authority in whose area it is situated to be in such a condition by reason of substances in, on or under the land that:

- significant harm is being caused or there is a significant possibility of such harm being caused;
- pollution of the water environment is being or is likely to be caused.

In determining whether land appears to be contaminated, regard should be paid to guidance which is issued by central government.[40–42]

The main responsibility for implementing the legislation rests with local authorities. However, both the Environment Agency and SEPA have responsibility for land ('special sites') that pose particularly difficult problems.

WATER

The law relating to water in the UK has been heavily influenced by European Community water law that is now approximately 30 years old.[16] Indeed, water law represents an area of environmental law in which the EU has been particularly active. The most important Directive to date on the subject of water pollution is the Water Framework Directive (2000/60/EC). This Directive, which is aimed at the regulation of both inland water use and quality, consolidates earlier piecemeal legislation, entered into force on December 22nd, 2000 and had to be implemented by Member States by December 2003. The purpose of the Directive is to protect all surface freshwater, estuaries, coastal waters and groundwater. The Directive requires that a list of priority substances with harmful effects on water should be drawn up at European Community level and action taken to reduce the discharge of these substances (Article 16).

In November 2001, the Council of Environment Ministers formally adopted Decision 2455/2001/EC, which entered into force on December 16th, 2001 and established the list of priority substances in the field of water policy. Substances are classified as Priority Hazardous Substances, Priority Substances under Review and Priority Substances. Releases of those which are classified as Priority Hazardous Substances must be either ceased or phased out by 2020.

In England and Wales, the Water Framework Directive is being implemented by the Water Environment (Water Framework Directive) (England and Wales) Regulations 2003. In Scotland, the Water Environment and Water Services (Scotland) Act 2003 provides the framework for implementing the EU Water Framework Directive.

As far as the regulation of water-polluting activities is concerned, the Water Resources Act 1991 is the principal statute that governs both water quality and quantity in England and Wales. No one may discharge polluting substances to water without holding a discharge consent, which is granted by the Environment Agency, the majority of consents being given for sewage effluent. A separate regulatory system applies in Scotland. Under the Water Environment (Controlled Activities) (Scotland) Regulations 2005, it is an offence to carry out controlled activities without an appropriate authorization.

REFERENCES

1. Bird IL. *Notes on Old Edinburgh*. Edinburgh: Edmonston & Douglas, 1869.
2. Wohl A. *Endangered Lives*. London: Dent, 1983.
3. Sandwith H. Defective arrangements in large towns. *British and Foreign Medical Review* 1943: 22.
4. Burnett-Hall R. *Environmental Law*. London: Sweet & Maxwell, 1995.
5. Clapp B. *An Environmental History of Britain*. London: Longman, 1994.
6. Royal Commission on Environmental Pollution. *Setting Environmental Standards*, 21st Report. Cm 4053. London: RCEP, 1998.

7. McManus F (ed.). *Environmental Law in Scotland*. Edinburgh: Thomson/Green, 2007.

8. Best G. Another part of the island – some Scottish perspectives. In: Dyos HJ, Wolff M (eds) *The Victorian City*. London: Routledge & Kegan Paul, 1970: 394.

9. First Action Programme on the Environment [1973] OJ C1112/1.

10. Second Action Programme on the Environment (1977–1981) [1977] OJ C139.

11. Third Action Programme on the Environment (1982–1986) [1983] OJ C46.

12. Fourth Action Programme on the Environment (1987–1992) [1987] OJ C328.

13. Fifth Action Programme on the Environment (1993) [1993] OJ C138/1.

14. Sixth Action Programme on the Environment [2002] OJ L242/1.

15. Bell S, McGillivray D. *Environmental Law*, 6th edn. Oxford: Oxford University Press, 2006.

16. Thornton J, Beckwith S. *Environmental Law*, 2nd edn. London: Thomson/Sweet & Maxwell, 2004.

17. McManus F, Burns T. The impact of EC law on noise law. In: Holder J (ed.) *Impact of EC Environmental Law in the UK*. Chichester: Wiley, 1997.

18. Jans J. *European Environmental Law*. Groningen: Europa Law Publishing, 2000.

19. Kramer L. *EC Environmental Law*, 4th edn. London: Sweet & Maxwell, 2000.

20. Scottish Executive Environment Group. *Draft Noise Management Guide*. Paper 2005/24. Edinburgh: Scottish Executive, 20058.

21. National Society for Clean Air and Environmental Protection. National Noise Survey, May 22, 2006. Brighton: NSCA (now Environmental Protection UK).

22. Adams M, McManus F. *Noise and Noise Law*. London: Wiley, 1994.

23. *AG v Hastings Corp.* (1950) 94 Sol. Jo. 225 at 225.

24. http://www.noiseabatement.org.uk (accessed November, 2009).

25. *Rushmer v Polsue and Alfieri* [1906] 1 Ch. 234.

26. *Andreae v Selfridge and Co.Ltd* [1938] Ch. 1

27. *Motion v Mills* (1897) 13 TLR 427.

28. *London, Brighton and South Coast Railway v Truman* (1886) 11 App. Cas. 45.

29. *Smith v Scott* [1973] Ch. 314.

30. *Kennaway v Thompson* [1981] QB 88.

31. *Webster v Lord Advocate* 1984 SLT 13.

32. *Prinsloo v Shaw* [1938] AD 570.

33. *Walker v Brewster* (1867) 17 LT(NS) 135.

34. *Budd v Colchester BC*, The Times, April 14th, 1999.

35. *Report of the Committee on Air Pollution*, Cmd 9322, London: HMSO, 1954.

36. Bell S, McGillivray D. *Environmental Law*, 7th edn. Oxford: Oxford University Press, 2008

37. *The Air Quality Strategy for England, Wales and Northern Ireland*. Cmnd 7169 Norwich: TSO, 2007.

38. Tromans S, Poustie M. *Environmental Protection Legislation*, 4th edn. London: Thomson/Sweet & Maxwell, 2003.

39. Tromans S, Turrall-Clarke R. *Contaminated Land*. London: Thomson/Sweet & Maxwell, 2008.

40. Department of the Environment, Transport and the Regions. Circular 1/2006. Norwich: TSO, 2006.

41. Scottish Executive. *Environment Protection Act 1990: Part IIA Contaminated Land*. Circular 1/2000. Edinburgh: Scottish Executive, 2000.

42. National Assembly for Wales. *Remediation of Contaminated Land. National Assembly for Wales Guidance to Enforcing Authorities under Part IIA of the Environmental Protection Act 1990*. Cardiff: National Assembly for Wales, 2001.

Policy development

MARTIN WILLIAMS

This chapter illustrates policy development in environmental health using policy responses to air quality problems as an example. It is arguable that air quality policies and their scientific underpinning are probably among the most well developed and mature in the environmental field. The understanding of air pollution sources and their atmospheric processing is relatively well developed (although much still remains to be done), so that the exposure consequences of different policy options can be assessed quantitatively. Moreover, considerable advances have been made in the understanding of the health impacts of air pollutants, so that it is also often possible to quantify, and even place a monetary value on, the health outcomes of different policy options. This has allowed fairly comprehensive analyses of costs and benefits to be carried out, so that policies on air pollution can be based on a comprehensive evidence base.

This is, however, not always the case in other areas of environmental policy, and indeed, even in the air pollution field, the quantitative assessment of policies dealing with ecosystem effects is often less easy to quantify in terms of exposure, response and outcomes than are those directed at health effects. In this sense, the assessment of air pollution policies directed at improving public health is probably one of the best characterized areas of environmental policy assessment and provides a good example for this chapter.

This chapter illustrates the development of policies in the air quality area, and draws very heavily on experience in the UK and more recently in the European Union (EU). Nonetheless the principles underpinning the historical development of policy are common to many countries, but more recently developments have taken place in the EU that could point the way forward for improvements in air quality policy and public health.

Urban air quality in the UK and in most other areas in the developed world has improved significantly in the past 50 years. The policy responses have also changed profoundly during this period in many respects, and indeed are still developing, but over the past decades they have changed in one fundamentally important way. Prior to, and including, the 1956 Clean Air Act, pollution control in the UK had since the late nineteenth century been concerned with *emissions* at source and was predominantly focused on industrial sources. Even though the 1952 smog arose from widespread diffuse sources, there was no mention in the 1956 Act of air concentrations, standards or guidelines, nor was there any explicit recognition in policy instruments of any concept of exposure to people or the environment. Contrast this with the present day, where the emphasis of policy has shifted almost completely to air *quality* targets of one form or another, with legislation on emissions forming the means of *implementation* and the achievement of the agreed environmental quality.

Along the way, there have been many reasons for this change and many associated developments in policy. Not least among these have been the rise in importance of the EU and other international fora, and the much wider availability of information and data as well as the involvement of a much larger constituency of 'stakeholders' on both sides of the environmental debate, in business and in the environmental organizations. This chapter – which cannot be comprehensive in the space available – seeks to draw out the main events in the evolution of policy responses to improving urban air quality with examples drawn chiefly from the UK. The discussion will not simply concern itself with the policy instruments themselves, but will also address the significant steps taken to formulate the evidence, from atmospheric science, from epidemiology and toxicology, and from economics, which has informed and underpinned the policy developments over the past 50 years or so.

POLICY AND THE EVIDENCE BASE AFTER THE SMOG EPISODES OF 1952 AND 1962

The Clean Air Act of 1956 had several important elements. First, it relied on the devolution of action to local authorities, who were empowered to designate Smoke Control Areas requiring the use of authorized solid fuels or authorized appliances in homes. The authorization was – and still is – based on emission limits set nationally, such as to prohibit the emission of smoke at the levels of uncontrolled burning before the Act. The major cities of the UK became virtually completely smoke-controlled, and emissions of smoke and sulphur dioxide decreased significantly.

However, progress was not fast enough to prevent the smog episode of December 1962 from occurring when weather conditions similar to those in the 1952 episode prevailed, even though domestic coal consumption in London was half what it had been in 1952. Emissions decreased very quickly after that however, and by 1991, when similar meteorological conditions occurred in London in December, mean black smoke levels in London had dropped by almost 90 per cent of the 1962 levels. The effects of the 1991 air pollution episode were much less than those of the smog of 1952. In 1952, mortality rates in London, calculated over a 2-week period, rose by 230 per cent; the increase reported for 1991 was 10 per cent.

On its own, the Clean Air Act would not have led to as large a decrease in urban emissions of sulphur dioxide as occurred. The main solid fuel replacement for coal, so-called smokeless fuel, had a sulphur content not much lower than UK coal, even though most of the volatiles that formed black smoke on combustion had been removed. The other factor that occurred at around the same time was the move away from the use of solid fuel to the use of gas, or even electricity, to heat premises. Both resulted in significant reductions in smoke and sulphur dioxide concentrations in urban areas, although in the case of electric heating, the emissions were generated in power stations, most of which had been moved from city centres to rural areas. These large extra-urban power plants with tall stacks helped to reduce urban concentrations considerably, although before abatement technology was installed to reduce emissions, they contributed to problems via 'acid rain' in more remote areas, not just in Scandinavia, but also in the UK.

During this period, there was a large amount of activity on the scientific front. The National Survey of Air Pollution was set up in the early 1960s (with data still available on the Defra archive at www.airquality.co.uk from around 1962), with measurements of black smoke and sulphur dioxide being made by local authorities. This network used the simple smoke stain/bubbler method (which actually measured total acidity rather than specifically sulphur dioxide) and until the 1980s included over 1000 monitoring sites. In the 1960s, the Medical Research Council established the Air Pollution Unit to undertake research into the effects of air pollutants on health, and this unit established the first epidemiological and toxicological studies linking health effects with air pollution concentrations. This science base of air pollution concentrations covering the whole of the UK, and knowledge of their effects on health, represented the most important information resource on the effects of smoke and sulphur dioxide in Europe and probably the world.

This, however, proved to be a two-edged sword: as the 1970s drew to a close, the control of coal emissions was clearly being successful, and this was considered to have largely solved the problem of the health effects of urban air pollution. The Air Pollution Unit of the Medical Research Council was closed in 1978. In the USA, the US Clean Air Act was promulgated in 1970, and this set standards for other pollutants, mostly related to motor vehicle emissions, such as carbon monoxide, lead, oxides of nitrogen and ozone, as well as for sulphur dioxide and particles. In the mid 1970s, policy-makers in the UK also began to recognize the growing importance of pollution from motor vehicles, and monitoring stations were set up to measure traffic-related pollutants in a small number of locations. These used the newly emerging automatic monitoring techniques to record hourly data and also addressed lead, carbon monoxide, oxides of nitrogen and ozone. At this time, however, there was no further policy activity; no health effects studies were being carried out on vehicle-related pollutants, and there was no particular incentive to produce air quality management legislation to cover the 'newer' pollutants.

Indeed, attention was diverted from urban air pollution in the late 1970s and early 1980s by the recognition of the problems of acid rain and the effects on more rural and remote ecosystems. A considerable amount of policy-making resource was devoted to solving these problems. This is not the place to discuss the detailed history of that problem, but suffice it to say that international scale issues of long-range transboundary air pollution (LRTAP) dominated policy for most of the 1980s. The early Scandinavian work in the Organisation for Economic Cooperation and Development (OECD) was taken up by the UN Economic Commission for Europe leading to the signing of the Convention on LRTAP in 1979. There followed a series of Protocols initially addressing the acid rain issue but subsequently dealing with ozone and its precursors, and more recently heavy metals and persistent organic pollutants.

One outcome of this process with benefits for urban air quality was the fact that this development was instrumental in opening up information on emissions and air quality across Europe. To today's audience, where even the most detailed data are freely available, this may not sound a major achievement, but at the time of the negotiation of the Convention, even national emission totals were in some countries considered to be extremely sensitive and were treated almost as state secrets.

Notwithstanding the acid rain issue, the policy process in the European Community was during the late 1970s and early 80s beginning to formulate legislation based on health-related problems of air pollution. From this point onwards, the air quality policy-making process in Europe has been dominated by the production of legislation within the EU, and to some extent the United Nations Economic Commission for Europe, rather than nationally. Moreover, there has also been a considerable amount of cooperative activity to develop the atmospheric science base, the health effects and the economics underpinning these policy developments. It has been a long and often difficult process, and continues to be a challenge, as the Member States have had to adapt to the principles of collective decision-making in these international fora.

During the 1980s, a major initiative took place within the European Regional Office of the World Health Organization, culminating in 1987 with the publication of the World Health Organization Air Quality Guidelines for Europe.[1] This addressed the effects on human health from 28 air pollutants and recommended guideline concentrations for averaging times of relevance to the effect in question. From a policy perspective, it is very important to be clear about the nature of these guidelines. It would first help to distinguish between *risk assessment* and *risk management*.

In dealing with air quality problems, and many others, the process can be simplified to one where the risk from a particular pollutant is assessed. For an air pollutant, if sufficient health effect and air concentration information is available, this might take the form of an assessment of the total burden of a given health outcome over a country. This result is determined purely by science and does not include any consideration of how much pollution could or should be reduced. The management of this risk is the phase where these latter issues are decided and other factors come into play, such as the technical feasibility of reducing emissions, the costs, assigning a monetary value to the health effects and, in some regions, even whether this could be an ethical or moral issue. The policy-maker, and ultimately society as a whole, has to balance all these factors in managing the risk in terms of proportionate actions. Depending on the balance of the stringency of control measures, or costs, it is possible that the risk may not be completely eliminated, and society de facto accepts some residual adverse health effects.

The World Health Organization guidelines form part of the *risk assessment* process. They were formulated to indicate concentrations and averaging times that would not lead to adverse health effects from the pollutant concerned. They are thus different in nature from legally enforceable air quality standards or limit values, the agreement on which has to balance the costs and the risks

in formulating acceptable policy solutions. The guidelines, however, have been extremely influential in the European policy process as they have generally formed the starting point for negotiations on limit values for air pollutants in European legislation.

The activity in the EU resulted in the first air quality Directive being agreed in 1980, which dealt with particulate matter ('smoke') and sulphur dioxide. The limit values were based on the health effect work done in the UK at the Medical Research Council unit mentioned above. This Directive was followed by others dealing with lead and nitrogen dioxide. The evidence base for adverse effects from these pollutants was mixed. There was a considerable amount of epidemiological and toxicological work carried out on lead, and the issue generated much controversy. There was little need for very subtle science in analysing the causes and effects of the 1952 smog, but the lead debate in the 1970s was the first time that relatively sophisticated medical science and statistics had played a role in influencing public attitudes to air pollution and in influencing policy.

The Directive on nitrogen dioxide agreed in 1985 represented a milestone in air quality policy in the EU as it was the first to recognize explicitly (albeit in an Annex) the concept that limit values should apply only in locations where people were likely to be exposed over time periods over which adverse effects might occur. At the time of these Directives, there was much debate on this issue. The rationale for this 'exposure' criterion was to prevent breaches of the limit values alleged at locations that were clearly nonsensical in terms of public exposure, such as the central area between two carriageways of a major road, but which would be legally within the scope of the Directive if no such exposure criterion were invoked.

THE DEVELOPMENT OF STRATEGIES IN THE UK AND EUROPE

One of the main motivating forces behind the resurgence of interest in urban air quality during this period, in the late 1980s and early 90s, was that major advances in the elucidation of the adverse health effects of urban air pollution were being made. These advances arose chiefly from the epidemiological studies of Schwartz, Dockery and co-workers in the USA, who showed, in a series of influential papers, that levels of particulate matter that would previously have been considered harmless were in fact associated not only with ill-health but with mortality. These studies employed sensitive and sophisticated statistical techniques and were initially greeted with scepticism in some quarters. However, further studies by other groups and intensive reanalysis and scrutiny by independent researchers, notably the Health Effects Institute in the USA, have led to these studies being accepted and their findings used to inform policy development in the USA, the EU and elsewhere.

This strategic thinking led to the UK Environment Act of 1995, which among other things required the government to publish an Air Quality Strategy, which appeared in 1997.[2] Space does not permit an adequate appraisal of the immense amount of scientific and medical research and assessments that have underpinned the UK Air Quality Strategy and its successors. There have been a series of definitive synthesis reports from expert groups in both the environment and health departments. Reports produced by the Photochemical Oxidants Review Group, the Quality of Urban Air Review Group, the Airborne Particles Expert Group and the Air Quality Expert Group, as well as the series of reports from the Department of Health Committee on the Medical Effects of Air Pollutants (COMEAP) and its forerunner the group on the Medical Aspects of Air Pollution Episodes, in addition to the joint Department of the Environment/Department of Health Expert Panel on Air Quality Standards (EPAQS), have been immensely influential in the wider European and international arenas as well as in the UK, and have been highly regarded by both scientists and policy-makers.[3,4]

The reports of these groups provided an extremely useful steer to the policy-making process and, coupled with the advice from the EPAQS panel and the production of the major Air Quality Strategy, provided a degree of leadership in Europe that was subsequently built upon by the European Commission as discussed below. The other significant report from the COMEAP group was published in 1998 and quantified premature mortality and other health outcomes associated with exposure to air pollutants in Great Britain.[5] The report concluded that the premature deaths associated with levels of particles less than 10 μm in diameter were 8100, with sulphur dioxide at 3500 and ozone at 700–12 500 depending on whether or not one assumes a threshold for no adverse effects (in the COMEAP calculations, assuming a threshold of 50 parts per billion hourly average led to the lower estimate of mortality). This result was also extremely valuable in informing policy development.

In the UK, the Air Quality Strategy was revised and updated, and published in 2007. The revision analysed a series of potential measures to improve air quality, and it included an extremely comprehensive evidence base covering atmospheric modelling and projections, and a detailed economic analysis of the costs and benefits of the possible measures.[6]

Meanwhile, the EU was similarly formulating a more strategic approach to air quality policy through the so-called Air Quality Framework Directive (96/62/EC), which was agreed in 1996. This paved the way for 'daughter Directives' the first of which (99/30/EC) dealt with particles, sulphur dioxide, lead and nitrogen dioxide and was agreed during a UK presidency of the EU and adopted in 1999. Subsequent Directives have dealt with carbon monoxide and benzene (2000/69/EC), and with ozone (2002/3/EC). The latter Directive on ozone does not contain mandatory limit values like the other Directives,

reflecting the transboundary nature of ozone and the fact that a Member State would not necessarily have complete control over the sources of the ozone levels that were measured within its territory. The fourth in the series covered arsenic, nickel, cadmium, mercury and polynuclear aromatic hydrocarbons and, like the ozone Directive, did not set mandatory limit values but incorporated target values for the pollutants concerned.

The European Commission consolidated this earlier work in a Thematic Strategy on Air Pollution under the Sixth Environmental Action Programme, which was adopted on September 21st, 2005.[7] The objectives of the Thematic Strategy are achieving 'levels of air quality that do not give rise to significant negative impacts on, and risks to human health and the environment'. For the natural environment, this means no exceeding of critical loads and levels.

The most recent development in Europe has been the agreement of a revised Air Quality Directive that brought together for revision the first three 'daughter Directives'. The new Directive (2008/50/EC), which was published in May 2008, incorporated some significant developments including the concept of 'exposure reduction' as a new advance in air quality management, foreshadowed in the UK Air Quality Strategy. This is discussed in detail below.

POLICY INSTRUMENTS THAT REDUCE EMISSIONS

Among the many policies and regulations on air quality that have been promulgated over the past decades, it is worth distinguishing the more important among them which have required reductions in emissions as opposed to setting standards or strategic frameworks.

Other than the 1956 Clean Air Act, the one series of instruments that has in the UK led to the most important improvement in overall public exposure to harmful air pollutants has been the European regulations on motor vehicle emissions. The first EU Directive dated from 1970 (70/220/EEC) and applied to light-duty vehicles. This and subsequent amendments set a cap on emission performance rather than forced large reductions, and it was not until the amendment embodied in Directive (88/76/EEC) – the so-called 'Luxembourg Agreement' – that significant reductions were set in train. This Directive effectively mandated the use of three-way catalysts (so called because they reduced levels of all three regulated pollutants: carbon monoxide, hydrocarbons or volatile organic compounds, and oxides of nitrogen). A fully functioning catalyst was able to reduce emissions by more than 90 per cent compared with an uncontrolled vehicle. A parallel measure for heavy-duty vehicles was agreed in 1988 in Directive 88/77/EC.

A subsequent series of Directives limiting vehicle emissions, covering light- and heavy-duty vehicles, and extending to particles as well as gaseous emissions, has since been agreed, and successive standards have become known as the 'Euro X' standards. The 'Luxembourg Agreement' 88/76/EEC is designated Euro 1, and subsequent improvements are now up to Euro 5 and 6, Euro 5 having come into force in September 2009. The parallel series of heavy-duty standards are designated with Roman numerals; the most recent level in force is Euro V, which came into force (Directive 2005/55/EC) in October 2008. This set of regulations, beginning with the 1987 and 1988 Directives, has had the single most important influence on urban air quality in the UK and the rest of Europe in the past two decades.

Airborne lead concentrations are now extremely low because of the removal of lead from petrol – a prerequisite for the use of catalytic converters. Initially, however, the lead content of petrol was reduced because of concern over its toxic properties. At the end of 1985, the maximum permitted lead content of petrol was reduced from 0.4 to 0.15 g/L, and the airborne lead levels throughout the UK (and EC Europe) more than halved in a matter of weeks. This still probably represents the most abrupt improvement in measured air quality in present times in the UK. Levels reduced to almost zero over a longer period as lead was gradually removed from petrol.

Another prerequisite for the improvements in catalyst performance required by successive Euro standards is low sulphur fuel, and Directive 98/70 as amended by Directive 2003/17/EC contains the environmental fuel quality specifications for petrol and diesel fuels in the European Community with the main focus on sulphur, and for petrol on lead and aromatics. Since January 1st, 2005 the limit on the sulphur content of petrol and diesel is 50 parts per million, and Member States were required to start phasing in ultra-low sulphur fuel with a maximum 10 parts per million sulphur content. Since January 1st, 2002, all petrol sold in the EU has been unleaded.

Industrial emissions have also been regulated through a series of significant developments in legislation, drawing on a history of over a hundred years. Recent developments have seen the integration of controls on emissions to air with those to other media in the system of Integrated Pollution Control in the Environmental Protection Act of 1990. This extended and improved the concept of 'best practicable means', which had served industrial pollution control in the UK for over 100 years, and introduced the concept of 'best available techniques'. More recently, the system has developed to incorporate the EC Directive on Integrated Pollution Prevention and Control (96/61/EC).

An evaluation of the air pollution reduction policies was carried out on behalf of Department for Environment, Food and Rural Affairs in 2004.[8] Space does not permit an exhaustive discussion of this work, but some conclusions are of interest. Between the years 1990 and 2001, the study estimated that reductions in sulphur dioxide, nitrogen oxides and particles with a diameter less than 10 μm from road transport were respectively 96 per cent, 36 per cent and 48 per cent compared with the 'no policies' values, and

those from the electricity supply industry (ESI) were 77 per cent, 58 per cent and 78 per cent respectively. It was further anticipated that, by 2010, the corresponding reductions from road transport would be 96 per cent, 69 per cent and 76 per cent, and those from the ESI 93 per cent, 69 per cent and 93 per cent, respectively. The study concluded that all of the road transport reductions were attributable to air quality policies, but that between approximately 35 per cent and 100 per cent of the ESI reductions could be the result of air quality policies.

FUTURE DEVELOPMENTS IN AIR QUALITY MANAGEMENT POLICIES

New directions in air quality management systems

Recent experience in the UK has suggested that an air quality management system based *solely* on objectives, limits or standards expressed as a target concentration to be met in all locations, might be inefficient in terms of improving public health. As emission reduction policies bite and areas in excess of a legal limit become smaller, it will generally become necessary to impose increasingly costly measures to achieve full compliance. The problem is that the legal framework based on a single mandatory standard requires precisely this. This inefficiency requires a new approach to air quality management, outlined below.

For pollutants with (at the level of current knowledge) no threshold of effect at the population level, such as particulate matter, it will generally be more beneficial for overall public health to reduce concentrations across the whole of an urban area, even where they already meet existing legal limits, than to 'chase hotspots'. The fundamental problem, however, is that legal frameworks based on ambient concentration standards require complete compliance, and therefore exert pressures in the wrong direction from what would be required to optimize abatement strategies in terms of improving public health.

The one important benefit of ambient standards or limit values is that compliance ensures a common standard of air quality for all citizens, and this should not be discarded lightly. However, the problems with attaining the limits have been set out above, and if limits or standards were to be retained, another criterion would be needed to optimize the system to direct attention to improving public health in some optimal way. Work in the UK has been directed towards the concept of a target for policy framed in terms of reducing 'population exposure' to ambient levels of a pollutant such as particulate matter, and expressed as a target to reduce concentrations *averaged over a whole urban area or region*, by some given percentage over a defined period. This is illustrated in Figure 62.1, showing how the idea is to shift the whole distribution of the exposed population to lower concentrations, rather than simply to remove the small area above the standard or limit value in the 'old' system of air quality management. As noted above, this 'exposure reduction' approach illustrated in Figure 62.1 is appropriate only for pollutants with no threshold of adverse effects and a linear dose–response relationship that goes through the origin. The public health improvement from reducing area B in Figure 62.1 will in general then be greater than that from reducing area A.

One could therefore conceive of a system of air quality management that encompasses the two targets: an overall limit on ambient levels to ensure some basic quality of air that all citizens could experience, embodying the 'environmental justice' concept, and an additional commitment to reduce ambient levels by a given amount even in areas where the ambient limit might already be achieved. To improve the public health gains to be obtained from this new system, it is the latter 'exposure' criterion which should be the driver for policies, not the 'cap' or limit value, or else the inefficient status quo will be unchanged. The extent of this 'exposure' reduction could be determined by the balance of costs and benefits.

The practicability of such a system would depend crucially on the balance of stringency between the two commitments. To work most efficiently, the limit or standard would ideally be set at a level somewhat less stringent than might otherwise have been the case had the limit been the only driving factor in air quality improvement. This could clearly cause some initial difficulties in adding on an exposure-reduction target to an existing standard or limit value. However, if one is starting from scratch, as the EU was with legislation on particles with a diameter less than 2.5 µm ($PM_{2.5}$), the system is workable, and this concept was embodied in the revision of EU legislation resulting in the Air Quality Directive 2008/50/EC published in May 2008.

In principle, there are issues surrounding the precise metric for the exposure reduction target – should it be in terms of measured concentrations, or should it be some measure of population exposure determined by a combination of measurements and modelling? In practice, in the EU Directive, the exposure reduction concept was defined for $PM_{2.5}$ in terms of an average exposure indicator (AEI), defined as the average of annual mean concentrations at urban background locations, reflecting public exposure, over the whole territory of the Member State and averaged over three calendar years.

The Directive then required the AEI to be less than $20\,\mu g/m^3$ by 2015 (the 'exposure concentration obligation'), and required Member States to 'take all necessary measures not entailing disproportionate costs to reduce exposure to $PM_{2.5}$ with a view to attaining the national exposure reduction target', which was set as a percentage reduction, the size of which was dependent on the initial value of the AEI in a Member State. This is designed so that Member States that start from low AEI values do not have to make disproportionately large reductions compared with those starting from much higher values. The concept of the 'cap' referred to above has been incorporated in the Directive as a two-stage limit value for *concentrations* of $PM_{2.5}$ of $25\,\mu g/m^3$ to be met by 2015 (and a non-mandatory target value of the same value to be met by 2010), with an indicative second stage limit value of $20\,\mu g/m^3$ to be achieved by 2020.

It is interesting to note that the exposure reduction approach also embodies a form of environmental justice, although of a different kind from the ambient standards. As long as there are sources of emission in an urban area, there will always be differences in *exposures* due to dilution and dispersion, even if there is complete compliance with legal *standards*. If the exposure reduction approach is adopted, and if the reduction amount is required to be the same everywhere, there will be uniformity in the *improvement* in exposure, in percentage terms, if not in absolute amounts.

Air pollution and climate change

Up until now, reductions in emissions of air pollutants have been generated through technology. There are clearly diminishing returns to this approach – technologies for reducing emissions from motor vehicles can achieve very high reductions, often well over 90 per cent. Technologies are applied to individual emitters rather than collectively, so wider approaches are needed to solve continuing air pollution problems. Climate change is becoming increasingly important and is now the dominant driver for environmental improvements. Fortunately, there are significant synergistic solutions available that can not only

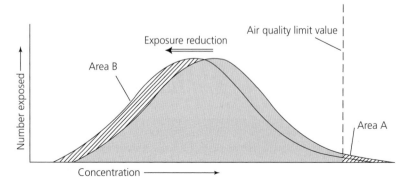

Figure 62.1 Illustration of the exposure reduction concept.

reduce greenhouse gas emissions, but also make large reductions in air pollution and generate correspondingly large improvements in public health. Space does not permit a full discussion here, but estimates of such potential public health benefits achievable by such synergistic approaches in London, UK, have been made.[9] In future, building on these 'win–win' solutions with climate change and managing the antagonisms (such as biomass use) will become increasingly important.

DISCLAIMER

The views expressed in this paper are those of the author and do not necessarily represent those of the Department for Environment, Food and Rural Affairs.

REFERENCES

● = Key primary paper

1. World Health Organization. *Air Quality Guidelines for Europe.* Copenhagen: WHO, 1987.
2. *The United Kingdom National Air Quality Strategy*, Cm 3587. London: Stationery Office, 1997.
3. Air Quality Expert Group. Ozone in the United Kingdom. Available from: http://www.defra.gov.uk/environment/quality/air/airquality/publications/ozone/documents/aqeg-ozone-report.pdf (accessed December 2, 2009).
4. Department of Health Committee on the Medical Effects of Air Pollutants. *Non-Biological Particles and Health.* London: HMSO, 1995.
5. Department of Health Committee on the Medical Effects of Air Pollutants. *The Quantification of the Effects of Air Pollution on Health in the United Kingdom.* London: HMSO, 1998.
6. Department for Environment, Food and Rural Affairs. *The Air Quality Strategy for England, Wales, Scotland and Northern Ireland.* London: HMSO, 2007.
●7. European Commission. Communication from the Commission to the Council and the European Parliament. Thematic Strategy for Air Pollution. Com(2005) 446 final. Available from: http://ec.europa.eu/environment/air/cafe/index.htm. http://eur-lex.europa.eu/LexUriServ/LexUriServ.do?uri=COM:2005:0446:FIN:EN:PDF (accessed December 1, 2009).
8. AEA Technology. *An Evaluation of the Air Quality Strategy.* Didcot, Oxon: AEA Technology, 2005.
●9. Williams ML. UK air quality in 2050 – synergies with climate change policies. *Environmental Science and Policy* 2007; **10**: 169–75.

Health impact assessment

FINTAN HURLEY, SALIM VOHRA

USING ENVIRONMENTAL HEALTH EVIDENCE TO INFORM POLICY DEVELOPMENT

There are many ways of summarizing and communicating scientific evidence for use in policy development when the aim is to protect public health and the evidence concerns risks from exposure to environmental pollutants. In the context of environmental medicine, one long-established approach involves developing health-based guidelines for specific pollutants. Typically, these guidelines are limit values, chosen so that if pollution is maintained at levels below these limits, the consequent risks to the health of even the most vulnerable individuals in the population are low.

Setting, implementing and maintaining health-based guidelines has proved very important in protecting human health. The approach has, however, some important limitations. First, it sometimes happens that, where pollutant levels are lower than guideline values, it is considered acceptable to allow a drift upwards towards those guidelines; or, in an equivalent manner, that policies or developments that imply an increase in pollution are considered acceptable as long as guideline levels are not exceeded. This ignores the possibility of effects at concentrations below guidelines, a problem especially with pollutants that have no threshold at population level.

Second, health-based guidelines do not per se take account of the difficulties and costs involved in achieving them, and therefore they are not amenable for comparing the costs and benefits of a new proposal. Third, measures to reduce pollution to conform with limits may have other unintended consequences, including health impacts

mediated through other environmental or social determinants of health. Attempts to overcome these limitations have contributed to the development and increased use of other methods of using science to inform the development of policy. One such set of methods is called health impact assessment (HIA).

HEALTH IMPACT ASSESSMENT

Health impact assessment is the systematic prediction of the potential positive and negative health and well-being impacts of new policies, plans, programmes and projects (hereafter referred to as proposals), including how these impacts are distributed across the population.[1] It was defined by the Gothenburg Consensus as 'A combination of procedures, methods and tools by which a policy, program or project may be judged as to its potential effects on the health of a population, and the distribution of those effects within the population'.[2]

It works within an explicitly stated ethical framework that promotes an impact assessment that is participatory, equitable, sustainable and ethical in its use of evidence and maximizes health opportunities for the affected population. It also generally provides a set of recommendations and/or a set of mitigation and enhancement measures so that positive health impacts are maximized and negative health impacts minimized within a given population. HIA is therefore about both protecting health by reducing exposures to harmful agents, and improving health by capitalizing on opportunities to promote and enhance health and well-being. HIA is also concerned with the inequalities/inequities generated by the uneven distribution of health impacts within an affected population.

DEFINITION OF HEALTH USED IN HIA

HIA tends to use both a biomedical and a social definition of health, recognizing that although illness and disease (mortality and morbidity) are useful ways of thinking about and measuring health, both health protection and health improvement need to be understood in ways that are wider than the reduction of illness and disease. HIA therefore generally uses the World Health Organization (WHO) definition that 'Health is a state of complete physical, social and mental wellbeing and not simply the absence of disease or infirmity',[3] or the more recent WHO psychosocial definition of health: 'the extent to which an individual or group is able to realize aspirations and satisfy needs, and to change or cope with the environment. From this viewpoint health is therefore a resource for everyday life, not the objective of living; it is a positive concept, emphasizing social and personal resources, as well as physical capacities.'[4]

THE HIA PROCESS

Key elements of the HIA process

There is a general consensus that the HIA process is made up of nine partially overlapping stages:

1. screening;
2. scoping;
3. baseline data-gathering and community profiling;
4. stakeholder involvement (this can be part of the other stages as well as occurring separately; it tends to involve different stakeholders at different points in time);
5. evidence-gathering and the identification of causal pathways;
6. an analysis of health impacts (identification, assessment of likelihood and magnitude);
7. making recommendations and/or developing a set of mitigation and enhancement measures, as well as how such recommendations/measures can be monitored and evaluated once introduced;
8. writing the HIA report or statement and presenting the findings to decision-makers;
9. follow-up of the HIA recommendations and of the HIA process (monitoring of the health impacts and evaluation of the HIA process).

Sources of evidence used in HIA

HIA uses a range of structured and evaluated sources of qualitative and quantitative evidence that includes public health, epidemiological, toxicological and medical knowledge, as well as public and other stakeholders' views and experiences. This means it uses both quantitative and qualitative peer-reviewed scientific evidence as well as community surveys and systematically collected and analysed anecdotal evidence based on the experiential knowledge and judgement of stakeholders (communities and professionals).

Rapid and in-depth HIAs

HIAs can generally be characterized as rapid or in depth depending on the level of detail of the analysis, the comprehensiveness of the scientific literature review and the breadth and depth of the community, and other stakeholder, engagement. However, any particular analysis can have both aspects because, although the nine stages outlined above are presented as linear, HIA tends to be an iterative process where findings and issues that emerge in later steps can lead to earlier steps being revisited with the scope and analysis being revised. For example, causal pathways may be identified and a rapid analysis of the important pathways undertaken to provide a first estimate of the likely impacts. This estimate is then refined with a more in-depth analysis of the pathways shown to have an important influence on the final answers, using better and more detailed baseline information and cause-and-effect relationship data.

Three practical considerations can and should have a major influence on the degree of rigour of any particular analysis:

1. *Proportionality*: It generally makes sense to put more resources into HIA where the expected health impacts are large or controversial.
2. *Timeliness*: Because the point of HIA is to inform the development of a proposal or policy, a timely albeit less in-depth analysis (but one whose strengths and weaknesses have been made explicit) will be more useful than a more comprehensive HIA that misses the decision points of proposal development and implementation. Meeting policy and decision-making deadlines can be a challenge even when an HIA is anticipated and planned well in advance.
3. *Limitations of evidence and data*: These can be to an extent overcome by making plausible assumptions and then checking how robust or sensitive conclusions are to changes in these assumptions; HIA lends itself well to sensitivity analyses along these lines.

Stakeholder involvement and community engagement

Actively listening to and involving people who may be affected by a proposal is an important part of HIA and its ethos of equity, participation, sustainability, accountability and transparency in the use of evidence and analysis. Involving the individuals and groups who are, or are likely to be, affected by a proposal is essential for obtaining a rounded picture of the actual and potential impacts on health and well-being. It can also reduce actual and potential concern, distrust and conflict, and so make an evidence-based decision more likely. Reasons why stakeholders should be, and generally are, actively involved in an HIA include the following:

1. Affected stakeholders will face the direct positive and negative health consequences.
2. Stakeholders have valuable experiential knowledge that can inform the analysis of health impacts.
3. Not adequately and appropriately addressing stakeholder concerns can lead to them experiencing social and psychological distress.
4. Allowing residents and others to have a voice and influence in decision-making processes reduces the sense of social exclusion, democratic deficit and inequity.

A range of community consultation and involvement methods can be used, from workshops and focus groups to one-to-one interviews and public meetings. The key issue is to be clear about the purpose of the activities and to communicate to stakeholders how the consultation findings have been used to inform the HIA.

HIA IN THE CONTEXT OF OTHER APPROACHES

HIA and other forms of impact assessment

HIA has its roots firstly in the healthy public policy movement of the 1970s and 80s, which recognized that non-health policies, for example housing, transport and welfare, are as important as, if not more important than, healthcare policy as determinants of public health. It has been rooted secondly in the environmental conservation and environmental impact assessment movement from the 1950s onwards and its perceived deficiencies in assessing the wider public health impacts of new projects, particularly infrastructure projects in the developing world;[5] thirdly in the sociology of health; and finally in epidemiology and quantitative health risk assessment.

HIA is increasingly carried out either in conjunction with or by being integrated into other forms of impact assessment at both policy/plan and project/programme levels; these include environmental impact assessment, strategic environmental assessment, sustainability appraisals, equalities impact assessment and policy appraisals.[6] This is increasingly being badged as integrated impact assessment or integrated policy appraisal.

HIA and evaluation studies

The purpose of HIA is to inform the development of new proposals in advance of their being put in place. Evaluation studies are empirical investigations that aim to assess the actual impacts of proposals that have been implemented; they are an elaboration of stage 9 of the HIA process. It is best that evaluation studies are designed, and baseline measurements taken, in advance of a proposal being put into place (cf. stage 7 of the HIA process).

HIA and evaluation studies are therefore different in tone and focus, and they play a different role in policy development and review. Both HIA and evaluation should, however, be considered as part of the overall process of developing a proposal, and there is a close and mutually supportive relationship between the two. For example, some of the data used in the HIA may be relevant to developing the baseline for an evaluation study. In addition, evaluation studies (if properly conducted and sufficiently powerful) will help show to what extent the HIA predictions have in fact been borne out by events (even though evaluation studies rarely aim to cover the full health impacts of a proposal).

HIA and health risk assessment

Health risk assessment is an established term for methodologies that aim to provide a quantitative assessment of the adverse health impacts of population exposure to single or multiple hazards, and in particular environmental and occupational exposure to chemical pollutants released or transferred into the air, water and soil and their direct physical health impacts. HIA includes health risk assessment as one of its component parts (within stages 5 and 6, as listed above). However, HIA is wider than health risk assessment in several ways.

- It takes a wider view of health.
- It considers health benefits as well as health hazards.
- It aims to assess the full health impacts of policies, and not only those which are mediated through changes in chemical and physical exposures.
- It examines the distribution of health impacts across a population.

Thus, HIA tends to be a broader and more holistic form of assessment that examines not only the effects of pollutants, but also the direct and indirect impacts on the wider determinants of health, for example: employment and economy; housing and shelter; transport and connectivity; learning and education; crime and safety; public and commercial services; social capital and community cohesion; culture, spirituality and faith; arts and leisure; lifestyle and daily routines; governance and institutional structures; energy and waste; and land and spatial factors.

AN OVERVIEW OF ENVIRONMENTAL HIA

Social HIA and environmental HIA

Given its historical roots, it is not surprising that HIA can in practice be seen as the fusion of two broad traditions of assessment – environmentally focused and socially focused HIA. 'Social' HIA has roots in the healthy public policy movement, sociology and environmental impact assessment. It tends to take a wide view of what constitutes health and, because of weaknesses in the evidence base, it has a strong focus on qualitative analysis of the wider determinants of health and a strong focus also on community participation, and other stakeholder engagement, as a key part of the process.

In contrast, 'Environmental' HIA (EHIA) has a narrower focus, on those health effects which are mediated by the environment and by environmental pollutants in particular, and has closer roots in health risk assessment and epidemiology. Consequently, it tends to interpret 'health' in traditional biomedical terms of adverse consequences – death, disease, use of health services, illness and some health-related behaviours such as days off work or off school. The analysis stages tend to be expert driven, especially where there is strong evidence of causal and quantifiable exposure–response relationships, and the stages are often time-consuming. The relatively strong evidence base for some environment and health pathways brings a danger of undue focus on what is quantifiable, at the expense of downplaying other health effects that are important but unquantifiable. This danger can be reduced through community and other stakeholder consultation, which, for environmentally focused HIA, is undertaken largely in the scoping phase where the question is framed, and in consultation on the results and recommendations, rather than in the intermediate stage of analysis of impacts.[7]

Environmental justice and health equity

Environmental burdens are often both geographically and socially located, thereby affecting the poorest, most vulnerable and already burdened members of a community or population. There is also some evidence that, over time, this becomes a systematic and institutionalized process that is very difficult to shift. There is therefore a call for both environmental justice and health equity in relation to new proposals.

Socially focused HIAs have an explicit value framework, in line with the Gothenburg Consensus, while environmentally focused HIAs tend not to; hence, one of the debates in the HIA community is whether it is the role of HIA to take a more overtly political and social stance, advocating health improvement and reductions in health inequalities/inequities. This has led to two broad stereotypes of how HIA is practised that are often seen in opposition to each other, with HIA being seen as either of the following:

1. a decision-support tool providing information and advice to the policy and decision-making process (an objective, technical, informing tool);
2. a decision-influencing tool providing support to communities to have their voice, and their views on what decisions should be made, heard within the decision-making process (a community advocacy and empowerment tool).

In reality, in most cases HIA is a mixture of the two. It does give voice to the most vulnerable by providing a structured approach to including their views and wishes and focusing on health equity/inequality. However, it also provides an evidence-based and systematic understanding of the potential positive and negative health impacts of the policy or measure under consideration – and this implies a role for subject matter experts. Part of the art of HIA is the ability to combine these two aspects in a transparent, credible and robust way. Indeed, from one point of view, there is no need to identify environmental HIA for special attention – all that applies to HIA and social HIA generally applies to EHIA also. In practice, however, EHIA has developed relatively independently from the wider socially focused HIA movement, and as noted it has some particular characteristics that give it a distinctive flavour within the HIA field. One such characteristic is a highly developed and often quantitative analysis stage, which will be the focus of much of the rest of this chapter.

A framework for EHIA analysis: the impact pathway or full-chain approach

There have been several attempts to develop a useful conceptual model for tackling the subject matter issues that are central to the analysis stage of EHIA and that form the basis for much EHIA work. The impact pathway[8,9] or full-chain approach is one way of systematically describing the various linked stages of an analysis that tracks the fate of pollutants from emissions through to monetary valuation. In terms of human health, this involves tracking the fate of pollutant emissions through a set of stages, for example:

1. from (changes in) policies in various sectors, insofar as they affect the environment; to consequent
2. (changes in) burdens, and emissions, to air, soil and water; to
3. (changes in) pollutant concentrations in microenvironments; to
4. (changes in) the exposure of individuals and populations (by inhalational, dermal and/or ingestional routes); to
5. (changes in) internal dose at target organs in the body; to
6. (changes in) the risks of health effects; to

7. (changes in) health impacts (overall and in subpopulations); to
8. (changes in) the monetary value of health effects

The linearity in this list, albeit somewhat artificial, helps to emphasize the importance of looking at the pathway as an integrated whole, focusing on the transitions between various steps of the pathway, as well as on the steps themselves (see also Chapter 1). It is essential to have an alignment between the output of one stage and the input of another. So, for example, in modelling the health effects of environmental tobacco smoke, the concentration-modellers and health experts need to agree on whether the analysis will be carried out with a simple exposure metric such as 'non-smoker, living with a smoker', or with a more complex one such as concentration of particulate matter with a diameter of 2.5 μm or less ($PM_{2.5}$), or with both (see also Chapter 5). There may also need to be an alignment in understanding a health end point – say, 'chronic bronchitis' or 'asthma attack' – between the epidemiological studies that provide evidence for risk functions and the willingness-to-pay studies that underlie monetary valuations.

It is important to check that what appears to be the same thing really is, and if necessary to make adjustments in order to ensure alignment. As a broad rule of thumb, it is usually worthwhile spending more time on alignments of this nature, and doing so as early as possible, than might at first sight seem necessary or even reasonable. It helps if the analysis is initially done more than once, rapidly, to identify alignment issues and data–evidence gaps, and to identify what matters before deciding where to focus the detailed effort.

A more realistic and less linear description is given in Figure 63.1, from the Health and Environment Integrated Methodology and Toolbox for Scenario Assessment (HEIMTSA) project's representation of the full-chain approach.[10] The left-hand side of the diagram is a representation of the full chain as described earlier in the text. Note, however, that the estimation of health effects may arise from studies that examine the relationships between health and (1) background concentrations, as with ambient air pollution; (2) exposures, as in most occupational studies; or (3) dose (or biomarkers), as for lead in the blood. It may also not be necessary, or even useful, to work through all stages of the pathway from concentration through to dose. This can also be compared with the Driving Forces–Pressures–State–Exposure–Effects–Actions model described in Chapter 1.

Some aspects of implementing a full-chain analysis

THE TARGET POPULATION, INEQUALITIES AND POPULATION DISAGGREGATION

Underlying the analysis as a whole is the key component of the 'target population'. Logically, this is the entire population whose health may be affected by the proposal under consideration. In practice, some analyses may, in framing the question, decide to focus on a more limited population, for example the effects within a particular region, country or group of countries, where the policy under consideration is targeted. In those circumstances, we think it is important that the wider health effects should at least be indicated. Here as elsewhere, how the HIA question is framed can have a major impact on the methods used and the results.[7]

The estimation of health effects has three component parts:

- exposure (concentration or dose);
- a risk function (concentration–response, exposure–response or dose–response), typically expressed as the

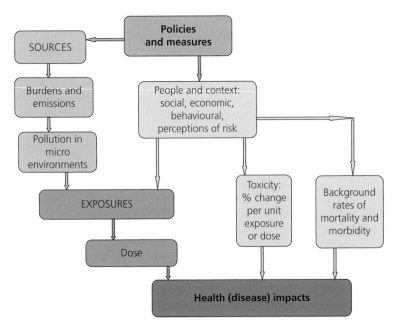

Figure 63.1 Schematic representation of the full-chain approach. (Adapted from Health and Environment Integrated Methodology and Toolbox for Scenario Assessment,[10] with permission.)

percentage change in (risk of) a specific health end point per unit exposure (concentration or dose);

- background rates of that health end point in the target population.

Issues of environmental justice/health equity/inequalities are relevant to all three components. That is, it is likely that there are differences between population subgroups in terms of (1) environmental exposures; (2) risk functions, per unit exposure; and (3) background rates of morbidity and mortality, and that together these differences may imply important differences in health impacts by population subgroup. In principle, the size and nature of such differences should influence the extent to which the population is disaggregated for any particular analysis, for example by age, gender, social class/socioeconomic status, current health status/pre-existing disease, geographical area or other relevant factors. In practice, however, the level of disaggregation is influenced strongly by limitations on resources needed for the analysis, such as data availability.

EXPOSURE ASSESSMENT

There are many definitions of environmental exposures, but they all include the key idea that exposure is a measure of the interaction (usually in a given time period) between people, or populations, and the environment(s) where they spend time. Exposure involves the interaction of two components – the state of the environment, and the time–activity patterns of people in relation to that environment. Note that a policy or measure may affect environmental exposures by affecting either (or both) the state of the environment and how people interact with that environment; and while pollution reduction might be considered the preferred option, there is a role also for the avoidance of exposure. Although the language of 'exposure' and 'risk function' generally carries negative connotations, suggesting adverse health effects, the concept as described here (of an interaction between a population and its environments) may also be life-enhancing. Therefore, for example, 'exposure' may be a measure of proximity or ease of access to greenspace or open space, for recreation, physical activity or conviviality.

This very simple overview does not do justice to what in practice may be a very detailed and time-consuming aspect of an analysis, i.e. identifying what microenvironments need to be considered (e.g. at home, at work, outdoors in or near traffic, and outdoors elsewhere) and how the proposal may affect both pollutant concentrations and the time–activity patterns of the target population and its relevant subpopulations. A fuller development of this area can be found in Chapter 5.

CAUSALITY AND STRENGTH OF EVIDENCE

The various 'pathways' or 'chains' of an analysis carry the implicit assumption that the environmental exposures being analysed are causes of the health effects being estimated, in the sense that changes in exposures will result in changes in health impacts. The evaluation of causality can be difficult and is best done as a multidisciplinary exercise including as a minimum exposure assessment, toxicology, epidemiology and clinical expertise, even though an elaboration of a full-chain analysis following the acceptance of causality may draw on some of these disciplines much more than on others.

Effects should be included if, on the basis of the available evidence, the chains leading to them are more likely than not to express relationships that are causal (the balance of probabilities). This is a weaker criterion than that of 'beyond reasonable doubt', often applied in science. Some favour it in HIA assessments because it is relevant to the aim of providing best estimates, and thus of giving a fair and unbiased assessment of the overall impacts: restricting assessments to impacts and risk functions that are practically certain gives an analysis that is biased towards underestimating overall health impacts, and so is in practice (although usually not intentionally) antiprecautionary.[11] The issue of evaluating strength of evidence in relation to different policy needs has been addressed more systematically and more comprehensively elsewhere.[12]

Causality is sometimes accepted for a pollution mixture, or for pollution from a source such as road traffic, but the particular agents responsible, or more generally the role of the components of the mixture, may be unknown or contested. This is not necessarily a barrier to HIA. It may be possible to quantify relationships based on proximity to source (the presence or lack of a gas cooker, living or not living with a smoker, or closeness of residence to roads). This gives a crude model in that it does not reflect the effects of changes in intensity of exposure that would follow from reduced emissions without elimination of the source. It is nevertheless a model that may be useful.

Alternatively or in addition, one pollutant of a mixture may be taken as a marker of or surrogate for the mixture as a whole, with health effects being estimated for that component and taken as expressing the effects of the mixture as a whole. For example, the health effects of outdoor air pollution as a whole are generally expressed via relationships in PM, represented as $PM_{2.5}$ and/or PM_{10}. Opinions vary on the extent to which PM measured as $PM_{2.5}$ or PM_{10} is the causal agent of the mixture; it is widely accepted, however, that it is the single best marker. It is also possible to quantify in terms of other pollutants, for example nitrogen dioxide, where the associated risk functions are generally understood as expressing the effects of traffic-related air pollution, rather than of whatever causal role nitrogen dioxide as a gas plays within the mixture as a whole. This can work well as long as changes in traffic-related nitrogen dioxide reflect changes in the mixture as a whole. Such quantification would be seriously misleading, however, in estimating the health effects of proposals that reduce traffic-related nitrogen dioxide without concomitant reductions in the other components of the pollution mixture.

This emphasizes a more general point – that there are not any universally best EHIA models. Rather, there are models of different complexity, with different assumptions and different data needs, and different strengths and weaknesses in the context of different applications. We support the concept of 'fit for purpose', not least because it pushes for early-stage clarification of what the purpose is, what degree of accuracy and precision is envisaged for the EHIA, and whether the resources (evidence, data, time and money) available are at all realistic in relation to the envisaged purpose.

RISK FUNCTIONS

Estimates of risk functions vary between studies, and this leads to interesting questions about which functions to use when 'local' estimates (i.e. those relating to the target population of the EHIA) are available, and about the transferability of functions from elsewhere. The key issue is whether the variability between estimates from different times and places arises from real known factors or from the complexity of issues we call 'chance'. If the former, it may be possible to adjust for differences in these factors when transferring relationships from one context to another. If the differences are best understood as chance effects, the use of random effects methods in meta-analyses will give better estimates of effects and of the uncertainties with which they are estimated. In either case, we think that the wider international evidence should weigh strongly relative to a particular, and possibly not large, local study, although stakeholder pressure to use local evidence may be strong.

For an informative discussion of these and many other relevant issues, see the reports of two WHO workshops,[13,14] the more recent focusing on outdoor air pollution but including many points of wider interest.

BACKGROUND RATES

For some health end points, relevant data may be collected routinely to a high standard across the target population, and be available for use. Often, background rates need to be estimated, for example by extrapolating from a small number of locations for which reliable data have been collected as a result of special exercises at specific times and places as, for example, was done by the Air Pollution and Health: A European Information System (APHEIS) HIA team with respect to hospital admissions in several European cities.[15] Alternatively, it may be possible to get good-quality data on background rates from specific research studies carried out by others. Because the focus here is on a health end point, these studies do not need to be limited to those investigating the environmental factors under consideration in the HIA.

In general, both analysts and stakeholders tend to be drawn to paying much more attention to the choice of risk functions than to the estimation of background rates, and while there is some rationale to this in terms of the influence on final estimates, more attention on estimating background rates would be worthwhile.

AGGREGATION ACROSS HEALTH END POINTS

It is rare that the HIA of a proposal implies effects on only one health end point. In the more usual situation of multiple health end points, there is often an interest in aggregating results across health end points into a single composite index. The two most commonly used approaches are disability-adjusted life–years, as used, for example, in the WHO Global Burden of Disease analyses, and monetary valuation.[16,17] Insofar as any aggregation of this kind can be done meaningfully, the results facilitate the comparison between studies and between the effects of different measures. Monetary valuation in addition allows a cost–benefit analysis of the proposal, which some decision-makers find particularly informative.

When aggregation is used, as it is widely, we recommend that the underlying separate health effects estimates also be presented. This not only increases the transparency of the final aggregated values, but also allows stakeholders to apply their own weighting factors. Indeed, the range and diversity of health effects, and not just their aggregated value, may be a spur to action to protect or improve health.

ISSUES OF SPACE AND TIME

Any full-chain analysis needs to consider issues of space and time in an integral way, from framing the question (e.g. what are the boundaries in space and time of the environmental exposures that are considered relevant, of the population at risk, and of the health effects?) through to the detailed linkage of information across the full chain. Estimates of one component of the chain (e.g. a dispersion-modelling of pollutants) may be carried out on quite a different spatial scale from estimates of other components (e.g. background rates of morbidity or mortality). However, the full-chain analysis will require linkage of all the data spatially, and it is helpful to be aware of this from the outset. The detailed work of any component may need to be adapted so that the analysis as a whole becomes workable. Similar issues apply to the time dimension, and this is greatly facilitated by going through the full chain more than once, first very approximately and then in more detail.

An important issue is the extent to which results may be sensitive to the spatial scale of the analysis; this is an area where sensitivity analyses may be helpful.

REPRESENTATION AND ASSESSMENT OF UNCERTAINTY

Any EHIA, indeed any full-chain analysis, implies uncertainties at different stages and in the final estimated health impacts, whether reported individually or in aggregated form. It is not practicable to pay close attention to all of these. It is, however, both possible and necessary to be explicit about what these are, and to get some perspective on which of these matter in terms of their impact on the final answers. This also helps with identifying what aspects of the full chain could most benefit from more attention and improvement.

There are many more-or-less sophisticated approaches to the assessment and representation of uncertainty. We suggest that they should begin with identifying and describing the various sources, and with some qualitative assessment of their size and importance to the final answers. This seems an essential precursor to more sophisticated methods, be these qualitative or quantitative, that attempt to assess and aggregate uncertainties across the full chain, for example by assuming particular distributional forms for the individual components, and using Monte Carlo methods to explore how they combine.

AN EXAMPLE: ENVIRONMENTAL HIA OF OUTDOOR AIR POLLUTION

Policies affecting outdoor air pollution are amenable to HIA

Some of the history of the development of environmentally focused HIA and several of its interesting characteristics can be illustrated with reference to the HIA of outdoor air pollution, the context within which EHIA is most strongly established both methodologically and in terms of its use in policy development. There are several reasons why the HIA of outdoor air pollution has gained this position:

- The impact pathway from emissions to health is relatively simple, with emissions to air and exposure by inhalation (although there are of course major complexities in modelling the fate of relevant emissions to air).

- There is a very substantial body of research evidence – epidemiology, toxicology and human experimental studies – for the assessment of causality and for estimating relationships between exposure and the risk of adverse health effects (mortality and morbidity).

- The main epidemiological studies are based on concentrations of outdoor air, as measured by fixed-point samplers located at background sites, rather than on personal exposures. This in effect removes one of the steps of the impact pathway and leads to a simpler schematic representation, as shown in Figure 63.2.[11]

Early HIA analyses of outdoor air pollution: effects of daily variations in air pollution

Early examples of what were in effect this approach were developed by Ostro and colleagues in the early 1990s, in a series of analyses about the effects of air pollution from electricity generation and in burden of disease estimates for the World Bank.[18] The basic framework has changed little since then. The essentials of the methodology can be found elsewhere.[11,19]

Those early analyses were based principally on studies of daily variations in mortality and morbidity. In principle, it was necessary: (1) to construct the full annual pattern of daily concentrations of ambient pollutants, and how these would change with changes to policy; (2) to apply the relevant concentration–response functions and background rates in order to estimate daily impacts; and then (3) to aggregate these impacts over days in the year to reach estimated annual impacts. In practice, however, the concentration–response functions used were linear, with no threshold, and an equivalent answer could be provided by the simpler method of applying concentration–response functions and background rates to annual average (changes in) ambient pollution, and then scaling appropriately.

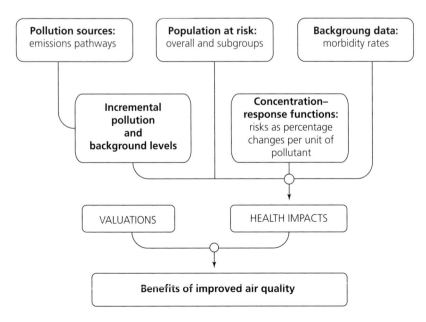

Figure 63.2 Schematic diagram of the health impact assessment of outdoor air pollution. Reproduced with permission from ref. 11.

The simplification, which is substantial, is a consequence of how the various component parts of the overall HIA process fit together; it is not a consequence of any one part of the process, viewed in isolation. This illustrates the benefits of doing an HIA using the impact pathway approach, not as a once-and-for-all pass through the various stages, but rather as an iterative process, i.e. in outline form initially, and then in more detail as the shape of the component parts becomes evident. This has several benefits:

- It allows aspects of integration to be properly addressed. For example, with ozone, the modelling of ambient concentrations may be in terms of 8 hour daily maximum ozone concentrations, whereas epidemiology uses other metrics, such as 1 hour daily maximum or 24 hour average concentrations. An initial scoping exercise will identify the need to join these up, for example by focusing on concentration–response functions in the metric of the 8 hour daily maximum, by carrying out the ozone modelling in the metric of 1 hour daily maximum or 24 hour daily average, or by scaling the relevant concentration–response functions according to the average relationships between 1 hour daily maximum, 8 hour daily maximum and 24 hour daily average.
- Initial scoping should help identify the most important uncertainties and evidence gaps, i.e. those which most affect the final answers; this helps in prioritizing further work.
- Viewing the process as a whole can lead to simplifications, as described earlier.

This period also saw an important debate about who was at increased risk of mortality from higher daily values of outdoor air pollution, i.e. where the focus was on daily values within the 'normal' range of variation in Europe and North America, rather than during specific episodes of unusually high air pollution. The emerging consensus was that the associated 'extra' deaths attributable to air pollution were among people with already severe (albeit possibly undiagnosed) cardiorespiratory disease. The implication was that, on average, the life expectancy of those at risk was less, and maybe very substantially less, than that of the general population of similar age; air pollution was viewed as 'bringing forward' a death that might in any case have occurred before very long.[20]

This was helpful in focusing attention on the fact that death is unavoidable – air pollution does not lead to 'extra' deaths, but rather it leads to earlier deaths. A complication was that the time series studies that quantified the risk of earlier deaths (attributable to daily variations in air pollution) were not directly informative about the degree of life-shortening. The debate, however, led to a questioning of the practice, until then current, of associating with the earlier ('extra') deaths attributable to air pollution a 'value of a statistical life' that ignored the likelihood of pre-existing

serious cardiorespiratory disease among those effectively at risk. This debate has not yet been fully resolved.

Some more recent developments: effects of long-term exposures

The emerging evidence in the mid-1990s, from two cohort studies in the USA,[21,22] showed associations between long-term exposure to outdoor air pollution, specifically PM, and mortality. Earlier studies had suggested such associations; the cohort studies provided stronger evidence because they adjusted for confounding factors at the individual level. Whether or not these studies expressed a causal relationship was disputed. It was clear, however, that if they did – and it is now widely accepted that they do – they implied substantially greater public health effects than did the mortality studies of daily variations in air pollution. This was partly because the estimated relative risks of mortality across the adult population were much higher than those implied by time series studies, and partly because the whole adult population – and not just those with pre-existing cardiorespiratory disease – was considered to be at risk. Together, these implied much greater effects, especially when expressed in terms of accumulated life expectancy rather than 'attributable deaths'.

Despite the caveats about causality, the effects of long-term exposure, as expressed via these cohort studies, were included quite soon in some HIA assessments as part of sensitivity analyses or as a central part of the assessment.[8,9] With growing epidemiological evidence[23] and a better understanding of possible mechanisms, a consensus has emerged that the HIA of outdoor air pollution should include the mortality impacts of long-term exposure as not to do so implies a possibly serious underestimation of mortality impacts. The overall evidence has been reviewed by various expert groups, including the UK Expert Committee on the Medical Effects of Air Pollutants.[24]

Using the results of cohort studies for the HIA of outdoor air pollution has highlighted a number of methodological issues that have been resolved only in part.[25] There are at least three.

First is *how to express mortality impacts, in terms of life expectancy or as 'attributable deaths'?* A simple approach yielding estimates of 'attributable deaths' was used in ExternE,[8] and has continued to be used until recently. The use of life tables was proposed by Brunekreef[26] and developed and recommended by others, for example ExternE, Leksell and Rabl, and Miller and Hurley.[9,27,28] Both approaches were used in the HIA and associated cost–benefit analysis of the Clean Air for Europe (CAFE) programme.

However, methodological work using life table methods has shown that estimates of attributable deaths – which in HIA analyses are treated as reproducible year on year – do in fact change over time, as the different mortality patterns imply differences in the size of the underlying population at risk.[29,30] Specifically, if the same population is analysed under two scenarios – lower and higher age-specific death rates – there will initially be more deaths per year in the population with higher death rates, but the situation will reverse in due course as the size of the surviving population at risk (under higher death rates) decreases more rapidly than when death rates are lower. Currently and in general, HIA analyses of 'attributable deaths' do not take this effect into account.

The second issue is *the time lag between reductions in air pollution and the associated or consequent changes in risks of mortality* – a concept sometimes known as cessation lag. It is linked to, but is not identical with, the latency period between exposure to ambient air pollution and the associated risk of mortality. Studies in Dublin[31] and Hong Kong[32] have shown that substantial reductions in air pollution can have clear and immediate benefits in terms of lower death rates. There may, however, also be delayed effects, for example effects on birth weight or on lung function in childhood, which may affect mortality risks in later life. How cessation lag is treated within an HIA can have substantial effects on the final results, especially if monetary values are linked with health impacts and if the discount rate is large.

The final issue is *the time frame for an analysis*. When an HIA of outdoor air was focused on the effects of daily variations, the associated health effects were more or less immediate, and so there was a concordance between the time frame of emissions and of effects – the two could be considered as concurrent, and effects 'within a year' was an unambiguous concept. With the effects of longer-term exposure, however, this identification was broken. It now became necessary to distinguish between (1) the health impacts in a given year, arising from emissions, whenever they occurred, and (2) the health impacts, whenever they occur, arising from emissions in a given year. The latter of these is more consistent with the HIA as a prospective exercise, and is what is generally used.

There are, however, other time frame issues to consider. While looking at the health effects of emissions in a given year may be helpful, for comparing with the costs of emission control in that same year, there is something artificial about an evaluation focused on one year's emissions given that policies to control air pollution are intended to be long-lasting, rather than reverting to the status quo after a single year. Consequently, how the HIA is framed in terms of time scale remains an issue that is very relevant to the analysis and to the results, but which does not have an obvious solution.

HIA of the Clean Air for Europe programme

The HIA within the CAFE programme was carried out as part of a wider cost–benefit analysis, commissioned by Directorate-General for the environment.[33] This shows, inter alia, how the methods and results of the HIA and cost–benefit analysis were used by the Commission to inform its policy development on outdoor air pollution. Briefly, results showed that the estimated benefits of a 20 per cent reduction in fine particulate air pollution (PM with a diameter of 2.5 μm or less [$PM_{2.5}$]) across the European Union far outweighed the estimated costs. The benefits were largely attributable to the effects on mortality risks of long-term exposure to outdoor air pollution, expressed as $PM_{2.5}$.

CURRENT TRENDS AND FUTURE PROSPECTS

There is renewed and growing interest in both socially and environmentally focused HIA globally, as policies and measures are developed to tackle two major health issues of the present period – the adverse effects of climate change, and of poverty and income inequality. Successfully tackling either of these issues requires policy-makers and others to draw on the main strengths of both traditions that underlie HIA: the strengths of socially focused HIAs in analysing the wider, social determinants of health and giving a voice in decision-making to all stakeholders, particularly those who are socially disadvantaged, and of environmentally focused HIA in providing precise numerical estimates of health impact that can be linked to monetary cost–benefit analyses which can support fine-grain decision-making between the costs and benefits of a range of proposal options.

All HIA, whether socially or environmentally focused, draw on both these traditions and, we see, methodologically, move towards a convergence, with an increasing focus on quantifying health impacts in socially focused HIA and on including wider health impacts (including positive health impacts) and on community engagement in environmentally focused HIA. Socially focused HIA is reaching the limits of what can be described and analysed qualitatively, and environmentally focused HIA is seeing the limits of focusing on tangible, chemical environmental exposures. This seems to show a coming together of the two approaches and an increasing integration of the methodologies between the two traditions of HIA, a direction that many strongly welcome and support.

ACKNOWLEDGEMENTS

Work on this chapter was supported in part by HEIMTSA, an Integrated Project, funded under the European Union Sixth Framework Programme – Priority 6.3 Global Change and Ecosystems, and draws on discussions with many HEIMTSA colleagues, whose help we acknowledge.

REFERENCES

● = Key primary paper

◆ = Major review article

1. Quigley R, den Broeder L, Furu P, Bond A, Cave B, Bos R. *Health Impact Assessment International Best Practice Principles.* Special Publication Series No. 5. Fargo: International Association for Impact Assessment, 2006.

●2. World Health Organization European Centre for Health Policy. *Health Impact Assessment: Main Concepts and Suggested Approach*, Gothenburg consensus paper. Geneva: WHO, 1999.

3. World Health Organization. *Health Promotion: A Discussion Document on the World Health Organization.* Preamble to the Constitution of the World Health Organization as adopted by the International Health Conference, New York, 19–22 June 1946, and entered into force on 7 April 1948. Geneva: WHO, 1946.

4. World Health Organization. *Health Promotion: A Discussion Document on the Concepts and Principles.* Copenhagen: WHO, 1984.

◆5. Kemm J, Parry J, Palmer S. *Health Impact Assessment: Concepts, Theory, Techniques and Applications.* Oxford: Oxford University Press, 2004.

6. Quigley R, Cavanagh S, Harrison D, Taylor L, Pottle M. *Clarifying Approaches to Health Needs Assessment, Health Impact Assessment, Integrated Impact Assessment, Health Equity Audit, and Race Equality Impact Assessment.* London: Health Development Agency, 2005.

●7. Briggs D. A framework for integrated environmental health impact assessment of systemic risks. *Environ Health* 2008; **7**: 61.

8. ExternE. DGXII (JOULE Programme). *Externalities of Energy, ExternE Project.* Report No. 2: *Methodology.* Prepared by ETSU and others. ExternE Luxembourg: Office for Official Publications of the European Communities, 1995.

9. Holland MR, Forster D, for ExternE: DGXII (JOULE Programme). *Externalities of Energy, ExternE Project.* Report No. 7: *Methodology.* Luxembourg: Office for Official Publications of the European Communities. Update 1998, 1999.

10. Hurley JF, Loh M, Sarigiannis D, van den Hout D *et al.* (In preparation) *Report on fundamental methodology and conceptual issues*; to be web-published www.heimtsa.eu.

11. Sanderson E, Hurley F (eds). *Air Pollution and the Risks to Human Health – Health Impact Assessment.* Available from: http://airnet.iras.uu.nl/products/pdf/airnet_wg4_hia_ report.pdf (accessed December 13, 2009).

●12. Gee D. Establishing evidence for early action: the prevention of reproductive and developmental harm. *Basic Clin Pharmacol* 2008; **102**: 257–66.

13. World Health Organization. *Quantification of the Health Effects of Exposure to Air Pollution. Report of a WHO Working Group.* 20–22 November, Bilthoven, Netherlands. Geneva: WHO, 2000.

14. World Health Organization. *International Expert Workshop on the Analysis of the Economic and Public Health Impacts of Air Pollution*, 6 September, 2001.

15. Air Pollution and Health: A European Information System; 2004). *Health Impact Assessment of Air Pollution and Communication. Third Year Report 2002–2003.* Available from: http://www.apheis.net/Apheis3NEW1.pdf (accessed December 13, 2009).

16. Lopez AD, Mathers CD, Ezzati M, Jamison DT, Murray CJL. *Global Burden of Disease and Risk Factors.* Geneva: World Health Organization, 2006.

17. Hanley NSCL. *Cost–Benefit Analysis and the Environment.* London: Edward Elgar, 1993.

18. Ostro BD. *Estimating the Health Effects of Air Pollutants: A Method with an Application to Jakarta.* World Bank, Policy Research Department Working Paper No. 1301. World Bank, 1994. Accessible from www-wds.worldbank.org.

19. Ostro BD. *WHO Air Quality Guidelines: Global Update 2005.* Geneva: World Health Organization, 2006.

◆20. Committee on the Medical Effects of Air Pollutants. *The Quantification of the Effects of Air Pollution on Health in the United Kingdom.* London: HMSO, 1998.

21. Dockery DW, Pope CAI, Xiping X *et al.* An association between air pollution and mortality in six US cities. *N Engl J Med* 1993; **329**: 1753–9.

22. Pope CA III, Thun MJ, Namboodiri MM *et al.* Particulate air pollution as predictor of mortality in a prospective study of US adults. *Am J Resp Crit Care Med* 1995; **151**: 669–74.

●23. Pope CA III, Burnett RT, Thun MJ *et al.* Lung cancer, cardiopulmonary mortality, and long-term exposure to fine particulate air pollution. *JAMA* 2002; **287**: 1132–41.

◆24. Committee on the Medical Effects of Air Pollutants. *Long-term Exposure to Air Pollution: Effect on Mortality.* London: HMSO, 2009.

◆25. Hurley F, Hunt A, Cowie H *et al. Methodology for the Cost–Benefit Analysis for CAFE. Volume 2: Health Impact Assessment.* Didcot: AEA Technology Environment, 2005.

26. Brunekreef B. Air pollution and life expectancy: is there a relation? *Occup Environ Med* 1997; **54**: 781–4.

27. Leksell L, Rabl A. Air pollution and mortality: quantification and valuation of years of life lost. *Risk Analysis* 2001; **21**: 843–57.

28. Miller BG, Hurley JF. Life table methods for quantitative impact assessments in chronic mortality. *J Epidemiol Commun Health* 2003; **57**: 200–6.

29. Miller BG, Hurley JF. *Comparing Estimated Risks for Air Pollution with Risks for Other Health Effects.* IOM Report TM/06/01. Edinburgh: Institute of Occupational Medicine, 2006.

●30. Brunekreef B, Miller BG, Hurley F. The brave new world of lives sacrificed and saved, and deaths, attributed to and avoided. *Epidemiology* 2007; **18**: 785–8.

31. Clancy L, Goodman P, Sinclair H, Dockery DW. Effect of air-pollution control on death rates in Dublin, Ireland: an intervention study. *Lancet* 2002; **360**: 1210–14.

32. Hedley AJ, Wong CM, Thach TQ, Ma SLS, Lam TH, Anderson HR. Cardiorespiratory and all-cause mortality after restrictions on sulphur content of fuel in Hong Kong: an intervention study. *Lancet* 2002; **360**: 1646–52.

33. Commission of the European Communities. *Commission Staff Working Paper. Annex to The Communication on* *Thematic Strategy on Air Pollution, and The Directive on 'Ambient Air Quality and Cleaner Air for Europe'. Impact Assessment.* COM(2005)446 final. COM(2005)447 final. Available from: http://ec.europa.eu/environment/air/pdf/ sec_2005_1133.pdf (accessed December 13, 2009).

Index

Note: page numbers in **bold** refer to figures; page numbers in *italics* refer to tables and/or boxes